PSYCHIATRIC MENTAL HEALTH NURSING

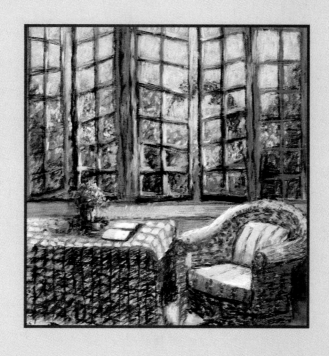

About the
ONLINE COMPANION™

Delmar Publishers offers a series of Online Companions.™ Through the Delmar site on the World Wide Web, the Online Companions™ let readers access updated information for our books.

To access the *Psychiatric Mental Health Nursing* site simply point your browser to:

http://www.DelmarNursing.com

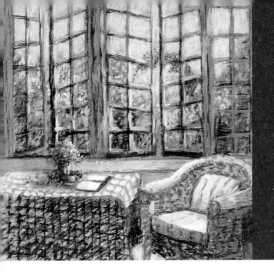

CONTENTS

UNIT 1: FOUNDATIONS FOR PRACTICE   1

"I am a student nurse. I am dying. I write this to you who are, and will become, nurses in the hope that by my sharing my feelings with you, you may someday be better able to help those who share my experience."—Anonymous student nurse, Chapter 14

This book is dedicated to the anonymous student nurse whose words have touched our lives and hearts. May there always be "someone there" to hold her hand and share her "lonely silent void."

NOTICE TO THE READER

Cover Art: Lea Barbato Gaydos
Cover Design: Brucie Rosch

Delmar Staff
Publisher: William Brottmiller
Acquisitions Editor: Greg Vis
Developmental Editor: Elisabeth F. Williams
Project Editor: Marah Bellegarde
Production Coordinator: Barbara A. Bullock
Art and Design Coordinator: Carol Keohane
Editorial Assistant: Diane Biondi

COPYRIGHT © 1998
By Delmar Publishers
a division of International Thomson Publishing Inc.

The ITP logo is a trademark under license.

Printed in the United States of America

For more information, contact:

Delmar Publishers
3 Columbia Circle, Box 15015
Albany, New York 12212-5015

International Thomson Publishing Europe
Berkshire House 168-173
High Holborn
London, WC1V 7AA
England

Thomas Nelson Australia
102 Dodds Street
South Melbourne, 3205
Victoria, Australia

Nelson Canada
1120 Birchmont Road
Scarborough, Ontario
Canada, M1K 5G4

International Thomson Editores
Campos Eliseos 385, Piso 7
Col Polanco
11560 Mexico D F Mexico

International Thomson Publishing GmbH
Königswinterer Strasse 418
53227 Bonn
Germany

International Thomson Publishing Asia
221 Henderson Road
#05-10 Henderson Building
Singapore 0315

International Thomson Publishing—Japan
Hirakawacho Kyowa Building, 3F
2-2-1 Hirakawacho
Chiyoda-ku, Tokyo 102
Japan

2 3 4 5 6 7 8 9 10 XXX 04 03 02 01 00 99 98

Library of Congress Cataloging-in-Publication Data
Frisch, Noreen Cavan.
    Psychiatric mental health nursing: understanding the client as
well as the condition / Noreen Cavan Frisch, Lawrence E. Frisch;
consulting editor, Lynn Keegan.
        p. cm.
    Includes bibliographical references and index.
    ISBN 0-8273-7233-7
    1. Psychiatric nursing. I. Frisch, Lawrence E. II. Keegan,
Lynn. III. Title.
    [DNLM: 1. Psychiatric Nursing. 2. Mental Disorders—nursing.
RC440.F75 1998
610.73'68—dc21
DNLM/DLC
for Library of Congress   97-42749
                                          CIP

PSYCHIATRIC MENTAL HEALTH NURSING

Understanding the Client as Well as the Condition

Noreen Cavan Frisch, RN, PhD, FAAN
Humboldt State University
Arcata, California

Lawrence E. Frisch, MPH
Humboldt State University
Arcata, California

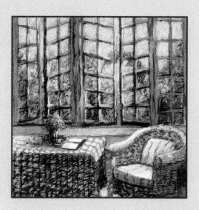

Consulting Editor
Lynn Keegan, RN, PhD, HNC, FAAN

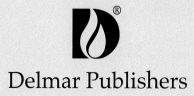

Delmar Publishers

an International Thomson Publishing company

Albany • Bonn • Boston • Cincinnati • Detroit • London • Madrid
Melbourne • Mexico City • New York • Pacific Grove • Paris • San Francisco
Singapore • Tokyo • Toronto • Washington

UNIT 5: CARING FOR THE NURSE 731

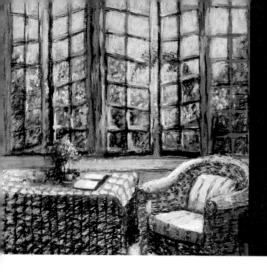

CONTRIBUTORS

Genevieve M. Bartol, RN, EdD
Professor
School of Nursing
University of North Carolina at Greensboro
Greensboro, North Carolina

Julia B. George, RN, PhD
Professor of Nursing
Chair, Department of Nursing
California State University—Fullerton
Fullerton, California

Lea Barbato Gaydos, RN, CS, MSN, HNC
Faculty
Beth-El College of Nursing
Colorado University-Springs
Colorado Springs, Colorado

Wanda Horn, RN-C
Psychiatric Unit
Southeast Missouri Hospital
Cape Girardeau, Missouri

Dorothea Hover-Kramer, RN, EdD
Licensed Psychologist in Private Practice
Director, Behavioral Health Consultants
Poway, California

Brenda P. Johnson, RN, MSN
Assistant Professor
Southeast Missouri State University
Cape Girardeau, Missouri
and
Doctoral Candidate
School of Nursing
University of Colorado Health Sciences Center
Denver, Colorado

Ruth W. Johnson, RN, EdD, FAAN
Campus Director
Coop City Campus
School of New Resources
College of New Rochelle
Bronx, New York

Jane Kelley, RN, PhD
Professor
Department of Nursing
Southeast Missouri State University
Cape Girardeau, Missouri

Nicki Potts, RN-C, PhD
Associate Professor
Abilene Intercollegiate School of Nursing
Abilene, Texas

Lynn Rew, RN-C, EdD, FAAN, HNC
Associate Professor
School of Nursing
The University of Texas at Austin
Austin, Texas

Karilee Halo Shames, RN, PhD, HNC
Psychiatric Clinical Specialist in Private Practice
Director, Nurse Empowerment Workshops and
    Services
Mill Valley, California

Marshelle Thobaben, RN-C, MS, FNP, PHN
Professor
Department of Nursing
Humboldt State University
Arcata, California

Wayne Wilson, PD, RPh
Pharmacist
Student Health Center
Humboldt State University
Arcata, California

Wendy Woodward, RN, PhD
Professor
Department of Nursing
Humboldt State University
Arcata, California

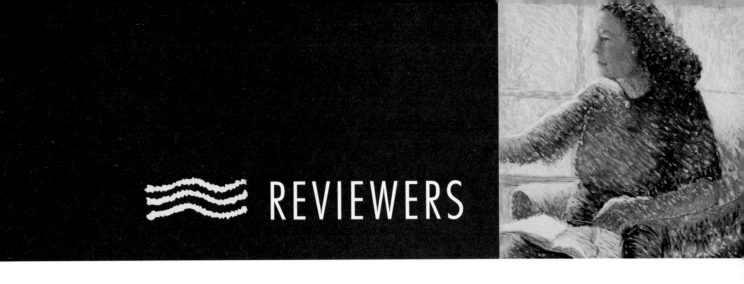

REVIEWERS

Deanah Alexander, RN, CS, MSN
Instructor
School of Nursing
West Texas A & M University
Canyon, Texas

Noreen Brady, RN, CS, MSN, LPCC
Teaching Assistant, ND Program
Frances Payne Bolton School of Nursing
Case Western Reserve University
Cleveland, Ohio

Patsy Britting, RN, MSN
Instructor, Psychiatric Nursing
West Texas A & M University
Canyon, Texas

Teresa S. Burckhalter, RN-C, MSN
ADN Faculty
Technical College of the Lowcountry
Beaufort, South Carolina

Pamela Carr, RN
Professor
Virginia Baptist Hospital
Lynchburg, Virginia

Carol Ann Coles, RN, MSN
Assistant Professor
Westmoreland County Community College
Youngwood, Pennsylvania

Carolyn Cooper, RN, PhD
Clinical Assistant Professor
University of North Carolina at Chapel Hill
Chapel Hill, North Carolina

Lois G. Cressman, RN
Senior Nurse Counselor
Chronic Fatigue Patient Management
Evergreen Medical
Deptford, New Jersey

Regina Cundall, MSN, BSN
Instructor
Lutheran Medical Center School of Nursing
St. Louis, Missouri

Susan Dewey-Hammer, RN, CS, MN
Associate Professor
Suffolk County Community College
Selden, New York

Elissa Emerson, RN, CS, PhD, FNP
Assistant Professor
Georgia Southern University
Statesboro, Georgia

Sandra K. Foltz, RN, MSN
Associate Professor of Nursing
Sinclair Community College
Dayton, Ohio

Rauda Gelazis, PhD, MN ED, BSN, CS, CTN
Associate Professor
Ursuline College
Pepper Pike, Ohio

Jeanne Gelman, RN, MA, MSN
Associate Professor
School of Nursing
Widener University
Chester, Pennsylvania

JoAnn Glittenberg, RN, PhD, FAAN
Professor
College of Nursing
University of Arizona
Tucson, Arizona

Nancy Green, RN, MSN
Nursing Instructor
Victor Valley Community College
Victorville, California

Nancy J. Hogan-Grover, BSN, MSN, CS
Associate Professor
Husson College
Bangor, Maine

Sarah Kersey, RN, MSN
Adjunct Nursing Instructor
Rowan College
Glassboro, New Jersey
and
School Nurse/Health Educator
Parkview School
Stratford, New Jersey

Jeanne B. Kozlak, RN, CS, MSN
Professor of Nursing
Humboldt State University
Arcata, California

Joanne Lavin, RN, CS, EdD
Associate Professor
Kingsborough Community College
Brooklyn, New York

Doris Lesseig, RN, CS, MA, MSN
Assistant Professor
Truman State University
Kirksville, Missouri
and
Clinical Nurse Specialist
Private Practice

Netta Moncur-Bowen, RN, MS
Instructor
Seminole Community College
Sanford, Florida

Cheryl Palmer, BScN, M Ed
Professor of Nursing
Humber College of Applied Arts and
    Technology
Etobicoke, Ontario, Canada

Lenora Richardson, PhD
Assistant Professor
University of North Carolina
Greensboro, North Carolina

Michael J. Rice, PhD, ARNP, CS
Associate Professor
Intercollegiate Center for Nursing
    Education
Spokane, Washington

Mary Rode, RN, MSN
Associate Professor
University of Evansville
Evansville, Indiana

Sandra Schuler, RN, MSN
Professor
Montgomery College
Tacoma Park, Maryland

Jaclene A. Zauszniewski, RN-C, PhD
Associate Professor of Nursing
Frances Payne Bolton School of Nursing
Case Western Reserve University
Cleveland, Ohio

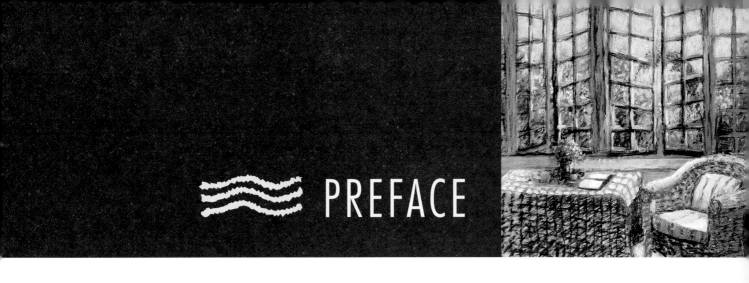

PREFACE

Psychiatric Mental Health Nursing is a comprehensive text for nurses and nursing students that provides a fresh and innovative approach to understanding the often intriguing yet disturbing world of individuals suffering from psychiatric conditions. Today's nurses are faced with many challenges, such as health care reform and shortened stays in inpatient units, that place increased demand on their nursing skills and professional competence. A growing emphasis on psychobiology, community care, and the ever-heightening importance of the technology age, are all factors that nurses will face in their every day care of clients with psychiatric conditions.

Truly understanding the client who is living with a psychiatric disorder is key to nurses' success in meeting the needs of these clients within the rapidly changing health care arena. A goal of this text is to help nurses humanize health care and disease treatment by preserving the best of the caring tradition of nursing and reintegrating this with expanding biomedical science and technology. Empowering readers as educated decision makers and developing skills of analysis and critical thinking, while encouraging excellent clinical and nursing skills, are all goals forming the foundation for this text.

CONCEPTUAL APPROACH

Psychiatric Mental Health Nursing was written and designed with the reader in mind. Like no other text currently available, *Psychiatric Mental Health Nursing* will draw readers into the subject matter in a way that is interesting to them. This text conveys the real-life experiences of clients suffering from psychiatric conditions in a manner that will stimulate and keep the reader's attention. Disorders are illustrated through literature, film, and art, then followed by a didactic explanation from the nursing and psychiatric literature, covering etiology, nursing perspectives, theory, nursing process, and sample case studies/care plans. Recurring features and an easy-to-follow format offer an approach that is friendly and delivers a wealth of information.

The conceptual approach to this text is based on the following:

◆ Dual focus combines the best of nursing as the art and science of caring. The use of literature, art, and the human experience, coupled with qualitative and scientific research, emphasizes the need for compassionate nursing care and respect for the lived experience of others. Nursing theory helps readers learn to provide caring and nurturing as part of all interventions, while maintaining an emphasis on living with mental illness. The importance of science is evident through the theoretical and epidemiological base underlying conditions.

◆ Chapter opening reflection boxes help the reader develop critical thinking skills and the ability to deal with moral dilemmas by enticing the reader to enter the world of the mentally ill, and by introducing issues of the social and moral implications of treatment. Emphasis is placed on considering first what the client feels and then what the client wants.

◆ Balanced nursing and medical approach (NANDA, DSM) underscores the importance of nurses working collaboratively with other health care team members with the mutual goal of providing the most appropriate and effective care to clients.

◆ Focus on self-care encourages nurses to think about and care for themselves as well as their clients. This reflects a fundamental premise that caring for others can be done only if the caregiver is balanced and well-centered.

Readers of *Psychiatric Mental Health Nursing* will need an understanding of basic nursing skills and the nursing process.

ORGANIZATION

Psychiatric Mental Health Nursing is composed of 32 chapters contained in five units. **Unit 1** outlines the foundations for practice that underlie the psychiatric nursing process. Fundamental principles of nursing, which help the reader understand the importance of the nurse/client partnership in the care of those with psychiatric conditions, are discussed. A unique chapter (Chapter 4) on diagnostic systems outlines scientific bases for care and explains NANDA, DSM-IV, ICD-9, and NIC, and how they are all used in practice. Chapter 6 on cultural and ethnic considerations highlights the holistic view of the client, and Chapter 7 on epidemiology outlines the scientific and research base for nursing care.

Unit 2 highlights specific psychiatric conditions clients may experience. These chapters explore conditions through use of illustrative literature, art, and movie clips, which give riveting examples of clients living with certain psychiatric conditions. These chapters are also key in encouraging the reader to be aware of personal feelings and biases towards mental health and illness, and how these personal opinions may affect interactions with both coworkers and clients.

Unit 3 introduces the reader to special populations needing mental health care. These chapters highlight the needs unique to these populations and discuss how to adapt nursing care to meet these special needs. A unique chapter on treating homeless and incarcerated clients will open doors for many nurses who may not previously have considered these special populations.

Unit 4 covers the diverse interventions and treatment modalities nurses may choose to employ, including psychopharmacology; individual, family, and group psychotherapy; complementary or somatic therapy; and community-based care.

Unit 5 is designed specifically to teach the reader how to care for self. In Chapter 31, self-help modalities are discussed in a way that is inviting and uplifting. Chapter 32 offers an annotated review of numerous films that can be viewed to help foster understanding of mental health and illness.

SPECIAL FEATURES

There are numerous special features in *Psychiatric Mental Health Nursing* designed to stimulate critical thinking and self-exploration, and to encourage readers to synthesize and apply knowledge presented in the text:

- ◆ **Literary excerpts** invite the reader to enter the client's world to better understand the process and impact of a psychiatric condition on an individual's overall health and functioning.
- ◆ **Movie boxes and classic art pieces** make the text come alive and help students understand what their clients are experiencing.
- ◆ **Chapter opening reflection boxes** set the stage for the chapter by inviting the reader to consider personal experiences with a given topic or to begin thinking about a certain psychiatric condition and the effects it may have on those experiencing it.

- ◆ **Reflective Thinking** features encourage readers to examine their own personal views on given topics in order to get and stay in touch with their own feelings, and to understand the varying viewpoints they may encounter in clients and coworkers. These boxes are designed to encourage reflection on an issue from a personal context, to raise awareness, and to stimulate critical thinking and active problem solving.
- ◆ **Nursing Tip** boxes encourage the reader to apply basic knowledge to real-life situations and offer helpful hints and shortcuts that will benefit new and experienced nurses alike.
- ◆ **Nursing Alert** features indicate life-threatening or serious indications, drug reactions or interactions, or critical precautions that need immediate attention.
- ◆ **Research Highlight** features outline findings from current research and offer discussion of their impact on nursing practice.
- ◆ **Exploring the Web** boxes are interactive tools that encourage readers to broaden their knowledge base and enhance their skills by searching the Internet for additional information and resources on specific psychiatric conditions or situations.
- ◆ **Case Study/Care Plan with Critical Thinking Band** features offer an opportunity for the reader to apply the material presented in the chapter to a real-life scenario, with an eye to encouraging extrapolation and intuitive thinking. Several case studies are based on the literary excerpts presented in the chapters and invite the reader to apply knowledge presented in text to an actual case example. Case studies are followed by a care plan based on the nursing process, and each concludes with a critical thinking band, which challenges readers to revisit the case study to determine what else should be considered in terms of providing thorough, quality care to a client in need.

PEDAGOGICAL TOOLS

Psychiatric Mental Health Nursing also includes numerous pedagogical features to promote learning and readability:

- ◆ **Competencies** open each chapter and introduce the main areas targeted for mastery in the chapter. They provide a checkpoint for study and tie in to crucial aspects of nursing care.
- ◆ **Chapter Outlines** are listed at the start of each chapter and serve as an overview and quick reference for the material to be covered.
- ◆ **Key Terms** with definitions are listed at the opening of each chapter and are boldfaced and defined at their first use in text.

- **Review Questions and Activities** afford an opportunity for readers to assess their acquisition of material and better define areas needing additional study.

- **References and Suggested Readings** underline the theoretical basis of each chapter with strong academic documentation.

- **Glossary** at the end of the book offers definitions of key terms used in text and serves as a comprehensive resource for study and review.

- **Appendices** offer important reference information, including American and Canadian Standards of Practice, DSM-IV and NANDA listings, a critical pathway, and a description of psychological tests in common use.

- **Index** facilitates access to material and also indicates tabular, illustrated, literary, film and art entries.

EXTENSIVE TEACHING/LEARNING PACKAGE

The complete supplements package was developed to achieve two goals:

1. To assist students in learning the essential skills and information needed to secure a career in the area of nursing.

2. To assist instructors in planning and implementing their programs for the most efficient use of time and other resources.

The Classroom Manager
(Order # 0-8273-7234-5)

This comprehensive, resource-packed, three-ring binder includes:

Instructor's Guide

- **Teaching Methods and Strategies** (Helpful Hints): Ideas and concepts to help educators manage different presentation methods. Suggestions for overall approach to studying and presenting the chapter material are included.

- **Lesson Plans:** Guidelines for incorporating psychiatric nursing into one-semester courses. These are tied into the chapter competencies, and include suggestions for different content delivery methods.

- **Learning Experiences:** Categories include theory application, individual activities, group activities, clinical activities, community application, and internet activities.

Computerized and Printed Testbank with Electronic Gradebook

- **Electronic Testbank** in IBM format and a printed testbank include approximately 1000 NCLEX style questions with rationales, with text page references for remediation.

- **Electronic Gradebook** automatically calculates grades, tracks student performance, prints student progress reports, organizes assignments, and more, to simplify administrative tasks.

- **On-line Testing** feature of the computerized testbank allows exams to be administered on-line via a school network or stand-alone PC.

The Companion Web Site

http://www.DelmarNursing.com will have high appeal to both educators and students. Features include:

- Updates to book content on quarterly basis

- Internet activities

- Periodic discussion forums with authors and contributors

- Frequently asked questions

- Comprehensive listing of pertinent URLs

- Focus on nursing research; updated every six months by RNdex™

- Expanded section on "self-care for the caregiver"

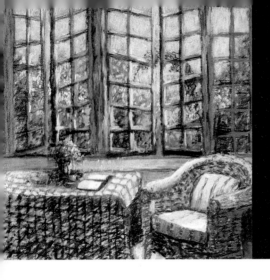

ACKNOWLEDGMENTS

The authors are indebted to many individuals and institutions for two lifetimes of learning, stimulation, and challenge. Only a few can be acknowledged in the brief space available to us.

Beth Williams, Greg Vis, Marah Bellegarde, Carol Keohane, Barb Bullock, Danya Plotsky, Margo Quinto, Bea Ruberto, Pat Gillivan, and Hilary Schrauf have been an unbeatable team at Delmar Publishers. Their constant enthusiasm and assistance have moved this book on a steady path from idea to reality.

We join every reader of this book in thanking Lea Barbato Gaydos, our remarkable psychiatric nurse-artist, for the original paintings that grace the book's front cover and open each chapter. Lea is one of many vibrant members of the American Holistic Nurses Association—an ongoing source of professional inspiration and renewal.

Each of our many contributing authors has brought a unique background and perspective to this book. We greatly appreciate the wisdom with which their efforts have enriched the text. Numerous colleagues offered ideas and support for this project throughout its gestation: Jeanne Kozlak proposed several important clarifications and content enhancements; Wendy Woodward contributed case studies and nursing care plans; Ellen Weiss, Nathan Copple, Alan Liu, Vincent Puzick, and fellow Internet webmates from the National Council of Teachers of English led us out of one particularly dark place and into Tennessee (Williams, that is); Alfred Guillaume, Jack Turner, and Beth Amen ably translated correspondence from faraway places. Finally, Ton Van Wageningen and his Amsterdam-based sister provided invaluable Dutch-speaking access to museums and art collections in the Netherlands.

Drawings, paintings, and images from movies and drama contribute greatly to this text. We appreciate contributions from the Kobal Collection, the Oregon Shakespeare Festival, and the Folger Shakespeare Library, and from numerous art museums throughout Europe and North America. We owe a special thanks to movie aficionado Ann Kimbrow, who did extensive viewing of many of the films discussed in this text.

No acknowledgment page would be complete without offering our deepest thanks to the authors, poets, artists, dramatists, and filmmakers whose works bring all of us closer to an understanding of the most profound depths of human experience. The great Russian author and dramatist Anton Chekhov once wrote that "both (the study of) anatomy and (the study of) literature are of equally noble descent; they have identical goals." Following Chekhov, we have tried to include equal measures of literature and anatomy as we pursued our own goal; making both the science and the experience of mental illness come alive for the reader.

For the numerous anatomic images (CT, MRI, and PET) that we have been privileged to include throughout the text, we owe thanks to Drs. John Homan (Mad River Community Hospital), Alex Habibian (St. Joseph's Hospital of Eureka), Scott Rauch (Massachusetts General Hospital), David Silbersweig (Cornell University Medical Center), Debbye Yurgelun-Todd (McLean's Hospital and Harvard Medical School), and Nancy Andreasen (University of Iowa). Jacqueline Spiegel-Cohen, M.S., of Mount Sinai School of Medicine was uniquely helpful and transferred to us by anonymous FTP more PET scan images than we have been able to use.

Finally, our appreciation goes to Barbara Georgiana, who spent endless months tracing copyrights and obtaining permissions for the literary excerpts, artistic reproductions, and scientific illustrations that give this book its unique character. Like Shakespeare's Puck, Barbara put many "a girdle around the earth," but more by Internet and fax than by magic (though her skills and perseverence often seemed magical to us).

And by way of conclusion, the inevitable worry; if we have missed someone important in this lengthy acknowledgment, we offer our humblest apologies. And to our many readers; thank you for choosing this text as you grow as a nurse and refine your skills in caring and healing.

Noreen and Larry Frisch

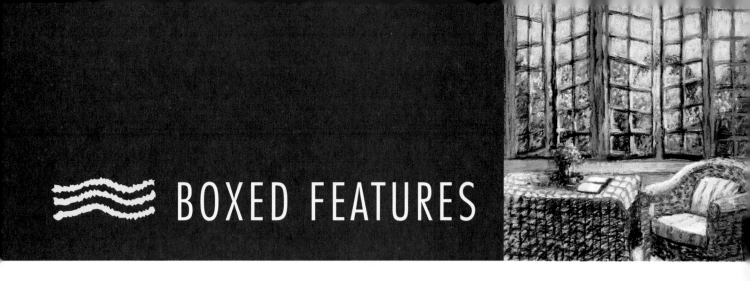

BOXED FEATURES

Nursing Tip

Reflective Thinking

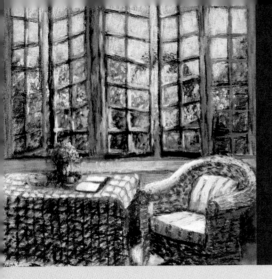

HOW TO USE THIS TEXT

Subject matter is presented in an innovative, interesting, and engaging manner throughout the text. The following suggests how you can use the features of this text to gain competence and confidence in psychiatric mental health nursing.

Chapter Opener Boxes

Each chapter opens with questions or statements that challenge you to examine your personal understanding of the topic or psychiatric condition under discussion. These boxes invite you to reflect on your own views of psychiatric nursing and of those individuals who are personally affected by psychiatric conditions.

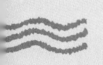

Reflective Thinking

These boxes deal with self-reflection and opinions on various topics. It may be useful to keep a journal in which you write down your immediate response to each box on a chapter-by-chapter basis. At the end of each chapter, review your journal entries and ask yourself how your values will affect your nursing care.

Chapter

10

THE CLIENT EXPERIENCING ANXIETY

Noreen Cavan Frisch
Lawrence E. Frisch

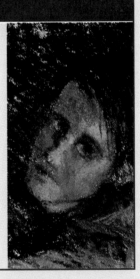

Anxiety in Everyday Life

Modern life is filled with tension and anxieties. Philosophers have stated that anxiety is a part of the human condition, both unavoidable and necessary for persons to seek to understand themselves and define their goals. However, each person tries to find balance within his or her own existence.

Consider the anxieties of your own life:
- What are the objects of your worries?
- Are there personal worries stemming from your societal roles and duties?
- Do you have personal fears associated with activities or objects? Are you able to avoid those situations that are anxiety provoking for you?

How do you find peace:
- What does a personal sense of peace mean to you?
- What can you do to find peace in your life?

As you read this chapter, which focuses on anxiety in illness, remember that all persons, well or ill, experience anxiety. The nurse must understand that anxiety can become an overpowering experience for many persons, and care must focus on a very personal understanding of anxiety, fear, and sense of loss of control.

☾☽ REFLECTIVE THINKING

Are We Overmedicating Children?

Sometimes medication is requested by a caregiver or teacher in order to make a child more manageable or to enhance cognitive development. Do you think this is an appropriate request? Why or why not? In your opinion, what situations would merit medicating a child in order to achieve behavior control?

The Man Who Mistook His Wife for a Hat

I found an extreme and extraordinary loss of recent memory—so that whatever was said or shown to him was apt to be forgotten in a few seconds' time. Thus I laid out my watch, my tie, and my glasses on the desk, covered them, and asked him to remember these. Then, after a minute's chat, I asked him what I had put under the cover. He remembered none of them—or indeed that I had even asked him to remember.

(Sacks, 1987, p. 27)

I wrote in my notes, "isolated in a single moment of being, with a moat or lacuna of forgetting all round him . . . He is a man without a past (or future), stuck in a constantly changing, meaningless moment" . . . I kept wondering, in this and later notes—unscientifically—about "a lost soul," and how one might establish some continuity, some roots, for he was a man without roots, or rooted only in the remote past.

(Sacks, 1987, p. 29)

Literary Excerpts

Literary excerpts invite you to enter the client's world to better understand the process and impact of a psychiatric condition on an individual's overall health and functioning. You may want to browse through a chapter and read the excerpts prior to reading the chapter in its entirety, to get an umbrella view of a given disorder. You may also want to practice writing care plans based on the characters presented through the literature.

Movie Clips

We've added photos from popular movies that accurately depict characters who are experiencing the situations you are studying. If you haven't seen these movies already, this is a perfect opportunity to become acquainted with them. Whenever possible, view these films while you are studying the chapter so you can determine what symptoms of a given disorder are embodied in the film's characters.

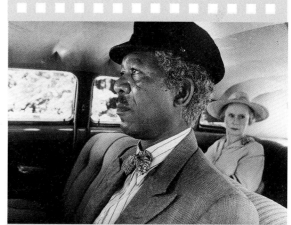

Driving Miss Daisy. Source: Warner Brothers/Courtesy Kobal.

Old age is a time of transition. In *Driving Miss Daisy,* Jessica Tandy's Daisy has to come to an accommodation with her increasing loss of independence and a world that changes greatly in 25 years.

🌀 NURSING ALERT!

Warning Signs of Delirium

- ◆ Rapid fluctuation in level of consciousness (agitated to lethargic)
- ◆ Difficulty in maintaining attention span
- ◆ Illusions or hallucinations
- ◆ Unfocused speech and disorganized thinking
- ◆ Disorientation to place or time
- ◆ Strong emotional reactions
- ◆ Memory problems

Nursing Alerts

In some situations, you must act immediately in order to ensure the health and safety of your clients. This feature will help you to begin to identify and respond to critical situations on your own, both efficiently and effectively.

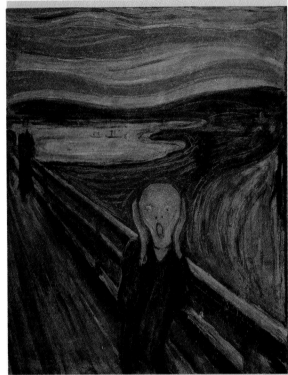

The Scream by Munch. Source: Erich Lessing/Art Resource, NY.

Almost an icon of anxiety, this work reflects the life experiences of a man who was haunted by mental illness—both his own and his sister's. Caught between land and sea, and isolated from the only other humans in sight, the screaming figure occupies a landscape whose unstable shapes and colors are both the source and the expression of unbearable anxiety.

Classic Art

Classic paintings allow you to experience through works of art the fascinating and disturbing worlds of those suffering from psychiatric conditions. The works of many famous artists beautifully illustrate the wide range of emotions and reactions of persons living with psychiatric conditions. As you view these, ask yourself what characteristics of the given disorders seem to be represented in the artwork.

Nursing Tips

In any profession, there are many helpful hints that assist you in performing more efficiently. As a nurse, you will also need to embrace sensitivity in your practice. The wide variety of hints, tips, and strategies presented here will help you to apply your basic knowledge as you work towards professional advancement. Study, share, and discuss these tips with your colleagues.

 NURSING TIP

Helping Children Who Exhibit Unacceptable Behavior

- Praise accomplishments through touch, verbal affection, or small rewards such as stickers or stars on an activity calendar.
- Model desirable traits, such as sharing and honesty.
- Acknowledge positive or desirable behaviors.
- Correct unacceptable or undesirable behaviors immediately and calmly.
- Communicate that the behavior, not the child, is unacceptable.
- Have the child help determine acceptable behavior parameters.
- Explain expectations in clear terms.
- Ensure that the child understands expectations by asking the child to repeat instructions.
- Be certain that expectations are within the child's developmental parameters.
- Clearly outline consequences for unacceptable behaviors, and follow through on their implementation.

Case Study/Care Plans

The Case Study/Care Plan will guide you as you apply the principles of nursing learned in each chapter to a client with the condition under study. Featuring real-world scenarios, the case study feature helps you make the connection between theory and practice more easily. This boxed element will reinforce your knowledge of the nursing process and the steps in the process of assessing, planning care, performing interventions, and evaluating the success of your course of care.

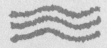

CASE STUDY/CARE PLAN

Penny is a young woman, 17 years old, who was brought to the emergency department by her mother. Penny had ingested an unknown quantity of medications from the family's medicine cabinet and was found unresponsive by her mother when the mother returned home from work. Penny was treated medically and has been referred to the mental health unit for hospitalization.

ASSESSMENT

Jane is a psychiatric nurse who will be Penny's primary nurse. Jane observes that Penny is withdrawn. Penny's physical appearance is disheveled; her eyes are reddened as if she has been crying recently. Penny avoids eye contact and does not speak much. Penny tells Jane that she is tired, that she has not slept. Penny does not answer the question "Do you feel you could or would harm yourself again tonight?"

NURSING DIAGNOSIS *Risk for injury*, related to psychological dysfunction (suicide attempt)

Outcomes	Planning/Interventions	Evaluation
◆ Penny will not harm herself further while in the hospital.	◆ Initiate suicide precautions to ensure Penny's safety.	Penny did not harm herself during the hospital stay.
◆ Penny will make a verbal contract to not harm herself for the next 4 days.	◆ Begin to establish trust with Penny by approaching her in a nonjudgmental manner.	Penny did make a verbal contract with the nurse by the second hospital day that she would not harm herself while in the hospital.
◆ Penny will sign a written contract to not hurt herself at any time in the next 4 months.	◆ Establish in each 24-hour period Penny's verbal contract to not harm herself.	
	◆ Offer positive encouragement to Penny for remaining free of injury and/or for taking a positive interest in herself.	Penny did sign a written contract to call a hotline number rather than make another attempt.

NURSING DIAGNOSIS *Ineffective individual coping*, related to situational crisis (suicide attempt), as evidenced by destructive behavior and inability to ask for help

Outcomes	Planning/Interventions	Evaluation
◆ Penny will verbalize one positive statement about herself.	◆ Permit Penny to be herself.	Penny did respond to the nurse and entered into a relationship with the nurse. Penny began to describe her interests, her feelings.
◆ Penny will begin to examine her coping skills and consider alternatives.	◆ Promote Penny's control by giving her choices of daily activities and of conversation topics.	
	◆ Develop a positive relationship with Penny by remaining caring and truthful in interactions, by actively listening when Penny wants to talk, and by remaining attentive when Penny wishes to be silent.	Penny accepted individual therapy and agreed to weekly sessions.
	◆ Encourage Penny to view others as a source of support and assistance.	
	◆ Encourage Penny to enter therapy on an ongoing basis.	

CRITICAL THINKING BAND

ASSESSMENT
Would you also assess Penny's family situation for possible clues into her present psychological state? What other contacts (friends, school, boyfriend) would you pursue?

NURSING DIAGNOSIS
What family-oriented diagnoses might be uncovered in Penny's case?

Outcomes
What outcomes would you identify for a longer term period (perhaps 2 weeks and beyond)? Are there family-oriented outcomes that you would include?

Planning/Interventions
Identify family interventions that might help in Penny's situation.

Evaluation
How would you plan follow-up care and evaluation for Penny and her family once she is discharged?

Critical Thinking Band

A Critical Thinking Band highlights each of the nursing process steps in the Case Study/ Care Plan. This element will teach you to look critically at the methods of care suggested in each nursing process section and to look for new ways to provide thorough, quality care to the client under study.

🌀 RESEARCH HIGHLIGHT

Worries of School-Age Children

STUDY PROBLEM/PURPOSE

To determine how worrisome some situations are for school-aged children and if their caregivers can identify how worrisome the situations would be for their children.

METHODS

A convenience sample of 48 children (7 to 11 years old), 40 mothers, and 8 fathers completed a 27-item questionnaire titled "What Worries You (Your Child) the Most." The child was asked to rate the events on a Likert scale using a facial drawing with a broadly smiling affect (1 = no worry at all) to a tearing affect (5 = most worry possible) and then to rank order the items. The questionnaire for caregivers contained the same items as the child questionnaire.

FINDINGS

For the most part, caregivers knew what would worry their children the most. Having a caregiver die and not being able to see were worries that both children and caregivers recognized. However, caregivers underestimated the importance of pets and adequate family income to the child. There were significant differences in child and caregiver perceptions of three items ranked among the most worrisome: being asked to take drugs, being in a war, and hearing caregivers quarrel.

IMPLICATIONS

Findings indicate that considerable discrepancies can exist between what the caregiver and the child perceive as worrisome. Nurses can help caregivers and children become more aligned in their perceptions and actions to counteract childrens' worries.

From "Worries of School-Age Children," by J. A. Neff and J. Dale, 1996, *Journal of the Society of Pediatric Nurses*, *1*(1), 27–32.

Research Highlights

The Research Highlights emphasize the importance of research in nursing by linking theory to practice. A useful learning tool, these boxes focus attention on current issues and trends in nursing.

〰 KEY CONCEPTS

- *Altered thought processes* is a nursing diagnosis representing the human response to situations where a person has lost ability to use rational mental processes.

- Schizophrenia is a major debilitating disease where the client loses rational thought and/or ability to interpret the environment.

- An individual experiencing schizophrenia may present with disordered thoughts, incomprehensible language, loss of function, delusions, and hallucinations.

- Positive symptoms of schizophrenia include outward behaviors that clearly display pathology.

- Negative symptoms of schizophrenia include behaviors that represent a change from the individual's prior personality and lead to social isolation and anhedonia.

- There is no predictable clinical course for any individual person diagnosed with schizophrenia.

- With about one new case of schizophrenia per 10,000 persons, the social costs are exceedingly high.

- Schizophrenia is an organic disease with a strong genetic component.

- Psychosocial treatment includes individual and family support services as well as socially directed rehabilitation.

- Pharmacological treatment is primarily through neuroleptic drugs.

- Nursing theory focusing on the nurse-client interactions are most helpful.

- The five aims of intervention provide a framework for nursing care.

Key Concepts

Key Concepts highlight the main points presented in each chapter and are ideal for study and review.

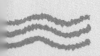

〰 REVIEW QUESTIONS AND ACTIVITIES

1. Differentiate between unipolar and bipolar depression.

2. Identify those who are at risk for developing depression.

3. Describe the characteristics of major depression, minor depression, and dysthymia.

4. Describe bereavement or grief; identify the stages of normal grieving.

5. Consider a client diagnosed with major depression. Explain the depression from the perspective of each of the following theories: psychoanalytic, object loss, learned helplessness, cognitive, and physical/biological.

6. Watson's nursing theory guides practice with depressed persons. How would her theory suggest you initiate interaction with a client?

7. What nursing interventions for a depressed person are consistent with Orem's theory?

8. List assessment parameters for nursing care of one who is at risk for depression.

9. What are the cultural considerations related to nursing care of one who is depressed?

10. Suggest the process needed to validate nursing diagnoses associated with depression.

11. Describe independent nursing interventions for depression. How are these interventions evaluated in practice?

12. Describe the nurse's role in monitoring clients on tricyclic antidepressants and other drugs.

Exploring the Web

These end-of-chapter boxes are interactive tools that encourage you to broaden your knowledge base and enhance your research skills by searching the Internet for additional information and resources on specific psychiatric conditions and situations. Bookmark the Delmar site in your computer for quicker entry.

Review Questions and Activities

At the end of each chapter, questions and exercises that encourage independent thinking assist you with the learning process and help you assimilate the information presented in the text.

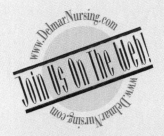

⚛ EXPLORING THE WEB

- Visit this text's "Online Companion™" on the Internet at **http://www.DelmarNursing.com** for further information on anxiety and anxiety disorders.

- What sites could you recommend to clients and families experiencing anxiety who are looking for self-help, chat rooms, or other electronic information sources?

- What resources are listed for caregivers and health care professionals?

- Is there a listing on the Internet of books, videos, or other media on anxiety and anxiety disorders? Are these resources available in your local library or through purchase over the Web?

- What other key terms might you search (e.g., phobia, Panic Disorder, Obsessive-Compulsive Disorder, Post-Traumatic Stress Disorder)?

- What organizations or professional journals could you search for information on anxiety?

Unit

FOUNDATIONS FOR PRACTICE

What is psychiatric mental health nursing? Where does it take place? Does it have a theoretical base? What is the language of psychiatry? How can nurses relate to mentally ill clients? How does culture affect our response to persons with mental illness? What do we know about why a person becomes mentally ill? What are the laws and ethical problems unique to mental health care and psychiatric nursing?

These questions outline some of the *Foundations for Practice* that will be addressed in the next eight chapters of this text.

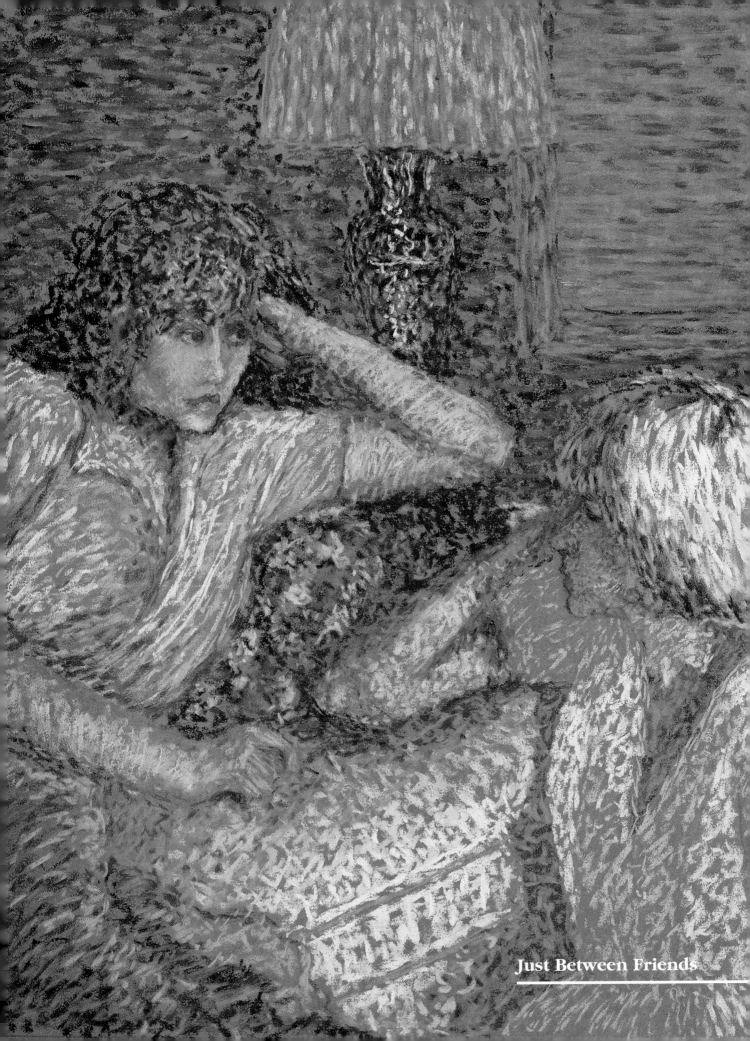

Just Between Friends

Chapter

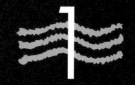

THROUGH THE DOOR

Your First Day in Psychiatric Nursing

Noreen Cavan Frisch

Your Own Experience and Feelings

- ◆ What has been your experience with and exposure to psychiatric care? What are your ideas and images of psychiatry and mental health care? Where do they come from?
- ◆ What are your feelings about taking a course in psychiatric mental health nursing? Are you anxious? Interested? Curious?

Read this chapter to help prepare you for the first day in an exciting and extremely rewarding nursing specialty.

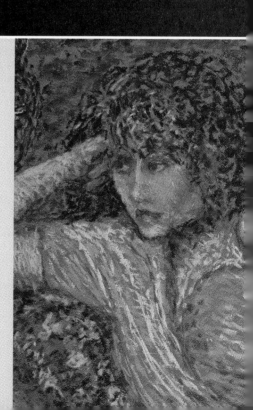

〜 CHAPTER OUTLINE

RITES OF PASSAGE

MENTAL HEALTH AND MENTAL ILLNESS

THE PSYCHIATRIC SETTING

QUESTIONS STUDENTS USUALLY ASK

Why and How Do Persons Seek Care?

Will I Be Able to Know the Staff from the Clients?

Will Clients' Behaviors Make Me Uncomfortable?

Are Psychiatric Clients Violent?

How Will I Feel Without My Regular Nursing Uniform?

What Do Psychiatric Clients Think of Student Nurses?

ADVICE FROM PRIOR STUDENTS

BEGINNING A NEW COURSE

〜 COMPETENCIES

Upon completion of this chapter, the reader should be able to:

1. Reflect on the experience of a psychiatric nursing course as a rite of passage in the process of becoming a nurse.
2. Describe basic information about the nature and practice of psychiatric mental health care, including:
   ◆ The nature of mental health and mental illness
   ◆ A sense of why a person is hospitalized for psychiatric care
   ◆ Basic job descriptions and education of various mental health workers
   ◆ Concerns and advice from prior students
3. Interpret the goal of psychiatric care as that of strengthening the healthy portion of the client.

〜 KEY TERMS

Depression State in which an individual feels very sad and despondent and has no energy or sense of future.

Disability Impairment in one or more important areas of functioning.

Distress Negative response to stimuli that are perceived as threatening.

Hallucination State in which an individual hears voices or sees images of things that others cannot hear or see.

Mania Psychiatric condition characterized by excess energy, abnormal excitability, and an exaggerated sense of well-being.

Mental Disorder Behavior or psychological syndrome or pattern associated with distress or disability or increased risk of suffering, death, pain, or loss of freedom.

Mental Health State in which a person has knowledge of self, meets basic needs, assumes responsibility for behavior and self-growth, integrates thoughts and feelings with actions, resolves conflicts, maintains relationships, respects others, communicates directly, and adapts to change in the environment.

Mental Illness State in which an individual shows deficits in functioning, cannot view self clearly or has a distorted image of self, is unable to maintain personal relationships, and cannot adapt to the environment.

Psychosis State in which an individual has lost the ability to recognize reality.

You are about to begin your course in psychiatric mental health nursing, an exciting and emotionally rewarding nursing specialty. But, despite the rewards and excitement that we are confident you will find in your psychiatric nursing experience, we would be surprised if you did not feel a bit anxious about what lies immediately ahead. Psychiatric nursing facilities seem very different from the medical-surgical units, from the maternity care units, and from the other clinics students have previously used for their clinical rotations. When you enter the psychiatric unit, often through a locked door, you enter a world significantly different from other health care settings. At first, the differences may seem overwhelming, but there are also many similarities between psychiatric nursing and other areas of nursing. You may find the same initial experience when you first enter day treatment centers and outpatient clinics. You will learn about similarities and differences between psychiatry and other areas as you experience your course, read the material in the various chapters of this book, and then complete the assignments your instructor has planned for you. A psychiatric course is a good time for reflection and self-examination, so as you begin this new course, take a few moments to reflect with us on what is going to happen and how you feel about it.

RITES OF PASSAGE

Nursing school is a time of growth and learning. Much of the growth is professional; you begin as a very new, novice nurse and leave school with enough background to take a position as a beginning professional. Some of the growth is personal; in nursing, you are exposed to very intimate human experiences, unlike any that are commonly experienced by other college or university students. Many nurses reflect on their time in school as a time of great transitions, of immense learning, and of bonding with other students. Along your path through nursing school and in the transition from new, novice nurse to beginning professional, you will encounter (or perhaps already have encountered) a number of important "rites of passage." Nursing students don special clothing and enter the closed doors of an operating suite to witness the dramatic ritual of modern surgery. They care for persons in pain and offer themselves and their treatments as comfort and support. Each experience marks a significant event, an achievement on the path to becoming a nurse.

For us, the first course in psychiatric mental health care was an experience with many dimensions: anxiety, learning, failure, and growth. We felt, years ago, that something significant happened when we passed through the door separating the psychiatric ward from the rest of the world—not quite sure yet who we really were or what we could do for anyone on the other side. Although locked wards exist today, the majority of clients now are treated through a variety of services in their homes, halfway houses, and clinics. Unfortunately, many chronically mentally ill people are homeless or incarcerated behind prison walls. You will encounter those who are fortunate enough to be treated within a health care service. What you learn from this experience should prepare you to be an advocate for mentally ill people throughout the community and especially for those within your responsibility of care as a nurse.

Caring for the mentally ill and growing from student to practicing caregiver is a transitional experience that anthropologists call a rite of passage. A rite of passage occurs when there is a role change; it is often accompanied by a series of accepted rituals, which can reduce the anxiety related to the change in role. Rites represent life transitions; the person going through a rite of passage is transformed and different for having had the experience. As you enter your work in a psychiatric unit, you are going to experience a rite of passage similar to some you have already encountered on your path to becoming a nurse. Remember when you first saw the birth of a baby? This is an experience surrounded by emotion—joy, wonder, the awe of creation. Remember when you first cared for one who was dying? Emotions surround this experience as well—sorrow, solemnity, the spiritual sense of grief, of parting.

The authors believe the experience of caring for and working with persons who are mentally ill to be just as moving, as transformational, as the experiences of birth and death. While caring for the mentally ill you may confront persons who have great difficulty in communicating and are desperately in need of care. Frequently the tools you have with which to give care—yourself and your ability to communicate with others—will not work for you as in your past nursing experiences. Approaching and talking with someone who is psychotic or sitting with someone who is profoundly depressed, you will experience a new dimension of nursing that will enrich your abilities to be an effective nurse. You will be challenged to reflect on your own behavior, your own methods of communication, and your own personality. You will have the chance to use this course to study human behavior in general and your own behavior in particular. You may emerge with different views of yourself, of nursing, and of mental health and illness.

But, you may be thinking, "I never wanted to be a psychiatric nurse! I'm taking this course because I have to." That is how many of us started, including most of us who became psychiatric nurses. However, psychiatric nursing opens up a new world, one that most students have never seen or experienced before, a world of human-to-human interaction, with much room for caring and compassion and excellent nursing. Enter the passage with an open mind and let the experience guide you, and always remember to be yourself.

☯ *REFLECTIVE THINKING*

Expectations

◆ What do you expect to see on a psychiatric unit? (List your ideas of what will be there.)

◆ From where do you think your perceptions came (i.e., what is your source of information about mental illness and psychiatry)?

◆ Do you have a definition of mental health and mental illness? What influenced your definition?

By way of advice, many former students report that the bonding and support of other students is particularly important in a psychiatric nursing course. Interestingly enough, in many cultures, persons go through rituals or rites of passage as social (rather than solitary) experiences. Like student nurses, people throughout the world often undertake initiation into new roles in the company of valued comrades or friends. In many cultures, people who go through rites of passage together "are considered to be linked by special ties which persist long after the rites have been concluded" (Farb, 1978, p. 406). Value those ties—they are special—and they will be of special help to you when the experiences of the psychiatric unit become intense and challenging.

We have prepared this chapter as a "crash course" to provide you with basic information needed to feel confident and somewhat knowledgeable on your first day(s) in psychiatric mental health work. Of course, information is only a part of what you need. Start by taking an inventory about what you now know about mental illness and where your knowledge came from.

MENTAL HEALTH AND MENTAL ILLNESS

A good introduction will begin with some basic definitions and descriptions of concepts of mental health and mental illness. Mental health and mental illness are relative concepts, defined and described in relation to a person's ability to function and, basically, to have a positive self-view.

There is no clear, singular definition of **mental health**. In general, a person is mentally healthy when he possesses knowledge of himself, meets his basic needs, assumes responsibility for his behavior and for self-growth, has learned to integrate thoughts, feelings and actions, and can resolve conflicts successfully. In relation to others, a mentally healthy person maintains relationships, communicates directly with others, and respects others. Lastly, a mentally healthy person adapts to change

in his environment. These characteristics provide a description of mental health but do not fully define mental health. Persons who are mentally ill often possess many of the characteristics of well persons, and mentally healthy persons not infrequently experience symptoms similar to those of mental illness. The difference between sickness and health can be quite arbitrary and is often based on the degree to which characteristics or behaviors affect a person's functioning. Above all, the mentally ill show deficits in functioning; it is usually these deficits that bring them to the facilities where you will encounter them.

Mental illness occurs when an individual is not able to view herself clearly or has a distorted view of self; is unable to maintain satisfying personal relationships; and is unable to adapt to her environment. The American Psychiatric Association defines **mental disorder** as "clinically significant behavior or psychological syndrome or pattern that occurs in an individual and is associated with

---

POSSIBLE SIGNS OF MENTAL ILLNESS

◆ Marked personality change over time

◆ Confused thinking; strange or grandiose ideas

◆ Prolonged severe depression, apathy, or extreme highs and lows

◆ Excessive anxiety, fear, or suspiciousness; blaming others

◆ Withdrawal from society; friendlessness; abnormal self-centeredness

◆ Denial of obvious problems; strong resistance to help

◆ Thinking or talking about suicide

◆ Numerous, unexplained physical ailments; marked changes in eating or sleeping patterns

◆ Anger or hostility out of proportion to the situation

◆ Delusions (false beliefs that are firmly maintained even though they are not shared by others), hallucinations (perceptual distortions, arising from any of the senses—hearing voices or seeing images that others do not hear or see)

◆ Abuse of alcohol or drugs

◆ Growing inability to cope with problems and daily activities such as school, job, or personal needs

From "Possible Signs of Mental Illness," by J. Kozlak, 1996, personal communication. Reprinted with permission.

REFLECTIVE THINKING

Mental Health

Consider your own behavior and personality. Which traits would you classify as representing mental health? Which seem more representative of mental illness? Are you satisfied with the balance between the two?

present **distress** (i.e., negative response to stimuli that are perceived as threatening) or **disability** (i.e., impairment in one or more important areas of functioning) or with a significantly increased risk of suffering, death, pain, disability, or an important loss of freedom" (1994, p. xxi). The accompanying display presents possible signs of mental illness. It is important to note that none of these signs, taken in isolation of the individual and his context or life experiences, *necessarily* indicates the presence of mental illness. These signs, however, assist a nurse to begin to understand the nature and experience of mental illness.

Knowing something about symptoms and signs of mental illness is important, but that knowledge represents only the beginning of your passage. To really give nursing *care*, you will need some sense of what it feels like to be mentally ill, some way to see at least a little way into the suffering within another human being's mind. During your course you will begin to develop the necessary tools of listening, watching, and *being present*. As you interact with clients, some of what you see and hear will seem strange, crazy, and maybe at times a little frightening. If you start from a place of awareness and openness, your skills and confidence will grow each day. Give those skills a try as you read the following excerpt from the writing of a psychiatric client. The writer is responding to the questions, "How did you become mentally ill? What is it like?"

The Parallel Universe

People ask, How did you get in there? What they really want to know is if they are likely to end up in there as well. I can't answer the real question. All I can tell them is, It's easy.

And it is easy to slip into a parallel universe. There are so many of them: worlds of the insane, the criminal, the crippled, the dying and perhaps of the dead as well. These worlds exist alongside this world and resemble it, but are not in it.

My roommate Georgina came in swiftly and totally. She was in a theater watching a movie when a tidal wave of blackness broke over her

head. The entire world was obliterated—for a few minutes. She knew she had gone crazy. She looked around the theater to see if it had happened to everyone, but all the other people were engrossed in the movie. She rushed out, because the darkness in the theater was too much when combined with the darkness in her head.*

And after that? I asked her.

A lot of darkness, she said.

But most people pass over incrementally, making a series of perforations in the membrane between here and there until an opening exists. And who can resist an opening?

In the parallel universe the laws of physics are suspended. What goes up does not necessarily come down, a body at rest does not tend to stay at rest, and not every action can be counted on to provoke an equal and opposite reaction. Time, too, is different. It may run in circles, flow backward, skip from now to then. The very arrangement of molecules is fluid: Tables can be clocks, faces, and flowers.

These are facts you find out later, though.

Another odd feature of the parallel universe is that although it is invisible from this side, once you are in it you can easily see the world you came from. Sometimes the world you came from looks huge and menacing, quivering like a vast pile of jelly; at other times it is miniaturized and alluring, a-spin and shining in its orbit. Either way, it can't be discounted.

Every window on Alcatraz has a view of San Francisco.*

(Kaysen, 1993, pp. 5-6)

The woman writing this excerpt describes mental illness as a parallel universe from which one can see the world of the sane, a place where the predictable laws of our world do not hold, a frightening place. She writes from her current position in "our" world, but the borders between sanity and insanity seem to her only a "membrane" thick. As she reflects on her voyages back and forth across that membrane, it is easy to feel her ambivalence about which world she wants to stay in. There is both fear and a sense of entrapment in the "crazy" world, but it is hard not to sense that a part of her

---

*From GIRL, INTERRUPTED by Susanna Kaysen. Copyright © 1993 by Susanna Kaysen. Reprinted by permission of Random House, Inc.

prefers to be there: "most people pass over incrementally, making a series of perforations in the membrane between here and there until an opening exists. And who can resist an opening?" She is describing her experiences, but at the same time she is challenging you, perhaps to see how you will react, whether she can scare you a little. Can you resist an opening? she asks. Come on over, "it's easy." It is not actually easy. Most of us have little chance of becoming psychotic during our lifetimes, but it *is* easy to get caught up by the expressiveness of her language. This is one way experienced nurses can recognize persons with disordered thought: their own feelings of attraction or intrigue for the world their client reveals to them. While others may not experience mental illness in this highly verbal way, Susanna Kaysen's reflections offer remarkable insight into how a person may feel and may react to the experience of mental illness.

THE PSYCHIATRIC SETTING

Most students want to know who they will encounter in a psychiatric setting (be it a psychiatric unit, clinic, short admission, outpatient/community care, crisis admission, or home care setting), what the setting will look like, and what they can expect from it. Let us begin, then, by describing both clients and staff the student is likely to encounter.

Clients on an acute psychiatric unit are there because they are ill and in need of supervision. Some, like Susanna, are thought disordered and psychotic. Some are depressed and suicidal; some have been admitted to the unit after an attempt on their lives. Some are manic: They do not sleep, and their energy is boundless. Some have been admitted for drug detoxification or because of a drug-induced depression or psychosis. Each is a unique human being whose mental illness keeps him or her from functioning effectively in society.

Before we go on, we need to introduce some important concepts that will be considered in more depth in subsequent chapters. **Psychosis** means that the individual has lost the ability to recognize reality. A psychotic person may experience **hallucinations**, where he hears voices or sees images of persons or things that others cannot see or hear. A psychotic person is frequently unable to care for his basic needs of safety, security, nutrition, and so on. Such an individual is hospitalized for his own safety and to initiate treatment (usually involving some form of medication) to bring his symptoms under control. A psychotic person may slip into and out of reality much as Kaysen described in her metaphor of parallel universes separated by an easily crossed membrane.

Persons who are profoundly **depressed** (feeling very sad, despondent, and with no energy and no sense of the future) are in treatment for their own safety, and it is the responsibility of the nursing staff to keep a depressed or suicidal patient from harming himself. Almost every student has some idea of how it feels to be depressed, to be "down," to have no energy and no enthusiasm for activities, but few of us ever reach the profound depths of suicidal depression. Many hospitalized depressed persons are too despondent to talk or communicate except by occasionally echoing the words of others; some are catatonic, holding bizarre and rigid postures despite all attempts to move them. Depression of this degree seems untouchable, unreachable, and its treatment needs all the nurse's resources of presence, patience, and caring.

Other clients may be on the psychiatric unit because they are exhibiting manic behaviors. **Mania** is a condition where the person has excessive energy, exhibits abnormal excitability, and has an exaggerated sense of well-being. The manic client also may exhibit disturbed thinking, most often racing thoughts where she may not be able to concentrate on any one thing for very long. If inadequately supervised, manic clients may injure themselves or others. The manic client is at risk for exhaustion, as is the student assigned to watch, protect, and care for her.

Psychotic, depressed, manic, and drug-dependent clients are generally acutely ill. Their psychiatric illnesses may continue after discharge, but as their symptoms improve, they will likely leave the ward or hospital for the world outside. Other individuals under psychiatric care have long-term chronic mental illnesses. Many of these individuals cannot live outside highly protected environments, and some spend their entire lives in institutions for the mentally ill. These persons may be in touch with reality, but often their cognitive skills or coping mechanisms have been severely disrupted. Most have chronic schizophrenia and are unable to work or make choices required for independent living. Some of these persons may have unpredictable behaviors and difficulties controlling aggressive or sexual impulses.

During your psychiatric course you will meet individuals with a variety of acute and chronic psychiatric conditions, and we suspect that some will leave a lasting impression, as they did for us many years ago. You will also meet a variety of staff who work on the psychiatric unit, and hopefully some of these will be among your best teachers and role models. Some of these individuals will have familiar titles and responsibilities, but others may represent unfamiliar disciplines. Table 1-1 presents a brief description of the various persons working in psychiatric facilities. Each person has a different background, and each contributes something different to client care. You are encouraged to learn the specific roles of the various professionals and staff in the facilities

Table 1-1   Mental Health Professionals

MENTAL HEALTH STAFF	EDUCATIONAL BACKGROUND	ROLE
Psychiatric nurse	Registered nurse	Manages the inpatient or outpatient nursing care of clients; administers medications; completes assessments on clients, establishes outcomes, writes nursing diagnoses, and implements plan of care, including client/family teaching
Psychiatric nurse, advanced practice, psychiatric nurse practitioner	MSN with psychiatric nursing specialty	Provides psychotherapy; prescribes psychotropic medications (in most states); manages and coordinates client care
Psychiatrist	MD, has completed a residency program in psychiatry	Manages patient care; admits patients to hospital; prescribes psychotropic medications; may provide in-depth psychotherapy
Psychologist/clinical psychologist	PhD in psychology, with an internship in clinical work	Manages care; provides individual or group therapy; skilled in behavioral assessment and interventions
Psychiatric social worker	MSW with background in psychiatric care	Provides care that integrates hospital and community services; skilled in individual and group work
Activity therapist/recreational therapist	Has completed at least a baccalaureate degree in recreational therapy	Provides recreation, diversional activity aimed at increasing socialization and activity
Occupational therapist	Has completed at least a baccalaureate degree in occupational therapy	Provides vocational counseling and activities designed to prepare clients for job-related skills
Certified addictions counselor	Has completed training and passed a certification exam in addictions-related work	Provides counseling; facilitates group work; gives support to persons with chemical dependency
Psychiatric technician, aide, or assistant	Has completed course work in psychiatric technician work; in some states is certified to work in psychiatric facilities	Provide supervision of clients on inpatient and outpatient units under the supervision of an RN
Student nurse	In school for an RN license	Provides care to selected and assigned clients

where you are assigned to complete your psychiatric rotation in order to better function as a member of an interdisciplinary team.

QUESTIONS STUDENTS USUALLY ASK

Each psychiatric unit and its staff are unique. Your actual experience will be determined by factors unique to the setting in which you work and study. Still, students frequently ask some basic questions as they enter their psychiatric mental health course. We have answered these questions frequently enough that we think many of you may have similar concerns and we thus address them here.

Why and How Do Persons Seek Care?

Persons with mental illnesses often seek care for reasons very similar to those who seek care for physical illnesses: They are uncomfortable, in pain, and in need of help. Others seek care because a member of their family or a close friend encourages them to get professional help for problems such as chemical addiction or depression. Still others obtain treatment because they have lost touch with reality and are unable to make judgements. Their deficits in self-care skills bring them to medical or police attention. Some persons become disoriented to person or place and may be brought to a psychiatric hospital or an emergency department for evaluation and treatment.

Will I Be Able to Know the Staff from the Clients?

In most psychiatric facilities nurses and other staff do not wear uniforms, but, rather, wear street clothes. This surprises some students, who are used to the hospital and clinical settings in which uniforms are commonly worn. Students are often concerned about whether they will recognize which persons on a unit are clients and which are caregivers. In almost all settings, the staff wear name tags and can be identified as staff members in this way. You will have an orientation to the unit to which you are being assigned, and after your first day you should feel comfortable that you know who the staff are who will be working with you.

Will Clients' Behaviors Make Me Uncomfortable?

Perhaps yes. In our society, you can walk down the streets of any major city and encounter persons who are mentally ill. You see people actively hallucinating, having conversations with people who are not there, and gesturing wildly. On the streets most of us are made a little anxious by such behaviors and, even if we do not make a point of crossing to the other side, we tend to mind our own business and avoid eye contact. Not so in the psychiatric hospital. No matter how bizarre a client's behavior is, the nursing goal is to establish contact and treat the individual with understanding and compassion. Most nursing students enter psychiatric classes with little or no previous experience working with the mentally ill. Fortunately, staff and instructors are present to offer guidance regarding what to do, what to say, and how to approach a person who is mentally ill. Some ill individuals will prove remarkably approachable; others will resist all efforts. For example, a client experiencing hallucinations may not respond to the nurse's efforts at communication. With time and experience, you will learn how to provide the needed care and grow in your abilities to participate in treatment.

Are Psychiatric Clients Violent?

Yes, some psychiatric clients are violent or have the potential for violence. While there is a risk for violence in psychiatric settings, studies have shown that the incidence of violence among persons with psychiatric disorders is not significantly different from that of the general population. In a psychiatric facility, the staff are experienced in assessing potential for violence and are skilled at recognizing those situations where violence may occur. Also, psychiatric staff know how to remove a client from a setting in which anger is escalating and know how to control a violent client. This experience in management of

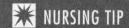

NURSING TIP

Suggestions for Conversing with a Psychotic Client

The following will help you in interactions with clients who are psychotic or out of touch with reality:

- ◆ Introduce yourself to the client.
- ◆ Talk to this person as you would other clients.
- ◆ Keep conversations concrete (rather than abstract).
- ◆ Help the client to stay in touch with reality by focusing on the immediate environment (elements and people in the room).

anger and violence is highly applicable to other settings and is one of the important skills to learn in a psychiatric course. Do be aware that there is a potential for violence in any health care setting, but also be assured that violent outbreaks are not a common occurrence on psychiatric wards and that experienced staff members, not the students, will handle such occurrences.

How Will I Feel Without My Regular Nursing Uniform?

It is interesting to observe how closely one can become attached to a nurse's uniform that identifies one as a professional nurse. The uniform provides an identity; to appear on a unit without wearing a uniform makes many feel like something was left behind. Further, nursing in nonpsychiatric settings is easily focused on "doing" things. A nurse takes a blood pressure and uses the need for a blood pressure reading to initiate a conversation with a client. In psychiatric mental health nursing, you must initiate the conversation without the need to take a blood pressure reading. On a psychiatric ward nurses cannot hide behind their uniforms or the physical "tools of the trade." Again, remember that the tools of psychiatric nursing are listening, watching, and being present. As you develop these therapeutic skills, you will come to identify yourself more with your abilities and less with the outward trappings of your nursing identity.

What Do Psychiatric Clients Think of Student Nurses?

Some clients are too absorbed in their own worlds or troubles to give any special thought to student nurses.

However, many clients are very aware of who is coming and going on the psychiatric ward. Susanna Kaysen provides an interesting description of the regular "influx" of student nurses to the hospital unit where she was hospitalized for many months:

Student Nurses

The student nurses were about nineteen or twenty: our age. They had clean, eager faces and clean, ironed uniforms. Their innocence and incompetence aroused our pity . . . it was because when we looked at the student nurses, we saw alternate versions of ourselves. They were living the lives we might be living, if we hadn't been occupied with being mental patients. They shared apartments and had boyfriends and talked about clothes. We wanted to protect them so that they could go on living these lives. They were our proxies . . . For some of us, this was the closest we would ever come to a cure.

(Kaysen, 1993, pp. 90–91)

Kaysen gives us a unique description of nursing students in that she is the same age and sex as many nursing students and was hospitalized for a long enough time period to see students come and go on her unit. Kaysen describes students as different from other hospital staff, as somewhat special. The fact that students are seen as living the lives the clients might live (or want to live) is a powerful idea. Perhaps this description helps you to put your role as a student in perspective.

ADVICE FROM PRIOR STUDENTS

Having taught psychiatric mental health nursing courses for many years, the authors pass along the following recommendations from prior students who wish to provide a bit of advice:

◆ Get used to a slower pace. You will not be running around a unit trying to get everything done in time for noon medications. Rather, you will be sitting with patients and interacting with them. If you feel you are not being a nurse if you are not busy with activities, you will have an adjustment. Keep in mind the side of nursing that listens, that cares, and that provides presence.

◆ Be yourself, and interact with clients as real people. The most important tool you have to use as a psychiatric nurse is yourself. If you see yourself as a caring nurse and show respect for other people, both staff and clients will eventually give you their trust.

◆ Take time to reflect on how you come across to others. You have a unique chance in a psychiatric mental health course to examine your own behaviors. If you sit close to a fellow student, what do they do? If you laugh, how do others respond? Catalog your strengths and weaknesses. What interpersonal situations are you most comfortable in? Which make you most anxious? Do some persons or situations evoke recollections of childhood experiences? How do these recollections affect the way you respond to the persons or situations?

◆ Emphasize and learn communication skills. Do not be afraid to say the wrong thing. Try out the communication skills you are learning. If you say the wrong thing, you will learn how to do it differently next time. Communication is a skill, and it takes practice to improve and master it. Use this course to practice these skills.

◆ Use the experience to learn about yourself. When you study psychiatric nursing, you will learn about yourself. For instance, you will read about defense mechanisms in this textbook and subsequently may find yourself using them in a conversation with someone you know! You have probably used such defense mechanisms all your life but perhaps never recognized them before. Defense mechanisms are normal human responses; it is OK to be normal and to recognize *how* you are normal. You will also read about mental illness and may begin to wonder if you or someone you are close to has some symptoms or characteristics of a certain condition. You probably do: Remember that mental illness is a matter of degree; the vast majority of us are healthy but also have a few characteristics of one psychiatric condition or another. Do not be surprised to find some "abnormal" characteristics in your personality makeup. But *do* seek help if you find any of your discoveries disturbing.

BEGINNING A NEW COURSE

Beginning this class, you are in a new phase in your nursing education. Hopefully, you will find this experience challenging and will emerge with different experiences and tools to use in nursing. Enter the course with an open mind and take information about human behavior and about yourself that is useful to you. Psychiatric care differs from other areas of health care. In order to work as a psychiatric nurse, you must be able and willing to live with a certain amount of ambiguity. Learn and grow from the experience!

Listen to, talk with, and *be* with the clients on your unit. They will be your best teachers; after a decade or more you may find them as vivid in your memory as they will be the first week. Above all, take time to "smell the flowers." Do not let hard work keep you from connecting with friends, family, nature, music, and the other experiences that make for rich, mentally healthy, and deeply satisfying lives. Now, put your hand on the doorknob, take a deep breath, and walk in.

≋ KEY CONCEPTS

- ◆ The study of psychiatric nursing affords an opportunity for the student nurse to perform self-examination of values, feelings, and beliefs.

- ◆ Rites of passage in psychiatric nursing refer to expected transitions and learning experiences linking the world of the student and the world of the practicing nurse.

- ◆ Mental health is a general concept referring to an individual's positive view of self, others, relationships, and the environment; it must be viewed in terms of degree, as all individuals experience varying degrees of mental health at different times in their lives.

- ◆ A mental disorder is presentation of clinically significant behavior or psychological syndrome or pattern as defined by the American Psychiatric Association.

- ◆ Familiarity with psychiatric settings and the different types of mental health professionals will ease the transition for the new nurse into the world of psychiatric nursing care.

≋ REVIEW QUESTIONS AND ACTIVITIES

1. Differentiate mental health from mental illness and from mental disorder.

2. Reflect back on a time when you experienced a severe threat to your mental health. What were the circumstances? Who was involved? What was your reaction, and what was the resolution?

3. Describe some of the reasons an individual might seek psychiatric care.

4. Discuss some of the professional options for individuals wanting to work in the mental health field and the educational requirements and general scope of practice of each.

≋ REFERENCES

American Psychiatric Association. *Diagnostic and Statistical Manual of Mental Disorders* (Fourth edition) Washington, DC: American Psychiatric Association, 1994.

Farb, P. (1978). *Humankind*. New York: Bantam Books.

≋ LITERARY REFERENCES

Kaysen, S. (1993). *Girl, interrupted*. New York: Turtle Bay Books.

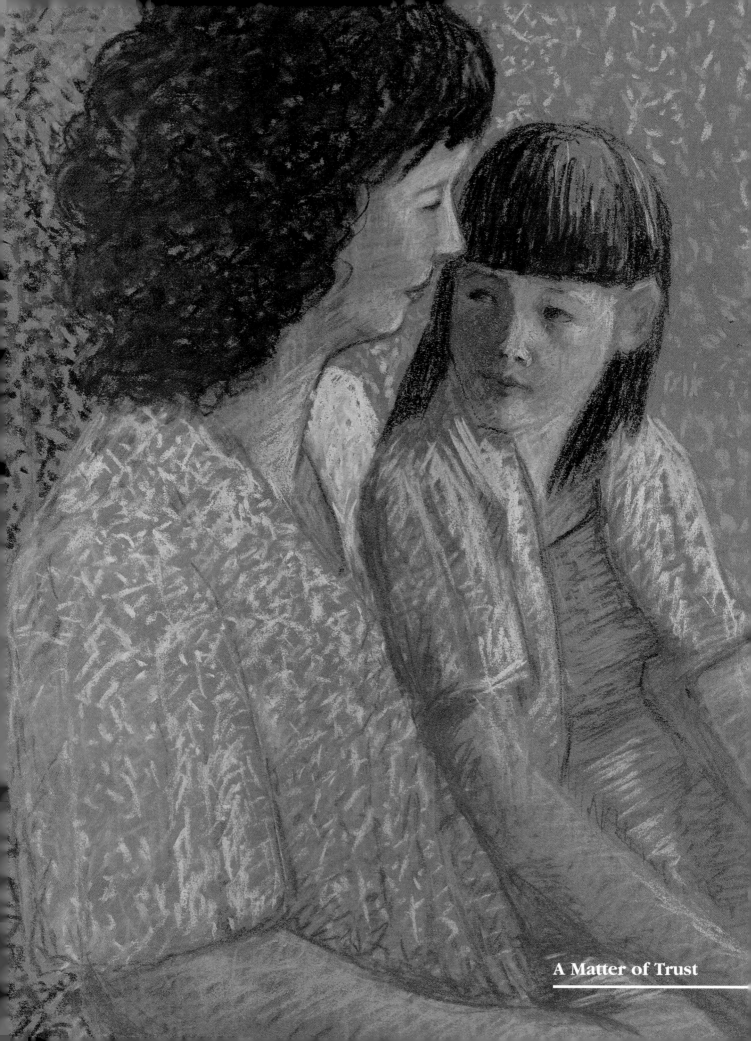

A Matter of Trust

Chapter 2

PSYCHIATRIC NURSING

The Evolution of a Specialty

Noreen Cavan Frisch

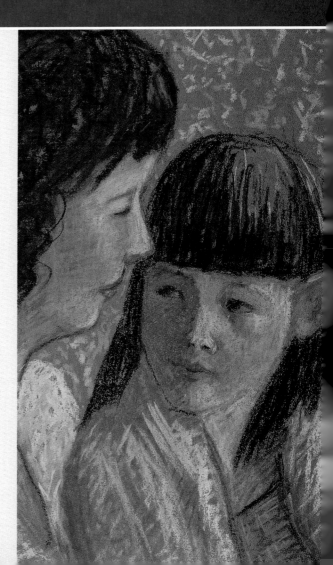

Your View on Psychiatric Nursing

Consider the following statements:

◆ Psychiatric nursing is very different from other nursing specialties.
◆ Psychiatric nursing has much in common with all areas of nursing practice.

Both of these statements are true. Learning about the history and development of psychiatric nursing may help to put these ideas in perspective. Reflect on both as you read this chapter.

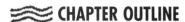 **CHAPTER OUTLINE**

CARE OF THE MENTALLY ILL

Early Civilization

Middle Ages and Renaissance

Eighteenth and Early Nineteenth Centuries

Nineteenth Century

NURSING EDUCATION

Eighteenth and Nineteenth Centuries

Twentieth Century

The Role of Nursing Theory and Scholarship

CURRENT TRENDS AND ISSUES

FUTURE DIRECTIONS

KEY TERMS

Asylum Large public hospital of the 18th century that provided for treatment of the insane.

Brown Report A 1948 report authored by Esther Lucille Brown on the future of nursing. This report advised that psychiatric hospitals be used as agencies for affiliation in teaching nurses.

National Mental Health Act Provided federal funds for research and education in all areas of psychiatric care. Act was passed in 1946. Established NIMH.

Psychiatric Mental Health Advanced Practice Registered Nurse A licensed nurse educationally prepared at the master or doctoral level and nationally certified as a clinical specialist in psychiatric and mental health nursing.

Psychiatric Mental Health Nurse A licensed nurse who has passed a certification exam and is thereby certified within the specialty.

COMPETENCIES

Upon completion of this chapter, the reader should be able to:

1. Describe societal changes in attitudes toward mental illness, leading to identification of mental illness as a disease.

2. Discuss the medicalization of mental illness in the 18th and 19th centuries.

3. Explain the reasons why nurses working with the mentally ill in the 19th century did not identify with nurses providing physical nursing care.

4. Identify factors that brought nursing of the physically ill and nursing of the mentally ill together.

5. Describe psychiatric nursing's role today as a core subject and content of nursing practice.

6. Identify the evolving role of psychiatric nursing in community settings.

Psychiatric nursing in the United States is currently so strongly integrated with the rest of nursing practice it may be hard to believe that 100 years ago general nursing and care of the mentally ill were completely separated. Readers of this textbook have probably assumed that a course in psychiatric mental health nursing would be part of their professional nursing education. Today, we have come to value the basic skills of mental health nursing as important for the nurse in the general hospital or clinic; and we have come to value the basic skills of physical assessment and management of physical health needs as important skills for nurses in both inpatient and outpatient psychiatric settings. However, as nursing schools developed in the 19th century, a distinct difference arose between those who studied care for general patients in hospitals and graduated as "nurses" and those who studied care for the mentally ill and graduated to be "mental nurses." Only after several decades of separate education, schools, and employment did the notion that every nurse must have a background in psychiatric mental health care become fully realized in the United States. The purpose of this chapter is to provide a brief history of the evolution of psychiatric nursing and to track the major developments that led to the recognition of psychiatric mental health nursing as an important nursing specialty in the United States. A brief historical overview of the treatment of mentally ill persons will be presented, with a discussion of how this treatment evolved to the point where there was recognition that the mentally ill were indeed ill and required both medical and nursing care.

CARE OF THE MENTALLY ILL

Early Civilization

Throughout history, those who were mentally ill have attracted the attention of others. In some societies the mentally ill or the insane were viewed with reverence, in some they were viewed with repulsion and anger. In primitive cultures where medicine, magic, and religion were not distinct, the insane were treated through magical rituals, prayer, and exorcism. Beliefs in the causes of mental illness ranged from the idea that the ill person was possessed by demons or was ill because of breaking some taboo to the notion that the affected person had had some harmful substance enter his body. Early civilizations, such as the Greek and Roman cultures, developed ideas of body "humors"—blood, black bile, yellow bile, and phlegm—which could influence emotional stability. Hippocrates believed that excesses of black bile caused melancholy and that blood-letting could remove this excess.

Middle Ages and Renaissance

In Europe during the middle ages and the Renaissance, mental illness was viewed with fear. Affected persons were thought to be influenced by the moon, thus the term "lunatic" emerged to refer to one controlled by the lunar body. In Europe during this time period, treatment of the mentally ill was influenced by beliefs that the mentally ill were evil, witches, or heretics. The mentally ill were excluded from community life, and eventually, in order to secure such seclusion, the mentally ill were confined to institutions that housed all those deemed not fit to live in society. Persons were treated as criminals and punished for their behaviors. Care was custodial, and inmates were poorly fed and clothed and were frequently restrained.

Eighteenth and Early Nineteenth Centuries

Throughout the latter part of the 18th and early 19th centuries, mentally ill persons who were insane were committed to asylums; those who committed crimes were put in prison. Care of the mentally ill, by and large, was provided by persons without training or interest in helping others and was often lacking in compassion. In both the United States and England, however, there were a few physicians who began to view the insane as persons suffering from disease and needing some kind of treatment. For example, English physician William Battie had a scientific background and a high social position. His interest in work with the insane ultimately served to elevate mental services to something respectable physicians could do. He believed that there is something powerful about a caring environment and recommended that those who work as attendants and nurses to the insane be carefully selected and trained (Nolan, 1993). Given the very positive influence of his work, it is somewhat ironic that the term "going batty" was derived from his name.

✆ *REFLECTIVE THINKING*

Society's Treatment of Those Who Are Different

All societies have means of dealing with those who are deemed "different" from the norm.

◆ When reflecting on a society's treatment of the mentally ill, what do you learn about that society?

◆ Who are the "deviants" in our current society?

◆ How are our deviants treated? What does that tell you about our modern culture?

During this time period, there were several theories regarding the cause of mental illness, as described in Table 2-1. No one theory was widely accepted, and the views of the physician in charge of an asylum dictated the nature of the care and treatment provided within (Nolan, 1993). Important, however, was the medicalization of the care of the insane. Physicians became those in charge of care; insanity was increasingly viewed as a disease, not a condition of character. In the 19th century physicians began their first attempts to classify mental disorders, and they so described both moral causes of illness (such as jealousy, religious excitement, and disappointment in love) and physical causes (such as epilepsy, injury to the head, overwork, and intemperance or drunkenness) (Nolan, 1993).

In 1846, the term *psychiatry* was first used by asylum doctors in England to identify their work and to further define the medical role in the treatment and cure of the insane. These physicians began to publish *The Journal of Mental Science* to further the legitimacy of psychiatry as a medical specialty (Nolan, 1993).

These physicians in England and their counterparts in the United States were part of a move to build asylums for the treatment and cure of the insane. The **asylums** were large, public institutions that were to provide humane and rational methods of treatment. The asylums were self-sufficient communities, having their own gardens for food production, their own kitchens, laundry facilities, carpentry shops, and the like. Everything needed for daily living could be found on the asylum grounds. Inmates (as the patients were called) had rigorous daily schedules that included work, time for reading and fresh air, and other activities. These asylums were designed and constructed as short-term hospitals for individuals who were expected to recover and return to society.

Nineteenth Century

Before long, however, the optimistic idea that the mentally ill would recover quickly and return to society broke down. The asylums required productive workers. Therefore, inmates who were "good" workers were not likely to be let go: They were needed to maintain the institution. Those who could not participate in the vigorous schedules had to be "controlled" by the asylum attendants. In many cases, physical restraints were used as the only means of controlling inmates. It became increasingly difficult to find persons willing to work in asylums, and many who did were not of sound character. Inmates were ill-treated, neglected, and taken advantage of by those who were supposed to care for them. Also, the asylums soon became overcrowded, making matters of control even more difficult.

Many individuals—physicians, private citizens, and recovered patients alike—called for reform. In the United States, Dorothea Dix, a private citizen who had provided nursing care to soldiers during the Civil War, became a crusader for reform in the treatment of the mentally ill (Figure 2-1). She advocated for humane treatment as well as safe and comfortable environments (which included heat in the winter). She fought for activities, such as dances, that would relieve the monotony of asylum life.

Table 2-1   Early Nineteenth-Century Theories on Causes of Mental Illness

THEORY	PREMISE
Inheritance theory	Belief that "insanity" is transmitted from one generation to another.
Moral degeneracy theory	Belief that persons are mentally ill by virtue of having bad character.
Miasmic theory	Belief that dirt and putrefaction are the principal causes of ill health. This theory provided justification for removing the ill and insane from the rest of society.
Germ theory	Belief that those who are ill can contaminate others; the insane, therefore, should be segregated.
Septic foci theory	Belief that there is a source of infection that causes insanity; removal of the infection (frequently through surgery) can cure the person.

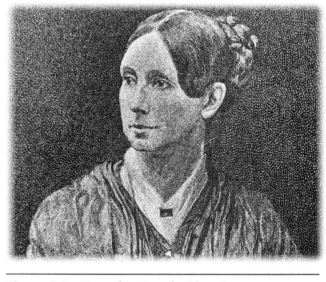

Figure 2-1   Dorothea Lynde Dix. *Courtesy American Nurses Association.*

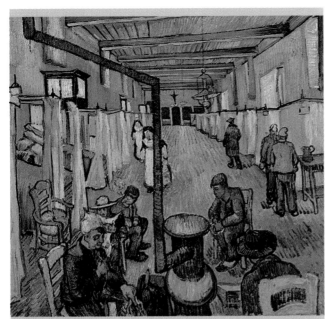

Men's Ward at Arles by Van Gogh
Courtesy of Oskar Reinhart Collection "Am Römerholz," Winterthur

V an Gogh was hospitalized for depression and psychosis twice between 1888 and 1889. The nearly empty long hall (leading to a distant and out-of-reach crucifix), the stovepipe separating the sisters from the inmates, and the strong sense of boredom characterize this picture, which makes both the mentally ill and their surroundings look far more depressing than frightening. Van Gogh probably suffered from manic depression (Chapter 13), but his epilepsy and suicide (see painting in Chapter 14) were probably greatly influenced by abuse of the drug "absinthe" (see painting by Degas in Chapter 15).

Through her efforts, care was improved throughout the United States and in Canada and Scotland as well (Dolan, Fitzpatrick, & Herrmann, 1983).

With the establishment of a reformed approach to care, it became increasingly clear that persons working in asylums (or what were then beginning to be called hospitals) needed training, a certain willingness to care for others, and a strong sense of compassion. How were such persons to be found? One physician wrote that women were to be more highly valued in this work than men, for women who were "of a kind and sensible disposition, could not fail to be of great comfort to those patients who require gentle and sympathetic attention" (Maudley, 1879, as quoted in Nolan, 1993). Still, how were women to be recruited into such work? One way was to set up training schools for persons to attend to the mentally ill and to provide education for respectable women and men who were willing and able to enter such schools.

NURSING EDUCATION

Eighteenth and Nineteenth Centuries

In 1882 the McLean Asylum in Somerville, Massachusetts, opened the first training school in the world for mental health nurses (Church, 1987). This school graduated its first class of 15 students in 1886 (Figure 2-2). Edward Cowles was the physician superintendent of McLean, and his effort to train nurses was part of his campaign to medicalize care of the insane. He proclaimed

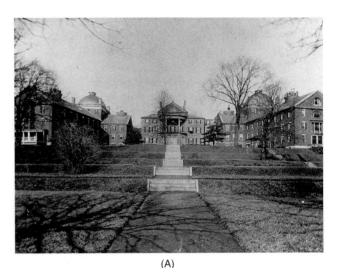

(A)

(B)

Figure 2-2 (A) Rear view of McLean Asylum, Somerville, Massachusetts, circa 1980. (B) America's first trained psychiatric nurses: The first class of 15 women graduated from the McLean Asylum Training School for Nurses in 1886. *Photos courtesy of McLean Hospital, Belmont, Massachusetts.*

that inmates would be called "patients" and that ward attendants would be called "nurses." He believed that the presence of a "nurse" indicated not only that the patient was ill but also that there was a hope for recovery.

During this same time period, other schools of nursing were opening in the United States. The most notable of these were the Bellevue Training School in New York and the Connecticut Training School in New Haven. These were the first in the country to operate primarily under the Nightingale model, where the training of nurses was accomplished via the tutelage of nurses (rather than physicians). These programs were granted autonomy from the hospital itself, and the education was securely in the hands of the matron or superintendent, who was herself a "trained nurse."

The programs to train the mental nurses were not autonomous in this way. Physicians like Dr. Cowles were in charge of the programs and established the curriculum. Dr. Cowles believed that these nurses needed skills in both physical and mental care and attempted to prepare nurses who could provide both. Ultimately, he designed a program where nurses studied physical nursing for the first year of training and studied skills in mental care in the second year (Church, 1987).

The year 1893 marked the first meeting of organized nursing in the United States. Nursing leaders met in Chicago at the World's Fair and participated in a formal conference on the state of nursing and nursing training. Various individuals presented papers on these topics,

and speakers included national leaders such as Isabel Hampton and Lavina Dock (Figures 2-3 and 2-4). These women called for clear standards for nursing education and for a clear definition of what it meant to be a "trained nurse" (Hampton, 1949/1893; Dock, 1949/1893). However, care of the mentally ill was not addressed in their proposals. Only one paper at this conference addressed the issues of asylum nursing (May, 1949/1893), and nurses providing care to the physically ill and those providing care to the mentally ill seemed to focus more on their differences than on any similarities that could be identified.

Mental nurses continued to be trained at asylums, and their training evolved to keep up with new approaches in psychiatric care. These nurses had to care for a wide range of patients. Much of the work still included custodial care and supervision of ward attendants. Staff had to make sure that patients did not harm themselves and did not escape. Treatments such as cold dressings, poultices (hot packs, often made with herbs, applied to a sore or inflamed part of the body), fomentations (lotions or compresses), and enemas were given. Manic behaviors were managed by packing patients in wet sheets (Nolan, 1993). Baths of different kinds were popular treatments: Hot baths were used for melancholy, cold for mania, and various positive claims were made about Turkish baths. Few drugs were available; however, sedatives such as alcohol and opium might be used sparingly for violent patients (Nolan, 1993).

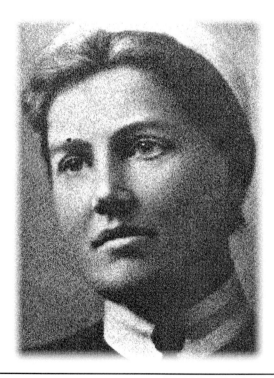

Figure 2-3   Isabel Hampton Robb. *Courtesy American Nurses Association.*

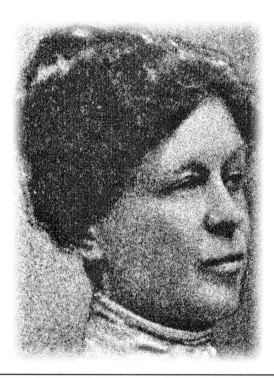

Figure 2-4   Lavina Lloyd Dock. *Courtesy American Nurses Association.*

Twentieth Century

The American Psychiatric Association established a committee on Training Schools for Nurses. This committee submitted a report in 1907 outlining the standards required for nursing, thus marking the physicians' official assumption of control over mental nursing care. In 1913, however, the Johns Hopkins Hospital School, under the leadership of Effie J. Taylor, the nursing director of the Phipps Clinic, included psychiatric nursing in the training of general nurses. This was the first time a hospital program offered training in psychiatric care to all of its students. Taylor's goal was to provide a standard knowledge base for all nursing so that there would be no arbitrary division of the patient's mind and body (Church, 1987). Her reasoning today comes across as the foundation of holistic care.

Over time, other nursing programs adopted a similar model to that of the Johns Hopkins program. Also, other programs developed exchanges where students who were studying to be mental care nurses spent a certain amount of time studying and practicing various aspects of general nursing. The time during and immediately after World War I increased the demand for nurses to provide care to mentally stressed persons. Mental hospitals were overcrowded and understaffed, and the national attitude was to develop increased services to meet the needs of veterans undergoing "shell shock" and other psychiatric disturbances. By 1920, the first psychiatric nursing textbook was published, *Nursing Mental Diseases*. This text was authored by Harriet Bailey, the Assistant Superintendent of Nursing at the Johns Hopkins School.

In the 1930s, new approaches to psychiatric care were emerging: mostly somatic therapies that involved treatments such as deep sleep therapy, insulin shock therapy, and ultimately electroshock therapy. The need for nurses trained in the physical care of patients became clearer, and by 1937 the National League for Nursing recommended that all nurses obtain education in psychiatric nursing as part of their basic nursing coursework.

In 1946, the United States Congress passed the **National Mental Health Act**, which established the National Institutes of Mental Health (NIMH). This act provided federal funds for research and education in all areas of psychiatric care. This act also provided funds for graduate nursing, assisting universities to establish graduate programs for psychiatric nurses.

During the late 1940s, nursing leaders joined together in a council of 14 nursing organizations and commissioned a study regarding the status of nursing education. Esther Lucille Brown, director of the Department of Studies in the Professions at the Russell Sage Foundation, was selected to carry out this work. She published her findings in 1948 in a document called "The Future of Nursing," better known through the years as the **Brown Report**. Among other recommendations, she advised that psychiatric hos-

pitals be used as agencies for affiliation in nursing programs, rather than having psychiatric hospitals conduct their own schools (Dolan et al., 1983). It was not until 1955, however, that the National League for Nursing required that nursing programs include classroom and clinical experiences in psychiatric nursing in order to receive national accreditation.

The Role of Nursing Theory and Scholarship

Nursing science and scholarship continued to advance in all aspects of nursing. In 1952 nurse theorist Hildegard Peplau published *Interpersonal Relations in Nursing*. This book presented the first nursing theoretical framework for the practice of psychiatric care. The framework is grounded in the interpersonal philosophy of psychiatry and is discussed in some detail in Chapter 3 of this text. Other nursing theorists followed, and some emphasized the interpersonal nature of all nursing care. Ida Jean Orlando published *The Dynamic Nurse-Patient Relationship* in 1961. This work was the result of a five-year project funded by the NIMH that attempted to identify factors that enhanced or impeded the integration of mental health principles into basic nursing curricula (Leonard & George, 1995). Orlando's theory suggests that all nursing care must be concerned with a patient's need for help (real or perceived) in an immediate situation. She suggested further that nurses help patients through disciplined interaction.

Psychiatric nurses established their own journals to further their work and to share their developing ideas. Two new journals were established in the early 1960s: *Perspectives in Psychiatric Care* and *Journal of Psychiatric Nursing and Mental Health Services*. Both are still published today, with the latter having changed its title to *Journal of Psychosocial Nursing and Mental Health Services*. In the 1970s specialty certification in psychiatric nursing became available through the American Nurses Association (ANA). With the establishment of certification, the ANA published the first standards of psychiatric and mental health nursing practice. Table 2-2 summarizes the important events in psychiatric nursing history.

CURRENT TRENDS AND ISSUES

Today, scholarship, research, and evaluation of psychiatric nursing have advanced to the point where there is no question that psychiatric nursing is a specialty within nursing. Other, more modern, nursing theories all address the holistic nature of people and emphasize the need to care for a person's mind and body (see Chapter 3). The ANA issued the current Standards of Psychiatric-Mental Health Clinical Nursing Practice in 1994. These standards document the scope of current practice and two levels of practice (basic and advanced). The accompanying display

Table 2-2 Important Events in Psychiatric Nursing History, 1773–1955

1773	First mental hospital in the United States established in Williamsburg, Virginia
1846	First use of the term *psychiatry* by physicians attempting to upgrade the status of their work with the mentally ill
1882	First school for psychiatric nurses (or mental nurses) established at the McLean Asylum in Somerville, Massachusetts
1913	Johns Hopkins Hospital included psychiatric nursing in the course of study for general nurses
1920	Publication of the first psychiatric nursing textbook, *Nursing Mental Diseases*, by Harriet Bailey
1946	Passage of the National Mental Health Act, which established the National Institutes of Mental Health (NIMH)
1948	Publication of the Brown Report, which recommended that psychiatric nursing be included in general nursing education
1952	Publication of *Interpersonal Relations in Nursing* by nurse theorist Hildegard Peplau
1955	National League for Nursing made psychiatric nursing a requirement for accreditation of basic nursing programs

PSYCHIATRIC MENTAL HEALTH NURSING: AREAS OF PRACTICE

BASIC LEVEL FUNCTIONS

- Health promotion
- Intake screening
- Case management
- Milieu therapy
- Self-care activities
- Psychobiological interventions
- Health teaching
- Crisis intervention
- Counseling
- Home visiting
- Community action
- Advocacy

ADVANCED LEVEL FUNCTIONS

- Psychotherapy
- Psychobiological interventions
- Prescriptive authority for drugs (in most states)
- Clinical supervision/consultation
- Liaison nursing

summarizes the scope of practice at these two levels. At the basic level of practice, the nurse works with individuals, families, communities, and groups to promote health, assess dysfunction, assist clients to regain or improve coping, and prevent further disability. At the advanced level, the nurse may focus on the full range of activities from mental health promotion to illness care, with additional skills in the diagnosis and treatment of mental disorders.

In the definition of psychiatric nursing, the ANA standards state that "psychiatric-mental health nursing is the diagnosis and treatment of human responses to actual or potential mental health problems. Psychiatric-mental health nursing is a specialized area of nursing practice, employing theories of human behavior as its science and purposeful use of self as its art" (ANA, 1994, p. 7). The accompanying display lists psychiatric mental health nursing's phenomena of concern.

The preparation for certification at the basic level of practice is a Registered Nurse, who has a baccalaureate degree in nursing and has demonstrated clinical skills within the specialty. The designation **Psychiatric Mental Health Nurse** applies to such a person who has passed a certification exam and is thereby certified within the specialty. At the advanced level is a **Psychiatric Mental Health Advanced Practice Registered Nurse** (APRN), who is a licensed Registered Nurse educationally prepared at the master or doctoral level and nationally certified as a clinical specialist in psychiatric and mental health nursing.

In addition to these levels of practice, there are also clear subspecialties within psychiatric nursing practice. Subspecialization requires education at the graduate level and currently can be categorized by age group addressed (such as child, adolescent, adult, and geriatric) or by a specific disorder (such as addictions, depression, or chronic mental illness). These categories are not mutually exclusive, but they provide a means of identifying a nurse's particular specialization. In some cases, certification is available for the subspecialty; in some cases, it is not. Currently, however, as long as an advanced practice nurse is certified as a specialist in psychiatric nursing, she may practice in a subspecialty.

FUTURE DIRECTIONS

In an introductory statement on the contemporary issues in psychiatric nursing, the ANA addresses the fact that the 1990s have become a time of increasing interest

PSYCHIATRIC MENTAL HEALTH NURSING'S PHENOMENA OF CONCERN

Actual or potential mental health problems of clients pertaining to:

◆ The maintenance of optimal health and well-being and the prevention of psycho-biologic illness.

◆ Self-care limitations or impaired functioning related to mental and emotional distress.

◆ Deficits in the functioning of significant biological, emotional, and cognitive systems.

◆ Emotional stress or crisis components of illness, pain, and disability.

◆ Self-concept changes, developmental issues, and life process changes.

◆ Problems related to emotions such as anxiety, anger, sadness, loneliness, and grief.

◆ Physical symptoms that occur along with altered psychological functioning.

◆ Alterations in thinking, perceiving, symbolizing, communicating, and decision making.

◆ Difficulties in relating to others.

◆ Behaviors and mental states that indicate the client is a danger to self or others or has a severe disability.

◆ Interpersonal, systemic, sociocultural, spiritual, or environmental circumstances or events which affect the mental and emotional well-being of the individual, family, or community.

◆ Symptom management, side effects/toxicities associated with psychopharmacologic intervention and other aspects of the treatment regimen.

From *ANA Statement of PMH Clinical Nursing Practice and Standards of PMH Practice*, 1994. Reprinted with permission.

COMMUNITY-BASED ROLES IN PSYCHIATRIC NURSING

HOME HEALTH PSYCHIATRIC CARE

◆ Case management for persons who live alone and are in need of supervision; care of the elderly and demented (see Chapter 23)

◆ Care for individuals with medical illnesses for which there is a strong emotional response (see Chapter 19)

◆ Ongoing care for the chronic mentally ill who live at home or in alternative care settings such as group homes/halfway houses (see Chapters 10 and 11)

◆ Participation in crisis response teams (see Chapter 9)

COMMUNITY-BASED CARE

◆ Family preservation, care of families at risk for violence, abuse, and dysfunction (see Chapters 21, 22, and 24)

◆ Care of the homeless (see Chapter 20)

◆ Care of the incarcerated (see Chapter 20)

◆ Psychiatric nursing in the community (see Chapter 29)

associated with aging, grief, and other serious illnesses or stressful events.

Mental health services are delivered today within a developing philosophy of managed care and cost containment. Today, many persons may be underdiagnosed and untreated. Those who are severely ill may be hospitalized for a very limited time, stabilized on medication, and discharged with unrealistic plans for follow-up care. There is an increasing need for psychiatric specialists in home care; it is the "fastest growing new area in the home health care industry" (Thobaben, 1996, p. v). At the same time, the notion of prevention is not being fully realized in most aspects of health. Mental health is no exception, and programs such as those that promote healthy parenting, stress reduction, or avoidance of addictive substances are underfunded and/or nonexistent in many communities. Contemporary issues such as domestic violence, addiction, homelessness, and poverty create environments where psychiatric care cannot remedy individuals' problems without addressing larger social issues. It appears that much of the delivery of mental health care and almost all of preventive mental health care must be done in community-based settings such as schools, homes, religious institutions, or halfway houses. As a majority of nursing care moves from the hospital to the community, there will be an increasing need for

and knowledge in biological, genetic, and pharmacological treatments of psychiatric disease (ANA, 1994). While these advances hold great promise for treatment, they have also raised concerns that advancing medical treatments could minimize the recognition of the continued need for psychotherapeutic interventions. Nurses in psychiatric care are called upon to lead the way for reintegration of physical and psychosocial care for persons with mental illness. Further, there is an unquestioned and rather urgent need for nurses with psychiatric nursing skills to provide service to individuals coping with acute and chronic illnesses, terminal diagnoses, effects of stress, societal problems (such as violence), and problems

psychiatric nurses to use all of their creativity and skill to provide needed services in the most effective way possible. Psychiatric nurses are taking on many additional roles in the community, including psychiatric home health care, prevention of mental illness and stress, and direct services to specific populations. The display on the preceding page presents many of the psychiatric nurse's community-based roles and lists the chapters in this text that present detailed information on each.

There are several nursing organizations that support psychiatric nursing, and these will continue to play a role in public education and forming professional alliances to advocate for individuals' access to care. The resource list at the chapter's end provides information on each.

✺ RESEARCH HIGHLIGHT

Home-Based Psychiatric Services

STUDY PROBLEM/PURPOSE

Evaluate the development and implementation of a home-based psychiatric program (which aims to off-set clients' anxiety and stress by providing a seamless system of health care delivery) as a continuum of care.

METHODS

A client is admitted to the psychiatric home care program when it is assessed that the client can be an active participant in a goal-oriented program and when the client demonstrates significant functional disability resulting from recent onset or diagnosis of an acute condition or the exacerbation of a chronic condition. The client is discharged when initial planning goals are met or when services could be provided in a different setting.

FINDINGS

The findings of these authors regarding an established psychiatric home-based program indicate that the average length of stay per admission to the program is 38 days; the average number of visits from a psychiatric nurse is 7.25 per case, with an additional 2 visits per case by a psychiatric social worker. Fifty-eight percent of the cases had fewer than 10 total visits from admission to discharge.

IMPLICATIONS

The study provides evidence that selected clients can benefit from psychiatric home-based services. Home-based services can assist in meeting planning goals.

From "Home-Based Psychiatric Services: A Continuum of Care for Hospitals, Home Health Care, Community Care and Physicians," by S. L. Spoelstra and M. Fitzgerald, 1996, *Home Health Care Management and Practice*, 9(1), pp. 40–48.

≋ KEY CONCEPTS

- ◆ Mental illness was not always viewed as illness, which led to inhumane treatment of the ill until the mid-1900s.

- ◆ In the 18th and 19th centuries a number of physicians became interested in the care of the mentally ill. Their work served to medicalize mental illness such that mental illness could be seen as a disease requiring medical treatment and nursing care.

- ◆ In the 19th century, nurses who were trained to work with the mentally ill were educated by physicians; nurses who were trained to work with the physically ill were educated by nurses.

- ◆ Several factors in the 20th century led to the integration of psychiatric mental health nursing with general nursing.

- ◆ Psychiatric mental health nursing today is a core subject upon which the professional practice of nursing is based.

- ◆ The current shift to community-based care has created new roles for the psychiatric nurse in managed care, primary and secondary prevention, and care of vulnerable populations.

≋ REVIEW QUESTIONS AND ACTIVITIES

1. Explain the reasons early societies did not view the mentally ill as ill.

2. Describe the process by which care of the mentally ill was medicalized.

3. What was the original purpose of constructing large asylums to care for the mentally ill?

4. How did Dorothea Dix reform services and care?

5. What was nursing training like for those who became mental nurses in the 19th century?

6. What factors led to the integration of general nursing and mental nursing?

7. Examine the current standards and scope of practice for psychiatric mental health nursing and suggest how this work supports the development of nursing as a profession.

8. Describe the community-based role of psychiatric nursing in your home community.

⚛ EXPLORING THE WEB

◆ Visit this text's "Online Companion™" on the Internet at **http://www.DelmarNursing.com** for further information on nursing history.

◆ Search for psychiatric nursing discussion groups as a topic; what can you find?

◆ The American Association for the History of Nursing (AAHN) is an organization offering information on the history of nursing; locate its site and review its offerings.

〰 REFERENCES

American Nurses Association (ANA). (1994). *A statement of psychiatric-mental health clinical nursing practice and standards of psychiatric-mental health nursing practice.* Washington, DC: Author.

Church, O. M. (1987). The emergence of training programmes for asylum nursing at the turn of the century. In C. Maggs (Ed.), *Nursing history: The state of the art* (pp. 107–123). London: Croom Helm.

Dock, L. L. (1949/1893). Relation of training schools to hospitals. In I. A. Hampton et al. (Eds.), *Nursing of the sick* (pp. 13–23). New York: McGraw-Hill.

Dolan, J. A., Fitzpatrick, M. L., & Herrmann, E. K. (1983). *Nursing in society: A historical perspective* (15th ed.). Philadelphia: WB Saunders.

Hampton, I. A. (1949/1893). Educational standards for nurses. In I. A. Hampton et al. (Eds.), *Nursing of the sick* (pp. 1–12). New York: McGraw-Hill.

Leonard, M. K., & George, J. (1995). Ida Jean Orlando. In J. George (Ed.), *Nursing theories, the base for professional nursing practice* (pp. 159–178). Norwalk, CT: Appleton & Lange.

May, M. E. (1949/1893). Nursing of the insane. In I. A. Hampton et al. (Eds.), *Nursing of the sick.* New York: McGraw-Hill.

Nolan, P. (1993). *A history of mental health nursing.* London: Chapman & Hall.

Orlando, I. J. (1961). *The dynamic nurse-patient relationship: Function, process and principles.* New York: GP Putnam's Sons.

Peplau, H. (1952). *Interpersonal relations in nursing.* New York: Putnam Press.

Spoelstra, S. L., & Fitzgerald, M. (1996). Home-based psychiatric services: A continuum of care for hospitals, home health care, community care and physicians. *Home health care management and practice, 9*(1), 40–48.

Thobaben, M. (1996). From the issue editor [editorial]. *Home Health Care Management and Practice, 9*(1), p. v.

〰 RESOURCES

ORGANIZATIONS

American Psychiatric Nurses Association
Association of Child and Adolescent Psychiatric Nurses
National Consortium of Chemical Dependency Nurses
National Nurses Society on Addictions
Society for Education and Research in Psychiatric-Mental Health Nursing

JOURNALS

Archives of Psychiatric Nursing
Hospital and Community Psychiatry
Journal of Psychosocial Nursing and Mental Health Services
Perspectives in Psychiatric Care

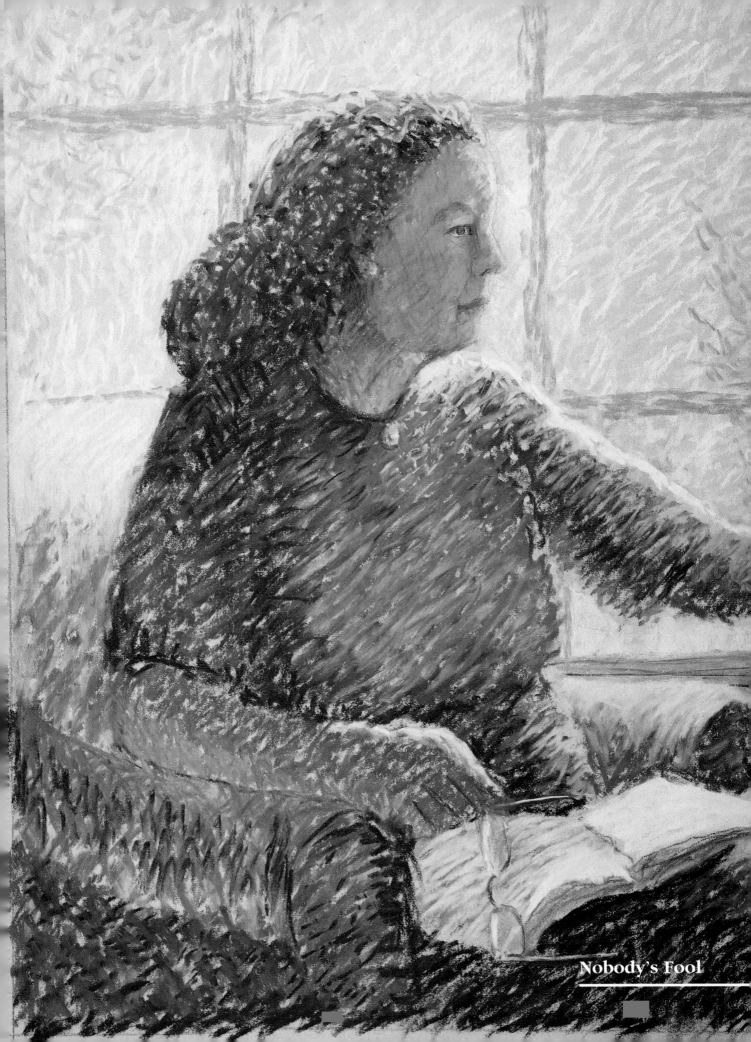

Nobody's Fool

THEORY AND NEUROSCIENCE AS BASIS FOR PRACTICE

Julia B. George

Lawrence E. Frisch

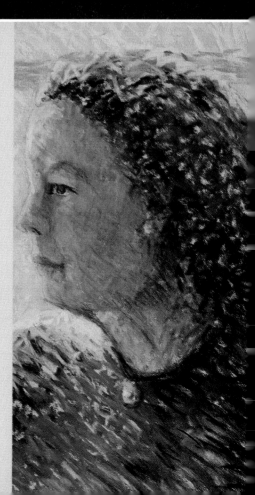

What is a Theory?

There is a common usage of the word *theory*; for example, a person might say, "I have a theory about why Cordelia didn't come to class today." What does a person mean when she makes such a statement?

What do you think the word "theory" means in a discipline?

Having your own answers to these questions may be helpful before thinking about how theory might influence nursing practice.

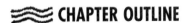 **CHAPTER OUTLINE**

WHAT IS THEORY?

THEORY AND PRACTICE

NURSING THEORY

Nursing Theories Based on Relationships
    Hildegard Peplau
    Helen Erickson, Evelyn Tomlin, and Mary Ann Swain

Nursing Theories Based on Caring
    Jean Watson
    Madeleine Leininger
    Anne Boykin and Savina Schoenhofer

Nursing Theories Based on Energy Fields
    Martha Rogers
    Rosemarie Rizzo Parse
    Margaret Newman

Nursing Theories Based on the Concept of
"When Nursing Is Needed"
    Dorothea Orem
    Callista Roy
    Betty Neuman

PSYCHIATRIC/PSYCHOLOGICAL THEORY

Psychoanalytic Theory
    Freud and Psychosexual Development
    Psychosocial Development
    Sullivan's Interpersonal Theory

Cognitive Development Theory
    Jean Piaget
    Adult Cognition

Humanistic Theory
    Basic Needs Theories
    Existential Philosophy

Behavioral Psychology

Sociocultural Theory

BIOPSYCHOPHYSIOLOGICAL THEORY

Brain Anatomy and Function
    The Diencephalon
    The Cortex

Brain Imaging
    Computerized Tomography
    Magnetic Resonance Imaging
    Positron Emission Tomography

Electrophysiology and Neurochemistry
    Neurotransmitters
    Membrane Receptors
    Neuropeptides and Intracellular Modification of Synaptic Signals

Genetics
    DNA
    Chromosomes and Genes
    Genetic Linkage
    Chromosome Mapping
    DNA Sequencing

Summary

COMPETENCIES

Upon completion of this chapter, the reader should be able to:

1. Discuss the relationship between psychiatric mental health nursing practice and theory.

2. Define terminology related to theory.

3. Identify the major components of selected nursing theories.

4. Discuss psychosocial theories from other disciplines useful in psychiatric nursing practice.

5. Discuss the emerging model of biopsychophysiological theory as an explanation of emotions and behavior.

6. Consider various theories as a guide to nursing practice.

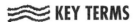
KEY TERMS

Adaptive Potential   Capacity of a person to respond to stressors—to utilize resources to cope.

Cognition   Process of thinking, knowing, and perceiving.

Concept   Basic building blocks of a theory.

Conceptual Framework   Group of concepts that are linked together to provide a way of organizing or viewing something.

Created Environment   Mobilization of all system variables.

Cultural Care   Facets of culture that deal with individual and group health and well-being, including efforts to improve upon the human condition or to deal with illness, handicaps, or death.

Cultural Care Accommodation/Negotiation   Nursing actions and decisions that involve reshaping the way in which care values are enacted so the actions will better support well-being, dealing with handicaps, recovering from illness, or facing death.

Cultural Care Preservation/Maintenance   Nursing actions and decisions that help people of a cultural group keep or preserve those care values that are applicable to the current situation to maintain well-being, deal with handicaps, recover from illness, or face death.

Cultural Care Repatterning/Restructuring   Change in culturally based care practices.

Culture   Values, beliefs, norms, and lifeways that are learned and shared within a particular group.

Ego   Conscious mind governed by the reality principle; controls the impulses of the id.

External Environment   Forces, factors, and influences that occur outside the boundaries of a system.

Extrapersonal Stressor   Stimuli from a great distance outside the system boundary.

Fixation   Preoccupation with pleasures associated with a previous developmental stage.

Folk System   Culturally based acts for responding to apparent or anticipated needs related to living, health, well-being, handicaps, or death.

Genetic Marker   Identifiable patterns of DNA structure that can be readily confirmed by laboratory analysis.

Genome   Entire complement of heritable information.

Id   Unconscious mind; the reservoir of psychic energy or libido.

Internal Environment   Forces, factors, and influences that occur completely within the boundaries of a system.

Interpersonal Stressor   Stimuli from outside the system boundary but proximal to the system.

Intrapersonal Stressor   Stimuli from within the system boundary.

Modeling   Assessment with the goal of understanding the client's world from the client's perspective.

Neurotransmitter   Chemical messenger.

Nursing   Learned humanistic and scientific profession focused on human care phenomena and activities designed to assist, support, facilitate, or enable individuals or groups to maintain or regain their well-being in culturally meaningful and beneficial ways or to help people face handicaps or death (Leininger, 1991).

Nursing Agency   Characteristic that allows nurses to act for others in meeting therapeutic self-care demands.

Nursing Situation   Context in which nursing occurs.

Professional System   Acts based on formal preparation for dealing with health, illness, and wellness.

Regression   Reversion to pleasures of a previous developmental stage.

Role-Modeling   Developing an individualized plan of care based on the client's world model.

Self-Care   Activities that humans perform for themselves.

Self-Care Agency   Ability to perform self-care in light of gender, age, socioeconomic status, developmental level, health, family, environment, living patterns, and availability of resources.

Self-Care Deficit   State that occurs when an individual's therapeutic self-care demand is greater than the individual's capacity to meet that demand.

Superego   Conscious mind governed by conscience and ego ideal.

Synapse   Structure formed where axons and dendrites come together.

Therapeutic Self-Care Demand   Activities needed to meet self-care requisites to fulfill self-care agency.

Nursing differs from other health care professions such as medicine, physical therapy, and pharmacy in many important ways; among these is the prominent place given to theory, both in the teaching and the practice of nursing. If you have friends who are pharmacy students, medical students, or occupational therapy students, you may find them surprised to hear you talking about theory, because it is uncommon for theoretical concepts to be explicitly discussed in these fields. In contrast, many nursing curricula and practicing nurses consistently use theory on a daily basis to help them understand and explain the basis for nursing care. Nurses are by no means alone in their adoption of theory-based practice: Theory is very important to the work of anthropologists, sociologists, and psychologists. Most scientists, in both the natural sciences and the social sciences, use theory to help guide their daily work. Physicists are, of course, among the best known theory users: Even as nonphysicists, most of us have heard of the big bang theory, the grand unified theory, and the theory of relativity, to name only a few. We may not know much about the details of any of these physical theories, but we do know enough about the enterprise of physics to believe that theories are important for guiding thought and experimentation. Theory is also important to nursing and perhaps especially so to psychiatric nursing. The authors of this book believe strongly in the usefulness of theory for nursing practice, but they also recognize that acquiring a theory base is hard for beginning nurses. This is true for several reasons:

♦ The meaning and use of theory are not fully intuitive, and it can be difficult for a nurse to reach an understanding of what theory is and precisely how it can be useful. Courses in theory often come near the end of nursing studies, so that the nursing student finishes almost all of his clinical courses, such as this one, before acquiring a formal grounding in theory.

♦ Individual theories are often difficult to understand, at least initially. The language is technical, and it frequently contains a variety of new words.

♦ Theory may seem highly abstract in contrast to work with clients in one's clinical rotation, where there are real individuals with pressing physical and emotional needs. It is sometimes hard to see how the abstractions of theory can be of practical help in providing care to individual clients, especially in the real world, where there never seems to be enough time to complete the day's pressing tasks.

Theory really is understandable and practical. However, learning and applying theory are not things that can happen quickly. Rather, they are like learning a new language: First comes the vocabulary, then the grammar, then simple applications, and only after all of these are assimilated does the whole structure become easy to use. The purpose of this chapter is not to make the reader an expert in either theory or any of the individual theories that are briefly discussed. This will take time and further study. Instead, the chapter provides an overview of theory and theories. The authors have tried to show throughout the chapter how a nurse might use the individual theories to better understand a specific client, who has been called Mr. James. In each of its clinical chapters, this text incorporates examples from a variety of these nursing theories. The reader may wish to return to this chapter or to some of the chapter's references when encountering the application of theory later in the course.

WHAT IS THEORY?

First, what is theory, and how is it used? Theory is a way to abstract or generalize knowledge so that it can be applied to a variety of individual circumstances. In this way, theories can be tested by empirical observation and experimentation. Theory might be defined as a set of interrelated concepts that are testable and provide direction or prediction. As abstractions, theories generate further hypotheses that can take the form of a series of logical propositions: "If this theory is true, then we predict that A follows. We have shown that A is true, so then theory predicts that B should also follow. Is B true? Let's try to find out." Theories are highly tentative structures and are constantly open to modification or replacement. A theory that correctly predicts a variety of phenomena is certainly strengthened by such predictions, but it can never be proven "true." To understand this better, consider a theory predicting that "all clovers have three leaves." While every three-leaf clover we find may seem to strengthen this theory, it should not be long before we find a two-leaf clover. On close examination we conclude that this clover began its life with three leaves but subsequently lost one. We may need to modify our theory as a result of finding a two-leaf clover, but the theory need not be abandoned. In contrast, finding a four-leaf clover, while lucky in folk belief, represents a potentially disastrous problem for the three-leaf theory. Theories are somewhat strengthened by observations that seem to confirm their validity, but they are seriously threatened or disproven by any observation that contradicts them.

Theories are not discovered but are instead created by experienced practitioners and scientists who can make abstractions from a large store of facts, concepts, and conceptual frameworks. **Concepts** are the basic building blocks of theory. Concepts are words and abstractions that represent reality. For example, the word *nurse* is a concept that represents the reality of the person who is being identified as a nurse. Concepts may be grouped together to form conceptual frameworks. A **conceptual framework** is a group of concepts that are linked together to provide a way of organizing or viewing something. The conceptual framework for this chapter includes the concepts of theory, nursing theory, psychiatric/psychological theory, and psychobiological and sociocultural theory. The major difference between a conceptual framework and a theory is that a theory is more precise and developed such that one can test the relationships contained within the theory. A theory is used in practice to describe what happens, to explain relationships or responses, to predict results of nursing actions, or to control outcomes through the selection of appropriate nursing actions. The nurse whose practice is based in theory can identify why certain behaviors are more appropriate in a given situation than other behaviors would be, can transfer knowledge and experience from one circumstance to another, and can communicate about nursing practice to others.

THEORY AND PRACTICE

Theory-based nursing practice may use both theories of and theories for nursing (Barrett, 1991; Phillips, 1990). Theories of nursing are theories basic to nursing, about nursing, and derived for nursing. They are original to nursing and deal with the phenomena of interest to nursing. Theories for nursing are theories that are developed in other disciplines but that inform and are applicable to nursing practice. Examples of theories of and for nursing are included in this chapter.

A word about the relationship among theory, practice, and research. Nursing is a practice discipline in which the practice is derived from theory that has been developed through or tested by research. The relationship among theory, practice, and research is continuously intertwined. We have already defined theory as a set of testable interrelated concepts. Theory provides a systematic way of looking at the world in order to describe, explain, predict, or control it. Practice, in terms of this text, is the delivery of nursing care to those who have psychiatric or mental health needs. Research is the planned and organized search for knowl-

🌀 *REFLECTIVE THINKING*

About Theory

- ◆ Why is theory important to nursing practice?
- ◆ What is the difference between theory of and theory for nursing?
- ◆ How does the approach to practice vary when using different theories as a base for practice?

edge, either new knowledge (basic research) or knowledge whose implementation has been tested in practice (applied research). Research is conducted to answer research questions or test hypotheses. Both questions and hypotheses can be derived from practice situations or from relationships suggested by theory. The results of research may provide direction to practice and may lead to the development of new theory or modification of existing theory. Practice may be based on theory and may be modified by the application of research results. Theory may be derived from practice or from research. Thus, practice may be shaped by theory or research, theory may be developed from practice or research, and research may grow from practice or theory. Or all of these may occur simultaneously! Theory, practice, and research are forever linked together.

NURSING THEORY

Nursing theory may guide and inform specific steps of the nursing process in psychiatric care or may supply a general approach to providing care. The nursing theories to be summarized include those of Hildegard Peplau, Dorothea Orem, Martha Rogers, Callista Roy,

CASE EXAMPLE *Mr. James*

The following case study will be used in examples of application of theory to practice. As several nursing theories are discussed, each will be applied to the situation of Mr. James, a 60-year-old man whose company downsized 4 months ago. In the process of downsizing, Mr. James's position of consulting engineer was eliminated; he was given a golden handshake and early retirement. He had no plans for retirement, having thought he would not retire until between ages 65 and 70 and "there was plenty of time to plan what he would do." His golden handshake provides him with the income he would have had should he have retired at

the planned time. Mrs. James continues with her full-time employment. They own their own home and at the present time have no serious financial concerns. Both of their children are married and live with their spouses and children in other cities in the same state. The entire family gets together three or four times a year and keeps in touch via telephone and e-mail.

Mr. James reports that since his retirement he is not sleeping well, he feels tired all the time, and he does not really have much interest in food. In fact, he has lost 10 pounds in the last 4 months. He says he feels useless and, at times, hopeless.

Betty Neuman, Jean Watson, Rosemarie Rizzo Parse, Madeleine Leininger, Helen Erickson, Margaret Newman, and Anne Boykin and Savina Schoenhofer. Nursing theories have been classified in a variety of ways. For the purposes of this text, the nursing theories discussed will be classified as focusing on relationships (Peplau, Erickson), caring (Watson, Leininger, Boykin and Schoenhofer), energy fields (Rogers, Parse, Newman), or when nursing is needed (Orem, Roy, Neuman). In discussing these theories, the term *patient*, rather than *client*, will be used when that is the term used by the theorist.

Nursing Theories Based on Relationships

Some nursing theorists have recognized that relationship is central to the practice of nursing. For some clients the relationship with a nurse may extend over years, whereas for others it may occupy only a few moments. Theories based on relationship recognize that no matter how lengthy or brief the human interaction and no matter what the content is of that interaction, a relationship is inevitably established between nurse and client. The form and content of that relationship may have a significant and long-lasting effect on both individuals.

Hildegard Peplau

Hildegard Peplau was a psychiatric nurse who was also an important early leader in the development of nursing theory. Peplau describes nursing as a therapeutic interpersonal relationship that provides a growth opportunity for both the nurse and the patient. The primary components of this relationship are two persons (a nurse and a patient, or client), professional expertise, and client need (Peplau, 1992). The interpersonal relationship identified by Peplau (1988) has four distinct phases: orientation, identification, exploitation, and resolution. During orientation, the nurse and patient meet, get to know each other, identify and clarify the patient's need(s) (previously felt but not necessarily identified by the patient), and progress toward patient comfort in a helping environment. The second phase is identification, in which the patient begins to respond selectively to those who can help meet the felt need. In this phase, the patient begins to experience an increased sense of belonging as well as a developing capability for problem solving alone and with others. In the third phase, exploitation, the patient takes advantage of available services to meet the felt needs and begins to gain a greater sense of control. Patients in the exploitation phase have not yet been fully restored to health and may manifest varying degrees of both independence from and dependence on their nursing caregivers. The exploitation phase is a transition period and may at times be difficult for both patient and nurse. It is important that the nurse maintain the therapeutic relationship in a nonjudgmental atmosphere while

this exploration is occurring. In the fourth and final phase, resolution, the therapeutic relationship is terminated after the patient's needs have been met. Conflicts and uncertainties found in the exploitation phase have been resolved, and the patient is ready to gain full independence, at least for the time being. Both nurse and patient will have gained from the experience.

Peplau (1992) indicates that her theory of interpersonal relations is particularly appropriate for psychiatric nursing practice because psychiatric patients often have problems with communication and with relating to others. Psychiatric nurses in particular may find that tracking their position in Peplau's scheme may help them understand both how to help their clients and how to respond to frictions that develop between them and their clients, especially in the exploitation phase. Peplau's theory is relatively simple and accords easily with commonsense notions of human relationships. This simplicity and lack of complex concepts and terms makes empirical testing of the theory difficult, but a number of psychiatric nurses have found Peplau's theory useful in generating testable hypotheses.

Helen Erickson, Evelyn Tomlin, and Mary Ann Swain

Helen Erickson, Evelyn Tomlin, and Mary Ann Swain (1983) developed the theory of Modeling and Role-Modeling. This theory owes some of its key concepts to the work of psychiatrist Milton Erickson and as a consequence is also easily adapted to working with psychiatric clients. Like Peplau's theory, Modeling and Role-Modeling emphasizes the nurse's interpersonal and interactive skills. The theory provides a formalized process through which those interpersonal skills can be applied in daily practice. The process begins with the concepts of modeling and of role-modeling.

Modeling involves nursing assessment (Erickson et al., 1983). The goal is for the nurse to develop an understanding of the client's world from the client's perception of that world—to understand the client's subjective experience. Modeling requires empathy to understand the client's view of the current situation, and in this way it differs substantially from the nursing assessment as traditionally incorporated in the nursing process. Traditional nursing assessment is factually oriented: The nurse's role is to obtain details of the client's life, illness, and perceived needs so that these can be synthesized into a care plan. Modeling requires a more holistic approach in which the nurse attempts to explicitly understand how the client sees his world. This worldview may be very different from the nurse's own and may be importantly influenced by cultural perceptions, prior experiences, and, for psychiatric clients, even thought disorders such as delusions or hallucinations. In the modeling process, it is the nurse's role to avoid objectification and judgment and instead to develop a clear concept of how the client views his life and personal needs. **Role-modeling** consists of developing an individualized plan of care based on the client's worldview. Role-modeling proposes that nursing interventions be guided not by the nurse's abstract perceptions of what the client needs but by the model that she has formed of the client's worldview. Role-modeling is not based solely on the nurse's model of the client's world but also incorporates a variety of theoretical constructs that are further aspects of the theory. Among these are aims of intervention, self-care knowledge, affiliated-individuation, and adaptive potential.

Erickson et al. (1983) identified five principles and associated aims of intervention that relate to similarities among human beings. The first principle is that of building trust: "The nursing process requires that a trusting and functional relationship exist between nurse and client" (p. 170) with the associated aim of building trust through the use of therapeutic communication skills. The second principle is that of promoting a positive orientation to increase the client's self-worth and hope: Modeling and Role-Modeling assumes that a healthy state "is dependent on the individual's perceiving that he or she is an acceptable, respectable and worthwhile human being" (p. 170). The third principle is that of promoting perceived control. Modeling and Role-Modeling theory postulates that individuals do not readily achieve physical or emotional health unless they have a sense of control over their lives: "Human development is dependent on the individual's perceiving that he or she has some control over his or her life, while concurrently sensing a state of affiliation" (p. 170). The fourth principle is that of focusing on client strengths. Every individual, no matter how ill or troubled, has a repertoire of strengths that can be called upon to lead to a healthier state. Modeling and Role-Modeling postulates that "there is an innate drive toward holistic health that is facilitated by consistent and systematic nurturance" (p. 170). Such holistic health is achieved by emphasizing the client's strengths so that ill health can be overcome or compensated for. The fifth principle is based on the concept that, working together, nurse and client can set mutual goals directed toward health enhancement. Modeling and Role-Modeling assumes that each individual has an innate drive toward health. The nurse's role is to work with her client to develop goals so that the innate drive can move the individual as rapidly as possible toward an enhanced state of health: "Human growth is dependent on satisfaction of basic needs and facilitated by growth-need satisfaction" (p. 170).

Having established a model of the client's world, the nurse working in this theory will attempt to focus care in a way such that each of the five aims of intervention is given an emphasis. That emphasis is further influenced by three related concepts: self-care knowledge, affiliated-individuation, and adaptive potential. Self-care knowledge is perhaps the most intuitive of these three concepts: Modeling and Role-Modeling theory postulates that most clients know what they need to do to improve their health.

The nurse's job is to help the client express that knowledge and to act on it through the development of personalized self-care resources. The Beatles were by no means the first to express the Modeling and Role-Modeling principle of affiliation when in the late 1960s they sang about the importance of wanting and needing "somebody to love." Modeling and Role-Modeling uses the concept of affiliated-individuation to emphasize that humans have the need to feel both attached to other individuals and individuated or separate from those individuals. Wanting and needing to love are important aspects of affiliated-individuation, but health also requires an element of independence from entangling relationships.

Adaptive potential is the capacity of a person to respond to stressors—to utilize resources to cope. Erickson et al. (1983) propose the Adaptive Potential Assessment Model (APAM), which includes equilibrium (adaptive or maladaptive), arousal, and impoverishment. Arousal is a stress state in which the individual has difficulty mobilizing resources. Impoverishment is a stress state in which the individual's resources are diminished or depleted. Equilibrium is a nonstress state. In adaptive equilibrium, all of the client's subsystems are in harmony. In maladaptive equilibrium, one or more of the client's subsystems are placed in jeopardy to maintain equilibrium. In either state of equilibrium, the client perceives no need to change. The client in maladaptive equilibrium requires interventions that help create a desire to change. The client who is impoverished requires help in meeting affiliation needs, promoting internal strengths, and identifying or accessing external resources. The client in the arousal state requires more support for individuation than for affiliation. Assistance for this client is directed at helping mobilize resources through guidance, direction, and teaching in relation to self-care.

The theory of Modeling and Role-Modeling can be very useful in the practice of psychiatric nursing as well as in a variety of nonpsychiatric nursing settings. Nurses may practice modeling a client's world as an empathic therapeutic technique without employing the entire theory. The concepts of adaptive potential may be found useful in conceptualizing a client's adaptive state even if the nurse is not explicitly using other aspects of the theory. Modeling and Role-Modeling is sometimes criticized for being overly simple and lacking explicit definitions and theoretical constructs. Some view this simplicity as one of the theory's strengths, others as a weakness. In this chapter, the student will find the theory applied to the case of Mr. James. Modeling and Role-Modeling is also used to analyze several other cases later in the book. From these analyses, the student can begin to decide whether relative simplicity, the theory's major strength, is also a significant liability.

See Table 3-1 for a summary of relationship nursing theories as related to the case example of Mr. James, presented earlier.

Table 3-1   Relationship Nursing Theorists and Mr. James

	PEPLAU
Orientation	Nurse explores with Mr. J. what his felt need is. After discussion, they conclude that he needs to feel needed and useful and has not felt this way since his forced retirement. Since his wife has continued working and has essentially not changed her lifestyle, he is uncertain how to continue feeling useful to others and an important part of his wife's life.
Identification	The nurse and Mr. J. explore how he can communicate these needs to his wife; they also explore where in the community he could use his skills to provide assistance to others and increase his sense of usefulness.
Exploitation	Mr. J. initiates a conversation with his wife in which she assures him that she values his ability to do repairs around the house and loves him for himself, not for the job he held. He also contacts community agencies about volunteer work and selects two to visit. In the process, he learns about a community organization of retired business people who provide support and advice to persons beginning new business ventures; he contacts them and discovers they have been seeking someone with his background and skills.
Resolution	Mr. J. reports that he is sleeping better, his appetite is back, he is exercising regularly, and he has been called to consult with two new businesses. It is time to conclude the nurse-patient relationship.

	ERICKSON, TOMLIN, AND SWAIN
Trusting and functional relationship	Nurse seeks to learn about Mr. J. to model his world. He shares that he had not planned to retire and had no plans for what to do after he retired. He feels at loose ends and is depressed.
Affiliated-individuation	Mr. J. states he feels that he is a burden to his family now; he used to feel that he was a productive member of society. He felt good about what he did and saw himself as the provider for his family.
Sense of control	The nurse explores with Mr. J. what activities might help him feel useful again (self-care knowledge).
Nurturance	The nurse explores what would reassure Mr. J. that his family still cares for him. He identifies that feedback from others that he has been helpful makes him feel good (self-care knowledge, self-care resources).
Growth	With encouragement from the nurse, Mr. J. identifies and explores opportunities to use his professional skills in helping others through volunteering and consulting (self-care action).

Nursing Theories Based on Caring

Theories based on caring do not deny the importance of relationship between nurse and client, but they emphasize the nurse's role in providing support through the means of human caring. This chapter considers three caring-based theories: those of Jean Watson, Madeleine Leininger, and Anne Boykin and Savina Schoenhofer. These three theories have substantial differences, and Leininger's theory is uniquely focused on caring across cultural boundaries. Each theory has elements that the nurse may find useful in approaching clients both in the practice of psychiatric and mental health nursing and in the broader domain of nursing practice.

Jean Watson

Jean Watson (1979) posited that curing disease is the domain of medicine, while caring is the domain of nursing. She proposed seven assumptions about the science of caring:

1. Effective caring is based on an interpersonal relationship.
2. Caring can be described through carative factors that lead to satisfying certain human needs.
3. Effective caring promotes health and growth.
4. The principle of caring accepts a person as he is both now and in the future.
5. A caring environment helps develop potential while supporting personal choice.
6. Caring is healthogenic and integrates biophysical and human behavior knowledge in a way that makes it complementary to the more medical role of curing.
7. The practice of caring is central to nursing.

From these assumptions, Watson developed a theory based on carative factors that allow the nurse to deliver integrated healthogenic care. The theory is itself based on three carative factors: the formation of a humanistic-altruistic system of values, the instillation of faith-hope, and the cultivation of sensitivity to one's self and to others. These three factors form the philosophical foundation for Watson's theory. In Watson's view, first, the nurse must be a developed humanist who is able to express altruism across cultural and other differences. Second, the nurse's role is to express hope for healing and to promote the concept that healing includes not just that of the body but that of the human spirit as well. Finally, the nurse must specifically cultivate personal skills of sensitivity so that an authentic contact with the client becomes possible. In Watson's view, only distinctly human and personalized relationships between nurse and client can lead to growth and healing. From these three principles—humanism/altruism, faith-hope, and sensitivity—are derived the seven carative principles on which Watson's theory is based:

1. The development of a helping-trust relationship. This relationship should be built on openness, empathy, and personal warmth. These factors all derive from interpersonal sensitivity and together allow the nurse to relate therapeutically to the client.

2. The promotion and acceptance of the expression of positive and negative feelings. Watson recognizes that nurses and clients alike tend to prefer the abstraction of thought to the experience of feeling. Based on humanism and sensitivity, she would have the nurse help her client to express real feelings.

3. The systematic use of the scientific problem-solving method for decision making. Although a theorist whose domain includes spirituality and the soul, Watson is also strongly grounded in empiricism. She emphasizes the importance of using logical and scientific thinking to understand and respond to clients' needs.

4. The promotion of interpersonal teaching-learning. In Watson's theory, communication of feelings from client to nurse is important, but of equal importance is the learning that takes place as nurse and client interact.

5. The provision for a supportive, protective, and (or) corrective mental, physical, sociocultural, and spiritual environment. In Watson's view, clients are often threatened or injured by their illnesses and need protection, support, and nurturance. These factors need to be seen as more than just physical and emotional; they must extend even to the sociocultural and the spiritual aspects of life. The client's environment should, where possible, promote health by being attractive, clean, and private.

6. Assistance with the gratification of human needs. Watson has characterized human needs as those related to survival, functional needs, integrative needs, and growth-seeking needs. She has developed a hierarchical description of these needs, but despite this ordering, she recognizes that all human needs are important and worthy of attention. Watson's theory recognizes the important reciprocal relationships between psychological needs and physical illness.

7. The allowance for existential-phenomenological forces. Watson recognizes that human experience includes both irrationality and arbitrariness. Illness and death occur unpredictably and can rarely be explained or accounted for in human terms. Human experiences often seem phenomena or existential accidents; there may be no better way to view them.

Watson's emphasis on caring is not unique. Many find her holistic emphases compelling. She sets a very high standard for nurses to follow and brings into her theory a number of important concepts: human needs, empathic human interactions, assessment of the spiritual aspects of health, and the importance of physical environment for health. Watson's carative approach becomes deeply involved with philosophical concepts of existentialism and phenomenology, subjects more abstract than many nurses wish to pursue. The theory continues to attract the attention of many, as nurses are drawn to the holistic nature of the theory. Watson's theory is studied by nurse researchers and is often subjected to tests, particularly of a qualitative nature.

Madeleine Leininger

Madeleine Leininger's (1991) theory is titled Cultural Care Diversity and Universality. She bases this theory on the belief that across cultures there are health care practices and beliefs that vary (diversity) and that are similar (universality). A nurse must have an understanding of the client's culture in order to give care. **Culture** includes values, beliefs, norms, and lifeways that are learned and shared within a particular group. These guide the thinking, decisions, and actions of members of that group in a way that creates patterns specific to the group. **Cultural care** involves those facets of culture that deal with individual and group health and well-being, including efforts to improve upon the human condition or to deal with illness, handicaps, or death. The practices for culturally related care are shaped by a number of aspects of the culture, including kinship, cultural values, political and legal factors, and language. Leininger (1991) identified three concepts involved in providing care. These are folk systems, professional systems, and nursing. **Folk systems** are those culturally based acts for responding to apparent or anticipated needs related to living, health, well-being, handicaps, or death. **Professional systems** are those acts based upon a formal preparation for dealing with health, illness, and wellness, generally within a multidisciplinary setting that is designed to serve consumers. **Nursing** is "a learned humanistic and scientific profession and discipline which is focused on human care phenomena and activities in order to assist, support, facilitate, or enable individuals or groups to maintain or regain their well-being (or health) in culturally meaningful and beneficial ways, or to help people face handicaps or death."

Nursing care decisions and actions are defined as **cultural care preservation/maintenance** (actions that help people keep and preserve their culture, for example, supporting one's need for prayer), **cultural care accommodation/negotiation** (reshaping the way in which values are enacted to support well-being, for example, supporting the use of a culturally based healing ritual as complementary to biomedical recommendations for treatment), and **cultural care repatterning/restructuring** (encouraging change in culturally based practices, for example, the way in which food is prepared) (Leininger, 1991). Any nursing decisions or actions should be sensitive to the beliefs, values, norms, and lifeways of the culture with which the individual, family, group, or institution identifies. Leininger warns against cultural imposition, in which the nurse functions as though the client's culture is the same as the nurse's. She also alerts us to the possibility of culture shock, in which the nurse is so surprised by cultural differences that she cannot function appropriately.

Madeleine Leininger forces us to begin by having an understanding of the client's culture. Nurses need to recognize that illness, and especially mental illness, occurs within a cultural framework. Culturally related issues are further considered in Chapter 6 of this text.

Anne Boykin and Savina Schoenhofer

Anne Boykin and Savina Schoenhofer (1993) developed an abstract theory of Nursing as Caring, which may be used in combination with other theories, for example, Watson's Theory of Human Caring, with which it shares many basic concepts. The details of this theory are complex and derive in part from the study of philosophical existentialism (Boykin & Schoenhofer, 1993). In psychiatric nursing, Boykin and Schoenhofer's theory calls upon the nurse to empathize with clients and to provide unconditional acceptance to clients who may not express caring or consideration of others in return. The nurse is challenged to provide nurturing and express caring so that the client may accept human care and initiate growth of self.

See Table 3-2 for a summary of caring nursing theories as related to the case example of Mr. James, presented earlier.

Nursing Theories Based on Energy Fields

A variety of nursing theories are based on the concept of a human energy field. The reader will recall a prior definition of the term *concept* as "words and abstractions that represent reality." The reality represented by the concept of a human energy field is that human interactions are complex beyond our ability to understand them fully.

While there is little doubt that we respond directly to others through our senses of sight, hearing, smell, and touch, many highly intuitive persons feel that human interaction involves more subtle and intangible factors. The concept of human energy fields tries to capture this intangible essence in a way that allows it to fit into a theory of nursing practice. Theories based on energy fields share a common view of the person as an irreducible whole comprising a physical body surrounded by an aura. Some persons claim to be able to see auras, but the concept of energy fields does not require an aura to be visible (or perhaps even that it really exist in the way that the reality of a magnetic field can be shown by bringing a compass into its path). The concept represents theorists' assumption that humans are more than their physical bodies and that their interpersonal influence extends beyond the scope of sight or sound. Accepting the concept of energy fields demands that the nurse take on a broader and highly holistic view of human existence than is implicit in the more traditional biopsychosocial view. Three nursing theories based on the concept of energy fields are described below. These theories are highly abstract and are presented in brief. The reader wishing more detail is referred to other readings cited at the chapter's end.

While energy-based theories have not generally been applied in psychiatric care, the complementary intervention of Therapeutic Touch (Krieger, 1979) is grounded in the concept and has been used to produce a relaxation response that can be helpful in psychiatric mental health nursing (see also Chapter 30).

Martha Rogers

According to Martha Rogers (1990, 1992), the science of nursing is the Science of Unitary Human Beings. In this theory, humans are irreducible, indivisible, pan-dimensional energy fields bearing recognizable patterns and are greater than the apparent sum of their physical parts. In Rogers's view, humans are in constant interaction with the environment. Human life is a continual interplay between an individual and his environment, though in stating this one must remember that Rogers's view of both an individual and the environment is energy based and not solely what is commonly meant by these words. Rogers views the human energy field as having a kind of physical resonance (her term is resonancy) that interacts constantly with the environmental field. Rogers further views these changing interactions as a homeodynamic process characterized by an inevitable movement toward increasing complexity. From these concepts, Rogers presents five assumptions about human beings:

1. Humans are unified wholes that are indivisible and cannot be identified as a sum of their parts.

2. Humans and their environments are in a constant exchange of energy and matter.

Table 3-2   Caring Nursing Theorists and Mr. James

WATSON	
Lower order needs	
Biophysical, or survival	Food and fluid: losing weight, reports no appetite.
	Elimination: occasional constipation.
	Ventilation: occasional rapid breathing.
Psychophysical, or functional	Activity-inactivity: Does not know what to do with self. Basically sits around the house all day.
	Sexuality: frequency of intercourse has gradually decreased over the last 10 to 15 years; only once or twice over the last 4 months. Does not really feel like a man anymore since not really the breadwinner.
Higher order needs	
Psychosocial, or integrative	Achievement: What's left? Mr. J. worked for that company for 35 years and they just decided he wasn't worthwhile anymore!
	Affiliation: Mr. J. knows his wife and kids are busy. He feels isolated and cut off from others.
Intra-interpersonal, or growth seeking	Self actualization: Mr. J. feels just dried up on the vine, not useful to anybody.
Using the carative factors, the nurse will assist Mr. J. with the following:	
System of values	Recognizing the value he places on feeling needed.
Faith-hope	Identifying how he can help others and meet his value to be needed.
Sensitivity to self/others	By exhibiting sensitivity to Mr. J., the nurse can help him regain his sensitivity to others.
Helping-trusting relationship	Developing a trusting relationship with Mr. J. will help him regain his confidence in his ability to trust in and help others.
Expression of feelings	Mr. J. has made a first step in expressing his feelings to the nurse; he needs to consider how to express his feelings to his family.
Scientific problem solving	Mr. J. has scientific problem-solving skills but needs assistance in applying them to himself and his situation, e.g., where can his skills be used to help others so he will once again feel needed and useful?
Interpersonal teaching-learning	Mr. J. has knowledge to share: Where and how can he share it most effectively?
Supportive, protective environment	Nurse supports Mr. J. in seeking answers to questions raised above.
Gratify human needs	Finding ways to feel useful: volunteering, consulting.
Existential-phenomenological forces	Nurse recognizes the choices are Mr. J.'s; he must be the one to make decisions about what he will seek to do.

LEININGER	
Gather information about:	
Technology	Mr. J. is an engineer; he is comfortable with a variety of technologies, including business use of computers.
Philosophy	The man of the household should be the provider.
Society	Mr. J. lives in a society that values self-care and self-direction.
Political/legislative	Policies allowed for forced early retirement.
Education	Mr. J. has a master's degree in business administration.
Environment	Mr. J. was in a busy office; now he is primarily home alone during the day.
Religion	Protestant; Mr. J. does not attend church regularly.
Kinship	Most important family members are his wife, children, and grandchildren. He has no living siblings..
Cultural values	He considers himself true blue American.
Economic	Mr. J. has no major financial concerns but still would like to see self as primary provider for his family.
Language	English is Mr. J.'s primary language.

Continued

Table 3-2   Caring Nursing Theorists and Mr. James   *Continued*

Folk system practices	Mr. J. takes 2 tsp of Grannie (Golden raisins soaked in gin) daily for arthritis; believes pain and constriction of motion have decreased significantly since he began this practice.
Professional health system practices	Mr. J. had an annual physical while working and has no major health problems; now relies on health insurance from his wife's employment.

Nurse identifies Mr. J's need to feel useful again. Chooses to provide culturally congruent care through repatterning/restructuring. The goal is to assist Mr. J. in changing from seeing his work as the primary source of his feeling useful to gaining a sense of usefulness from other sources. Ways in which he can use his engineering and business skills would be culturally congruent.

BOYKIN AND SCHOENHOFER	
Nursing situation	Being: The nurse meets and talks with Mr. J., encouraging him to direct the conversation as he wishes. Knowing: The nurse seeks to understand and to help Mr. J. understand what his concerns are. Living: The nurse and Mr. J. together explore the avenues of opportunity that are available to him (such as volunteering). Valuing: Mr. J. decides what he wants and chooses ways in which he can feel useful (care).
Nurture him in living caring, and growing in caring	Identify Mr. J.'s ways of living caring (helping others and feeling useful).
Enhance personhood of both	Both the nurse and Mr. J. grow and change as they explore the choices available to him and as he chooses volunteer activities in the community.
Response to call for nurturance	The nurse, in aspiring to grow in caring, has a commitment to recognize and nurture caring. Mr. J.'s caring is demonstrated in his concern for his family and his desire to help others.

3. The life process of humans evolves irreversibly but unpredictably in one direction only.

4. The wholeness of humans is reflected in their energy patterns.

5. Humans are capable of imagery, thought, abstraction, language, sensation, and emotion.

Unlike some other theorists, Rogers neither makes nor implies a specific definition of health or of the process of nursing. Nursing participates in the process of human individual evolution and tries to understand how a person and his environment have previously interacted. Since life evolves in one direction only, nursing interventions cannot return a client to his previous state of health but can only work to move him forward toward more complex human states. The nurse is viewed as part of the client's environmental energy field, as the nurse is external to the client. Because of the mutual interaction between the individual and the environment, the nurse works *with* the client to achieve maximum potential, as opposed to working *to* or *for* the client, as in many other theories.

Rogers's theory can seem divorced from reality, but for many nurses it serves as a stimulus to rethink simplistic assumptions about human nature and, in consequence, to understand the client and self in clinically useful ways.

Rosemarie Rizzo Parse

Rosemarie Rizzo Parse (1981, 1992) developed her Theory of Human Becoming from existential phenomenology and the work of Martha Rogers (1970). Parse (1995) extends Rogers's theory and gives it much more dense philosophical underpinning. Parse's assumptions are that the human is "an open being, freely choosing meaning in situation, bearing responsibility for decisions" and "coexisting while coconstituting rhythmical patterns with the universe." Becoming is "an open process, experienced by the human" as "an intersubjective process of transcending with the possibles" (pp. 5–6). The reader can see both how existential ideas mix with concepts derived from Martha Rogers and how difficult Parse's theory is to decode. Parse believes that people create reality for themselves through the choices they make at many levels. People reflect their reality through spoken words, silence, movements and being still (languaging), living based upon personal beliefs (valuing), and knowing both specifically and implicitly (imaging).

Parse sees paradoxes within human interactions: revealing-concealing, enabling-limiting, and connecting-separating. For example, as a person chooses to reveal something, he must also conceal something else. As one enables another's action, one also limits choices at the same time. As two people connect, they also must separate. In practice, the nurse does not seek to control or shape the actions of the client or family but, rather, helps them recognize their own experience through a process of equal partnership—two individuals coming together to examine and understand the meaning of life's experiences. Parse's theory can help link theories of energy fields with theories of caring, but only for the nurse who relishes a very high degree of philosophical and linguistic complexity.

Margaret Newman

Margaret Newman grounds her theory in an attempt to understand the concept of Health as Expanding Consciousness (Newman, 1994). As noted previously, the abstract idea of health is not found in Rogers's work, and Parse is far more concerned with open-ended human becoming than with health. Newman (1994) supports a view of health that fuses disease and nondisease into a paradoxical formulation that some may find perplexing. Health, Newman assumes in her theory, includes both the condition of being well (which commonsense usage also associates with the definition of health) *and* the condition of being ill. Because health is seen, in ideas deriving from Rogers, as the evolving process of expanding consciousness, becoming ill may paradoxically be a manifestation of health. Newman proposes that those states that we identify as sickness may be needed to achieve something an individual has desired but been unable to achieve otherwise—an idea that may derive from classical psychoanalysis. She further adopts from Rogers the concept of unitary human beings and concludes that if beings are truly unitary, they cannot be either ill or well but instead must at all times manifest some synthesis of the two conditions.

Newman's view of health has strong implications for how nursing is practiced. The client is not seen as having an illness to cure or care for but as manifesting patterns that themselves provide information about the whole person. Recognizing these patterns, the nurse then seeks to relate to the unfolding of the individual's life pattern. Newman (1994) indicates that one's flexibility in responding to one's own illness or stress determines whether or not the result will be disabling. She strongly encourages that we accept our experiences as ours no matter how they differ from what we had planned or wished for: "The important factor is to be fully present in the moment and know that whatever the experience, it is a manifestation of the process of evolving to higher consciousness" (p. 68).

Newman's theory is, of course, far more complex than outlined here and includes extensive consideration of the role of time and rhythms in human experience. Like other theories grounded in phenomenology and the philosophy of Hegel, Newman's theory is difficult to understand and apply. Nurses who are attracted to paradox and complexity may find themselves especially interested in Newman's work.

See Table 3-3 for a summary of nursing theories based on the concept of energy fields.

Nursing Theories Based on the Concept of "When Nursing Is Needed"

Several nursing theories have evolved to answer questions something like the following: How do we know that any specific individual needs nursing care? These theories offer the attraction of addressing fairly concrete and practical questions and providing answers that attempt to assess the specific needs that people have that, not being able to meet for themselves, they must meet through nursing care.

Dorothea Orem

Dorothea Orem (1991) proposed a general Self-Care Deficit Theory of Nursing, which is composed of three interrelated concepts—self-care, self-care deficit, and nursing systems—which are themselves based on six central and one peripheral concept. The central concepts are self-care, self-care agency, therapeutic self-care demand, self-care deficit, nursing agency, and nursing system. The peripheral concept is that of basic conditioning factors (Orem, 1991). **Self-care** includes those activities that human beings perform for themselves (or for dependent others) to maintain life, health, and well-being. **Self-care agency** is the ability to perform self-care and is influenced by the basic conditioning factors of gender, age, socioeconomic status, developmental level, and health; health care system factors such as available diagnostic and treatment facilities; family; environment; living patterns; and availability of adequate resources. Health deviation self-care needs are those that arise from illness, injury, or disease or from medical measures taken to diagnose or treat such. **Therapeutic self-care demand** consists of all the activities needed to meet self-care requisites to fulfill self-care agency. **Self-care deficit** occurs or exists when the therapeutic self-care demand is greater than the person's capacity to meet the demand (Orem, 1991). Thus, nursing is needed when the person can no longer provide self-care. Nursing activities to help the person may include doing for the person, teaching, guiding, supporting, or managing an environment to be developmentally supportive. **Nursing agency** is that complex characteristic gained through formal preparation and experiences that allows nurses to act for others in meeting therapeutic self-care demands through exercising or developing self-care agency.

After a self-care deficit is identified, the nurse designs the appropriate nursing system (Orem, 1991). The type of

Table 3-3   Energy Field Nursing Theorists and Mr. James

ROGERS	
Integrality	Mr. J. is in continuous exchange with his environment; change in his environment from business to home has changed the environment from a mix of office and home to primarily home.
Resonancy	The length and frequency of Mr. J.'s wave patterns have changed; his level of activity was much higher and changed more often when he was working. His own description of himself indicates much slower change.
Helicy	The direction of change for Mr. J. continues to be toward increasing diversity and complexity. He has not lost the business knowledge he had, but he has not been using it for the last 4 months.

Mr. J. needs to balance his exchange with his environment (integrality) to regain a wave pattern (resonancy) that is acceptable to him and supports his increasing diversity and complexity (helicy). One way he can do this is to volunteer in the community, thus increasing the diversity of the environments in which he functions, causing more frequent change in his patterns, and providing additional learning for him, which will increase his diversity and complexity.

PARSE	
Explicating	The nurse and Mr. J. explore the meaning of the situation to him and attempt to make a connection between his current feelings of despair and his forced retirement.
Dwelling with	The nurse and Mr. J. become involved in the struggle of connecting-separating. Mr. J. was forced to separate from his employment and has not experienced equivalent connecting. What connecting would be of interest to him?
Moving beyond	The nurse supports Mr. J. in planning for changing patterns, identifying choices for connecting (volunteering), and making choices.

NEWMAN	
Choice point	Mr. J. was forced to retire and does not have past experience in how to handle the situation. He has identified that staying at home does not meet his needs and he needs to find new ways of behaving.
Movement	Mr. J.'s movement is less than it was 4 months ago; he seeks new ways to increase his movement.
Time	Time is moving slower in association with decreased movement.
Space	The space Mr. J. has been occupying has been smaller.
Consciousness	Mr. J. has experienced a decreased exchange of new information.
Patterns	His patterns have changed without his control; he seeks a transformation in which he regains control of his choices and activities.
Health	As a reflection of the whole and examples of underlying patterns, Mr. J. indicates his current patterns are not satisfactory to him.
Search for patterns	Mr. J. has had a change in pattern from Monday–Friday, work to retirement; he is searching for new acceptable patterns.
Information	Mr. J. provides information about his feelings of uselessness.
Body–dynamic energy field	Sleeplessness and weight loss indicate reaching a choice point.

Data indicate Mr. J. has reached a choice point. Selecting volunteer activities that get him out of the house and allow him to feel useful again will change his patterns and indicate expanding consciousness.

nursing system needed is defined by the type of self-care deficit that exists. A wholly compensatory system is needed when the patient is incapable of or should not be engaging in deliberate actions focused on meeting self-care needs. Incapability may be physical, mental, emo- tional, or some combination of these. In contrast, those who can perform some but not all aspects of self-care activities require a partially compensatory nursing system. In this system, both nurse and patient are active partici- pants. Finally, those who can perform all self-care actions but need assistance with gaining new knowledge or skills, making decisions, or achieving behavior control require a supportive-educative or supportive-developmental system.

Orem's theory has proven popular with both practicing nurses and academicians. Many studies have tested hypotheses derived from Orem's work. In contrast to Newman's theory discussed preceding, Orem's concept of health is highly static, and her view of the nurse-client intervention may seem somewhat one-sided when viewed from the perspective of a theory like Modeling and Role-Modeling. Further, Orem's theory has little explicitly to say about psychiatric care or the issues of caring addressed in Watson's theory. Nonetheless, because it is concrete and widely known, Orem's theory has potential utility in approaching the unique challenges of psychiatric nursing care.

Callista Roy

The four essential elements of the Roy Adaptation Model, developed by Callista Roy, are the person or system (recipient of nursing care), environment, health, and nursing (Roy & Andrews, 1991). The recipient of nursing care is seen as a holistic adaptive system that responds to stimuli from the environment. When adaptation occurs, health may be present. Health is defined as "a state and a process of being and becoming an integrated and whole person" (p. 19) and is apparent when the person is able to meet goals of survival, growth, reproduction, and mastery.

The person processes the environmental stimuli through coping mechanisms identified as the cognator and regulator subsystems. The cognator subsystem processes are related to higher brain functions such as information processing, judgment, emotion, and perception. The regulator subsystem processes are related to chemical, neural, and endocrine responses such as those of the autonomic nervous system. The processes within these subsystems are not seen directly but, rather, are identified through psychomotor behaviors within four adaptive modes (Roy & Andrews, 1991).

These modes are named physiological, self-concept, role function, and interdependence (Roy & Andrews, 1991). The physiological mode includes oxygenation, nutrition, elimination, activity and rest, protection, senses, fluids and electrolytes, neurological function, and endocrine function. The self-concept mode relates to the spiritual and psychological aspects of the person and includes the physical self (body sensation, body image) and the personal self (self-consistency, self-ideal, moral-ethical-spiritual self). The interdependence mode includes interpersonal relationships with both individuals and groups. Affectional needs are met in this mode.

Responses to environmental stimuli may be either adaptive or ineffective (Roy & Andrews, 1991). Adaptive responses are those that support the integrity of the person and help fulfill goals of survival, growth, reproduction, and mastery. Ineffective responses are those that do not support integrity or help fulfill goals.

Roy's nursing process has six steps: first-level assessment, second-level assessment, nursing diagnosis, goal setting, intervention, and evaluation (Roy & Andrews, 1991). The first-level assessment focuses on behaviors that are responses to environmental stimuli and results in identifying those behaviors that are adaptive and those that are ineffective. The second-level assessment focuses on ineffective behaviors and those adaptive behaviors that need nursing support. This assessment includes identifying the stimuli that have led to the behaviors.

After assessment comes diagnosis, and according to Roy and Andrews (1991), there are several methods of making a nursing diagnosis. The first is to use Roy's typology of diagnoses that relate to specific adaptive modes. An example of such a diagnosis would be *anxiety* in relation to the personal-self component of the self-concept mode. The second is to state the response observed in one mode along with the associated stimuli. An example would be *anxiety* caused by concern about ability to deal with results of impending surgery. The third is to provide a summary of responses in one or more adaptive modes that are related to the same stimuli. An example representing the self-concept and physiological modes would be *anxiety* and *sleep disturbance* related to concern about impending surgery.

The goal of nursing is to promote adaptive responses (Roy & Andrews, 1991). Thus, goal setting will include identifying those behaviors that, when observed, will indicate the person has achieved adaptive responses. Nursing interventions will seek to alter or manage the environment so adaptive responses can occur. Evaluation requires that patient behaviors be compared to goal behaviors to identify whether adaptive responses are present.

Roy's model is discussed here as a theory of when nursing is needed, but in reality it is both more and less than this. Roy presents her work as a model rather than a theory, and technically this makes her work somewhat less than a theory. The distinction is somewhat arbitrary, but models are often taken to be descriptions of practice out of which theories are abstracted. Like theories, models may be used to generate testable hypotheses, so Roy's model has many of the features of other theories considered in this chapter. In addition to considering when nursing is needed, Roy's model presents a comprehensive view of the overall nursing process. Roy challenges the nurse to follow assessment with a nursing diagnosis using specific qualifiers and offers opportunities for assessing diagnostic accuracy between observers. She further challenges the nurse to assess clinical outcomes by setting and monitoring desired behavioral outcomes. With Roy's emphasis on diagnosis, qualifiers, and observed outcomes, her model may have considerable applicability to psychiatric care.

Betty Neuman

Betty Neuman's Systems Model is based on concepts related to stress and reaction to stress (Neuman, 1995). The system in the model may be an individual, a family, a group, a community—any of which can be identified as an open system. Open systems function with repeating cycles of input, throughput, output, and feedback exchanges with the environment. Forces, or stressors, from both within and outside of the system seek to disrupt system balance or stability. Stability is present when the energy available to deal with these forces exceeds that which is being used by the system. Neuman indicates that reactions to stressors may be positive or negative and either possible (not yet occurring) or actual (identifiable).

The Neuman Systems Model includes the various aspects of the model. The core of the system is the basic structure or central core and represents basic survival factors, including the physiological, psychological, sociocultural, developmental, and spiritual variables of the system (Neuman, 1995). The physiological variable deals with the body and its structures and functions. The psychological variable deals with mental relationships and processes. The sociocultural variable deals with those functions of the system that involve social and cultural interactions and expectations. The developmental variable deals with developmental processes and needs that vary as the system matures. The spiritual variable deals with the system's spiritual beliefs and their influence and is, according to Neuman, the least understood despite its importance.

The system core is surrounded by the lines of resistance (Neuman, 1995). The function of the lines of resistance is to protect the system core and basic functions. These lines are activated when stressors invade the normal line of defense. Effective responses by the lines of resistance protect the system and allow for reconstitution, or return to system stability. Reconstitution is apparent through an increase of energy in reaction to the stressor. Ineffective responses lead to depletion of energy resources and even to death. The next layer of protection is the normal line of defense. The normal line of defense represents the system's usual level of wellness, or system stability. This stability is not fixed but dynamic; it changes over time as the system copes with various stressors. When stressors invade the normal line of defense, the system reacts in the form of illness. The outer boundary of protection is the flexible line of defense. This is the initial protection, the portion of the system that is first encountered by the stressor. Neuman describes the flexible line of defense as an accordion-like cushion or buffer that protects the normal line of defense. The greater the distance between the flexible line of defense and the normal line of defense, the greater the protection available to the system.

The system has an environment. Neuman (1995) defines three types of environment—internal, external, and created. The **internal environment** consists of those forces, factors, and influences that occur completely within the boundaries of the system. The **external environment** consists of those forces, factors, and influences that occur outside the system boundary. The **created environment** symbolizes system wholeness, exemplifies the exchange between the internal and external environments, and represents the unconscious mobilization of all system variables, particularly the sociocultural and psychological variables.

Stressors are those factors or stimuli that place a demand upon the system, create system tension, and have the potential for leading to system instability (Neuman, 1995). Stressors may be **intrapersonal**, or from within the system boundary; **interpersonal**, or from outside the system boundary but proximal to the system; or **extrapersonal**, or from a greater distance outside the system boundary. At any moment, the system may be dealing with one or more stressors.

Neuman (1995) labels the interventions that may be taken to assist the system in retaining, attaining, or maintaining system stability as primary, secondary, or tertiary prevention. Primary prevention occurs before stressors invade the normal line of defense and seeks to strengthen the flexible line of defense through prevention or reduction of risk factors. Examples of primary preventions include health promotion activities and immunizations. Secondary prevention occurs after the system has reacted to the invasion of a stressor; secondary prevention deals with existing symptoms. The focus of secondary prevention is to strengthen the internal lines of resistance to protect the system core and energy resources. Tertiary prevention occurs after secondary prevention has begun to be successful and seeks to support system reconstitution through protecting client strengths and conserving client energy.

Neuman's theory was not explicitly derived from a mental health perspective, but its emphasis on stressors and on psychological, sociocultural, developmental, and spiritual variables would certainly seem to suggest psychiatric applicability. Neuman claims that her theory is useful over the entire range of nursing practice and even outside the field of nursing. This would further suggest applicability to psychiatric mental health nursing.

See Table 3-4 for a summary of nursing theories based on the concept of when nursing is needed as related to the case example of Mr. James.

PSYCHIATRIC/PSYCHOLOGICAL THEORY

Just as nurses need to identify the theoretical bases of their practice, it is helpful to understand the theoretical bases of practice of others in health care. In psychiatric nursing, the interdisciplinary team is of particular importance and may include psychiatrists, psychologists, social workers, and counselors as well as nurses. Each of these

Table 3-4   When Nursing Is Needed: Nursing Theorists and Mr. James

	OREM
Basic conditioning factors	Gender: male Age: 60 Socioeconomic status: middle class Development: retired (not by choice) Health: generally good by history; currently not sleeping well, losing weight Health care system factors: has insurance and a primary physician Family: wife; two married children, four grandchildren Environment: lives in own home Living patterns: change in these in last 4 months
Universal self-care requisites	Air: occasional rapid breathing Food: available, decreased appetite Water: met Elimination: occasional constipation Activity/rest balance: significant decrease in activity in last 4 months, sleep disturbed Solitude and social interaction: decreased social interaction, increased solitude over last 4 months Promotion human functioning: decreased functioning last 4 months Hazard prevention: no identified environmental hazards; potential hazards related to feelings of uselessness
Developmental self-care requisites	Retired, not by own choice; had made no plans for activities postretirement
Health deviation self-care requisites	None identified at this time
Therapeutic self-care demand	Need to feel useful greater than current ability to meet the need; thus self-care deficit exists
Nursing system design	Supportive-educative nursing system needed. Key components are to help Mr. J. identify skills he has to offer others and ways in which he can use these skills: work at home, community volunteering, connecting with programs at church.

	ROY
First-level assessment	Physiologic mode: oxygenation, protection, senses, fluids and electrolytes, neurologic, endocrine, all show adaptive responses. Ineffective responses seen in nutrition (lack of appetite and 10-lb weight loss over 4 months), elimination (occasional constipation), and activity and rest (sleeplessness). Self-concept mode: Body image shows adaptive responses. Ineffective responses in personal self (feels useless and worthless). Role function mode: Secondary roles show adaptive responses. Primary roles show ineffective responses in relation to development stage of retirement. Tertiary roles show ineffective responses in lack of development of hobbies and other non-work-related activities. Interdependence mode: may have ineffective responses in interdependence with wife; more data needed.
Second-level assessment	Focal stimulus: forced retirement Contextual stimuli: no plans for retirement, major changes in his life with little apparent change in lives of family members Residual stimuli: concerns that he will die if he is not employed
Nursing diagnosis	Stress and depression related to early retirement
Goal setting	Establish activities that are effective in enhancing sense of self within 2 months.
Intervention	Nurse and Mr. J. identify activities in which he would be interested and locate places where he can carry out these activities. For example, serving as a consultant to new small businesses.
Evaluation	Successful if Mr. J. is once again sleeping well, his appetite has returned, his weight has stabilized, and he is feeling useful and needed.

Continued

Table 3-4 When Nursing Is Needed: Nursing Theorists and Mr. James *Continued*

NEUMAN	
Person	Physiological: loss of system stability seen in change in eating and sleeping patterns
	Psychosocial: loss of system stability demonstrated in feelings of uselessness
	Sociocultural: loss of system stability seen in lack of contact with previous business associates
	Developmental: loss of system stability seen in view of retirement as unplanned and forced
	Spiritual: loss of system stability seen in feelings of uselessness
Flexible line of defense, normal line of defense	Both flexible and normal lines of defense invaded
Lines of resistance	Activated as seen by symptoms of sleeplessness, loss of appetite, weight loss, feelings of uselessness, and in his seeking help with these
Stressor	The major stressor identified is Mr. J.'s change in employment status (an interpersonal stressor).
Primary prevention	Planning for retirement did not occur.
Secondary prevention	Symptoms are present, this level of prevention is needed. Plan and seek ways to be occupied and useful—volunteering, home repairs, church activities.
Tertiary prevention	Once sleeping and eating well again and feeling useful (system stability restored), develop plans for continued involvement, potentially including development of hobbies that he and his wife can enjoy together when she retires.

individuals, including nurses, may use psychological theories as the basis for their practice. Knowledge of representative psychological theories will enhance the nurse's ability to communicate with other members of the team.

Psychoanalytic Theory

The psychoanalytic theories to be reviewed are those of Freud, Erikson, and Sullivan. Freud's focus was on psychosexual development, Erickson's on psychosocial development, and Sullivan's on the development of interpersonal relationships. All are stage theorists, that is, the developmental process they each describe is envisioned as occurring in discrete stages or steps rather than continuously.

Freud and Psychosexual Development

Sigmund Freud is best known for two sets of concepts: those related to personality (id, ego, and superego) and those related to stages of psychosexual development (oral, anal, and phallic or oedipal). Freud initially described the **id** as the unconscious and identified it as the most primitive part of the personality. The goal of the id is to minimize pain and maximize pleasure—otherwise known as the pleasure principle. Freud (1965a) viewed pleasure as the release of tension and suggested that frustration and psychological symptoms might occur when the release of tension was repressed, or blocked. The id also contains impressions and impulses that have been repressed into it

and thus are not accessible to the conscious mind. Because the goal of the id is to release tension, it also includes forces of aggression and destruction. The id is not logical; thus, when it seeks to reduce tension, it does not consider the consequences of pleasure-seeking actions, even when those might result in serious harm to someone or something the person needs or loves.

The **superego**, or conscience, serves to delay the immediate impulse generated by the id and to bring rationality into consideration before the **ego**, or self, acts. In Freud's view, the ego both represses and derives its own energy from the id; consequently it seeks to achieve a balance among the demands of three masters—the id, reality, and the superego. The ego is subject to anxiety associated with concerns about meeting the demands of each of these masters. Anxiety occurs when there is concern about mastering the impulses of the id. Moral anxiety is associated with meeting the expectations of the superego and realistic anxiety occurs in response to dangers in the external world.

Freud's theories of personality remain of interest to psychoanalysts, literary critics and writers, and some nurses. They seem to accord fairly well with the way we perceive our behavior to be influenced by conscience and impulse. It is not clear to what extent these theoretical concepts explain common psychopathology, and many psychologists believe that Freud's theories of personality have very little empirical support. They have remained influential because until recently, Freudian psychoanalysis was the dominant model of treatment for mental illness. As a more biomedical model has evolved in recent years, the Freudian viewpoint has lost influence. This loss of influence also extends to Freud's concepts of psychosexual development, a topic that is taken up in the following paragraphs.

The stages of development, according to Freud (1905), are based on sexual feelings (defined as anything that produces pleasure) and occur in a sequence of stages. Freud's general term for sexual energy is libido, and when this energy becomes focused on a part of the body through the process of cathexis, that area of the body is known as an erogenous zone. The stage sequence occurs as the zone that is the focus of the child moves from the mouth (oral) to the anus (anal) and finally to the genital region (phallic or oedipal). The oral stage is divided into two parts. The first part occurs during the first 6 months of life, in which sucking provides not only nutrition but also pleasure in its own right. Freud (1905) called finding gratification through one's own body autoerotic and described the young infant as objectless, or having no conception of differentiation between self and others. The infant's focus is primarily inward and was identified by Freud as a state of narcissism. At about 6 months of age, the infant enters the second part of the oral stage and begins to be aware of the mother as a separate being. Because the infant identifies the mother as necessary, anxiety is often exhibited when she leaves the room or house. The infant is at this time developing teeth and the urge to bite. Few mothers will tolerate being bitten during nursing, so the infant is faced at this early stage with two conflicting urges: biting and feeding.

The anal stage occurs between approximately ages 1½ and 3 years when, according to Freud, children become increasingly aware of pleasurable sensations associated with bowel movements. As they gain maturational control, Freud felt, children might deliberately delay having a bowel movement in order to heighten the pleasure through increasing pressure on the rectal mucosa (Freud, 1905). There is little evidence that such delay actually occurs, but this has not kept the concept of anality from enjoying popular recognition. Toilet training does require that the child delay defecation, but the reward for this outcome is probably praise or a sense of mastery rather than anal pleasure. In the conflicts that arise around the period of toilet training, Freud saw the origins of certain personality characteristics, one of which he termed anal compulsivity (1959). Freud saw the anal compulsive personality as manifesting excessive interest in cleanliness, order, and reliability along with resentment of authority that is often expressed passive aggressively. While some psychoanalysts still adhere to such Freudian descriptions of personality types and disorders, many other psychiatrists separate out the obsessive-compulsive and the passive-aggressive personalities as distinct (but indeed related) entities. It is by no means universally agreed on that personality aberrations derive from early toileting experiences. This book discusses common disorders of personality in Chapter 16.

The phallic, or oedipal, stage occurs between about 3 and 6 years of age and applies primarily to boys. According to Freud, an oedipal crisis begins with a boy's interest in his penis. This interest leads to a desire to compare his organ to those of other males, of animals, and of girls and women. His fantasies often involve being the heroic lover of his primary love object—his mother. He quickly learns that the behaviors required to carry out his fantasies are not viewed by others as acceptable. He discovers that he cannot marry his mother and may even be offered less physical contact with the mother than before, either because (likely more in Freud's time than now) such contact was felt to be developmentally inappropriate or because other children have subsequently been born and require more of the mother's time. In Freud's view the boy observes that his father has seemingly unlimited access to physical contact with the mother, and this observation leads to the Oedipus complex, in which the little boy views his father as a rival for his mother's affection. (The reader will remember that in ancient Greek tradition, Oedipus unwittingly killed his father and married his mother.) The young boy may become frightened by his wishes to see his father out of the way since, after all, he loves and needs his father too. More importantly, the boy may also begin to fear castration, especially if threatened when caught masturbating. Freud associated the fear of castration with the boy's realization that females do not have penises and the boy's belief that they once had penises that were cut off. If this happened to females, it could happen to him. These predicaments are typically resolved through a series of defensive actions (Freud, 1960). Repression, or burial of any sexual feelings toward the mother, is used to fend off incestuous desires and to identify his love for his mother as a higher, purer love. Resolving the Oedipus complex, the boy seeks to identify with his father, to join him rather than fight him. He also internalizes a superego or takes on his parents' moral prohibitions as his own. In this way, Freud was able to explain a striking range of psychological phenomena, especially the emergence of conscience, or the superego.

Freud was less specific about the Oedipus complex for girls. He stated that at about the age of 5, girls become disappointed in their mothers (Freud, 1965b). He associated this disappointment with feelings of deprivation since she no longer receives the level of love and attention she received as a baby (especially if another baby has entered the family); irritation about her mother's prohibitions, especially in relation to masturbation; and anger that she does not have a penis (penis envy). Feminine pride is regained as the little girl begins to appreciate the attentions of her father. As with the little boy, she will discover that she cannot lay sole claim to her father and may see her mother as a rival (Freud termed this the Electra complex). While the boy's primary motivation to resolve the Oedipus complex is the fear of castration,

Freud was unable to find a comparable motivator for girls but did not deny that women also develop superegos. Freud believed, however, that a girl's superego is weaker than the boy's because the girl's motivation to resolve the conflict is weaker. This belief accorded with popular 19th-century views that women were morally inferior to men and were less capable of repressing sexual impulses. Freud seems to have based his view of woman's superego on theory alone rather than on any empirical data. This is a good example of the ability of a theory to gain acceptance even when evidence might be obtained that would call it seriously into question.

With the development of the superego and its associated defenses against oedipal impulses, the child enters the latency stage. This stage lasts from ages 6 to 11. Freud (1905) described this stage as one in which the sexual feelings and memories from the previous three stages are repressed. Thus, the latency period is relatively calm, and energies are directed into socially acceptable activities.

Latency has been described as the lull before the storm. Puberty begins around age 11 in girls and 12 in boys. In puberty, sexual energy rises to adult levels and threatens the previously established defenses. Freud (1965a) described the individual's task from now onward as that of "freeing himself from the parents" (p. 345). This task involves releasing the tie to the parent of the opposite sex and finding a mate of one's own. Freud (1905) noted that human struggles for independence from parents are never easy and rarely result in complete independence.

While Freud carefully described each of the stages of normal psychosexual development, he also recognized (1905) that not all persons pass uneventfully through each. He concluded that an individual might become fixated at a stage or regress from one stage to a previous one. **Fixation** occurs when we maintain a preoccupation with the pleasures associated with a stage, even though we have advanced beyond that stage. For example, in the Freudian model, those who are fixated at the oral stage are often preoccupied with food or suck or bite on objects such as pencils. **Regression** occurs when one reverts to the pleasures of an earlier stage during times of frustration. For example, a child may seek comfort in thumb sucking when very upset, or an adult may seek comfort in food when depressed. Freud (1965a) believed that more serious fixations and/or regressions resulted in serious emotional disorders. For example, the psychotic individual with delusions of grandeur who believes him- or herself to be God may be considered as having regressed to a primary narcissism in which the boundaries between self and the external world are once again blurred. While an excellent example of Freud's imaginative inventiveness, no empirical evidence supports this contention. Even many supporters of Freudian psychoanalysis feel that Freud's theories apply better to the minor psychological abnormalities than they do to major

Table 3-5	Freud's Stages of Development	
STAGE	**AGE**	**CHARACTERISTICS**
Oral stage	0–12 months	Oral gratification, sucking
Anal stage	1–3 years	Rectal gratification, control of bowel movements
Phallic/oedipal stage	3–6 years	Genital fixation and concentration
Latency stage	6–11 years	Repression of sexual feelings and memories
Puberty	11 years on	Rise in sexual energy, independence from parents

psychotic illness. A summary of Freud's theories can be found in Table 3-5.

This text discusses psychoanalysis in Chapter 26, where more of Freud's ideas are considered along with his therapeutic techniques. His ideas have exerted a huge influence on 20th-century culture and society. While Freud continues to have many adherents over 50 years after his death, nurses should regard his theories as fascinating but still largely unproven.

Psychosocial Development

Erik Erikson developed a theory of child development that emphasizes social growth over Freud's sexually related conflicts. Also a stage theory, Erikson's description took from Freud the concept of a series of personal crises that led the child from stage to stage. In Erikson's view, the successful resolution of one stage will have a positive effect on the person's ability to be successful in the next stages. Biological maturation and social forces compel the individual to move through all of the stages whether or not a given stage has been resolved successfully (Crain, 1985). As in Freud's theory, the failure to resolve a stage may lead to psychological symptoms either in childhood or subsequently in adulthood.

The first stage deals with trust versus mistrust and occurs between birth and age 1½ years. The focus here is to develop a healthy ratio between trust and mistrust. Infants seek to meet their needs through interactions with caregivers. When the caregiver's responses are consistent, predictable, and reliable, the baby begins to develop a basic trust in the caregiver. The alternative is a sense of mistrust that develops based upon unpredictable and inconsistent responses from the caregiver (Erikson, 1950). Infants also must learn to trust in themselves. Erikson (1950) states that when the teething child learns to regulate chewing and biting urges to suck without nipping, that child begins to view him- or herself as "trustworthy enough so that providers will not to be on guard lest they be nipped" (p. 248). The developing sense of trust is demonstrated in the infant's behavior. Erikson states the first sign of trust in the mother is seen when the infant is willing "to let her out of sight without undue anxiety or rage" (p. 47). Trust must be balanced with an appropriate amount of mistrust: "The human infant must experience a goodly measure of mistrust in order to trust discerningly" (Erikson, 1976, p. 23). Erikson (1950) emphasized that the development of trust in the infant is dependent on the confidence of the caregivers and indicates that it is culturally important that we believe that what we do for our children is good. Trust is seen as an ego strength that enables the delay of gratification, which is an important psychological tool for success in adolescence and adulthood.

The second stage, autonomy versus shame and doubt, occurs between 1½ and 3 years of age. Erikson identified the basic modes of this stage as holding on and letting go, thus exercising choice. This exercise of choice is associated with a sense of autonomy. The developing sense of autonomy is further supported by developing abilities to walk, feed oneself, and talk. It is a common experience that a 2-year-old says "no" much more frequently than "yes," thus seeking to exercise self-determination. Autonomy comes from within as the child grows and develops. Shame and doubt occur as a result of social pressures—the efforts of parents and family to teach the child culturally defined proper behavior. Shame occurs with concern about being looked upon favorably by others; doubt is associated with questioning one's ability to perform. This conflict between autonomy and shame and doubt is successfully resolved when the child's experiences with shame and doubt do not overwhelm the initial sense of autonomy. Those who do not resolve this conflict successfully are likely to have life-long feelings of shame and doubt when they seek to respond to their urges towards self-determination.

The third stage, initiative versus guilt, occurs between the ages of 3 and 6 years. Erikson's (1950) term for the primary mode of this stage is intrusion, which he uses to describe the sense of exploration and daring exhibited by children of this age. Developing physical and mental abilities allow the child to intrude physically and verbally through activity, locomotion, talking, and other methods of exercising curiosity. Initiative is also intended to indicate forward movement. In developing initiative, the child demonstrates the ability to plan, set goals, and seek to carry out the plans to meet the goals. The crisis occurs when children realize they cannot achieve their biggest goals, those described by Freud in the oedipal phase as the desire to possess one parent and thus rival the other. The discovery of the social taboos associated with these goals leads to the development of the superego and the production of guilt. Erikson (1950) recognizes the necessity of the superego for socially acceptable behavior but views the development of a superego also as a loss since it often stifles imagination and initiative.

The fourth stage, industry versus inferiority, occurs from about 6 to 11 years of age. This is a period of mastery of social and cognitive skills. Socially, the child now focuses skill development outside of the family to the wider culture. This is a time of development of peer relationships. It is also a time fraught with the danger of failure, which may result in feelings of inadequacy and inferiority. Erikson felt that such a sense of inferiority is likely to be greatest in those who developed more doubt than autonomy and in those who believe themselves to be viewed as inferior by those outside of the family.

The fifth stage, identity versus role confusion, is associated with adolescence (11 to 12 years to 18 to 20 years). Erikson's theory was one of the first to recognize the developmental stage of adolescence and to emphasize its association with the growth of personal autonomy. Erikson claimed that the conflicts in this stage are related to the adolescent's great increase in energy, dramatic physiological changes, and the evolution of new social conflicts and demands. The primary task is to develop identity—a sense of who one is and how one fits into the larger social order. The physical changes that occur in adolescence are dramatic and visible. These changes can lead the adolescent to identity confusion— a sense of hardly recognizing oneself. This, in turn, leads to concerns about looking attractive to others, meeting others' expectations, and establishing a vocational role. Erikson observed that adolescents often delay making commitments in an effort to avoid "identity foreclosure" or, instead, make decisions before all of the options are known. The uncertainty about who they are leads adolescents to associate with groups, which helps provide them with identity and clear-cut good/bad views of the world. In Erikson's view, identity is developed through identification with those whom we admire as well as through our accomplishments. The search for identity, and thus the time spent in role confusion, may be a long and painful one but can lead to higher levels of personal integration and to social innovations (Crain, 1985).

The Eriksonian period for young adulthood (ages 18 to 25) is labeled intimacy versus isolation. The adolescent is too self-absorbed to develop real intimacy with another. This becomes the task of the young adult who has developed enough of a sense of identity to be able to lose him- or herself in mutuality with another (Crain, 1985). Those who are unable to attain such mutuality experience isolation and, often, self-absorption. Adulthood (ages 21 to 45) is described as involving generativity versus stagnation. Once two people have achieved intimacy, they are ready to look beyond themselves. Generativity involves the production of both children and success at work. Erikson focused more heavily on the creation of and care for children than on the contributions made at work. Note that in Erikson's theory the mere creation of children does not satisfy the definition of generativity. Generativity involves productivity through caring for and guiding children, whether one's own or those of others. Those who do not achieve generativity will experience stagnation and impoverishment of the personality. Erikson suggested that the person who cannot achieve generativity may have had such an empty childhood that he or she cannot envision parenting in a more enriched fashion. In contrast with the general social view of old age as a period of decline, Erikson (1950) sees this period (ages 45 years to death) as one with potential for growth and wisdom. He labeled the crisis of this period ego integrity versus despair. Rather than focus on the external adjustments related to the series of physical and social losses experienced by the elderly, Erikson focused on an internal struggle. As death approaches, people begin a life review that involves deciding whether or not their lives have been worthwhile. This opens them to the ultimate despair—the view that their lives have not been what they could or should have been and now it is too late to do anything about it. The resulting disgust is actually contempt for themselves (Erikson, 1959). Facing such despair invokes the search for ego integrity. Ego integrity involves "the acceptance of one's one and only life cycle as something that had to be and that, by necessity permitted no substitutions" (Erikson, 1950, p. 268). It includes accepting that mistakes were made (perhaps unavoidably) while recognizing the good things that were accomplished, developing a sense of the inevitable order of the past. It also involves a feeling of companionship "with the ordering ways of distant times and different pursuits" (p. 268) or a detached, philosophical wisdom about life in general rather than only one's own in particular. See Table 3-6 for a summary of Erikson's stages of development.

Half a century after its publication, Erikson's theory seems at times a bit dated, and, like Freud's, it was developed with relatively little formal empirical basis. Erikson was, however, among the first popular psychologists to recognize that human development did not stop in childhood but proceeded over an entire lifetime. Whether or not Erikson's stages are real milestones that apply to every individual, they still offer a relatively useful view of the challenges that each of us pass as we move from childhood to productive adult roles.

Sullivan's Interpersonal Theory

Harry Stack Sullivan was a leader in emphasizing the importance of interpersonal relationships. He sought to decrease what he perceived to be an emphasis on heredity in assigning cause to psychiatric conditions and to increase recognition of the importance of environment, especially the sociocultural environment. His approach has been described as holistic and interactional (Mullahy, 1970). In Sullivan's view, no one can become fully human without "the support and nurture of the social environment" (Mullahy, 1970, p. 128). All human processes occur in interrelationships; none occur in isolation. Sullivan identified three life processes: genetic organization, communal existence, and functional activity. Genetic organization determines the type of organism, innate individual differences, instincts, and the general course of development. Genetic organization provides the possibilities and boundaries for development and in general prescribes the sequence for maturation but does not determine the development itself. Communal existence includes those processes that connect the human with his or her environment. The interaction between human and environment is ever present although the boundaries between human and environment are often not clear-cut. Functional activity in general is associated with the accumulation of "free energy" and activity to maintain life.

Table 3-6   Erikson's Stages of Development

STAGE	AGE	CHARACTERISTICS
Trust versus mistrust	0–18 months	Development of trust
Autonomy versus shame and doubt	18 months–3 years	Exercise of choice and self-determination
Initiative versus guilt	3–6 years	Exploration and daring
Industry versus inferiority	6–11 years	Mastery of social and cognitive skills
Identity versus role confusion	11–20 years	Development of identity
Intimacy versus isolation	18–25 years	Mutuality and intimacy with another person
Generativity versus stagnation	21–45 years	Productivity through caring for and guiding children
Ego integrity versus despair	45 years to death	Internal struggle and life review

Mentally, functional activity represents mental processes such as imagining, learning, desiring, thinking, perceiving, and sensing.

Sullivan viewed humans as essentially social beings and believed childhood development should be understood in terms of interpersonal relations as influenced by culture. In earliest infancy, the prevailing activity is sleeping followed by the taking of nourishment and those activities associated with relieving distress not connected to hunger. Like Freud, Sullivan viewed sucking as a form of oral behavior, which he thought both met the need for nourishment and helped to use excess energy.

Infancy ends and childhood begins with the development of articulate speech. The variety of total activities increases as cultural forces begin to make themselves felt. The juvenile period begins as the child develops the need to interact and play with other children. This is "the period of growth of egocentric sociality and of the elaboration of social personality. If real playmates are not available, the youngster creates imaginary playmates" (Mullahy, 1970, p. 125).

The next interpersonal relation that develops is the beginning of a new kind of attachment to another; this attachment, when it prospers, is love. A new need, the need for interindividual affection, arises and replaces the egocentricity of the juvenile. The ability to love, according to Sullivan, moves the development of the personality into its "ultraimportant phase" of growth. During this phase of early adolescence (initially termed preadolescence by Sullivan) boys and girls tend to participate in gender-specific organized groups or gangs. Those whose personal or social circumstances do not support the development of these interpersonal relationships will not experience this phase of development and may never experience love.

In Sullivan's view, true adolescence begins with the development and psychosocial management of overt sexual impulses. This stage is followed by adulthood, a life situation that includes one or two other persons in "a total activity, prevailingly sexual in character, the resolution of which is complete, in the sense that it does not proceed into disturbing situations, which in turn would require resolution" (Mullahy, 1970, p. 126). Entering adulthood requires successfully passing through all the previous stages.

Each stage or phase of development prepares the personality for the principal development of the next stage. In Sullivan's view, failure to successfully achieve the activities of a stage can severely limit one's personality development and chances for a normal, successful life. Sullivan shared this determinative view of stage theory with Erikson and Freud. Clearly, Sullivan had much in common with Erikson but tended to emphasize social and interpersonal determinants more than strictly psychological ones. Both were concerned with the factors that lead to healthy psychological development from infancy into adulthood.

Cognitive Development Theory

Cognition, the process of thinking, knowing, and perceiving, is of particular interest to psychiatric nursing, as alterations in this ability are often the first indications of psychiatric concerns. Jean Piaget was among the first psychologists to describe and define stages of child cognitive development. Piaget's pioneering work was expanded by Perry and, with regard to females, by Belenky, Clinchy, Goldberger, and Tarule. Together, these writers have offered a still largely valid view of the way in which cognitive skills come to maturation. These cognitive skills are thought to develop in much the same staged way as do the more explicitly interpersonal or psychodevelopmental skills described by Freud, Erikson, and Sullivan.

Jean Piaget

Piaget developed a stage theory of cognitive development largely by empirically observing the sequence in which infants and young children acquire skills. While Erikson, Freud, and Sullivan were careful observers of childhood development, Piaget designed psychological experiments to try to assess when and how children become able to make specific cognitive distinctions. Piaget established what he felt to be an accurate sequence of cognitive stages that all children progress through on their way to maturity. He believed that children moved through each of these stages at various paces but will always do so in the same order. Piaget's stages are based on the belief that children themselves develop their cognitive structures. They must interact with the external environment to do so, but neither the environment nor anything in it construct the changes in cognition (Crain, 1985). This interaction with environment comprises what Piaget termed assimilation, accommodation, and organization. Assimilation involves taking in the experiences from the environment. Accommodation occurs when what is taken in from the environment does not match a person's existing structure and thus changes the structure to match the new information. Organization is the process of placing one's ideas into a coherent state or order.

Piaget proposed several multistaged periods of development. The first period of development is entitled the sensorimotor intelligence period and occurs approximately from birth to 2 years of age. During this period, babies organize their physical actions and reactions to deal with the environment that immediately surrounds them. The first stage, from birth to 1 month of age, deals with the use of reflexes; the inborn reflexes are the first pattern of action. The most conspicuous reflex is sucking, which occurs whenever the infant's lips are touched or brushed. These reflexes begin as passive activity but soon develop into self-initiated activity. The second stage, from ages 1 to 4 months, is called primary circular reactions. A circular reaction is when an infant seeks to repeat a new experience. Piaget's (1974) example is that of thumb sucking. The infant encounters the experience of thumb in mouth and seeks to repeat this experience. Coordination is such that initial efforts to again insert thumb in mouth are not successful—body movements are not yet coordinated by individual parts. Instead, the entire body moves as a whole. In Piaget's terms, the infant is not yet able to make the accommodations needed to assimilate the hand into the sucking scheme. Eventually, after many efforts, the infant is successful and thumb sucking becomes part of the scheme. The third stage, from ages 4 to 10 months, is identified as secondary circular reactions. These reactions involve repeating an event that occurs outside the infant's body, such as making a mobile move. This typically involves a single action and a single result: The baby kicks and the mobile moves. Awareness of objects as separate from self is beginning in this stage. Children will look where an object has fallen and can find partly hidden objects. They can also find objects they have put aside but cannot find something that has been completely hidden by another person.

The fourth stage, from ages 10 to 12 months, involves the coordination of secondary schemes. In this stage, the infant learns to coordinate two schemes to achieve a desired result. For example, the child may push aside a cereal bowl to reach a piece of fruit that is behind the bowl. This involves the schema of pushing and grasping. It also demonstrates some understanding of space and time, as the infant has demonstrated a sense that some objects are in front or back of others and some events or actions must precede or follow others (Ginsberg & Opper, 1979). In this stage, object permanence begins. The child can find a completely hidden object, for example, a toy covered by a blanket or cushion. The fifth stage, from ages 12 to 18 months, is designated tertiary circular reactions, which involve using different actions for different results. In this stage, the child explores the world without adult teaching, encouraged by an intrinsic curiosity. Examples include pounding upon a hollow object with varying levels of intensity to obtain different sounds or splashing water from different angles to direct the water toward different objects. In Stage 5, a child can follow a series of displacements so long as he or she has observed those displacements. The sixth stage, from ages 18 months to 2 years, marks the beginning of thought. In Stage 5, the child explores the world through physical action; in Stage 6, there is more apparent thinking before acting. Piaget's (1974) example involved his daughter and her efforts to remove a chain from a matchbox. Her initial, and unsuccessful, efforts were to turn the box over and to try to stick her finger in a slit in the box. She then paused, concentrated on the slit, and opened and closed her mouth several times. After this "thought process," she proceeded to open the box and remove the chain.

In Stage 6, the child can follow invisible displacements such as detouring around a chair to find a ball that has rolled under the chair.

The second and third periods are those of preoperational thought, from ages 2 to 7, and concrete operations, from 7 to 11 years of age. Preoperational thought marks the beginning use of symbols and requires reorganization of thinking. This reorganization takes some time and effort, as is evidenced by the child's thinking being unsystematic and illogical during this stage. The use of symbols allow make-believe play and rapid development of language. While some believe language mastery enhances the development of logic, Piaget disagrees. His belief is that a child organizes his or her world from the beginning in a logical manner. To demonstrate the organization, Piaget used a series of scientific tasks with children as young as 4. The most famous of these relates to the conservation of continuous quantities of liquid. The child is shown two tall, slender glasses that are filled to the same level. When asked if they contain the same amount, the child usually agrees that they do. Then, the liquid from one glass is poured into a shorter, wider glass and the child is again asked if the two contain the same amount of liquid. The child in the preoperational stage answers in two substages. In the first substage, the child fails to conserve and states that the amounts are not equal; one or the other has more because it is higher or because it is wider. The use of a single dimension of measurement overcomes the logic that they must still be the same. In the second substage, the child is moving toward but has not yet reached conservation. The child's response may first be that one has more because it is taller, and then the response is changed to that the other has more because it is wider. Finally, the child becomes confused. This demonstrates intuitive regulations—a beginning consideration of two dimensions that does not yet include reasoning about both dimensions at the same time. About the age of 7, the child enters the period of concrete operations and recognizes that equal amounts of liquid are in both glasses.

A second task relates to the conservation of number. In this task, Piaget gave children a row of egg cups and several eggs. The children were asked to take just enough eggs to fill the cups. Preoperational children in the first substage made rows that were equal in length with no consideration for the number of cups or the number of eggs. They were consistently surprised they had more eggs than cups when asked to place the eggs in the cups. At the second substage, children lined one egg up with each cup. However, if either row was bunched up or spread out, the children claimed that now one row had more in it, as they equated length with quantity. Some did begin to waver in their reasoning between there was more because a row was longer and there was more in the other row because it was denser. In concrete operations, children again recognized the number did not change with changes in length.

Table 3-7   Piaget's Stage Theory of Cognitive Development

STAGE	AGE
Sensorimotor intelligence	0–2 years
Preoperational thought	2–7 years
Concrete operations	7–11 years
Formal operations	11 years to adulthood

Just as preoperational children seem unable to take into consideration two dimensions of an object simultaneously, they seem unable to consider a perspective other than their own. Piaget called this inability egocentrism. An interesting example can be found when listening to preoperational children talking. Two preoperational children may appear to be having a conversation, but if you listen closely, you will discover that each is talking about what is of personal interest. These "conversations" are known as collective monologues. As children enter concrete operations, they become more concerned about and interested in the viewpoints of others, and conversations with an exchange of ideas begin.

Piaget's fourth period is entitled formal operations and begins at about age 11 and continues through adulthood. The child operating at the level of concrete operations can think systematically and logically as long as the thought is related to tangible objects. Formal operations involves the ability to organize and work with ambiguity and multiple meanings.

Piaget's theories are complex, challenging, and of abiding interest to the study of childhood cognitive development. New theories about language acquisition have called into question some of Piaget's work, but his efforts remain among the important contributions of 20th-century developmental psychology.

See Table 3-7 for a list of the stages of Piaget's theory of cognitive development.

Adult Cognition

While differing with each other and with Freud in significant details, Erikson and Sullivan carried Freud's view of stage theory beyond adolescence and into adulthood. Perry accomplished much the same task by expanding on Piaget's conceptions. Unsatisfied with the idea that formal operations represents the final stage of human cognitive development, Perry (1970) studied young men during their years as undergraduate students at Harvard. His focus was on how their perception of nature and the nature of knowledge evolved during their college experience. As a result of his study, Perry identified positions, or stages, of knowing that he described as linear, or occurring in a specific order, with each succeeding position dependent upon the previous one. The first position

is dualism, in which the knower sees him- or herself as passive and authorities as all-knowing. The view of the world is one of dichotomies—right or wrong, black or white, good or bad. The student perceives that there is one right answer to every question or human dilemma. The next position is multiplicity, in which the knower recognizes that authorities may not always have the right answer and that the knower can have his own opinion. There is a tendency to believe that any one opinion is as good as any other opinion. The third position is relativism, in which the individual comes to understand that any apparent truth is valid primarily in a particular context. As the context changes, so may the likelihood of a given position being true. In this position, the knower recognizes that knowledge is constructed rather than given, contextual rather than absolute, and mutable rather than fixed. This recognition extends into all aspects of life. While Perry's theory was first developed in a longitudinal study of men, the theory has been tested and used by others in numerous college populations of both men and women (Knefelkamp, Widick, & Parker, 1978). These studies confirm that Perry's studies, while derived from a unique Harvard male sample, are probably applicable to a wide range of young adults. Clearly, not all adults complete the transition from dualism to relativism, and perhaps even a majority of adults remain concrete dualistic thinkers. This has important implications for nursing teaching in all disciplines as well as for the psychiatric nurse trying to convey difficult or novel information to a client.

Belenky, Clinchy, Goldberger, and Tarule (1986), concerned that Perry's positions may not reflect the ways in which women learn, conducted a similar study with a group of women drawn from academic institutions and the "invisible colleges"—human service agencies that serve women who are parents. Building on Perry's scheme, they identified five perspectives from which women know or view the world. These perspectives are not linear and the knower may shift from one perspective to another. The first perspective is silence, in which the knower sees self as mindless, voiceless, and subject to authority in all its whims. The second perspective is received knowledge, in which the knower sees self as capable of receiving knowledge as well as of reproducing it. This knowledge comes from authorities, and the knower is not capable of creating knowledge. The received knower listens to the voices of others. The third perspective is subjective knowledge, in which the knower sees knowledge as personal, private, and intuitive. The subjective knower listens to an inner, intuitive, subjective voice and seeks to know self. The fourth perspective is procedural knowledge, in which the knower is invested in learning and applying information empirically; information is both obtained and communicated. The procedural knower seeks a voice of reason and experiences knowledge as that which is both autonomous (separate)

᎒᎒ *REFLECTIVE THINKING*

Developmental/Psychoanalytic Theories

How do developmental/psychoanalytic theories help you understand the behavior of people of various ages?

See Table 3-8 for a summary of developmental theories as related to the case example of Mr. James, presented earlier.

and in relationship with others (connected). The fifth perspective is constructed knowledge, in which knowledge is seen as contextual; the knower views self as capable of creating knowledge, and both objective and subjective strategies for knowing are valued. The constructed knower seeks to integrate the voices and blend both that knowledge that is intuitively considered personally important and that which is learned from others.

Belenky et al. (1986) have made a potentially important contribution to the study of adult development by suggesting that women's cognitive maturation develops differently from that of men. Their conceptualization is clearly different from that of Perry, and it remains to be seen how useful the Belenky model will prove for understanding how women come to see the adult world.

Humanistic Theory

Other schools of thought that are applicable to psychiatric nursing include basic needs theories, existential philosophy, and behavioral theories. Basic needs

theories are represented by Maslow, general propositions of existential philosophy are presented, and the work of psychologist B. F. Skinner is summarized to represent the behavioral theories he pioneered.

Basic Needs Theories

Maslow (1970) proposed a hierarchy of needs to explain motives for human behavior. His hierarchy has five levels. The bottom two levels represent basic needs, and the upper three represent growth needs. The first level is physiological needs for food, air, water, sleep, sex, and so on. The second is safety and security. The third level (the first growth need level) is love and belonging. The fourth level is esteem and self-esteem. The fifth level is self-actualization. Maslow indicated that persons seek levels 3 to 5 only after more basic needs have been satisfied. The primary focus of his work was on the highest level, self-actualization. He identified the characteristics of the self-actualized person as being tolerant, even welcoming, of uncertainty; self-accepting, with an inner-directedness; spontaneous; creative; autonomous; caring for others; capable of intense interpersonal relationships; having a sense of humor and an open attitude to life as well as needing solitude and privacy. Maslow's work is frequently cited by other theorists, and his hierarchy of needs has been a consistently useful conceptual framework for thinking about human sociocultural development.

Existential Philosophy

Many authors have contributed to the development of existential philosophy, a philosophical movement of the latter half of the 20th century that has strongly influenced

---

Table 3-8   Developmental Theories and Mr. James

Freud	No stage beyond puberty.
Erikson	Ego integrity versus despair: involves external adjustments associated with physical and social loss. Mr. J.'s current loss is primarily social in the loss of his status as an employed person and of the social interactions associated with that employment. Mr. J. is involved in life review: what has been worthwhile in his life (primary identification with his work); how his life can continue to be worthwhile. He experiences despair and self-contempt if he views himself as no longer capable of doing worthwhile things. If he faces any despair associated with his change in status, accepts his mistakes (e.g., not planning for retirement and not seeking other activities during the last 4 months), and recognizes his capacity for good (ability to contribute to others), he will regain ego integrity.
Sullivan	Adulthood: a total situation that involves one or two others. Mr. J. has isolated himself from his wife in seeing his retirement as primarily creating change for him. He needs to resolve the changes with his wife, not by himself.
Piaget	No stage beyond age 11.
Adult Cognition	If thinking is relativistic, he will see situations as contextual. Retirement could be seen as good or bad. If seen as the end of productive life, then it is bad. If seen as an opportunity to be productive in new and different ways, then retirement is good.

the language and content of several important nursing theories. The basis of existential philosophy, sometimes referred to as existentialism, is a view of human beings as continually changing or becoming. Corey (1991) presents a summary of six major existential propositions. The capacity for self-awareness allows us to reflect and make choices. As our awareness increases, so do the possibilities for freedom. Increasing awareness includes being cognizant of a series of apparent human realities. Among these are the realizations that:

- Life is finite (there is a limit to the time we have to accomplish what we want to do).
- We have the potential to act or not to act (taking no action is a decision).
- We choose our actions and thus influence our destiny.
- Existential anxiety is essential to living.
- As awareness of choice increases, so does our sense of responsibility for the effects of these choices.
- We are subject to multiple feelings (loneliness, meaninglessness, emptiness, isolation, guilt).
- We are basically alone while having the opportunity to relate to others.

We have freedom and responsibility. While we did not choose to be born, the choices we make shape the way in which we live. This freedom for making choices is connected to the need to accept responsibility for the outcomes of those choices. Existential guilt occurs when we evade a commitment, choose not to make a choice or take an action, or allow others to make choices for us.

The third proposition is that we are striving for identity and relationship to others. This involves the courage to be, the experience of aloneness, and the experience of relatedness. As humans, we are simultaneously seeking to maintain our uniqueness and establish relationships with others and with nature. As humans, we depend on relationships with others as part of our fulfillment. Once we are comfortable with our aloneness, we can seek the fulfillment associated with interaction with others.

The fourth proposition relates to the search for meaning, which includes discarding old values, experiencing meaninglessness, and creating new meaning. This creative act continues throughout our lives; it is never finished. Meaning is not found by searching for it directly; rather, it is found through an activity known as engagement. Engagement is the person's commitment to creating, loving, working, building—to living a fully involved life.

The fifth proposition is that anxiety is a condition of living. The efforts to survive, to have personal identity and relationships with others, and to identify meaning lead to normal anxiety. This anxiety can be a stimulus for growth. In fact, Corey (1991) states: "One construc-

REFLECTIVE THINKING

The Stranger

In Albert Camus' classic work *The Stranger*, the narrator begins by telling us that his mother died today or perhaps yesterday, he can't remember when. This opening air of indifference sets the tone for the entire novel and ultimately leads to the narrator's demise at the hands of a society that, in effect, eventually punishes him for not appropriately mourning his mother's death.

- Does this statement of confusion or indifference about the time or circumstances of a parent's death seem unusual to you?
- What reaction would you have to an individual who seems indifferent to what is generally perceived as a significant life event, the death of a parent?
- What theoretical foundations could help you frame care for such an individual?

tive form of normal anxiety, existential anxiety, can be a stimulus for growth in that we experience it as we become increasingly aware of our freedom and the consequences of accepting or rejecting that freedom" (p. 183).

The sixth proposition is that we have an awareness of death and nonbeing. Such recognition makes the present, and our activities in it, more crucial. Living life to the fullest now tends to negate the fear of death that is often associated with feelings of having never really lived.

Existentialism is an attempt to provide a comprehensive life philosophy, primarily for individuals who find they can no longer believe in traditional moral and religious values. It has been influenced by and attracted the attention of some of the 20th century's most profound ethical and religious thinkers. Students interested in contemporary nursing theory will find their understanding enhanced by a careful reading of existential philosophy, including authors such as Martin Heidegger, whose writings may prove quite difficult.

See Table 3–9 for a summary of humanistic theory as related to the case example of Mr. James, presented earlier.

Behavioral Psychology

Behavioral psychology forms the basis for a number of approaches to psychotherapy. B. F. Skinner was among the first psychologists to promote a behaviorally oriented approach to psychological problems. Skinner's orientation was as an experimentalist, and he worked more with pigeons and rats as subjects than he did with humans.

Table 3-9 Humanistic Theory and Mr. James	
BASIC NEEDS	
Physiological	Sleep and food needs not fully met.
Safety and security	Threatened by unplanned retirement.
Love and belonging	Threatened by Mr. J.'s withdrawal from his usual level of interaction with his wife; has not adjusted to the change in his situation.
Esteem and self-esteem	Mr. J. needs to revise his sources of esteem and self-esteem since he is no longer employed.
Self-actualization	Cannot reach this level until he resolves the other levels.
EXISTENTIAL	
Self-awareness	Needs to reflect on changes in his life and the possibilities created by these changes. Needs to make choices.
Freedom and responsibility	Mr. J. has been freed to make choices about the direction of his life; currently must take responsibility for having chosen to sit at home.
Striving for identity and relationship with others	Needs to redefine identity as retired and to recognize that his relationship with his wife and children is changing.
Search for meaning	What is the meaning of life now that he is retired? What meaning does he wish to create?
Anxiety as a condition of living	Anxiety about need to make decisions he had not planned to make for several years has paralyzed him; Mr. J. needs to use this as a stimulus for growth.
Awareness of death and nonbeing	Mr. J. needs to recognize death is inevitable and he needs to develop plans to use his limited time productively to be able to live life to the fullest.

He was also more concerned with getting these animals to perform specific tasks through a system of rewards than with understanding specific human behavioral motivations. Nonetheless, Skinner's work provided a framework for subsequent efforts that have changed the way in which psychotherapy is done. One of the most successful current therapeutic approaches is titled cognitive behavioral therapy, in acknowledgment of the debt its conception owes to the work of Skinner and his followers.

Skinner believed that the focus of psychological study should be behavior and the ways in which behavior is affected by environment. He rejected psychological studies and theories about developmental stages, perception, cognition, personality, and a number of other areas that had tended to interest psychologists. Instead, he focused exclusively on operant behavior, or behaviors that are repeated by experimental subjects who have been rewarded for that repetition. For example, a rat who successfully runs through a maze and is then fed will be likely to work hard to repeat its maze-running success. Behaviorists call this process of modifying behavior by providing rewards operant conditioning. Skinner defined a variety of terms and concepts describing elements of conditioning as he observed them in a variety of experimental studies. These elements included reinforcement, extinction, discriminative stimuli, shaping, behavior chains, schedules of reinforcement, and negative reinforcement, or punishment.

Reinforcement occurs, Skinner taught, when the consequence of the behavior is satisfying to the person. Primary reinforcers are those that have "natural" reinforcing properties, for example, food or comfort. Conditioned reinforcers develop in association with primary reinforcers and are usually connected to responses from others—smiles, approval. The closer in time the reinforcement occurs to the behavior (immediacy), the greater the reinforcement effect. Extinction of undesirable behaviors is a result of withdrawal of attention from those behaviors. Behaviors that have been extinguished may show spontaneous recovery and need to be extinguished again. While the emphasis is on behavior and consequences rather than on stimulus and response, Skinner does recognize that there are discriminative stimuli that will encourage or discourage a behavior. For example, we are more willing to approach someone who is smiling than someone who is frowning. Shaping of behavior is the process of reinforcing closer and closer approximations of the desired behavior. This process happens bit by bit as each new aspect is developed. The child learning to play the piano may first gain approval for proper posture, then for appropriate hand placement, then for identifying the correct key for the desired note, and so on. Behavior chains develop as each step in such a bit-by-bit sequence begins to serve as a reinforcer for the previous step as well as a stimulus for the next one (Crain, 1985).

Behavior is rarely reinforced continuously but, rather, receives intermittent reinforcement. Skinner discovered by experiments with animals that certain patterns of intermittent reinforcement were associated with very good long-term adherence to the desired behavior. Behavior that has been intermittently reinforced appears to be harder to extinguish than that which has been continuously reinforced. These observations suggest that the best way to achieve a desired behavior quickly is to begin by reinforcing the behavior continuously; after the behavior has been well established, switching to an intermittent schedule of reinforcement will increase the likelihood of persistence.

Positive reinforcement strengthens responses by providing positive consequences. Negative reinforcement, or punishment, is an effort to extinguish behavior rather than reinforce it and does not always work. Punishment, according to Skinner (1953), typically provides only a temporary suppression of the undesired behavior and often produces unwanted side effects. While Skinner's experiments were largely involved with animals, he also spoke and wrote about child rearing. His and his followers' ideas about punishments and rewards have greatly influenced contemporary views of managing human behavior.

See Table 3-10 for a summary of behavioral theory as related to the case example of Mr. James, presented earlier.

Table 3-10	Behavioral Theory and Mr. James
Observation of behavior	Mr. J. has been sitting at home since his retirement.
Operant conditioning	His wife does not like his behavior change and chooses to use operant conditioning to improve the situation. She uses extinction by no longer commenting on his staying at home and discriminating stimuli by smiling when he makes an effort to do something new. She provides pamphlets on community agencies that could use his skills and reinforces his positive behavior of seeking more information about an agency by telling him how pleased she is.
Example	A behavior chain she might reinforce by positive comments, smiles, and such would be Mr. J. reading a pamphlet about a community agency, calling the agency for information, visiting the agency, agreeing to go back one day to help out, and gradually increasing his volunteer time at the agency. Mr. J. will also gain reinforcement from the satisfaction he receives from once again being helpful to others.

Sociocultural Theory

While the influence of social factors on personal behavior has been recognized for many years, the movement of social psychiatry has only recently provided a conceptual framework for understanding the relation of society and culture to human behavior. Schwab and Schwab (1978) suggest that the following eight questions or concepts are important for understanding the basis of social psychiatry:

1. Social causation: How much do sociocultural processes (i.e., poverty, child abuse) alone and intertwined with genetic and other influences contribute to mental health or illness?

2. Community and family causation: How much do group and familial processes, including an individual's social role and economic status, contribute to mental illness?

3. Treatment and rehabilitation: Should the individual be treated alone or must the family and other social groups be involved?

4. Prevention: Involves interdisciplinary efforts to deal with "political, economic, environmental, and ethical issues" (p. 18) that influence the protection or attainment of mental health.

5. Governmental and community programs: How do these provide treatment and rehabilitation for mental illness?

6. Cultural influences: How does culture (of the therapist as well as the person being treated) influence both the definition of mental illness and the treatment outcome?

7. Social control mechanisms: What are the means used by society to maintain social order?

8. The possible existence of a sick society: Is it possible that it is society rather than the person that is ill?

⊚⊚ *REFLECTIVE THINKING*

Sociocultural Perspectives

◆ What theories in this chapter reflect, include, or are congruent with a sociocultural perspective?

◆ What theories focus so completely on the individual that they ignore the potential influence of society and culture?

◉◎ *REFLECTIVE THINKING*

Is Mental Illness Real?

Not all agree with the concept of psychiatric diagnoses. One author in particular, Thomas Szasz (1974), argues that mental illness is a myth. His arguments are summarized as follows:

◆ Strictly speaking, disease or illness can affect only the body; hence, there can be no mental illness.

◆ Mental illness is a metaphor. Minds can be "sick" only in the sense that jokes are sick or economies are sick.

◆ Psychiatric diagnoses are stigmatizing labels phrased to resemble medical diagnoses and applied to persons whose behavior annoys or offends others.

◆ Those who suffer from and complain of their own behaviors are usually classified as "neurotic"; those whose behaviors make others suffer and about whom others complain are usually classified as "psychotic."

◆ Mental illness is not something a person has but something he or she does or is.

◆ If there is no mental illness, there can be no hospitalization, treatment, or cure for it. Of course, people may change their behaviors or personalities with or without psychiatric intervention. Such intervention is nowadays called "treatment," and the change, if it proceeds in a direction approved by society, "recovery" or "cure."

◆ The introduction of psychiatric considerations into the administration of criminal law —for example, the insanity plea and verdict, diagnoses of mental incompetence to stand trial, and so forth—corrupts the law and victimizes the subject on whose behalf they are ostensibly employed.

◆ Personal conduct is always rule following, strategic, and meaningful. Patterns of interpersonal and social relations may be regarded and analyzed as if they were games, the behaviors of the players being governed by explicit or tacit game rules.

◆ In most types of voluntary psychotherapy, the therapist tries to elucidate the inexplicit game rules by which the client conducts himself and to help the client scrutinize the goals and values of the life games he plays.

◆ There is no medical, moral, or legal justification for involuntary psychiatric interventions. They are crimes against humanity.

What do you believe and why?

BIOPSYCHOPHYSIOLOGICAL THEORY

The biopsychophysiological theory of mental illness is quite different from the other theories described previously, for it assumes that mental illness occurs because something has gone wrong with fundamental physiological processes in the brain. What actually "goes wrong" can vary widely depending on diagnosis. In some instances, the problem may stem from a fixed anatomical abnormality such as a loss of brain cells; in others, it may stem from a maldistribution of critical neurotransmitters; while in yet others, it may derive from abnormal functioning of some critical enzyme or biochemical pathway. The biopsychophysiological theory does not place any limits on how such specific brain abnormalities came to be: They may be due to genetics, acquired brain injury, interpersonal/psychological experiences, or some combination of the above. The theory does not exclude an interpersonal, psychodevelopmental, or environmental causation of mental symptoms. It does say, however, that, in whatever way mental illness is originally caused, the resultant symptoms can be associated with some abnormality in neuroanatomy or neurophysiology (or both).

The word *biopsychophysiology* seems relatively intuitive: Psychological phenomena are explained by neurobiological events within the brain. While it is unlikely that anyone actually claims the entire title of biopsychophysiologist, in recent years the study of mental disorders has been greatly enriched by the convergence of research interests that this word implies. Psychiatrists, physiologists, and neuroscientists have grown more sophisticated in their biochemical understanding as biologists have brought exceptionally powerful new tools to bear on the various neurotransmitters, receptors, and genetic encodings relevant to healthy and diseased brain functioning. In conditions like schizophrenia, bipolar disorder, and obsessive-compulsive disorder (all addressed in this book), there is an evolving certainty that the illnesses result from specific biochemical, neuroanatomical, or genetic processes.

At the root of the current strong interest in exploring the neurobiology of mental illness is a basic assumption that we sometimes forget to see as a theoretical assumption: the concept that our minds and our consciousness are phenomena that arise out of the complex neurochemical workings of the brain. For hundreds of years, philosophers and theologians have believed that the mind (or what Aristotle and others have termed the soul) had some sort of unique existence. It certainly feels to us as if our minds are real entities, quite independent of our brains: That is more or less what the philosopher Descartes meant more than 350 years ago when he wrote, "I find myself thinking, therefore I must exist." (In reality, he wrote more simply: *cogito ergo sum*, "I think, therefore I am.") Francis Crick, best known for his discovery with James Watson of the DNA double helix, summarizes the biopsychophysiological position as follows: "'You,' your joys and your sorrows, your memories and your ambitions, your sense of personal identity and free will, are in fact no more than the behavior of a vast assembly of nerve cells and their associated molecules" (Searle, 1995, p. 62).

In some ways, Crick has reversed Descartes' epigram: *sum ergo cogito*, "I am, therefore I think." But however one interprets Crick's statement (and in one form or another, his ideas are shared by many leading neuroscientists), he is making a particularly important claim: Mental phenomena —how we feel and act—are somehow caused by an array of biochemical and neurophysiological processes that take place from moment to moment in the brain. In this view, the mind is most decidedly not a soul and not fundamentally distinct from the body itself. In Crick's view, consciousness owes its existence to processes or forces that someday will be described in a physiology laboratory. While the biopsychophysiological view does not mean that we will necessarily ever have a "brain in a box" or in a test tube, it does say that the processes giving rise to consciousness, mental life, and mental illness are open to investigation using the tools of modern biology.

The great 20th-century Anglo-Irish poet William Butler Yeats once asked rhetorically, "Who can distinguish darkness from the soul?" Yeats believed that the goals of art and poetry are to elevate human thought toward the rarified spiritual realm in which the soul was conceived, nurtured, and finally—with death—returns. Yeats believed that poetry and art were the "star-lit . . . flames begotten of flame" that distinguished the soul from darkness. Neuroscientists might assign a comparable role to electrical action potentials in neurons of the brain, but most neuroscientists are neither poets nor philosophers, and few think of themselves as developing or even working with a biological macrotheory. Most practicing scientists resist speculation, restricting their investigative efforts to observable phenomena: for example, the interaction between membrane proteins and cyclic AMP, the distribution of haloperidol among the various brain pathways, and the measurement of hippocampal size in brain scans from individuals with different psychiatric disorders. Observations based on such studies may generate their own theories (strictly speaking, hypotheses) such as the theory that the hippocampus of schizophrenic individuals is smaller than that of unaffected persons. Such "microtheories" require some belief in the larger assumptions underlying the biopsychophysiological theory, whether or not this dependency is explicitly acknowledged by scientists.

There are several concepts and ideas underlying the biopsychophysiological theory. These are summarized following, both to provide a reference to neuroanatomy and physiology and to acquaint the reader with modern techniques for studying brain function and the relationships between the brain and behavior. The following areas are addressed: brain anatomy and function, brain imaging, electrophysiology and neurochemistry, and genetics.

Brain Anatomy and Function

Of the four major divisions of the central nervous system (spinal cord, brain stem, diencephalon, and cerebral hemispheres, see Figure 3-1), this review will focus only on the last two because virtually all major functions having to do with consciousness can be localized to the diencephalon and cortex.

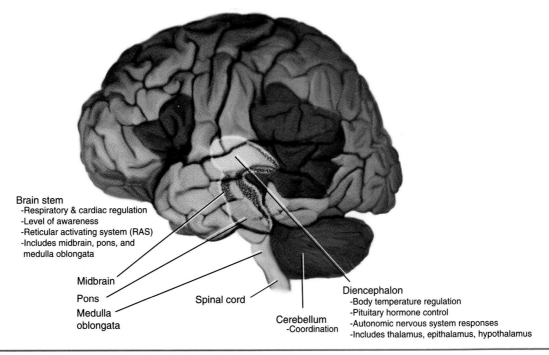

Brain stem
-Respiratory & cardiac regulation
-Level of awareness
-Reticular activating system (RAS)
-Includes midbrain, pons, and
  medulla oblongata

Midbrain
Pons
Medulla
oblongata

Spinal cord

Cerebellum
-Coordination

Diencephalon
-Body temperature regulation
-Pituitary hormone control
-Autonomic nervous system responses
-Includes thalamus, epithalamus, hypothalamus

Figure 3-1   Locations and functions of the cerebral lobes, brain stem, and cerebellum. *From* Health Assessment & Physical Examination, *by M. E. Estes, 1998, Albany, NY: Delmar Publishers.*

Psychiatric disorders generally involve emotional experience, and through many years of experimentation on animals and humans, emotions have been closely mapped to specific brain regions. Most of us have a commonsense view of how emotions develop: For example, we generally assume that people cry because they experience something sad, we expect that people get angry because someone offends them, and we believe that people become sexually aroused because they see (or think about, or remember, or otherwise focus their attention on) someone who attracts them. As with many such "commonsense" views, careful scientific study shows that this intuitive understanding of emotional responses is not quite correct. Stated most simply, we do not experience our emotions solely because of events in the "real world"; instead, we experience the internal signals of emotional responses and then associate them with those outside events. The difference is subtle but important. Let us look at an example. Someone who rear-ends us when we have stopped our car at an intersection of course makes us angry. But this experience of anger is generated deep in the brain and is then cognitively associated with the car accident only in the highest areas of the association cortex. The brain assembles the two experiences (the visceral sense of anger and the sights and sounds of the collision) in such a way that it seems to us that the accident has caused our emotion.

In the example just discussed, a car accident has set off the biologically programmed anger response, but sometimes the response occurs without a real-world cause and for no clearly understood reason. This phenomenon is commonly seen in a number of mental disorders, perhaps more clearly with emotions other than anger or rage. For example, depressed persons (see Chapter 12) frequently assume they feel sad because something bad has happened to them or feel guilty because they have done something wrong when in truth nothing bad has happened and they have done nothing wrong. The bio-psychophysiological theory suggests that in these persons, the association cortex takes the "raw" emotional perception of sadness or guilt and associates it with previously learned behavior ("at other times when I felt guilty I had done something bad, so this time . . ."). The resulting inaccurate perception of guilt or misfortune is, for many, a fundamental experience of depression. Other psychiatric conditions may involve similar cognitive misperceptions, such as in panic disorder (see Chapter 10), where for no discernible reason, diencephalic and limbic "fear centers" produce such strong autonomic stimuli that the conscious cortex falsely assumes some terrible physical catastrophe has taken place. Having explored some of the general features of the biopsychophysiological theory (including its relationship to some aspects of depression and panic), it is time to look more explicitly at relevant brain anatomy.

The Diencephalon

The diencephalon consists of two major structures: the thalamus and the hypothalamus. The hypothalamus is a single midline organ. The thalami (there are two, one on each side) are exceptionally important brain regions that serve to relay a wide range of sensory inputs to the cerebral cortex. The thalamus is a critical structure for maintaining consciousness, but its function is still incompletely understood. In contrast, it has long been known that the hypothalamus participates in a wide range of regulatory functions, especially those that relate to emotion. These are discussed in the following paragraphs.

The brain has been shown to possess a set of stereotyped emotional responses that may be triggered by a variety of factors: drugs, environmental or interpersonal stimuli, or even electrical stimulation. These responses are produced in and adjacent to the hypothalamus and are communicated to higher brain centers, where cortical association systems attempt to link the emotional responses to perceived or remembered stimuli. The hypothalamus, while only a tiny part of the brain, also exerts control over both the autonomic nervous system and the endocrine system, both of which significantly affect the way we perceive emotion. For example, most of the symptoms of anxiety are mediated through the autonomic nervous system: rapid heart rate, racing thoughts, increased respiration. Direct stimulation of the hypothalamus can change vital signs of pulse, respiration, and blood pressure. More important, Hess's Nobel Prize–winning investigations on animals showed that highly localized hypothalamic stimulation evoked not only changes in vital signs but also a range of stereotypical physical and behavioral responses: for example, rage or sexual excitement. Hess's work is fundamental to the biopsychophysiological theory in its claim that the diencephalon is able to generate stereotypical states of feeling, emotion, and even "primitive" behavior on its own, quite independent of any external stimulus.

The hypothalamus also controls pituitary function by releasing hormones that flow through the pituitary portal venous system. While psychiatrists still disagree on precisely how this endocrine control affects emotions, depressed individuals sometimes have measurable abnormalities of the hypothalamic-pituitary axis, often manifested as elevations of serum cortisol (from hypothalamic-pituitary stimulation of the adrenal glands) or of thyroid-stimulating hormone (directly from hypothalamic stimulation of the pituitary). These mild endocrine abnormalities have no clinical significance apart from their effect on emotions; however, persons with profound endocrine derangements (such as Cushing's disease or hyperthyroidism) may have significant psychiatric symptoms as part of their illnesses. Without a doubt, the hypothalamus has a powerful direct and indirect effect on the way we feel and behave.

The Cortex

Most of the brain is composed of cortex, which is, in turn, divided into four lobes: frontal, temporal, parietal, and occipital. The best understood cortical functions are the processing of sensory data and the organization of motor behavior; much of the parietal, temporal, and occipital lobes is devoted to sensory and motor functioning. A great deal of the remainder of the cortex is made up of association areas, of which the temporal association cortex and the closely related limbic cortex are by far the most important for the present review.

Temporal association areas are strongly involved with emotion and with memory. Memory clearly is of great importance to normal mental health: Persistent unpleasant memories, as in post-traumatic stress disorder, can play a central role in psychopathology. Such recollections represent long-term memories, whereas short-term memory (lost in many dementias) is essential for conducting activities of daily life. Memory is not highly localized in the brain, but the temporal association areas play a major role in organizing the process of long-term memory storage.

Deep in the temporal lobe is a complex set of structures known as the limbic system. The limbic system is intimately connected with the hypothalamus and consists of several highly important structures: the amygdala, the hippocampus, and the cingulate gyra. These are all very near the center of the brain, and together they form a loop encircling the thalamus. The limbic system seems to be important in the first weeks of memory storage; after this period, memories are either lost or are transferred back into the cortex for very long-term storage. While memory processing is clearly a highly important limbic and temporal lobe function, the limbic system has an equally significant role in the experiencing of emotion.

Recent research on the generation of emotions assigns an increasingly major role to a previously little-known member of the limbic system: the amygdala. The word *amygdala* means "almond," referring to the appearance of this small but critical brain region. Experiments confirm that the amygdala is involved in a wide variety of emotions and emotionally mediated behaviors: for example, fear, apprehension, sexual response, and feeding and sucking behaviors. The amygdala has direct connections to and from the hypothalamus, and many of the hypothalamic responses discovered by Hess may actually have their origins in the amygdala.

Brain Imaging

Imaging is a generic word to describe a range of remarkable techniques to visualize internal organs. While

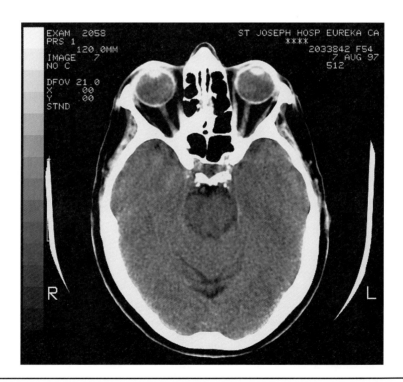

CT scan of the normal human brain. This CT scan reproduces a "slice" of the human brain at the level of the orbits. The eyes (with the tip of the nose visible in between) can be clearly seen at the top of the illustration. The lens of the eye appears white, and the optic nerves are clearly visible passing superiorly and medially from the rear of each eye. The small black areas between the orbits are portions of the sinuses. The white and gray matter of the brain form a large mass within the (white) margins of the skull. Some brain detail is visible on this particular slice, and greater contrast of structures can be obtained by injecting "contrast material" into the client's vein. The CT scan can easily delineate a tumor or bleeding within the homogeneous brain substance. A full CT study includes many separate "slices" taken at intervals of several millimeters and in different orientations. *Courtesy of Alex Habibian, MD, St. Joseph Health System, Humboldt County, California.*

imaging can be applied to nearly any structure from the knee to the eye, this section focuses on imaging of the brain.

Computerized Tomography

Computerized tomography (CT) scanning was among the first of the current techniques to be developed. The CT scan uses conventional x-rays to form an image, but the image is reconstructed from hundreds of x-rays taken at varying angles. Since x-ray beams are absorbed differently by different body structures, averaging this absorption over many angles can allow very powerful computers to generate an image of the underlying tissue. Prior to CT scanning, x-rays could generally give useful information only about bones or about soft tissues that were highlighted by radio-opaque "contrast material." The CT scan allowed remarkable views of soft tissue structures, especially of the brain. While CT images are reconstructions from multiple x-ray images, modern scanners record images at very low radiation levels so that the total dose is not much different (or may even sometimes be lower) than that of conventional x-rays.

Magnetic Resonance Imaging

Magnetic resonance imaging (MRI) is an imaging technique that uses no ionizing radiation (x-rays) at all. Instead, a portion of the body, such as the head or the knee, is placed into a very powerful magnetic field. Hydrogen atoms respond strongly to magnetic fields, and the body has many magnetically active hydrogen atoms, primarily in water molecules. If a brief pulse of radio-frequency energy is passed through water-containing tissue exposed to a strong magnet, the hydrogen atoms will release energy that can be measured by detectors. Through a complicated series of computer reconstructions, this energy can be converted into visual images that bear a remarkable resemblance to true tissue anatomy. The MRI images often can separate out features, especially in the brain, that cannot be visualized by CT scans.

Positron Emission Tomography

Positron emission tomography (PET) has been a major advance in research studies on a variety of psychiatric disorders. The PET scanning techniques are not fundamentally different from those used in CT

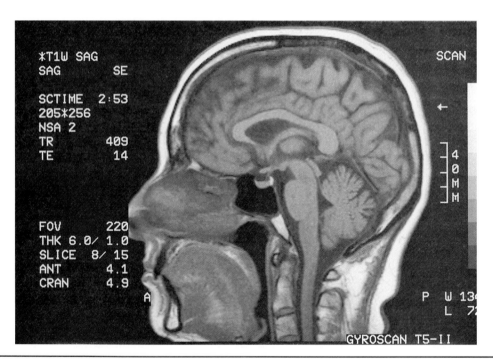

MRI scan of the normal human brain. This MRI image is a "saggital" view taken as if the client's brain had been sliced from top to bottom by a sharp knife. The "slice" has occurred at about the midline. The mouth is visible at the lower front just above the lowest letter "A." To the right of this "A" is the large gray mass of the tongue. The brain structures are seen in remarkable detail. Students familiar with neuroanatomy will easily recognize the midbrain, pons, cerebellum, diencephalon, corpus callosum, and cerebral hemisphere. Even the pituitary gland is visible, extending slightly into the black nasopharyngeal cavity, which is seen just behind the tissues of the nose. The eyes cannot be seen on this midline slice, but would be imaged in a full MRI study, which includes a dozen or more similar images taken in different planes and orientations. *Courtesy of Alex Habibian, MD, St. Joseph Health System, Humboldt County, California.*

scanning, with one important addition: The PET scan requires the injection of a small amount of radioactive isotope that is localized in brain tissue. The PET scan allows the location of that isotope to be traced while a subject performs certain tasks. This emphasis on task is critical because, unlike CT and MRI, which largely focus on brain structure, PET scanning assesses brain function.

As implied in its name, PET scanning uses positrons as radioactive tracers, or, more precisely, uses positron-generating tracers that are bound to molecules (including glucose and certain neurotransmitter analogues). Positrons are a form of antimatter: electrons with a positive charge. When antimatter and matter (in this case, an electron) meet, they are both annihilated and produce two gamma particles traveling in nearly opposite directions. This production of two diverging particles allows the precise location of the original collision to be determined. Since human tissues (like nearly all matter) are full of electrons, the collision occurs very close to the site that the positron-generating substance was concentrated. The PET scan allows scientists to map functions like the flow of blood within the brain, the uptake of glucose, or the binding of neurotransmitters to synaptic membranes, all in response to *specific real-time behaviors*. For example, studies with PET show that in normal individuals, there are major differences in where brain functions localize depending on whether an individual:

- ◆ Looks at a word: The metabolic activity is limited to the visual cortex.
- ◆ Listens to a word: The metabolic activity is limited to parts of the temporal cortex.
- ◆ Speaks a word: The metabolic activity is limited to the medial frontal cortex.
- ◆ Thinks about word meaning: The metabolic activity is widely spread over areas of the association cortex.

The PET scan provides a remarkable confirmation of aspects of the biopsychophysiological theory: Brain functions do link to mental processes and are highly localized within the cortex. Throughout this text, the nurse will see how PET scanning can provide images of brain functioning, not just in health, but in various psychiatric disorders.

Electrophysiology and Neurochemistry

A defining characteristic of higher organisms is that they consist of numerous cells that have highly complex interconnections with each other. This is especially true for neural tissue, whose primary purpose is to pass signals from cell to cell. The brain consists of billions of cells (neurons) arranged in complex anatomical structures and connected by axons, dendrites, fibers, and tracts. Most nerve cells have axons, relatively long fibers that serve to conduct electrical impulses from the body of the cell to

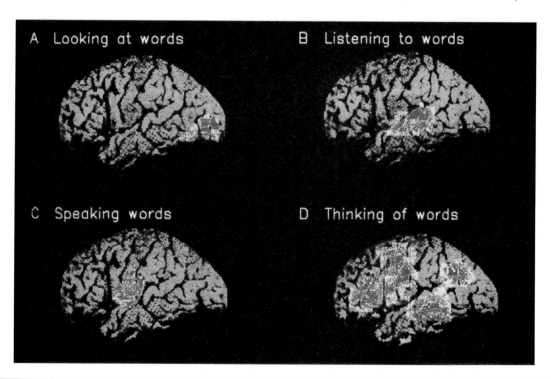

PET scans illustrating changes of blood flow within the brain based on subject's activities: looking at a word, listening to words, speaking words, and thinking of words. *From* Essentials of Neural Science and Behavior, *by E. R. Kandel, J. H. Schwartz, and T. Jessell, 1995, Stamford, CT: Appleton Lange. Reprinted with permission of Appleton Lange and Dr. Eric R. Kandel, M.D., Center for Neurobiology & Behavior, New York, NY.*

some other cell lying as close as 0.1 mm and as far away as a person's full height. Dendrites receive signals from the axons of other nerve cells and may be short, long, single, or very richly branched, depending on their locations within the nervous system. Fibers and tracts are collections of axons all traveling together as in an electrical cable. Tracts usually connect areas of the nervous system that are physically separated. Tracts travel within nerve substance but are clearly devoted to one function. Tracts differ from nerves in that the latter typically pass out of the nervous system into adjacent connective tissue, whereas tracts stay within the brain. The nervous system contains many nonnerve cells known as glial cells, which protect, nourish, and sheathe neural tissue so that it can effectively carry on its communication and signaling functions. (Figure 3-2 illustrates parts of a nerve cell.)

Physiologists have learned that electrical impulses called action potentials travel down the substance of neural axons. When the action potential reaches the end of the axon, communication is made with the body of another cell, usually through that cell's dendrites (if it is a nerve cell) or through a motor end plate (if it is a muscle cell). Within the central nervous system, virtually all axons end on the dendrites of other nerve cells. Communication between those cells occurs in one of two ways. Occasion-

ally, the axons of one cell lie very close to the dendrites or the cell body of another. The connection between these cells is termed a gap junction and is formed so that the membranes of each cell come close together and form a point of contact. When an action potential builds up electrical charge on one side of a gap junction, multiple hexagonal pores in the membranes open up and allow the free flow of a wide range of chemical compounds between the cells. Simple ions such as sodium, potassium, and chloride flow freely, but pores are also large enough that relatively large organic molecules can occasionally get through as well. After the action potential passes, the pores close and the cells are once again physically isolated. This kind of direct depolarization through a gap junction is usually bidirectional and is most frequently seen in motor nerves where very rapid muscle responses are required. In the human brain, most nerve cells communicate with each other through **synapses** rather than gap junctions. Synapses are special structures formed where axons and dendrites come together. The separation between cells across synapses is much wider than at gap junctions, and, as a result, no direct flow of ions or other nonspecific cellular chemicals occurs across synapses. Instead, the synapse is specialized to allow a unique chemical messenger, called a **neurotransmitter**, to pass

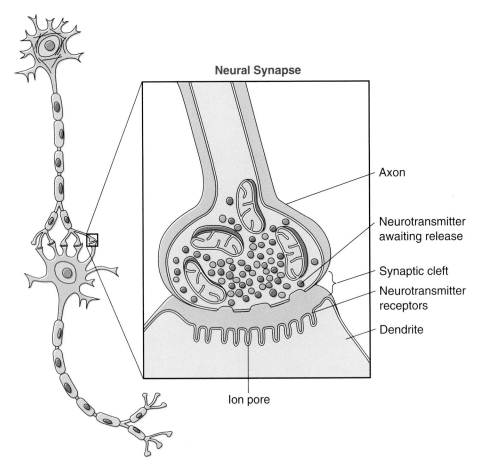

Neural Synapse

Axon

Neurotransmitter awaiting release

Synaptic cleft

Neurotransmitter receptors

Dendrite

Ion pore

Figure 3-2   Microanatomy of a neuron.

from the axon of one cell to the dendrite of the other across the synaptic cleft separating the cells. Once on the other side of the cleft, the neurotransmitter interacts with the dendrite's cell wall to cause the opening of channels, which, in turn, allows ions (typically sodium) to pass into the dendrite. Finally, the neurotransmitter returns to the axon from which it was originally released; cellular processes lead to reuptake of the neurotransmitter back into the cytoplasm of the axon. When the neurotransmitter is taken back up out of the synaptic cleft, the channel pores close and ion flow stops. Signaling across synapses is in one direction only and can be very precisely controlled by a range of factors including the mix of neurotransmitters released: Some *stimulate* the dendrite, others *inhibit* it. In summary, direct conduction across a gap junction is a physiologically simple process, but synaptic transmission is far more complex, involving neurotransmitter release, channel opening, ion flow, and, finally, neurotransmitter reuptake. Since most psychiatric medications exert their pharmacological effects directly at the nerve synapse, it is particularly important for nurses to develop an understanding of synaptic transmission and of neurotransmitters. Neurotransmitters and their receptors are discussed in the following sections.

Neurotransmitters

Neurotransmitters are substances that:

1. Are released by presynaptic axon membranes
2. Cross the synaptic cleft
3. Interact with receptors on an adjacent postsynaptic neuron
4. Are quickly removed from the synaptic cleft by a biochemical process specific to the individual neurotransmitter

Neurotransmitters have yet another important property: Their actions at postsynaptic neurons are directly mimicked when they are given as drugs, most commonly by parenteral injection. The doses required for such systemic action are generally quite large, but the effects are indistinguishable from those that occur during natural synaptic release.

All known neurotransmitters belong to one of a limited number of chemical families: biogenic amines, amino acids, acetylcholine, and purines. Each of these chemical substances or families contains an active nitrogen group that facilitates binding to the appropriate neurotransmitter receptor in the postsynaptic membrane (see the section on receptors, following).

- ◆ Biogenic amines are a group of substances (dopamine, epinephrine, histamine, norepinephrine, and serotonin) synthesized either from a common amino acid (tyrosine or histadine) or from one of the other biogenic amines.

- ◆ Amino acids: While tyrosine and histadine are neurotransmitter precursors but not themselves neurotransmitters, two other amino acids (glycine and glutamic acid) do function as neurotransmitters. GABA, a very important neurotransmitter widely distributed throughout the nervous system, is closely related to glutamic acid.

- ◆ Acetylcholine is the major neurotransmitter in all muscles; it also is widely distributed at synapses throughout the brain.

- ◆ Purines include adenine, guanine, and adenosine triphosphate (ATP). Most of these chemical substances should be familiar to the nurse from past biochemistry studies.

All neurotransmitters function in essentially the same manner: An action potential propagated along an axon causes release of the neurotransmitter across the synaptic cleft. After receiving a neurotransmitter "message" across the synaptic cleft, the postsynaptic neuron has two choices: It can either fire its own action potential to communicate with other cells to which it is connected or it can fail to respond to the message. Which of these two "choices" the postsynaptic cell makes depends on whether it receives an excitatory or an inhibitory stimulus across its membrane. Excitatory stimulation will continue the action potential on its way to the next cell(s), whereas inhibitory stimulation will decrease the likelihood that the postsynaptic cell will fire its own action potential. Most cell-to-cell communication is very complex, and cells may receive synaptic signals from up to 10,000 other neurons, some excitatory, others inhibitory. The receiving cell sums up all its inhibitory and excitatory inputs and then "decides" to fire its own action potential depending on the overall balance of excitation and inhibition. Inhibitory synapses are often located near the receiving cell's body, where their effects are more pronounced. In contrast, excitatory synapses are more likely to be relatively far out along dendrites. As a result, whether or not a given cell "fires" is not just a "counting" of the number of inhibitory and excitatory signals it receives; some signals are given more "weight" than others. Inhibitory and excitatory synapses function very similarly, but they are actually distinguishable when viewed through an electron microscope. Not only are there structural differences between these synapses, but their neurotransmitters are typically different: GABA and glycine are the commonest brain inhibitory transmitters, whereas glutamic acid (very closely related to GABA) is an excitatory transmitter. Most, if not all, neurotransmitters consistently act either in an inhibitory or in an excitatory role, but not both. Nothing is more important to understanding how the brain works than recognizing that each neuron continuously receives hundreds upon thousands of competing inputs; it then fires (or fails to fire) its own action potential to multiple other cells (depending on whether excitatory or inhibitory stimuli were more strongly expressed on its membrane).

Membrane Receptors

For nearly 100 years scientists have recognized that the specific functions of neurotransmitters, hormones, and other biologically active molecules occur because these molecules interact with receptors that "recognize" one specific hormone or neurotransmitter. Recognition occurs through a direct chemical bond between the receptor and its stimulating molecule. The relationship of neurotransmitter to receptor is just like that of key and lock; usually only one fits. (There is another important similarity: Just as a locksmith can often make a "master key" that opens a lock without being exactly the same as the usual key, so pharmacologists can make drugs that act on receptors even though the drugs are not chemically identical with the natural neurotransmitter or hormone. Without such an ability to produce useful receptor-active drugs, modern nursing practice would be very different.) Receptors recognize only one specific molecule, and binding of that molecule to the receptor site sets up a chain of other chemical reactions analogous to the opening of a door when a key is turned in a lock. When a neurotransmitter binds to a specific receptor, either of two outcomes may result:

◆ An influx of ions or other small molecules into the cell: Ion influx occurs because nearly all membrane receptors are protein molecules that bridge the cell membrane, partly outside the cell and partly inside. Some such receptors have central "ion channels" that open when a neurotransmitter is bound and close when the neurotransmitter leaves to return to its presynaptic site. This direct gating results in very rapid interneuron signaling, as ion flows are very quick.

◆ The activation of another signaling system—the "second messenger." Other receptors are more complex: These receptors activate another signaling system that brings about intracellular changes. Neurotransmitters interact with receptors that, in turn, bind to a G protein on the inside of the membrane. The G protein turns on an enzyme called adenyl cyclase, which quickly produces a large quantity of the substance cyclic AMP. Cyclic AMP itself activates other intracellular enzyme systems that bring about metabolic change within the cell. The "first messenger" in this system is the neurotransmitter; cyclic AMP is the second messenger and is activated indirectly by the interaction of neurotransmitter and cell-surface receptor. Second-messenger effects are somewhat slower than those produced by direct gating, and they may continue briefly after the neurotransmitter dissociates from the membrane receptor. Cyclic AMP is the best-understood second messenger, but other substances may act as second messengers within cells.

Many of the neurotransmitters important in psychiatric disorders act through second messengers, including the biogenic amines, GABA, glutamate, and many neuropeptides (see section on neuropeptides, following). However, GABA is one of a number of neurotransmitters that has both directly gated receptors (GABA$_A$) and G-protein-type receptors (GABA$_B$).

Neuropeptides and Intracellular Modification of Synaptic Signals

Most neurons receive simultaneous signal inputs from a number (sometimes thousands) of other neurons. Some inputs are excitatory, others inhibitory. The receiving cell sums its many input signals, and when the sum is excitatory, it responds with an action potential; when the sum is inhibitory, there is no action potential sent on to the next cell. Nerve cells share with computers this basic "binary" function: they are either *on* or *off*; the action potential either fires or does not. While the sum of inhibitory and excitatory synapse inputs is a major factor in determining whether any particular cell fires, there are other important influences on the firing behavior of neurons. Among the most important of these influences is a group of chemicals called neuropeptides.

Peptides are relatively small chains of amino acids that are generally smaller than proteins and so typically lack the folded configuration that gives most proteins their functions. Nurses are very familiar with many common biological peptides, including insulin, vasopressin, ACTH, thyrotropin (TSH), and calcitonin. While better known as hormones, each of these peptides has been shown to act on the nervous system as well. There are several dozen neuropeptides that, like the examples given, either are hormones or are active within the gastrointestinal tract (or both).

Neuropeptides seem to have an important effect on the way in which emotions and sensations are perceived. Stress responses and perception of pain are strongly influenced by neuropeptides. The neuropeptide endorphins act to moderate the perception of pain and emotion in the central nervous system; synthetic opiates such as morphine, heroin, and methadone act at endorphin receptor sites. Prolactin seems to have an effect on maternal behavior, and cholecystokinin may mediate the sensation of "being full" after a large meal.

Genetics

DNA

Deoxyribonucleic acid (DNA) is a highly variable molecule that consists of two strands that wrap around each other so that they resemble a pair of entwined ladders (Figure 3–3). The ladder sides are made up of sugars, whereas the rungs connecting the two sides

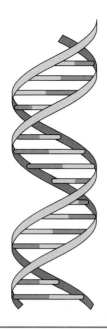

Figure 3-3   Deoxyribonucleic acid (DNA)

consist of matched pairs of "bases." Bases, in turn, are either purines or pyrimidines, relatively simple organic molecules that contain nitrogen rings. The DNA carries a "genetic code" in its sequence of bases: The base adenine pairs only with thymine, and cytosine pairs only with guanine. From this very simple set of rules, the entire genome is generated.

Chromosomes and Genes

The human **genome** (the entire complement of heritable information) contains at least 100,000 genes,

each of which is formed from a defined length of DNA localized to one of 24 chromosomes. Chromosomes typically contain a hundred million or more base pairs, and the entire human genome consists of about three billion base pairs. Amazingly, only about 10% of the genome is actually genetic information. Ninety percent of all human DNA is contained in intron sequences that separate genes. Some introns clearly serve to provide signaling functions so that DNA can be accurately transcribed into RNA for the production of proteins. Remarkably little is known about the function (if any) of the majority of human intron DNA.

A great deal is known, however, about the 10% of DNA that codes for genetic material. Nurses will be familiar with the transcription and translation processes that lead to unfolding of DNA, transcription into RNA, and, finally, translation into protein on the surface of cytoplasmic ribosomes. The primary purpose of DNA is to code for the amino acid structure of proteins. Three base pairs are required to code unambiguously for each amino acid, and as a result, the average protein of about 1,000 amino acids requires 3,000 base pairs to code.

Chromosomes are far from mere collections of DNA; rather, they contain nearly identical quantities of DNA and protein. When chromosomes are stained with certain dyes, a complex banding pattern is revealed (Figure 3-4). This banding reflects large-scale variations in the number of base pairs. Sometimes banding studies can be used to identify mutations in DNA, particularly where chromosomes have been broken and rejoined (translocations) or where pieces of chromosomes are missing (deletions). Most mutations result from subtle DNA changes, often at the level of a single base pair, and cannot be detected by visual examination of chromosomes.

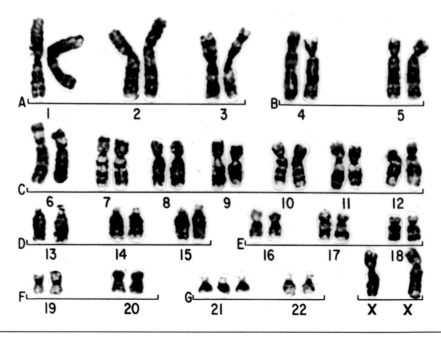

Figure 3-4   Chromosomes

Genetic Linkage

While some mutations have been identified by directly sequencing proteins, the major recent breakthroughs in genetic understanding have come from studies of genetic linkage. Linkage studies require the identification of one or more **genetic markers**. Markers are identifiable patterns of DNA structure that can be readily confirmed by laboratory analysis. In most cases, markers are unambiguous sequences of DNA base pairs, but certain highly repetitive areas of DNA allow other characteristics (such as DNA length) to occasionally be used as markers. Linkage studies are done by observing how frequently two markers are inherited together. Since recombination (breakage and reassembly of DNA occurring between two DNA chains, one from each of two parents) is a common genetic process, the farther apart two markers are on a chromosome, the more likely it is that a recombination process will separate them. (This separation leads, for example, to a maternal marker sequence being replaced by a paternal sequence through the process of recombination.) When two markers are located very close to one another on a chromosome, they are very likely to be passed together from a parent to the offspring. When markers are very close and nearly always passed together, this is termed *tight linkage*. Two markers are defined as being 1 cM (cM = centimorgan, named after Thomas Morgan, a famous geneticist) apart if they are separated by recombination 1% of the time. Further studies show that a separation of 1 cM is roughly equal to a million base pairs. (The reader should note that a centimorgan bears absolutely no direct relationship to the similarly abbreviated centimeter. While the centimorgan is functionally a measurement of DNA length, it is not a physical measurement and is in no way related to the metric system.)

At present, the human genome has been mapped to a resolution of about 5 million to 7 million base pairs. While this is much finer resolution than is possible with banding studies on chromosomes, it is still quite crude compared to the basic mutation level of one base pair. Nonetheless, linkage has proven a very powerful tool for genetic understanding.

Chromosome Mapping

More precise understanding of chromosome structure has come from techniques of physical mapping. Chromosome banding, discussed earlier, is a crude form of physical mapping that can provide gross detail of the microscopic appearance of chromosomes but is limited in its resolution to identification of regions visible in the light microscope, about 10 million base pairs (10 cM). Increasingly precise mapping can be done using the techniques involving DNA restriction enzymes. Restriction enzymes can be thought of as miniaturized "DNA choppers" able to cut the large molecules of DNA found in chromosomes into much smaller fragments. Many different restriction enzymes have been isolated (mostly from bacteria, where they serve to protect against invading viruses by destroying foreign DNA), and each is able to reduce DNA to fragments of differing size. Depending on the choice of restriction enzymes, large strands of DNA can be converted to a few long fragments containing millions of base pairs or, usually more usefully, a myriad of small fragments each containing merely hundreds or thousands of base pairs.

For restriction analysis to be useful, it is first necessary to separate individual chromosomes from each other. This is accomplished via a remarkable technique known as flow sorting, in which laser-guided equipment successfully identifies and separates individual chromosomes from each other. Once the chromosomes are separated, restriction enzymes can reduce them to a "library" of different-sized fragments (each size produced by a different interaction with a separate restriction enzyme). The process of building DNA fragment libraries is laborious, but once fragments have been produced, they can be amplified by processes such as polymerase chain reaction to produce quite large quantities of each fragment. The fragments can then be ordered by matching regions on different overlapping fragments. Once again, the process is tedious, but the results are quite powerful, at least for understanding small areas of chromosomes.

DNA Sequencing

Even more powerful mapping strategies come from techniques of DNA sequencing. Sequencing requires that very large quantities of DNA fragments be produced, often by splicing these fragments into the genome of microorganisms, growing the microorganisms in large quantities, and then extracting the microbial DNA containing the fragments of human (or other higher animal) DNA. This procedure can provide nearly limitless quantities of specific DNA, as can the process of polymerase chain reaction, mentioned in the previous paragraph. Polymerase chain reaction (PCR) is a remarkable technique that can produce very large quantities of any DNA fragment in a "test tube" after only a few hours incubation. Current PCR techniques can amplify a single DNA target by 1 million times in only an hour.

Once large quantities of the desired DNA have been produced, automatic analyzers are capable of analyzing the base-pair sequences of the DNA. While often fully automated, this sequencing process remains slow and costly.

The result of all this effort may be a detailed physical map of the human genome. Such a map would tell scientists where the genes for specific inherited disorders are located and would potentially allow further understanding of—and perhaps therapy for—genetically related disorders. Since many psychiatric and mental health disorders have important inherited components, understanding the human genome better may have highly important implications for the diagnosis and treatment of psychiatric conditions.

Summary

Biopsychophysiological theory is based on the premise that consciousness (and the whole range of mental and emotional activity that accompanies it) is not merely a psychological phenomenon but derives in some as-yet-unknown way directly from processes of brain functioning. The processes that "produce" consciousness rely on the complexities of brain anatomy and on the principles of neurophysiology. Among the most important neurophysiological principles is the concept that neurons receive input from a variety of cells and that the neuron's "decision" to discharge an action potential results from summation of a range of excitatory and inhibitory stimuli and modulatory factors such as the effect of one or more neuropeptides released into synaptic clefts along with neurotransmitters. Brain structure can be imaged with remarkable detail by CT and MRI scanning, but PET scanning allows function to be localized within the brain. The PET scan offers the potential for important insights into brain functioning in psychiatric disorders. Finally, many psychiatric mental health disorders have important genetic components. Some are inherited in precisely known genetic patterns; others just "tend to run in families." There have been great advances in genetics in the past decades, and these have allowed the localization of some psychiatric disorders to specific points on a chromosome. Regardless of whether such discoveries will truly lead the way to revolutionary forms of "gene therapy," they certainly allow increasingly more profound understanding of the brain and its function in health and disease.

- Theories based on the notion of when nursing is needed include Orem's Self-Care Deficit Theory, Roy's Adaptation Theory, and Neuman's Systems Model.

- Each nursing theory gives the nurse a different way of perceiving, interpreting, and understanding her client's condition.

- Psychiatric and psychological theories also inform psychiatric nursing practice; these theories were developed to assist in understanding human behavior.

- Theories grounded in psychoanalysis include Freud's theory of psychosexual development, Erikson's theory of psychosocial development, and Sullivan's Interpersonal Theory.

- Theories of human cognitive development include Piaget's stage theory of the cognitive development of children, Perry's theory of young adult cognitive development, and Belenky's theory of the way women think.

- Humanistic theories are exemplified by basic needs theory and existential philosophy.

- Behavioral theory focuses on overt behavior and ways in which the environment and changes in it affect behavior.

- Sociocultural theory suggests that all human behavior must be understood from within the society and culture in which the person lives.

- Biopsychophysiological theory claims that science can ultimately understand the mind through studying the brain.

〰 KEY CONCEPTS

- A theory is a group of concepts linked together that give a nurse a way of understanding phenomena.

- Nurses use theories of nursing and theories for nursing.

- Nursing theories can be grouped as those focusing on relationships, caring, energy fields, or the notion of when nursing is needed.

- Relationship theories include Peplau's Theory of Interpersonal Relationships and Erickson, Tomlin, and Swain's Modeling and Role-Modeling Theory.

- Caring theories include Watson's Theory of Human Caring, Leininger's Cultural Care Theory, and Boykin and Schoenhofer's Theory of Nursing as Caring.

- Energy field theories include Rogers's Science of Unitary Human Beings, Parse's Theory of Human Becoming, and Newman's Theory of Expanding Consciousness.

〰 REVIEW QUESTIONS AND ACTIVITIES

1. What is theory?

2. How are theory, practice, and research related in a practice discipline such as nursing?

3. What are the phases of interpersonal relationships described by Peplau?

4. How and why does the nurse model and role-model according to Erickson, Tomlin, and Swain?

5. What is the difference between caring and curing?

6. What is culturally congruent care? Can you provide an example?

7. What are Boykin and Schoenhofer's assumptions about persons as caring?

8. According to Rogers, what is the relationship between the person and the environment?

9. How does Newman define health?

10. According to Orem, when is nursing needed?

11. In the Roy Adaptation Model, what is the goal of nursing?

12. Describe primary, secondary, and tertiary prevention.

13. Select an age between birth and 12 years and compare the developmental expectations of that age as outlined by Freud, Erikson, Sullivan, and Piaget.

14. In what ways are the two theories of adult cognition alike and in what ways are they different?

15. What is the basis of existentialism? What are the major propositions of existentialism?

16. What is the difference between positive and negative reinforcement?

17. Why is culture important in understanding mental illness?

18. Describe how emotions and behavior can be understood in terms of physiological processes in the brain.

⚛ EXPLORING THE WEB

◆ Visit this text's "Online Companion™" on the Internet at **http://www.DelmarNursing.com** for further information on theory and research.

◆ What organizations or professional journals could you search for information on nursing and psychiatric theories?

◆ Try searching under the names of some of the theorists and theories discussed in this chapter. What do you find?

〰 REFERENCES

Barrett, E. A. M. (1991). Theory: Of or for nursing? *Nursing Science Quarterly, 4,* 48–49.

Belenky, M. F., Clinchy, B. M., Goldberger, N. R., & Tarule, J. M. (1986). *Women's ways of knowing: The development of self, voice, and mind.* New York: Basic Books.

Boykin, A., & Schoenhofer, S. (1993). *Nursing as caring: A model for transforming practice.* New York: National League for Nursing.

Brown, J. F. (1940). *The psychodynamics of abnormal behavior.* New York: McGraw-Hill.

Corey, G. (1991). *Theory and practice of counseling and psychotherapy.* Pacific Grove, CA: Brooks/Cole.

Crain, W. C. (1985). *Theories of development: Concepts and applications* (2nd ed.). Englewood Cliffs, NJ: Prentice-Hall.

Erikson, E. H. (1950). *Childhood and society* (2nd ed.). New York: Norton.

Erikson, E. H. (1959). Identity and the life cycle. *Psychological Issues* (Vol. 1). New York: International Universities Press.

Erikson, E. H. (1976). Reflections on Dr. Borg's life cycle. *Daedalus, 105,* 1–28.

Erickson, H. C., Tomlin, E. M., & Swain, M. A. P. (1983). *Modeling and role modeling: A theory and paradigm for nursing.* Lexington, SC: Pine Press

Ferguson, M. (1980). *The aquarian conspiracy: Personal and social transformation in the 1980s.* Los Angeles: JP Tarcher.

Freud, S. (1905). Three contributions to the theory of sex. *The basic writings of Sigmund Freud* (A. A. Brill, Trans.). New York: The Modern Library.

Freud, S. (1959). Character and anal eroticism. In *Collected papers* (Vol. II, J. Riviere, Trans.). New York: Basic Books (original work published in 1908).

Freud, S. (1960). *The ego and the id* (J. Riviere, Trans.). New York: Norton (original work published 1960).

Freud, S. (1965a). *A general introduction to psychoanalysis* (J. Riviere, Trans.). New York: Washington Square Press (original work published 1920).

Freud, S. (1965b). *New introductory lectures on psychoanalysis* (J. Strachey, Trans.). New York: Norton (original work published 1933).

Ginsberg, H., & Opper, S. (1979). *Piaget's theory of intellectual development* (2nd ed.). Englewood Cliffs, NJ: Prentice-Hall.

Knefelkamp, L., Widick, C., & Parker, C. (Eds.). (1978). Applying new developmental findings. In *New directions in student services* (No. 4). San Francisco: Jossey-Bass.

Krieger, D. (1979). *Living the therapeutic touch: Healing as a lifestyle.* New York: Dodd, Mead.

Leininger, M. M. (1991). *Culture care diversity and universality: A theory of nursing.* New York: National League for Nursing.

Maslow, A. (1970). *Motivation and personality* (Rev. ed.). New York: Van Nostrand Reinhold.

Mullahy, P. (1970). *Psychoanalysis and interpersonal psychiatry: The contributions of Harry Stack Sullivan.* New York: Science House.

Neuman, B. (1995). *The Neuman Systems Model* (3rd ed.). Norwalk, CT: Appleton & Lange.

Newman, M. A. (1994). *Health as expanding consciousness* (2nd ed.). New York: National League for Nursing.

Orem, D. E. (1991). *Nursing: Concepts of practice* (4th ed.). St. Louis: Mosby.

Parse, R. R. (1981). *Man-living-health: A theory of nursing.* New York: Wiley.

Parse, R. R. (1992). Human becoming: Parse's theory of nursing. *Nursing Science Quarterly, 5,* 35–42.

Parse, R. R. (Ed.). (1995). *Illuminations: The Human Becoming Theory in practice and research.* New York: National League for Nursing.

Peplau, H. E. (1988). *Interpersonal relations in nursing.* New York: Springer (original work published in 1952, New York: GP Putnam's).

Peplau, H. E. (1992). Interpersonal relations: A theoretical framework for application in nursing practice. *Nursing Science Quarterly, 5,* 13–18.

Perry, W. G. (1970). *Forms of intellectual and ethical development in the college years.* New York: Holt, Rinehart, & Winston.

Phillips, J. R. (1990). Nursing: A basic or an applied science? *Nursing Science Quarterly, 3,* 144.

Piaget, J. (1974). *The origins of intelligence in children* (M. Cook, Trans.). New York: International Universities Press (original work published 1936).

Rogers, M. E. (1970). *The theoretical basis of nursing.* Philadelphia: Davis.

Rogers, M. E. (1990). Space-age paradigm for new frontiers in nursing. In M. E. Parker (Ed.), *Nursing theories in practice* (pp. 105–113). New York: National League for Nursing.

Rogers, M. E. (1992). Nursing science and the space age. *Nursing Science Quarterly, 5,* 27–34.

Roy, C., & Andrews, H. A. (1991). *The Roy Adaptation Model: The definitive statement.* Norwalk, CT: Appleton & Lange.

Schwab, J. K., & Schwab, M. E. (1978). *Sociocultural roots of mental illness: An epidemiologic survey.* New York: Plenum.

Searle, J. R. (1995). The mystery of consciousness. *New York Review of Books, 42*(17), 60–67.

Skinner, B. F. (1953). *Science and human behavior.* New York: Macmillan.

Szasz, T. S. (1974). *The myth of mental illness* (Rev. ed.). New York: Harper & Row.

Watson, J. (1979). *Nursing: The philosophy and science of caring.* Boston: Little, Brown.

SUGGESTED READINGS

Barnum, B. J. S. (1994). *Nursing theory: Analysis, application, and evaluation* (4th ed.). Philadelphia: Lippincott.

Chinn, P. L., & Kramer, M. K. (1991). *Theory and nursing: A systematic approach* (3rd ed.). St. Louis: Mosby.

Fawcett, J. (1993). *Analysis and evaluation of nursing theories.* Philadelphia: Davis.

George, J. B. (Ed.). (1995). *Nursing theories: The base for professional nursing practice* (4th ed.). Norwalk, CT: Appleton & Lange.

Meleis, A. I. (1991). *Theoretical nursing: Development and progress* (2nd ed.). Philadelphia: Lippincott.

Piaget, J., & Inhelder, B. (1969). *The psychology of the child* (H. Weaver, Trans.). New York: Basic Books (original work published 1966).

Watson, J. (1988). *Human science and human care, a theory of nursing.* New York: National League for Nursing (originally published 1985 by Appleton & Lange).

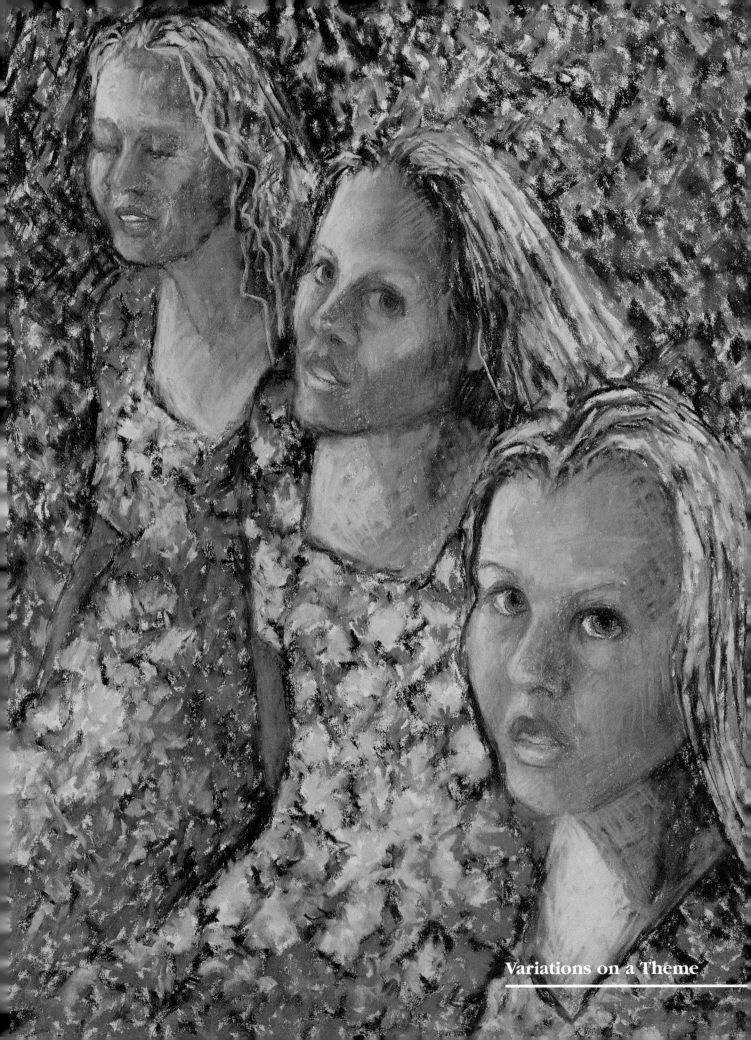

Variations on a Theme

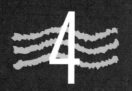

Chapter

4

DIAGNOSTIC SYSTEMS FOR PSYCHIATRIC NURSING

Noreen Cavan Frisch

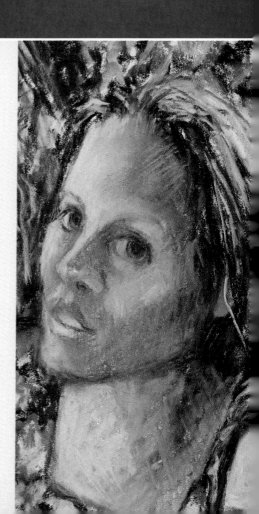

What's in a Name?

Consider the following phrases:
- Type 1 diabetes
- Carcinoma in situ
- Risk for infection
- Sleep pattern disturbance
- Upper respiratory infection
- Decreased cardiac output
- Major depressive disorder

These words are labels that clearly identify certain signs, symptoms, or client conditions. For nurses, these labels bring to mind specific physiological, emotional, or environmental conditions.
- Imagine if or how we could practice nursing without such language.
- Try to identify how you learned the language of health care professionals and how knowing that language affects your thinking and behavior.

This chapter focuses on the languages used in psychiatric practice. Think about how our language affects communication and care.

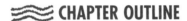

CHAPTER OUTLINE

ICD-9

DSM-IV

NANDA TAXONOMY OF NURSING DIAGNOSES
Collaborative Problems
Development of Psychiatric Nursing Diagnoses

CHOOSING A DIAGNOSTIC SYSTEM

NURSING INTERVENTIONS CLASSIFICATION

DIAGNOSTIC SYSTEMS AND COMPUTERIZED HEALTH RECORDS
Issues of Privacy and Confidentiality
Diagnostic Coding

ADVANCES IN DIAGNOSTIC NOMENCLATURE

COMPETENCIES

Upon completion of this chapter, the reader should be able to:

1. Define a diagnostic system and the meaning of a diagnostic taxonomy.

2. Explain the ICD-9 system of medical diagnoses.

3. Explain the DSM diagnostic system, including the meaning of each axis.

4. Explain the use of the NANDA taxonomy in psychiatric mental health nursing practice.

5. Explain the use of the current *Nursing Interventions Classification.*

6. Describe how information systems affect psychiatric nursing care.

KEY TERMS

Classification System of categorization that allows useful distinctions to be established.

DSM-IV *Diagnostic and Statistical Manual,* 4th edition: classification system for mental disorders.

ICD *International Classification of Diseases*: a comprehensive listing of clinical diagnoses, each associated with a unique numerical code.

NANDA North American Nursing Diagnosis Association prepared a taxonomy of nursing diagnoses, which are statements of the phenomena of concern to nurses.

NIC *Nursing Interventions Classification*: outlines list of nursing interventions designed to identify activities that nurses perform to assist client status or behavior.

NMDS Nursing Minimum Data Set: grouping that identifies the minimum information necessary to meet information demands of nursing practice.

SNOMED Systematized Nomenclature of Medicine: coding system that includes nursing diagnoses, nursing interventions, multiple axes that identify causative factors of illness, and related functional deficits and social factors.

UMLS Unified Medical Language System: thesaurus of all terms included in existing taxonomies.

ascination with naming and classifying has been part of human experience from earliest times. Noah was careful to include representatives of all animal species on his Ark, and by Aristotle's time, the passion for categorization had reached seemingly modern proportions. In a 1964 essay, Jorge Luis Borges seems gently amused by such human efforts to impose order on a stubbornly chaotic world. Borges invents a "comprehensive" classification of animals that he fancifully attributes to an ancient encyclopedia, the *Celestial Emporium of Benevolent Knowledge*. He offers his readers a selection from the *Emporium*:

Celestial Emporium

On those remote pages it is written that animals are divided into (a) those that belong to the Emperor, (b) embalmed ones, (c) those that are trained, (d) suckling pigs, (e) mermaids, (f) fabulous ones, (g) stray dogs, (h) those that are included in this classification, (i) those that tremble as if they were mad, (j) innumerable ones, (k) those drawn with a very fine camel's hair brush, (l) other, (m) those that have just broken a flower vase, (n) those that resemble flies from a distance.

(Borges, 1964, p. 123)

It doesn't take much effort to see that Borges's intriguingly imaginative categories are completely arbitrary: Category (h) adds no new animals to the list, whereas category (l) seems to add an exceedingly large number. And then there is the seeming irrelevance of flower vases and flies. At their core, are all classification schemes as absurd as the *Celestial Emporium*? Borges might wish us to think so, but few modern experts would agree. Good classification is not easy, and many categories *are* arbitrary, perhaps sometimes almost as arbitrary as the *Celestial Emporium*'s. However, despite such shortcomings, classification has important uses in clinical practice, especially in psychiatric and mental health nursing.

Classification is a system of categorization that allows useful distinctions to be established, distinctions that may lead to deeper understanding of natural phenomena. Colors and shapes are part of the ways in which we perceive differences among persons and objects around us. These differences can be investigated further through observation and experiment. Assessing similarities and differences can help us understand the nature of

objects and phenomena. For example, acute viral hepatitis, liver failure from isoniazid, and cirrhotic end-stage liver disease all share jaundice as a major manifestation. This jaundice identifies them each as diseases of the liver, but not all conditions resulting in jaundice are liver disease; in fact, hemolytic disease of the newborn is typically associated with profound jaundice in the presence of completely normal liver function. Increasingly sophisticated understanding of pathophysiology has allowed medical phenomena to be categorized in ways that bring out *differences* between superficially similar categories and *similarities* between conditions that superficially seem unrelated.

In recent years, the science of epidemiology has contributed greatly to such knowledge of health and illness. Epidemiology is the study of factors that lead to the occurrence of disease in a population of people. Epidemiological investigation begins with a careful definition of clinical phenomena so that their incidence and prevalence can be compared between groups of individuals who differ in defined ways. While epidemiological investigations have given rise to many important insights into human health and illness, enthusiasm for classification and for the epidemiological approach to understanding human experience is not universal. Many modern scientists share Borges's mistrust of epidemiological methods based on categorization and description; they prefer to seek causes of phenomena in molecular and neurochemical processes that can be measured in the laboratory. Fortunately, the study of mental illness today benefits from both laboratory insights and insights that derive from classifications. Take, for example, Borges's category (i), "those that tremble as if they are mad": Some of these trembling animals in Borges's *Celestial Emporium* (the human ones, at least) may have hyperthyroidism, whereas others will have anxiety disorders (generalized, post-traumatic, panic, and phobias). There is much to be gained from establishing and steadily refining such categories.

This chapter discusses important formal categorizations relevant to psychiatric nursing practice, particularly the *International Classification of Diseases* (ICD), each associated with a unique numerical code; the *Diagnostic and Statistical Manual*, 4th edition (DSM-IV); the North American Nursing Association (NANDA) taxonomy; and the *Nursing Interventions Classification* (NIC). To illustrate each of these classification systems, the case example on the following page will be used.

The reader will see that each of the diagnostic classification systems will provide a different view of Maria's case. Each system gives one a perspective from which to think and from which to plan Maria's care.

CASE EXAMPLE *Maria*

Maria is a 28-year-old woman who has recently been divorced from her husband of 5 years. She has the history of one admission to a psychiatric hospital at age 22 years for depression and suicidal ideation. She was followed after that hospitalization for 6 months of individual and group therapy. She works as a teller in a bank, where she has been employed for 7 years.

She is now seeking care in a mental health clinic because of feelings of severe depression, sadness, and inability to concentrate at work. She is having increasing trouble thinking of herself as independent; she states, "I can't handle life alone." She reports that her coping style had been such that her former husband would "take care of things" and "tell me what to do."

She did not want the divorce and identifies the divorce as the event that precipitated her current state.

Past medical history indicates adult-onset asthma, which she controls with inhaled medication. Other medical history is unremarkable.

She lives alone, reports feeling isolated from others, and states she wishes she had more social contact with others. She has very few friends and has begun to experience conflicts with others at work because she isn't "doing her share." She has lost her appetite and doesn't prepare meals for herself at home. She has lost about 10 pounds over the past few weeks. Her parents are a source of support to her, but her parents live in the family home, about 2 hours drive from the city in which Maria lives.

ICD-9

The **ICD** consists of a comprehensive listing of clinical diagnoses, each associated with a unique numerical code. The codes resemble library book call numbers and serve to uniquely identify each of many possible physical and psychiatric diagnoses. ICD codes are most commonly three-digit numbers followed by a decimal point and a single digit. A typical ICD-9 code might be 296.2 (Major Depressive Disorder—single episode). Similar disorders are grouped together so that similar-appearing codes usually refer to closely related conditions. For example, 296.2 and 296.3 are, respectively, Major Depressive Disorder—single episode and Major Depressive Disorder—recurrent. ICD utilizes codes so that diagnoses can be evaluated by computer and closely related diagnostic categories can be "lumped" for data analysis. Because ICD codes are so valuable for epidemiological analysis, it is very important that they be both specific and descriptive. There was strong feeling in the United States that the original ICD-9 codes were not fully applicable to American medicine and its specialist-oriented diagnostic categories. In consequence, soon after the release of ICD-9, the U.S. National Center for Health Statistics published a "clinical modification" of ICD-9 (ICD-9-CM). This modification added a fifth digit to many codes in order to accommodate more complex diagnostic codings. The four basic ICD digits were unchanged so that ICD-9-CM is more detailed than its international predecessor but otherwise compatible. Despite the subsequent release of ICD-10 in 1992, it is probable that ICD-9-CM will remain the diagnostic standard in the United States through the end of the century. ICD-9-CM and ICD-10 differ relatively little so that the cost and effort involved in changing such a widely used

standard is felt by most experts not to be justified by the small benefits.

The ICD classification lists the name of the clinical condition, for example Major Depressive Disorder, without further definitions of the diagnostic label. Therefore, as a coding system, ICD can be used to label a diagnosis but has limited ability to describe clinical symptoms (such as sleep disturbances), laboratory abnormalities, or other nondiagnostic information (such as client lifestyle or social conditions such as homelessness). Current versions of ICD have been expanded to include health status, disability, and some clinical procedures. Despite these additions, ICD is strongest in the coding of diagnoses. Its primary uses have been for epidemiological studies and tracking of illnesses. Insurance coverage and reimbursement for services are linked to ICD, in that services rendered must be consistent with an ICD diagnosis.

For Maria's case, the appropriate ICD-9 diagnosis would be Major Depressive Disorder—recurrent (296.3). Her asthma could be identified according to ICD-9 as well, with indication that her asthma is controlled at the present time.

DSM-IV

The first version of a diagnostic classification for mental disorders, **DSM**, was published in 1952 as *Diagnostic and Statistical Manual: Mental Disorders*. DSM-IV, the fourth revision, appeared 42 years after its parent. The first version, now known as DSM-I, was adapted from the post–World War II edition of *International Classification of Diseases* (ICD-6), one of the first such classifications to include psychiatric diagnoses (American Psychiatric Association, 1994). The first version of DSM offered little guidance on making accurate and reproducible psychiatric diagnoses, as it was patterned after the model of ICD. The authors of DSM-I assumed that psychiatrists knew how to diagnose mental disorders and that no further guidance was necessary for diagnostic success. There was little real change between DSM-I and DSM-II, but by the time DSM-III was published in 1980, much had changed. DSM-III included explicit criteria for making psychiatric diagnoses, and these criteria have been increasingly validated by careful epidemiological study. Thus, DSM-III was the first classification system to clearly define the criteria needed to confirm a diagnosis. New to DSM-III was a multiaxial system that allowed developmental and other disorders to be considered along with psychiatric diagnoses of more recent onset. This axial system involves assessment of different domains that help the mental health clinician understand an individual client's situation and plan appropriate care. There are five axes:

- Axis I identifies clinical disorders.
- Axis II identifies personality disorders and conditions of mental retardation.
- Axis III identifies general medical conditions.
- Axis IV identifies psychosocial and environmental problems.
- Axis V identifies a global assessment of functioning.

In practice, the axial system facilitates comprehensive evaluation and provides a format for organizing clinical information and for describing the unique character of a client's condition. The axial system requires that the clinician evaluate all five domains and record information regarding each. The DSM manual clearly presents diagnostic criteria that must be met for a client to receive a diagnosis on Axis I or II. Axis III conditions, that is, general medical conditions, are diagnosed according to ICD-9. Axis IV is used for reporting psychosocial and environmental problems that may affect the diagnosis, treatment, and outcome of the mental disorders diagnosed on Axes I and II. For example, homelessness is a social and environmental problem that would undoubtedly affect the treatment of Major Depressive Disorder. Therefore, should the condition of homelessness exist, it would be documented in Axis IV. Axis V, the global assessment of functioning, is based on the clinician's judgment. DSM-IV provides the Global Assessment of Functioning (GAF) Scale, which suggests criteria for assigning points on a scale of 0 to 100. Table 4-1 presents the GAF Scale, so the reader may see how the numbers on Axis V are assigned.

For the case example of Maria, the DSM-IV diagnoses are listed in the accompanying display. The reader is encouraged to examine these diagnoses and to consider how the multiple axes provide comprehensive information. Compared to the ICD-9 diagnosis, it is clear

DSM AXIAL DIAGNOSES FOR CASE EXAMPLE: MARIA

Client is a 28-year-old female:

- Axis I: 296.3 Major Depressive Disorder—recurrent
- Axis II: 301.6 Dependent Personality Disorder
- Axis III: asthma
- Axis IV: recent divorce
- Axis V: GAF = 60

that DSM-IV provides an expanded view of the client's situation.

A very important advantage of DSM is the avoidance of controversies about what causes psychiatric conditions. Much of American and British psychiatry in the middle 20th century had been dominated by psychoanalysis, and psychoanalytic theories of etiology were complex and rooted in subjective interpretations of reported memories, experiences, and dreams. The great achievement of DSM-III was to describe the *phenomena* of mental disorder without taking sides in the controversies of causation. This neutrality opened the way both for the widespread acceptance of

GENERAL PSYCHIATRIC DIAGNOSTIC CATEGORIES OF DSM-IV

- Disorders usually first diagnosed in infancy, childhood, or adolescence
- Delirium, dementia, amnestic, and other cognitive disorders
- Mental disorders due to a general medical condition
- Substance-related disorder
- Schizophrenia and other psychotic disorders
- Mood disorders
- Anxiety disorders
- Somatoform disorders
- Factitious disorders
- Dissociative disorders
- Sexual and gender identity disorders
- Eating disorders
- Sleep disorders
- Impulse-control disorders
- Adjustment disorders
- Personality disorders

Table 4-1 Global Assessment of Functioning Scale

Consider psychological, social, and occupational functioning on a hypothetical continuum of mental health–illness. Do not include impairment in functioning due to physical (or environmental) limitations.

Code (**Note:** Use intermediate codes when appropriate, e.g., 45, 68, 72.)

91–100 **Superior functioning in a wide range of activities, life's problems never seem to get out of hand, is sought out by others because of his or her many positive qualities. No symptoms.**

81–90 **Absent or minimal symptoms** (e.g., mild anxiety before an exam), **good functioning in all areas, interested and involved in a wide range of activities, socially effective, generally satisfied with life, no more than everyday problems or concerns** (e.g., an occasional argument with family members).

71–80 **If symptoms are present, they are transient and expectable reactions to psychosocial stressors** (e.g., difficulty concentrating after family argument); **no more than slight impairment in social, occupational, or school functioning** (e.g., temporarily falling behind in schoolwork).

61–70 **Some mild symptoms** (e.g., depressed mood and mild insomnia) **OR some difficulty in social, occupational, or school functioning** (e.g., occasional truancy or theft within the household), **but generally functioning pretty well, has some meaningful interpersonal relationships**.

51–60 **Moderate symptoms** (e.g., flat affect and circumstantial speech, occasional panic attacks) **OR moderate difficulty in social, occupational, or school functioning** (e.g., few friends, conflicts with peers or co-workers).

41–50 **Severe symptoms** (e.g., suicidal ideation, severe obsessional rituals, frequent shoplifting) **OR any serious impairment in social, occupational, or school functioning** (e.g., no friends, unable to keep a job).

31–40 **Some impairment in reality testing or communication** (e.g., speech is at times illogical, obscure, or irrelevant) **OR major impairment in several areas, such as work or school, family relations, judgment, thinking, or mood** (e.g., depressed man avoids friends, neglects family, and is unable to work; child frequently beats up younger children, is defiant at home, and is failing at school).

21–30 **Behavior is considerably influenced by delusions or hallucinations OR serious impairment in communication or judgment** (e.g., sometimes incoherent, acts grossly inappropriately, suicidal preoccupation) **OR inability to function in almost all areas** (e.g., stays in bed all day; no job, home, or friends).

11–20 **Some danger of hurting self or others** (e.g., suicidal attempts without clear expectation of death; frequently violent; manic excitement) **OR occasionally fails to maintain minimal personal hygiene** (e.g., smears feces) **OR gross impairment in communication** (e.g., largely incoherent or mute).

1–10 **Persistent danger of severely hurting self or others** (e.g., recurrent violence) **OR persistent inability to maintain minimal personal hygiene OR serious suicidal act with clear expectation of death.**

0 Inadequate information.

Note: The rating of overall psychological functioning on a scale of 0–100 was operationalized by Luborsky in the Health-Sickness Rating Scale in "Clinicians' Judgments of Mental Health," by L. Luborsky, 1962, Archives of General Psychiatry, 7, pp. 407–417. Spitzer and colleagues developed a revision of the Health-Sickness Rating Scale called the Global Assessment Scale (GAS) in "The Global Assessment Scale: A Procedure for Measuring Overall Severity of Psychiatric Disturbance," by J. Endicott, R. L. Spitzer, J. L. Fleiss, and J. Cohen, 1976, Archives of General Psychiatry, 33, pp. 766–771. A modified version of the GAS was included in DSM-III-R as the Global Assessment of Functioning (GAF) Scale.

Reprinted with permission from the *Diagnostic and Statistical Manual of Mental Disorders*, Fourth Edition. Copyright 1994. American Psychiatric Association.

DSM and for new, increasingly "biological" approaches to the understanding of mental illness.

DSM-IV defines a set of general psychiatric diagnostic categories. Within each of these categories is a group of psychiatric diagnoses, each typically characterized by explicit diagnostic criteria. The display on the next page is presented as an example of diagnostic criteria; it lists the criteria for major depressive disorder. For many DSM-IV diagnoses, there are more diagnostic criteria given than are necessary to make the diagnosis. This means that individuals with any given diagnosis may differ signifi-

cantly in their clinical presentations. Some diagnoses have a set of *required* criteria followed by optional ones. In most cases, a number (usually the majority) of the optional criteria must be present for a diagnosis to be made. Some criteria are strongly influenced by culture and are said to apply only to some cultural groups and not necessarily to others.

DSM-IV is far from perfect: Persons with mental disorders may not fit clearly into a diagnostic category and, at the same time, different DSM users may classify individuals in differing ways. These problems of diagnostic accuracy, reproducibility, sensitivity, and specificity are inherent in any clinical test used to separate individuals into categories. Despite its imperfections, DSM-IV does offer a current language for mental health care. It provides a tested set of diagnostic criteria for common psychiatric disorders. It attempts to recognize the potential for cultural, gender, and other bias in assessment and diagnosis. DSM-IV continues to be important to all mental health professionals. While not a substitute for clinical judgment and diagnostic skill, DSM-IV serves as the current "gold standard" for making mental health diagnoses. Few health care fields have such a gold standard, and for the foreseeable future, DSM makes a landmark contribution to progress in mental health care.

EXAMPLE OF DSM-IV DIAGNOSTIC CRITERIA

296.3x MAJOR DEPRESSIVE DISORDER, RECURRENT

A. Presence of two or more Major Depressive Episodes.

Note: To be considered separate episodes, there must be an interval of at least 2 consecutive months in which criteria are not met for a Major Depressive Episode.

B. The Major Depressive Episodes are not better accounted for by Schizoaffective Disorder and are not superimposed on Schizophrenia, Schizophreniform Disorder, Delusional Disorder, or Psychotic Disorder Not Otherwise Specified.

C. There has never been a Manic Episode, a Mixed Episode, or a Hypomanic Episode.

Note: This exclusion does not apply if all of the manic-like, mixed-like, or hypomanic-like episodes are substance or treatment induced or are due to the direct physiological effects of a general medical condition.

Specify (for current or most recent episode):
   Severity/Psychotic/Remission Specifiers
   Chronic
   With Catatonic Features
   With Melancholic Features
   With Atypical Features
   With Postpartum Onset

Specify:
   Longitudinal Course Specifiers (With and Without Interepisode Recovery)
   With Seasonal Pattern

Reprinted with permission from the *Diagnostic and Statistical Manual of Mental Disorders*, Fourth Edition. Copyright 1994. American Psychiatric Association.

⚡ NURSING ALERT!

Cultural Sensitivity and DSM

The DSM manual alerts the clinician to carefully evaluate the nuances of each individual's cultural frame of reference whenever performing an assessment. The following factors constitute the information to be gathered as part of a culturally sensitive assessment:

◆ Cultural identity of the individual

◆ Cultural explanations of the individual's illness

◆ Cultural factors related to psychosocial environment and levels of functioning

◆ Cultural elements of the relationship between the individual and the clinician

◆ Overall cultural assessment for diagnosis and care

---

෯ *REFLECTIVE THINKING*

Pros and Cons of a Psychiatric Diagnostic System

PROS

◆ Observable behaviors are identified as necessary to make a diagnosis.

◆ Diagnoses are standardized and bias is removed.

◆ Practitioners are held accountable for language used.

◆ Records can be computerized.

CONS

◆ Human experience is reduced to a diagnostic label.

◆ Some clients will not easily fit into a predefined category.

◆ Some persons with differing presentations and differing needs will carry the same diagnosis.

Given the above:

◆ What do you think the nurse's role should be in using psychiatric diagnoses?

◆ Evaluate the use of DSM diagnoses in a clinical facility. What are the benefits you can observe?

◆ Can you identify an alternative to our current system?

NANDA TAXONOMY OF NURSING DIAGNOSES

Most nurses are familiar with the **NANDA** nursing diagnoses. This list has been developed and published by NANDA and has been in general use in nursing since its first publication in the 1970s. While the DSM system is specifically designed for use with the psychiatric mental health client, the NANDA nursing diagnoses are a statement of phenomena of concern to nurses and can be used in conjunction with DSM criteria. Therefore, the NANDA diagnoses can be used as a tool in naming and describing phenomena of concern to all nurses and in all of nursing's specialties.

In 1973, a group of nurses met in St. Louis, Missouri, and organized the First National Conference for the Classification of Nursing Diagnoses. This meeting began a formal effort to develop a list of diagnoses that addressed the independent role of the professional nurse in client care. Nurses were acutely aware of the fact that without diagnoses to name the phenomena of concern specifically to nursing, the nurse's role in client care was largely identified as one of carrying out physician's orders and working in collaboration with other health care professionals. Nurses observed that much of what we might call the "essence" of nursing remained undocumented and unnoticed. For example, a nurse understood that certain nursing care was considered critical in preparing a client for surgery (preoperative medications had to be given and vital signs needed to be taken and recorded), but the *caring* aspect of nursing was unnoticed and undocumented. In a hypothetical situation, a preoperative nurse might well assess that the client who is to receive the preoperative medications is anxious and/or fearful of the surgical procedure. Upon making a further assessment of the client's fear, the nurse might learn that the client is waiting for his aunt to arrive and that this aunt is the primary support person for the client. Before surgery, then, the nurse assesses that the client expresses anxiety and fear, is in a state of isolation from support persons, and wants to ask the nurse questions about the surgical procedure and outcome itself. These aspects of nursing care—care of the client experiencing anxiety, fear, sense of isolation, and need for information—would have been met by a professional nurse in the 1960s or 1970s (or earlier), but without a nursing language to communicate and document these aspects of care, they would very likely have gone unnoticed in the work setting.

Nurses began to recognize that without language to state the "essence" of nursing, such aspects of nursing care would be known and understood only by nurses. Further, nurses realized that without such language it would be difficult to communicate nursing knowledge about a client to another nurse. Thus, the group meeting in St. Louis began the process of naming that which "is" nursing for the purpose of giving nursing a language of its own.

In 1974, Gebbie and Lavin identified four steps that

@@ *REFLECTIVE THINKING*

What Is Unnamed Is Unnoticed

Psychiatric nurse Wendy admits a client, Harold, to her unit at 2:00 AM. Harold is depressed, with suicidal ideation. He has been homeless for about 6 weeks. He is fatigued, with no affect. He is in touch with reality. He was brought to the hospital for evaluation because the police found him wandering the city streets. He is crying and states he is at the "end of his rope." The psychiatrist's evaluation includes the DMS-IV diagnosis of Major Depressive Episode with suicidal ideation.

Nurse Wendy assesses Harold during the night, and she determines that Harold is demonstrating the defining characteristics of the nursing diagnoses of *self-esteem disturbance, powerlessness,* and *sleep-pattern disturbance.*

◆ What if Wendy provides care for all three diagnoses but does not label and document the nursing diagnoses? Does that affect the care Wendy gives?

◆ Will her nursing care be valued more or less through such documentation?

◆ In the facility in which you work, is Wendy's care for above-noted nursing problems expected? Reinforced? How do you know?

they believed were necessary for the development of a classification system for nursing:

1. Identify all those things that nurses locate or diagnose in patients.

2. Reach some agreement about consistent language that can be used to describe the domain of nursing as identified in step 1.

3. Group the identified diagnoses into classes and subclasses so that patterns and relationships among them can emerge.

4. Substitute numbers or abbreviations for the terminology that evolves so that data related to the various diagnoses can be assessed and manipulated easily.

In one way or another, each of these steps has been followed to devise the current NANDA list.

There have been 12 biannual conferences on the development and classification of nursing diagnoses. The process for accepting new diagnoses has been refined over the years. Currently, there are written guidelines for the submission and review of diagnoses, and a new diagnosis is now accepted based on information presented formally to the Diagnosis Review Committee. Diagnoses are staged (see the display on the next page) on the basis of how well developed they are, so that diagnoses reach-

STAGES OF NANDA DIAGNOSES

STAGE 1.0: RECEIVED FOR DEVELOPMENT

1.1 Diagnostic label only.

1.2 Label and definition.

1.3 Label, definition, and defining characteristics or risk factors.

1.4 Label, definition, and defining characteristics or risk factors, with references.

Throughout Stage 1, content must demonstrate consistency with current nursing knowledge base.

STAGE 2.0: ACCEPTED FOR CLINICAL DEVELOPMENT

2.1 Label, definition, defining characteristics, and literature review for diagnosis and related factors.

2.2 In addition to criteria for 2.1, a case study is presented.

2.3 In addition to criteria for 2.1, there are clinical studies with at least 10 cases described that exhibit the diagnoses. Risk factors, related factors, and interventions are documented.

STAGE 3.0: CLINICALLY SUPPORTED

Diagnoses have supporting validation and clinical testing.

STAGE 4.0: REVISION

Diagnoses have been revised, based on clinical testing.

From *Nursing Diagnoses: Definitions and Classifications 1997–1998*, by the North American Nursing Diagnosis Association, 1996, Philadelphia: Author. Reprinted with permission.

HUMAN RESPONSE PATTERNS

◆ Exchanging: mutual giving and receiving

◆ Communicating: sending messages

◆ Relating: establishing connections between people

◆ Valuing: assigning relative worth

◆ Choosing: selecting alternatives

◆ Moving: activity

◆ Perceiving: receiving information

◆ Knowing: meaning associated with information

◆ Feeling: subjective awareness

From *Nursing Diagnoses: Definitions and Classifications 1997–1998*, by the North American Nursing Diagnosis Association, 1996, Philadelphia: Author. Reprinted with permission.

There is currently a list of 128 approved diagnoses that have been placed within the taxonomy under a human response pattern. A NANDA diagnosis consists of a name (or diagnostic label), a definition, a statement of etiology, and defining characteristics. The definition is simply a statement of what the label means. The etiology provides information on the cause and settings in which the diagnosis will be found. The defining characteristics provide the observable criteria that must be present to make the diagnosis. For example, for the nursing diagnosis *hopelessness*, the defining characteristics include "passivity, decreased verbalization, decreased affect, and verbal cues (such as "I can't" and sighing)" (NANDA, 1996, p. 71); for the nursing diagnosis of *self-esteem disturbance*, the defining characteristics include "self-negating verbalization; expressions of shame and guilt, evaluates self as unable to deal with events, rationalizes away positive feedback, exaggerates negative feedback about self, hesitant to try new things, denial of problems obvious to others, projection of blame/responsibility for problems, rationalizing personal failures" (NANDA, 1996, p. 68).

In examining the NANDA list, it is important to note that over half of the approved/accepted nursing diagnoses address nursing concerns in the psychosocial-spiritual realm of client care. This fact underscores that the essence of nursing has been defined over a 20-year period to include meeting the mental health, emotional, and spiritual needs of clients. Whether or not a nurse works in a psychiatric mental health setting, attention to these needs and concerns stands out as nursing's unique contribution and nursing's unique role. The display on the next page lists the human response patterns of communicating, relating, valuing, choosing, perceiving, and feeling with diagnoses most likely to be used by the nurse in psychiatric mental health practice.

ing the third and fourth stages have research bases that document the relevance and applicability of the diagnoses to nursing practice.

Organization of the diagnoses was first proposed after a series of conferences with nurse theorists. After some time, the concept of human response patterns was adopted as a means of organizing the diagnoses. To date, the human response patterns are still used as a means of organizing or grouping a series of diagnoses. Clearly, the notion of human response patterns was derived from the American Nurses Association (ANA, 1960) definition of nursing as "the human response to actual or potential health problems," first introduced in the 1960s. This concept of the "human response" assisted nurses in their thinking about what nursing is and how nurses could identify that which was truly important in their work. The accompanying display lists the human response patterns.

SELECTED HUMAN RESPONSE PATTERNS WITH NANDA DIAGNOSES USED IN PSYCHIATRIC MENTAL HEALTH NURSING

COMMUNICATING

- *Impaired verbal communication*

RELATING

- *Impaired social interaction*
- *Social isolation*
- *Risk for loneliness*
- *Altered role performance*
- *Altered parenting*
- *Caregiver role strain*
- *Altered family process: alcoholism*
- *Parental role conflict*
- *Altered sexuality patterns*

VALUING

- *Spiritual distress*
- *Potential for enhanced spiritual well-being*

CHOOSING

- *Ineffective coping* (individual/family/community)
- *Impaired adjustment*
- *Defensive coping*
- *Ineffective denial*
- *Ineffective management of therapeutic regimen*
- *Decisional conflict*

PERCEIVING

- *Body image disturbance*
- *Self-esteem disturbance*
- *Personal identity disturbance*
- *Sensory perceptual alterations* (visual, auditory, kinesthetic, gustatory, tactile, olfactory)
- *Hopelessness*
- *Powerlessness*

KNOWING

- *Knowledge deficit*
- *Impaired environmental interpretation syndrome*
- *Confusion* (acute, chronic)
- *Altered thought processes*

FEELING

- *Grieving* (anticipatory, dysfunctional)
- *Risk for violence* (directed at self, directed at others)
- *Risk for self-mutilation*
- *Post-trauma response*
- *Anxiety*
- *Fear*

Collaborative Problems

As work in nursing diagnosis progressed, the concept of nursing diagnosis versus "collaborative problems" was introduced into the nursing literature as a means of distinguishing that which was the independent nursing role and that which was professional nursing practice carried out only in collaboration with another professional (Carpenito, 1997). A nursing diagnosis represented that part of nursing practice that the nurse was licensed to address independently; a collaborative problem represented that part of nursing practice for which the nurse required a physician's order or collaboration with another to perform. For example, a psychiatric nurse is licensed to assess that a client is experiencing *impaired social interaction* and *anxiety* and initiate nursing interventions to assist the client to increase the nature and quality of social interactions. However, if the same client requires medication to assist him to feel less anxious, the nurse cannot give an antianxiety medication without a physician's order. The administration of the medication is a collaborative nursing role; the nursing intervention to invite the client

to a socialization group is an independent nursing role. These concepts have been widely recognized and have served to further identify the nature of nursing and to further develop needed nursing diagnoses to name all aspects of nursing care.

Development of Psychiatric Nursing Diagnoses

In the 1980s the ANA authorized and supported its Division of Psychiatric and Mental Health Nursing Practice to identify specific concerns and diagnostic labels for psychiatric mental health nursing practice. A group of psychiatric nursing experts worked to develop a classification system that was then called the ANA Classification of Phenomena of Concern to Psychiatric and Mental Health Nursing, or simply, Psychiatric Nursing Diagnoses, first edition (PND-1) (Loomis, Brown, Pothier, West, & Wilson, 1986). PND-1 evolved to become a list of 113 diagnostic labels, many of which overlapped with the existing NANDA diagnoses. In 1994, the entire PND-1 list was presented to and adopted by NANDA for incorporation into NANDA's taxonomy (Rantz & LeMone, 1995).

These diagnoses were presented as diagnostic labels, without definitions, statements of etiology, or defining characteristics. Thus, these additional diagnoses appear in the NANDA taxonomy as diagnoses accepted for further development (NANDA, 1996).

Many nurses have been concerned over the years that the nursing diagnosis model has been overly focused on problems, cures, disease, and illness. There have been several attempts to define "wellness" diagnoses and to identify how the evolving nursing language system could document the preventive and carative nursing roles. A trifocal model of nursing diagnosis has been proposed to augment the existing concepts of nursing diagnosis to allow for the use of the current diagnostic labels in preventive work (Kelley, Frisch, & Avant, 1995). The trifocal model identifies that there are three levels of nursing practice: care of an identified nursing problem, care to prevent the problem when the nurse assesses that there is a clear risk, and care directed toward enhancing the client's current level of effective functioning. Any diagnostic label may be used at each of the three levels. For example "individual coping" is a NANDA label, and a nurse may assess that a client has difficulty in use of coping mechanisms or that the client's current patterns of coping are ineffective for the client's present situation. Thus, the nurse may make a diagnosis of *ineffective individual coping* to address that there is an identified problem. On the other hand, if the nurse assesses that a different client is in a situation of crisis or stress such that current coping patterns may be inadequate to meet client needs, the nurse may assess that there is a *risk for ineffective coping* due to the extraordinary stress or upheaval in the client's life. Lastly, the nurse may assess that yet a third client has entered a time in her life where she is reflecting on her patterns of coping and relating to others. This client is functioning effectively in aspects of her life but is embarking on a journey of personal growth and self-reflection. Here, the nurse may make the diagnosis of *opportunity to enhance coping patterns*. The phrase "opportunity to enhance" reflects two ideas: (1) that the client is in a state of effective functioning and (2) that, for some reason, there is a willingness and/or readiness on behalf of the client to enhance his functioning.

Figure 4-1 illustrates the trifocal model as the movement toward health and wellness through a pyramid. Health and wellness are defined as a state of harmony and balance in a person's being. Each person is recognized as having three components of being—body, mind, and spirit—that together and in harmony make the whole. A state of wellness is a state wherein the individual is comfortable with his physical body, is satisfied with relationships, is content with personal cognitive abilities and achievements, and is developing a higher self. Positive resolutions of all human responses came together to achieve the harmony. Use of this model and of the language "problem, risk for . . ." and "opportunity to enhance . . ." gives the nurse a framework to use the diagnostic language in all aspects of nursing care.

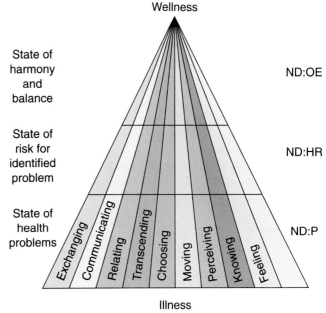

Integration of Human Response Patterns to the State of Harmony and Wellness

Legend
ND: Nursing diagnosis
OE: Opportunity for enhancement
HR: High risk
P: Problem

Figure 4-1 Trifocal model of nursing diagnosis.
From "A Trifocal Model of Nursing Diagnosis: Wellness Revisited," by Kelley, J., Frisch, N., and Avant, K., 1995, Nursing Diagnosis, *6, pp. 123–128. Reprinted with permission.*

Returning to the case of Maria, use of nursing diagnoses provides a clear and concise statement of nurses' focus on her care. The accompanying display lists the NANDA diagnoses that could be made for Maria. Note that use of the NANDA list places emphasis on particular

---

NURSING DIAGNOSES FOR CASE EXAMPLE: MARIA

◆ *Social isolation,* related to absence of satisfying personal relationships, as evidenced by expressed feelings of loneliness and statements that she feels removed from others and wishes more social contacts

◆ *Self-esteem disturbance,* related to feelings that she cannot function on her own, as evidenced by self-negating verbalizations

◆ *Altered nutrition: less than body requirements,* related to psychological factors, as evidenced by loss of appetite and recent weight loss

⊚⊚ *REFLECTIVE THINKING*

Are Nursing Diagnoses Useful?

Consider the following comments, made by experienced nurses:

◆ "I work in a home health agency following mental health clients. We only get paid for what we can document by ICD-9 codes. I don't use nursing diagnoses because it only takes up my time and doesn't help us with reimbursement."

◆ "I work in psychiatric home health care, too. I do much more than provide care based on medical problems described in ICD. When I document that my client has *hopelessness*, I remind myself and others to care for the whole person and to provide true nursing care."

◆ "I'm a holistic nurse, and I think diagnosis is putting labels on real people; it reduces human experience to a title. I don't make any diagnoses."

◆ "I'm a member of NANDA, and I joined the organization to promote the development of diagnoses. I think nurses need to identify what they do that is nursing's unique contribution to care."

◆ "I'm a psychiatric nurse, and I need to communicate with other mental health professionals—DSM-IV is our common language. I have no use for nursing diagnoses."

◆ "At the mental health clinic where I work, the focus is on outcome of care. We are developing critical pathways and care maps that identify what must be done within a certain amount of time. Nursing diagnoses aren't needed, because we only care about outcome of care."

◆ "My hospital administrator said we don't need the number of registered nurses we have, because the tasks of care can be provided by psychiatric technicians."

Each of these comments represents a different perspective on the use and benefit of nursing diagnoses. In many discussions with nurses across the country, the authors have heard nurses making such comments.

◆ What do you think affects the use of nursing diagnoses? The decisions to use or not use them?

◆ Describe how the use of nursing diagnoses can both help and hinder professional nursing.

aspects of care (e.g., social isolation) that might not be addressed by using only the ICD or DSM labels.

CHOOSING A DIAGNOSTIC SYSTEM

A clear question that emerges from the information presented thus far is which diagnostic system a nurse should use. Table 4-2 presents the diagnoses made for the case example of Maria. One can see that each system provides a different perspective on Maria's care. Examine the table and reflect on how each system allows the nurse to document and think about the client's condition.

In many settings, the psychiatric nurse uses the DSM-IV diagnoses because the clinical setting requires that care be documented by all care providers in the same manner. Because DSM was developed for use by all mental health workers, nurses certainly find that it is a useful means of identifying client problems and planning appropriate care. However, the DSM-IV diagnoses do not take into account all of the activities that may be specific to nursing, for example, assistance with self-care deficit or interventions directed at enhancing client communication. The nursing classifications are clearly more specific to the realm of what a nurse actually assesses and does.

In making a decision about which classification system to use, the nurse must remember that each of these systems was developed with one major purpose in mind. Any classification system should facilitate understanding and enhance communication about its content area. If we are to enhance communication between nurses, the NANDA system is helpful, simply because diagnoses are discipline-specific and advance communication within the discipline. If we are to enhance communication among nurses, psychologists, psychiatrists, and psychiatric social workers, the DSM system is the common language. If we are to enhance communication between the psychiatric nurse and a medical internist who is called in to evaluate a physically ill client, the ICD-9 diagnoses are clearly appropriate. Advice from the authors is to use each of these diagnostic systems as tools to enhance

Table 4-2   Diagnoses from Three Systems for Case Example: Maria

ICD-9	DSM-IV	NANDA
Major Depressive Disorder, recurrent	Axis I: Major Depressive Disorder, Recurrent	*Social isolation*
Asthma, controlled	Axis II: Dependent Personality Disorder	*Self-esteem disturbance*
	Axis III: asthma	*Altered nutrition: less than body requirements*
	Axis IV: recent divorce	
	Axis V: GAF = 60	

communication and understanding. Practicality of current health care reimbursement systems has dictated that, in many instances, ICD-9 must be used in order to establish diagnoses and document care consistent with the diagnosis to gain reimbursement for care. A nurse must gain an appreciation for each of the diagnostic systems and use the tool or tools that are most effective to accomplish nursing's work. Further, institutional requirements may dictate that a nurse use, for example, the ICD-9 system simply because that system is clearly linked to reimbursement.

Throughout this text, the authors have presented information from both the DSM-IV and the NANDA classifications. DSM-IV is of major importance in understanding psychiatric diagnoses for clients who are admitted into care. The NANDA diagnoses have been used to identify that part of care that is unique to nursing. It is hoped that the case studies presented using NANDA diagnoses will assist the nurse who is already familiar with nursing diagnoses to move her practice into the specialty of psychiatric mental health nursing.

NURSING INTERVENTIONS CLASSIFICATION

A discussion of classification systems in a nursing text is not complete without reference to the **NIC**. First published in 1992, the NIC is a list of nursing interventions. The purpose of such a classification is to identify and document those activities that nurses carry out to assist client status or behavior. The widespread use of the nursing diagnostic language has increased nurses' awareness of the need for standardized classifications of nursing activities (McCloskey & Bulechek, 1996), for if nurses can identify those situations for which nursing care is needed, the next step is to clearly define what nurses actually do in providing that care.

The current NIC is the second edition, and there are 433 interventions on this list. This list serves as a public statement that the activities described are widely accepted within the nursing profession as being within the domain of nursing practice. Further, the NIC provides the standardized language for nurses to use when researching which interventions are most likely to produce positive outcomes in particular client situations.

Of interest to psychiatric nurses is the wide range of nursing interventions dealing with psychosocial interventions with clients. A selection of these is presented in the accompanying display. The NIC itself provides the reader with the name of the nursing intervention, its definition, and the nursing activities involved in carrying out the nursing care (McCloskey & Bulechek, 1996).

In addition to this work on nursing interventions, a research team at the University of Iowa has developed a classification of patient outcomes sensitive to nursing treatment. The Nursing Outcomes Classification (NOC) provides another tool to assist nurses to relate three aspects of nurses' work: diagnosis, interventions, and outcomes.

SELECTED NURSING INTERVENTIONS ADDRESSING PSYCHOSOCIAL NEEDS

- Active listening
- Anger control assistance
- Anxiety reduction
- Assertiveness training
- Behavior management
- Body image enhancement
- Caregiver support
- Communication enhancement
- Delusion management
- Eating disorders management
- Grief work facilitation
- Hallucination management
- Impulse control training
- Milieu therapy
- Mood management
- Patients' rights protection
- Role enhancement
- Sleep enhancement
- Smoking cessation assistance
- Spiritual support
- Substance abuse: prevention and treatment
- Suicide prevention
- Teaching

DIAGNOSTIC SYSTEMS AND COMPUTERIZED HEALTH RECORDS

Several important developments promise to significantly affect diagnostic practice during the next century and will likely have an impact on the practice of mental health nursing. First, there is an increased interest in computerized health records. Computerized records permit documentation of diagnoses and outcomes of care, permit epidemiological evaluation of populations, and facilitate the management of care based on data. All computerized records require use of a diagnostic or classification system coded in a manner that allows one to trace diagnoses knowing that the diagnoses have been made using clear criteria. Computerized records will make use of one or all of the diagnostic and classification systems described preceding. Further, there is currently work being completed that attempts to link all of these systems together, both for use in computerized records and for use in a universal medical/health care data base that will allow a comprehensive literature search to obtain current information on any condition. Some highlights of this work are summarized in the following discussion.

In 1991 the Institute of Medicine released its landmark report strongly endorsing the universal adoption of computerized patient records in health care (Dick & Steen, 1991). The Institute's report highlighted numerous deficiencies in United States health care that directly or indirectly derived from the inefficiencies of paper-based records systems. These included the frequent unavailability of records either within a single institution or between health care institutions. This unavailability results in unnecessary delays, costly and unneeded repetition of tests when data are inaccessible, complete loss of important information, and inability to provide appropriate coordination and continuity of care.

Preventive health care (such as immunizations or Pap smears) is difficult to trace and document in cumbersome paper records and, following the course of chronic physical or mental illness, is frequently impossible. The American population at the century's end is characterized both by high mobility and by an increasingly large number of elderly. Paper-based records cannot easily be transferred as individuals move, and health care documentation becomes complex for an aging population due to the greater number of health problems identified in this population. Both of these factors add to the urgency of finding automated record-keeping solutions. As the Institute report observed, technology to implement automated records has been available at least since the 1980s. Missing have been leadership, motivation, and an adequate set of diagnostic and coding standards to incorporate into new records systems. Since *managing* care requires hard data, the dramatic growth of managed-care organizations has increased motivation for automated records.

Widespread adoption of computerized clinical records will likely come within the first decade of the 21st century, and most readers of this text will find their professional lives much influenced by automated records systems. For this reason, important definitions and issues are described following.

Information systems are typically computer-based systems used by managers to assess the efficiency or effectiveness of their activities and to increase their strategic advantage in a competitive market. Hospital information systems may be used to optimize patient flow, length of stay, reimbursement, staffing, and resource utilization. These types of information systems are typically regarded as management investment, and their goal is to reduce costs or increase revenue.

Computer-based records are systems for recording and storing on computers important aspects of the clinical encounter. These systems may be as "simple" as scanning existing records and storing them as images on large computer discs. Such storage increases availability, ensures that multiple users can access records when needed, and usually prevents loss or tampering. Imaging of records does not allow easy searching for data, does not improve problems of readability, and does not allow

data to be readily graphed or otherwise presented in useful summary form. But because such imaging solves some of the problems of paper records, it is being adopted as an interim system by many hospitals and medical centers.

True computer-based patient records utilize direct data entry, often by the primary caretaker at the point of service. For example, nurses will often use computers on a ward, or even in a client's home, to enter data about the individual's course and care. In some systems, data may be dictated or entered as "free-text" narrative, but in most applications, the care provider enters discrete information (most often specific observations, diagnoses, or interventions). These are then coded and stored for later display or analysis. In most cases, preexisting coding schemes such as ICD or NIC are used to classify diagnoses or interventions. When the automated record is used both in the hospital and in primary care practice, it is sometimes referred to as the computer-based *health* record to reflect its more general basis. The principles remain the same: structured data entry based on diagnostic and procedural coding, longitudinal record-keeping throughout an individual's lifetime, and widespread access for authorized users in multiple settings.

Issues of Privacy and Confidentiality

Clearly, such widespread access to health records raises important issues of confidentiality and privacy. Clients are currently concerned about the privacy of their records, particularly when these reflect some of the highly sensitive personal disclosures that may occur in mental health and psychiatric practice. Inappropriate disclosure of medical or psychiatric data may threaten individuals' employment, community status, or general future prospects. Inappropriate disclosure may occur when data are shared for reasons other than a client's personal interest or the protection of others, and, of course, any disclosure without the client's consent is inappropriate. Issues of privacy and confidentiality are being addressed by experts who are designing systems with password-protected access to records and strictly enforced policies regarding access and use of information.

Diagnostic Coding

The primary focus of diagnostic coding is to ensure that all descriptions make maximum use of a "controlled vocabulary." A controlled vocabulary means the use of words that have well-established descriptive and diagnostic meaning. Readers of this text will recognize that *depression*, while a useful informal clinical term, is not a DSM-IV concept. DSM-IV refers to mood disorders, depressive symptoms, and depressive disorders, but it does not formally use the term *depression*. The goal of diagnostic coding is to ensure that clinical encounters can be described using controlled (and hence codeable) terms.

ADVANCES IN DIAGNOSTIC NOMENCLATURE

In recent years there have been major developments in coding and computer tools for organizing clinical terms and codes. These developments are complex and beyond the scope of this text; however, three ideas merit mention. The **UMLS** is the Unified Medical Language System being developed by the national Medical Library (Humphreys, 1994). The core of UMLS is a "Metathesaurus," a listing on CD-ROM of all terms included in existing taxonomies. Terms from the ICD, DSM, NANDA list, and NIC are included. The purpose of UMLS is to organize codes into a semantic network so terms can be linked and relationships identified. For example, terms such as Major Depressive Disorder can be linked to terms such as *hopelessness* and *powerlessness*, so that one could ultimately evaluate in what situations (or in how many cases) individuals diagnosed with Major Depressive Disorder are also treated by nurses for the condition of *hopelessness*. In another example, a medical diagnosis such as "cancer" could be linked to the nursing diagnosis of *powerlessness* to further study

and evaluate the nursing contribution to a particular aspect of client care.

A related effort is called **SNOMED**, the Systematized Nomenclature of Medicine (Henry, Holzemer, Reilly, & Campbell, 1994). SNOMED is a coding system that is more inclusive than ICD-9, as it includes nursing diagnoses and nursing interventions as well as multiple axes that identify causative factors of illness and related functional deficits and social factors. To one way of thinking, SNOMED is a system that patterns ICD after the axial system in DSM and includes nursing taxonomies as well. While SNOMED is not currently used in documentation or billing, nurses need to follow its development closely so that the impact of keeping data under this system can be realized with nursing taking a knowledgeable role in this comprehensive system.

Lastly, nurses should be aware that there is a recognized Nursing Minimum Data Set (**NMDS**) that identifies the minimum information necessary to meet information demands of nursing practice (Werley & Lang, 1988). The accompanying display lists the items included in the NMDS. This list is nursing's attempt to clarify the factors that must be recorded to show nursing's contributions to client care. For psychiatric nurses, use of the NMDS on computerized records permits evaluation of the unique aspects of care provided under a strictly nursing model. If psychiatric nurses choose to document their care under a DSM model, nursing's contributions become incorporated into a larger set of contributions made by all mental health professionals. While there may be benefits to this interdisciplinary approach, some are concerned that nursing could be undervalued by systems that do not identify nursing. Over the next decade, the challenges facing psychiatric nursing will be threefold: providing the best care possible; documenting and evaluating that care; and maintaining a presence amidst computerized systems so that nursing contributions can be noticed, valued, and remunerated.

ELEMENTS IN THE NMDS

1. NMDS: identifies the minimum set of data items necessary to meet information demands of nursing practice

2. Nursing care items
   - Nursing diagnosis
   - Nursing interventions
   - Nursing outcomes
   - Intensity of care

3. Client demographics
   - Personal identification
   - Date of birth
   - Sex
   - Race or ethnicity
   - Residence

4. Service time
   - Unique facility or service agency number
   - Health record number
   - Registered nurse provider number
   - Episode admission or encounter date
   - Discharge or termination date
   - Disposition of client
   - Expected payer of bill

From *Identification of the Nursing Minimum Data Set*, edited by H. Werley and H. Lang, 1988, New York: Springer.

∞ *REFLECTIVE THINKING*

Where Will Nursing Be in an Era of Computerized Records?

If computerized records do not include nursing classification systems:

- ◆ Will professional nursing be needed?
- ◆ Who will notice if nursing care is provided or not?

If computerized records do include nursing classification systems:

- ◆ Are nurses ready to measure outcomes of care based on defined categories of diagnoses?
- ◆ Are nurses ready to be accountable for measuring the outcomes of their care?

≋ KEY CONCEPTS

◆ Classification systems provide language by which to define, describe, and record phenomena and allow health professionals to document the differences and similarities between conditions.

◆ ICD is a classification system of medical diagnoses. The coding of ICD-9 permits computerized data entry and tracking.

◆ DSM defines mental disorders and is multiaxial, allowing the classification system to take several domains into account.

◆ The NANDA taxonomy is a listing of phenomena of concern to nursing and permits one to identify client concerns as nursing diagnoses.

◆ The trifocal model expands the concept of nursing diagnosis to include wellness/preventive diagnoses.

◆ The NIC is a classification of nursing interventions.

◆ DSM, NANDA, and NIC all have use in psychiatric mental health nursing practice.

◆ Evolving information systems that will ultimately track nursing diagnoses, interventions, and outcomes are based on the classification and coding systems that can be computerized and will influence how care is delivered, documented, evaluated, and reimbursed.

≋ REVIEW QUESTIONS AND ACTIVITIES

1. Examine three client records in a psychiatric mental health facility. Look for DSM diagnoses and explain the axial system and what information is provided.

2. Choose appropriate NANDA diagnoses for the same three clients. Write these nursing diagnoses, including the diagnostic statement with a "related to" clause.

3. Compare the information and nursing care planned on the basis of the DSM and NANDA diagnoses assigned for the same three clients.

4. Examine the use of coding systems in the psychiatric mental health facility. Inquire whether computerized records are being used or planned for use. Explain reasons behind the answer you receive.

⚛ EXPLORING THE WEB

◆ Visit this text's "Online Companion™" on the Internet at **http://www.DelmarNursing.com** for further information on diagnostic systems.

◆ Search the web under some of the organizations listed in this chapter (SNOMED, NMDS, NANDA, American Psychiatric Association, etc.); what information is available?

≋ REFERENCES

American Nurses Association (ANA). (1960). *A social policy statement*. Kansas City, MO: Author.

American Psychiatric Association. (1994). *Diagnostic and statistical manual* (4th ed.). Washington, DC: Author.

Carpenito, L. (1997). *Nursing diagnosis: Application to practice* (7th ed.). Philadelphia: JB Lippincott.

Dick, R. S., & Steen, E. B. (Eds.). (1991). *The computer-based patient record: An essential technology for health care*. Washington, DC: National Academy Press.

Gebbie, K., & Lavin, M. A. (1974). Classifying nursing diagnoses. *American Journal of Nursing, 74*, 250–253.

Henry, S. B., Holzemenr, W. L., Reilly, C. A., & Campbell, K. E. (1994). Terms used by nurses to describe patient problems: Can SNOMED III represent nursing concepts in the patient record? *Journal of the American Medical Informatics Association, 1*, 61–74.

Humphreys, B. L. (Ed.). (1994). *UMLS knowledge sources: Fifth experimental edition documentation*. Bethesda, MD: National Library of Medicine.

Kelley, J., Frisch, N., & Avant, K. (1995). A trifocal model of nursing diagnosis: Wellness revisited. *Nursing Diagnosis, 6*, 123–128.

Loomis, M., Brown, M., Pothier, P., West, P., & Wilson, H. S. (1986). *ANA classification of individual human responses*. Kansas City, MO: American Nurses' Association.

McCloskey, J., & Bulechek, G. M. (1996). *Nursing interventions classification (NIC)* (2nd ed.). St. Louis: Mosby.

North American Nursing Diagnosis Association (NANDA). (1996). *Nursing diagnoses: Definitions and classifications: 1997–1998*. Philadelphia: Author.

Rantz, M., & LeMone, P., (1995). *Classification of nursing diagnosis: Proceedings of the 11th conference*. Glendale, CA: CINAHL Information System.

U.S. Department of Health and Human Services. (1994). International classification of diseases (ICD-9-CM). (DHHS Publication No. PHS94-1260). Rockville, MD: Author.

Werley, H., & Lang, H. (Eds.). (1988). *Identification of the Nursing Minimum Data Set*. New York: Springer.

≋ LITERARY REFERENCES

Borges, J. L. (1964). In D. Yates & J. Irby (Eds.), *Labyrinths: Selected stories and other writings*. New York: New Directions.

≋ SUGGESTED READINGS

Coler, M. S. (1994). Achieving linguistic clarity: A model to aid translation. *Nursing Diagnosis, 5*, 102–105.

Fitzpatrick, J. J., & Zanotti, R. (1995). Nursing diagnosis internationally. *Nursing Diagnosis, 6*, 42–47.

Frisch, N. (1994). Nursing process revisited. *Nursing Diagnosis, 5*, 3.

Molzahn, A., & Northcott, H. (1989). The social bases of discrepancies in health/illness perceptions. *Journal of Advanced Nursing, 14*, 142.

O'Connell, B. (1995). Diagnostic reliability: A study of the process. *Nursing Diagnosis, 6*, 99–107.

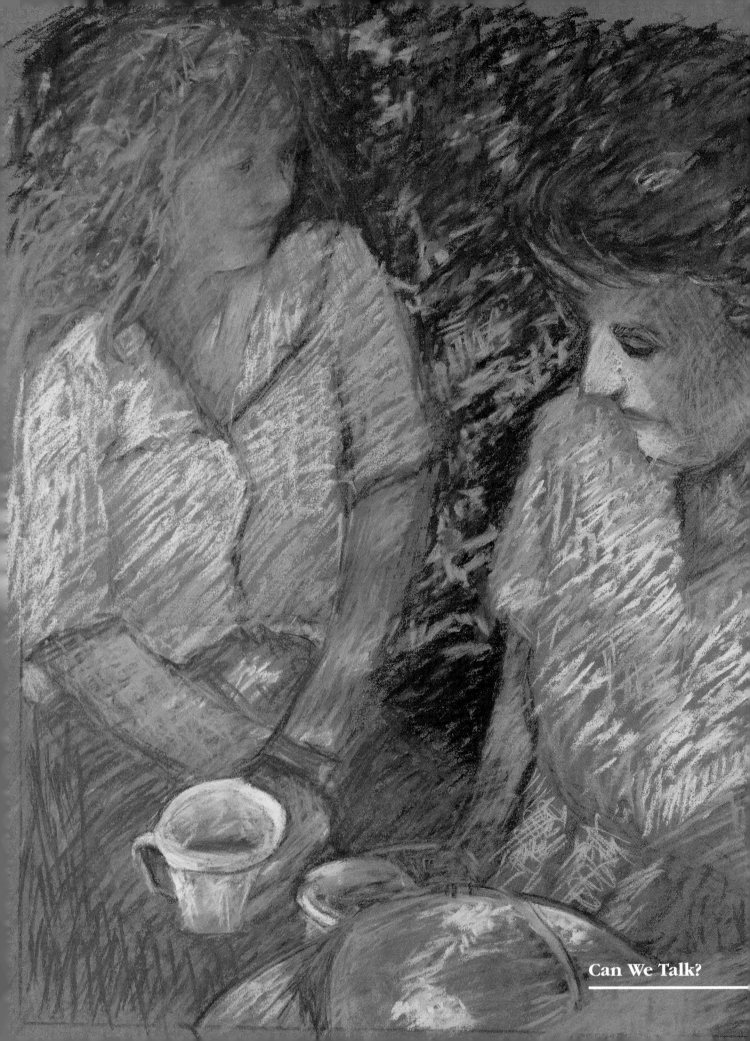

Can We Talk?

5

TOOLS OF PSYCHIATRIC MENTAL HEALTH NURSING
Communication, Nursing Process, and the Nurse-Client Relationship

Ruth W. Johnson

Noreen Cavan Frisch

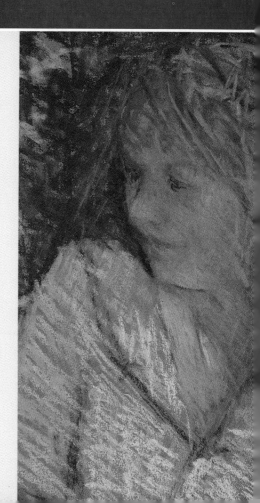

Using "Self" in a Therapeutic Manner

◆ Can you identify a time in your past when you wanted and/or needed the presence of another person to help you with something?

◆ How have you benefited from experiencing silence with another?

◆ Can you identify an individual you would seek out for support at a time of crisis? If yes, what qualities does that individual have?

◆ How do you see yourself in a helping role with others?

◆ Reflect on your activities when reaching out to others for the purpose of giving emotional support and/or comfort; which activities seem most effective?

◆ How do you express caring to others, especially those with different lifestyles, abilities, cultural backgrounds, and languages than your own?

Reflecting on answers to each of these questions will help you to understand how to give and receive support and how to develop a positive and supportive nurse-client relationship.

≋ CHAPTER OUTLINE

COMMUNICATION

Communication Theory

Nonverbal Communication
    Physical Space
    Actions or Kinetics
    Paralinguistic Cues
    Touch

Verbal Communication
    Listening
    Silence
    Broad Openings
    Restating
    Clarification
    Reflection
    Focusing
    Informing
    Suggesting
    Confronting

Defense Mechanisms

EVALUATING COMMUNICATION

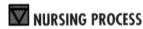 NURSING PROCESS

THE NURSE-CLIENT RELATIONSHIP

≋ COMPETENCIES

Upon completion of this chapter, the reader should be able to:

1. Describe what is meant by therapeutic use of self.
2. Define verbal and nonverbal communication, giving examples of each.
3. Utilize skill of therapeutic communication in interactions with clients.
4. Identify various techniques of therapeutic communication and state when each could be helpful in interactions.
5. Evaluate own communication with clients.
6. Apply the nursing process in psychiatric settings, emphasizing nursing diagnoses frequently seen in psychiatric care.
7. Identify phases of the nurse-client relationship.
8. Use the nursing process and a therapeutic nurse-client relationship to establish care.

≋ KEY TERMS

Defense Mechanisms Unconscious responses used by individuals to protect themselves from internal conflict and external stress.

Feedback Response of a receiver of a message to the communicator.

Nonverbal Communication Messages sent by means other than oral or written.

Orientation Phase First stage of a relationship, during which the nurse and client get to know one another, establish trust, and outline goals and boundaries.

Process Recording Verbatim account of a communication, with interpretation of techniques used and their effectiveness.

Termination Phase Third stage of a relationship, during which the nurse and client evaluate the progress made toward reaching goals and determine that the client is ready to move forward independently of the nurse.

Therapeutic Communication Purposeful use of dialog to bring about the client's insight, control of symptoms, and healing.

Working Phase Second stage of a relationship, during which the nurse and client implement interventions designed to bring about the outcomes identified during the orientation phase.

Nurses working in acute-care facilities have several "tools of the trade" (stethoscopes, thermometers and other measuring instruments, IV pumps, computers) that assist them in providing care. Further, nurses in acute-care facilities exert a great deal of control over the care environment: The clients are usually in bed, furniture in client rooms is arranged by the nursing staff, and nurses arrange objects/tools needed for necessary nursing care (bandages, bath basins, etc.). In acute-care nursing there is usually an immediate focus on the client's physical needs related to illness or injury. Many nurses find that when they go into a psychiatric or mental health facility or on a psychiatric home visit for the first time, they feel something is "missing." There are no physical objects to become the focus of care—dressings, IVs, blood pressure measurements. The psychiatric hospital environment is quite different from the general hospital setting: The staff and care providers do not wear uniforms; the clients are not confined to bed; and the environment may look more like a residence hall than a health care facility. New psychiatric nurses frequently report feeling somewhat "lost," sometimes with the sense of "I don't know what to do!" and "I don't know how to be here!" The purpose of this chapter is to review the tools of psychiatric nursing to help the novice psychiatric mental health nurse begin a new area of practice.

The psychiatric nurse uses tools of self and of knowledge as the basis for care. The psychiatric nurse needs well-developed communication skills, knowledge of nursing and psychological/psychiatric theory, and knowledge of resources for community referrals. The nurse, using this set of skills and knowledge, has the ability to offer interactions to the client that are compassionate and empathetic, that offer hope and a sense of future, and that provide clients with the ability to see their current situations in a new light and to focus on their strengths and abilities. These abilities help to meet the goals of psychiatric care: control of symptoms, provision of a therapeutic relationship, identification of nursing problems, and provision of nursing interventions that assist in returning the client to the best state of health that is possible. The chapter is divided into three sections: communication, the nursing process, and the nurse-client relationship.

COMMUNICATION

Nurses learn early in their careers that there are certain ways to communicate with clients, regardless of setting, and that they must present a professional and helpful stance in interactions. For example, the professional nurse will approach a new client, introduce herself, and then let the client know that she will be the nurse in charge of the client's care that day. Part of this professional communication includes the requirement that the nurse present both verbal and nonverbal cues that the nurse is kind, accepting of the nursing role to provide care, and competent to do so.

In psychiatric nursing, the nurse must build on already solid skills of professional communication and develop expertise in the techniques of **therapeutic communication**. Therapeutic communication is the purposeful use of dialog to bring about the clients's insight, control of symptoms, and/or healing. To accomplish therapeutic communication, the nurse needs a thorough understanding of communication theory and of how to build a positive nurse-client relationship; both of these are discussed below.

Communication Theory

Communication theory suggests that there are two roles in any interaction: the communicator (the person sending a message) and the receiver (the person receiving the message). For communication to be effective, the meaning of the message received should be the same as the meaning of the message sent. To evaluate communication skills and use communication as a therapeutic tool, the nurse must have knowledge of verbal and nonverbal communication and must know how to interpret feedback from clients regarding what is being communicated.

Feedback is the response of the receiver of a message to the communicator. Feedback serves to let the communicator know that his message was understood, or in the opposite circumstances, feedback is a clue that the message was not interpreted correctly. In interactions between two persons, there is always some type of feedback occurring. The nurse must become skilled in looking for and interpreting the client's feedback to her messages, so that she can deal directly and immediately with any misperceptions that may have occurred. Further, in psychiatric mental health nursing practice, many of the clients with whom nurses interact have a history of poor and ineffective communication with others. For example, some clients may not know that they are sending feedback to others that discourages interactions or that makes others feel intimidated. The nurse who is alert to understanding communication can use her observations of the communications sent, received, and interpreted to assist clients in developing better skills.

Nonverbal Communication

While most of us think of communication as a verbal interchange, there is much about communication that is nonverbal. **Nonverbal communication** refers to all of the messages sent by other than verbal or written means. It has been estimated that over half of all messages communicated are nonverbal, for they include behaviors, cues, and presence (such as proximity) that send a message. Consider the following two scenarios:

Student Alice goes to her instructor's office because she is having trouble completing an assignment. The instructor has given her the office building and room number and has told the class she has office hours today from 3 to 5 PM. Alice walks down the hall and finds the room number. The door to the room is barely open, but Alice can see into the room. Instructor Smith is sitting behind a rather large, dark, wooden desk that is situated in the middle of the room, almost directly in front of the door. Ms. Smith has a computer on the top of the desk and is busy reading something on the computer screen. Alice knocks on the door, but there is no answer. Almost immediately, the telephone rings, and Ms. Smith picks up the phone and begins to have a rather loud and animated discussion with someone. Alice waits about 5 more minutes, unnoticed, and then retreats to her dorm with a resolve to try and complete the assignment without help.

Across town, student Barry is having trouble with an assignment given him by his instructor. Instructor Jones has provided his class with his office building, room number, and office hours (which occur today). Barry finds the room and sees that the door is wide open. Mr. Jones has a desk pushed up against a wall, to one side of the door. Mr. Jones is sitting in a chair at the desk, allowing him to have a clear view of the door. Mr. Jones is talking on the phone and gestures immediately for Barry to wait a minute so the two can talk. Barry waits, and soon initiates discussion with his instructor.

In these student-instructor scenes, each instructor provided the student with nearly identical verbal cues (i.e., spoken and written communications) regarding office hours and availability. However, the nonverbal cues influenced interaction greatly. Which instructor met the needs of the student seeking help? Did each instructor purposefully set up the nonverbal cues? One finds that many persons (instructors included!) have little understanding of the nonverbal messages they send. The following components of nonverbal communication may greatly influence interactions.

Physical Space

The physical space between two individuals as well as the design of the room and the furniture that contributes to the environment have great meaning in communication. Space between two persons gives a sense of their relationship and, like all aspects of communication, is linked to cultural norms and values. In general, studies of interactions between and among people in North America indicate that a person has four zones of interaction defined by the space or distance between two persons (Hall, 1959). Public space, or approximately 12

꩜ REFLECTIVE THINKING

Nonverbal Communication in Your Life

Take time today to observe and reflect on the nonverbal communication of those around you:

- If at school, what nonverbal messages are sent to you by your classmates when you walk into your class?
- What nonverbal messages do students in your class send your instructor when it is 5 minutes before the end of the scheduled lecture time?
- When you have an informal conversation with a friend, what messages let you know that it is time to end the conversation and do something else?
- At home, what nonverbal messages are sent to you and your family members/housemates at the dinner table? At the end of the work day? Before people in the household leave for an activity?

Noticing nonverbal communication will help you develop skills in therapeutic communication.

---

feet, is comfortable for most persons in public activities, such as giving a talk in a classroom. Social space is about 9 to 12 feet and is a comfortable distance in social settings, for example, walking down a street or being seated at a restaurant. Personal space ranges from 18 inches to about 4 feet and refers to the space between persons with some sense of connection: fellow students seated in a classroom, for example. Intimate space is space closer than 18 inches and is reserved for those with whom a person has a close relationship, such as family and personal friends.

A nurse can use her knowledge of the meaning of space and distance between two persons to understand and interpret nonverbal behaviors. Some clients are comfortable sitting next to the nurse in "social" space, others may get up and walk away. The nurse can use these cues to understand that, for some, social interactions may feel too invasive and be uncomfortable, while for others the contact within social space may provide a source of comfort and be interpreted as support. In some situations, the nurse may find that a client moves in "too close" for the nurse to feel the interaction can be professional and appropriate. A nurse may find that a passive, dependent client always sits next to her on a couch such that the client chooses to be within 12 to 18 inches of the nurse. Further, the same client may follow the nurse this closely down the hall. In such cases, the nurse will understand that the client may need

✆⊚ *REFLECTIVE THINKING*

Physical Space and Interaction

1. Observe your own level of comfort on a psychiatric unit. For instance, when you sit next to a client, what seating arrangement is most comfortable for you?
   - At a table (e.g., playing cards)
   - On a couch
   - Other

2. In what settings are most clients likely to approach you?
   - When you are at the nurses' station
   - When you are at a meal table during dinner
   - When you are sitting in a day room

3. How do you interpret the social space on the unit?
   - How is the physical space in the unit arranged? Sketch the furniture/space arrangement.
   - How do you think the physical space contributes to communication and interaction between and among people?
   - What changes would you suggest to enhance communication?

speech have significant meaning, these actions are almost always culture-bound, and interpreted meaning must be understood within the socio-cultural context of the speaker.

Paralinguistic Cues

Vocal cues are parts of spoken language other than words. These include tone, pitch, emotions expressed verbally (such as anxiety or anger or fear), sounds of hesitation, nervous laughter, and nervous coughing. These cues provide the context in which the words are delivered, and they influence meaning directly. As the actions during speech convey messages based on social and cultural norms, so do paralinguistic cues. The nurse is cautioned to interpret vocal cues within the context of the client's cultural and social/familial norms.

Touch

Touch is a form of communication used almost daily by nurses providing direct physical care and support to clients. Touch can convey warmth, positive regard, support during silence, and reassurance that the nurse is fully present and caring. Touch has many meanings, however. Psychiatric mental health nurses often use touch—for example, reaching out and holding a client's hand—as a means to extend support. However, like other forms of nonverbal communication, touch may be interpreted many ways. The therapeutic value of touch is dependent upon the client perceiving the intended message. Nurses must always be aware of the meaning touch has for any particular client and use touch only in a way that is therapeutic (Figure 5-1).

to develop boundaries and a stronger sense of self in order to establish the social skills necessary to initiate communication with others. When appropriate in the nurse-client relationship, the nurse will use observations to let the client know how the client's nonverbal messages come across to others.

Room and space design (e.g., the design of an instructor's office) can also send messages about how inviting interaction may be. Chairs can be spaced to invite personal and social interactions. Desks can be placed to provide barriers to interactions. Observations of where persons choose to sit and where they put furniture provide many cues as to the desire and need for interactions.

Actions or Kinetics

Actions refer to movements, expressions, gestures, and posture that accompany interactions and influence communications. They convey messages of intent and mood and can support or contradict a verbal message. For instance, an instructor who is frequently glancing at a clock during a student conversation conveys a different message than one who is looking directly at the student. While actions during

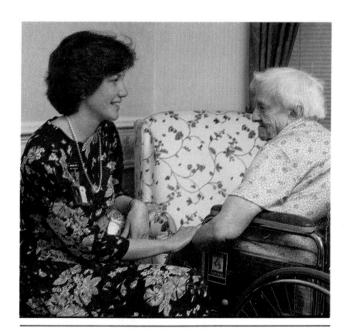

Figure 5-1 Touch can be a valuable means of extending therapeutic support and comfort to a client.

Verbal Communication

Verbal communication is the use of words, written and spoken, to send messages to another. For communication to be most therapeutic, it must convey a respectful attitude, one that supports the individuality and self-esteem of both the client and the nurse. There are identified techniques of communication that allow one to learn *how* to convey such an attitude and also allow one to step back and reflect on the nurse-client interaction. These techniques are summarized in Table 5-1 and will be discussed below.

Listening

Listening is perhaps the most important communication technique, for it involves being fully present for another while obtaining information needed to truly understand the client. While it is sometimes difficult to listen, it is essential that the nurse learn to give the client every chance to be heard.

Silence

Silence is the ability to wait, to pause, to refrain from using language, giving the client and nurse time to reflect, respond, and feel emotions. Silence is effective in letting the client lead the way, for silence is waiting for the client to direct the communication. The nurse's silence encourages the client to feel and explore emotions and may foster self-awareness.

Broad Openings

Broad openings are words that permit the client to decide the manner of the response. Comments such as "Tell me about that" or "What do you think about that?" or "What's on your mind today?" are all broad openings. Such statements let the client know the nurse wants to listen and permit the client a wide range of responses. The client will choose the topic, as well as the degree to which he will open up to disclose inner feelings. The broad opening allows the nurse to get the conversation started without making demands that the client talk about one particular subject.

Restating

Restating is a technique whereby the nurse repeats the main message the client has expressed. Restating permits the nurse to verify understanding of the client's message and also permits the client to reflect on the statement and emotion expressed. Restating lets the client know that the nurse is truly listening and making every attempt to understand.

Clarification

Clarification is a technique whereby the nurse tries to put the client's ideas into a simple statement. The nurse might say, "Are you saying that . . . " and fill in the messages she has heard to check her understanding and to make the client's thoughts or feelings explicit.

Table 5-1   Summary of Therapeutic Communication Techniques

TECHNIQUE	EXAMPLE	PURPOSE
Listening	Silence, eye contact, attitude of being fully present	Permits the client to be heard; conveys interest in what the client is saying
Silence	Not breaking the quiet	Provides time for nurse and client to gather thoughts, to reflect
Broad openings	"What's been going on?" "Tell me what's been on your mind."	Initiates conversation; puts the client in control of the content
Restating	"Are you saying you were angry when your wife had to work late?"	Provides feedback, letting the client know that the nurse understood the message; lets the client know that the nurse is attentive
Clarification	"Are you saying you want to move out of your apartment?"	Puts client's ideas into a simple statement; makes the client's ideas explicit
Reflection	"So you start feeling depressed when no one calls you over the weekend."	Presents themes that have emerged through a series of interactions
Focusing	"Let's go back to the situation at school, where you felt uncomfortable in class."	Directs conversation back to an area of importance; explores a topic in depth
Informing	"The medication must be taken every day."	Provides facts or recommendations
Suggesting	"Have you considered the alternative of a self-help group for weekly support?"	Presents new ideas; assists client to consider alternative options
Confronting	"You say you're upset, but you are laughing."	Presents contradictions and inconsistencies

Reflection

Reflection is, as its name implies, reflecting or interpreting back to the client what has been heard and understood. Reflection may be a statement like "It sounds like you got mad when your roommate left the kitchen dirty," reflecting on the situation and the client's feelings. Reflection is a powerful tool to bring out important aspects of the client's feelings and to put them in the context of when and where they occur. Different from restating, reflection allows the nurse to describe a theme that the client has not identified verbally. Therefore, reflection must be used when the nurse has a good understanding of what is important to the client, so that the nurse does not come across as implying that she knows the client's feelings better than does the client. Reflection must be used sparingly and works best in those situations where the nurse intends to underscore a theme that seems important to the client.

Focusing

Focusing is a technique in which the nurse directs the conversation to focus on a topic of particular importance or relevance to the client. Here, the nurse asks questions about one theme that has emerged or is emerging in the client interactions. The purpose is to draw the client's attention to the theme—its meaning and significance in the client's life and adjustments. An example of focusing would be "Let's talk some more about . . . "

Informing

Informing is the nursing skill of providing information, when needed. Informing, used by nurses in the nurse-client education role, refers to simply giving facts and information. In psychiatric mental health nursing, the client often needs information about his illness, the etiology and genetic basis of his disease, the legal aspects of care, and alternatives for medication and treatment. "The medication will not have an effect for two weeks . . . " is an example of informing.

Suggesting

Suggesting is used to encourage a client to consider alternatives, for example, suggesting or questioning whether the client has considered a specific option or asking the client to consider an alternate means of coping with a particular situation. For suggesting to be therapeutic, the nurse must not tell the client what to do or implicitly take responsibility for the decision and the outcome away from the client.

Confronting

Confronting is communication that points out inconsistencies or incongruencies between feelings, thoughts, and actions. For example, the nurse might state, "You say

you are upset about the degree of drinking in your family, but you smile as you say so and ask others to party with you on Saturday night." Used correctly, confrontation encourages clients to explore maladaptive behaviors. To use confrontation as a therapeutic tool, the nurse must use a friendly but firm approach and recognize that a client may deny or become angry with the suggestion that something in his life in inconsistent. Nonetheless, in using confrontation, the nurse must remain patient and know that confrontation may be the only way to encourage the client to examine his own dysfunctional behaviors.

In addition to these techniques of communication, the nurse should also evaluate her choice of words and whether or not the messages she has sent are being understood by the client. Clear, precise language is always preferable. Simple words that convey the meaning intended are better than complicated phrases and difficult vocabulary.

Defense Mechanisms

Defense mechanisms are unconscious responses used by persons to protect themselves from internal conflicts and external stressors. A nurse skilled in therapeutic communication will notice when a client is using one or more of these mechanisms. When a nurse concludes that her client is using a defense mechanism to avoid dealing with certain subjects, the nurse can use this knowledge to guide interactions, knowing that the defense mechanism indicates the presence of psychologically significant material. In interviews, the nurse may choose to pursue additional information on the topic, but the nurse will also realize that the client may not be able to answer direct questions about related issues. Table 5-2 presents examples of common defense mechanisms.

EVALUATING COMMUNICATION

The nurse must always evaluate whether communication was therapeutic or nontherapeutic. A course in psychiatric nursing is a time for self-examination, a time to look carefully at how one as a nurse comes across to others, and a time to look at how one's own communication and behaviors impact others.

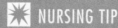 **NURSING TIP**

Communication Skills Awareness

Psychiatric mental health nursing offers a chance to explore one's communication skills. Use this time to grow and learn. Be kind to yourself and understand that all nurses find aspects of their communication skills that need improving!

Table 5-2 Common Defense Mechanisms

MECHANISM	DESCRIPTION	EXAMPLE
Denial	Negation of reality of threatening situations, despite factual evidence	The client refuses to admit to anger, even though the situation warrants it and the client's voice indicates anger.
Projection	Attribution of one's own thoughts, feelings, or impulses to others	"I'm not attracted to him. My best friend is."
Repression	Unconscious blocking from awareness material that is threatening or painful	"I never got angry at my father; our family lived in harmony and love" (when such descriptions of the family life would not fit with anyone else's interpretation of the events).
Rationalization	Intellectual explaining away of threatening circumstances	"The test had too many trick questions; I really know all the material; our instructor was out to get me."
Introjection	Incorporating, without examination or thought, the qualities or attitudes of others	The adolescent who takes on all the values and styles of an admired teacher.
Displacement	Transfer of feelings or reactions evoked by one topic or event to another that is less threatening	The husband who is angry at his wife and yells at the family dog rather than dealing directly with his anger.
Reaction formation	Expression of a feeling that is the opposite of one's authentic feeling or of feelings that would be appropriate in the situation	A client who brings gifts to the nurse at whom he is really mad.
Regression	Retreat to a previous developmental level	A child starts to suck his thumb (after 2 years of not thumb sucking) when admitted to the hospital.
Suppression	Conscious or unconscious attempt to keep threatening material out of consciousness	Failure to remember a significant childhood event, like the death of a grandmother.
Sublimation	Channeling of socially unacceptable impulses into socially acceptable activities	A young man who is dealing with aggression by playing football.
Symbolization	Use of an object, idea, or act to express emotion that is not expressed directly	The client who leaves the nurse a flower rather than directly saying she cares about the nurse.

Use of therapeutic communication techniques does not, in and of itself, mean that communication will be therapeutic. There is judgment involved in deciding when to be silent, when to probe or question, when to restate, when to ask for clarification. After the communication has taken place, one can determine if it was therapeutic. A therapeutic communication is one that builds a trusting relationship and helps to give the client insight and tools to become independent and regain or attain health.

There are several ways of evaluating communication. First and foremost, the nurse should take the time to get feedback from the client that he understands what the nurse has said. Second, the nurse should provide feedback so that the nurse can know that what she has understood is what the client intended. Many nurses will keep some form of a process recording that documents their interactions with clients. A **process recording** is a verbatim account of the communication, with the nurse's interpretation of the specific communication technique used and an evaluation of whether or not the communication was therapeutic. A process recording gives the nurse information upon which to reflect. When the nurse discovers that some aspect of communication was not therapeutic, a process recording gives the nurse a chance to consider and suggest another means of communication that might be preferable. A sample process recording is presented in Table 5-3.

Process recordings may be done in several ways. Videotape recordings of interactions are, of course, the best documentation of interactions, for on tape both verbal and nonverbal messages can be observed. Next to a video recording, an auditory recording is most accurate. When neither of these is feasible, a nurse may have a conversation with a client and immediately afterward write down all that she can remember from the interaction. While a written account from memory may not be the most accurate, it is probably the most frequently used method of documenting interactions between nurses and clients. Issues of permission, confidentiality, and

Table 5-3 **Sample Process Recording**

INTERACTION	COMMUNICATION TECHNIQUE USED	EVALUATION
Nurse: What's been going on this week? Client: I've been thinking a lot about my job. I just don't like my boss. In fact, I can't stand working with her.	Broad opening	Permits client to begin with what is important at the moment.
Nurse: You don't like her? Client: No. She doesn't value me or anyone else. She always tells us all about what is wrong, but never says anything good.	Restating	Provides a chance for client to expand, which he does.
Nurse: So you would like to feel valued? Client: Yes! It's like when I was in school and no one thought I did well enough.	Reflection	Returns the client to feelings. The client is able to talk about experiences from his past.
Nurse: No one? Client: Yeah, my parents, friends, they made me feel like I was no good.	Clarification	Allows the nurse to seek information, yet encourages client to go on.
Nurse: This current situation at work, it is similar to feelings you've had before.	Reflection	Returns focus to current situations and the theme of feeling devalued.

anonymity must be addressed with any recording of a client's person or voice. Sometimes it is counter-therapeutic to even ask to videotape a client, for example, if the client is paranoid or in an excitable state. Therefore, nurses will determine the best means of documenting interactions to evaluate use of communication techniques. Over time, the process of reflecting on the communication will become easier for the nurse, and techniques of therapeutic communication will become part of the nurse's tools of practice.

NURSING PROCESS

The nursing process is a way of thinking that allows nurses to reflect on nursing care and work in an organized, systematic manner. In recent years, many nurses have criticized the nursing process as unhelpful in providing holistic care (Jones & Brown, 1993). It is important, however, to remember that there are, and have always been, two definitions of the nursing process (Erickson, Tomlin, & Swain, 1983). The first is that the nursing process is a step-by-step, linear process of assessment, diagnosis, outcome identification, planning/interventions, and evaluation. As such, it is a problem-solving technique. The second, more basic definition is that the nursing process is a means of reflecting on the entire process of the nurse-client interaction. In this second definition, one is reminded that *process* means a series of actions leading to an end. If one views nursing as an interactive encounter, the nursing process is the means by which the nurse-client interaction takes place (Frisch, 1994). Experienced nurses know that one never really applies the nursing process in a step-by-step fashion. One does not assess, then diagnose, then devise outcomes, then plan, provide, and evaluate care in that order. One is diagnosing while one is assessing. As soon as a nurse begins an interaction with a client, the nurse is intervening, because the nurse's words, actions, and presence serve as an intervention and are part of nursing care. A nurse is constantly evaluating; one knows that evaluation does not come only at the end of a detailed care plan. As a nurse provides care in the psychiatric mental health setting, it is important to recognize that the nursing process is a complex process—it is more circular than linear—and that the idea of the step-by-step analysis of the nursing process can help one to understand and reflect on the nursing care more than it actually reflects activities as they are experienced in real life. Figure 5-2 presents two views of the nursing process, the linear view and the circular view. The nurse is encouraged to consider the meaning of the nursing process in a setting in which interaction and use of self are the most important nursing tools.

For purposes of learning, it is useful to consider the steps of the nursing process in order and then apply the

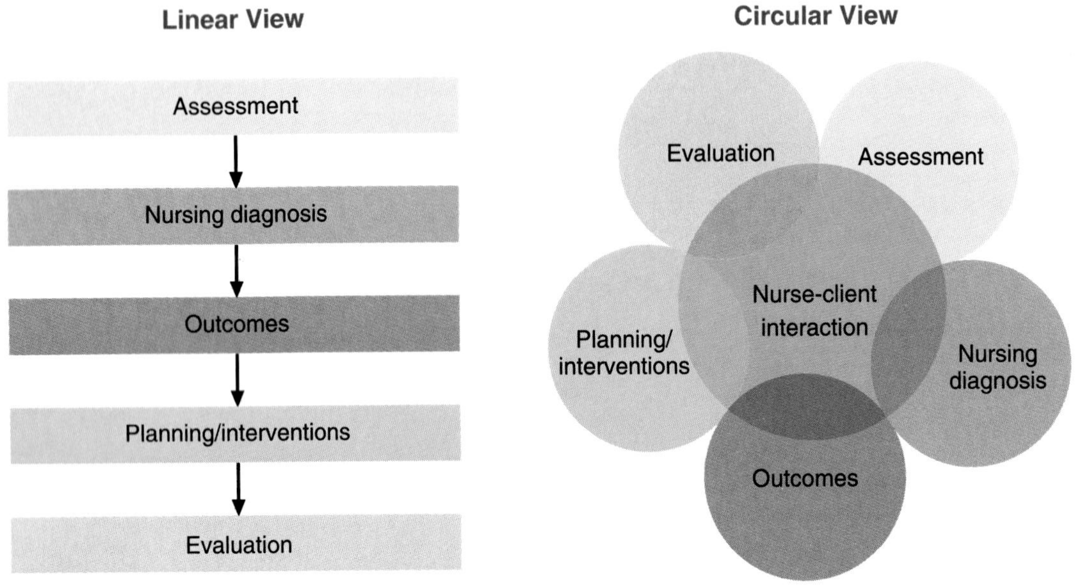

Linear View

Circular View

Figure 5-2   Two Views of the Nursing Process

steps to the psychiatric mental health setting. A discussion on each step follows.

ASSESSMENT

A nurse will always begin by gathering data from the client (and his family/significant others) to develop an understanding of the client's reason(s) for seeking help and to determine the client's specific needs. Assessment in psychiatric nursing begins with knowledge obtained from a basic psychiatric history and a mental status assessment. The purpose of such an initial assessment is to:

1. Document the client's presenting problem and/or the precipitating event (mental health history).

2. Evaluate whether the client is in touch with reality (mental status examination).

3. Determine whether the client is in danger such that he needs protection or whether the client is likely to injure others (critical decisions related to safety).

In many cases the initial evaluation will be done by a psychiatrist, and results of the evaluation will be available to the nurse. The nurse can complete her own assessment, based on a nursing model; that is, the nurse may gather data relevant to a nursing theory or functional health patterns (Gordon, 1994) or on the basis of the human response patterns (NANDA, 1996). Table 5-4 lists the elements contained in a psychiatric history (Mabbett, 1996). While all mental health professionals use data obtained to write DSM diagnoses, the nurse will also use information to identify specific nursing problems that can be written as nursing diagnoses.

NURSING DIAGNOSIS

More often than not, the nurse will obtain data over a period of time. Most clients will not be willing to disclose very personal information to a nurse they do not know. Further, many clients will present in a state of emotional excitement or depression such that they are unable to sit and answer many questions. The nurse must focus on the client's immediate needs, take steps to develop trust, and build a positive nurse-client relationship. Over time and the course of interactions, it will become clear that a client has particular needs that the nurse will be able to address.

Many of the nursing diagnoses in the human response patterns emphasized in psychiatric care cannot be made on the basis of direct observation or objective evidence alone. For example, the nursing diagnosis of *social isolation* cannot be made unless the client provides subjective evidence that he experiences feelings of aloneness imposed by others (NANDA, 1996). Similarly, the nursing diagnosis of *self-esteem disturbance* is made only by assessing that the client has negative feelings about self or self-capabilities (NANDA, 1996). Thus, the nurse must have a rapport with the client to the degree where the client will disclose information about his perceptions and feelings. Further, the nurse can make diagnoses and address these as nursing concerns only after discussion with the client that these are areas the client wishes to pursue with the nurse. When the nurse and client agree that a particular area is a nursing concern, the nurse can make a nursing diagnosis and begin to plan care directed toward the concern. Table 5-5 lists the NANDA diagnoses most frequently seen in psychiatric care.

Table 5-4   Elements of a Psychiatric History

ELEMENT	DESCRIPTION	EXAMPLE
Identifying data	Summarizes the case, including information about previous hospitalizations or treatment and some indication of the current problem.	This is one of numerous psychiatric admissions for this 45-year-old woman, who is readmitted at this time for recurrence of paranoia, auditory hallucinations, and suicidal ideation.
Chief complaint	Describes the client's perception of the current problem.	"The voices are telling me to kill myself and I can't get away from them."
Present illness history	Describes events leading to admission or seeking of psychiatric help.	The client was discharged from hospital 1 month ago. She attended day treatment but took her medication inconsistently. Over the past 3 days, she has become preoccupied with suicide. She states she has recently discovered that her husband is having an affair, and she thinks he wants to leave her. She blames herself for difficulties in her marriage.
Past medical history	Outlines medical conditions, including laboratory or diagnostic data	There are no known medical conditions.
Developmental and psychosocial history	Outlines circumstances that are significant for understanding the current problems. Includes such information as marital status, children, significant relationships, work or school history, relationships with family members, and developmental stage.	Client was the middle child in a family of three children. Her parents had an intact marriage, although there was a great deal of hostility between them. She has flashbacks of her mother and father yelling at each other in the night. She is currently married, with no children. She has completed college, with a liberal arts degree. She is employed part time in a local decorating business.
Mental status examination	Evaluates the client's mental and emotional functioning, including appearance, behavior, and attitude; characteristics of speech; affect and mood; thought content (delusions, illusions, ability to concentrate); orientation (oriented to person, time, place, and self); memory; intellectual level; and suicidal ideations	The client is cooperative with the interviewer. Her mood and affect are depressed and anxious. She became tearful throughout the interview. Her flow of thought is coherent, and her thought content reveals feelings of low self-esteem as well as auditory hallucinations that are self-demeaning. She admits to suicidal ideas but denies having a plan or intent. Her orientation is good. She knows the current date, place, person. Recent and remote memory are good. She shows some insight and judgment regarding her illness and need for help.
Critical Decisions	Assesses client's immediate status and risk factors:	• Is the client suicidal? • Is there a potential for suicide in the near future? • Is the client violent?

Note: *The content of examination for suicide and violence is covered in detail in Chapter 14.*

From *Delmar's Instant Nursing Assessment: Mental Health*, by P. D. Mabbett, 1996, Albany, NY: Delmar Publishers. Adapted with permission.

▽ OUTCOME IDENTIFICATION

For every nursing diagnosis, the nurse must identify specific outcomes that can reasonably be expected as a result of nursing and psychiatric care. Outcomes will be both short term and long term. Outcomes should be clearly stated and be discussed with the client so that the nurse and client have a stated, mutual goal of their work together.

For example, if the initial assessment indicates that the client is feeling depressed, alone, and isolated and that he wishes more interactions with others, the nurse may list the following as a short-term outcome: The client will form a one-on-one relationship with the nurse such

that the client will talk with the nurse for 30 minutes daily. A more long-term outcome might be: The client will build relationships with others in his environment and will interact socially with others at least two times throughout the day by 3 month's time. Further, another longer term goal for this client might be: Within 1 month, the client will interact in a social setting with another person, at least twice per week. With these specific outcomes in mind, the nurse will plan interventions with this client aimed at establishing a nurse-client relationship first and extending that relationship to others by increasing the amount of social interaction the client will have with others in his environment.

Table 5-5 NANDA Diagnoses Frequently Seen in Psychiatric Care

HUMAN RESPONSE PATTERNS	DIAGNOSES
Exchanging	Risk for injury
Communicating	Impaired verbal communication
Relating	Impaired social interaction Social isolation Risk for loneliness Altered role performance Altered parenting Sexual dysfunction Altered family process Altered family process: alcoholism Caregiver role strain
Valuing	Spiritual distress
Choosing	Ineffective individual coping Impaired adjustment Defensive coping Ineffective denial Ineffective family coping Ineffective management of therapeutic regimen Decisional conflict
Moving	Self-care deficit
Perceiving	Body image disturbance Self-esteem disturbance Personal identity disturbance Hopelessness Powerlessness
Knowing	Knowledge deficit Acute confusion Chronic confusion Altered thought processes Impaired memory
Feeling	Dysfunctional grieving Risk for violence: self-directed or directed at others Risk for self-mutilation Post-trauma response Rape trauma syndrome Anxiety Fear

▽ PLANNING/INTERVENTIONS

After the nurse has made nursing diagnoses and identified outcomes of care, the nurse will plan interventions directed at each nursing diagnosis. For example, if the client is admitted to an inpatient unit and the nurse has made the diagnosis of *social isolation*, the nurse will plan interventions to help alleviate the client's feelings of aloneness, planning a certain amount of time to be with

the client one on one and then assisting the client to engage in interaction with another client over a game of cards. The nurse may then support the client in social activity by inviting him to participate in a ward activity with a different client. In these interactions, the nurse is attempting to teach the client a means of becoming socially involved and is meeting the client's affiliation needs so that his feelings of aloneness and isolation can be diminished.

Collaborative Nursing Interventions

In addition to the independent nursing role, psychiatric nurses will participate in a multidisciplinary treatment plan. This is a collaborative nursing role whereby the nurse will collaborate with other health professionals to meet clients' needs (Carpenito, 1995). Two major areas of collaborative care arise in the care of most clients: (1) medication/direct services provided by other professionals such as occupational therapists and (2) services in the community provided by identified volunteer or self-help groups. The nurse has an important collaborative role in each (Figure 5-3).

To administer medications, the nurse must be fully aware of the drugs used, the reasons for their prescription, the dose, and the client's individual response. As in all situations of administering medications, the nurse is fully responsible for the safe administration and the evaluation of the client's response. Chapter 25 provides a detailed description of the major medications used in psychiatric care; the nurse will also need to consult with appropriate drug references for medications, as needed. Managing and evaluating the safe administration of psychotropic drugs and teaching the client and family about the medications ordered are critically important

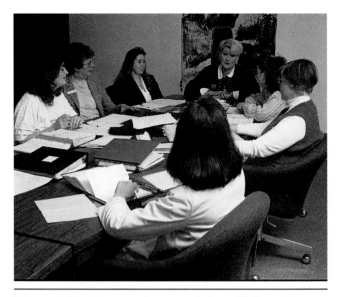

Figure 5-3 Nurses often work in collaborative teams to plan client care.

nursing interventions. Given that a majority of chronic psychiatric clients are readmitted to inpatient units as a result of poor compliance and/or inappropriate knowledge of medications, nurses must consider their role in medication administration of very high priority.

When the individual client is receiving care from another professional, for example an occupational therapist (OT), the nurse has a role to know and understand the goals the OT has for the client's care and to support those goals in her own interaction with the client. Chapter 1 details the roles of various health professionals. It will suffice here to reaffirm that the nurse will support the work of other professionals during their interactions with the client. Lastly, because a nursing goal is to return the client to the community and to help the client achieve a maximum state of health, the nurse will almost always have a role in referring the client to community resources.

Nursing Theory to Guide Interventions

Some nurses still find it difficult to initiate interventions with psychiatric clients. Following guidelines of established nursing theory will help the new nurse feel confident in initiating care. The authors recommend basing interactions on the five aims of intervention described by Erickson, Tomlin, and Swain (1983), listed in the accompanying display. The five aims help one to focus interventions on goals that are universal and appropriate for psychiatric clients. (The Modeling and Role-Modeling Nursing theory is described in detail in Chapter 3.) The nurse may find that she needs additional assessment data to meet the five aims; for example, she may need to know more about the client's strengths. Thus, following the five aims gives the nurse insight as to when additional information is needed and provides goals that nursing interventions can address.

FIVE AIMS OF INTERVENTION

◆ Build trust
◆ Promote positive orientation
◆ Promote perceived control
◆ Promote strengths
◆ Set mutual goals that are health directed

From *Modeling and Role Modeling: A Theory and Paradigm for Nursing*, by H. Erickson, E. Tomlin, and M. Swain, 1983, Englewood Cliffs, NJ: Prentice-Hall.

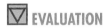 EVALUATION

The final step of the nursing process is to evaluate the outcomes of the nursing actions. As all health care moves to outcome-based evaluations, psychiatric nurses need to demonstrate that their interventions with clients result in positive outcomes. Returning to the example cited previously, consider that the client expresses social isolation, feels aloneness that he perceives to be imposed by others, and tells the nurse this is uncomfortable for him. The nurse plans specific interventions and implements them. The nurse must seek the client's evaluation of his own feelings of social isolation to monitor the degree of success achieved, as every diagnosis and intervention must be clearly evaluated. Further, when all health care must account for outcomes achieved, nurses will need to demonstrate that there is some significance in the outcomes of nursing care. For example, nurses may be asked to explain why it is important for clients to feel engaged with others rather than isolated. While it may appear self-evident that social interactions are positive, nurses will be challenged to explain why and how that is so. Evaluating care, then, means documenting that care had or did not have intended outcomes and demonstrating that the outcomes of care had significant positive effects.

THE NURSE-CLIENT RELATIONSHIP

A nurse-client relationship evolves over time, as do relationships between any two individuals. There is an **orientation phase**—a time for getting to know one another, for establishing trust; a **working phase**—implementing nursing interventions to achieve outcomes; and a **termination phase**—an end to the relationship because the client has achieved independence from the nurse and can maintain health or stability without the nurse's care.

In the orientation phase, the nurse assumes responsibility for initiating and sustaining the relationship. To establish trust, the nurse must demonstrate caring and consistency. The nurse must keep all appointments or promises and will always follow through on any activity she said or implied she would do. Further, the nurse will provide an environment in which the client can feel free to express his feelings and thoughts. The nurse's attitude is accepting and nonjudgmental.

In the working phase, the nurse identifies and implements interventions that facilitate positive changes for the client. The client accepts the nurse's caring and may discuss concerns with the nurse that he has been unable to discuss with others. He listens to the nurse's reactions and, with the nurse's guidance, explores his methods of interaction and coping. He may tentatively try out new ways of responding to situations, and evaluate the effects. The working phase of the relationship can become extremely rewarding, and it is not uncommon for the client to become emotionally attached to the nurse during this time.

The termination phase occurs when the nurse and client evaluate progress and determine that the client is ready to move on, to establish new patterns of interacting without the nurse. Termination is part of a professional relationship, because there is no expectation that the nurse and client will become friends or continue a relationship beyond that period of time when the client needs the nurse's assistance. Successful termination may mark the beginning of other relationships for the client. Peplau referred to this termination phase as a "freeing process," in which the client can let go and move on with other aspects of his life and with other relationships.

CASE EXAMPLE *Mrs. Rose M.*

Rose M. is a 50-year old woman who was married for 27 years. She has one grown son in college. She and her former husband have just obtained a divorce. Her husband has moved out of their home, and Rose now lives alone. Rose has become depressed, finds herself crying often, and lacks energy. She came to a mental health clinic for help and was assigned to nurse Maria.

Maria initiates interactions so to build trust and establish a working relationship with Mrs. RM. On their first encounter, the interactions included the following:

Nurse: I understand that you came here to the clinic because you have been troubled recently. Tell me about your situation.

Rose: I am at the end of my rope. I cry a lot and don't feel that I can function on my own. I feel ugly; I've never been strong, and now I don't know what I will do. This is worse than I've felt before.

Nurse: Tell me about what's happened before and how this is different.

Rose. You don't really want to know all about me. It doesn't matter.

Nurse: I have time to talk with you. I'm interested in exploring how I might assist you. You are upset now. That's why you came in. I am here to listen to you.

During this initial phase, the nurse offers herself to the client, lets the client know she has time and interest to speak with her, and demonstrates patience. Through her nonverbal messages Nurse Maria demonstrates she is attentive and concerned; she looks at Rose, offers herself by leaning toward the client, and waits for the client to respond.

Later, as the relationship between Rose and Nurse Maria evolves, they are in the working phase.

Rose is telling the nurse about experiences within her life that contributed to self-doubt:

Rose: I always had to be independent as a young girl. I never could rely on anyone, but I wanted to.

Nurse: What does that mean to you in terms of your current life?

Rose: If I am divorced, I have to be independent. I have to rely on myself, and I'm not so sure.

Nurse: Not so sure of what?

Rose: Not so sure I can take care of myself.

Nurse: What does it mean to take care of yourself?

In the working phase, the nurse assists Rose to identify feelings and to explore her life. Nurse Maria presents the reality of the situation to Rose. Maria learns that Rose is successfully employed as a secretary, is able to live on her own, but feels emotionally vulnerable. Rose is searching for stability and support. With Maria's referral, Rose joins a women's support group in the community. Rose continues to see Maria for several weeks, as her social supports in the community increase. At this point, Maria and Rose enter into the termination phase:

Nurse: Rose, you seem to have built many supports in the community. How are you feeling about this?

Rose: I am better. I have a friend to call if I am lonely. I have people who will listen to me and care about me.

Nurse: Perhaps now you need only come and see me once a month—to check in. You are quite independent now, compared to when we first met.

Rose: Yes, I think that is good. We can meet the first week of next month; then we'll see what I need.

Nurse: I have enjoyed getting to know you, and I am pleased that you seem happier than you were a few weeks ago.

Maria suggests that Rose may not need the nurse-client relationship on an ongoing basis. By suggesting that Rose come to see her next month, Maria is terminating the relationship over time to prevent any sense of abandonment. Rose's response indicates that she, too, feels that termination is appropriate.

The phases of the nurse-client relationship follow the steps of the nursing process. The orientation phase is also the assessment phase—the time of getting to know each other and gathering information. The working phase begins with establishing goals and setting plans for nursing care. The termination phase comes about during evaluation, when it becomes clear that initial goals are met and there are no further goals that need to be established to continue the work. Table 5-6 illustrates the relationship.

The case example illustrates the phases of the nurse-client relationship.

The nurse must use all of the skills described in this chapter to initiate client care in the psychiatric setting. First, skills of therapeutic communication are needed to establish interactions with client, and good communication skills are necessary to begin the nursing process. The nurse must be able to communicate in a manner that puts the client at ease and gives the client enough comfort to disclose information about self. The nurse-client relationship is based on trust and caring. All communications (verbal and nonverbal) must demonstrate this caring and show that the nurse is trustworthy. New psychiatric nurses find that the best way to begin their work is to approach a client sincerely and begin interactions. With experience, nurses find that positive nurse-client relationships require time and energy; some clients are easier for some nurses to engage than for others. Continual self-exploration helps the nurse assess her own limitations and abilities. The nurse-client relationship helps both nurse and client to grow, to engage, and to learn about self.

KEY CONCEPTS

- ◆ Psychiatric mental health nurses use tools of self and tools of knowledge in their work.

- ◆ Well-developed skills in communication are essential to effective psychiatric nursing care. These include awareness of verbal and nonverbal communication techniques.

- ◆ The nurse should evaluate her own communication skill, identifying therapeutic and nontherapeutic techniques.

- ◆ The nursing process can be viewed in both a linear and a circular fashion as a tool to help nurses evaluate clients, identify appropriate outcomes, and plan and implement effective care.

- ◆ Several NANDA nursing diagnoses are seen frequently in the psychiatric mental health setting and help to identify the nursing role in care.

- ◆ Nursing interventions are grounded in a positive nurse-client relationship and address specific nursing diagnoses.

- ◆ The nurse-client relationship can be viewed as having three phases: orientation, working, and termination.

Table 5-6 Relationship of the Nursing Process with the Phases of the Nurse-Client Relationship

STEPS OF THE NURSING PROCESS	PHASES OF THE NURSE-CLIENT RELATIONSHIP
Assessment	Orientation phase
Diagnosis	
Outcome identification	Working phase
Planning/interventions	
Evaluation	Termination phase

REVIEW QUESTIONS AND ACTIVITIES

1. Identify ways that you can approach a client with the intention of establishing a positive nurse-client relationship.

2. Describe nonverbal interactions between yourself and another over a 5 minute period (or between two other persons you can observe).

3. Complete a process recording.

4. Explain the value of the nursing process in understanding client needs.

5. Use the NANDA diagnostic categories for a psychiatric mental health client; identify the independent nursing role and the collaborative nursing role.

6. Identify the phases of the nurse-client relationship as you initiate interaction with clients, as you enter the working phases, and as you plan for termination.

REFERENCES

Carpenito, L. J. (1995). *Nursing diagnosis: A handbook for practice*. Philadelphia: Lippincott.

Erickson, H., Tomlin, E., & Swain, M. (1983). *Modeling and role-modeling: A theory and paradigm for nursing*. Englewood Cliffs, NJ: Prentice Hall.

Frisch, N. (1994). The nursing process revisited. *Nursing Diagnosis, 5*, 51.

Gordon, M. (1994). *Nursing diagnosis: Process and application*. St. Louis: Mosby.

Hall, E. (1959). *The silent language*. New York: Doubleday.

Jones, S., & Brown, L. N. (1993). Alternative view on defining critical thinking through the nursing process. *Holistic Nursing Practice, 7*, 71–75.

Mabbett, P. D. (1996). *Instant nursing assessment: Mental health*. Albany, NY: Delmar.

North American Nursing Diagnosis Association (NANDA). (1996). *Nursing diagnoses: Definitions and classification 1997–1998*. Philadelphia: Author.

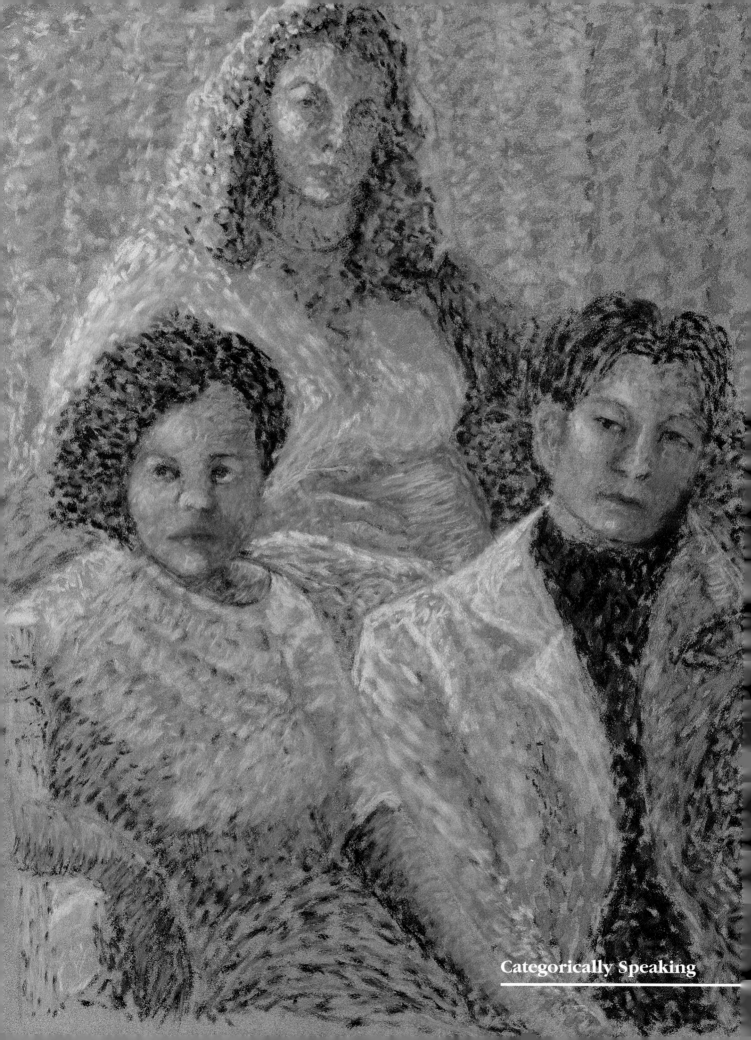

Chapter

6

CULTURAL AND ETHNIC CONSIDERATIONS

Jane Kelley

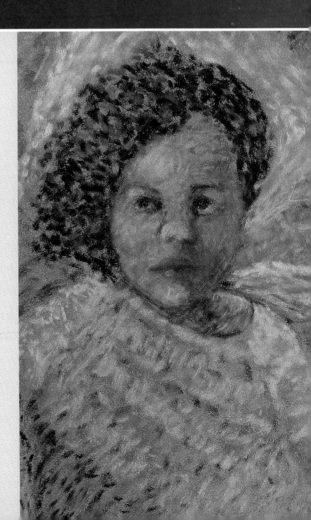

Know Your Own Culture

To understand the culture of others, what do I have to know about myself? We can see the culture of others because of the different behaviors, customs, and beliefs. But we do not see our own culture unless we learn about it. Why? Because we experience our own culture as the way things *really are*. Our reality is an exotic *other culture* to others! So, what must you know about yourself to provide skillful care to persons of different cultures? You must examine those aspects of your own behaviors, customs, and beliefs that are drawn from your culture: "Such self-knowledge is critical to realizing which cultures or groups one tends to favor or avoid and which groups one negatively or unrealistically . . . stereotypes" (Andrews & Boyle, 1995, p. 271). Think about your own culture as you study this chapter.

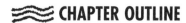 **CHAPTER OUTLINE**

CULTURE DEFINED

CULTURAL SENSITIVITY

Beliefs about Mental Illness and Care
  Normal Versus Abnormal Behavior
  Care Seeking and Acceptable Care

Interpersonal Interaction

Verbal and Nonverbal Communication
  Eye Contact
  Proxemics
  Touch
  Silence
  Social Behavior
  Time Orientation

Diet and Food Habits

Biological Variation

THE CULTURALLY COMPETENT MENTAL HEALTH NURSE

COMPETENCIES

Upon completion of this chapter, the reader should be able to:

1. Define *culture* as it applies to psychiatric mental health nursing.

2. Discuss the importance of understanding cultural variation when planning and implementing care.

3. Recognize, when caring for clients, ways in which clients may vary in their beliefs about the health care system and their attitudes about seeking appropriate care, especially mental health care.

4. Analyze verbal and nonverbal communication factors that affect transcultural interactions between nurse and client.

5. Describe the effect of cultural and ethnic variation on therapeutic management of psychiatric mental health care, including pharmacologic and behavioral elements.

KEY TERMS

Cultural Blindness Attempt to treat all persons fairly by ignoring differences and acting as though differences do not exist; misguided attempt to achieve "fairness" by ignoring real cultural differences.

Cultural Facilitator/Broker Person who can interpret the language, culture, and health care culture of another as a means to bridging the communication barriers between people from different cultures.

Culture The complex whole, which includes knowledge, belief, art, morals, law, custom, and any other capabilities and habits acquired by a person as a member of society (Tylor, 1871).

Culture Shock State in which a person is overwhelmed or even immobilized by cultural differences in expectations, communication, and general habits between an individual's culture of origin and a new culture to which the individual is trying to assimilate.

Ethnicity Identification with a socially, culturally, and politically constructed group that holds a common set of characteristics not shared by others with whom its members come in contact (Lipson, 1996b).

Ethnocentrism Perception that one's worldview is the only acceptable truth and that the beliefs, values, and behaviors sanctioned by one's culture are superior to those sanctioned by all others.

Norms Learned behaviors that are perceived to be appropriate or inappropriate in a culture.

Stereotyping Assumption that people sharing certain characteristics will think and act similarly.

Values Learned beliefs about what is held to be good or bad in a culture.

The role of culture in mental health is difficult to isolate because every human lives within a cultural context. However, our beliefs and behaviors and the way we communicate these interpersonally are culturally based. The variation among cultures can create misunderstandings and misinterpretation of behaviors and communications when interacting individuals are unfamiliar with each other's culture. The purpose of this chapter is to identify the components of culture that can affect the therapeutic relationship and to determine how psychiatric mental health nurses can incorporate this knowledge to provide culturally competent care.

Interpersonal relationships, verbal and nonverbal communication, value orientations, religion, social systems, diet, and health and illness-related beliefs are all culturally based and directly or indirectly affect psychiatric mental health care. Given that culture affects our thoughts and behaviors to such a pervasive extent, it can be concluded that nurses who deal with peoples' thoughts and/or behaviors must understand the role of culture.

Culture and its expression through group and individual norms, values, and behaviors must be understood and used to assess client status and to plan and implement appropriate care. The primary tool of the psychiatric mental health nurse is interpersonal communication. Because culture is intrinsic to communication, and because interpersonal communication is an interaction of two cultures (client's and nurse's), it is essential that the nurse understand how culture affects verbal and nonverbal communication and how to modify communication skills to appropriately interact with a variety of clients.

CULTURE DEFINED

Culture has been defined in many different ways but is still not well understood. One classic and comprehensive definition is that of Tylor (1871), which describes culture as the complex whole, including knowledge, belief, art, morals, law, custom, and any other capabilities and habits acquired by man as a member of society. Culture comprises every verbal or behavioral system that transmits meaning. Culture is learned, shared, and ever-changing. It is learned through socialization, shared by all group members, and associated with adaptation to the environment.

The traditional definition of culture describes it to be static or near static. Agar (1994) has proposed a different definition that incorporates the ever-changing, dynamic nature of culture. He proposes that culture is malleable like clay, and any interaction by persons from different cultures modifies the cultures of both participants.

For Agar, culture serves as an ever-changing frame for interpreting information and understanding how the world works. Agreeing with Hermans, Kempen, and Van

Loon (1992), Agar sees the self as "dialogical," a product of all past stories and multicultural experiences, producing multiple identities interacting within the same individual. In this view, psychological processes are influenced by and develop from this dynamic interaction of culture and history. Therefore, in Agar's view, one cannot talk about a person's culture as though it can be shared by all members of a group and transmitted as a whole from one generation to the next, as is implied in more traditional definitions of culture.

Culture, itself, is universal in that humans cannot exist apart from culture. In this traditional view of culture, the culture defines **values** (learned beliefs about what is held to be good or bad in a culture) and **norms** (learned behaviors that are perceived to be appropriate or inappropriate in a culture). Therefore, in a given society, culture defines the roles, relationships, rights, and obligations of its members. It is through the lens of culture that profound questions of existence and being are addressed, such as the essence of human nature, the purpose of human existence, and the relationship of humans to each other, to nature, and to the divine or eternal. The worldview is drawn from and reflects the total integration of the group's beliefs and practices, flowing from the culture.

The worldview that each of us forms based on our own culture becomes for us reality. Unless we have come to recognize that many cultures have different worldviews, we are often not aware that other people might have a different perception about what is right and true. This perception that our worldview is the only acceptable truth and that our beliefs, values, and sanctioned behaviors are superior to all others is called **ethnocentrism**.

Many individuals are aware that other cultures exist and that they have different beliefs, values, and accepted behaviors. However, many persons do not understand that great variation exists within any cultural group. When this variation is not recognized, individuals tend to **stereotype** all members of the particular culture, expecting the group members to hold the same beliefs and behave the same way.

CULTURAL SENSITIVITY

Much has been written on the need for nurses to become skilled at incorporating transcultural concepts into nursing care. Campinha-Bacote (1994) has proposed a conceptual model for developing cultural competence in psychiatric mental health nurses. She describes four elements as being essential to cultural competence: (1) cultural awareness, (2) cultural knowledge, (3) cultural skill, and (4) cultural encounter (see Figure 6-1).

Cultural assessment assumes that the nurse adopts a cultural perspective for providing nursing care. Such a cultural perspective includes three interacting viewpoints: objective, subjective, and contextual (Lipson, 1996a). The

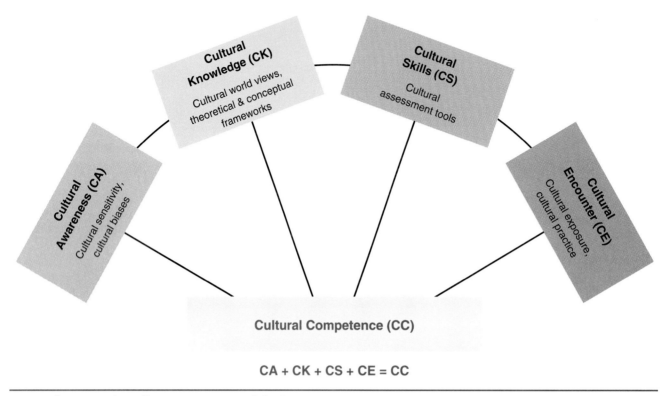

Figure 6-1 A Culturally Competent Model of Care. *From Campinha-Bacote, "Cultural Competence in Psychiatric Mental Health Nursing: A Conceptual Model," Philadelphia, W.B. Saunders Company, 1994. Printed with permission from Transcultural C.A.R.E. Associates and W. B. Saunders Company.*

context referred to is the context of the cross-cultural encounter, which includes the broader cultural, socioeconomic, and political influences operating within the health care system and affecting the client and nurse. Objective components include the client's, family's, nurse's, and community's cultural and social characteristics, communication patterns, and worldviews. The subjective components are the nurse's personal and cultural characteristics and cultural self-awareness.

Cultural assessment can only be accomplished skillfully when the nurse has acquired sufficient knowledge of his or her own and a variety of other cultures to avoid

⊙⊙ *REFLECTIVE THINKING*

Cultural Identity

Consider the dominant culture in which you live. What are the values and beliefs (i.e., time, money, family, honesty, productivity, wisdom, and the like) that seem most important in this culture? Which of these values do you most closely espouse? If your values come into conflict with those of the dominant culture or with the value system enforced by the institution where you work, how do you decide which set of values to follow?

stereotyping and ethnocentrism. Leininger (1978, 1991) urges nurses to avoid seeing all individuals as being alike and to adopt a broad, open, objective attitude toward cultural variation and toward individuals from the various cultural groups. Another behavior to avoid is **cultural blindness**, which is the attempt to treat all persons fairly by ignoring differences and acting as though the differences do not exist. Such cultural blindness can be perceived as insensitivity just as readily as are stereotyping and ethnocentrism.

Cultural assessment in any health care setting must address the many sources of within-group variation that result from influences other than culture. First, cultural assessment usually includes elements often identified as racial, based on biological differences such as disease susceptibility and genetic variation. (Incidentally, studies of biological variation show no clustering of characteristics that would support a biological basis for race.) Cultural assessment includes variation resulting from **ethnicity**, which is identification with a "socially, culturally, and politically constructed group of individuals that holds a common set of characteristics not shared by others with whom its members come in contact" (Lipson, 1996b, p. 8). Such characteristics as common ancestry, sense of historical continuity, common language, religion, and intergroup interaction are elements of ethnicity. These characteristics may not be shared by any but one subgroup of a larger cultural group.

Other cultural assessment components not directly related to culture are socioeconomic status and social class. Circumstances of minority status or recent immigration may be thought to be inseparable from low socioeconomic status and social class, but much variation can be found within any cultural or ethnic group. However, a challenge for the nurse undertaking a cultural assessment is separating the effects of these four influences on health and health care. Often, the effect of low socioeconomic status on health and seeking care is greater than that of other cultural or ethnic influences (Williams & Collins, 1995). Careful assessment will seek to distinguish between cultural and socioeconomic influences or the interactions of the two. It is important to note that most cultural or ethnic groups within the United States have some members who are in high socioeconomic categories and high social class. The nurse must recognize that variation within cultural groups may be great.

Several approaches to cultural assessment have been developed by and for nurses. A tool by Giger and Davidhizar (1991) addresses six cultural variables having an effect on health and illness behaviors: (1) communication, (2) space, (3) social organization, (4) time, (5) environmental control, and (6) biological variations.

Andrews and Boyle (1995) provide a comprehensive guide for transcultural nurses to assess cultural manifestations relevant to nursing. Categories to be assessed include (1) value orientations, (2) interpersonal relationships, (3) communication, (4) religion and magic, (5) social systems, (6) diet and food habits, and (7) health and illness belief systems. The importance of these two sets of cultural variants to psychiatric mental health nursing will be examined. For purposes of this chapter, categories to be assessed and around which culturally sensitive mental health care can be planned will include (1) beliefs about mental illness and related care, (2) interpersonal interaction, (3) verbal and nonverbal communication, (4) diet and food habits, and (5) biological variation.

Beliefs about Mental Illness and Care

Health and illness states are not universally perceived. Culture defines what is considered to be normal or abnormal with regard to physical and psychological health: "It is culture not nature that defines disease, although it is usually culture and nature which foster disease" (Hughes, 1978, p. 153).

Many variations in culturally based beliefs and behaviors affect care, specifically care for clients with mental aberrations. Beliefs about causation of illness or disease vary greatly across cultures. There is a close integration of these beliefs with other institutions of the society, such as religious and social structures (Hughes, 1978). In less industrialized societies, and to some extent in fully industrialized societies, these beliefs about causation fall into

five basic categories: (1) sorcery, (2) breach of taboo, (3) intrusion of a disease object, (4) intrusion of a disease-causing spirit, or (5) loss of soul (Clements, 1932, as discussed in Hughes, 1978). Usually the major belief pattern in a society will emphasize one or more of the categories. For instance, Eskimos emphasize soul loss or breach of taboo as causes of illness, while many African groups attribute disease to sorcerers or witches. The ancient Greeks emphasized the role of interaction with others and the environment. They attributed illness more to a disharmony in the relationship with the universe. The Native American belief system is more aligned with the Greek belief in that illness is believed to result more from moral transgression (thought or action) against the norms of society, creating an imbalance in mind, body, spirit, and environment (Hughes, 1978).

If the client's belief system differs from that of the usual Western psychomedical beliefs, then the effect of the type of treatment and its method of delivery must be considered before interventions can be determined. Otherwise there may be no therapeutic effect or the intervention could actually produce harm for the client or for the client's family.

To provide culturally safe and effective care, the nurse needs to understand the potential variations in the who, what, and when of care seeking. In a given cultural group, and specifically for a particular client, the nurse needs to determine:

1. What behaviors, feelings, or states would be considered abnormal, depending on subgroup (age, gender, or other designation).

2. At what point or in what circumstances the individual would seek care and from whom care would be sought.

3. What care or treatment would be acceptable.

Normal Versus Abnormal Behavior

One behavior often cited as an example of cultural variation in the perception of normal versus abnormal behavior is *pibloktog*, seen in Eskimo women. Also called "Arctic hysteria," under certain circumstances the women exhibit unrestrained, bizarre behavior such as running naked through the snow. The condition is not considered to represent abnormal behavior in the Eskimo culture (Parker, 1977).

Even in cultures as closely related as the American Anglo culture and the British culture of England, what is considered normal and abnormal behavior differs. The behaviors that lead to the diagnoses of depression and anxiety differ enough for an American who is vivacious, talkative, and energetic to be diagnosed as anxious or manic in England and for an English man or woman who is only slightly more reserved in demeanor than is average to be diagnosed as depressed in the United States (Dasen, Berry, & Sartorius, 1988).

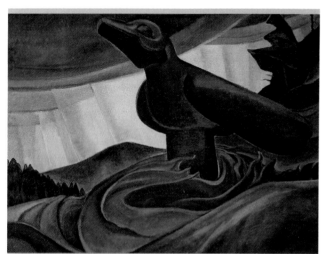

Big Raven by Emily Carr
Courtesy: Vancouver Art Gallery; photo: T. Mills. VAG #42.311

This well-loved Canadian painter returned throughout her long life to paintings and carvings of the Northwest Indian villages. Of this painting she wrote: "Here I wanted to paint not so much . . . what they looked like as what they felt like." It is unlikely that Carr ever saw totems of this monumental size, but the Raven's spiritual power—and that of the culture that created him—stirred the painter's imagination. The painting is a powerful depiction of a culture's physical and psycho/spiritual environment as seen through the sympathetic eyes of an outsider.

Care Seeking and Acceptable Care

As noted in the following chapter on epidemiology of mental illness, even within the dominant cultures of the United States, there is variation in care seeking for mental illness. Often, immigrant and minority individuals seek mental health care only or initially from a traditional practitioner such as a Medicine Man, herbalist, curandero or santero, Voodoo priest, or other traditional healer. Sue and Sue (1990) reported studies that found that Native Americans, Asian Americans, African Americans, and Hispanics use mental health services substantially less or terminate therapy after only one contact at a rate much higher than European Americans. Reasons for the differences are thought to be: few minority professionals; a one-to-one counseling style in the counselor's office; an emphasis on social-emotional needs rather than on vocational and educational needs; and the verbal focus, which is difficult for those with nonstandard English or an accent. Other suggested barriers include:

1. Monocultural assumptions of mental health
2. Negative stereotypes of pathology for minority lifestyles

3. Ineffective, inappropriate, and antagonistic counseling approaches to the values held by minorities

Another example of cultural beliefs producing a barrier to professional care seeking for mental illness is described by Ho (1987). Ho noted that a central Asian belief is that "the best healing source lies within the family" and seeking help from outside (like counseling and therapy) is nonproductive and against dictates of Asian philosophy. Since balance is the Asian ideal, and mental as well as physical illness is thought to be associated with imbalance, traditional healers and Chinese medicine would be the care options of choice to many Asians: "The Chinese have characteristic ways of dealing with mental illness in the family, starting with a protracted period of intrafamilial coping with even serious psychiatric illness, followed by recourse to friends, elders, and neighbors in the community, consultation with traditional specialists, religious healers, or general physicians, and finally, treatment from Western specialists" (Andrews & Boyle, 1995).

Other ethnic groups within the United States seek folk or popular health care systems before entering the Western, institutionalized system. Many do so out of contrasting beliefs about cause of illness. Others do so because they are intimidated by the impersonal and technological environment, lengthy history taking, and invasive diagnostic procedures. Traditional, alternative, or complementary health care techniques are also rapidly increasing in popularity among members of the educated mainstream United States culture.

The role of spirituality and religion cannot be omitted from a discussion of mental illness and care. Modern psychology and psychiatry have developed mostly in Western cultural settings, and, therefore, many of the concepts and ideas for achieving psychological health are based on Western culture and theology. However, beliefs about the role of psychic forces in mental status have a cultural and theological basis. Because spiritual concerns are deeply entwined with self-perception and perception of the world around us, the nurse providing care must understand the client's beliefs with regard to self, others, and God or a transcendent being and how these beliefs may affect care. As noted by Andrews and Boyle (1995), "use of psychiatric resources is discouraged by professionals' intolerance for magical and religious orientations and practices, which is common when science and systems of symbolic beliefs and faith compete."

Interpersonal Interaction

Culture is an important variable to be incorporated into therapeutic interpersonal interactions. In addition to verbal and nonverbal communication, to be discussed in the next section, other components of interpersonal interaction vary across cultures and affect personal relationships, therapeutic relationships, and care for psychiatric mental health clients. Examples of cultural values that may be reflected in interpersonal interaction include (1) acceptance of inequality of status and power among its members, (2) acceptance of collectivism versus individualism, (3) favoring of masculine versus feminine cultural traits, and (4) the level of need to avoid uncertainty (Pedersen & Ivey, 1993).

Differences in these cultural values relative to interpersonal interaction can affect care. For instance, persons from cultures that accept inequality of status and power among its members may expect different levels of care for more or less powerful persons, and they may specify decision makers among family or group members who will need to be consulted. Persons from collectivist cultures will determine the individual to be less important than the group, and dependent or self-sacrificing behaviors must be interpreted within the cultural belief system. In group-oriented societies, the concept of self is not well defined; self-actualization as a goal or psychoanalysis as a therapy would not be acceptable in such a cultural setting. Persons from cultures valuing masculine traits will focus on achievements, assertiveness, competitiveness, and toughness, and social gender roles will be distinctly separated. Such persons will be less likely to seek health care, especially mental health care, because of its association with weakness.

Pedersen and Ivey (1993) noted that within a given culture, certain behaviors are interpreted to communicate attributes, such as being friendly, unfriendly, trusting,

---

★ NURSING TIP

Storytelling

Could storytelling be used as a way of bridging the cultural gap for persons from cultures in which self-disclosure is not acceptable or is not valued? Narayan (1991), in a chapter entitled "According to Their Feelings: Teaching and Healing with Stories," tells of the use of folklore stories to heal, to decrease pain, or to increase endurance. These stories are well-known folklore transformed to meet the needs of the occasion. He describes the use of symbols and symbolic meaning in Hindu, Oriental, Islamic, and Amerindian stories. Perhaps sharing the story with input from the client may elicit feelings and provide understanding without the client having to directly reveal personal details or emotions. (Read Narayan in Witherell and Noddings, 1991, *Stories Lives Tell: Narrative and Dialogue in Education*, pp. 113–135.)

---

mistrustful, interested, or bored. However, the associated behaviors that clearly communicate given attributes will differ across cultures. When people of two quite different cultures interact, the behaviors exhibited may not be the behaviors expected in each other's culture to convey the attribute. For instance, in one culture, interest is conveyed by direct eye contact, while in another culture, no eye contact is interpreted to indicate interest and direct eye contact may indicate boredom (Pedersen & Ivey, 1993).

Because we tend to assume that others are similar to us, differences such as these can result in enormous communication barriers. People from outside a cultural group may not know the cultural rules of that group. It is easy to see where a client and nurse or counselor from different cultures may misunderstand each other. One may be restrained and formal, the other animated. One may be soft-spoken, the other loud. One may internalize stress, the other externalize it. In each case, the person is likely behaving in a manner appropriate to his or her culture but may be conveying a very different meaning because the behaviors do not meet the expectations of the other's culture.

It is important for a nurse to communicate effectively with a client; to do so, the nurse must be able to interpret the meaning of more than the words used. The nurse must be conscious of the patterns, expectations, meanings of behaviors, and the likely barriers to communication: "When two culturally different parties misattribute each other's behavior, this misattribution is likely to result in a negative chain reaction of escalating hostility" (Pedersen & Ivey, 1993).

Verbal and Nonverbal Communication

When the client and nurse do not speak the same language, a potentially challenging communication barrier must be overcome. As can be surmised from the discussion preceding and from the discussion to follow about nonverbal communication, more than mere words must be interpreted if effective communication is to occur. It is for this reason that persons designated as "translators" or "interpreters" must know more of the culture than just the oral or written language to adequately meet the need in a health care setting. A **cultural facilitator** or **broker**, who can interpret the language, the client's culture, and the health care culture, is the ideal person to serve as interpreter (Jezewski, 1993). If such a person is unavailable and a language interpreter must be used, then certain criteria should be considered. Avoid selecting an interpreter from a rival faction or group; from a sex, age, or socioeconomic group that would prevent open communication; or from among family members when status would affect disclosure. When using an interpreter, the nurse should speak in his or her own language directly to the client, not to the interpreter. This direct approach conveys much more than just the content of the words.

If no interpreter is available even for word translation, then approach the client in a calm, friendly manner using pantomime as necessary and construct a picture board to which the client can point to communicate basic needs until an interpreter can be found. One source of interpreters is the telephone companies. Some telephone companies, such as AT&T, offer immediate interpreting services.

Communication is the primary tool of psychiatric mental health nursing. In order to understand the client's situation as the client does, the nurse needs to be able to understand the meaning of the words used and the implication of the behaviors demonstrated or described by the client. Mutually understandable communication between nurse and client will facilitate a working, collaborative relationship.

There are many components of communication that may serve as barriers to conveying the message intended by the sender. Nurses must recognize the areas of verbal and nonverbal communication that can serve as barriers and use this knowledge to facilitate understanding. Andrews and Boyle (1995) divide nonverbal components of communication into four categories: vocal cues (pitch, tone, and quality of voice); action cues (posture, facial expression, and gestures); object cues (clothing, jewelry, and hair style); and care of belongings and use of personal and territorial space and touch. In addition to oral and written language, the relevance of tone of voice, eye contact, facial expressions, use of gestures, use of silence, proxemics (touch and comfortable distance), courteous social behavior, dress, and associated gender differences will be discussed as areas of potential miscommunication.

An example of variation in the cultural norm for tone of voice is described by Thiederman (1991, video). A Middle Eastern mother and baby were passengers on an airplane. The mother approached Dr. Thiederman and said, "Give me your newspaper." The woman's voice was relatively harsh, forceful, and to the point, not asking "please" or "may I." As an American raised in the predominant culture of the American middle class, Dr. Thiederman's first reaction was negative and resentful. But as a consultant for cultural variation, Dr. Thiederman recognized that the Middle Eastern woman was using the polite and normal requesting style of her culture. Had the woman asked in the American style of "Could you let me have your newspaper, please?" it would have sounded to her as if she were saying, "Would it be possible for you to graciously let me have your newspaper, please?" This would sound overly solicitous to our ears, just as our courteous request would sound overly solicitous to a Middle Easterner.

Eye Contact

Eye contact has many implications in different cultures and is probably the most variable of the nonverbal communicators. Whether or not to maintain direct eye contact, with whom, and for how long are all variables to consider. Gender differences are also to be considered, because eye contact is tied to expression of modesty and intimacy. Persons from certain Middle Eastern, Asian, Native American, and Appalachian backgrounds consider direct eye contact to be impolite or aggressive, and Hispanic Americans may use downcast eyes to indicate appropriate deference and respect toward others based on age, sex, social position, economic status, or position of authority (Andrews & Boyle, 1995). As clients, these individuals may avert their eyes when talking, but in their cultures, such behavior indicates paying close, respectful attention to what is being said. Often African Americans will avert their eyes when being spoken to but use direct eye contact when speaking, and some use eye rolling when asked a question that is perceived to be ridiculous (Andrews & Boyle, 1995). This pattern is perceived by European Americans to represent inattention or disrespect. The effect of differences in rank or gender may result in reluctance to maintain direct eye contact or to interpret the nurse's eye contact pattern to be insulting or disrespectful. If the nurse maintains the level of direct eye contact considered professionally therapeutic in American nursing, the client may interpret the behavior to be sexual in nature. In many cultures, the only women who smile at men in a public place are prostitutes (Andrews & Boyle, 1995).

Proxemics

Proxemics, or how close we stand to another individual for social or professional conversation and what is considered to be culturally appropriate regarding touch, varies greatly across cultures. Social events that include guests from a variety of cultures are often used to illustrate social distance. When European Americans and persons of Arabic, European, or Hispanic origin begin a conversation, the American tends to take a step back, the person from the other culture moves closer, the American moves back, the other moves closer, and on and on, until the American is against the wall! In international circles, this has been referred to as the "cocktail party two step."

Touch

Touch is such an important part of the therapeutic role of the nurse, in providing hands-on care, in healing through therapeutic or healing touch, and in conveying comfort. Extreme care must be exercised when using touch with persons from different cultures. For instance, whether or not to touch a baby has major implications. Touching or examining a baby's head requires parental permission or should not be done at all in some Southeast Asian cultures. Eighty percent of the world's Hispanic population believes in *mal ojo*, whereby a child is thought to become ill if given excessive admiration by another person (Andrews & Boyle, 1995). However, there is even variation within cultures. In some parts of Mexico, looking at and admiring a child without touching is considered to be the source of illness; in other parts of Mexico, touching itself if done by a stranger is considered to be the source of illness. And then there is touch between adults. Physical touch by health care professionals is acceptable only between clients and professionals of the same sex in some Islamic and Hispanic societies. Even within middle-class American society, some individuals (caregivers or clients) are uncomfortable with touching or being touched by another. It may be necessary to discuss expectations of touch with a client to prevent misunderstanding and miscommunication.

Silence

Silence is both a nonverbal behavior and a component of the qualities of verbal expression patterns. In both senses, the use of silence varies across cultures. Trompenaars (1993/1994) contrasted speech patterns of European Americans, Hispanic Americans, and Asian Americans and described the discomfort of each group with the alternate patterns of the other two. In a conversation between two European Americans, when one stops speaking, the other starts. Among Hispanic Americans, there is overlap so that before one is finished, the other person begins. Among Asian Americans, when one stops speaking, the other waits in silence for a few moments before beginning to speak. These patterns are characteristic of polite, interested conversation in the respective cultures. If a European American interrupts or

REFLECTIVE THINKING

Use of Silence

Have you ever been caring for a client from a cultural background different from your own and experienced awkwardness with the use of silence? In the dominant American culture, silence is often viewed as uncomfortable, and you may feel an urge to jump in and fill the silence. As a nurse, you must remember that silence can be a very valuable therapeutic tool when used to allow a client to gather thoughts, reflect on statements or situations, or check emotions.

remains silent when the other person stops speaking, it usually indicates rudeness or disinterest or some other undesirable intent. If a Hispanic American either does not enthusiastically jump in with comments before the other person finishes or remains silent, disinterest or distrust is being conveyed. The Asian American remains silent in order to allow processing of the comments and to formulate a thoughtful, respectful reply.

Other uses of silence also convey meaning. For instance, silence may convey respect for privacy among English and Arabs; a sign of agreement among French, Spanish, and Russians; or a sense of absurdity if asked what is perceived to be a ridiculous or senseless question (Andrews & Boyle, 1995). But silence used in a manner not considered positive in the respective culture produces discomfort or other negative feelings.

Social Behavior

Behavior is culturally based. The level of formality in human relationships varies markedly, from the informality of American social interaction, wherein people of different age groups and economic or social positions often call each other by first name, to the formality of Asian cultures, wherein a rigid system exists for interactions between people of different ages or ranks. Accepted methods for greeting each other are defined by the culture as well. In Latino cultures and some European cultures, kissing on both cheeks is expected for females who know each other

NURSING TIP

Cultural Awareness

Analyze a conversation with another person, preferably one from a culture different than your own, and list the similarities and differences in your approaches to silence, time, proxemics, body language, and eye contact.

and, often, for males who know each other, and hugs between same-sex friends or colleagues are expected. Handshaking is the norm and may accompany cheek kisses in some cultures. Who offers a hand first and to whom also varies among cultures.

Time Orientation

Orientation to time is another cultural factor that influences interpersonal behavior. There are two aspects of time orientation that can affect psychiatric mental health care: (1) emphasis on past, present, or future time orientation and (2) organization of activities either sequentially or synchronically.

In cultures emphasizing the present, for instance, keeping appointments may be a low priority. Whatever is going on in the present is perceived to be of greater importance than a future good, so if one is involved in something pleasing or important, then the appointment will be dealt with later. Delaying gratification is not perceived to be of great benefit because future outcome is not the focus. In some cultures, such as American and Northern European ones, time is perceived to move in a straight line. In other cultures, time is often perceived to be moving in a circle, with the past and present mixed together with future possibilities (Trompenaars, 1993/1994).

The expected way of organizing activities varies across cultures and can produce miscommunication. Sequentially organized persons complete a task before moving to the next one. Synchronically organized persons can skillfully carry out two or more tasks at the same time. Trompenaars (1993/1994) describes this difference and the misunderstanding that can result. An example describes major misunderstanding resulting from a Korean man entering an office when his American colleague is talking on the telephone. Having just arrived in America, the Korean expects the American to be able to continue the conversation while eagerly welcoming him. Instead, the American barely acknowledges his entrance until ending the telephone conversation, at which time he enthusiastically greets the Korean. But the greeting is perceived to be too late and, therefore, insincere.

Sequential people tend to be punctual and keep to an agenda, characteristics less common among synchronous people. Again, several other cultural values compete with punctuality. Obviously, sequentiality and synchronicity are associated with the different time orientations of past, present, or future.

Diet and Food Habits

There is much variation in diet and food habits across cultures. These differences are readily noted in the many ethnic cookbooks at bookstores. Many variations exist even in the United States. New England food differs from Southern food, and both differ from California cuisine. But of greatest importance to psychiatric care is the interaction of certain foods with medications or mood. More detail is provided on these variations in the chapters where conditions and medications are discussed.

Biological Variation

Biological variation is important to consider for psychiatric mental health care because certain physical and genetic characteristics affect the epidemiology of diseases and the effects of medications. The epidemiology of psychiatric conditions is discussed in another chapter. A brief overview of ethnopharmacology is included here.

The effects of genetic, environmental, and behavioral differences across cultural groups must be considered when administering medications. Differences in pharmacokinetic and pharmacodynamic properties of medications have been compared for individuals of Asian, African, Hispanic, Native American, and European descents. Important findings suggest that Asian Americans are slow metabolizers as compared to African Americans and European Americans (reviewed in Andrews & Boyle, 1995). The basis for this finding may be the association between smoking, drinking alcohol, and increased drug metabolism (evident in African Americans and European Americans) and between a low-protein, high-carbohydrate diet and slow metabolism (characteristic of Asian Americans).

The misdiagnosis and overmedication of African Americans for psychosis is thought to be associated with cultural behaviors that are diagnosed as abnormally violent by non–African American caregivers (Andrews & Boyle, 1995). Further, as noted by Lin (1986), "Asians, especially Chinese, require significantly smaller doses of neuroleptics, tricyclic antidepressants (TCAs), and lithium than do whites, sometimes one-half the dose. Similar dif-

---

✴ NURSING TIP

Time Orientation

In the mainstream American culture, time is a very valued commodity (after all, "time equals money!"). When caring for clients of different cultural backgrounds, be sensitive to the fact that they may well place a different value on time than what you are accustomed to. If a client is late for an appointment or seems to want to spend more time discussing a certain topic than you feel is warranted, be careful not to jump to the conclusion that the client is lazy or disrespectful of your time. Instead, take a moment to step back from the situation and ask yourself what value this client might place on time and consider how you might meet the client's needs as well as your own.

ferences have been reported between Indian or Pakistani clients and white clients" (Andrews & Boyle, 1995). Because of these metabolic and behavioral differences, care should be taken to base medication dosages on serum levels and culturally relevant clinical observations rather than on culturally biased norms.

THE CULTURALLY COMPETENT MENTAL HEALTH NURSE

When a client enters a mental health facility, the culturally competent nurse will have some knowledge of the central beliefs and behaviors of the client's culture of origin. The nurse will verify the client's level of integration and identification with that culture and with the dominant culture of the society where care is being given. The nurse will be aware of similarities and differences among the dominant culture, the client's culture, and the nurse's culture; will assess areas that may produce miscommunication or conflict; will discuss these areas with the client; and will work with the client to plan culturally sensitive care.

If the client has only recently arrived in the country or entered a cultural setting different from her culture of origin, the nurse will assess for signs of culture shock. **Culture shock** occurs when a person is overwhelmed or even immobilized by cultural differences in expecta-

☜☜ *REFLECTIVE THINKING*

Institutional Culture Shock

There is a culture in every work environment. Persons not a part of the work group culture can experience the same reactions as they would to negotiating a foreign culture, with its own language, meanings, and assumptions about acceptable behavior. Employees and clients who have to learn the routines and language of an institution often experience this culture shock. Since all clients who have not previously been admitted to a mental health facility are subject to institutional culture shock, how would you modify the assessment for a client from a culture different from your own? What approaches would convey caring and sensitivity, despite cultural differences?

tions, communication, and general habits between the culture of origin and a new culture to which the individual is trying to assimilate. Feelings of helplessness, anger, or acute discomfort are usual. Entry into an institution of the health care culture can produce this reaction in persons who share the culture of origin of the caregivers but who do not share the institutional or

CASE EXAMPLE *Clash of Cultures*

Anita, a 26-year-old female from Honduras, was traveling by bus to visit relatives in the United States. While travelling through the Midwest, Anita began to demonstrate mannerisms that concerned other passengers. They reported to the bus driver that Anita was reaching into the air and talking unintelligibly. At the next stop, the bus driver called the police, who took Anita to the emergency room of the local hospital for an evaluation.

A psychiatrist and a psychiatric nurse attempted to interview Anita but recognized that Anita spoke limited English; an adequate psychiatric examination was not possible without an interpreter. Because of her unexplained mannerisms, the psychiatrist and the nurse determined that Anita might not be in touch with reality and might not be able to safely care for herself. The psychiatrist decided to admit Anita to the psychiatric unit on an emergency admission and to request that an interpreter be called to assist with further evaluation.

The hospital staff learned that Anita was responding to and interacting with "spirits." She denied seeing the spirits but reported that she knew they were present. The staff also learned that Anita's aunt lived in the

vicinity, and the aunt was notified of Anita's admission and asked to come to the hospital to assist.

Anita's aunt attended a staff conference. After assisting with interpretation among the psychiatrist, nurse, and Anita, Anita's aunt explained that Anita had become exhausted from traveling and was communicating with spirits, asking their assistance to relieve the stress and anxiety of travel in a strange land where she could hardly make herself understood to meet even basic needs. The idea of spirits was part of her cultural background, and the behaviors she demonstrated were appropriate and expected in her culture. The staff quite readily decided to discharge Anita.

This case example illustrates the idea that there is no universal definition for mental illness. Each society defines what it will accept as "normal." In the assessment of any client, cultural background has to be considered. The behaviors being evaluated must be examined from the client's cultural perspective. Obviously, cultural differences and poor English language skills are not appropriate reasons for admission to a psychiatric setting. They are not symptoms of mental illness.

professional culture. The professional routines and language differ substantially and can result in culture shock. For persons whose cultures differ from the caregivers' cultures of origin, the culture shock will be that much greater, and the culturally competent nurse will take this into consideration as diagnoses, status, and care are assessed and planned.

Understanding broad cultural patterns is a good first step ·to providing sensitive care, but broad generalizations about any client based on his or her culture of origin can lead to cultural misunderstanding. It is not the culture of origin but the person's level of integration into or identification with the culture that influences beliefs and behaviors (Helman, 1990). Within any culture there are groups that differ from the broader culture in one or many ways. There are differences even among group members who have a high level of identification with the culture. And constant fluctuations and small variations of culture in the individual based on personal experiences must be considered. For culturally competent care to be provided, the client's level of integration and identification with both the culture of origin and the dominant culture of the society in which he or she is residing must be determined.

KEY CONCEPTS

◆ Culture (classic definition) comprises all that is learned through socialization, shared by all group members, and associated with adaptation to the environment. Culture includes knowledge, beliefs, art, morals, law, and customs.

◆ Culture, as used by those facilitating intercultural communication, is defined to be malleable and changes slightly during interpersonal interactions between persons from different cultures.

◆ Stereotyping clients from different cultures can lead to unsafe care.

◆ Culture pervades thoughts and behaviors associated with value orientations, interpersonal relations, communication, religion, social systems, diet and food habits, and health and illness beliefs.

◆ When assessing and providing care, the nurse must consider cultural and ethnic influences on beliefs about mental illness and care, interpersonal interaction, verbal and nonverbal communication, diet and food habits, and biological variation.

◆ All aspects of verbal and nonverbal communication are culturally based and often serve as barriers to communication.

◆ A cultural facilitator or culture broker is the best person to assist with interpreting for a non–English-speaking client. A translator or interpreter who translates only words is unable to interpret the many cultural components of the communication.

◆ What are considered to be normal versus abnormal behaviors, feelings, or states reflecting mental status vary across cultures.

◆ Genetic, environmental, and behavioral differences affect pharmacological and behavioral aspects of medicating clients of different cultures.

◆ There is much variation in the level of integration into or identification with a specific culture among members of that cultural group. Careful assessment of the level of integration and identity is necessary.

REVIEW QUESTIONS AND ACTIVITIES

1. Define culture.
2. Describe the importance of integrating concepts of cultural variation into planning and implementing psychiatric mental health nursing care.
3. Discuss ways in which clients may differ in beliefs about what are normal or abnormal behaviors, feelings, or states associated with mental status.
4. What are the dangers of stereotyping, ethnocentrism, and cultural blindness? What steps should nurses take to ensure that they provide sensitive nursing care?
5. Plan methods for adapting communication skills to effectively communicate with a client from a culture other than your own. Begin by verifying the client's level of identification with the culture, then work to find out the values held by the client and how they may complement or differ from your own.

EXPLORING THE WEB

◆ Visit this text's "Online Companion™" on the Internet at **http://www.DelmarNursing.com** for further information on cross-cultural or transcultural nursing.

◆ Are there specific Web sites listed under these topics?

◆ Check the sites of some of the major nursing organizations such as NANDA and National League of Nurses (NLN). Do they include pages that might offer you information on cultural sensitivity?

≋ REFERENCES

Agar, M. (1994). The intercultural frame. *International Journal of Intercultural Relations, 18*(2), 221–237.

Andrews, M., & Boyle, J. (1995). *Transcultural concepts in nursing care* (2nd ed.). Philadelphia: Lippincott.

Campinha-Bacote, J. (1994). Cultural competence in psychiatric mental health nursing: A conceptual model. *Nursing Clinics of North America, 29*(1), 1–8.

Dasen, P., Berry, J., & Sartorius, N. (Eds.). (1988). *Health and cross-cultural psychology.* Newbury Park: Sage.

Giger, J., & Davidhizar, R. (1991). *Transcultural nursing.* St. Louis: Mosby.

Helman, C. G. (1990). *Culture, health and illness: An introduction for health professionals* (2nd ed.). London: Wright.

Hermans, H., Kempen, H., & Van Loon, R. (1992). The dialogical self: Beyond individualism and rationalism. *American Psychologist, 47*(1), 23–33.

Ho, M. K. (1987). *Family therapy and ethnic minorities.* Newbury Park, CA: Sage.

Hughes, C. (1978). Medical care: Ethnomedicine. In M. Logan and E. Hunt (Eds.), *Health and the human condition.* Belmont, CA: Wadsworth.

Jezewski, M. (1993). Culture brokering as a model for advocacy. *Nursing and Health Care, 12*(2), 78–85.

Leininger, M. (1978). *Transcultural nursing: Concepts, theories and practices.* New York: John Wiley & Sons.

Leininger, M. (1991). *Culture care diversity and universality: A theory of nursing.* New York: National League for Nursing.

Lipson, J. (1996a). Culturally competent nursing care. In J. Lipson, S. Dibble, & P. Minarik (Eds.), *Culture & nursing care: A pocket guide* (pp. 1–6). San Francisco: UCSF Nursing Press.

Lipson, J. (1996b). Diversity issues. In J. Lipson, S. Dibble, & P. Minarik (Eds.), *Culture & nursing care: A pocket guide* (pp. 7–10). San Francisco: UCSF Nursing Press.

Narayan, K. (1991). "According to their feelings": Teaching and healing with stories. In C. Witherell & N. Noddings (Eds.), *Stories lives tell: Narrative and dialogue in education* (pp. 113–135). New York: Teachers College, Columbia University.

Parker, S. (1977). Eskimo, psychopathology in the context of Eskimo personality and culture. In D. Landy (Ed.), *Culture, disease and healing: Studies in medical anthropology* (pp. 349–358). New York: Macmillan.

Pedersen, P., & Ivey, A. (1993). *Culture-centered counseling and interviewing skills: A practical guide.* Westport, CT: Praeger.

Sue, D., & Sue, D. (1990). *Counseling the culturally different* (2nd ed.). New York: John Wiley & Sons.

Thiederman, S. (1991). *Bridging cultural barriers: Managing ethnic diversity in the workplace* (videotape). Irwindale, CA: Barr Films.

Trompenaars, F. (1993, 1994). *Riding the waves of culture: Understanding diversity in global business.* Burr Ridge, IL: Irwin.

Tylor, E. B. (1871). *Primitive cultures* (Vols. 1 and 2). London: Murray.

Williams, D., & Collins, C. (1995). US socioeconomic and racial differences in health: Patterns and explanations. *Annual Review of Sociology, 21,* 349–387.

Witherell, C., & Noddings, N. (Eds.). (1991). *Stories lives tell.* New York: Teachers College Press.

≋ SUGGESTED READINGS

American Academy of Nursing. (1992). Culturally competent health care. *Nursing Outlook, 40*(6), 277–283.

Burk, M., Wieser, P., & Keegan, L. (1995). Cultural beliefs and health behaviors of pregnant Mexican-American women: Implications for primary care. *Advances in Nursing Science, 17*(4), 37–52.

Foster, S. (1990). The pragmatics of culture: The rhetoric of difference in psychiatric nursing. *Archives of Psychiatric Nursing, 4,* 292.

Galanti, G. (1991). *Caring for patients from different cultures.* Philadelphia: University of Pennsylvania Press.

Gaw, A. (1993). *Culture, ethnicity, and mental illness.* Washington, DC: American Psychiatric Press.

Hofstede, G. (1991). *Cultures and organizations: Software of the mind.* London: McGraw-Hill.

Lipson, J., Dibble, S., & Minarik, P. (Eds.). (1996). *Culture & nursing care: A pocket guide.* San Francisco: UCSF Nursing Press.

Meleis, A., Isenbery, M., Koerner, J., & Stern, P. (1995). *Diversity, marginalization, and culturally competent health care: Issues in knowledge development.* Washington, DC: American Academy of Nursing.

Quershi, B. (1994). *Transcultural medicine: Dealing with patients from different cultures.* Newbury, UK: Kluwer Academic Publishers.

Rooda, L. (1992). Attitudes of nurses toward culturally diverse patients: An examination of the social contact theory. *Journal of National Black Nurses Association, 6*(1), 48–56.

Spector, R. (1996). *Cultural diversity in health & illness* (4th ed.). Stamford, CT: Appleton & Lange.

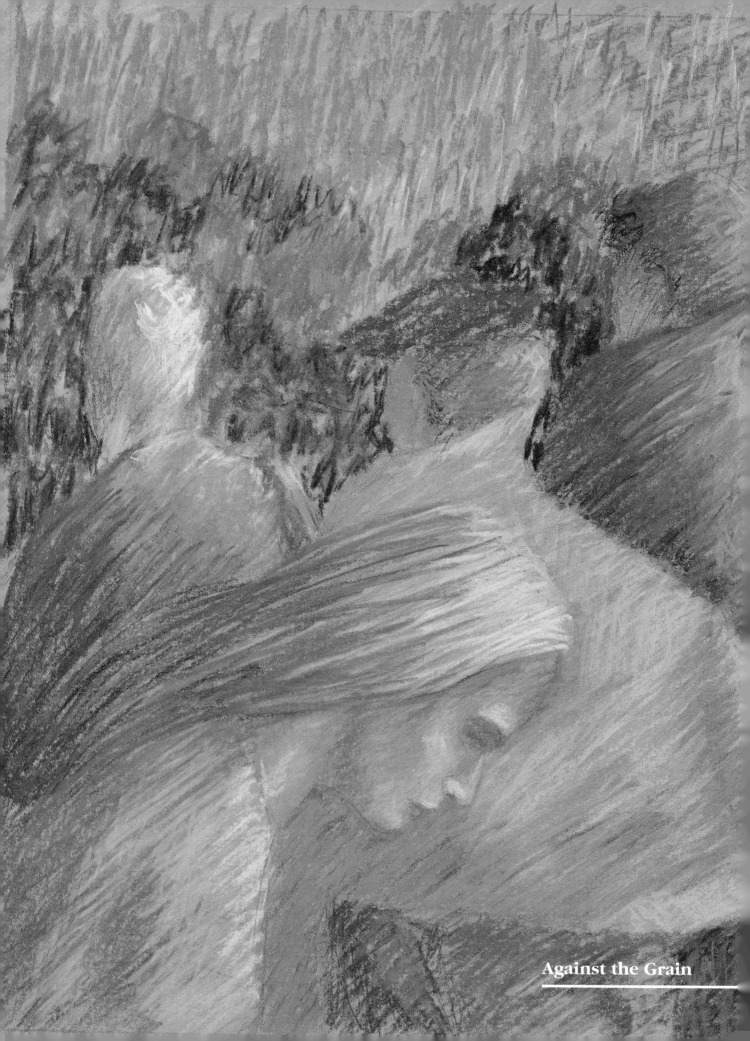

Against the Grain

Chapter

7

EPIDEMIOLOGY OF
MENTAL HEALTH AND ILLNESS

Lawrence E. Frisch

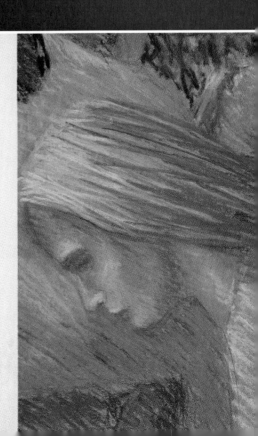

Planning Services and Guiding Public Policy

◆ If you had to tell your city planners what services were needed in
   your community to care for those with mental disorders, what would
   you say?
◆ As a nurse, you will have opportunities to be involved in helping
   plan policy (writing letters, serving on committees, being involved in
   civic organizations); think about what areas of nursing care and
   public policy interest you the most.
◆ There is specific information required to intelligently guide decisions
   regarding care facilities and servicing clients. Have you ever considered how health professionals gather this information?

Epidemiology is important for all public health policy. In this chapter you
will explore its role in mental health.

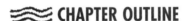

CHAPTER OUTLINE

WHY STUDY EPIDEMIOLOGY?

HOW IS EPIDEMIOLOGY DONE?

EPIDEMIOLOGY AND MENTAL DISORDERS: DEFINING DISEASE

The Diagnostic and Statistical Manual of Mental Disorders
    Assessing the Epidemiology of Mental Disorders
    Disorders in DSM-IV

EPIDEMIOLOGICAL STUDIES OF MENTAL DISORDERS

Early Studies

The Carter Commission and the Epidemiologic Catchment Area Study
    Planning and Execution
    General Results

The Tip-of-the-Iceberg Phenomenon

Importance of the ECA and Other Related Studies

COMPETENCIES

Upon completion of this chapter, the reader should be able to:

1. Define epidemiology and describe the major types of epidemiological studies related to mental health.

2. Explain the basic tools of epidemiology, including research tools of descriptive studies, case-controlled studies, and meta-analysis.

3. Discuss the challenges of standardized definitions in mental health.

4. Describe the development of the *Diagnostic and Statistical Manual* as a means to standardize definitions of psychiatric diagnosis.

5. Present data from early epidemiological studies and the Epidemiologic Catchment Area Study to provide insight regarding the incidence and prevalence of mental disease in the United States.

KEY TERMS

Blinded Clinical Trial Study in which subjects do not know whether they are receiving an active treatment or a placebo.

Case-Control Study Study comparing two groups: the cases (all members have the given disease or condition) and the controls (all members are free of the disease or condition).

Cohort Study See Longitudinal Study.

Control Group Persons receiving no treatment or being free of a given condition or disease under study.

Controlled Clinical Trials Evaluations in which neither the clients nor their caregivers are allowed to know exactly what treatment is being given.

Descriptive Study Survey to determine the incidence and prevalence of a disease or condition.

Double-Blinded Trial Study in which neither subjects nor persons evaluating the outcome know whether subjects are receiving treatment or a placebo.

Endemic Descriptor for a disease or condition that is constantly or regularly found in the population.

Epidemic Descriptor for a disease or condition that spreads or circulates within a population.

Epidemiology Study of the causes and distribution of injuries and diseases in a population.

Experimental Group Persons receiving treatment or having a given condition or disease under study; also known as Case Group.

Incidence Number of new cases of an illness, condition, or injury that begin within a certain time period.

Interrater Agreement Accord on diagnosis between individuals evaluating the same condition.

Interrater Reliability Accord on diagnosis between different evaluators on the same examination.

Intrarater Reliability Accord on diagnosis on different examinations by the same evaluator.

Longitudinal Study Population-based study conducted over a period of time, typically years; also known as Cohort Study.

Meta-analysis Statistical analysis that combines the results of several separate clinical studies.

Placebo Treatment that has no intended effect on the expected outcome of a trial.

Prevalence Number of persons in a population who are living with a disease or disorder at any time; includes both new and old cases.

Quasi-Experimental Study Analytical study in which a population is studied before and after a given event; usually includes both a case and a control set.

Reliability Measurement of reproducibility of a testing instrument.

Risk Factors Traits that predispose an individual to a disease.

Validity Measurement of accuracy of a testing instrument.

Epidemiology is the study of the causes and distribution of injuries and diseases in a population. Many people think that epidemiology is the study of epidemics, but this is only partly true. The word **epidemic** is well known in nursing practice and describes a disease or condition that spreads or circulates within a population. In 1861 Florence Nightingale, referring to the spread of diseases like diphtheria and scarlet fever, wrote of "children's epidemics," and similar use of the word can be traced back to Shakespeare's time. While the tools of epidemiology are very important in understanding epidemics, most diseases that we face in modern life are not epidemic. More typically, they are **endemic**, meaning that they are constantly or regularly found in the population. Epidemiology also includes the study of such endemic diseases: their causes, their treatment, and their prevention and control.

Most mental disorders are endemic or sporadic: while they may be common in most communities, they seem to occur largely without pattern. This lack of pattern has ensured that the causes and treatment of mental illness have been of continuing concern in history and imaginative literature. In the Old Testament, only the music of David's harp could rouse Saul from his deep depression. Robert Burton's *Anatomy of Melancholy* is an important 17th-century work filled with classical quotations on mental illness and written to keep its lonely author's mind off his own severe depression. It is now more clearly understood that Alexander the Great suffered from alcoholism. As one of the greatest soldiers and conquerors of the ancient world, surely Alexander's struggles with alcohol have profoundly influenced history. While epidemiology rarely concerns itself directly with the illness or struggle of an individual, epidemiology is very much the study of how diseases of all kinds manifest themselves in populations. Depression, alcoholism, and other mental disorders are important epidemiological concerns that affect both individuals and populations. The epidemiologist's goal is to better understand how frequently diseases occur in a population, in whom they are most likely to occur, and what their natural history is.

WHY STUDY EPIDEMIOLOGY?

Epidemiology is of value because it allows one to understand how illnesses affect a population. Only through epidemiology can we know accurately how many cases of a given illness occur, who is likely to become ill, and what the impact of that illness is likely to be. Through epidemiological study, researchers may be better able to determine possible causes for disease and can often detect **risk factors**, such as age, race, or gender, that predispose persons to a disease. Epidemiology may guide public policy that leads to the prevention of illness. For example, national and international programs for immunization grew out of classic epidemiological investigations and are among the greatest public health successes of the modern era.

In addition to exploring disease causation and prevention, epidemiology can also examine health care outcomes. Effective health care is now available for many

---

WHAT IS A CONTROLLED CLINICAL TRIAL?

Controlled clinical trials are epidemiological studies conducted like true experiments. Each trial has at least one **experimental group** (persons receiving treatment or having a given condition or disease under study) and at least one comparison or **control group** (persons receiving no treatment or being free of a given condition or disease under study). Controlled trials are usually conducted to test a type of treatment, and treated individuals are assigned to the experimental group while untreated individuals make up the controls. A true clinical trial is **blinded**, which means that the subjects in the trial do not know whether they are receiving the active treatment or a **placebo** treatment that is thought to have no specific effect on the expected outcome. In a **double-blinded trial**, neither the subjects nor the persons evaluating the outcome know whether any subject is receiving active treatment or placebo.

EXAMPLE

To determine the effect of treatments for depression, cognitive-behavioral therapy, interpersonal psychotherapy, antidepressant medication (imipramine), and placebo treatments were compared in a study of 155 clients. Clients were assigned to one of four groups: Group 1 received cognitive behavioral therapy, group 2 received interpersonal psychotherapy, group 3 received medication with clinical management, and group 4 received a placebo with clinical management. Study findings indicated that 40% of the clients recovered with placebo and 60% recovered with one of the specific treatments. Also, the study results suggested that the specific treatments were more powerful in the more severely affected clients. It was noted that cognitive and interpersonal therapies are of benefit and particularly helpful for persons who cannot or do not wish to take drugs.

Example taken from "National Institute of Mental Health Treatment of Depression Collaborative Research Program: General Effectiveness of Treatments," by I. Elkin, T. Shea, and J. Watkins, 1989, *Archives of General Psychiatry, 46,* 971–983.

illnesses, but often at great cost. It is essential to know what the natural, or untreated, course of an illness is likely to be if no treatment is given. The outcome of differing treatments can then be compared to see which treatment is better and whether any offer improved outcome over the untreated course of the disease. Many studies of outcomes are done as **controlled clinical trials**, evaluations in which neither clients nor their caregivers are allowed to know exactly what treatment is being given. The display on the preceding page provides an example of a controlled clinical trial. Epidemiology allows us to study the outcomes both of disease and of treatment. In this way the study of illness in a population may translate to improved health care for an individual who is ill with a disease.

HOW IS EPIDEMIOLOGY DONE?

Epidemiologists may be equally at home studying insects in a tropical rain forest as poring over century-old records of births and deaths. They may use pencils and pocket calculators or the latest techniques in molecular biology and computerized biostatistics. Some epidemiologists interview and examine clients; others look only at medical records or at public archives. Important epidemiological work may be done through written or telephone-based questionnaires. Epidemiologists may measure concentrations of toxins and pollutants, they may examine the latest data on genetic linkages, or they may read and analyze already published data using complex statistical tools such as **meta-analysis**, a form of statistical analysis in which the results of several separate clinical studies are combined. The epidemiologist is concerned both with the phenomena of disease, illness, and treatment and with public policy. Epidemiologists study natural occurrences of illness, but they also study the effectiveness of treatments and the effects of political and social decisions on the health and living circumstances of groups and individuals.

Epidemiologists use a specific vocabulary to define aspects of their work. They typically begin their work by defining the condition or disease of interest, the population at risk for illness, and the potential risk factors to be examined. They then decide what data to collect and how to examine it. In some cases the data are preexisting, either in public archives or in medical records. Often new data collection is required, either by interviews with clients or in some other manner. When new data are needed from clients, the epidemiologist must decide whether to use a previously established data instrument (often a questionnaire) or to develop a new instrument specifically for the purpose. Established instruments generally have known **validity** and **reliability** (they determine accurately and reproducibly what the epidemiologist believes them to measure), but they may not be designed to answer the question needing investigation. For this reason and despite the extra work required to pretest and validate questionnaires, new instruments are often developed for major epidemiological research undertakings.

Many epidemiological studies are **descriptive**. This means that the study documents and describes the condition under study. Often the goal of descriptive work is to determine the incidence or prevalence of a disease or condition. **Incidence** refers to the number of *new* cases of an illness, condition, or injury that begin within a certain time period. **Prevalence** refers to the number of persons in a population who are living with a disease or disorder at any time. Prevalence measures both new cases *and* old cases, whereas incidence measures only new cases. Incidence is the most important measurement for serious acute problems such as heart attacks; prevalence may be a more important measure for disorders such as depression, which may begin almost unnoticed but may cause severe symptoms for many years.

While descriptive studies are important, other epidemiological studies are analytical or **quasi-experimental**, meaning that a population is studied before and after some event such as the introduction of a new service or a new law. In these studies the epidemiologist usually studies both a set of cases and a set of controls. **Case-control studies** compare two groups: In one group (the cases) all members have the given disease or condition; in the other group (the controls) all members are free of the disease or condition. By comparing these groups, the epidemiologist tries to determine what factors are likely causes of the condition. Sometimes cases and controls come from the same population, and this population is observed over time to see who develops a disease or other outcome. These population-based studies are known as **longitudinal** or **cohort** studies. Some cohort studies have followed specific groups of clients for 25 years or longer: This long follow-up is difficult to achieve when clients (or epidemiologists) move periodically from place to place, change interests, or drop out of the study.

Once data are collected, epidemiologists may use complex biostatistical analysis to interpret their data. However, much epidemiological data are presented using simple rates and percentages. Many important epidemiological questions can be answered with basic descriptive statistics; other questions require complicated mathematical modeling or techniques. Thus, many epidemiologists maintain a high level of mathematical proficiency.

EPIDEMIOLOGY AND MENTAL DISORDERS: DEFINING DISEASE

One of the important contributions that epidemiology makes to the understanding of diseases and disease processes is its insistence on standardized definitions. The question of case definition is so important that a complete book entitled *What Is a Case?* has been written on this question alone (Wing, Bebbington, & Robins, 1981). Defining a case when studying mental disorders initially proved difficult for epidemiologists for two reasons. First, psychiatrists tended to diagnose mental disorders without using any standardized criteria. Consequently, two psychiatrists seeing the same client may disagree completely on diagnosis, echoing the confusion faced by Alice in the Looking-Glass world: "'When I use a word,' Humpty Dumpty said, 'it means just what I choose it to mean—neither more nor less.'" While obviously troubling for the client, any difficulty in getting **interrater agreement** between psychiatrists evaluating the same client meant that epidemiologists could never accurately determine the incidence or prevalence of the conditions the psychiatrists were diagnosing. This problem of nonstandardized definitions was found to be serious wherever epidemiologists studied mental disorders.

Second, at one time many psychiatrists and therapists felt that for a variety of mental disorders there was no clear dividing line between normal and disease. This too was troubling for epidemiologists who usually do not have much trouble defining diseases: It is generally not difficult to know whether or not a person has measles, for example. It would seem nonsensical to say that "she's just a little more 'measley' than normal" when we mean she has a mild case of measles. The diagnosis of a mental disorder is much more complicated, however. Most persons feel blue or depressed some days, or after a personal disappointment, and nearly all normal persons have a period of profound mourning after the death of close friends or family. How does the disease "depression" differ from these normal feelings? Or, as an epidemiologist might put it, "What is a *case* of depression?" Many psychiatrists felt that they could best answer this question by carefully interviewing an individual, but often two psychiatrists would interview the same client and still disagree on whether or not the person was depressed.

The Diagnostic and Statistical Manual of Mental Disorders

Fortunately for epidemiology, psychiatrists and other therapists were also troubled by these difficulties with definition, and in the 1950s, leaders in the American Psychiatric Association began to develop a standardized set of criteria on which to base psychiatric diagnosis (American Psychiatric Association, 1994). After lengthy discussion and debate, the first version of these criteria, DSM-I, was published in 1952. By 1980 the third edition (DSM-III) had been published, and the validity of using DSM to make standardized diagnostic assessments had been widely accepted. In 1987 DSM-III was further revised, and in 1994 DSM-IV was released. The *Diagnostic and Statistical Manual* offers a series of diagnoses, and for each diagnosis it provides a list of symptoms and diagnostic criteria. To be diagnosed, a client must meet a specified minimum number of the listed criteria or symptoms. The number of criteria (and their type) varies for each diagnosis, but the process is similar and similarly standardized. Multiple studies have established that when made by trained professionals, DSM diagnoses have substantial agreement between different evaluators (**interrater reliability**) and on different examinations by the same evaluator (**intrarater reliability**) (American Psychiatric Association, 1994). While the multiple revisions since DSM-I suggest that there has been much to improve in DSM, the widespread adoption of DSM criteria among mental health providers has allowed standardized case definition.

Assessing the Epidemiology of Mental Disorders

One of the reasons for DSM's success is that despite being authored by the American Psychiatric Association, DSM does not require diagnoses to be made only by a psychiatrist. The level of acceptance that DSM has achieved has been remarkable in large part because DSM can be effectively used by all well-educated mental health professionals. More important from the epidemiological perspective, many of the psychiatric disorders listed in DSM have diagnostic criteria that can be readily assessed by asking persons a series of questions on a standardized questionnaire. These questions need not be asked by a highly trained mental health professional. This means that specially trained nonprofessionals can survey large numbers of persons using standardized written questions, and while the results may not have full psychiatric validity, they are likely to correspond fairly closely to diagnoses that would have been made by a skilled psychiatrist or psychiatric nurse directly interviewing the same patient.

Disorders in DSM-IV

In DSM-IV there is an extensive number and range of diagnoses, many of which are treated in more detail throughout this textbook. To understand the epidemiology of mental disorders, it is necessary to have some

✿✿ REFLECTIVE THINKING

Labeling Diseases

Some professionals are concerned over the consequences of giving clients labels, such as "depressed" or "schizophrenic." Labels seem to stigmatize clients and turn them from real human individuals into objects of scientific description. The ANA standards of performance require a nurse to be nonjudgmental and nondiscriminatory. How do you respond to this concern, knowing there is a need for standardization in language?

understanding of psychiatric terms. The following discussion is very brief and touches on only a few general DSM diagnoses. For more detail, the reader can consult either the appropriate chapter in this text or a copy of DSM-IV (American Psychiatric Association, 1994).

Mood disorders. Mood disorders are most often characterized by feelings of depression. The most common mood disorder in DSM is Major Depressive Disorder, which is diagnosed when a set of symptoms associated with depression (feeling "blue, sad, or depressed," losing interest in previously pleasurable activities, and/or having thoughts about death or suicide) have been present for 2 weeks or more. Other important diagnostic criteria may include weight change and sleep disturbance. In addition to Major Depressive Disorder, important mood disorders include Dysthymia (characterized by significant sadness most days for at least 2 years) and Bipolar Disorder (commonly called manic-depressive disorder and characterized by episodes of excitement and racing thoughts, often, but not always, alternating with episodes of depression).

Schizophrenia. Schizophrenia is a major psychiatric disorder characterized by symptoms of psychosis or loss of touch with reality. These symptoms include delusions (such as beliefs that other persons can read one's mind or are controlling one's thoughts or movements) and hallucinations (most commonly hearing "voices"). The diagnosis of Schizophrenia also requires that a person have deteriorated from a previously more normal level of functioning and that symptoms have been present for at least 6 months.

Substance abuse disorders. This category includes abuse of both alcohol and a variety of other substances. The DSM-IV criteria require that a person show evidence of dependence on drugs or alcohol to be classified as having a drug- or alcohol-related disorder. Substances considered potentially abusive in DSM-IV include sedative drugs (among them Valium and other benzodiazepines), opioid drugs (including heroin), amphetamines, cocaine, hallucinogens, marijuana, and alcohol.

Anxiety disorders. The common DSM-IV diagnoses in this category include Obsessive-Compulsive Disorder, phobias, Generalized Anxiety, and Panic Disorder. In DSM-IV, obsessions are defined as "persistent ideas, thoughts, impulses, or images that cause marked anxiety or distress." A common obsession might be that one's hands are dirty even though they have been recently washed. Compulsions are "repetitive behaviors the goal of which is to prevent or reduce anxiety or distress . . . that accompanies an obsession or to prevent some dreaded event or situation." Common compulsions include washing hands repeatedly or counting objects ritually. Phobias are "unreasonable" fears of specific situations such as heights, closed spaces, or going out of the house alone. Since most people are afraid of dangerous situations, to qualify as phobic such fears need to be severe and to occur in situations where the average person would probably not have any significant anxiety. Generalized Anxiety is defined as "unrealistic or excessive anxiety or worry . . . about two or more life circumstances" in the absence of other DSM-IV diagnoses that can cause anxiety. Symptoms must also be present for a specified period of time. Panic Disorder is a condition in which one experiences brief, intense feelings of anxiety associated with physical symptoms (such as rapid heart rate, sweating, dizziness) in the absence of a definable physical diagnosis. The diagnosis is made only when a certain number of episodes occur within a specified period of time.

There are numerous other DSM-IV diagnoses, and the diagnostic criteria listed above are also far from complete. Nonetheless, this very brief introduction to psychiatric terminology should allow the reader to understand some of the actual accomplishments of recent studies of the epidemiology of mental disorders.

EPIDEMIOLOGICAL STUDIES OF MENTAL DISORDERS
Early Studies

As early as the 1950s, three important studies were carried out (Robins & Regier, 1991): the Stirling County Study in Nova Scotia, Canada; the Midtown Manhattan Study in New York; and the Baltimore Morbidity Study. Each of these studies interviewed about 1,000 residents of a community for evidence of mental disorder and made important contributions to the understanding of mental illness in the community. These studies are all considered groundbreaking efforts because they marked the first actual studies of entire communities. They were all carefully designed by sophisticated epidemiological thinkers, they used highly trained interviewers and carefully researched interview protocols, and each tried to assess the prevalence of psychiatric symptoms and disorders. Previous investigations had looked only at persons under psychiatric or psychological care, but the Nova Scotia, Manhattan, and Baltimore studies chose people at random living in the community and interviewed them for the presence (or absence) of psychiatric symptoms.

In some ways the most important outcome of these three studies was the highly different conclusions that they reached (Robins & Regier, 1991). The Stirling County Study found that 57% of the persons interviewed had at some time in their lives met DSM-I diagnostic criteria for a mental disorder and 24% of people had at one time had severe impairment of the ability to function at work and home as a result of mental disorder.

Strikingly, 90% of all these people were experiencing symptoms of mental disorder and severe functional impairment at the time of the Stirling County interviews. In contrast, the Baltimore study found only 11% of the population to qualify for a current DSM-I diagnosis and only 2% to have moderate to severe functional impairment. The Midtown Manhattan Study reported findings much closer to those of rural Nova Scotia, with significantly impaired functioning in 23% of the population. These three studies suggested that some form of mental illness was widespread in the general population. Because of the differences in findings among the studies and the difficulties in directly comparing any of them, epidemiologists and psychiatrists recognized the need for solid epidemiological data to determine the true national prevalence of mental illness and functional impairment due to mental disorder.

The Carter Commission and the Epidemiologic Catchment Area Study

Concerns about the results of these important studies led President Carter's Commission on Mental Health to push for a multisite comprehensive epidemiological survey in 1978. One of President Carter's first official actions was to appoint a President's Commission on Mental Health under the supervision of his wife, Rosalyn. Among the achievements of this commission was the recognition that many important basic epidemiological facts about mental illness were unknown. The President's Commission listed the following questions it thought important:

1. What is the prevalence of mental illness in the overall United States population?

2. Does the prevalence and type of illness vary in differing parts of the country?

3. Is there variation in type and severity of illness depending on race or socioeconomic status?

4. Among people who have ever had mental illness, how many are currently affected by this illness?

5. How much difficulty does mental illness cause?

6. What is the outcome of mental illness?

7. What percentage of persons with past and current mental illness are receiving treatment, and from what sources?

8. Does treatment for mental illness change outcome?

9. What are the causes of mental illness?

10. Can mental illness be prevented?

In reviewing these and similar questions, the President's Commission and the National Institutes of Mental Health (NIMH) recognized that there was a more important question underlying epidemiological study of mental health: How is mental illness to be defined? Studies in the 1960s had shown marked differences between the United States and England in frequency of hospitalization for several psychiatric diseases. Further evaluation of these studies showed, however, that these differences in hospitalization rates had little to do with real differences between clients or services but were explained almost completely by consistent differences between how clients were diagnosed in the two countries. The certainty sought by the President's Commission required that the definition of mental disorders be sufficiently standardized so that information collected was equivalent and comparable regardless of in which city or state it was collected. This led to a landmark project known as the *Epidemiologic Catchment Area (ECA) Study*.

Planning and Execution

The ECA Study had several purposes (Robins & Reiger, 1991). One purpose was to establish prevalence data for major psychiatric diagnoses. By 1980 DSM-III had been published, but as DSM had come to maturity, there were no data on how frequently the increasingly sophisticated DSM-III diagnoses were found in the population at large. A second purpose was to seek out subgroups in the United States population who had unusually high or low rates of mental disorder. It was hoped that finding any such differences might provide useful clues to the causes of these disorders.

The first ECA task was to design a screening questionnaire based on DSM-III. This questionnaire had been completed by 1981 and was called the *NIMH Diagnostic Interview Schedule (DIS)*. The DIS was 25 pages long and consisted of several sections. The first section included general information about education, work, household income, and marital status/family structure. The next section included questions about use of health and mental health treatment services. The remainder of the DIS asked questions designed to suggest probable diagnoses of a range of mental disorders perceived likely to be most common and selected from among the 122 included in DSM-III. Questions were designed to elicit diagnoses of mood disorders (called affective disorders in DSM-III), schizophrenia, substance use disorders (including alcohol abuse or dependence), and anxiety disorders. Eight other diagnoses including Pathological Gambling, Tobacco Use Disorder, and several disorders of sexual functioning were also covered in the questionnaires. While DSM does not specifically include the diagnosis of "cognitive impairment," questions designed to determine an individual's level of intellectual functioning were also included in the DIS.

The next step in carrying out the ECA Study was to decide how many subjects needed to respond to the DIS questionnaire. Determining needed sample size is one of the most important tasks in epidemiology because if too few people participate in a study, it may not be valid to apply results to a larger population, and its results may not be convincing enough to justify its cost; however, large sample sizes greatly increase cost. The ECA Study planners decided that the DIS should be given to 20,000 persons in communities throughout the United States. Because some of the conditions about which the DIS asked were rare enough that even a sample of 20,000 would likely turn up few affected persons, the ECA Study planners decided that a small number of the persons studied would be residents in institutions (including nursing homes, psychiatric hospitals, and prisons). The rarer disorders were thought likely to occur more commonly among institutionalized individuals.

While no professional credentials were required of DIS interviewers, all interviewers were trained uniformly. Five sites were selected: St Louis, Missouri; Durham, North Carolina; Los Angeles; Baltimore, Maryland; and New Haven, Connecticut. The DIS was tested for inter-rater reliability using studies in which the test was given by an interviewer and by a psychiatrist; the same client was then freely interviewed by a second psychiatrist. Reliability was said to be "much better than chance." By the time the "first wave" of the ECA Study was completed, a total of 19,182 persons had been interviewed; 17,803 were living at home or had lived at home during the preceding year, and the remainder were living in institutions (primarily nursing homes or prisons).

General Results

The ECA Study results (Robins & Reiger, 1991) showed that 32% of all persons surveyed had, at some time in their lives, symptoms that would have assigned them a DSM psychiatric diagnosis. More strikingly, 20% of persons had symptoms that would have qualified them for some kind of psychiatric diagnosis within the preceding year:

◆ Alcohol abuse/dependence and phobias were by far the most common diagnoses discovered by the ECA Study, with anxiety, depression, and drug abuse also fairly prevalent.

◆ In the year preceding the ECA Study 3% to 4% of people reported symptoms that would qualify for a DSM diagnosis of anxiety, depression, or drug abuse.

One of the most important ECA findings was that gender correlated strongly with the types of symptoms found:

◆ Women were overall twice as likely as men to suffer from phobias, depression, or panic disorder.

◆ In contrast, men were five times more likely to receive a diagnosis of alcoholism.

Another major ECA Study finding was that mental disorders are significant problems for young and middle-aged Americans:

◆ Cognitive impairment (not a DSM diagnosis) was, not surprisingly, much more common in persons over 50 years of age. However, nearly all other symptoms of psychiatric disorder were evident in young persons.

◆ For those whose symptoms indicated a psychiatric diagnosis sometime in their lives, the median age of onset of symptoms was 16 years.

◆ Over 75% of those with psychiatric diagnoses had developed their symptoms by age 24, and over 90% by age 38.

Social factors were also shown to be related to symptoms of mental disorder:

◆ Almost all diagnoses studied were more common among persons who were less well educated or who had been multiply divorced or separated.

◆ Persons unemployed or on welfare had significantly higher rates of diagnosed disorder, although it was not possible to say how financial and mental states were related. For example, researchers could not determine whether poor financial status was a stress that led to mental illness or whether the impairments of mental symptoms made an individual less able to get and hold employment.

The contributions of race were more complex. The study had relatively few Hispanic participants (nearly all were in the Los Angeles catchment area) and virtually no participants who were Native American or of Asian origin. In contrast, African Americans were well represented among study participants, and though their rate of mental disorder did exceed that of whites, the difference was largely attributable to excess cognitive impairment in older males. What role earlier educational deficits and social deprivation may have played in skewing these men's responses was not determined by the study.

In some ways, the most striking ECA Study findings involved the relationship between symptoms and treatment (Robins & Reiger, 1991):

◆ Only 20% of persons who reported symptoms diagnostic of a psychiatric disorder within the preceding year reported receiving any kind of treatment.

◆ Only 2.4% of the population had ever been hospitalized for psychiatric reasons.

The Tip-of-the-Iceberg Phenomenon

The Stirling County Study was explicitly based on a "tip-of-the-iceberg" concept (Leighton, 1985). The study's authors recognized that many more persons in a community have symptoms of mental disorder than actually seek health care. This concept that *many persons have symptoms but few seek help* became known as the tip-of-the-iceberg phenomenon, because an iceberg may show only

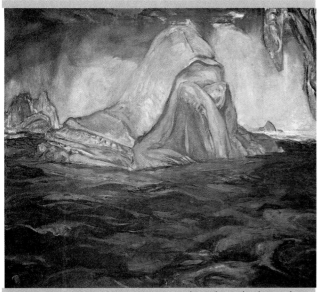

Arctic Landscape by Frederick H. Varley
Source: National Gallery of Canada, Ottawa

Epidemiologists like to talk about the tip-of-the-iceberg phenomena. Canadian F. H. Varley illustrates an iceberg in his painting *Arctic Landscape.*

a small tip above water, while the majority is invisible below the waterline. The Stirling County Study estimated that 20% of the population had significant symptoms of mental illness and hence were "part of the iceberg." The ECA Study findings seemed to corroborate these earlier conclusions:

◆ In the ECA Study sample, 20% had symptoms of a DSM psychiatric disorder within the preceding year, yet only one in five of these reported having sought professional help.

A concern related to the tip-of-the-iceberg phenomenon is that many people who *do* seek mental health care may be less troubled or ill than their neighbors who "tough out" their symptoms without looking for, or at least without finding, help.

◆ Of the people who completed the ECA Study and *had no evidence of a psychiatric diagnosis,* 4% were currently receiving some form of mental health treatment.

◆ Ten percent of persons with a past history of mental disorder *but with no present symptoms* were currently in treatment. (It is of course possible that without treatment they would have significant symptoms.)

This tip-of-the-iceberg concept is of the utmost importance to nursing and to the general delivery of health care.

◆ While much education for mental health professionals takes place in inpatient and outpatient facilities for mental health care, the majority of persons

✪ REFLECTIVE THINKING

The Tip of the Iceberg

One finding of the ECA Study is that many people who have severe symptoms of mental disorders do not seek help:

◆ What are the barriers to obtaining psychiatric help in your community?

◆ How can a nursing organization influence availability of services? The acceptance of services?

◆ How are nurses and other mental health professionals reaching the needy population?

◆ What do you think should be done to ensure that psychiatric care is available to those who need it?

with symptoms of significant mental disorders do not seek care for these symptoms. They are more likely to be encountered at home while giving care to ill friends or family members or in general medical facilities. Some clients who seek mental health care have symptoms of mental illness but may not meet criteria for a psychiatric diagnosis. Some of these may be less "sick" than clients not receiving care or services.

◆ Clients hospitalized for mental illness represent only the tip of the iceberg of those with symptoms. The ECA Study found that even for schizophrenia, among the most serious of all psychiatric diagnoses, only 40% of sufferers had ever been admitted to a hospital. Only about 1% of schizophrenic persons were hospitalized at the time of the study. Twice as many were in nursing homes. In the ECA Study sample, as many schizophrenic persons were found in prisons as in mental hospitals.

◆ Because of the high prevalence of mental symptoms, most persons will have one or more friends, acquaintances, or family members with significant mental illness.

◆ Alcohol and substance abuse are pervasive problems in our society and are generally underrecognized by health care providers.

◆ While not a specific DSM diagnosis, cognitive impairment is common and often unrecognized in older individuals.

◆ Anxiety (including phobias) and depression are among the most common of mental disorders. Many clients suffer from anxiety, fear, and despair without revealing their suffering to caregivers. Unless nurses explicitly ask about these symptoms, clients are unlikely to reveal them or to seek help.

Importance of the ECA and Other Related Studies

The ECA Study was a costly undertaking, and it is unlikely that a comparable effort to define the prevalence or causes of mental illness will be made again for many years. This chapter has discussed only the most general conclusions of the ECA Study. The ECA Study findings have been reported for many specific DSM diagnoses, and summaries of this epidemiologic data along with more detailed consideration of these diagnoses can be found later in this text. Knowing how common a disorder is and who is most likely to be afflicted can certainly help nurses in performing assessments and providing care. This is undoubtedly one of the contributions of the ECA Study and of psychiatric epidemiology in general. There are differences between DSM-III (the diagnostic criteria used by the ECA Study) and DSM-IV. These differences make it somewhat more difficult to apply the ECA Study to the diagnostic categories that are currently accepted. Nonetheless, the ECA Study remains important both for what it has taught us and for what it failed to determine.

As various psychiatric conditions are considered in this text, it will be seen that effective treatments are currently available for mood disorders, obsessive-compulsive disorder, and some other manifestations of anxiety disorders. The ECA Study showed that each of these conditions is widespread in the population and probably both underrecognized and largely untreated. This underrecognition and undertreatment are major health care challenges that, at least for depression, have begun to be addressed.

For many other high-prevalence conditions, such as substance abuse, treatment is costly and of unproven benefit. The ECA Study clearly shows the prevalence of these conditions, but it does not point the way to effective treatment. In addition, the ECA Study has not offered new insights into the prevention of mental disorders. Like many other major accomplishments, the ECA Study has taught much but leaves many questions unanswered. Both these questions and the partial answers gained from the ECA Study will surface many times in the remaining chapters of this book.

≋ KEY CONCEPTS

◆ Epidemiology is the study of causes and distribution of diseases in a population.

◆ The goal of epidemiology is to better understand how frequently diseases occur in a population and in whom they are most likely to occur, and to document the natural history of the diseases.

◆ Many epidemiological studies in mental health are descriptive, that is, they seek to evaluate the incidence and prevalence of a disorder.

◆ Standardization of definitions of mental disorders posed challenges to any significant epidemiological study, as there were no standard or agreed-upon definitions of mental disorders until the *Diagnostic and Statistical Manual,* 1st ed. (DSM-I), was published in 1952.

◆ The *Diagnostic and Statistical Manual,* 4th ed., is now widely recognized and used and has served to standardize definitions.

◆ Three early epidemiological studies in mental health were the Stirling County Study in Nova Scotia, Canada, the Midtown Manhattan Study, and the Baltimore Morbidity Study. These early studies suggested that some form of mental illness might be widespread in the general population.

◆ In 1978, President Carter commissioned the Epidemiologic Catchment Area (ECA) Study, a multisite comprehensive study in the United States, which showed that mental illness was more common than most people were aware of; for example, 32% of persons surveyed had symptoms that would have assigned them a psychiatric diagnosis according to DSM.

◆ The most common diagnoses discovered by the ECA were alcohol abuse/dependence and phobias, with anxiety and depression also being fairly common.

◆ The ECA also indicated that only 20% of persons who reported symptoms diagnostic of a psychiatric disorder reported receiving any kind of treatment.

REVIEW QUESTIONS AND ACTIVITIES

1. Define epidemiology.

2. Differentiate between epidemic and endemic.

3. Provide an example of how one could conduct a controlled clinical trial for some aspect of mental health care.

4. Differentiate between incidence and prevalence.

5. Discuss the challenges of standardization of definitions in psychiatric care.

6. Describe the most prevalent mental conditions in the United States.

7. All epidemiological studies indicate a large number of Americans are suffering from mental illness. How does this information impact nursing in the general hospital? In mental health care clinics? In home health care?

EXPLORING THE WEB

♦ Visit this text's "Online Companion™" on the Internet at **http://www.DelmarNursing.com** for further information on epidemiology.

♦ Is there any information available from the government concerning the ECA Study? Is information on any other government research studies available on line?

♦ What sources can you locate that deal with epidemiology?

REFERENCES

Leighton, A. (1985). The initial frame of reference of the Stirling County study: Main questions asked and reasons for them. In J. E. Barrett & R. M. Rose (Eds.), *Mental disorders in the community: Progress and challenge.* New York: Guilford.

Robins, L. N., & Regier, D. A. (Eds.). (1991). *Psychiatric disorders in America.* New York: Free Press.

Wing, J. K., Bebbington, P., & Robins, L. N. (1981). *What is a case? The problem of definition in psychiatric community surveys.* London: Grant McIntyre.

SUGGESTED READINGS

American Psychiatric Association. (1994). *Diagnostic and statistical manual* (4th ed.) (DSM-IV). Washington, DC: Author.

Elkin, I., Shea, T., & Watkins, J. (1989). National Institute of Mental Health treatment of depression collaborative research program: General effectiveness of treatments. *Archives of General Psychiatry, 46,* 971–982.

Last, J. M. (Ed.). (1988). *A dictionary of epidemiology.* New York: Springer-Verlag.

Templer, D. I., Spencer, D. A., & Hartlage, L. C. (1993). *Biosocial psychopathology: Epidemiological perspectives.* New York: Springer.

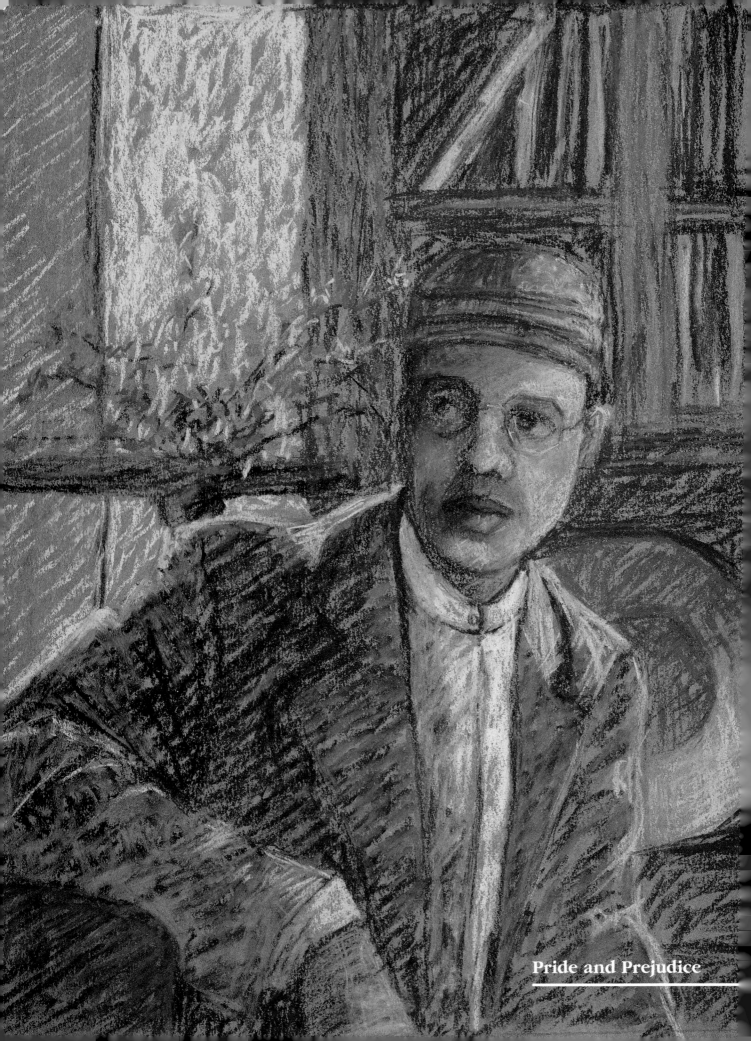

Pride and Prejudice

ETHICAL AND LEGAL BASES FOR CARE

Lawrence E. Frisch

Power and Control

Individuals usually seek nursing care when they are ill, at risk for illness, or dependent in some way. Thus, nurses continually encounter clients who are vulnerable and in need of protection. Consider the following:

◆ When you provide care to compensate for a client's self-care deficit, what kind of power do you have over that client?

◆ When you participate in decisions regarding a psychiatric client's treatment plan, what kind of control do you have over the client?

Professional nurses are in a position of power and control over other human beings, those clients under their care. The nurse is generally regarded by the public as compassionate—the health care professional who is present to care for and support others.

Nurses must forever maintain the public trust and, to do so, must continually examine the roles of power and control in nursing practice. As you read this chapter, take time to reflect on these issues in your day-to-day work. Keeping a journal that identifies situations of either power or control may be particularly helpful in encouraging you to reflect on moral, ethical, and legal behaviors.

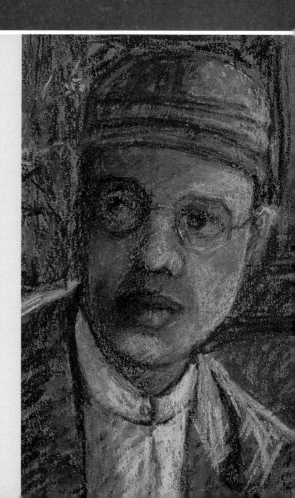

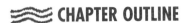

CHAPTER OUTLINE

ETHICAL ISSUES IN PSYCHIATRIC MENTAL HEALTH NURSING

Normative Ethics

Ethical Theories

Ethics and the Law

Making Ethical Decisions

Ethical Actions for the Social Good

LEGAL ISSUES IN PSYCHIATRIC MENTAL HEALTH NURSING

Clients' Rights
    Right to Privacy
    Right to Keep Personal Items
    Right to Enter into Legal Contracts
    Right of Habeas Corpus
    Right to Informed Consent
    Right to Refuse Treatment

Legal Issues in Hospitalization and Inpatient Treatment

Legal Issues Related to Care in the Community

Professional Negligence
    Failure to Prevent Dangerous Client Behavior
    Sexual Involvement with Clients
    Breaching Confidentiality
    Failure to Honor Individual Rights

Control of Violent or Self-Destructive Behaviors

COMPETENCIES

Upon completion of this chapter, the reader should be able to:

1. Describe the legal parameters and nursing responsibilities related to:
   - Clients' rights
   - Confidentiality
   - Psychological competence
   - Informed consent
   - Right to refuse treatment
   - Involuntary hospitalization
   - Professional negligence
   - Violent or self-destructive clients

2. Define the ethical theories of utilitarianism and deontology.

3. Identify the principles that guide practice decisions in psychiatric mental health nursing, including autonomy, beneficence, fidelity, justice, and non-maleficence.

4. Use the Value Analysis Model for evaluation of ethical dilemmas.

KEY TERMS

Abandonment   Negligence in which a client is left in need without alternatives for treatment.

Autonomy   Individual's right to self-determination and independence.

Beneficence   Belief that all treatments must be for the client's good.

Civil Commitment   Period of hospitalization requested by a mental health provider following an emergency hospitalization.

Code of Ethics   Positive statements and guidelines of what persons should do.

Competency to Stand Trial   Judgment that an individual is able to understand the nature of legal proceedings and is able to tell his or her own story to an attorney and the court.

Conservator   Person appointed to handle the estate of another person who is judged incompetent.

Deontology   Theory founded on human duties to others and the principles on which these duties are based.

Emergency Hospitalization   Power of states to detain a person in an emergency situation for a limited time until further evaluation and court proceedings can occur.

Ethics   Branch of philosophy that considers how behavioral principles guiding human interactions can be analyzed and set.

Fidelity   Individual's obligation to honor commitments and contracts.

Incompetence State of an individual with a mental disorder that causes inability to make judgments and renders the person unable to handle his or her own affairs.

Justice Principle ensuring fairness, equity, and honesty in decisions.

Least Restrictive Alternative Legal principle requiring that clients be treated with the least amount of constraint of liberty consistent with their safety.

Malpractice Negligence in the medical field that results in harm.

M'Naghten Test Legal definition of lack of guilt of a crime by virtue of insanity.

Negligence Behaving in a way in which a prudent individual would *not* have behaved or failing to use the diligence and care expected of a reasonable individual in similar circumstances.

Nonmaleficence Belief that care providers must do no harm.

Normative Ethics Guidelines and procedures useful in establishing moral decisions and actions.

Physical Restraint Use of an apparatus that significantly inhibits mobility.

Probate Proceedings Judicial hearing to determine the competence of an individual to manage personal affairs.

Seclusion State of a client being put in an isolated room or cell.

Tarasoff Duty to Warn Legal obligation of health care professionals to advise potential victims of violence so that the potential victim may seek protection.

Utilitarianism Theory based on the principle that an ethical decision serves to produce the greatest good for the greatest number of persons.

Every working day, nurses confront a variety of ethical and legal issues that arise in the course of providing care that respects each client as an individual. Nursing actions in psychiatric care must be consistent with the Nurse Practice Act of the state in which the nurse is practicing and also with laws governing clients' rights and society's interests should the two come into conflict. The purpose of this chapter is to review ethical principles and legal issues applied to psychiatric care so that the nurse will have additional tools to analyze situations and make considered and defensible judgments. The chapter is divided into two parts, covering first the ethical and then the legal perspectives on practice.

ETHICAL ISSUES IN PSYCHIATRIC MENTAL HEALTH NURSING

Many real-life situations are highly emotional and people cannot always assess their options and choices dispassionately. Even when truly dispassionate reflection is possible, reasonable individuals do not always come to the same decision. Philosophers have long recognized the difficulties posed by complex decisions involving alternative courses of action and competing personal and group interests. Such decisions, difficult as they are, must be made every day in health care as well as in other fields. In recent years ethicists have tried to define rules and procedures useful in providing guidance for human decisions and actions. This philosophical effort is often called the study of **normative ethics**. Normative ethics is a core discipline for nursing education, and nowhere is it more important than in the field of psychiatric mental health nursing.

Normative Ethics

Ethics is the branch of philosophy that considers how behavioral principles guiding human interactions can be analyzed and set. Normative ethics tries to establish parameters and guidelines for making human moral decisions. The study of ethics can help uncover guiding principles that allow one to describe and value differing human interactions, but individuals must still rely on moral and religious guidance as they decide how to react when confronted with various ethical dilemmas. While many persons may live most of their lives without confronting a major ethical dilemma or decision, this is not true for nurses, who typically confront such issues on virtually any working day. Nurses are sometimes frustrated to discover that ethical study cannot tell them precisely how to behave in any given situation, but understanding the basic principles of ethics can help with responsible ethical decision-making.

✪ *REFLECTIVE THINKING*

Considerations of Homelessness and Well-Being

Harold is a man about 30 years old who lives in a small community in California. He is homeless and lives on the streets, in camps in a forest outside of town, or on the beach. He is frequently seen pacing in town during the day; many in the community know him by name. He often responds to voices that others do not hear and talks and gestures as if someone is present although there is no one with him. He gets food from a food bank some of the time, but he is often observed picking through discarded food in public garbage cans.

Harold has never committed an act of violence (to anyone's knowledge). He appears to have no family or friends, as he is always alone. A community social worker has been able to arrange for Harold to receive support from various community agencies from time to time. She has offered to take Harold to see a mental health worker for evaluation and possible treatment, but Harold refuses to go. The district public health nurse has also approached Harold and offered basic health care services, including a physical assessment. Again, Harold has refused treatment.

The social worker and nurse are both concerned for Harold's well-being. They would like to have him evaluated and treated. The nurse has stated that she believes any moral society would ensure that Harold had treatment, care, shelter, and food.

- ◆ What ethical principles come into conflict when considering Harold's case?
- ◆ What do you think is the best action for society to take in a case such as this?

Many of the dilemmas that nurses face are encountered as legal problems; for example, the nurse wanting to mandate treatment for a homeless person finds that there are laws prohibiting her from forcing the individual into treatment. Legislators have already confronted these dilemmas and in an effort to ensure "right" behavior have constructed laws. While laws often originate as an attempt to promote ethical behavior, law and ethics are quite separate concepts. Law most commonly involves what are called negative duties, which dictate what persons must *not* do. Ethical principles dictate positive duties—those activities one *should* do. The familiar "golden rule" is a generalized statement of the importance of positive duties: "Do unto others as you would have them do unto you." These kinds of positive statements of what persons should do are more commonly found in **codes of ethics**.

The American Nurses Association (ANA) published a code of ethics for nurses in the 1960s, covering all aspects of nursing practice. This code is currently being revised and updated. In 1994 the American Holistic Nurses' Association published the *Code of Ethics for Holistic Nurses* (see the accompanying display), which includes many of the principles of other nursing ethical codes (responsibilities toward clients and coworkers and protection of the client from harmful acts). In addition, this code adds provision for nurses' responsibilities toward self and the environment and their behavior toward other nurses.

The ANA Council on Psychiatric and Mental Health Nursing has set standards of professional performance, which guide psychiatric nursing practice (ANA, 1994). The core of these standards is that the relationship between a nurse and client is therapeutic and professional. The standards further specify that the nurse maintains confidentiality, functions as a client advocate, and is nonjudgmental and nondiscriminatory. Other standards specify the importance of reporting illegal or unethical practices, obtaining informed consent, and maintaining appropriate personal boundaries with clients. Standard V of the Council on Psychiatric and Mental Health Nursing Standards specifically deals with ethics by stating: "The psychiatric-mental health nurse's decisions and actions on behalf of clients are determined in an ethical manner." The purpose of the following discussion is to highlight how nurses in psychiatric mental health practice can maintain behaviors that are both professional and ethical.

Ethical Theories

There are two broad ethical theories that can guide the development of professional ethics: the theories of utilitarianism and deontology. **Utilitarianism** is based on the principle that an ethical decision serves to produce the greatest good for the greatest number of persons involved. While many ethical theorists endorse utilitarian thinking, many nursing ethicists find deontological analysis more helpful in approaching common clinical dilemmas. **Deontology** looks at human duties to others and tries to analyze the principles on which these duties are based. The basic deontological principles are autonomy, beneficence, fidelity, justice, and nonmaleficence. **Autonomy** refers to the client's right to self-determination and independence. **Beneficence** is the view that all treatments must be for the client's good. **Fidelity** is an individual's obligation to be faithful to commitments and contracts. **Justice** is the principle ensuring fairness, equity, and honesty in decisions. **Nonmaleficence** is the view that, above all, care providers must do no harm.

Ethical principles assert that mental health professionals adopt an attitude of respect for persons, ensure that clients make their treatment decisions without coercion (the principle of autonomy), and work for their

AMERICAN HOLISTIC NURSES' ASSOCIATION CODE OF ETHICS

We believe that the fundamental responsibilities of the nurse are to promote health, facilitate healing and alleviate suffering. The need for nursing is universal. Inherent in nursing is the respect for life, dignity and right of all persons. Nursing care is given in a context mindful of the holistic nature of humans, understanding the body-mind-spirit connection. Nursing care is unrestricted by considerations of nationality, race, creed, color, age, sex, sexual preference, politics or social status. Given that nurses practice in culturally diverse settings, professional nurses must have an understanding of the cultural background of clients in order to provide culturally appropriate interventions.

Nurses render services to clients who can be individuals, families, groups or communities. The client is an active participant in health care and should be included in all nursing care planning decisions.

In order to provide services to others, each nurse has a responsibility toward him/herself. In addition, nurses have defined responsibilities towards the client, co-workers, nursing practice, the profession of nursing, society and the environment.

NURSES AND SELF

The nurse has a responsibility to model health behaviors. Holistic nurses strive to achieve harmony in their own lives and assist others striving to do the same.

NURSES AND THE CLIENT

The nurse's primary responsibility is to the client needing nursing care. The nurse strives to see the client as a whole, and provides care which is professionally appropriate and culturally consonant. The nurse holds in confidence all information obtained in professional practice, and uses professional judgment in disclosing such information. The nurse enters into a relationship with the client that is guided by mutual respect and a desire for growth and development.

NURSES AND CO-WORKERS

The nurse maintains cooperative relationship with co-workers in nursing and other fields. Nurses have a responsibility to nurture each other, and to assist nurses to work as a team in the interest of client care. If a client's care is endangered by a co-worker, the nurse must take appropriate action on behalf of the client.

NURSES AND NURSING PRACTICE

The nurse carries personal responsibility for practice and for maintaining continued competence. Nurses have the right to utilize all appropriate nursing interventions, and have the obligation to determine the efficacy and safety of all nursing actions. Wherever applicable, nurses utilize research findings in directing practice.

NURSES AND THE PROFESSION

The nurse plays a role in determining and implementing desirable standards of nursing practice and education. Holistic nurses may assume a leadership position to guide the profession toward holism. Nurses support nursing research and the development of holistically oriented nursing theories. The nurse participates in establishing and maintaining equitable social and economic working conditions in nursing.

NURSES AND SOCIETY

The nurse, along with other citizens, has responsibility for initiating and supporting actions to meet the health and social needs of the public.

NURSES AND THE ENVIRONMENT

The nurse strives to manipulate the client's environment to become one of peace, harmony, and nurturance so that healing may take place. The nurse considers the health of the ecosystem in relation to the need for health, safety and peace of all persons.

From *Code of Ethics for Holistic Nurses*, by American Holistic Nurses' Association, 1995, Raleigh, NC: Author. Reprinted with permission.

clients' well-being (the principle of beneficence). Ethical standards typically endorse the importance of professional behavior and responsibility (the principle of fidelity). Certain activities—for example, sexual relationships with clients—are prohibited as being explicitly unethical because these activities could bring harm to the client (the principle of nonmaleficence). The principle of justice is less prominent in professional codes of ethics than are the other principles. Perhaps this is because in

American society, neither health nor mental health care has been defined to be a universal right.

Ethics and the Law

Nurses should recognize that conflict between the law and ethics may be unavoidable. Involuntary psychiatric commitment, a seemingly essential means to prevent harm to a mentally ill individual or others around him, is

⊚⊚ *REFLECTIVE THINKING*

Autonomy

Your neighbor has been judged to be unable to make rational decisions. He is 80 years old, lives alone, and has appeared "forgetful" to you. He is about to be placed in a nursing home against his expressed wishes.

◆ How do you feel about this situation?

◆ At what point is commitment acceptable to you? What behaviors make it so?

STEPS OF VALUE ANALYSIS MODEL

1. Identify and clarify the value question.

2. Assemble purported facts.

3. Assess the truth of purported facts.

4. Clarify the relevance of the facts.

5. Arrive at a tentative value decision.

6. Test the value principle implied by the decision.

◆ Does the value principle fit in the current situation?

◆ Does the value principle fit in other, similar situations?

◆ Would the value principle fit if the client were your mother? Your father? Your spouse? Your child?

◆ Would the value principle fit if you were the client?

---

provided for by the laws of every state but flagrantly violates the principle of autonomy. Autonomy establishes that a person can make free choices even if those choices result in personal harm. Commitment law is based on the premise that if there is reason to doubt an individual's ability to make fully rational decisions, the principle of beneficence takes priority over that of autonomy.

Ethical conflicts and dilemmas are often accompanied by highly emotional circumstances that may not be fully conducive to patient and rational consideration. The very presence of conflict or emotion suggests the likelihood of an ethical dimension. When faced with such a crisis, the nurse should reflect on the ethical principles: Autonomy, beneficence, and nonmaleficence are usually the critical principles to consider. When doubt arises, nurses often use techniques in helping them consider all aspects of the ethical dilemma. One such technique, the Value Analysis Model, is discussed below.

Making Ethical Decisions

The Value Analysis Model is a classic model for use in evaluating a dilemma (Coombs & Meux, 1971; Frisch, 1987). This model is a formal method of analysis to assist individuals in making value judgments when facing ethical dilemmas. The model emphasizes the need for careful evaluation and weighing of facts prior to drawing conclusions regarding ethical problems. The model requires the nurse to complete six steps of analysis before drawing conclusions regarding the issue. The steps are presented in the accompanying box. The initial steps of the analysis force the nurse to articulate the value questions and assemble facts regarding the question. Thus, the nurse must search for data supporting claims regarding action. Next, the nurse must judge assembled facts according to their truth or validity as well as determine whether the arguments presented by others have relevance for the situation at hand. The nurse must give plausible and rational arguments for each decision. Completing the analysis of facts, the nurse must arrive at a tentative value

decision and go on to test the value principle implied in that decision by hypothetically putting self in the position of all persons involved by the decision. It is recommended that the nurse complete the entire process before attempting conclusions about the issue. The reader is encouraged to think about moral and ethical judgments that arise in psychiatric mental health practice and use this model in analyzing the dilemmas that arise, as the model has proved helpful to many (Frisch, 1987).

Ethical Actions for the Social Good

Nurses may occasionally disagree with specific laws or with the ethical analysis underlying them. For example, the nurse may believe that health professionals should have the right to medicate clients who are delusional and unable to function fully in society because the nurse believes that medication will lead to a more positive adjustment and quality of life for the client. In such a case the nurse may choose to work actively to identify those specific situations where the nurse believes the law should change and may take action to bring about a change in the law. There are certainly instances in which nurse activists and nurse legislators have brought about legal changes that greatly benefit their clients. Occasionally, such changes may require actions of civil disobedience. Nurses and other mental health professionals risk being judged guilty of unethical behavior if they violate laws, even laws they judge to be against the interests of their clients.

LEGAL ISSUES IN PSYCHIATRIC MENTAL HEALTH NURSING

Law has relevance in nearly all aspects of nursing practice, but in no other area of nursing is the law more intimately involved than in psychiatric mental health nursing. Psychiatric clients may:

◆ Be placed in treatment against their will

◆ Pose a risk to themselves

◆ Have been judged to have committed a crime while legally insane

◆ Be unable or unwilling to consent to treatment

◆ Be incapable of fully understanding medication risks

◆ Require restraint for their safety or that of others

◆ Make threats that obligate their caretakers to warn potential victims

◆ Undergo forensic evaluation that requires the nurse to testify in court

In each of these circumstances, the client's rights and society's interests may, and often do, come into conflict. In such cases, laws are often designed to clarify the conflicting interests involved. Unfortunately, at times the laws themselves seem contradictory on the subject of mental health treatment. Some statutes ensure that clients cannot be forced into treatment; others require that treatment be offered to certain subgroups of the mentally ill but not to others. To a nurse practicing psychiatric mental health nursing, such contradictions are visible every day. For example, in most communities, the practicing mental health nurse will find no shortage of untreated mentally ill clients who have access to care but choose to exercise their legal right of refusal. At the same time, most nurses encounter individuals actively seeking mental health assistance who are denied care because they lack satisfactory insurance coverage. Laws attempt to provide for the public good and public safety, but rarely do the laws offer comprehensive solutions to social problems such as how a community is to support a homeless individual who is mentally ill and refusing treatment. Instead, laws set out series of rules and procedures and often penalize those who fail to follow those procedures. The following sections, while not intended to make the reader an expert in mental health law, will provide a general introduction. Experience in local clinical placements will help nurses become acquainted with the specific regulations and procedures that apply in their communities.

Clients' Rights

While the law is based on the complementary social concepts of responsibilities (duties) and rights (privileges), many 20th-century Americans have come to view laws almost exclusively in terms of rights rather than responsibilities. The last half of the 20th century saw a remarkable extension of legal rights to groups and individuals who had previously been inadequately protected. Among the groups who benefited most from this extension of rights were the mentally ill. Not only has national and local legislation been drafted to protect the mentally ill from unwanted treatment and other loss of personal liberty, but a number of voluntary agencies have attempted to define appropriate treatment standards. For example, the American Hospital Association has issued a statement of Patients' Bill of Rights, which many health care agencies have adopted. The combination of legal protection and voluntary codes has had an important impact on the practice of psychiatric mental health nursing. In the following sections, specific client rights and legal protections will be discussed.

Right to Privacy

Privacy is the right of any client to keep personal information secret. Thus, any client has the right to keep the fact that he is in treatment to himself. He may not wish for his spouse, employers, friends, or others to know that he is receiving care. In honoring that right, professional codes of behavior frequently state that confidentiality must not be breached. Laws, however, rarely state that the nurse *must* maintain confidentiality, as laws more commonly define negative rather than positive duties. Thus, it is generally recognized that the nurse has an obligation to maintain confidentiality, and in any situation where a client can show that a breach of confidentiality has caused the client damage (e.g., damage to his reputation), the client may sue the nurse in civil court for inappropriate disclosure of professional, confidential information.

∽ *REFLECTIVE THINKING*

Releasing Information

You are a nurse working on a chemical dependence unit, and you answer the telephone at the nurses' station. A woman who tells you she is Mrs. Anderson is calling. Mrs. Anderson states that her son, Joe, was admitted to your unit last night, and she is very concerned about his condition. She is asking you for an update on his status. Joe Anderson is a 20-year-old young man who was admitted during the night.

◆ What do you tell Mrs. Anderson?

◆ What do you say if the caller says, "I'm from the Police Department and need to know if Joe Anderson, who is wanted for arrest, is at the hospital"?

While laws in every state differ, most states have laws that do allow the nurse to discuss a client case with a supervisor or with other members of the treating team. However, nurses and other mental health providers cannot release information to a client's family members without explicit permission, and this information includes disclosing that their family member is in the hospital or is being seen at the mental health clinic. Further, nurses may not disclose client information to other nurses or other health professionals who are not involved with direct care or service to that client. If such disclosure occurs, the nurse is legally liable for any resulting harm experienced by the client. For example, a psychiatrist was successfully sued for revealing information to a client's spouse when that information appeared to contribute to a subsequent divorce (*MacDonald v. Clinger*, 1982).

Best clinical practice dictates that in order to release client information, the nurse should have written consent (a signed release-of-information form), and the consent should be specific as to the information to be released. In some cases, however, the nurse may release information without written consent, for example, if the nurse has the client's verbal consent to discuss information with a specific person. Caution should always be taken when requests come to the nurse to release information over the telephone, as it is not possible to identify the caller. A nurse should never disclose information to a person who cannot be positively identified.

Mental health information may have detrimental effects if it is released to employers, insurance carriers, or others whose interest is not primarily therapeutic. Nurses must ensure and document that their clients have considered (and are able to understand) any risks that might occur as a result of the client's authorization for records release. In most cases the client should be allowed (or even encouraged) to see the contents of any records being released. If for some reason this cannot be done, it is important that the nurse be certain of the client's intent that specific records be released and to document the reason for that certainty.

There are several situations, however, in which laws related to privacy and confidentiality allow different actions than discussed in the previous paragraph. These are described following:

1. Mental health evaluations done for reasons other than direct client care: Examples of such evaluations include court-ordered exams, disability determinations, and employment physicals. These examinations are done for the benefit of a third party, and the reports are sent to this third individual or agency. By agreeing to participate in the evaluation, the client waives some confidentiality rights. The client should be told at the onset of the evaluation who will see the completed report and that confidentiality may not be fully ensurable.

2. The case of minors: Parents can usually be given details of their child's mental health treatment. However, older adolescents living on their own are usually considered "emancipated," and parents may not have a right to information concerning their mental health. These issues are usually treated in mental health statutes, which vary from state to state. Nurses should be sure they understand laws that apply to the care of minors in their respective states and can usually obtain information from the administrators and/or legal counsel of the psychiatric facility in which they work.

3. Issues of violence and safety: Confidentiality can (and *must*) be breached in certain situations where the nurse has reason to suspect child abuse, elder abuse (see Chapter 24), or that an individual may be at risk to harm specific other persons. The latter situation, involving "duty to warn," is discussed in more detail later in this chapter.

Right to Keep Personal Items

When a client enters treatment in a facility—hospital, board-and-care home, halfway house, or nursing home—the client still maintains rights to his personal property. When storage of items becomes difficult, the client can be asked to leave some of his items at home. However, if a client has items of value, the nurse is obligated to document the items and store them in the safe or other secure place. Removing items from a client may be considered theft if the nurse takes them away and either loses them or refuses to return them. In situations where the nursing staff have professional justification to remove potentially harmful objects such as knives, guns, or scissors, the nurse must recognize that the objects are still owned by the client and can be removed only during the time of hospitalization or treatment.

Right to Enter into Legal Contracts

A client maintains his legal rights as a citizen. Thus, if an adult, the client has a right to vote, get married, sign for a mortgage, write a personal last will and testament, and manage personal financial affairs or control personal funds.

There are some situations, however, when a client is deemed not responsible (hence not accountable) for his own actions. In these cases, mental health professionals are often called upon to assess individuals' competence both in and outside of mental health care settings. Judgments of competence may have important consequences in determining whether an individual can continue to manage his own finances, whether he should be placed in a nursing home or other supervised living environment against his will, or whether he can appropriately make decisions about his own medical and psychological treatment. At times, competence judgments are required to assess whether an accused person can stand trial or was sane at the time a crime was committed. While the issues in each of these situations are similar, the details of competency assessments vary between them and from individual to individual.

Probate proceedings are often carried out to establish a judicial ruling that an individual is or is not competent to manage activities. These are court proceedings wherein a judge hears evidence on the individual's ability to function and makes a judgment of "competence" or "incompetence." **Incompetence** is a legal term reflecting that the individual has a mental disorder, the disorder causes inability to make judgments, and the disorder renders the person unable to handle his or her own affairs. Such probate proceedings can result in the appointment of a **conservator** of the person or a conservator of the estates for persons whose mental status makes them unable to care for their daily needs or to handle their financial affairs. Many mentally ill, retarded, or demented individuals will need conservators, and some states allow an individual to select his or her own conservator (subject to court approval). Limited conservatorships may be defined to act in certain specific areas, leaving the person some residual personal or financial responsibilities without explicit oversight. Nurses may be asked to testify in such proceedings.

A ruling of incompetence means that the individual cannot enter into contracts and further deprives the person of rights such as voting and, in some cases, driving. Such rights may be restored to the individual only through another court hearing.

A related concept of relevance to the psychiatric nurse is **competency to stand trial**. Competence to stand trial requires that an individual be able to understand the nature of legal proceedings and be able to cogently tell his own story to his attorney and the court. At times mental health professionals must assist the court in judging whether an individual was sane at the time a crime was committed. While successful insanity defenses are often highly publicized, less than 1 percent of criminal defendants are judged legally insane (Swenson, 1993, p. 214). Such judgments usually involve the **M'Naghten test**, sometimes also called the M'Naghten rule. This legal definition was put forth after a famous 19th-century murder trial in which Daniel M'Naghten was found not guilty by virtue of insanity. As any reader of Charles Dickens knows, public opinion in Victorian England was strongly in favor of vigorous punishment for wrongdoing. M'Naghten's commitment to a mental hospital, in lieu of execution, caused a huge public outcry, and the Queen ordered a judicial reexamination of the basis for the insanity defense (Swenson, 1993, p. 215). This judicial review established two criteria for legal responsibility that are still used over 150 years later. The M'Naghten test requires that if a defendant either does not know the significance of her action or does not know it was wrong,

then she cannot be held legally accountable. While the M'Naghten test remains important and useful, it fails to apply to the mentally ill individual who, for any of a variety of reasons, lacks the ability to control his behavior even if he knows that behavior is wrong and harmful. In recent years courts have expanded the "insanity defense" to apply also to acts seemingly not within an individual's control.

Right of Habeas Corpus

Habeas corpus is a right protected by the U.S. Constitution that permits a speedy legal hearing and evaluation for any individual who claims he is being detained illegally. In such a hearing, a judge (and at times a jury as well) hears evidence and makes a determination of whether or not the individual may be released or detained for psychiatric treatment.

Right to Informed Consent

Informed consent is fundamental to all medical treatment and must be obtained whenever there is a potential for harm from any therapeutic intervention. Clients have the right to be given clear information about treatment options, risks, benefits, and alternatives. They may have the right to refuse treatments that are offered to them. Informed consent presumes that clients are mentally competent, as defined above. It is important to recognize that individuals may be judged legally competent to consent to (or refuse) treatment despite elements of irrational thought or behavior (Merz & Fischoff, 1990). To give consent, an individual must be alert and oriented, must understand the procedure or treatment being offered, and must freely (without coercion) accept the treatment. Courts frequently regard consent as informed when clients can actively communicate their choice of therapies and can show that they understand information provided to them (Simon, 1992, p. 126).

To obtain informed consent, the standards of communication of risk to psychiatric clients do not differ from those applying to any other clients; that is, major risks need to be described, but there is no need to be exhaustive in listing all possible harms from a therapy (DHHS, 1982). The importance of communicating risks is greatest when alternative treatments are available that may be safer.

Informed consent is a legal requirement in all states, but the nature of the required consent may differ among states. Under some circumstances the law requires written consent, and in most cases it is highly prudent for clinicians to obtain written consent for treatments that have any risk of adverse outcome. There are several situations in which the requirement for consent may be waived or significantly modified. For example, in a genuine emergency, physicians and other licensed caregivers are obligated to do whatever is required to treat or protect a client. For example, if any individual is brought to an emergency room comatose and in need of life-saving treatment, the emergency department staff are expected to provide immediate care. It is important to define emergencies with accuracy. Some states have statutory definitions of emergencies that clarify when informed consent can be dispensed with. Even in the absence of such definitions, it is risky to forego informed consent unless the client's safety and/or well-being would be threatened by any necessary delay in treatment.

Documented consent is of utmost importance for somatic treatments, especially hospitalization, the prescription of drugs, and the administration of electroshock.

Right to Refuse Treatment

Of clients' legal rights, the right to refuse treatment is among the most important. No different than other clients, psychiatric clients have the right to consent to treatment, to refuse specific treatments, and, where consent has been given, to withdraw consent. To threaten to give treatment or to actually force treatment without consent leaves the nurse criminally liable for charges of assault and battery.

An issue of particular importance to psychiatric nursing is consent to take medications. There are legally identified situations where clients may not have the right to refuse psychiatric hospitalization. However, once hospitalized, the law generally gives individuals the right to decide whether or not to be treated with medication. Psychiatrists have, not surprisingly, expressed their concern about a "legal system that orders people into mental hospitals and then orders psychiatrists not to treat them" (Stone, 1981, p. 358). This concern is made even more acute because not only do mental health providers risk liability if they treat a client against his wishes, but they may also (rarely) be sued for *not* treating a client who refuses such treatment (*Whitree v. State*, 1968).

Most treatment refusals focus on antipsychotic medications and are based on real concerns that use of these medications may lead to permanent neurological disability (most commonly tardive dyskinesia, discussed in Chapters 12 and 25). In a well-known case, the New York Supreme Court ruled that under certain conditions, medication could be given to clients against their will when four considerations were explicitly taken into account:

1. The client's liberty interests (freedom to travel, right to autonomy)
2. The client's best interests
3. The benefits of treatment
4. The available less intrusive alternative treatments (*Rivers v. Katz*, 1986)

These considerations may not apply in other states, but do provide fairly clear guidelines for medication decision-making.

☯ *REFLECTIVE THINKING*

Right to Refuse Treatment

Mrs. Wenzel is a middle-aged woman diagnosed as having schizophrenia, paranoid type. She lives with her daughter Wendy and son-in-law and is generally happy with her living arrangement. She is independent in her daily activities. She does take medication for her schizophrenia and has monthly visits with her psychiatrist. She helps with the housework and cooking and volunteers some of her time to do filing and office work at a local community recreational center.

Over the past month, Wendy has noticed that Mrs. Wenzel has a skin lesion on her left forearm that is raised and dark in color and had not been noticed before. At Wendy's urging, Mrs. Wenzel agrees to see the family doctor about this lesion. Dr. Percens immediately raises strong concerns that the lesion could be a melanoma and recommends that the lesion be biopsied and removed. Dr. Percens explains that the lesion could be a form of skin cancer and that without treatment this cancer could lead to metastases and death.

Mrs. Wenzel refuses treatment, stating, "I don't like needles!" She and Wendy go home, and Wendy again urges her mother to reconsider having the lesion treated. At this point, Mrs. Wenzel becomes agitated and anxious and says, "This spot is nothing. Doctors just want money and tell us to do things we don't need to do!" She goes on to say, "If you take off this spot, I will lose my soul—I don't want to lose my soul." The more Wendy raises the issue, the more upset and agitated Mrs. Wenzel becomes.

Wendy, concerned for her mother's health, makes an appointment to talk with Dr. Percens regarding her mother's refusal of the treatment. Dr. Percens explains that the lesion very likely is a melanoma, but also explains that Mrs. Wenzel has the right to either consent to or refuse the biopsy.

Wendy then contacts Mrs. Wenzel's psychiatrist regarding her mother's refusal of treatment, her agitation, and her delusion that removing the lesion is connected with her soul. Psychiatric evaluation indicates that Mrs. Wenzel is alert and oriented, able to talk coherently about her reasons for refusing treatment, and able to state that she understands that Dr. Percens believes this "spot" could be a cancer.

- ◆ Does Mrs. Wenzel have a life-threatening condition?
- ◆ What do you think Wendy and the physicians should do?
- ◆ Do you think there are grounds for court-ordered treatment?

RESEARCH HIGHLIGHT

Medication against the Client's Will

STUDY PROBLEM/PURPOSE

To uncover client attitudes after involuntary medication.

METHODS

Researchers interviewed a group of 24 individuals who had been confined involuntarily to psychiatric hospitals and medicated against their will; the interviews took place after discharge.

FINDINGS

Seventeen of the 24 persons (70.8%) felt that the decision to medicate them was correct and that if a similar situation arose again, they would want to be given medication, even if they once again refused it vehemently.

IMPLICATIONS

After the fact, a majority of clients indicated that they believed that the medication was in their own best interests, regardless of their feelings at the time of medication administration.

From "Autonomy and the Right to Refuse Treatment: Patients' Attitudes after Involuntary Medication," by H. I. Schwartz, W. Vingiano, and C. B. Perez, 1988, *Hospital and Community Psychiatry, 39*, pp. 1049–1055.

Another very difficult situation in psychiatric care occurs when a client refuses treatment for a physical condition based on thought processes that are part of the psychiatric illness, for example, a client who refuses to go to the dentist because the client believes that dental tools carry evil radio waves harmful to the client. In such cases, the client's family can petition a court for power of attorney to give consent for treatment. In all cases, however, the much-preferred approach is to work with the client over time so that he may give consent for care himself.

Individuals committed for psychiatric care because of criminal behavior raise a particularly difficult societal problem. Such persons would seem to lose some liberties because the purpose of their commitment should be rehabilitative. Some court decisions have allowed involuntary medication of committed persons following crimes (*Stensvad v. Reivitz*, 1985). A more recent United States Supreme Court case, *Washington v. Harper* (Applebaum, 1990), allowed medication against an incarcerated person's will when the individual was a danger to himself or others and when the proposed medications were clearly in the person's best interests. In this decision, the court seemed to endorse the use of professional review panels within the hospital to decide whether or not to medicate against a client's wishes. The court observed that such panels generally provide adequate constitutional protection and are more likely to decide in the client's interest than are medically naive judges. This argument may eventually have some impact on procedures for decision-making in medication refusal situations, but at present these decisions almost always end up being made in a courtroom.

Legal Issues in Hospitalization and Inpatient Treatment

A client may be admitted to a hospital voluntarily or through a court-ordered commitment. About half of the admissions to psychiatric hospitals are voluntary and occur when a client seeks treatment of his own free choice. For admission to be voluntary, the client must have knowledge of the facility, its appearance, and the conditions of his hospitalization there and must be informed of alternatives to hospital care.

For the other half of admissions to psychiatric hospitals, clients are admitted involuntarily through proceedings of emergency hospitalization or civil commitment. **Emergency hospitalization** is the power of states to detain a person in an emergency situation for a limited time until further evaluation and court proceedings can occur. Emergency hospitalization is usually for a short period only, typically 48 to 72 hours, and allows the need for longer inpatient treatment to be assessed. In most jurisdictions, emergency hospitalization is legally based in police powers and can generally be invoked only when an individual is judged potentially harmful to himself or others.

After the 48- to 72-hour period has lapsed, legally empowered mental health providers (usually psychiatrists) can petition the court for a lengthier period of hospitalization. This lengthier involuntary hospitalization is known as **civil commitment**. Procedures for approving or denying civil commitment vary from state to state but almost always involve a court hearing. In such hearings the court may use a standard of "clear and convincing evidence," which is lower than the "beyond a reasonable doubt" standard used in criminal cases. Once an individual is committed to involuntary mental hospitalization, periodic judicial case reviews are required on a regular basis but no less than yearly. Long-term commitment almost always requires evidence that the individual remains dangerous either to self or to others (Simon, 1992, p. 157).

Depending on where they work, psychiatric nurses may also encounter clients who have been involuntarily hospitalized through the criminal justice system. These individuals have been judged either guilty of crimes or not guilty by reason of insanity, and they have been criminally committed for treatment. This form of involuntary hospitalization is very different from involuntary commitment initiated by a psychiatrist, as the client is in the criminal justice system, not the health care system. (Refer to Chapter 20 for specific information on care of the incarcerated.)

REFLECTIVE THINKING

Informed Consent

Mrs. Roebuck is a 50-year-old, married woman with a history of depression. Today, she was brought to the emergency room by her husband, who found her at home this afternoon. She has self-inflicted, superficial cuts on each wrist and states she has been drinking both beer and wine today. She is crying, stating, "I don't care what happens to me." She requires treatment (stitches) for the wounds on her wrist, although the bleeding has stopped. The emergency room physician has requested a psychiatric consult for possible admission to the mental health unit.

Mrs. Roebuck is oriented to reality and states that she understands the hospital staff and her husband want to help her, but she says, "I'm too much trouble—I don't want your help." Further, she states, "I don't want anything! Just let me be, I don't want to live."

Mr. Roebuck says, "Please help us, she is not herself today."

◆ Under the circumstances, do you think Mrs. Roebuck gave informed consent for her treatment?

◆ Can the emergency room staff provide treatment for the wounds on her wrists, given her comment that she does not want help?

◆ Can the hospital staff and Mr. Roebuck hospitalize Mrs. Roebuck on the mental health unit without her consent?

REFLECTIVE THINKING

Informed Consent and the Community Health Nurse

At a team meeting, a group of community health nurses were discussing client families they had been visiting in their maternal-child program. Several of the families they were seeing had stress in the home following the birth of a baby, and the nurses offered education, support, and counseling during the home visit.

Community health nurses in this setting visit any mother with a new baby, and they frequently continue visiting during the postpartum period. When a nurse's assessment indicates stress in the home, increased numbers of visits are offered. Nurses keep records in the health department office to document the visits.

Janette, a new nurse to the health department, inquired if the families were all informed that records were kept at the health department office. Further, she asked if the clients knew the content of the records.

◆ Do nurses need to inform clients that written records are kept in this situation?

◆ How can conditions of informed consent be met in this situation?

Involuntarily hospitalized clients do not lose their civil rights and are not presumed legally incompetent solely because they have been committed. As noted earlier, most clients retain their right to refuse treatment, especially with potentially dangerous psychiatric medications. However, the law also provides that judicially committed individuals have a right to receive psychiatric treatment. Applicable state laws stipulate very little about the content or quality of mandated treatment in the community, and often the right to treatment applies only to inpatient settings. Hospitalized clients have a variety of other rights, such as those to visitation, control of funds, and privacy, that can only rarely be abridged and then only in the client's interests.

Legal Issues Related to Care in the Community

There are specific legal obligations for psychiatric nurses practicing in the community. These involve both informed consent and the concept of professional abandonment.

Many experts feel informed consent is required for individuals beginning psychotherapy (Simon, 1992, p. 135), for psychotherapy is a treatment, and a client must understand what psychotherapy is before granting consent. Informed consent to begin psychotherapy requires that the client be provided information about what is to be expected in the therapy sessions, how long the therapy may take, the fact that there will be records kept of the therapy visits, and how the bill for service is expected to be handled. Some clinicians assume that consent requires a client's signature on specially prepared consent forms, and indeed such a signature may document informed consent. However, a chart note describing what the clinician told the client and the clinician's perception of the degree of understanding and free choice involved is probably more important than a client's signature. In ideal practice, both a signature and a chart note would be completed.

All mental health professionals have an obligation to provide continuing care to their clients and to arrange appropriate follow-up care in the provider's absence. These clinicians make an implicit contract with their clients at the time of initiating care that they will provide

꩜ *REFLECTIVE THINKING*

Abandonment

Psychiatric nurse Linda has been providing individual and group therapy to clients in her community for 5 years. Linda is moving to another city and will be closing her practice.

◆ How do you think Linda should make this move, leaving about 20 active clients in her practice and many others whom she has not seen in several months?

◆ How does Linda leave her clients in a manner that is ethically and legally responsible?

continuing service. Failure to do so constitutes a breach of contract and could lead to accusations of **abandonment**, a form of negligence that stems from leaving a client in need without alternatives for treatment. At times, clinicians may choose to terminate care for one or more clients, either because the clinician is changing jobs or affiliations or because she finds the course of the client encounter unsatisfactory. Codes of conduct require that in such circumstances the clinician provide clear interpretation of her intent to the client and continue to see the client for a reasonable time until other care arrangements have been worked out. Failure to ensure such follow-up can leave the clinician open to a legal charge of abandonment. Nurses providing group or individual psychotherapy in any setting potentially risk an accusation of abandonment by the nature of their contract to provide continuing care to their clients.

Professional Negligence

Professional negligence in mental health care is a problem that all nurses need to understand and prevent. **Negligence** means either behaving in a way that a prudent individual would *not* have behaved or failing to use the diligence and care expected of a reasonable individual in similar circumstances. In situations where negligence has occurred, the nurse may be faced with a **malpractice** lawsuit, that is, a lawsuit where the client seeks recovery for damages caused by the nurse's negligent actions. It is probable that all health care providers are negligent on occasion, but most negligent events do not lead to serious client harm either through good fortune or because a colleague recognizes and corrects the negligent error. Negligence that results in harm to a client or that allows a client to harm someone else may involve the nurse in a lawsuit. Although lawsuits against psychiatrists and psychotherapists may be more common than those against nurses, certain situations likely pose a particular risk for all mental health professionals.

Failure to Prevent Dangerous Client Behavior

Mental health professionals have increasingly been held to high standards of accountability in predicting and preventing client danger. Thus, in situations where a client discloses that he is likely to inflict harm on himself or on others, the mental health professional is obligated to take action to prevent that harmful action.

All nurses should be aware of the **Tarasoff Duty to Warn** potential victims of violence that might be directed against them. If a mental health professional has any reason to believe that a client harbors thoughts of harm toward a specific individual or individuals, then she has a legal obligation to ensure that the potential victim is warned so that protection may be sought. In the Tarasoff case, a client informed his psychologist that he intended to kill a young woman acquaintance. The psychologist informed the police, who interviewed the man, but neither psychologist nor police warned the woman of the potential risk to her life. She was subsequently murdered by the client, and her parents brought successful suit for failure to warn. The Tarasoff Duty to Warn potential victims takes precedence over the duty to protect client confidentiality. Even if the client does not name a specific victim, warning is required if the therapist can reasonably deduce who is at risk. Lawsuits continue to occur over failure to warn, and while few if any have involved nurses, there is no reason to believe the Tarasoff Duty does not extend to the psychiatric nurse.

One of the corollaries of the Tarasoff Duty is that therapists are held accountable for their ability to correctly predict when a client is likely to be lethally violent. Prediction of any behavior is difficult, and clinical predictions of violence are generally not particularly accurate (Bednar, Bednar, Lambert, & Waite, 1991). The clinician is legally required to take threats very seriously and to be alert for historical data, such as poor impulse control, use of stimulant drugs, and prior violence, that might substantially increase the likelihood of recurrent violence. While courts do not require unreasonably accurate prediction, they may judge a nurse or other clinician negligent if due caution is not taken to assess, record, and act on potential warnings and risk factors for subsequent violent behavior.

Clinicians may also be held negligent if they fail to recognize suicidal risk. As with violence, this is a particularly difficult task because suicidal behavior is notoriously difficult to predict. Relatively few successful malpractice lawsuits are brought because of a client's suicide. Nonetheless, the nurse will always use her best skills to assess suicidal risk (see Chapter 14) and to contract with a potentially suicidal client. Providing and documenting information about 24-hour telephone support (usually through community hotlines) are helpful to clients and serve as evidence of careful clinical practice. Periodically assessing and documenting a client's mental competence will help detect delusions or other bizarre thought processes that might lead to suicide and will help provide evidence regarding the client's competency and state of mind in the event of a subsequent accusation of negligence.

Lawsuits are not an inevitable consequence of negligent care. Many clinical errors are not followed by lawsuit, even when considerable damage results. Suits seem to occur more frequently when clients fail to develop close, therapeutic relationships with their caregivers and feel residual anger, anger that is increased by unfavorable clinical occurrences. The nurse who cultivates professionally appropriate but close and nurturing relationships with clients very likely reduces the risk of being sued while at the same time increases satisfaction with the practice of psychiatric mental health nursing.

Sexual Involvement with Clients

The ANA (1994) *Standards of Psychiatric-Mental Health Clinical Nursing Practice* explicitly discourage intimate or sexual relationships with present or former clients. Such prohibitions are part of virtually all codes of behavior for other mental health professionals, and sexual liaisons between therapist and client are prohibited by statute in a number of states. Violation of such statutes may result in loss or suspension of one's professional license. Despite this widespread prohibition, sexual relationships between client and therapist do occur. Popular novels and films such as *Prince of Tides* continue to portray romantic attachments between therapist and client even as such involvement seems to be decreasing in frequency (Borys & Pope, 1989).

Breaching Confidentiality

Issues related to confidentiality have been discussed in a previous section. Whether purposely or by accident, if a nurse reveals information given to her in clinical confidence, the client may bring suit. Clearly, the nurse must avoid any release of confidential information without explicit authorization from the client.

Failure to Honor Individual Rights

Clients may bring suit against mental health professionals for wrongful commitment to a psychiatric hospital, failure to obtain appropriate consent, wrongful restraint, or a variety of other perceived assaults on personal autonomy. Following appropriate guidelines for commitment, restraint, and medication treatment can significantly protect against successful lawsuit.

Control of Violent or Self-Destructive Behaviors

Violent or self-destructive clients are frequently committed involuntarily to psychiatric hospitals. When violent or self-destructive behavior is overt or thought highly probable, the nurse's primary focus is on protecting the client and those around him. Suicidal or potentially violent individuals may refuse medication or other potentially useful treatments. Under conditions of true emergency, treatment without permission is occasionally justified. When urgency is less but treatment is clearly in a refusing individual's best interest, an attempt should be made to obtain court-ordered treatment, usually through a declaration of judgmental incompetence.

Either because appropriate treatment is refused or because insufficient time has elapsed for treatment to be effective, hospital staff must sometimes make special efforts to ensure a client's safety. These efforts may include one-to-one staffing, use of on-site police or other guards, **seclusion** (putting someone in a usually empty or padded room or cell by themselves), or **physical restraints** (apparatus that significantly inhibit mobility). Seclusion and restraints are treatments that could violate the important treatment principle of the **least restrictive alternative**. This principle is a legal doctrine that requires that clients be treated with the least amount of constraint of liberty consistent with their safety. Clearly, seclusion and restraints should be used only when required to prevent imminent harm to self or others (Lion & Soloff, 1984). While some institutions may use restraints to prevent agitated individuals from inflicting physical damage on hospital facilities, this use of restrictive treatments is hard to justify unless all other options for behavioral control have been exhausted.

Some states have explicit laws regulating or prohibiting the use of restraints and seclusion. Nurses should be aware of the laws that apply in their respective states and be careful to ensure that care complies with these regulations. It is

---

✳ NURSING TIP

Prudent/Appropriate Nursing Behaviors

1. Present self as trustworthy to clients:
   - Tell the truth
   - Establish rapport
2. Know your state laws.
3. Use techniques to deescalate client anger (speak in a calm voice, acknowledge that anger is an appropriate emotion but that it must be controlled, remove the client who is getting angry from excess stimulation).
4. Do not rush in your interactions with clients or your explanations to clients.
5. Carefully document all assessment data.
6. Carefully record all treatments, interventions, and procedures followed when giving care.

of course important that seclusion and restraint not be used as substitutes for close nursing attention and supervision. Since seclusion and restraint are often used for agitated clients, the nurse should be absolutely confident that the agitation is not due to some undiagnosed medical condition for which treatment is necessary, perhaps urgently.

Many institutions still use neuroleptic medications as "chemical restraints" to sedate agitated individuals. This use of medication has historically been particularly common in the elderly. Chemical restraint is currently regarded as unethical unless antipsychotic medication is used to treat a diagnosed psychotic disorder that is causing agitation. While there are undoubtedly justified exceptions that allow the cautious use of neuroleptics in the nonpsychotic, these are rare. The short-term and well-monitored use of physical restraints is generally preferable to medicating clients with either neuroleptics or respiratory-depressing sedatives.

Other risks for negligence that psychiatric nurses face are similar to those confronted in nonpsychiatric nursing practice: errors in medication administration, failure to prevent nonintentional physical injury, violation of privacy, and failure to provide needed treatment. Nurses who practice psychotherapy or prescribe medications may be found negligent in these activities in much the same way as a physician.

KEY CONCEPTS

- Nurses are responsible for knowing and following all laws relevant to their work.

- There are specific legal issues central to psychiatric mental health nursing: confidentiality, clients' rights, psychological competence, informed consent, involuntary hospitalization and treatment, violent or self-destructive behaviors, and professional negligence in mental health care.

- Ethical theories of utilitarianism and deontology give the nurse a moral guide to practice.

- Ethical principles of autonomy, beneficience, fidelity, justice, and nonmaleficence may be used to guide decisions.

- The Value Analysis Model gives the nurse a method of evaluating an ethical dilemma before drawing conclusions about an issue.

REVIEW QUESTIONS AND ACTIVITIES

1. You are working in a geriatric psychiatric unit where a client who is in touch with reality is yelling at others for hours at a time. His behavior is disruptive to the overall unit environment. At what point do you think the client's right to autonomy is overriden by the utilitarian notion of greater good for the greater number? How do you decide? What is your state law? Could you or would you administer chemical restraints?

2. Give an example of a situation where you would violate a client's right to confidentiality and disclose psychiatric information to another person. Explain why.

3. Does your psychiatric institution have a client bill of rights? If yes, how does this bill of rights ensure that clients' legal rights are being met?

4. What procedures are taken at your psychiatric facility to obtain informed consent for hospitalization, medications, treatments, and outpatient care?

5. Identify a client who has been hospitalized under 48/72 hour emergency hospitalization proceedings. What were the factors that led to commitment?

6. Define the concept of least restrictive alternative.

7. What is the Tarasoff Duty to Warn?

8. Apply the Value Analysis Model either to a situation you have observed in practice or to a hypothetical situation in which you think it would be difficult to decide what to do.

⚛ EXPLORING THE WEB

- Visit this text's "Online Companion™" on the Internet at **http://www.DelmarNursing.com** for further information on ethical and legal issues of concern to nursing.

- Search the web sites of certain law schools, such as Harvard or University of Virginia, to see what information is available.

- What organizations or professional journals could you search for information on nursing and ethical/legal issues?

- What resources are available through the Internet for families and/or health care professionals needing legal advice? Are phone numbers and addresses given?

REFERENCES

American Holistic Nurses' Association. (1995). *Code of ethics for holistic nurses*. Raleigh, NC: Author.

American Nurses Association (ANA). (1994). *A statement on psychiatric-mental health clinical practice and standards of psychiatric-mental health clinical nursing practice*. Washington, DC: Author.

Applebaum, P. S. (1990). Washington v Harper: Prisoners' right to refuse antipsychotic medication. *Hospital and Community Psychiatry, 41*, 731–732.

Bednar, R. L., Bednar, S. C., Lambert, M. J., & Waite, D. R. (1991). *Psychotherapy with high-risk clients: Legal and professional standards.* Pacific Grove CA: Brooks/Cole Publishing.

Borys, D. S., & Pope, K. S. (1989). Dual relationships between therapist and client: A national study of psychologists, psychiatrists, and social workers. *Professional Psychology: Research and Practice, 20,* 283–293.

Coombs, J. R., & Meux, M. (1971). Teaching strategies for values analysis. In L. Metcalf (Ed.), *Values education* (pp. 29–74). 41st Yearbook, Washington DC: National Council for the Social Studies.

Department of Health and Human Services (DHHS). (1982). *President's Commission for the Study of Ethical Problems in Medicine and Biomedical and Behavioral Research: Making health care decisions: A report on the ethical and legal implications of informed consent in the patient-practitioner relationship.* Vol 1: Report. Washington DC: Superintendent of Documents, October.

Frisch, N. (1987). Value analysis: A method for teaching nursing ethics and promoting the moral development of students. *Journal of Nursing Education, 26,* 328–334.

Lion, J. R., & Soloff, P. H. (1984). Implementation of seclusion and restraint. In K. Tardiff (Ed.), *The psychiatric uses of seclusion and restraint* (pp. 19–34). Washington DC: American Psychiatric Press.

Merz, J. F., & Fischoff, B. (1990). Informed consent does not mean rational consent: Cognitive limitations on decision-making. *Journal of Legal Medicine, 11,* 321–350.

Schwartz, H. I., Vingiano, W., & Perez C. B. (1988). Autonomy and the right to refuse treatment: Patients' attitudes after involuntary medication. *Hospital and Community Psychiatry, 39,* 1049–1055.

Simon, R. I. (1992). *Clinical psychiatry and the law.* Washington, DC: American Psychiatric Press.

Stone, A. A. (1981). The right to refuse treatment. *Archives of General Psychiatry, 38,* 358–362.

Swenson, L. C. (1993). *Psychology and law for the helping professions.* Pacific Grove, CA: Brooks/Cole Publishing.

COURT CASES

MacDonald v. Clinger, 84, A.D.ed 482, 446, N.Y.S.2d 801 (N.Y. App. Div. 1982).

Rivers v. Katz, 67 N.Y.2d 485, 504 N.Y.S.2d 74, 495 (N.E.2d 337, 1986).

Stensvad v. Reivitz, 601 F Suppl. 128 (W.D. Wisc. 1985).

Whitree v. State, 56 Misc. 2d 693, 290 N.Y.S.2d 485 (N.Y. Sup. Ct. 1968).

2

CLIENTS WITH PSYCHIATRIC DISORDERS

What are the different mental illnesses that may afflict clients seeking nursing care? How can nurses help heal life's crises? How does anxiety differ from psychosis? How does depression differ from normal grief? How can the nurse help someone who is suicidal? Is there really a difference between dependence on cocaine and dependence on tobacco?

These questions highlight some of the many issues raised in the ten chapters included in this unit on *Clients with Psychiatric Disorders*.

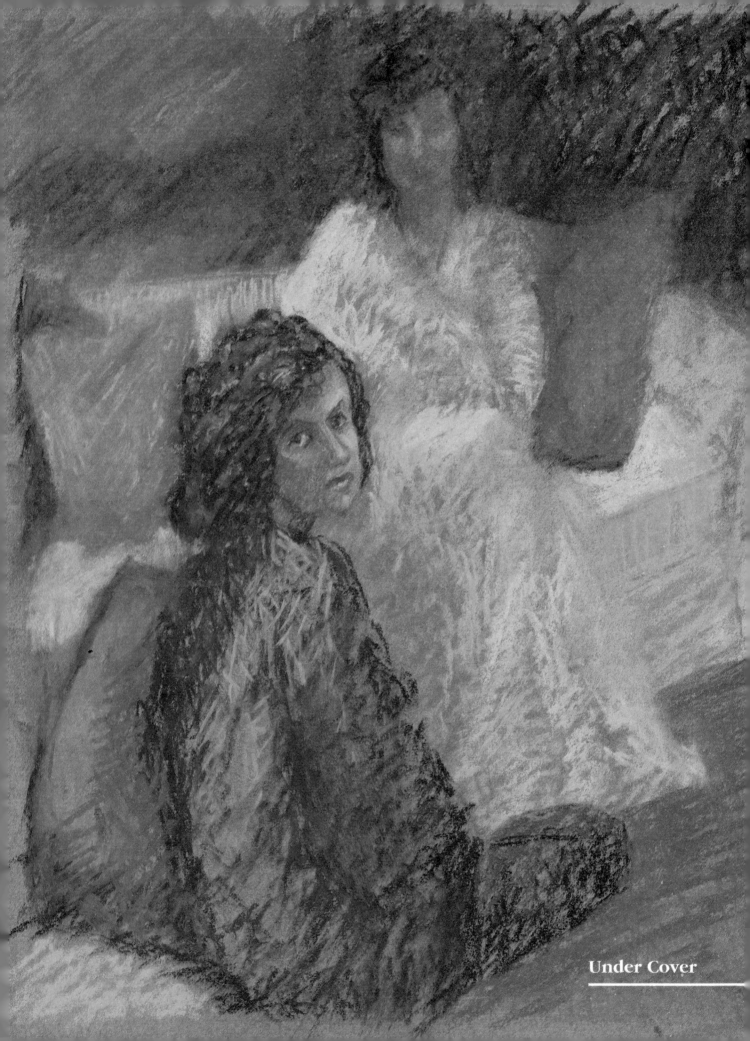

Under Cover

Chapter

9

THE CLIENT
UNDERGOING CRISIS

Noreen Cavan Frisch

Lawrence E. Frisch

What Have Been the Crises in Your Life?

Consider a time when you had to make a change in your living, for example, graduation, a family move, a death of a family member or loved one, divorce/separation, significant illness, loss of employment, loss of housing, or some other change.

- ◆ Did you believe that you had many choices?
- ◆ What did you do?
- ◆ Where did you go for help?
- ◆ Did you discuss your situation with anyone? if yes, whom?
- ◆ What did you do to cope with the emotions?
- ◆ Can you identify the coping mechanisms that have worked for you?

Use your answers to these questions to develop an understanding of your personal methods of responding to life's challenging events. As you read through this chapter, continue to examine your own responses to those discussed.

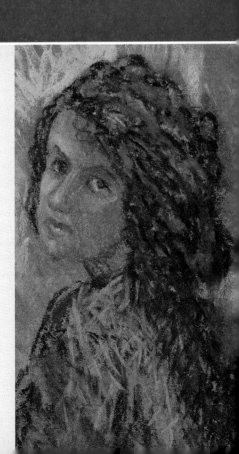

⩰ CHAPTER OUTLINE

WHAT IS CRISIS?

Kinds of Crisis

Stages of Crisis

Personal Development and Crisis

Stress Theory

NURSING THEORY AND CRISIS

Adaptation Theories

Caring Theories

Cultural Care Theory

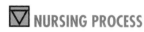 NURSING PROCESS

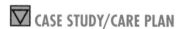 CASE STUDY/CARE PLAN

⩰ COMPETENCIES

Upon completion of this chapter, the reader should be able to:

1. Identify crises as part of life and describe situations that bring on crisis for many individuals.

2. Describe situational, maturational, cultural, and community crises.

3. Identify four phases of a person's experience of crisis.

4. Use stress theory to interpret an individual's response to crisis.

5. Identify daily stressors in modern life that produce personal stress and require adaptive responses.

6. Use the adaptation nursing theory of Roy and Erickson's Modeling and Role-Modeling theory to evaluate the crisis response, adaptation, and return to an equilibrium state.

7. Use the caring, interpersonal nursing theories of Watson and Peplau to seek to understand the client's subjective experience of the crisis event and provide unconditional, humanistic care.

8. Use cultural care theory to obtain knowledge of the client's culture and to understand the meaning of life's events from within that culture.

9. Apply the nursing process to clients in crisis by:

   ◆ Performing nursing assessments for crisis

   ◆ Analyzing data in terms of nursing and crisis theories

   ◆ Formulating individual nursing diagnoses

   ◆ Deriving a plan of care

   ◆ Evaluating care based on resolution to the precrisis state

〰 KEY TERMS

Adaptive Energy Individual's ability to respond to a stressor.

Adaptive Potential Assessment Model Erickson and colleague's model describing three states of coping potential: arousal, equilibrium, and impoverishment.

Arousal Stress state in which an individual possesses coping resources.

Community Crisis Threat of a proportion to affect an entire group of people.

Conservative-Withdrawal State Psychological response to stress; stage of exhaustion.

Crisis Stressor or life challenge that requires an individual to adjust to the unexpected and to adapt to an upredicted situation or event.

Cultural Crisis Situation of shock resulting from an individual's adaptation to a new culture or return to a previously experienced culture; also known as Culture Shock.

Culture Shock See Cultural Crisis.

Equilibrium State of balance following a stress state.

Fight-Flight Response Psychological response to stress; state of high anxiety and energy.

General Adaptation Syndrome Specific, predictable, physiological response to stress, involving an alarm reaction, a resistance stage, and an exhaustion stage.

Impoverishment Stress state in which an individual's coping resources are depleted.

Maturational Crisis Stage in an individual's life requiring adjustment or adaptation to new responsibilities or life patterns.

Psychological Development Continuum of milestones from infancy through adulthood showing evolution of personal history.

Situational Crisis Event that poses a threat or challenge to an individual.

Stress Stimulus that an individual perceives as challenging or harmful.

A crisis is one of the many of life's challenges that call upon people to adjust to the unexpected and to adapt to a situation or event that is unpredictable and, more often than not, unwanted. Nurses encounter crises daily in their work. For example, in any given day a nurse may face a crisis in the staffing schedule, a crisis for the client who has just been given a disturbing diagnosis, a crisis for the family victimized by assault, a crisis for a teenager suffering from an accidental injury, or a crisis for a patient contemplating suicide. Nurses themselves face their own individual crises of everyday living, such as failed babysitting arrangements, cars that do not work, health problems, and inability to complete a day's work in a day. Nearly everyone knows something of what it means to live through a crisis.

In many ways, understanding the significance and management of the crises in clients' (and one's own) lives is the essence of learning to be a nurse. While central to all nursing practice, the understanding of crisis is particularly important in psychiatric and mental health nursing. Why is this? A crisis stresses the individual's coping resources, and each person responds differently to seemingly identical situations: Faced with similar adversity, one person may redouble her efforts to achieve success while another may retreat into despondency. Crisis requires that an individual call on all of her personal skills as well as on the outside social and familial supports that she has built through her life. Each individual has personality strengths, interpersonal networks, and socioeconomic resources that offer some protection against the threat of crisis. When any (or all) of these protections are weak, a person's response to crisis may be dysfunctional, and the result may be one or more symptoms of mental illness. While theories differ in their definitions of crisis and stress, it is generally accepted that most psychiatric problems result from or are strongly influenced by the interaction of stress and overwhelmed coping mechanisms.

The purpose of this chapter is to explore the nature of crisis. Later chapters will discuss specific forms of mental illness typically encountered by a nurse. While crisis can (and does) occur in every life, mental illness affects only a minority of persons. Even though significant mental illness can occur in the absence of crisis, crisis management skills are very important in psychiatric practice, as they are in all nursing care. For many clients, thoughtful nursing intervention early in a crisis may make the difference between mental health and mental illness.

WHAT IS CRISIS?

In psychological terms, a crisis is a stressor that forces an individual to respond and/or adapt in some way. As illustrated in the examples preceding, each nurse faces personal crises of living and comes in daily contact with clients and families undergoing their own crises. Is a crisis always a bad thing? Common usage suggests that it is: No one would wish for a crisis. No one would ask to be out of control, to have an unexpected demand placed on them. But by searching definitions of the word *crisis*, it is clear that crisis itself is neither bad nor good, and the outcome may be positive or negative.

The *Oxford English Dictionary* (1971) defines crisis as the turning point in a disease, the decisive stage in the progress of anything, a state of affairs in which change for the better or worse is imminent. The original usage of the term was the turning point in an illness. *Webster's New World Dictionary* (1994) defines a crisis as a turning point, or a decisive or crucial time, stage, or event. In nursing, a crisis is a critical situation, stage, or event in which a person is called upon to respond to the unexpected. Thus, a crisis calls for one to face a challenge, to initiate adaptive patterns, and to adjust.

The following example of life-threatening illness as a crisis is presented to illustrate the challenges of crisis and the way in which past coping mechanisms influence responses.

Learning one has a fatal illness would seem to be among the most profound crises possible. In the following essay, entitled "Death," the Chinese writer Lu Xun (1881–1936) reflects on his own soon-to-be-fatal illness. Lu Xun died a few weeks after writing this essay.

Death

Not till my serious illness this year did I start thinking distinctly about death. At first I treated my illness as in the past, relying on my Japanese doctor, S_____. Though not a specialist in tuberculosis, he is an elderly man with a rich experience who studied medicine before me, is my senior, and knows me very well—hence he talks frankly. Of course, however well a doctor knows his patient, he still speaks with a certain reserve; but at least he warned me two or three times, though I never paid any attention and did not tell anyone. Perhaps because things had dragged on so long and my last attack was so serious, some friends arranged behind my back to invite an American doctor, D_____, to see me. He is the only Western specialist on tuberculosis in Shanghai. After his examination, although he complimented me on my typically Chinese powers of resistance, he also announced that my end was near, adding that [if] had I been a European I would already have been in my grave for five years. This verdict moved my soft-hearted friends to tears. I did not ask him to prescribe for me, feeling that since he had studied in the West he could hardly have learned how to prescribe for a patient five years dead. But Dr. D_____'s diagnosis was in fact extremely

accurate. I later had an X-ray photograph made of my chest which very largely bore out his findings.

Though I did not pay much attention to his announcement, it has influenced me a little: I spend all the time on my back, with no energy to talk or read and not enough strength to hold a newspaper. Since my heart is not yet "as tranquil as an old well," I am forced to think, and sometimes I think of death too. But instead of thinking that "twenty years from now I shall be a stout fellow again," or wondering how to prolong my stay in a cedarwood coffin, my mind dwells on certain trifles before death. It is only now that I am finally sure that I do not believe that men turn into ghosts. It occurred to me to write a will, and I thought: If I were a great nobleman with a huge fortune, my sons, sons-in-law, and others would have forced me to write a will long ago; whereas nobody has mentioned it to me. . . .

I remember also how during a fever I recalled that when a European is dying there is usually some sort of ceremony in which he asks pardon of others and pardons them. Now I have a great many enemies, and what should my answer be if some modernized person asked me my views on this? After some thought I decided: Let them go on hating me. I shall not forgive a single one of them either.

No such ceremony took place, however, and I did not draw up a will. I simply lay there in silence, struck sometimes by a more pressing thought: if this is dying, it isn't really painful. It may not be quite like this at the end, of course; but still, since this happens only once in a lifetime, I can take it. . . . Later, however there came a change for the better. And now I am wondering whether this was really the state just before dying; a man really dying may not have such ideas. What it will be like, though, I still do not know.*

(Xun, 1994, pp. 192–194)

Lu Xun's crisis comes when his doctors tell him he will soon die from his tuberculosis. He meets this crisis with the ironic humor that was likely also a feature of his healthy life: "I did not ask him to prescribe for me, feeling that since he had studied in the West he could hardly have learned how to prescribe for a patient five years dead." Although he acknowledges that the crisis of his impending death "has influenced me a little," he would have his readers believe that human uncertainty in the face of death is a natural part of life itself. For Lu Xun, the crisis of impending

---

*From *Silent China: Selected Writings of Lu Xun*. Edited/Translated by Gladys Yang. Beijing: Foreign Language Press.

death has no "good or bad" value; it is merely another life challenge to be met with equanimity and ironic curiosity.

Kinds of Crisis

Crises can affect individuals, families, or communities. Crises can be a result of an individual's personal growth and development, including the aging/maturing process. Crises can also be the result of situations external to the individual. Such external situations may affect only one person or may be such that they affect all persons in a community. It is useful to identify and name various kinds of crisis:

◆ A **situational crisis** is any event that poses a threat or challenge to an individual person. Accidental injury, loss of employment, receiving the diagnosis of a significant illness, and loss of one's possessions through theft or fire are all examples of situational crises.

◆ A **maturational crisis** is a stage in a person's life where adjustment and adaptation to new responsibilities and life patterns are necessary. Movement from childhood years to young adulthood presents the crisis of adolescence; movement from middle adulthood to old age poses the crises of aging and is often called the time of "midlife crisis."

◆ A **cultural crisis** is a situation where a person experiences culture shock in the process of adapting/adjusting to a new culture or returning to one's own culture after being assimilated into another.

◆ A **community crisis** is a crisis of a proportion to affect an entire community of people. Natural disasters, armed conflicts, and significant social ills are community crises.

Nurses deal with all types of crisis, and the more information one has in relation to the underlying dynamics of crisis, the better equipped one will be in assessing, diagnosing, and intervening in crisis situations.

Stages of Crisis

Crises have been conceptualized as progressing through four phases (Caplan, 1964). The first phase is a situation or threat to the individual, resulting in anxiety. The individual uses whatever coping mechanisms he has to overcome the anxiety. If anxiety is not reduced, the person enters the second phase, in which anxiety increases and the persons's ability to cope decreases. The person feels pressure and is unable to respond. Then, he enters the third phase, in which anxiety continues to escalate. During this third phase, the individual uses every means available to bring his anxiety level and the situation under control. He may use cognitive skills to redefine the crisis so his coping mechanisms can work; he may seek out counseling or support from others as a "last resort." If the person cannot bring his anxiety under control, he enters Caplan's fourth phase of crisis, which presents as a panic state. For some, fourth-phase symptoms may manifest themselves as anxiety or panic; for others, symptoms may include depression or even frank psychosis. How such symptoms manifest is probably determined in large part by an individual's personality as well as by a range of social support systems important to individual and group coping. Both personality development and social support have been extensively studied and are the subjects of numerous theories. The reader should not assume that the following brief summary is complete, but any understanding of the response to crisis requires some consideration of both personality and social support.

Personal Development and Crisis

Nurses are familiar with the process of normal **psychological development**. Each individual's life proceeds through a continuum from infantile dependency to adult autonomy (and then, for many, back through the dependency of old age and chronic illness). Although theories and cultures vary, important psychological milestones include self-differentiation (in which the infant recognizes itself as separate from the mother), basic trust (in which the infant comes to see the animate and inanimate worlds as consistent and trustworthy), and individuation (in which the child and adolescent develops a specific personality and set of aspirations). The psychologically healthy adult has appropriate levels of self-esteem, a sense of personal and social identity that guides interpersonal and vocational choices, and a spiritual identity that provides her with a sense of life-meaning. Crises may severely test any or all of these resources, and an individual's personal history may leave one or more of these resources incompletely established. This, in turn, may lead to vulnerability under crisis.

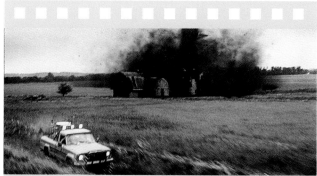

Twister. Source: Warner Brothers/Universal (Courtesy Kobal).

Natural disasters, such as tornados, floods, and earthquakes create severe crises in people's lives. Often, individuals and communities require support of mental health professionals to return to their precrisis level of functioning.

An individual uses his developmentally determined sense of self-esteem and identity to create a range of social supports and to meet basic life needs. Family ties often require maintenance through a lifetime but are usually established at birth. In many cultures individuals create extrafamilial networks of meaningful relationships as they mature, pass through schooling, and enter adult and vocational life. In most cultures, marriage is the most common way in which such networks are forged. Basic life needs include at least food, shelter, clothing, health care, and safety from natural and human disaster. While rarely equitably distributed, financial and social status are of great human importance. There is a strong and consistent empirical relationship between social status and physical well-being. Although possession of wealth rarely single-handedly leads to happiness, few individuals achieve fulfillment while living in abject poverty. Despite the presence of a highly complex relationship between these social factors and an individual's response to crisis, few doubt that those who have strong social supports (including adequate financial resources) can generally weather crises better than those who do not.

Stress Theory

Stress, a stimulus that an individual perceives as challenging or harmful, is intimately involved with crisis.

While experts may differ on precisely how to define both stress and crisis, that each leads to and/or enhances the other seems nearly certain. There is a well-developed theory of stress, and because of the close relationship between stress and crisis, stress theory is highly relevant to the nurse's understanding of crisis.

Selye, the originator of stress theory, suggested that persons have differing abilities to respond to life's stressors. Each person has resources that he called **adaptive energy**, which allow a response to any stressor. Through physiologic experiments, Selye demonstrated that there is a specific, predictable, physiologic response to stress, which he labeled the **General Adaptation Syndrome** (GAS) (Selye, 1974). This response involves an alarm reaction, a stage of resistance, and a stage of exhaustion. The first and third phases were broken down further to include stages of shock and countershock. Table 9-1 provides a summary of the biophysical phenomena of the GAS.

Selye likened the adaptive resources a person has to an inherited fortune. Each individual has adaptive energy; all persons have differing amounts. Once a person uses up whatever adaptive resources he has, there is nothing left from which to draw. The result of a drain of adaptive energy will be illness, disease, or even death. Any crisis can exhaust adaptive resources, but a crisis that is perceived as extremely threatening to life may be most likely to do so.

Table 9-1 Biophysical Phenomena: General Adaptation Syndrome

ALARM REACTION		STAGE OF RESISTANCE	EXHAUSTIVE STAGE	
Shock	**Countershock**		**Countershock**	**Shock**
Depressed nervous system	Excretion of epinephrine	Normal range systolic pressure	Excretion of epinephrine	Depressed nervous system
Decreased muscle tone	Elevated systolic blood pressure	Normal range diastolic pressure	Elevated systolic blood pressure	Decreased muscle tone
Hypotension	Equal or lower diastolic blood pressure	Normal range pulse	Equal or lower diastolic blood pressure	Hypotension
Leucopenia		Glyconeogenesis		Leucopenia
Eosinopenia	Increased pulse pressure	Transfer of free fatty acids to triglycerides	Increased pulse pressure	Eosinopenia
Hemoconcentration	Increased pulse rate	Protein anabolism	Increased pulse rate	Hemoconcentration
Decreased plasma glucose	Glycogenolysis	Normal range respiratory rate	Glycogenolysis	Decreased plasma glucose
Protein catabolism	Gluconeogenesis	Normal range temperature	Gluconeogenesis	Protein catabolism
Hypochloremia	Mobilization of free fatty acids		Mobilization of free fatty acids	Hypochloremia
Hypothermia	Protein catabolism		Protein catabolism	Hypothermia
	Increased respiratory rate		Increased respiratory rate	
	Hyperthermia		Hyperthermia	

From *Modeling and Role-Modeling: A Theory and Paradigm for Nursing*, by H. Erickson, E. Tomlin, and M. A. Swain, 1983, Lexington, SC: Pine Press. Reprinted with permission. Distributed by EST Co 7306 Anaqua, Austin, Texas 78750.

Other researchers, most notably Engel, observed and recorded psychosocial responses to stress. Engel (1962) observed two major responses to stress: the **fight-flight response**, which is a state of high anxiety and energy, and the **conservative-withdrawal state**, which is one of exhaustion.

Stress theory provides a means to understand the following example of an extreme crisis that affected an entire community.

In 1972 an ill-constructed dam broke and sent a deluge of floodwater and debris down Buffalo Creek near the town of Man, West Virginia. Over 100 people were killed, and many homes were destroyed. For many, the psychological impact of this flood was life-long and catastrophic. Sociologist Kai Erikson interviewed survivors more than a year later; here is the voice of one survivor:

Everything in Its Path

For the sake of a little cigarette, I guess, is the reason we're here today. I woke up to get me a cigarette and my pack was empty. I got up and just put on my trousers and went out of the bedroom—me and my wife was sleeping downstairs with the baby, and the rest of the girls were upstairs. I come through the living room, through the hall, into the kitchen, and got me a pack of cigarettes. For some reason, I opened the inside door and looked up the road—and there it came. Just a big black cloud. It looked like twelve or fifteen foot of water. It was just like looking up Kanawha River and seeing barges coming down four or five abreast.

Well, my neighbor's house was coming right up to where we live, coming down the creek. It was a row of houses, bringing everything as it came. It was coming slow, but my wife was still asleep with the baby—she was about seven years old at the time—and the other kids were still upstairs asleep. I screamed for my wife in a bad tone of voice so I could get her attention real quick—of course I never talk nasty to my wife, but I had to get her attention real quick—and when I screamed at her she knowed something was wrong. She sat up on the side of the bed, pulled the drapes apart, and it was washing cans and tires and everything right over into our yard. I don't know how she got the girls downstairs so fast, but she run up there in her sliptail and she got the children out of bed and downstairs.

Now I had a car parked in back of the house. I looked around. Everything above us was acom-

ing right on down, getting closer and closer, and we didn't have much time nohow. So we all got in that car and I was pulling out going up the valley. There was no way in the world out except going right into it. We had water in the yard all around, but none of the big stuff had got down there yet. We headed up the road. My wife was hollering, "Wilbur, you can't get through there," and my daughter Ann—she was twenty-one at the time—she said, "Yeah Daddy, you can." Well, all the time the water and all those houses was coming right at us in a row.

Well, I don't know what happened. I just turned the key off, left it in the car, and we all rolled out one side, got in the water, run across over to the railroad tracks. And there were cars for the Lundale mines sitting there to put coal in. My wife and some of the children went between the cars; me and my baby went under them because we didn't have much time. My neighbor's house hit the car that we was under while we were still under it and wrecked it, and that turned the big water down through the valley to give us a chance to get up into the woods. We got up into the woods and I looked around and our house was done gone. It didn't wash plumb away. It washed down about four or five house lots from where it was setting, tore all to pieces.

At that time, why, I heard somebody holler at me, and I turned around and saw Mrs. Constable. She lived up there above us. Her husband was a wheelchair patient, got hurt in the Lorado mines, and they had four kids. She had a little baby in her arms and she was hollering, "Hey, Wilbur, come and help me; if you can't help me, come get my baby." Well, there was a railroad car between me and her and I couldn't have got back to her anyway. But I didn't give it a thought to go back and help her. I blame myself a whole lot for that yet. She had her baby in her arms and looked as though she was going to throw it to me. Well I never thought to go help that lady. I was thinking about my own family. They all six got drowned in that house. She was standing in water up to her waist, and they all got drownded. . . .

The first five houses above me, there was about fourteen drowned, and I saw everyone of them in their homes as they floated by where I was at. Well,

I looked back on down the valley, and everything had done washed out and gone. I didn't know where my daughter was who lived down below me. And about that time I passed out. I just slumped down. It was around maybe nine o'clock, in that vicinity somewheres.

My house was washed down about five lots from where it had been setting. It had washed up against another big two story house, leaning on about a forty five degree angle, tore all to pieces. The whole back side of it was torn off, the porch was gone, the bathroom was gone, and mud and water and stuff up to the upstairs window. I decided to go over there. I had eight or nine hundred dollars of my money there at the house. I knew where I had it, and I thought maybe I could go in and maybe it wasn't washed away and maybe I'd get some valuable papers and so forth. I got over there and there was a little child had washed up in mine and my wife's bed and it was torn in half. It was laying there in the bed, looked like eight or ten years old by the size of it. There was a truck, a pickup truck, setting in our living room, and it had a dead body in it. There was two dead bodies washed up with the debris that was laying outside of our house, and I had to step over them to get into the house. I just turned and went back. . . .

A fellow by name of Willard Dingess, he asked us was we in the flood and we told him we was. And he asked us where we was going to stay and we said we didn't know. He said, "Well, I've got a little wash house up here, just one room, and you're welcome to it. I've got a little gas heater in it, and you can make your bed down on the floor." So we stayed in that man's wash house, six of us, for nineteen days—a one-room wash house about twelve by twenty. . . .

(Now) I have the feeling that every time it comes a storm it's a natural thing for it to flood. Now that's just my feeling, and I can't get away from it, can't help it. Seems like every time it rains I get that old dirty feeling that it is just a natural thing for it to become another flood.

Why, it don't even have to rain. I listen to the news, and if there's a storm warning out, why I don't go to bed that night. I set up. I tell my wife, "Don't undress our little girls; just let them lay down like they are and go to bed and go to sleep

and then if I see anything going to happen, I'll wake you in plenty of time to get you out of the house." I don't go to bed. I stay up.

My nerves is my problem. Every time it rains, every time it storms, I just can't take it. I walk the floor. I get so nervous that I break out in a rash. I'm taking shots for it now.

I live up on a hill now, but that doesn't take away my fear. Every time it rains or goes to come up a storm, I get my flashlight—if it's two o'clock in the morning or if it's three. Now it's approximately five hundred feet from my house to the creek, but I make me a round about every thirty minutes, looking at that creek. And then I come back to the house, light me a cigarette or maybe get me a cup of coffee, and carry my coffee cup with me back down the hill to see if the creek has raised any.

What I went through on Buffalo Creek is the cause of my problem. The whole thing happens over to me even in my dreams, when I retire for the night. In my dreams, I run from water all the time, all the time. The whole thing just happens over and over again in my dreams.

This just puts on me a load I can't carry. It seems like I just got something bulging on my chest. I can't breathe like I should, and it just makes me feel that my chest weighs a hundred pounds. Just a big bulge in there.

I can remember back from 1932 up till 1972 much plainer than I can the past two years. In other words I've got a mental block of some kind. In the past two years, there've been weeks or months went by, and I don't know where they went, what I've done, or what's happened to them.

I don't want to get out, see no people . . . I didn't even go to the cemetery when my father died. It didn't dawn on me that he was gone forever. And those people that dies around me now, it don't bother me like it did before the disaster . . . I don't have the feeling I used to have about something like death. It just don't affect me like it used to. . . .

Back before this thing happened, you never went up the road or down it but what somebody was ahollering at you. I could walk down the road on a Saturday morning or a Sunday morning and people would holler out their door at me, and maybe I would holler back at them, maybe go sit down and have us a cup of coffee or a cigarette or something. And there'd be half a dozen families would just group up and stand there and talk. But anymore you never see nobody out talking to one another. They're not friendly like they used to be. It's just a whole different life, that's all.*

(Erikson, 1976, pp. 138–147)

Clearly, the catastrophic nature of the flood exhausted the adaptive resources that many of the survivors had. Wilbur, the narrator of the story, describes his own alarm reaction and the fight-flight response during his escape from the water. He further describes his exhaustion immediately following the alarm phase: "I just slumped down." Presumably, he fell into exahustive state when all the adaptive energy he could summon had been used up. He goes on to describe less immediate reactions: his recurring guilt of having watched his neighbors die without his own attempts to save them, the devastation of his home, and the horror of the dead bodies that prevented him from rescuing any of his remaining belongings. The crisis

---

MODERN-DAY STRESSORS

◆ Death of a spouse or partner

◆ Death of a child

◆ Divorce or separation

◆ Death of a family member or close friend

◆ Major illness (self, family)

◆ Victimization—violence

◆ Victimization—theft

◆ Fired at work/laid off at work

◆ Legal battles/being called to court

◆ Marriage

◆ Change in living situation

◆ Change in eating habits

◆ Change in social activities

◆ Gain of a new family member, acquiring stepchildren or stepparents

◆ Merging two households

◆ Change in working conditions

◆ Significant debt

◆ Chemical abuse, drug dependency (self)

◆ Chemical abuse, drug dependency (family member/friend)

---

*Reprinted with the permission of Simon & Schuster. From EVERYTHING IN ITS PATH by Kai T. Erikson. Copyright © 1976 by Kai T. Erikson.

caused great stress for him. One year after the flood, he is living with anxiety and fears lasting well beyond the time of the immediate crisis. Further, he describes a change in his whole community, where people no longer talk to one another in quite the same way. Listening to this flood survivor helps the nurse understand the depth of tragedy people experience in severe situations.

Less severe than the flood, common life stresses can themselves become crises for many persons. The accompanying display provides a list of modern-day stresses in

⑨ RESEARCH HIGHLIGHT

Restructuring Life After Home Loss by Fire

STUDY PROBLEM/PURPOSE

Document the lived experiences of persons going through the crisis of home loss through fire. It is recognized that persons who have lost their homes experience helplessness, sadness, and depletion. The researchers questioned how these persons processed the experience of losing their homes. Further, they evaluated how social rituals served to meet the individuals' needs.

METHODS

The researchers used a grounded theory approach and interviewed fire victims. Data from interviews were examined, categorized, and presented back to selected fire victims for accuracy and fit with their own perceptions.

FINDINGS

Fire victims spoke of the loss as severe as losing family members. They described going through a period of disorientation and having to restructure their lives in a manner that forced them to "start from scratch." Much of the support the fire victims received from others in the form of ritual (or social) support was disconnected to the actual needs the victims had. At times, support offered by others was actually insulting to the victims. Statements such as "You're lucky no one was hurt" came across as uncaring and left the victims feeling neglected and misunderstood. In other situations, persons who wanted to help the fire victims had no idea of how. In general, loss of possessions was trivialized by others, and the victims were not given permission to display grief.

IMPLICATIONS

The researchers recommend use of support groups as a logical intervention for home fire victims.

From "Restructuring Life After Home Loss by Fire," by P. N. Stern and J. Kerry, 1996, *Image, the Journal of Nursing Scholarship, 28*(1), pp. 11–16.

American life. These stresses tax individuals daily and create a drain on their coping resources. Ultimately, such stress may result in physical illness or emotional instability. The nurse should remember that these events, unlike the flood or similar disasters, are private stressors. No one necessarily knows that the individual is under stress and coping with impending crises when the problem is personal financial debt. It is always important to allow clients to talk about their lives and to listen to their life challenges.

NURSING THEORY AND CRISIS

While psychological and stress theories are important, nursing theories provide further means of understanding behaviors. Of the many nursing models used in current practice, the models addressing adaptation fit best with ideas in general mental health work relating to crisis. Other nursing perspectives, particularly caring theories and cultural care theories, provide important alternative views to crisis. Therefore, each will be addressed in what follows.

Adaptation Theories

Nursing theories defining health in terms of successful adaptation and equilibrium are consistent with the general mental health approach to crisis. Roy's adaptation model (1980) and Erickson's theory of Modeling and Role-Modeling (Erickson, Tomlin, & Swain, 1983) fall into this category. For both of these theories, the person is seen as having component parts. For Roy these parts are biopsychosocial components; for Erickson these parts are biophysical, cognitive, psychological, and social. In both of these theories, health is defined in terms of an equilibrium or balance between the parts that promotes harmony or adjustment. Systems theory has influenced these ideas, such that these nursing theories posit that any event that serves as a stressor on one component of the person will have an effect on the other components.

In light of these theories of adaptation, it is clear that any crisis event serves as a stressor that threatens the balance. The individual undergoing a crisis is in a state of disequilibrium, and any intervention must serve to reestablish balance. The nurse can expect to see symptoms in any of the dimensions of the person; for example, the stress of the crisis may exhibit as an emotional instability, a physical illness, or an inability to concentrate. These reactions to the stress of crisis are highly individual; information from the client about past history and coping will assist the nurse to recognize and interpret the varied symptoms of crisis for an individual.

Erickson's Modeling and Role-Modeling theory provides an integrated view of stress by incorporating ideas of stress theory into a nursing, adaptation framework. Erickson and colleagues introduced the **Adaptive**

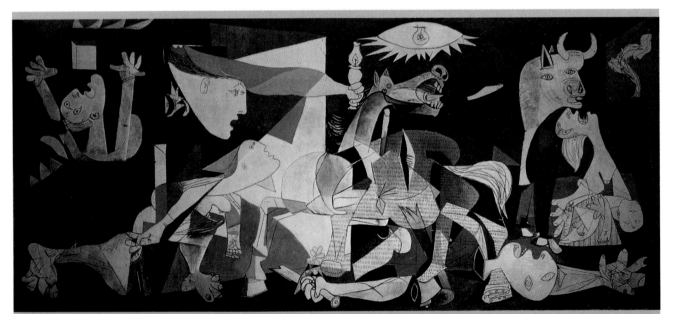

Guernica by Picasso.
Source: Archivo fotográphico Museo Nacional Centro de Arte Reina Sofía. © 1988 Estate of Pablo Picasso/Artists Rights Society (ARS), New York

An unarmed mountain village is bombed by Fascist airplanes during the Spanish Civil War. Picasso captures in stark black and white the horror and dehumanization of modern warfare. If any of the subjects of this picture, human or animal, survived the war, it would be hard to imagine lives unhaunted by their traumatic experience. *Guernica* is regarded by many critics and viewers as one of the greatest paintings of the 20th century. Many viewers have had their perceptions of war—and of painting—forever changed by viewing this monumental canvas.

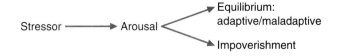

Figure 9-1   Adaptive potential assessment model.
From Modeling and Role-Modeling: A Theory and
Paradigm for Nursing, *by H. Erickson, E. Tomlin, and
M. A. Swain, 1983, Lexington, SC: Pine Press. Reprinted
with permission. Distributed by EST Co 7306 Anaqua,
Austin, Texas 78750.*

Potential Assessment Model (APAM) to describe three
states of coping potential (Erickson et al., 1983). These
states are **arousal**, **equilibrium**, and **impoverishment**.
Figure 9-1 depicts the APAM model. Figure 9-2 provides
a description of the phenomena specific to each state.
Arousal and impoverishment are both stress states. In
arousal the person has coping resources, while in impoverishment the resources are depleted. A stressful event
thrusts a person into a state of arousal. The person will
react, attempting to reestablish balance or equilibrium.
If the reaction is successful, the person will return to an
equilibrium state. If the reaction is unsuccessful, the
person will drop into a state of impoverishment, as it is
not possible to maintain a state of arousal indefinitely.

The theory further states that equilibrium may be
either adaptive, that is, a positive state of balance, as in
Lu Xun's essay on his impending death from tuberculosis,
or maladaptive, that is, a state of balance that provides
equilibrium at the expense of one of the individual's
dimensions. The flood survivor interviewed by Kai
Erikson was in a state of maladaptive equilibrium. One
year postcrisis, he was not functioning: He describes
being unable to recollect recent events and being unable
to tolerate storms and any slight indication of water and
flood. He is living in fear and anxiety.

All nursing theories provide suggestions to guide
practice. For example, Erickson's Theory of Modeling and
Role-Modeling directs the nurse to establish trust, identify
strengths, promote positive orientation, promote perceived control, and set mutual goals. Actions directed
toward these goals, with an understanding of crisis and
the individual client's responses to stress, will form the
basis of nursing care.

Caring Theories

Theories that emphasize caring, most notably
Watson's Theory of Human Care (1988) and Peplau's
theory of interpersonal relationship between nurse and
patient (O'Toole & Welt, 1989), provide a different understanding of crisis and crisis care. If caring and/or relationships are the most important aspects of nursing, a
nurse who encounters a person experiencing a crisis will
provide unconditional, humanistic care (Figure 9-3). The

Equilibrium (adaptive)
Normal blood pressure reading
Normal pulse
Normal respiration
Expression of marked hope and positive expectations
Absent or low feelings of tenseness and anxiousness
Normal motor-sensory behavior
Absent or low feelings of fatigue, sadness, and
depression

Arousal
Marked feelings of tenseness and anxiousness without
feelings of fatigue, sadness, and depression
Elevated motor-sensory behavior
Elevated systolic blood pressure
Elevated pulse
Elevated respiration
High score for verbal anxiety

Impoverishment
Marked feelings of tenseness and anxiousness with
feelings of fatigue, sadness, and depression
Elevated verbal anxiety
Elevated motor-sensory behavior
Elevated blood pressure
Elevated pulse
Elevated respiration

**Figure 9-2   Adaptive potential assessment model:
phenomena specific to each state.** *From* Modeling
and Role-Modeling: A Theory and Paradigm for
Nursing, *by H. Erickson, E. Tomlin, and M. A. Swain,
1983, Lexington, SC: Pine Press. Reprinted with permission. Distributed by EST Co 7306 Anaqua, Austin,
Texas 78750.*

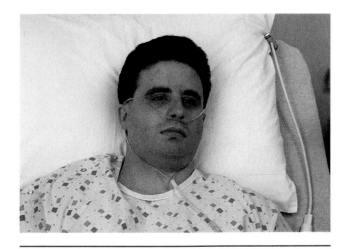

**Figure 9-3   Clients facing a crisis of physical
illness often feel lonely and abandoned.**

nurse will be interested in the client's subjective experience of the crisis. Therefore, the theory would direct the nurse to meet the client at the client's level with an attitude of sincere caring, accept the client's view as the important perspective of the event, seek to understand the client's subjective experience of the crisis, and interpret the meaning of the crisis to the client. As the client relates these personal meanings, the nurse will be able to assist the client to make sense of situations that seem random, unfair, and tragic. Nursing care would be planned mutually. Listening is among the most important skills for this type of assistance (Figure 9-4). All too often clients report that their caregivers do not listen to them. The following excerpt provides an illustration of how meaningful listening to another can be.

Listening to the client is one of the themes of Michael Cristofer's play *The Shadow Box*, in which several persons with an unnamed illness (presumably cancer) find themselves spending their last days in a country "hospice." In the play's opening lines Joe speaks of his reactions to learning he has a fatal illness. He is about to see his wife and son for the first time since his diagnosis.

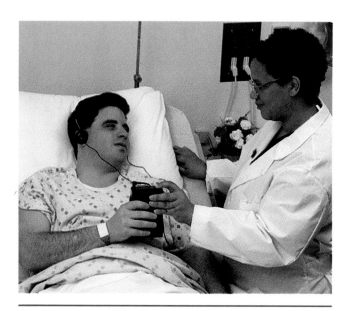

Figure 9-4 Listening to clients' feelings and responding to their needs will help you deliver compassionate and effective nursing care.

The Shadow Box

ACT I

Morning

A small cottage that looks like a vacation house, set in the trees, secluded. A front porch, a living room area and a large kitchen area.

The lights come up first on a small area downstage and away from the cottage. A stool is there. . . .

JOE is surprised by the light. He is a strong, thick-set man, a little bit clumsy with moving and talking, but full of energy.

He steps into the light and looks out toward the back of the theater. A MIKED VOICE speaks to him.

VOICE OF INTERVIEWER: Joe? Joe, can you hear me?

JOE: Huh? (Looking around) What . . . uh . . . ?

VOICE OF INTERVIEWER: Can you hear me?

JOE: Oh, yeah. Sure. I can hear you real good.

VOICE OF INTERVIEWER: Good. Have a seat, Joe.

JOE: (Still looking around, a little amused) What? Hey, where . . . uh . . . I can't see . . .

VOICE OF INTERVIEWER: We're out here.

JOE: What? Oh, yeah. I get it.

VOICE OF INTERVIEWER: Yes.

JOE: You can see me. Right?

VOICE OF INTERVIEWER: Yes. That's correct.

JOE: You can see me, but I . . .

VOICE OF INTERVIEWER: Yes.

JOE: . . . can't see you. Yeah (He laughs) I get it now. You can see me, huh?

VOICE OF INTERVIEWER: Yes, we can.

JOE: Far out.

VOICE OF INTERVIEWER: What?

JOE: (Smiling) Nothing. Nothing. Well, how do I look?

VOICE OF INTERVIEWER: Have a seat, Joe.

JOE: That bad, huh? I feel all right. Lost a little weight, but outside of that . . .

VOICE OF INTERVIEWER: Have a seat, Joe.

JOE: Sure. Sure. (He sits) What?

VOICE OF INTERVIEWER: Nothing special. We just wanted to talk. Give you a chance to see how we do this.

JOE: Sure.

VOICE OF INTERVIEWER: There's nothing very complicated about it. It's just a way we stay in touch.

JOE: Yeah. It's like being on TV.

VOICE OF INTERVIEWER: Just relax.

JOE: Right. Fire away.

VOICE OF INTERVIEWER: You seem to be in very good spirits.

JOE: *Never better. Like I said, I feel great.*

VOICE OF INTERVIEWER: *Good. (There is a pause. JOE looks out into the lights.)*

JOE: *My family is coming today.*

VOICE OF INTERVIEWER: *Yes. We know.*

JOE: *It's been a long time. Almost six months. They would have come sooner, but we couldn't afford it. Not after all these goddamn bills. And then I always figured I'd be going home. I always figured I'd get myself back into shape . . . (Pause)*

VOICE OF INTERVIEWER: *Have you seen the cottage?*

JOE: *Yeah. Yeah, it's real nice. It's beautiful. They're going to love it.*

VOICE OF INTERVIEWER: *Good.*

JOE: *Maggie always wanted a place in the mountains. But I'm an ocean man. So every summer, we always ended up at the beach. She liked it all right. It just takes her a while to get used to things. She'll love it here, though. She will. It's real nice.*

VOICE OF INTERVIEWER: *Good.*

JOE: *It just takes her a little time. (The lights slowly start to come up on the cottage area.)*

VOICE OF INTERVIEWER: *(To JOE) Then everything is settled, right?*

JOE: *What? Oh, yeah. Maggie knows the whole setup. I wrote to her.*

VOICE OF INTERVIEWER: *And your son?*

JOE: *Steve? Yeah. I told Maggie to tell him. I figured he should know before he got here.*

VOICE OF INTERVIEWER: *Good.*

JOE: *It's not an easy thing . . . I guess you know that. . . . You get used to the idea, but it's not easy.*

VOICE OF INTERVIEWER: *You seem fine.*

JOE: *Oh, me. Yeah, sure. But Maggie . . . You get scared at first. Plenty. And then you get pissed off . . . Plenty pissed off. I don't mind telling you that. In fact, I'm glad just to say it. You get tired of keeping it all inside. But it's like, nobody wants to hear about it. You know what I mean? Even the doctors . . . they shove a thermometer in your mouth and a stethoscope in their ears . . . How the hell are you supposed to say anything? But then, like I said, you get used to it . . . I guess . . . I mean, it happens to everybody, right? I ain't special.*

VOICE OF INTERVIEWER: *I guess not Joe.*

JOE: *I mean, that's the way I figure it. We could talk about that too.*

VOICE OF INTERVIEWER: *Yes, we can.*

JOE: *But maybe tomorrow . . . I'm a little nervous today.**

(Cristofer, 1977)

Joe is not able to express his experiences or his concerns. He is telling the interviewer that it is good to have an opportunity to talk. To this point, Joe has not received care based on the theory of human caring. The interviewer and audience in the play are willing to accept Joe as he is. The interviewer provides the unconditional acceptance that caring theory would have all nurses provide. Such individual attention, as opposed to the attitude that Joe is not special or worthy (*I ain't special*), might have helped to resolve the crisis of Joe's illness and its impact on his familial relationships. Simple as it may seem, listening to one in crisis is a caring intervention.

Cultural Care Theory

Nurses skilled in cultural care understand that there are important cultural perspectives in all life's events. Related to crisis, Cultural Care Theory guides the nurse in two matters: recognizing that crises are culturally determined and understanding that insensitive cross-cultural experiences can produce crisis and culture conflict for the nurse and client.

Leininger's theory (1991) directs the nurse to obtain knowledge of the client's cultural background and to understand the meaning of life's events from the client's perspective. It is readily apparent that crisis is highly individual: What is a crisis for one person may not be a crisis for another. The best way to learn of a client's culture and the meaning of events to the individual is to ask the client directly. Questions like "How does your family interpret this situation?" or "What is the meaning of this loss to you?" help the nurse to understand and help the client to articulate his own response to the crisis situation. It is easy for nurses to believe that all clients can and should be able to handle life's events in the same manner as the nurse or in the same manner as the dominant culture; therefore, talking to the client to gain understanding is extremely important.

To be in a situation where one does not understand the social rules, language, and other aspects of a culture is to be in crisis. Situations where there is a reordering of cultural rules and norms is known as **culture shock**; it could just as easily be called culture crisis. Travel can bring on culture crisis, as can reading to a limited degree.

---

*From THE SHADOW BOX by Michael Cristofer. Copyright © 1977 by Michael Cristofer.

⑤ RESEARCH HIGHLIGHT

Intercultural Assessment of Crisis

STUDY PROBLEM/PURPOSE

To document cultural similarities and differences in factors precipitating crisis.

METHODS

Researchers investigated the precipitating events leading to crisis for three groups of persons in different countries (the United States, Brazil, and Taiwan). The methods included use of an Intercultural Crisis Precipitant Assessment Tool, designed by the researchers, to sample 30 persons (10 from each country) seeking crisis intervention at facilities in their respective countries. The tool assessed the events leading to the crisis and the emotional intensity with which the event was felt by the individual.

FINDINGS

Results showed that five precrisis factors were present in persons from all three countries:

◆ Change in sleeping habits
◆ Change in familial relationships
◆ Realization of life's objectives
◆ Change in eating habits
◆ Change in personal habits

There was one factor unique to the Tawainese population:

◆ Change in life's philosophy

There were four unique factors to the United States population:

◆ Food less available
◆ Sense of victimization
◆ Separation from important persons
◆ Substance abuse

The Brazilian population had no unique factors, but this group had the highest intensity recorded for each factor. Researchers also noted that subjects in both the Tawainese and American groups had a focus on somatic, rather than psychological, stressors.

IMPLICATIONS

Researchers conclude that antecedent factors to crisis are different in kind and intensity among culturally distinct groups.

From "An Intercultural Assessment of the Type, Intensity, and Number of Crises Precipitating Factors in Three Cultures: United States, Brazil, and Taiwan," by M. S. Coler and L. P. Hafner, 1991, *International Journal of Nursing Studies, 28*(3), 223–235.

NURSING PROCESS

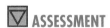ASSESSMENT

To provide care, the nurse must be able to assess the individual undergoing crisis and determine the severity of the crisis and the person's responses to it. There are five factors to assess:

1. Determine the event or situation that precipitated the crisis and what caused the individual to seek help.

2. Assess the person's subjective experience of the crisis.

3. Assess the person's level of anxiety.

4. Assess the person's coping style and strengths.

5. Assess the supports available to the person.

The accompanying display lists a series of questions that could be used in an initial interview when obtaining basic assessment data. In addition to these questions, it is important to determine whether or not the crisis situation has produced feelings of severe despair or anger that could lead to self-destructive, suicidal, or aggressive behavior. If any of these are present, interventions appropriate for such behaviors, such as nursing actions to prevent self-harm, as presented in Chapters 12 and 14, should be instituted immediately. Such a client is not a candidate for crisis intervention, but, rather, must be treated for potentially suicidal and/or violent conditions.

⚡ NURSING ALERT!

Crisis and Suicide

The client experiencing crisis who discloses that he is thinking of suicide or implies that he is contemplating self-destructive behaviors of any kind *must be evaluated for suicide risk*. This client needs more than short-term crisis intervention counseling. (See Chapter 14.)

ASSESSMENT QUESTIONS FOR A CLIENT IN CRISIS

- Tell me about the situation that troubled you.
- What was your immediate reaction?
- Were you alone or with others?
- Explain as best you can what you thought and how you felt.
- Have you ever felt like that before? If yes, when?
- Have you discussed this current situation with anyone else?
- Does anyone you know understand what you are going through?
- Are you feeling anxious now?
- Are you able to go to work? To concentrate on other things?

- Are you sleeping at night?
- How do you usually handle stressful events?
- Do you feel you are going out of control?
- Do you feel you are about to harm yourself or others?
- What would be the most supportive thing another person could do for you?
- Do you have anyone to turn to?
- If you were very anxious and afraid in the middle of the night, what would you do?
- Do you have someone you can call on for help?
- How do you usually cope?

Many nurses have found that the APAM provides a good means of understanding the client's perspective of a crisis event. Bowman (1992) developed a flow chart (presented in Figure 9-5) that assists both in assessing an individual's adaptive potential and forming appropriate nursing interventions.

Analysis of assessment data should lead to nursing diagnoses and to initiation of a nursing care plan that will guide interventions. In most cases, intervention for crisis is short term and provides support for the here and now, with a goal of restoring equilibrium as soon as possible. Typically, crisis intervention lasts for 1 month.

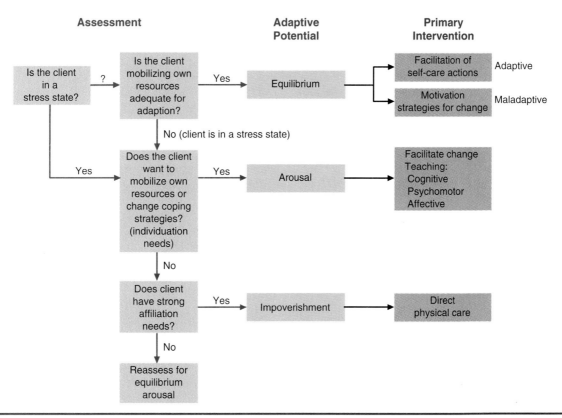

Figure 9-5 Adaptive potential as a guide to planning nursing interventions. *From S. Bowman, Humboldt State University 1997. Reprinted with permission.*

◻ NURSING DIAGNOSIS

Nursing diagnoses (NANDA, 1996) that are common in persons undergoing crisis are:

- *Anxiety* related to the sense of the unknown
- *Fear* related to the precipitating event
- *Ineffective individual coping* related to inability to handle the situation
- *Powerlessness* related to sense of being overwhelmed
- *Hopelessness* related to sense of inability to recover from the crisis
- *Sleep pattern disturbance* related to changes in daily patterns and state of excitement or arousal
- *Risk for violence* related to feelings of anger
- *Dysfunctional grieving* related to actual or perceived object loss

Anxiety and *fear* are diagnosed when the client reports continued concerns related to his own safety or ability to cope. The difference between the two diagnoses is that *anxiety* is diagnosed when the client experiences a general uneasiness and cannot attribute the feeling to any specific stressor. *Fear* is diagnosed when the client expresses anxiety, uneasiness, or fear directed at some specific object or occurrence. *Ineffective individual coping* would be diagnosed when the client's coping patterns, or defense mechanisms, do not serve to reestablish an equilibrium or balance in the person's life. Using the Modeling and Role-Modeling theory, any client in impoverishment or in maladaptive equilibrium could be diagnosed as having *ineffective individual coping*. *Powerlessness* and *hopelessness* are both subjective feelings that express the client's belief that he cannot control the events in his life. The nurse can make these diagnoses only when she has sufficient validation from the client that he, indeed, feels out of control and has given up. *Sleep pattern disturbance* is common postcrisis and for some individuals will be the only clue that they are still feeling stress. Thus, the nurse must ask questions related to sleep even when clients state there are no immediate stressors or crises in their lives. Assessment for *risk for violence* is always appropriate in situations where the client has experienced a crisis that will seem unfair and unjust. Likewise, *grieving* is to be expected whenever personal loss is involved. It is important for the nurse to remember that clients in crises may not recognize that crisis is at the root of their distress. It is not at all unusual for clients in crisis to present with physical symptoms, either new symptoms, such as shortness of breath, pain, or neurological symptoms (usually with no evident physical explanation for the symptom), or the activation of medical conditions associated with stress, such as headaches or peptic ulcer disease. At times, crises may present as acute psychiatric distress and may receive a DSM-IV diagnosis associated with crisis, such as Acute Stress Disorder. The principles of crisis management do not differ depending on whether the client presents with somatic or psychological symptoms; however, the content of the client's concerns and anxieties will likely be different in each case. It is important to recognize that, by definition, crises cannot last indefinitely: They must either resolve or become diagnosable psychiatric disorders. Depending on its seriousness, an unresolved crisis may lead to any of a variety of adjustment reactions in DSM-IV or even to the anxiety diagnosis Post-traumatic Stress Disorder (the diagnosis that a psychiatrist would likely give Wilbur 1 year after the Buffalo Creek flood).

◻ OUTCOME IDENTIFICATION

As in all nursing care, the nurse and client must jointly identify expected outcomes of nursing interventions. Dealing with those facing crisis, the nurse will consider both short-term and long-term objectives/goals of care. For example, when the immediate problem is *sleep pattern disturbances*, the nurse may identify the short-term outcome that, within 1 week, the client will feel safe enough to sleep through the night. When the problem is *grief* related to losses associated with the crisis situation, the expected outcomes will be more long term. For example, a nurse may identify the expected outcome that within 2 months the client will have resolved the grief and begin to make adjustments/adaptations to "get on with life." It is essential here that the nurse evaluate what can and cannot be accomplished within a predicted time frame and make clear to herself and to her client that crises take time to be resolved and the nurse is willing to assist for the necessary period. Recall that research has indicated that family members/significant others seem to expect the client undergoing crisis to have resolved the emotions long before the client is really able to do so (Stern & Kerry, 1996). Attention to outcomes and time needed to achieve them will help the nurse realistically plan for assisting the client through the duration of the crisis and its aftermath.

◻ PLANNING/INTERVENTIONS

The focus of crisis intervention is to deal with the here and now, to help put the crisis event in perspective of the individual's life, and to allow that life to move on quickly past the crisis. Crisis intervention does not deeply explore a person's past psychological history. Though the individual's personality is formed in large part by the past, and though personality certainly affects response to crisis, crises occur and *are managed* in the present.

Selecting a Nursing Theory

There are several nursing conceptual models or theories used in modern practice. Many of these are summarized in Chapter 3, and this chapter on crisis identifies three types of nursing perspectives that are useful in guiding care of the client undergoing a crisis. *How will you choose which to use?*

Begin by selecting one theory or approach that makes sense to you, whether or not it is one of the three the authors have outlined in this chapter. Next, take one of the cases presented in the beginning of the chapter that describes an actual experience of a crisis event. Ask yourself what you need to know and what you need to do as a nurse to assist that person from within your chosen framework. Write down your approach and your rationale for nursing actions.

Next, select a differing perspective and, taking the same case, answer the same questions.

Compare the nursing actions and the rationale underlying those actions. Were the actions different? Was the rationale for the actions different, depending on the theoretical approach?

Repeat the exercise using yet another perspective.

The ability to examine two or more options for care, with an understanding that both are helpful, will help you develop skills of critical thinking.

A goal of crisis intervention is to reestablish equilibrium or balance. It is imperative that the nurse understand the crisis event from the client's perspective; therefore, the first intervention is that of therapeutic listening. The nurse must establish trust with the client, ensure confidentiality, and seek to develop a good understanding of the client's experiences and feelings. For the client, describing emotions and reactions to the nurse serves to release feelings. The nurse encourages an honest disclosure and does not attempt to avoid emotional reactions such as anger or crying. The Interviewer's voice in the play *The Shadow Box* is abstract and impersonal: Joe can never see the interviewer, who remains offstage, but the voice is at least effective in encouraging Joe to tell some of his story instead of "keeping it all inside." In real life the voice would likely have been less effective at getting Joe to share his feelings. For example, after Joe admits "It's not an easy thing" (coping with a fatal illness), the interviewer responds, "You seem fine." But Joe does not really feel (or seem) fine. A more therapeutic response might have been, "No, it never is easy. Can you tell me about some of the things that seem particularly hard *for*

you?" Actively listening to clients (and friends and family) is a challenging but very important skill to learn.

If necessary, a change of physical environment may be indicated, as it may serve to alleviate stress and may produce a sense of comfort and/or safety. For example, if the crisis event was the death of a spouse, the client may be more comfortable staying at the home of a family member or close friend rather than returning to the family home on the day of the death.

The nurse should support the client in the use of defense mechanisms that support an adaptive adjustment. All clients will use defenses that they have established as coping mechanisms throughout life. Some will be more adaptive than others. The nurse should never criticize that client's method of coping at a time of crisis but may gently suggest ways that the client can face the reality of the situation. It is helpful to keep in mind that all defenses serve to maintain self-esteem and that a time of crisis is one when this maintenance is critical for the clients.

There are several means of providing crisis interventions. Individual interactions with the nurse or crisis counselor is one, but groups established for this purpose can be very helpful, particularly if the client can gain support from others who have faced or are facing similar crises. An example would be a support group for survivors of a flood. Nurses should become aware of crisis groups and support groups in their local communities to be able to refer clients as appropriate.

Crisis Intervention as Mental Health Prevention

Data exist that crisis intervention can prevent the need for psychiatric hospitalization and save money (Hoult, 1986; cited in Sartorius, DeGirdano, Andrews, German, & Eisenberg, 1986, p. 305). Crisis intervention is a very important aspect of primary prevention of more serious mental disorders. Crisis intervention at the primary level refers to the establishment of social, political, and environmental conditions that support health. Community mental health work that provides healthy support for families, schools, and identified community groups (such as the elderly) and helps a community and individuals within it to develop the trust, the skills, and the referral networks needed to cope with unexpected, tragic events is primary mental health at its best.

▽ EVALUATION

The nurse must assess the outcomes of the crisis work. The nurse and client together can determine whether there was a successful resolution of the crisis. Does the client feel he can return to a normal life? Does he have the skills and the confidence to return to work? To friends? To family? To carry on?

At times, a crisis opens up new ideas for the affected person and challenges him to examine life from a deeper perspective. For example, many persons who have experienced cancer indicate that receiving the diagnosis of a significant illness created a crisis in their lives. As these persons dealt with the immediate crisis, denial, and shock, they learned to accept the diagnosis and treatment. Because of the experience, they also reexamined their lives, their priorities, and their interactions with others. These persons became different because of having to deal with the crisis, and their personal growth was stimulated by the event. Thus, when a crisis is resolved but the client wishes to pursue continued therapy, group support, and development, the nurse should refer the client to available resources.

෨ *REFLECTIVE THINKING*

Crises as a Social Problem

1. What are the factors in your own community that contribute to the community's mental health or lack thereof?

2. Are there supports for identified groups?

   ◆ Children

   ◆ Young families

   ◆ Working parents

   ◆ Handicapped

   ◆ Elderly

   ◆ Poor

   ◆ Victims of abuse

   ◆ Sufferers of addictions

3. If yes, where are these services? Are nurses involved? How does one know where to find them?

4. If no, what is lacking? What would it take to initiate services?

5. To what degree do you believe it is a nurse's role to promote conditions in society that support individuals in their day-to-day lives?

6. Can a nurse be professional without being involved in community issues?

෨ *REFLECTIVE THINKING*

Your Own Approach to Significant Illness

Nurses frequently come in contact with others who are facing life-threatening illness. In order to truly empathize with clients, it is helpful for the nurse to reflect on her own experience and feelings about illness. The following questions are a guide:

◆ Have you ever confronted a significant illness or the threat of a significant illness in yourself? If yes, what were your feelings and your coping mechanisms at the time? If no, can you imagine how you might feel in such a situation?

◆ Have you ever supported a family member or close friend who was facing significant illness? What was it like for you to be the support person?

◆ How intense is the threat of disability for you?

◆ Do you find it difficult to talk with someone who has been diagnosed with a significant illness? If yes, examine what it is that makes this interpersonal contact difficult.

Use your answers to these questions to evaluate areas that are sensitive for you. Get to know your own coping style. Determine how you can best meet clients' needs when clients have issues that overlap with your own sensitive areas.

CASE STUDY/CARE PLAN

Stewart Alsop was a prominent newspaper columnist who developed an unusual form of leukemia. In the following passage from his book *Stay of Execution* he is in a state of arousal. By his own descriptions he is sometimes a difficult patient for doctors and nurses alike. He had (and expressed) a strong need for control over an illness and process that constantly denied him that control.

Continued

Stay of Execution

"Is there any chance I have aplastic anemia?" I asked. Aplastic anemia is a serious marrow disease, but it is not malignant.

Dr. Henderson hesitated for a moment. "No," he said.

"Then I do have some form of cancer, leukemia, or something else?"

"Yes," he said quietly.

He left, and . . . I began, for the first time in about fifty years, to cry. I was utterly astonished, and also dismayed. I was brought up to believe that for a man to weep in public is the ultimate indignity, a proof of unmanliness. Only my elderly roommate was in the room, and he hadn't noticed. I ducked into our tiny shared bathroom, and closed the door, and sat down on the toilet, and turned on the bath water, so that nobody could hear me, and cried my heart out. Then I dried my eyes on the toilet paper and felt a good deal better. . . .

When Dr. Henderson said "no" to my first question and "yes" to my second, a small light went out, a light of hope that I might not have cancer after all. . . .

I spent a lot of time reading—nothing very profound, since I was in a mood for escape, not profundity. I was enjoying . . . The Day of the Jackal, the best seller about an attempted assassination of de Gaulle . . . thoroughly when one of the characters told another that his girl friend had "luke-something." I closed the book hurriedly, sure that the girl friend would soon die. In fact, I'm told, she didn't, but I've never finished the novel.

When I wasn't reading for escape, I spent a lot of time trying to remember quotations . . . mostly from school and college days, and I almost always get them wrong. . . . For example, I kept trying to remember T.S. Eliot's eternal Footman. After much brain cudgeling, I scribbled in my notebook:

> *I have seen the moment of my greatness flicker.*
> *I have seen the eternal Footman hold my coat, and snicker.*
> *In short, I was afraid.*

. . . Then there were snatches of nonsense verse, for which I've always had a fondness. From Belloc's Cautionary Tales:

> *The chief defect of Henry King*
> *Was chewing little bits of string.*
> *At last he swallowed some which tied*
> *Itself in ugly knots inside.*
> *Physicians of the utmost fame*
> *Were called at once; but when they came*
> *They answered, as they took their fees,*
> *"There is no cure for this disease."*

. . . The thrust of these snippets of memory suggests a melancholy frame of mind, but I found it oddly comforting to dig into my small store of remembered quotations. It was a way of papering over misery. I always liked the story about Winston Churchill . . . in the Boer War when he had to spend a couple of days hiding . . . in a dark hole. He passed the time quite happily reciting to himself all the familiar quotations and Latin tags he could recall. This is at least a better way to spend the time than fearing death.[*]

(Alsop, 1973, p. 68)

Imagine that nurses are actually giving care to the client described above. His expressions of feelings and his behaviors are very similar to those seen by nurses when encountering clients who are life-threatened by illness. This is a fictionalized nursing care plan.

ASSESSMENT

The client is experiencing a crisis of learning that he has a significant illness. He is in a state of arousal—attempting to cope and using his love of books, reading, and quotations as a method of establishing equilibrium. He is mobilizing his resources. He cries and seeks privacy so that no one will know. His arousal has grown from a sense of denial—a coping mechanism that allows him to believe his tumor is benign. He hears the final declaration from his physician and knows and accepts that he has a malignancy.

---

[*]*Stay of Execution,* Alsop, S., 1973, HarperCollins Publishers. Used with permission.

NURSING DIAGNOSIS   *Fear*, related to the unknown course of a life-threatening illness, as evidenced by ability to identify object of fear.

Outcomes

Within 4 weeks, the client will acknowledge and discuss his fear about his illness with his primary care provider and will recognize both adaptive and maladaptive strategies he is using to cope.

Planning/Interventions

◆ Assist the client in dealing with his fears.

◆ Offer quiet, uninterrupted periods of time for listening and talking.

◆ Encourage the expression of feelings through use of therapeutic communication techniques (active listening, reflecting, restating).

◆ Explore what client sees as coping strategies, identifying which ones he believes are useful and which ones are not.

Evaluation

Within 4 weeks, the client was verbalizing his fear. Some of his fears were associated with a lack of information about his illness. The nurse provided extra information in oral and written form. He was also fearful that he would not be able to control his own emotions and behaviors when undergoing treatment. This fear was expressed.

NURSING DIAGNOSIS   *Powerlessness*, related to illness treatment regimen, lack of privacy, as evidenced by verbalizations of having no control over situation.

Outcomes

◆ Within 4 days of hospitalization, client will verbalize feeling in control of treatment choices and his own life activities.

◆ Client will allow himself to express his personal feelings in a variety of ways without self-criticism, particularly during the next 3 months.

Planning/Interventions

◆ Provide expert assistance to client by answering his questions and allowing him to discuss his various treatment options.

◆ Help client construct an activities schedule that acknowledges his need to read and write.

◆ Identify energy-saving activities that will permit client to both pace himself and do the things that are most important to him.

◆ Encourage expression of feelings by asking open-ended questions and listening actively.

◆ Attempt to limit client's self-critical messages, pointing out his personal strengths and affirming positive aspects of his coping.

◆ Provide for client's need for privacy: procure a private room, knock before entering the room, ask him if this is an acceptable time, arrange activities according to his needs.

◆ Inform client that many persons have the need to reflect and will feel emotional when facing significant illness. Offer to discuss these issues if he wishes.

Evaluation

Client said he particularly appreciated help that allowed him to reflect on the choices he did have.

His writing continues to be meaningful to him and should be encouraged.

Client began to express his feelings both alone and with others.

CRITICAL THINKING BAND

ASSESSMENT

What support mechanisms (family, friends, colleagues) should you include in your assessment?

NURSING DIAGNOSIS

What other diagnoses might apply?

Outcomes

What other mutual goals would be reasonable to explore for this client?

Planning/Interventions

What other strategies might we try with this client? Do you think a support group should be suggested?

Evaluation

What else should we have considered with this client? How could we revise this care plan to better meet his needs?

≋ KEY CONCEPTS

◆ A crisis is one of the many of life's challenges that call upon people to adjust to the unexpected and to adapt.

◆ Crisis stresses each individual's coping resources, and each person responds differently to seemingly identical situations.

◆ In nursing, a crisis is defined as a critical situation, stage, or life event in which a person is called upon to respond and adapt to the unexpected.

◆ There are several kinds of crisis: situational, an event posing a challenge to an individual; maturational, a stage in a person's growth and development when he must adjust and adapt to new life patterns; cultural, a situation where a person experiences culture shock; and community, a crisis of a proportion to impact an entire community.

◆ In experiencing crises, persons go through predictable stages in which coping methods used in the past are used to help bring the crisis under control.

◆ Stress theory provides a means to understand the human experience of crisis. Each person has resources, collectively called adaptive energy, that

are used in response to crisis. When all of a person's resources are used up, that person is left in a state of exhaustion.

◆ Psychosocial responses to stress include the fight-flight response, associated with high energy, and the conservative-withdrawal response, associated with exhaustion.

◆ The Modeling and Role-Modeling nursing theory includes the adaptive potential assessment model, which provides the nurse language to describe the client's adaptation to stress.

◆ Watson's Theory of Human Care suggests that listening to the client and understanding the person's subjective experience of the crisis is of the utmost importance.

◆ Cultural Care Theory points out that a crisis cannot be understood without knowledge of the client's culture.

◆ Assessment of the crisis and the client's past coping mechanisms and current strengths begin the process.

◆ Crisis intervention is considered short-term therapy, usually lasting 1 month.

◆ The goal of crisis intervention is to return the client to normal life, with adjustment at least at the precrisis level.

≋ REVIEW QUESTIONS AND ACTIVITIES

1. Identify kinds of crisis (situational, maturational, cultural, and community) and provide an example of each.

2. Describe Caplan's stages of crisis.

3. Explain how personal psychological development influences reaction to crisis.

4. Explain Selye's GAS response to stress.

5. Describe the fight-flight response and the conservative-withdrawal response.

6. Use a nursing adaptation theory to interpret a crisis event.

7. Explain how caring theories and the intervention of listening could be helpful for a person in crisis.

8. Describe how culture influences the perception of and reaction to crisis.

9. Use the flow sheet in Figure 9-5 to evaluate whether or not a client is in equilibrium, arousal, or impoverishment.

10. Explain crisis intervention as a form of mental health prevention.

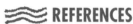 *EXPLORING THE WEB*

◆ Visit this text's "Online Companion™" on the Internet at **http://www.DelmarNursing.com** for further information on stress, crisis, and crisis management.

◆ What sites could you recommend to families undergoing crisis who are looking for self-help, chat rooms, or other electronic information sources?

◆ Is there a listing on the Internet of books, videos, or other media on stress and crisis management? Are these resources available at your local library or through purchase over the Web?

≋ REFERENCES

Bowman, S. (1992). *Adaptive potential as a guide to planning nursing interventions.* Paper presented at the Fourth National Modeling and Role-Modeling Conference, Boston, MA.

Caplan, G. (1964). *Principles of preventive psychiatry.* New York: Basic Books.

Coler, M. S., & Hafner, L. P. (1991). An intercultural assessment of the type, intensity and number of crisis precipitating factors in three cultures: United States, Brazil and Taiwan. *International Journal of Nursing Studies, 28*(3), 223–235.

Engel, G. (1962). *Psychological development in health and disease.* Philadelphia: Saunders.

Erickson, H., Tomlin, E., & Swain, M. A. (1983). *Modeling and role-modeling: A theory and paradigm for nursing.* Lexington, SC: Pine Press.

Leininger, M. (1991). The theory of culture care diversity and universality. In M. Leininger (Ed.), *Culture care diversity and universality: A theory of nursing* (pp. 55–68). New York: National League for Nursing.

North American Nursing Diagnosis Association (NANDA). (1996). *Nursing diagnosis: Definitions and classification 1997–1998.* Philadelphia: Author.

O'Toole, A. W., & Welt, S. R. (Eds.). (1989). *Interpersonal theory in nursing practice: Selected works of Hildegard Peplau.* New York: National League for Nursing.

Oxford English Dictionary. (1971). Oxford: Oxford University Press.

Roy, C. (1980). The Roy adaptation model. In J. P. Riehl & C. Roy (Eds.), *Conceptual models for nursing practice* (2nd. ed., pp. 179–188). New York: Appleton Century Crofts.

Sartorious, N., DeGirdano, G., Andrews, G., German, G., & Eisenberg, L. (Eds.). (1986). *Treatment of mental disorders.* Washington, DC: American Psychiatric Press.

Selye, H. (1974). *Stress without distress.* Philadelphia: JB Lippincott.

Stern, P. N., & Kerry, J. (1996). Restructuring life after home loss by fire. *Image, the Journal of Nursing Scholarship, 28*(1), 11–16.

Watson, J. (1988). *Nursing: Human science and human care: A theory of nursing.* New York: National League for Nursing.

Webster's New World Dictionary (2nd. College Ed.). (1994). New York: Simon & Schuster.

≈ LITERARY REFERENCES

Alsop, S. (1973). *Stay of execution.* Philadelphia: Lippincott.

Cristofer, M. (1977). *The shadow box.* New York: Drama Book Specialists.

Erikson, K. (1976). *Everything in its path.* New York: Simon & Schuster.

Xun, L. (1973). Silent China: Selected writings of Lu Xun. Edited/Translated by Gladys Yang. Beijing: Foreign Language Press.

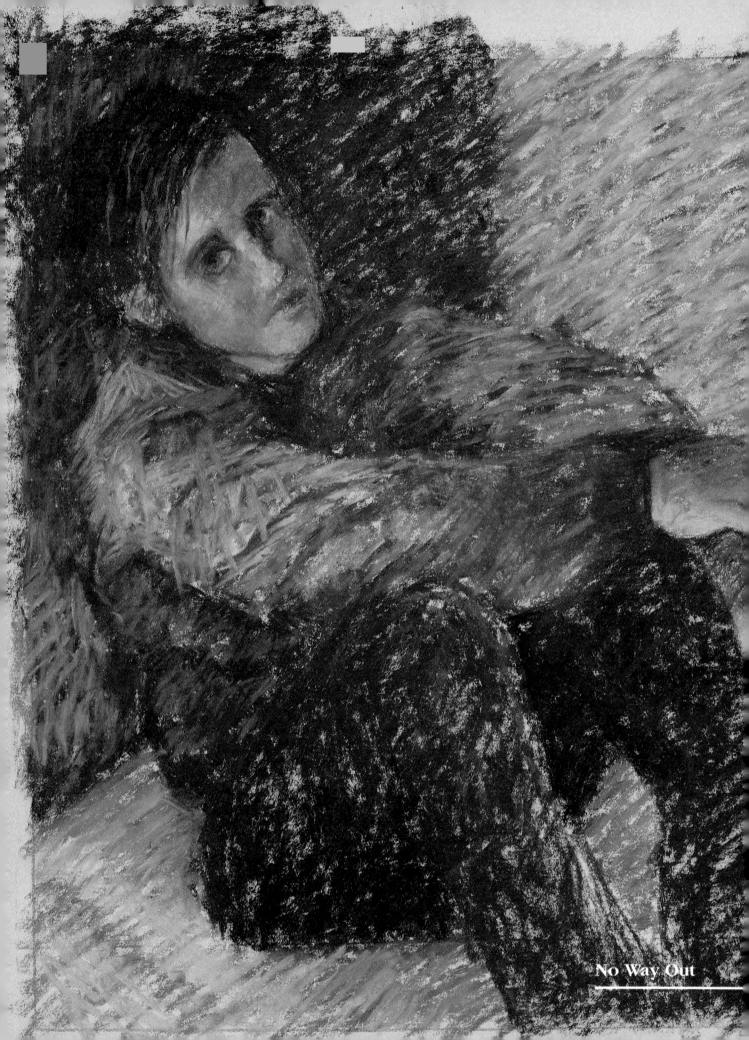

No Way Out

Chapter

10

THE CLIENT
EXPERIENCING ANXIETY

Noreen Cavan Frisch
Lawrence E. Frisch

Anxiety in Everyday Life

Modern life is filled with tension and anxieties. Philosophers have stated that anxiety is a part of the human condition, both unavoidable and necessary for persons to seek to understand themselves and define their goals. However, each person tries to find balance within his or her own existence.

Consider the anxieties of your own life:
- What are the objects of your worries?
- Are there personal worries stemming from your societal roles and duties?
- Do you have personal fears associated with activities or objects? Are you able to avoid those situations that are anxiety provoking for you?

How do you find peace:
- What does a personal sense of peace mean to you?
- What can you do to find peace in your life?

As you read this chapter, which focuses on anxiety in illness, remember that all persons, well or ill, experience anxiety. The nurse must understand that anxiety can become an overpowering experience for many persons, and care must focus on a very personal understanding of anxiety, fear, and sense of loss of control.

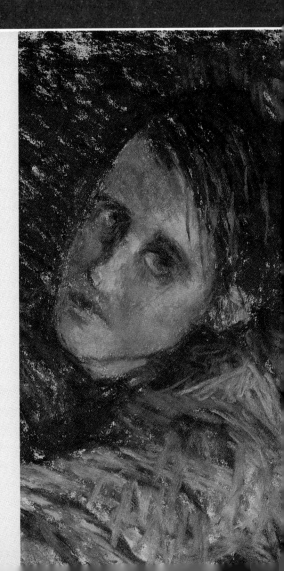

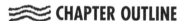 CHAPTER OUTLINE

THE EXPERIENCE OF FEAR AND ANXIETY

Autonomic Nervous System

Neurobiology of Anxiety

STAGES OF ANXIETY

ANXIETY DISORDERS

Generalized Anxiety Disorder
   Epidemiology

Panic Disorder
   Epidemiology

Agoraphobia
   Epidemiology

Phobias
   Epidemiology

Obsessive-Compulsive Disorder
   Epidemiology

Post-Traumatic Stress Disorder
   Epidemiology

CAUSES OF ANXIETY DISORDERS

TREATMENT OF ANXIETY DISORDERS

Psychotherapy
   Insight-Based Treatments
   Behaviorally Based Treatments

Pharmacotherapy

Combination Therapy

ANXIETY AND SPIRITUAL WELL-BEING

**NURSING THEORY AND CLIENTS
EXPERIENCING ANXIETY**

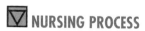 **NURSING PROCESS**

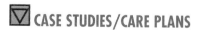 **CASE STUDIES/CARE PLANS**

COMPETENCIES

Upon completion of this chapter, the reader should be able to:

1. Understand the subjective experience of the emotion of anxiety.

2. Describe the differences between anxiety and fear.

3. Define and describe six major anxiety disorders (Generalized Anxiety Disorder, Panic Disorder, Agoraphobia, Phobias, Obsessive-Compulsive Disorder, Post-Traumatic Stress Disorder).

4. Relate the prevalence of anxiety disorders in the general population.

5. Participate in the major treatments of clients with anxiety disorders, including psychotherapy, medication therapy, and combination treatment.

6. Apply nursing theory and nursing diagnoses in the planning, implementing, and evaluating of nursing care of clients with anxiety disorders.

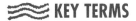

KEY TERMS

Adversity   Measure of the strength of a given stimulus for anxiety.

Agoraphobia   Fear of going out in public places.

Anxiety   State where a person has strong feelings of worry or dread, when the source is nonspecific or unknown.

Cognitive-Behavior Therapy   Treatment approach aimed at helping a client identify stimuli that cause the client's anxiety, develop plans to respond to those stimuli in a nonanxious manner, and problem-solve when unanticipated anxiety-provoking situations arise.

Compulsion   Repetitive behavior or act, the goal of which is to prevent or reduce anxiety or distress.

Fear   State wherein a person feels a strong sense of dread focused on a specific object or event.

Generalized Anxiety Disorder   Psychiatric illness characterized by excessive anxiety or dread.

Obsession   Recurrent thought, image, or impulse that is experienced as intrusive and inappropriate and that causes marked anxiety or distress.

Panic Disorder   Psychiatric illness characterized by discrete episodes of intense anxiety (panic attacks) that begin abruptly and peak within ten minutes.

Phobia   Persistent fear of a specific object or situation.

Positron Emission Tomography (PET)   Tool to accurately measure blood flow patterns in the brain.

Post-Traumatic Stress Disorder   Anxiety disorder resulting from a frightening event such as a crime, accident, or battle.

Trait Anxiety   Personality characteristic reflecting susceptibility to anxiety.

Anxiety is a nearly universal human experience that has long been of interest to both psychologists and creative writers. As will be seen throughout this chapter, the experience of profound anxiety can be severely disabling. In the short story "He?" by Guy de Maupassant, a young man finds his aversion to marriage overcome by the sudden development of a serious anxiety disorder. In this excerpt, he is talking to a close friend about his upcoming marital plans:

Isn't It Dreadful?

"Isn't it dreadful, to be in this state?"

My dear friend, you are completely baffled by it, aren't you? And I can easily understand why. I suppose you think I have gone mad. Perhaps I am a little insane—but not for the reasons you imagine.

Yes. I'm getting married. It's quite true.

And yet my ideas and convictions on the subject have not changed. I still consider legalized cohabitation to be foolish. . . . And yet I am getting married.

I might add that I hardly know the girl who will become my wife tomorrow. I have only seen her four or five times. I know that I do not find her displeasing—and that is sufficient for the purpose I have in mind. She is short, fair, and plump. After tomorrow I shall ardently wish for a woman who is tall, dark, and slender. . . .

"Then why on earth do you get married?" you will say.

I hardly dare to tell you the strange, incredible reason which is urging me to commit this senseless action.

I am getting married so I shall not have to be on my own!

I don't know how to tell you about it, how to make myself understood. I am in such a wretched state of mind that you will feel sorry for me, and also despise me.

I cannot bear to be alone any more at night. . . . I'm afraid of the walls, of the furniture, of familiar objects, which seem to take on a kind of animal life. Above all, I am afraid of the horrible confusion of my thoughts, of the way my reason becomes blurred and elusive, scattered by a mysterious, invisible anguish.

At first I feel a vague uneasiness which enters my soul and sends shivers all over my skin. I look all around me. There's nothing there. . . . I happen to say something aloud—and I'm frightened by the sound of my own voice! I walk about the room—and I'm afraid there might be something strange behind the door, behind the curtains, in the cupboard, under my bed. And yet I know very well that there is nothing there at all.

Sometimes I suddenly turn round because I'm afraid of what might be behind me—and yet there is nothing there, as I very well know.

I become agitated, feel the nervousness increasing, and so I lock myself in my room, bury myself in my bed and hide myself under the sheets. Then cowering there, all huddled up as round as a ball, I close my eyes in despair and stay like this for a long, long time. . . .

Isn't it dreadful, to be in this state?

I never used to feel in the least like this. . . . It all started last year in a very curious way . . . one damp evening in the autumn. . . .

Ever since that time I have been afraid when I have been alone at night. . . . It is ridiculous—but it's horrible. I'm sorry . . . I simply can't help it. . . . But if there were two of us in the place . . .

(de Maupassant, 1903/1990, pp. 136–142)

In this excerpt from the short story "He?" the French writer Guy de Maupassant captures the desperate experience of anxiety: "At first I feel a vague uneasiness which enters my soul and sends shivers all over my skin. . . . I'm afraid of what might be behind me—and yet there is nothing there, as I very well know. . . . Above all . . . I'm afraid of fear, afraid of my panic-stricken mind, afraid of that horrible sensation of incomprehensible terror." Paralyzed by fear, the narrator can only lie curled up in

---

✳ NURSING TIP

Difference Between Anxiety and Fear

- ◆ **Anxiety** is a state wherein a person feels a strong sense of dread, frequently accompanied by physical symptoms of increased heart rate, respiratory rate, elevated blood pressure (autonomic nervous system responses), without having a specific source or reason for the emotions.

- ◆ **Fear** is a state wherein a person feels a strong sense of dread, with autonomic nervous system responses that are focused on a specific object or event—fear of a tornado, fear of surgery, fear of failing in a job.

---

bed and wait until his terror passes. Not only does this excerpt give a vivid sense of what it is like to feel profound anxiety—knowing all along that there is no recognizable reason for fear—but, as will be seen later in this chapter, de Maupassant's story portrays vividly the psychiatric diagnosis of agoraphobia, one of the major categories of anxiety disorders.

Anxiety has a great deal in common with fear, and indeed de Maupassant's narrator freely uses the word "fear" to describe his experience. Still, he is quite careful to separate his anxiety experiences from ordinary fear. Here is another passage from "He?":

Oh, I don't suppose you will understand!

It's not that I'm afraid of any danger . . . if a burglar were to come into the room I would kill him without turning a hair. I'm not afraid of ghosts, and I do not believe in the supernatural. I'm not afraid of the dead. . . . I am afraid of myself!

(de Maupassant, 1990, p. 137)

It is perfectly natural to fear a stranger entering one's room at night and not at all unusual to be afraid of ghosts, or snakes, or the dead. Humans and chimpanzees both seem to have an innate fear of dead bodies, and baby chickens appear genetically programmed to respond with fear to hawklike shadows (Goodwin, 1986). De Maupassant's agoraphobic narrator denies having these "ordinary" fears. Instead, he is afraid of the creations of his own mind: of fear itself. He is truly a victim of anxiety.

THE EXPERIENCE OF FEAR AND ANXIETY

Both fear and anxiety are common experiences, and it seems likely that—no matter how distressing the experience is—appropriate fear is necessary for individual and species survival. In 1872 Charles Darwin wrote a still-influential book called *The Expression of the Emotions in Man and Animals*. He observed that fear may have two very different functions: to increase ability to fight—"a [frightened] man or animal . . . is endowed with wonderful strength, and is notoriously dangerous"—or to flee—"Fear . . . soon induces . . . the most violent and prolonged attempts to escape from the danger" (p. 81). Darwin also graphically described the degrees of human fear:

Expressions of Fear

[The] eyes and mouth are widely opened, and the eyebrows raised. The frightened man at first stands like a statue motionless and breathless, or crouches down as if instinctively to escape observation.

The heart beats quickly and violently, so that it palpitates or knocks against the ribs . . . the skin instantly becomes pale, as during incipient faint-ness. . . . That the skin is much affected under the sense of great fear, we see in the marvelous and inexplicable manner in which perspiration imme-diately exudes from it. This exudation is all the more remarkable, as the surface is then cold, and hence the term a cold sweat. . . . The hairs also on the skin stand erect; and the superficial muscles shiver . . . the breathing is hurried. The salivary glands act imperfectly; the mouth becomes dry, and is often opened and shut. I have also noticed that under slight fear there is a strong tendency to yawn. One of the best-marked symptoms is the trembling of all the muscles of the body; and this is often first seen in the lips. From this cause, and from the dryness of the mouth, the voice becomes husky or indistinct, or may altogether fail. . . .

As fear increases . . . the heart beats wildly or may fail to act and faintness ensue; there is a death-like pallor; the breathing is labored; the wings of the nostrils are wildly dilated; there is a gasping and convulsive motion of the lips, a tremor of the hollow cheek, a gulping and catching of the throat; the uncovered and protruding eyeballs are fixed on the object of terror; or they may roll restlessly from side to side. . . . The pupils are said to be enormously dilated. All the muscles of the body may become rigid, or may be thrown into con-vulsive movements. . . . As fear rises to an extreme pitch, the dreadful scream of terror is heard.

(Darwin, 1965/1872, pp. 289–292)

Autonomic Nervous System

In this striking description of fearful behavior, Darwin emphasizes the stereotyped patterns of movement and of what would now be termed responses of the autonomic nervous system. Seventy-five years after Darwin's descrip-tions, Walter Hess won the Nobel Prize for demonstrating in animals that electrical stimulation of the hypothalamus can reproduce complex behavioral patterns closely resembling what animals actually do when they exhibit fear or rage (Kupfermann, 1985). From this and other work, it seems likely that fear behaviors are organized in the limbic system (the subcortical or primitive brain of which the hypothalamus is one part) and are, as Darwin surmised from observation, expressed in patterns com-mon to many higher animals. As Darwin implied in the

title of his book, the expression of emotion (which can be observed by others) is not the same as the perception of emotion (which can only be directly studied by human reports). While de Maupassant's anxious narrator must have displayed many of the physical signs of fear, his extreme distress came from his feelings and not their physical expressions.

Neurobiology of Anxiety

Given what is currently known about brain function, it seems nearly certain that the cerebral cortex must be involved in the perception of fear. Studies using **positron emission tomography** (PET scanning—a powerful tool to accurately measure blood flow patterns in the brain) suggest that this hypothesis is likely correct. A PET scan-ner can identify and precisely localize rapid changes in blood flow that occur as the result of various mental and emotional stimuli. When susceptible persons are made anxious during PET scanning, blood flow increases signif-icantly both in the limbic system and in several specific areas of the cerebral cortex (Rauch et al., 1995). From what is currently known about the neurobiology of anxiety, it seems that the anxiety experience has its origins in the limbic system or even deeper in midline brainstem structures. Limbic connections to the autonomic nervous system produce the most striking physical manifestations of anxiety: heart rate changes, pallor, sweating, hair "standing on end." If Darwin's description is correct and postural changes (crouching, yawning, raising arms) are indeed part of the fear pattern, then they are likely directly patterned by connections from the limbic area to affected muscles. However, simultaneously with this autonomic activation and patterned muscle stimulation, neural messages from the limbic system travel through the nearby temporal lobe and up into the cortical association areas. These association areas are the brain centers where sensory experiences are linked, joined to memory, and somehow processed as thoughts. Only the involvement of these cortical association centers allows de Maupassant's narrator to feel so vividly his "sensation of incomprehen-sible terror."

As stated earlier, fear typically occurs in response to a real-life threat or danger. While excessive fear may be self-defeating, fear is commonly an adaptive response allowing an individual to successfully avoid or face dan-ger. In contrast, anxiety is an experience akin to fear but without a realistic source. Although perhaps the majority of anxious people can identify one or more factors that bring on their anxiety responses, most of these persons recognize that their feelings of anxiety are far out of proportion to any real dangers. Both fear and anxiety are common and have likely been part of the human expe-rience for thousands of years. The following passage from the *Book of Job* vividly describes the human experi-ence of fear:

The Human Experience of Fear

In thoughts from the visions of the night, when deep sleep falleth on men, fear came upon me, and trembling, which made all my bones to shake. Then a spirit passed before my face; the hair of my flesh stood up. It stood still, but I could not discern the form therof: an image was before my eyes, there was silence, and I heard a voice, saying, Shall mortal man be more just than God? Shall a man be more pure than his Maker?

(Job iv. 13)

Within the last century, anxiety has become a topic of considerable interest to philosophers. The Danish theologian Soren Kierkegaard taught that anxiety was inescapably part of the human condition. In the last decades of the 19th century the stresses of rapidly accelerating social and economic change no doubt contributed to the anxiety felt by many persons. In the first years of the 20th century, T. S. Eliot wrote a poem that seemed to capture the anxiety of a world that had seemingly become caught up in trivial daily concerns to the exclusion of larger spiritual values:

There Will Be Time

And indeed there will be time
To wonder, "Do I dare?" and, "Do I dare?"
Time to turn back and descend the stair,
With a bald spot in the middle of my hair—
(They will say: "But how his arms and legs are thin!")

Do I dare
Disturb the universe?
In a minute there is time
For decisions and revisions which a minute will reverse. . . .

Should I, after tea and cakes and ices,
Have the strength to force the moment to its crisis?
But though I have wept and fasted, wept and prayed,
Though I have seen my head (grown slightly bald) brought in upon a platter,
I am no prophet—and here's no great matter;
I have seen the moment of my greatness flicker,
And I have seen the eternal Footman hold my coat, and snicker,
And in short, I was afraid. . . .
I grow old . . . I grow old . . .

I shall wear the bottoms of my trousers rolled.
Shall I part my hair behind? Do I dare to eat a peach? *

(Eliot, 1970, pp. 3–4)

The narrator of Eliot's poem is overwhelmed by anxiety in the course of an uneventful life:

For I have known them all already, known them all—
Have known the evenings, mornings, afternoon,
I have measured out my life with coffee spoons. . . .

(Eliot, 1970, p. 6)

Eating a peach, parting his hair, asking a woman to marry him (the apparent subject of the poem)—these are all decisions that are too complex for the anxious Prufrock, decisions "that lead you to an overwhelming question . . . Do I dare disturb the universe?" And if he did dare propose marriage, and if in response she, "settling a pillow by her head, should say, 'That is not what I meant at all. That is not it, at all: . . .'" Prufrock asks "Would it have been worth it? . . ." and confesses "in short, I was afraid." (Eliot, 1970). For J. Alfred Prufrock, Job's fear and trembling before God has become anguished indecision over a life measured by nothing larger than coffee spoons.

More than a generation later, in and just after the closing days of World War II, W. H. Auden wrote a much longer poem called "The Age of Anxiety." Anxiety was also a central theme in the philosophy of existentialism, another creation of the years following World War II. Existentialists claimed that a person's major philosophical goal ought to be the choice of a life reflecting authentic personal and social commitment. Imperfect political structures and the fallibility of human nature inevitably made such choices difficult and anxiety-ridden. Seen from the standpoint of more recent history—Hiroshima, political assassinations, wars, refugees, ecological disaster—it is hard to see how any modern life could be lived in awareness and yet without anxiety. Surely the present era is, in Auden's memorable words, an "Age of Anxiety."

Without anxiety, according to Kierkegaard and other modern thinkers, humankind would lose its ability to find both spiritual direction and political freedom. Some psychiatrists disagree strongly, arguing that while mild fear is useful for negotiating truly dangerous situations, virtually *any* degree of anxiety is self-defeating (Goodwin, 1986). Whatever one's philosophical beliefs about the need for some anxiety in life, few would claim that the crippling

---

*From "The Love Song of J. Alfred Prufrock," *Collected Poems 1919–1962* (pp. 3–7), by T. S. Eliot, 1970, New York: Harcourt Brace & Company.

anxiety suffered by the narrator of de Maupassant's "He?" or the perhaps milder anxiety affecting Eliot's Prufrock serves any useful human purpose. At least in its extremes, anxiety clearly results in a serious limiting of human potential.

STAGES OF ANXIETY

Because anxiety exists as part of each person's everyday existence and also exists as a distinct psychiatric condition, there is general agreement that a continuum of anxiety responses exists ranging from mild anxiety to a panic state. These stages are presented in Table 10-1. In mild anxiety, the person experiences day-to-day tensions and is alert, with an increased perceptual field. In moderate anxiety, the person focuses only on the immediate concerns, with a narrowed perceptual field. In severe

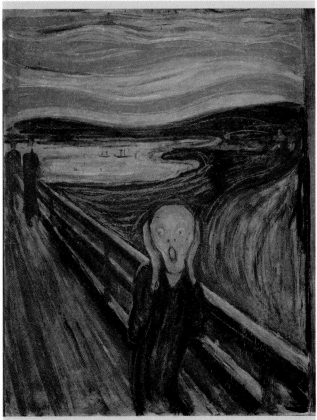

The Scream by Munch. Source: Erich Lessing/Art Resource, NY.

Almost an icon of anxiety, this work reflects the life experiences of a man who was haunted by mental illness—both his own and his sister's. Caught between land and sea, and isolated from the only other humans in sight, the screaming figure occupies a landscape whose unstable shapes and colors are both the source and the expression of unbearable anxiety.

Table 10-1	Stages of Anxiety
Mild	Tension of day-to-day living; individual has an alert perceptual field; can motivate learning. *Example:* anxiety felt when missing the bus.
Moderate	Focus is on immediate concerns; perceptual field is narrowed; individual exhibits selective inattention. *Example:* anxiety felt when taking an exam.
Severe	Focus is on specific detail; perceptual field is greatly reduced. *Example:* anxiety felt when witnessing a car accident.
Panic	Individual experiences a sense of awe, dread, and/or terror; individual loses control; there is a disorganization of the personality. *Example:* anxiety felt when experiencing an earthquake and being unable to cope.

anxiety, the person's perceptual field is greatly reduced and the individual focuses on a specific detail. In a panic state, the person has feelings of dread or terror and is unable to control his behaviors.

ANXIETY DISORDERS

The *Diagnostic and Statistical Manual*, third edition (DSM-III), and its successor, DSM-IV (American Psychiatric Association, 1994), made what was then a radical claim: that it was possible to categorize several varieties of anxiety as psychiatric disorders, distinct both among themselves and from "normal" existential anxiety. It is important for the nurse to be familiar with these. The DSM provides the current definitions for the distinction between anxiety in health and anxiety in illness; that is, it is recognized that all persons experience anxiety, but it is also recognized that some individuals experience anxiety to a degree that it interferes with ability to function in daily life. Thus, there exists anxiety in illness—the anxiety disorders. There is a general category of anxiety disorders and there are 14 subtypes that have been identified. Six of these are particularly important, distinct, and common. These subtypes of anxiety disorder are summarized in Table 10-2 and are discussed following.

Generalized Anxiety Disorder

The primary symptom of **Generalized Anxiety Disorder** is, not surprisingly, excessive anxiety or dread. Clients with Generalized Anxiety Disorder typically recognize that their symptoms are out of proportion to any real threat. According to DSM-IV definitions, anxiety is

Table 10-2 Summary of Major Anxiety Disorders

DISORDER	DEFINITION	SYMPTOMS	PREVALENCE (Percentage in Adult U.S. Population)
Generalized Anxiety Disorder	Anxiety focused on a variety of life events or activities	Restlessness, fatigue, difficulty in concentrating, irritability, muscle tension, sleep disturbances	5
Panic Disorder	Discrete episodes of intense anxiety that begin abruptly and reach a peak within about 10 min	Palpitations, sweating, trembling, shortness of breath, sensation of choking, chest pain, nausea, dizziness, fear of losing control, fear of dying, sense of altered reality	6
Agoraphobia	Acute anxiety in crowds; fear of being alone; fear in any physical setting from which the individual may have trouble escaping	Intense feelings of anxiety and/or fear of losing control that results in either refraining from going out or avoiding situations that may bring about anxiety	5
Phobia	Persistent, excessive, or unreasonable fear of a specific object or situation (examples: elevators, airplanes, dogs, spiders, injections, tunnels)	Fears that interfere markedly with life activities	10
Obsessive-Compulsive Disorder	Occurrence of recurrent thoughts, images, and/or impulses that are intrusive and inappropriate, causing anxiety (obsession) and coupled with repetitive actions or behaviors performed to reduce the anxiety (compulsions)	Individual recognizes that his thoughts and/or behaviors are unreasonable; for example, the person who wishes to stop checking and rechecking an alarm clock at night but feels unable to stop the repetitive behavior	2.6
Post-Traumatic Stress Disorder	After exposure to a significant, life-threatening event, the experience of anxiety symptoms in which the event is reexperienced through recollections	Recurrent recollections, dreams, hallucinatory-like flashbacks, impairment of social functioning	3–58 (for person exposed to serious danger)

considered excessive when it is present more days than not for a period of 6 months or more. Anxiety is "generalized" if it focuses on a variety of life events or activities. The focus of anxiety cannot be solely on certain specific topics, such as gaining weight or fearing illness. Persons anxious only about their weight may have eating disorders, and persons anxious only about their health may have hypochondriasis (one of the somatoform disorders). To meet DSM-IV criteria for a disorder, the anxiety must both be difficult to control and cause significant distress or impairment in functioning. Finally, DSM-IV requires that certain specific symptoms be present and not be caused by medications, drugs, or illness. These symptoms include three or more of the following: restlessness, easy fatigue, difficulty concentrating, irritability, muscle tension, and sleep disturbance. When symptoms are due to another psychiatric illness such as depression,

Generalized Anxiety Disorder is usually not diagnosed (American Psychiatric Association, 1994).

Epidemiology

It should be evident from the preceding description that Generalized Anxiety Disorder is very much a "diagnosis of exclusion." Clients are most commonly given this diagnosis when they have disabling symptoms of anxiety that do not fit any other pattern. In the Epidemiological Catchment Area study, 4% to 7% of individuals had met DSM-III criteria for Generalized Anxiety Disorder at some time in their lives (Blazer, Hughes, Swartz, & Boyer, 1991). Although the DSM-IV criteria for diagnosis have changed somewhat, 5% is still the best estimate for the lifetime incidence of generalized anxiety. Unlike persons with many psychiatric diagnoses (including a number discussed in this chapter), those with generalized

RESEARCH HIGHLIGHT

Generalized Anxiety Disorder in Stroke Sufferers

STUDY PROBLEM/PURPOSE

To assess the prevalence and outcome of Generalized Anxiety Disorder in clients having suffered a stroke.

METHODS

Cohort study of 80 stroke sufferers.

FINDINGS

The prevalence of the disorder in stroke sufferers was 28% in the acute stage of the stroke, and there was no significant decrease over a 3-year follow-up period. In 1 year, only 23% of those with early Generalized Anxiety Disorder had recovered, and those not recovered had high risk for development of chronic anxiety disorder. Comorbidity with major depression was high, which seemed to impair the prognosis with regard to depression.

IMPLICATIONS

Stroke is a significant illness that may be experienced as a life-threatening or life-changing event. The high incidence of Generalized Anxiety Disorder following stroke was previously unrecognized. The researchers conclude that Generalized Anxiety Disorder after stroke is a common and long-lasting affliction. Health care providers should evaluate individuals who have had strokes for presence of the disorder so that appropriate treatment can be offered.

From "Generalized Anxiety Disorder in Stroke Patients: A 3-Year Longitudinal Study," by M. Estrum, 1996, *Stroke, 27,* pp. 270–275.

anxiety often present in significant distress from their symptoms, which are frequently made harder to tolerate by a variety of social and situational stressors. For example, an individual experiencing daily severe anxiety may find it exceedingly difficult to participate in committee meetings required at work. If so, that person may seek treatment because the anxiety causes difficulty in job performance.

Panic Disorder

Panic Disorder is a condition characterized by discrete episodes of intense anxiety that begin abruptly and reach a peak within 10 min. They include at least four of a set of specified symptoms. These symptoms include palpitations or rapid heart rate, sweating, trembling, short-

ness of breath, sensation of choking, chest pain, nausea, dizziness, fear of losing control, fear of dying, numbness or tingling, chills or hot flushes, and some sense of altered reality. There is often a strong wish to run away or otherwise escape from the situation that provoked the attack. Compared to Generalized Anxiety Disorder, the anxiety of Panic Disorder is very much more severe and strikingly episodic. Most persons who experience panic attacks have little or no residual anxiety between attacks. In some individuals, the panic attacks are reproducibly provoked by exposure to certain stimuli (e.g., seeing a snake). In others, they may appear "out of the blue" or be most likely to occur in specific settings (such as the dentist's office).

Many years ago, William Leonard, a Professor of English at the University of Wisconsin, described his personal experiences with Panic Disorder. In the following excerpt from his book-length description, he emphasizes both the severity of the anxiety and the rapidity with which symptoms develop. (Both severity and rapid onset are highly characteristic of Panic Disorder.)

Let Me Assume

Let me assume that I am walking down University Drive by the Lake. I am a normal man for the first quarter of a mile; for the next hundred yards I am in a mild state of dread, controllable and controlled; for the next twenty yards in an acute state of dread, yet controlled; for the next ten, in an anguish of terror that hasn't reached the crisis of explosion; and in a half-dozen steps more I am in as fierce a panic of isolation from help and home and of immediate death as a man overboard in mid-Atlantic or on his window-ledge far up in a skyscraper with flames lapping his shoulders. The reader who can't understand why I have not whistled or laughed or ordered [the panic attacks] off my psychic premises, or who thinks that I must be grossly exaggerating a mere normal discomfort, like the initial dread in a dentist's chair, is not the reader for whom I am writing one line of this book. . . . I know that my [panic attacks] at their worst approach any limits of terror that the human mind is capable of in the actual presence of death in its most horrible forms. That I have never fainted away or died under them is due to two factors: first, my physical vitality; and, second, my skill in devising escapes. . . . The fools say nothing ever happened from one of these [attacks]—so why worry. Nothing ever happened? Well, here is what happens always. First, the [attack] happens—as well say, nothing happens if a red-hot iron is run down the throat, even though it should miraculously leave no after-effects. . . . Second, the [attack] leaves me always far more exposed to [panic attacks] for weeks or months [and] increases my fear of the Fear.

(Leonard, 1927, pp. 66–71)

Leonard's "fear of the Fear" is also a very characteristic aspect of Panic Disorder. Persons who suffer panic attacks often live in severe fear that the attacks will recur, and they often change their lives significantly in an effort to minimize recurrence. Recognizing this feature of panic attacks, DSM-IV defines the diagnosis of Panic Disorder, which in general can be made when panic attacks recur in association with worry about future attacks and/or behavior change related to these attacks. The diagnosis of Panic Disorder also requires that no other physical or psychological condition be present that better explains the panic attacks.

Epidemiology

The Epidemiologic Catchment Area study found that panic attacks occur in about 6% of persons (Robins & Regier, 1991). Multiple studies have demonstrated that between 1.5% and 3.5% of unselected individuals experience Panic Disorder during their lifetimes (American Psychiatric Association, 1994). Clearly, only about half of persons with panic attacks have Panic Disorder; most of the rest have other anxiety disorders in which panic attacks may be seen. There is a strong association between Panic Disorder and Major Depressive Disorder (Chapter 14), and over half of persons with Panic Disorder also suffer from significant depression (American Psychiatric Association, 1994). There is also a significant correlation between Panic Disorder and substance abuse. In many cases, the abuse problem may occur because individuals with Panic Disorder treat their symptoms with alcohol or other substances. Panic Disorder tends to occur in relatively young persons, with onset common some time between adolescence and the mid-30s. There is probably a genetic component to Panic Disorder in that persons are more likely to develop the disorder if their

> ### 🌀 NURSING ALERT!
>
> ### Panic Disorder and Suicide Risk
>
> Persons with Panic Disorder have a high risk of suicide; they think about death, feel as though they want to die, and consider or attempt suicide more than do individuals with any other psychiatric condition, including depression.

identical twin also has it. There is also a significant increased risk for Panic Disorder in children of individuals with the condition.

Persons with Panic Disorder often do not consult with mental health practitioners about their symptoms. Therefore, the diagnosis of Panic Disorder is never made or is made only after many years of suffering. Individuals commonly present to acute health care facilities (often emergency rooms) complaining of physical symptoms: palpitations, chest pain, shortness of breath, faintness, dizziness. Affected individuals are frequently evaluated repeatedly for cardiac, pulmonary, or neurological conditions, and they often undergo complex workups for endocrine problems: thyroid disease or pheochromocytoma. There is almost certainly a link between physical factors and panic attacks, because attacks can often be reproduced by hyperventilation.

The natural history of Panic Disorder is quite variable. However, three stages in the development of Panic Disorder have been described (Kanton, 1989). In the first stage, the panic attack is experienced after a variety of stressors and most often occurs during a routine task (such as driving a car). In stage 2, the individual begins to live in fear that he may have another panic attack, and out of fear, he may avoid an increasing number of events associated with prior panic attacks. Lastly, in the third stage, the person may develop intense avoidant behaviors and refuse to participate in social events. This condition is called **Agoraphobia** and refers to a fear of going out in public places. Most individuals with Panic Disorder will improve over long-term follow-up, but about 20% will continue to have the kind of ongoing moderate to severe disability that Leonard reports in the description of his own symptoms. Some studies have indicated that persons with Panic Disorder have a much higher risk of suicide than does the nonaffected population (Weissman, Klerman, Markowitz, & Ouelette, 1989).

Agoraphobia

Only a few years before de Maupassant wrote the story with which this chapter began, the German neurologist Karl Westphal described a group of persons who became acutely anxious both when in crowds and when walking through deserted areas. Westphal called this condition agoraphobia, a Greek term meaning fear of public places. More than 100 years later, this term is still in use for a strikingly common and often severe anxiety disorder. In current usage, Agoraphobia is a description applied to persons who are afraid of crowded public areas. The DSM-IV definition is actually somewhat broader and includes individuals who become fearful in any physical setting from which they might have trouble escaping or getting help in the event of an acute panic attack. Some agoraphobics—like de Maupassant's narrator—are afraid of being home alone. More commonly, the

NURSING TIP

Agoraphobia: Opposing Symptoms, Single Cause

- "I do not want to be alone any longer at night. . . . But if there were two of us in the place. . . ." (de Maupassant, 1903/1989)

- "Should I ever leave home, which is improbable, I will with much delight, accept your invitation." (Dickinson, 1955)

The various symptoms of Agoraphobia can sometimes seem contradictory. In Agoraphobia, the primary psychological need is to avoid panic; consequently, some persons stay fearfully at home while others experience an inability to remain alone at home. Although these symptoms might seem so opposite to one another that they must have different diagnoses, they do truly have a common root. The similarity comes from underlying motivation rather than behavior, in each case the intense desire to avoid recurrent panic episodes.

opposite situation occurs: Agoraphobic persons are afraid to leave their houses alone even if, as they leave, they have to walk through deserted (rather than crowded) areas. Since leaving home often results in panic attacks, many agoraphobic individuals are rendered virtually homebound by their fear.

Many agoraphobic persons stay away from public places because of fears they will do something embarrassing (scream uncontrollably, commit a sexual indiscretion) or be dangerous (assault someone). People with Agoraphobia do not actually behave in this way; however, they typically fear each of these consequences with great intensity. Goodwin describes some of the ways that agoraphobics use to mitigate their anxiety to maintain social functioning:

> Sometimes just carrying an umbrella helps. Other inanimate objects reported to provide relief include canes, shopping baskets on wheels, a bicycle pushed down the street, a folded newspaper carried under the arm. . . . Agoraphobics almost always are more comfortable in dark places than in sunlight. . . . If they go to theatres at all, they find an aisle seat near the back to make a fast getaway if necessary . . . the most reliable fear-reducer is a trusted companion. Many agoraphobics only venture out of the house when accompanied by someone they know and trust: a husband, friend, child, or even a dog.

(Goodwin, 1986, pp. 147–148)

Recall that in the opening literary selection, "He?" de Maupassant's narrator plans marriage to a woman he has barely met because any company is preferable to the fear he suffers when home alone. There are some symptoms of Agoraphobia that seem contradictory. The accompanying Nursing Tip helps to explain that differing and even opposite symptoms have a common root.

Many agoraphobics never seek medical or psychiatric treatment for their symptoms and accept a measure of social disability from them. The famous 19th-century American poet Emily Dickinson led a remarkably homebound life, which it appears was almost certainly caused by severe Agoraphobia (Garbowsky, 1989). Many of Dickinson's poems seem to describe experiences of intense anxiety, very likely panic attacks. Here, for example, is one poem, "I Felt a Funeral, in my Brain," that might be taken to describe the depersonalization and fear of a typical panic attack:

I Felt a Funeral, in my Brain

I felt a Funeral, in my Brain,
And Mourners to and fro
Kept treading, treading, till it seemed
That Sense was breaking through.

And when they all were seated,
A Service, like a Drum
Kept beating, beating, till I thought
My Mind was going numb.

And then I heard them lift a Box
And Creak across my Soul
With those same Boots of Lead, again,
Then Space began to toll,

As all the Heavens were a Bell,
And Being, but an Ear,
And I, and Silence, some strange Race
Wrecked, solitary, here

An then a Plank in Reason broke,
And I dropped down, and down
And hit a World, at every plunge,
And Finished knowing—then.

(Dickinson, 1955, pp. 199–200)

Yet another poem suggests an almost puzzled response to some kind of mental catastrophe, the puzzlement perhaps reflecting Goodwin's (1986) comment that "agoraphobics usually have difficulty explaining why they are afraid" (p. 146):

I Felt a Cleavage in My Mind

I felt a cleavage in my Mind
As if my brain had split;
I tried to match it, seam by seam,
But could not make them fit.
The thought behind I strove to join
Unto the thought before,
But sequence ravelled out of reach
Like Balls upon a floor.

(Dickinson, 1955, p. 358)

Garbowsky has made a strong case that Dickinson suffered from both Panic Disorder and Agoraphobia, taking the title of her book from a fragment of yet another of Dickinson's poems in which Dickinson seems to describe feeling trapped within a "House without the Door":

Doom is the House without the Door—
'Tis entered from the Sun—
And then the Ladder's thrown away,
Because Escape—is done.

As psychiatrist John Cody writes in a Foreword to Garbowsky's book (Garbowsky, 1989), "The difficult question is not whether there was a diagnosable [psychological] infirmity present—for it is clear that there was—but what was its essential nature." Garbowsky bases her case for Agoraphobia not just on the poetry but also on the details of Emily Dickinson's unusual life. At age 23 Dickinson wrote to a friend who had invited her to visit, "I thank you. Abiah, but I don't go from home, unless emergency leads me by the hand, and then I do it obstinately, and draw back if I can. Should I ever leave home, which is improbable, I will with much delight, accept your invitation" (Garbowsky, 1989, p. 37). In reality, she did make several brief trips in her 20s and 30s, but by the time she reached age 40, she had been completely housebound for five years and wrote to an admirer of her poetry: "I do not cross my Father's ground to any House or town" (Garbowsky, 1989, p. 29). Only after Dickinson died 20 years later did her sister discover the thousands of poems written in her agoraphobic seclusion. All exceedingly brief, some of these are among the most memorable in the English language.

While Agoraphobia likely created for Emily Dickinson the conditions under which she could become one of the 19th century's greatest poets, for most persons it creates nothing other than a life of misery. Agoraphobia is among the most disabling and difficult to treat of all the anxiety disorders (Goodwin, 1989). Unfortunately, cases like Dickinson's, lasting a lifetime and leading to total confinement in the house, still occur with some frequency.

Epidemiology

There is a very strong linkage between Panic Disorder and Agoraphobia. In some studies, 95% of individuals with Agoraphobia also have Panic Disorder, and up to half of all individuals with Panic Disorder also suffer from Agoraphobia. Agoraphobia occurs in about 5% of individuals in the community. Symptoms may develop gradually over years or, as in the story told by de Maupassant's narrator, begin suddenly and then persist.

Phobias

A **phobia** is a persistent fear of a specific object or situation. The fear occurs whenever the phobic individual is brought in contact with that object or situation. Phobias are categorized as Social Phobia (e.g., profound fear of public speaking) and Specific Phobia. Specific Phobia commonly involves fear of such things as airplane travel, high or exposed places, closed places, animals (often snakes or spiders), or seeing blood. To meet DSM-IV diagnostic criteria for Specific Phobia, the fear must be excessive or unreasonable, must be recognized as excessive or unreasonable by the phobic individual, and must result in significant social, occupational, or academic disruption. As the narrator observes in Erica Jong's novel *Fear of Flying*, multiple phobias are not at all uncommon:

Fear of Flying

Oh, I have phobias about practically everything you can think of: plane crashes, clap, swallowing ground glass, botulism, Arabs, breast cancer, leukemia, Nazis, melanoma.*

(Jong, 1973, pp. 253–254)

While most of these phobias get little attention elsewhere in the book, the novel's opening pages vividly describe intense fear of air travel:

My husband grabbed my hand therapeutically at the moment of takeoff. "Christ—it's like ice," he said. He ought to know the symptoms by now since he's held my hand on lots of other flights. My fingers (and toes) turn to ice, my stomach leaps upward into my rib cage, the temperature in the tip of my nose drops to the same level as the temperature in my fingers, my nipples stand up and salute the inside of my bra (or in this case, dress—since I'm not wearing a bra), and for one screaming minute my heart and the engines correspond as we attempt to prove again that the laws of aerodynamics are not the flimsy superstitions which, in my heart of hearts, I know they are. . . . I happen

---

*From *Fear of Flying*, by Erica Mann Jong. © 1973 by Erica Mann Jong. Reprinted by permission of Henry Holt & Co., Inc.

*to be convinced that only my own concentration
(and that of my mother—who always seems to
expect her children to die in a plane crash) keeps
this bird aloft. I congratulate myself on every successful takeoff, but not too enthusiastically because
it's also part of my personal religion that the
minute you grow overconfident and really relax
about the flight, the plane crashes instantly.*

(Jong, 1973, pp. 2–3)

Terrified as she is, Jong's narrator seems to find herself on
airplanes fairly frequently, and not always in her husband's company. By requiring that truly phobic fears
interfere markedly with life activities, DSM-IV attempts
to distinguish between common fears and true phobias.
In the following passage from the modern novel *Hotel du
Lac*, by Brookner, it appears that Jennifer has encountered a spider:

Hotel du Lac

*But a sharp scream from the corridor, and a
sound of running feet, startled her into an awareness of danger. She listened, motionless, ancient
fears awakening. Silence. Opening her door carefully, she saw light streaming from the Pusey's
suite, and heard voices. Oh, God, she thought.
A heart attack. And willed herself to take charge.*

*It was Jennifer's door that was open, and
Jennifer herself, the straps of a satin nightgown
slipping from her plump shoulders, laughing and
uttering little moans, was poised on her bed, her
legs drawn up. Her mother, in a pale pink silk
kimono, stood in the doorway, her hand to her
mouth. In the corner, crouching, Mr. Neville busied
himself with a newspaper, then went to the window
and flung something out.*

*"Quite safe now," he pronounced. "No more
spiders. . . ."*

*Mrs. Pusey came forward and laid a hand on
his arm. "How can we thank you?" she breathed.
"She's been terrified of spiders ever since she was
tiny."** *

(Brookner, 1984, pp. 77–78)

While spider phobias are common, screaming on seeing
a spider is not by itself an indication of either "excessive
or unreasonable" fear. Jennifer's laughter would suggest

---

*From *HOTEL DU LAC* by Anita Brookner. Copyright © 1984 by Anita
Brookner. Reprinted by permission of Pantheon Books, a division of
Random House, Inc.

that her response was far from "intense anxiety or distress," and there is nothing in the rest of the novel to suggest that anxiety about spiders affected any of Jennifer's
normal routine or social activities. Jennifer, like many
people, is fearful but not phobic.

Epidemiology

While neither Jennifer nor Jong (more accurately, her
novel's narrator) may qualify for a DSM-IV diagnosis of
Specific Phobia, millions of other individuals do. It is estimated that about 10% of Americans have symptoms of
Specific Phobia during any year (American Psychiatric
Association, 1994). Epidemiological studies bear out common stereotypes in showing that women are about twice
as likely to have symptoms of Specific Phobia as are men
(Eaton, Dyman, & Weissman, 1991). Phobias are notoriously private, and patients with phobic disorders rarely

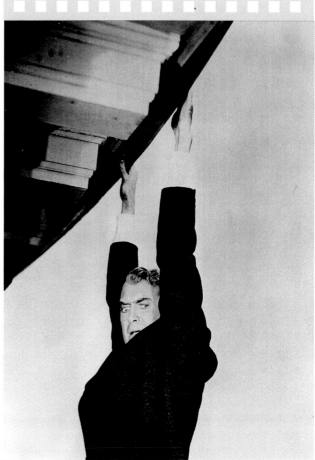

Vertigo. Source: Paramount/Courtesy Kobal.

In this movie the main character experiences danger in a chase episode involving a friend's fatal fall.
He is forced to retire from police work due to his
fear of heights—acrophobia.

disclose their symptoms, sometimes denying them when asked directly. Goodwin observes:

> Many people are embarrassed about their phobias and often keep them hidden from even their closest friends. This habit of secrecy may persist even when they see doctors and see them for psychiatric reasons. It is not unusual in psychiatric practice to see a patient for a long period and then have him describe, almost in passing, a phobia that has plagued him for years. In routine questioning of patients, phobias are not even asked about. Many non-psychiatrists seem unaware even of their existence.

> (Goodwin, 1986, p. 125)

Most phobias begin in early adulthood, typically before the age of 30. Animal phobias commonly begin even earlier, often in childhood. While phobic individuals sometimes become adept at avoiding situations that provoke their phobias, in many cases such avoidance is impossible. Elevators, cars, airplanes, dogs, spiders, injections, tunnels—all common foci of phobic anxiety—are remarkably hard to avoid in modern life. In most cases, repeated exposure significantly diminishes the anxiety brought on by the feared situation; in such cases, the phobia may vanish or at least recede to manageable proportions. Follow-up studies suggest that most phobias beginning in adolescence will be cured or much improved within 5 years (Goodwin, 1986). Phobias that begin later or persist into middle age tend to cause more difficulties with social functioning and may even worsen with time. Many individuals with Specific Phobia can maintain functionality by managing either to cure the disorder via continued exposure or to adapt to their anxiety and avoid the specific object.

Obsessive-Compulsive Disorder

Persons with Obsessive-Compulsive Disorder suffer from a combination of obsessions and compulsions. "**Obsessions** are recurrent thoughts, images, or impulses that are experienced as intrusive and inappropriate and that cause marked anxiety or distress" (American Psychiatric Association, 1994, p. 418). Common obsessions include fear of self-contamination (becoming infected by touching something or shaking hands), fear that one has forgotten to do something important (like lock a door or turn off an oven), or a need to have things in one's life (e.g., chairs in a room) in a particular physical arrangement. "**Compulsions** are repetitive behaviors . . . or mental acts . . . the goal of which is to prevent or reduce anxiety or distress" (American Psychiatric Association, 1994 p. 418). Persons who experience obsessions often find relief from these via repetitive ritualistic actions or compulsions. "For example, individuals with obsessions about being contaminated may reduce their mental distress by wash-

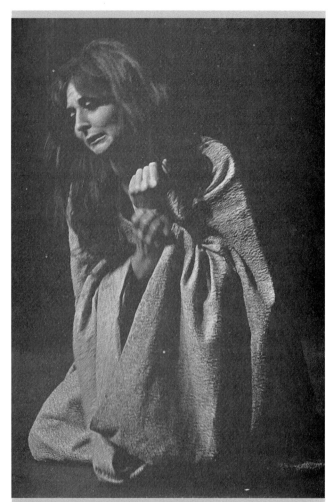

Lady Macbeth at the Oregon Shakespeare Festival. Courtesy of Oregon Shakespeare Festival. Martha J. Tippin as *Lady MacBeth* in the 1971 production of *MacBeth* at the Oregon Shakespeare Festival. Photographer: Carolyn Mason Jones, Director: Philip Davidson, Costume Designer: Jean Schultz Davidson, Scenic Designer: Richard L. Hay, Lighting Designer: Steven A. Maze.

"Out, damned spot! Out, I say." Lady MacBeth feels guilty for her role in a man's murder. This guilt results in extreme anxiety, and is displayed through obsessive-compulsive behavior. In this scene from Act V, Scene 1, she demonstrates compulsive handwashing—as if to cleanse herself of the deed.

ing their hands until their skin is raw; individuals distressed by obsessions about having left a door unlocked may be driven to check the lock every few minutes" (American Psychiatric Association, 1994, p. 418). While obsessions and compulsions are often experienced by the same individual, Obsessive-Compulsive Disorder refers to individuals who exhibit either obsessions or compulsions or both. In addition, individuals with this diagnosis recognize that their thoughts and/or behaviors are unreasonable.

In a thoughtful discussion of the challenges of practicing obstetrics in areas of the world with very high rates of human immunodeficiency virus (HIV) infection among young women, Douwe Verkuyl observed:

> Doctors have their own problems and private risks like everybody else and they lose colleagues and acquire extra family responsibilities. Professionally it is difficult to keep up morale when there are tragedies all around and to see the improvements in health indicators of a few years ago wiped out. Needle accidents are more than a 100 times riskier than in most of the first world where they are already cause for serious discussion. Tinkering with your car or even playing sport becomes dangerous because a resulting abrasion might be splashed by blood during the next breech delivery or soaked via a small puncture in a (re-sterilised) glove.
>
> Detecting a fungal infection between your toes, an infected mosquito bite, or an aphthous ulcer in your mouth brings on a cold sweat—and empathy with patients who do not want to be tested.

(Verkuyl, 1995, pp. 293–296)

While worries of contamination through touching unclean surfaces are common in Obsessive-Compulsive Disorder, it is hard to pass Verkuyl's concerns off as unrealistic anxiety. Practicing obstetrics in Zimbabwe probably *is* dangerous, and it is likely that any reasonable health care professional would have justifiable anxiety about becoming HIV infected. When concerns are in proportion to risk, the DSM-IV criteria for Obsessive-Compulsive Disorder are not met. Often, however, the fear of contamination greatly exceeds any real risk, a situation well illustrated by the following biographical excerpts from the life and writings of the late Howard Hughes.

Howard Hughes was one of the most successful and unusual Americans of the 20th century. Born in 1905, Hughes became a daring airplane pilot, the holder of numerous transcontinental and trans-Atlantic speed records, and, ultimately, the owner of several airlines. He also became a prominent Hollywood director, producer, and movie studio owner. Despite extraordinary wealth and fame (for years he was regarded as the world's richest man), his later life was lived in total isolation and was completely dominated by symptoms of Obsessive-Compulsive Disorder.

Howard Hughes

[By] December 24, 1958, his fifty-third birthday . . . Hughes spent almost all his time sitting naked in . . . the center of the living room—an area he called the "germ-free zone" . . . watching one motion picture after another. The furniture had been pushed back against the walls and the floor was piled high with stacks of old film cans, magazines, and newspapers. Although he rarely read anything, Hughes insisted on receiving every edition of the Los Angeles dailies. As newspapers accumulated, aides stacked them so as to leave aisles just wide enough for one person, criss-crossing the room. Each day Hughes painstakingly used Kleenex to wipe "dust and germs" from his chair, ottoman, side table, and telephone, going over the earpiece, mouthpiece, base, and cord with Kleenex, repeating the cleaning procedure again and again, tossing the used tissues onto a pile behind his chair.

. . . He dictated a torrent of memoranda aimed at preventing the 'backflow' or 'back transmission' of germs to him. In one, three pages long and single-spaced, he explained how he wanted a can of fruit opened: "The equipment used in connection with this operation will consist of the following items: 1 unopened newspaper, 1 sterile can opener, 1 large sterile plate, 1 sterile fork, 1 sterile spoon, 2 sterile brushes, 2 bars of soap, sterile paper towels."

Hughes outlined nine steps for opening the can: preparing a table, procuring a fruit can, washing of can, drying the can, processing the hands, opening the can, removing fruit from can, fallout rules while around can, and conclusion of operation. Hughes detailed how each step was to be accomplished. In Step No. 3, "Washing of Can," he wrote

> *The man in charge then turns the valve in the bathtub on, using his bare hands to do so. He also adjusts the water temperature so that it is not too hot nor too cold. He then takes one of the brushes, and using one of the bars of soap, creates a good lather, and then scrubs the can from a point two inches below the top of the can. He should first soak and remove the label, and then brush the cylindrical part of the can over and over until all particles of dust, pieces of paper label, and, in general, all sources of contamination have been removed. Holding the can in the center at all times, he then processes the bottom of the can in the same manner, being very sure that the bristles of the brush have thoroughly cleaned all the small*

indentations on the perimeter of the bottom of the can. He then rinses the soap from the cylindrical sides and the bottom of the can.

When the fruit was dished onto the plate, Hughes wanted "fallout rules" in effect: "Be sure that no part of the body, including the hands, be directly over the can or the plate at any time. If possible, keep the head, upper part of the body, arms, etc. at least a foot away from the can of fruit and the sterile plate at all times." During the procedure, there must be "absolutely no talking, coughing, clearing of the throat, or any movement whatsoever of the lips."

To make absolutely certain that, with a few authorized exceptions, no one would come in contact with any of the supplies stored in an adjoining bungalow for his use, Hughes issued explicit orders:

> *No matter how extreme the emergency, no matter how unusual the circumstances may be, no matter what may have arisen, it is extremely important to me that nobody ever goes into any room, closet, cabinet, drawer, bathroom or any other area used to store any of the things which are for me—either food, equipment, magazines, paper supplies, Kleenex—no matter what. It is equally important to me that nobody ever opens any doors or opening to any room, cabinet or closet or anything used to store any of my things, even for one-thousandth of an inch, for one-thousandth of a second. I don't want the possibility of dust or insects or anything of that nature entering.*

. . . There were even special procedures to be followed in removing his hearing-aid cord from the cabinet where it was stored.*

(Bartlett & Steele, 1979, pp. 232–235).

Unlike Hughes, few sufferers of Obsessive-Compulsive Disorder have the money to hire others to participate with them in the compulsive behavior that "protects" them from fears of contamination. Many persons with this disorder hide their symptoms and rituals from family and friends; others incorporate them into a troubled daily life:

> In a fanatic pursuit of cleanliness [one 49-year-old woman] uses up more than 225 bars of soap on herself every month, wears rubber gloves even to switch on a light—and makes her husband sleep alone so she won't be contaminated by him.

(Goodwin, 1986, p. 174)

Epidemiology

While few persons carry their obsessive-compulsive anxieties to the extreme reached by Hughes, the condition that affected this man is far from rare (Nymberg & Van Noppen, 1994). Obsessive-Compulsive Disorder is said to occur about as commonly as diabetes and asthma, and yet patients frequently hide their symptoms from family and health care providers. Most cases of this disorder begin in quite young individuals, often during young adulthood or before. While most obsessive-compulsive individuals improve with time, some require intensive treatment or hospitalization. As will be discussed in what follows, until recently Obsessive-Compulsive Disorder was very resistant to drug treatment.

Post-Traumatic Stress Disorder

Post-Traumatic Stress Disorder is an anxiety disorder that typically occurs after a frightening event, most often an accident, crime, or battle. This condition may follow natural disasters, as discussed in Chapter 9. Individuals with this disorder have been exposed to an event that threatened or caused either death or "a threat to the physical integrity of self or others" (American Psychiatric Association, 1994, p. 427). The response to this exposure must have been one of fear or helplessness, and the event needs to be persistently reexperienced through recurrent recollections, dreams, or hallucinatory-like flashbacks. Additionally, individuals with this diagnosis exhibit impairment of social functioning, the presence of specific anxiety symptoms, and "persistent avoidance of stimuli associated with the trauma and numbing of general responsiveness" (American Psychiatric Association, 1994, p. 428).

It is important to remember that illness and even medical care itself can be profoundly frightening experiences. For some persons, hospital memories can act as stimuli to true Post-Traumatic Stress Disorder. In the 1970s, several cases were reported of surgical patients who awoke out of general anesthesia only to find themselves still mentally undergoing surgery and fully paralyzed. None could remember the actual event, but each suffered marked and sometimes quite prolonged distress, with nightmares and a vague sense of the experience being more than just a dream:

---

*From *EMPIRE: The Life, Legend, and Madness of Howard Hughes* by Donald L. Bartlett and James B. Steele. Copyright © 1979 by Donald L. Bartlett and James B. Steele. Reprinted by permission of W. W. Norton & Company, Inc.

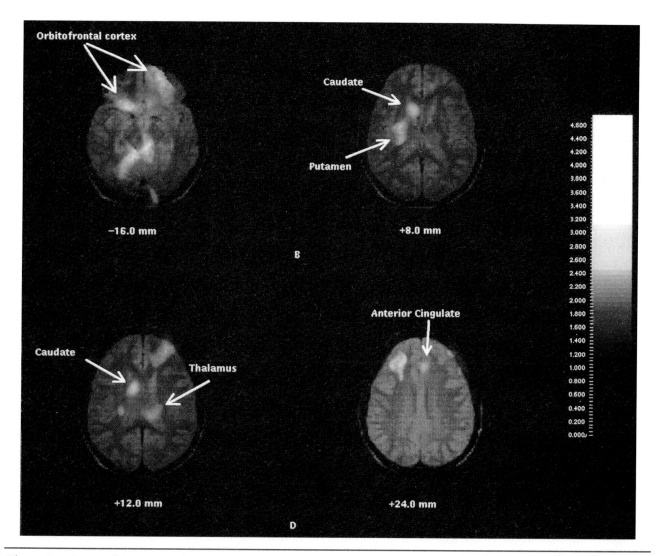

Obsessive-Compulsive Disorder: PET images. Four persons with Obsessive-Compulsive Disorder were exposed to images or objects that provoked severe anxiety related to obsessive-compulsive symptoms. PET images show increased blood flow (yellow, orange/red) in specific brain areas after exposure compared to exposure to "neutral objects." *From "Regional Cerebral Blood Flow Measured During Symptom Provocation in Obsessive-Compulsive Disorder Using Oxygen-15 Labeled Carbon Dioxide and Positron Emission Tomography," by Rauch, S. L., Jenike, M. A., Alpert, N. M., Baer, L., Breiter, H. C., Savage, C. R., and Fischman, A. J., 1994,* Archives of General Psychiatry, 51, *p. 66. Copyright 1994, American Medical Association. Reprinted with permission.*

Coronary Bypass Surgery

A 52 year old man was extremely anxious and irritable following coronary bypass. . . . He had repetitive dreams of being tied down and unable to move. He related his anxiety to a recollection of being sewn up at the end of surgery.

EXAMINER: Are you sure it wasn't a dream?
PATIENT: I'm positive!
EXAMINER: Are you sure?
PATIENT: I'm absolutely sure!

EXAMINER: I think you're right. You were awake at the end of surgery.
PATIENT: (With amazement) I was?*
(Blacher, 1975, pp. 67–68)

Each of the surgical patients described in this report had a remarkably rapid cure after recognizing that their symptoms originated from awakening paralyzed during surgery.

*From "On Awakening Paralyzed During Surgery," by R. S Blacher, 1975, *Journal of the American Medical Association, 234,* pp. 67–68. Copyright 1975, American Medical Association. Reprinted with permission.

Hysterectomy

A 25 year old hospital secretary underwent a hysterectomy. . . . [Later] she . . . disclosed that she had been plagued by a nightly nightmare of hearing voices and then seeing people floating over her. She would fight their taking her somewhere, and felt she was choking and couldn't defend herself. The prominent feeling was that she was dead or dying and she would awaken in terror and be unable to go back to sleep. She was constantly preoccupied with death.

She had not told of her symptoms in the hospital for fear she would be considered insane, but now she felt overwhelmed by them. When it was suggested that she must have been awake during surgery, she began to connect the dream with specific people. She recalled her surgeon giving orders; she related the choking to the endotracheal tube. . . . The night after this discussion, she had the dream again but instead of experiencing the usual terror, she rolled over and went back to sleep. The nightmare never recurred, her irritability disappeared, and she felt normal by the next day.

(Blacher, 1975 p. 67)

In none of the cases described by Blacher was there any independent corroboration that anesthesia had lightened. And while the explanations seemed to relieve all clients' symptoms, and midsurgical awakenings *have* previously been documented by anesthesiologists, there can be no absolute certainty that each client truly suffered paralysis while awake. Establishing the reality of a post-traumatic stress episode may not be critically important when surgery is the cause and reassurance brings about a rapid cure. However, in recent years there has been great interest in adult post-traumatic stress due to unrecalled childhood trauma, most commonly sexual abuse. In several highly publicized cases, individuals "remembered" sexual assaults that occurred many years before and brought criminal charges against alleged perpetrators (Crews, 1994). Psychologists are strongly divided as to where the truth lies in these complex stories, but there is little doubt that individuals can vividly remember events that did not happen and confess to crimes they did not commit. In fact, there is reason to believe that under some circumstances, a person who confesses to a crime may be more likely to be innocent than one who denies involvement (Cohen & Stewart, 1995). The psychological dynamics of Post-Traumatic Stress Disorder are exceedingly complex and interesting; truth is sometimes difficult or impossible to determine. While some apparently repressed memories may involve events that never truly happened, many, if not most, of the events giving rise to post-traumatic stress are well documented, violent, and all too real. A particularly famous example of Post-Traumatic Stress Disorder due to a disastrous flood is discussed in detail in Chapter 9.

Epidemiology

Post-Traumatic Stress Disorder is probably most commonly seen in military situations. The conditions of war are exceedingly frightening to civilians and soldiers alike. The

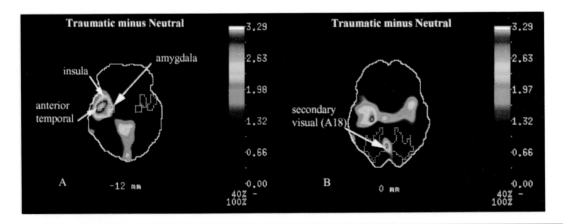

Post-Traumatic Stress Disorder: PET image. These PET scans depict brain blood flow changes in two clients with Post-Traumatic Stress Disorder who were asked to listen to a recorded "neutral voice" describing an episode of trauma similar to one that they had previously experienced. Listening to this script greatly increased heart rate and fear (as reported on a standardized scale). The PET results show marked increases in brain blood flow to specific areas. *From "A Symptom Provocation Study of Post-Traumatic Stress Disorders Using Positron Emission Tomography and Sight-Driven Imagery," by Rauch, S. L., Vanderkolk, B. A., Fisher, R. E., Alpert, N. M., Orr, S. P., Savage, C. R., Fischman, A. J., Jenike, M. A., Pitman, R. K., 1996, Archives of General Psychiatry, 53, p. 385. Copyright, 1996, American Medical Association. Reprinted with permission.*

more violence experienced, the more likely it is that post-traumatic stress will occur. The degree of anxiety and the duration of symptoms may be highly variable from person to person (Goodwin, 1986) and may depend importantly on pre-traumatic mental health and subsequent social support. There is an exceedingly wide prevalence range reported for this condition. In surveys of persons exposed to serious danger, Post-Traumatic Stress Disorder has been found in as few as 3% and as many as 58% of individuals (American Psychiatric Association, 1994). While persons with pre-traumatic psychiatric symptoms may be more likely to develop serious Post-Traumatic Stress Disorder, given a severe enough psychological stressor, virtually anyone seems likely to be susceptible. Half of individuals are completely recovered by 3 months, but the remainder may continue to be affected for a year or more (American Psychiatric Association, 1994).

CAUSES OF ANXIETY DISORDERS

While the symptoms of anxiety have their biological origins in the limbic system of the brain (or perhaps deeper in the brainstem), many forms of anxiety occur in response to environmental stimuli. Psychologists have developed a wide range of theories to explain anxiety. While psychoanalysis offers somewhat different explanations for each person's symptoms, psychoanalytic theories typically postulate the origin of anxiety as being infantile conflicts involving sexual development. The essence of psychoanalytic theory is that mental processes are unconscious and, as a result, only dimly accessible to personal understanding, most often through dreams. Anxiety, according to psychoanalysis, comes from unconscious processes that originate in early childhood experiences. Such psychoanalytic explanations are virtually impossible to validate, given how subjective and private an individual's unconscious experience really is. As one sympathetic critic has observed:

> The question is not whether Freud got it exactly right, or whether strong criticisms cannot be made of some of his case histories, but whether the types of explanation he introduced substantially amplify the understanding of ourselves and others that common-sense psychology provides.

(Nagel, 1994a, p. 34)

Recently, such "commonsense" theories have seemed more attractive to many psychologists than psychoanalysis. One such theory postulates two highly individual factors: adversity and trait anxiety. **Adversity** is a measure of how strong a given stimulus for anxiety is: A large earthquake or explosion is likely to make almost anyone anxious, whereas a small spider is unlikely to bother most individuals very much. **Trait anxiety** is an abstract but measurable personality characteristic based on the everyday observa-

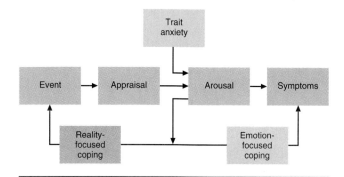

Figure 10-1   Model for anxiety. *From* Treatment of Anxiety Disorders: A Clinician's Guide and Patient Manuals, *by Andrews et al., 1994, New York: Cambridge University Press. Reprinted with permission of Cambridge University Press.*

tion that some quite normal individuals appear to experience more anxiety than do others. Persons who admit to feeling more anxious than others are said to have high levels of trait anxiety. A model for perceived anxiety based on these two concepts is illustrated in Figure 10-1.

In this model, the individual appraises an event based on its actual adversity and on inherent patterns of trait anxiety. The result is a degree of arousal that may or may not lead to symptoms. Arousal often also results in efforts to reduce anxiety. These can take the form of symptom-reducing activities such as deep breathing or stimulus-reducing activities such as getting out of a closet that has a spider in it. This model refers to these two coping methods as "emotion-focused coping" and "reality-focused coping," respectively.

This kind of commonsense model can be useful in understanding anxiety and in helping clients to improve their abilities to cope with anxiety symptoms. However, many psychologists are uncomfortable with ideas like trait anxiety, which do not seem to offer any deep explanation of why some people are more anxious than others. Some have sought biological explanations in neurotransmitters, brain blood flow, and brain receptors for tranquilizer-like substances. While much research has been reported, to date none of these biological explanations has provided a complete explanation for the mystery of anxiety. Fortunately, effective treatment for anxiety disorders seems not to require a full understanding of the causes of human anxiety.

TREATMENT OF ANXIETY DISORDERS

Psychotherapy

Psychotherapy continues to be widely used in the treatment of anxiety disorders. Psychotherapy can be viewed as falling into two general categories: those therapies based on helping individuals achieve insight into *why* they feel anxiety and those that emphasize behavioral means of controlling the anxiety.

Insight-Based Treatments

Psychotherapy based on insight into symptoms may sometimes be valuable, especially for highly motivated individuals whose symptoms are not disabling. Psychoanalysis is among the best known of the insight therapies and has been widely employed to assist persons with anxiety. The benefits claimed for psychoanalysis and other insight-based therapies in anxiety are entirely anecdotal:

> While I don't know whether psychoanalysis is more or less effective in eliminating unwanted symptoms than medication or behavior therapy, for example, I am quite sure that it has a different kind of effect on patients from more "external" forms of treatment. My observation is that psychoanalysis can confer a valuable form of self-knowledge which is deep though essentially perceptual and not theoretical, and that this self-understanding, whether or not it cures [anxiety] directly, can be used by those who have it to anticipate, identify and manage forms of irrationality that would otherwise victimize or even disable them. It also permits a subtler response to [anxiety] in others, through the enhancement of psychological imagination. For this reason I believe it will survive the development of simpler symptomatic cures.
>
> (Nagel, 1994b, p. 56)

Behaviorally Based Treatments

In contrast, there is strong empirical evidence that behaviorally based treatments are effective in treating at least some anxiety disorders. For example, studies consistently show that cognitive-behavior therapy results in significant benefit for persons suffering from panic attacks (Goldfried, Greenberg, & Marmar, 1990). **Cognitive-behavior therapy** assumes that clients can learn to identify the common stimuli that give rise to their anxiety, develop plans to respond to those stimuli with nonanxious responses, and problem solve when unanticipated anxiety-provoking situations arise. While insight is very much involved in this process, it is not insight into deep psychological causes, as in psychoanalysis, but, rather, practical commonsense problem solving. Data show that cognitive-behavior therapy is better than placebo in treating phobic disorders, Obsessive-Compulsive Disorder, and Generalized Anxiety Disorder (Andrews, 1993). Treatment appears both to be effective during the relatively brief course of therapy and to remain effective for some months after therapy finishes. It is still unclear, however, how long benefit from cognitive-behavior therapy truly lasts (Andrews, 1993). As a result,

there may be an important need for medical and psychological follow-up to ensure satisfactory improvement. Further information about cognitive-behavior therapy is found in Chapter 26.

Techniques for enhancing relaxation might seem to be of use in controlling acute symptoms of anxiety, but studies to date suggest relaxation alone may be no more beneficial than placebo in affecting long-term symptoms of Generalized Anxiety Disorder (Andrews, 1993).

Pharmacotherapy

Humans have known for centuries that certain drugs (alcohol in particular, but also opiates) are effective under some circumstances in significantly reducing anxiety. In recent years safer and more effective pharmacological treatments have been developed. The most common of these medications used for the treatment of anxiety include the benzodiazepine "minor tranquilizers" such as diazepam (Valium), alprazolam (Xanax), and chlordiazepoxide (Librium). Antidepressants can be effective in some forms of anxiety disorder, particularly Obsessive-Compulsive Disorder. Medications commonly used for this problem include clomipramine, fluvoxamine, and fluoxetine (Prozac). Buspirone, neither a tranquilizer nor an antidepressant, may also be effective for anxiety and appears to have very few side effects. Tricyclic antidepressants have proven effective in treating Panic Disorder.

Benzodiazepines have established short-term effectiveness in the control of anxiety symptoms. They are clearly the treatment of choice for acute episodes of anxiety, such as occur during crises. They are widely used to reduce anxiety responses to uncomfortable or frightening medical procedures such as colonoscopy. Their long-term effectiveness is more uncertain. In one study, 61% of 31 persons with Generalized Anxiety treated for 6 to 12 months with diazepam (Valium) sought additional psychological counseling (Power, Simpson, Swanson, & Wallace, 1990). One might conclude from these findings that benzodiazepines only partially relieve the symptoms of anxiety. What benefit these drugs do bring is often achieved at the expense of significant physical dependence. In one 40-month study, 65% of persons put on benzodiazepine medication were still taking the drug after the 40 months (Rickelsk & Schweizer, 1990). Withdrawal from benzodiazepines frequently produces moderate to severe symptoms of insomnia, anxiety, and even seizures. Benzodiazepines are controlled substances and should probably be used with more discretion than is currently the case. As Saraceno and colleagues observed in a World Health Organization review of psychiatric treatment:

> The recent literature concerning [benzodiazepines] has focused almost exclusively on their potential to produce dependence. . . . Their prescription is

widespread in general practice, and an important fraction of long-term consumers start off with symptomatic treatment irrespective of formal diagnoses of mental disorder and eventually become "cases" of formal psychiatric interest precisely on the grounds of their developing dependence.

(Saraceno, Tognoni, & Garattini, 1993, p. 63)

Combination Therapy

In many cases it would appear that the ideal treatment for anxiety disorders is a combination of medication and psychotherapy. For Generalized Anxiety Disorder, psychotherapy, particularly cognitive-behavior therapy, should likely be the main treatment, with benzodiazepines used as needed to control acute episodes not responding to learned cognitive skills. Post-Traumatic Stress Disorder is often treated with a combination of antidepressants and psychotherapy, although the effectiveness of antidepressant treatment has not been consistently shown (Andrews, 1993). This disorder often proves particularly difficult to treat, and patients frequently remain seriously impaired by their symptoms despite the best of current treatment efforts.

Panic Disorder without Agoraphobia usually responds effectively to drugs, but side effects (antidepressants) and dependence (alprazolam) often limit long-term use. Cognitive-behavior therapy has been shown to be quite effective, and addition of drug treatment apparently does not increase treatment effectiveness (Andrews, 1993). With or without associated Panic Disorder, Agoraphobia is often very difficult to treat. Antidepressants are of value in some persons and may be combined with behavior therapy. One effective behavior therapy for Agoraphobia may be "exposure therapy," in which clients are exposed for 2 hours or more to the stimuli that bring on their symptoms. Studies using nurses trained as behavior therapists show high levels of effectiveness (Marks, 1987). Exposure therapy is successful in reducing symptoms, but few clients experience full relief from their anxiety.

The best treatment for Specific Phobia is almost certainly some form of behavioral therapy, probably controlled exposure therapy (Cottraux, 1993). There is some evidence that adding benzodiazepines may increase effectiveness, but this has not been confirmed. In the absence of associated depression, tricyclic antidepressants have little benefit in this disorder.

As noted previously, Obsessive-Compulsive Disorder often responds well to selective serotonin reuptake inhibitor (SSRI) antidepressants such as fluvoxamine and clomipramine, but relapse is very common after medication is stopped. It is thought by some that combining cognitive-behavior psychotherapy and medication may be particularly effective (Mavissakalian & Jones, 1989), but there is no strong evidence that such combination

RESEARCH HIGHLIGHT

Partial Hospital Management of Severe Obsessive-Compulsive Disorder

STUDY PROBLEM/PURPOSE

To evaluate the effects of a partial-hospital program that combined behaviorial therapy, medication, and psychosocial intervention for 58 clients with severe Obsessive-Compulsive Disorder.

METHODS

Partial hospitalization involved attendance at the program 5 days a week, 6 hours a day, for at least 6 weeks, after which the time at hospital was tapered. Most clients completed the program in 12 weeks. Clients were assigned to a treatment team that consisted of a nurse, a psychologist, and a physician. Psychosocial intervention included individual and group work; clients were given education to recognize their obsessions and compulsions, to identify their own need for drugs, and to determine how work could improve their functioning. Medications included clomipramine or SSRIs. Behavioral therapy was given, designed to target each client's obsessive fears.

FINDINGS

Results indicated that a majority had successful outcome. Fifty-five percent completed the program with only mild symptoms of Obsessive-Compulsive Disorder. Most clients sustained their improvement at 6, 12, and 18 months after discharge.

IMPLICATIONS

Partial hospitalization is an effective treatment for clients with Obsessive-Compulsive Disorder.

From "A Preliminary Study of Partial Hospital Management of Severe Obsessive-Compulsive Disorder," by A. Bystritsky et al., 1996, *Psychiatric Services, 47,* 170–174.

treatment is better than either treatment alone. When Obsessive-Compulsive Disorder is extremely severe, as in the description of Howard Hughes earlier in this chapter, neurosurgical procedures may occasionally be the only effective treatment (Griest, 1990). This surgery involves making lesions to interrupt efferent tracts from the frontal cortex to the limbic and basal ganglia structures thought to be involved in Obsessive-Compulsive Disorder. Less than 0.5% of clients with Obsessive-Compulsive Disorder become surgical candidates, but for those that do, outcomes are particularly positive. In one study, 65% were symptom free without additional treatment; others were much improved (Griest, 1990).

ANXIETY AND SPIRITUAL WELL-BEING

While both medication and psychotherapy can provide relief for disabling symptoms, many persons manage to live creative and spiritually full lives despite moderately severe anxiety. E. B. White, perhaps best remembered today for his children's story *Charlotte's Web* about an anxious pig and a reassuring spider, was, like Mr. Trexler in the excerpt that follows, a victim of anxiety. For Mr. Trexler (and, one assumes, for the author who created him), gentle humor and a heart-felt appreciation of natural beauty provide a powerful and deeply spiritual antidote to the worries and fears of daily life:

The Second Tree from the Corner

"Ever have any bizarre thoughts?" asked the doctor.

Mr. Trexler failed to catch the word. "What kind?" he said.

"Bizarre," repeated the doctor, his voice steady. He watched his patient for any slight change of expression, any wince. It seemed to Trexler that the doctor was not only watching him closely but was creeping slowly toward him, like a lizard toward a bug. Trexler shoved his chair back an inch and gathered himself for a reply. He was about to say "Yes" when he realized that if he said yes the next question would be unanswerable. Bizarre thoughts, bizarre thoughts. . . . Let's see, bizarre thoughts. Trexler dodged back along the dreadful corridor of the years to see what he could find. He felt the doctor's eyes upon him and knew that time was running out. Don't be so conscientious, he said to himself. If a bizarre thought is indicated here, just reach into the bag and pick anything at all. A man as well supplied with bizarre thoughts as you are should have no difficulty producing one for the record. Trexler darted into the bag, hung for a moment before one of his thoughts, as a hummingbird pauses in the delphinium. No, he said, not that one. He darted to another (the one about the rhesus monkey), paused, considered. No, he said, not that.

Trexler knew he must hurry. He had already used up pretty nearly four seconds since the question had been put. But it was an impossible situation—just one more lousy, impossible situation such as he was always getting himself into. . . .

He looked straight at the doctor. "No," he said quietly. "I never have any bizarre thoughts." . . .

For several weeks thereafter he continued to visit the doctor. . . . Each session would begin with a resume of symptoms—the dizziness in the streets, the constricting pain in the back of the neck, the apprehensions, the tightness of the scalp, the inability to concentrate, the despondency and the melancholy times, the feeling of pressure and tension, the anger at not being able to work, the anxiety over work not done, the gas on the stomach. . . .

It was on the fifth visit, about halfway through that the doctor turned to Trexler and said, suddenly, "What do you want?" He gave the word "want" special emphasis.

"I d'know," replied Trexler uneasily. "I guess nobody knows the answer to that one."

"Sure they do," replied the doctor.

"Do you know what you want?" asked Trexler narrowly.

"Certainly," said the doctor . . . "I want a wing on the small house I own in Westport. I want more money, and more leisure to do the things I want to do." . . .

Trexler settled down again and resumed the role of patient for the rest of the visit. It ended on a kindly, friendly note . . . and the doctor followed along to let him out. It was late; the secretary had shut up shop and gone home. Another day over the dam. "Goodbye," said Trexler. He stepped into the street, turned west toward Madison, and thought of the doctor all alone there, after hours, in that desolate hole—a man who worked longer hours than his secretary. Poor, scared, overworked bastard, thought Trexler. And that new wing! . . .

Trexler felt invigorated. Suddenly his sickness seemed health, his dizziness stability. A small tree, rising between him and the light stood there saturated with the evening, each gilt-edged leaf perfectly drunk with excellence and delicacy. Trexler's spine registered an ever so slight tremor as it picked up this natural disturbance in the lovely scene. "I want the second tree from the corner, just as it stands," he said, answering an imaginary question from an imaginary physician. And he felt a slow pride in realizing that what he wanted none could bestow, and that what he had none could take away. He felt content to be sick, unembarrassed at being afraid; and in the jungle of his fear he glimpsed (as he had so often glimpsed them before) the flashy tail feathers of the bird courage.*

(White, 1954, pp. 97–103)

REFLECTIVE THINKING

Finding Peace by Knowing One's Values

The excerpt from E. B. White brings to mind the fact that knowing one's values and beliefs helps one to separate from the general anxiety in life and know what is important. Consider the meaning of wanting the second tree from the corner and identify what you want, that "inexpressible and unattainable" thing that would be your personal source of comfort or solace.

E. B. White implies that there is a transcendent sense of humanness that has much to do with finding peace in an anxiety-driven existence. Consider the issues raised in the accompanying Reflective Thinking box in relation to your own life.

NURSING THEORY AND CLIENTS EXPERIENCING ANXIETY

From a perspective of nursing care, two major ideas are relevant to caring for clients with anxiety disorders. First, providing such care requires great patience, trust, and intuition, and, second, the nurse must fully understand the nature of the client's anxiety and sense of being overpowered by the emotion. While no nursing theory directly addresses anxiety as a concept, the Modeling and

---

*All pages (edited) from *The Second Tree from the Corner* by E. B. White. Copyright 1947 by E. B. White. Copyright renewed. Reprinted by permission of HarperCollins Publishers, Inc.

Role-Modeling Theory gives clear direction in providing care to any client with anxiety disorders. Modeling and Role-Modeling suggests two nursing interventions critical to initiating care: building trust and modeling the client's world. Both of these interventions are effective but, for many nurses, difficult to accomplish when working with clients experiencing anxiety.

Building trust requires that the nurse accept the client as he is, without demands or judgments. The nurse must show the client that the nurse comes to the relationship in an atmosphere of caring. Supportive presence, then, is the first step in establishing trust. Modeling the client's world means entering into the client's perceptions, seeing the world from the client's perspective, and basing interactions on the nurse's understanding of the client's subjective experiences.

Building trust with a person overcome by anxiety will take patience. The nurse must have a true understanding that the client's emotions are real, overpowering, and not within the client's conscious control. It is easy for a nurse to assume that the client is exaggerating her emotions, because of the fact that the emotions themselves are an exaggeration of the situation. In anxiety disorders, the client knows that her emotions are extreme for the context; however, these emotions are still a very real part of her existence. Before trust can be established, the client needs assurance that the nurse is accepting and will not simply expect that the client can "snap out of it."

The best way for the nurse to show acceptance is to model the client's world—to understand the client's subjective experience, to consider what the outside world is like from the client's perspective, and to enter figuratively into the client's personal world. If the nurse understands the client's emotions, feelings, and needs, the nurse will be able to assist the client to use whatever resources available to reestablish balance.

N U R S I N G   P R O C E S S

▽ ASSESSMENT

Since all persons experience anxiety in everyday living and all persons seeking health care express at least some anxiety related to their need for care, it is essential that the nurse have the ability to make an assessment of anxiety and determine if the anxiety being expressed is healthy or not. One author states, "Recognizing anxiety and assessing its cause are as essential [to nursing care] as monitoring vital signs" (Spear, 1996, p. 41.) Another author cautions that nurses

in home care settings will see clients with anxiety and the nurses must be in a position to make careful assessment of that anxiety (Busch, 1996). In such an assessment, the nurse must be able to determine if the client's anxiety is a symptom of one of the anxiety disorders presented in this chapter or if the anxiety is a temporary response to a current stressor.

In making the assessment, the nurse should begin with the observable, physical signs of anxiety—increased pulse, blood pressure, and respiratory rate; a heightened startle response; and "gut symptoms" such as urinary frequency or abdominal distress. Then, the nurse should inquire about the client's cognitive responses—sense of disorientation, difficulty concentrating, and/or fear of losing control. When anxiety level rises, the client may become confused and/or distressed, may have difficulty thinking, and may not be able to cope.

The nurse may find that both the client and his family members can provide information on how he usually copes and what degree of stress he has been experiencing. Knowledge of the client's support system will also assist in determining to what degree the client's environment is able to support his own ability to cope. The accompanying display provides an excellent tool for use in screening for anxiety disorders. By asking these 13 questions, the nurse has a measure to assess if an anxiety disorder may exist.

Once data are collected and screening is completed, the nurse may assess that the client has anxiety to the level that psychiatric care need be initiated.

▽ NURSING DIAGNOSIS

Several nursing diagnoses are relevant to any of the anxiety disorders, and some are likely to be relevant to one of the specific disorders. The accompanying display lists diagnoses and related factors commonly assigned to clients with anxiety disorders. These diagnoses address not the anxiety disorder itself, but the *human response* to the disorder.

▽ OUTCOME IDENTIFICATION

Nursing care for any of the anxiety disorders must be based on achieving realistic outcomes of care. The nurse will set outcome goals in collaboration with the client and will recognize that it may take weeks for the client to feel a sense of control of his life or months to achieve a day-to-day perception of decreased anxiety. Realistic outcomes might be that the client's anxiety is decreased so that he may drive a car on the freeway without fear of panic attack or that he may leave the house in the morning at least 2 days without excessive anxiety regarding being out in public.

▽ PLANNING/INTERVENTIONS

The nurse's independent role in treating anxiety disorders is to plan interventions aimed at assisting the client to cope with subjective, human responses to the anxiety experienced. The nurse's collaborative role is to work with a psychiatric team to carry out a multidisciplinary treatment plan. Thus, the interventions discussed in what follows will include both the nurse's independent and collaborative roles.

As described in the section related to nursing theory, the nursing interventions of therapeutic listening, building trust, and establishing a positive nurse-client relationship are essential to providing care. The nurse must let the client know that he understands and accepts her symptoms of anxiety as real and important; the nurse knows the client feels she is about to lose control and does not make demands that the client is unable to meet. Nursing interventions for specific nursing diagnoses are directed toward alleviating symptoms, for example, identifying symptoms of an impending panic attack and administering medication. The nurse can use his understanding of the client's typical response to anxiety to help the client enhance her coping skills and social supports. The nurse may be able to help the client redirect activities so that there is less time and focus on the symptom and more time and focus on present, constructive activities. For example, the nurse may help a client with Obsessive-Compulsive Disorder to engage in satisfying activities—walking with others, going to movies, doing volunteer work—instead of directing attention to the client's particular symptoms. The nurse

---

NURSING DIAGNOSES AND RELATED FACTORS COMMON IN CLIENTS WITH ANXIETY DISORDERS

◆ *Anxiety*, related to a subjective sense of uneasiness and tension

◆ *Fear*, related to a specific object, for example, a phobic fear of heights

◆ *Sleep-pattern disturbance*, related to anxiety of being alone, fear of the dark, or flashbacks associated with post-traumatic stress

◆ *Social isolation*, related to restriction of travel away from home or places felt to be "safe"

◆ *Altered family processes*, related to adjustments family members must make to accommodate compulsive and/or phobic behaviors of one of their members

◆ *Powerlessness*, related to feeling out of control of one's own thoughts and behaviors

◆ *Post-trauma response*, related to anxiety felt following a significant, life-threatening event

◆ *Dysfunctional grieving*, related to inability to cope with grief following significant losses associated with a significant, life-threatening event.

North American Nursing Diagnosis Association (1996) *NANDA Nursing Diagnoses: Definitions and Classification 1997–1998.* Philadelphia: NANDA.

ASKING CLIENTS ABOUT SYMPTOMS OF ANXIETY DISORDERS

Here are questions that have been useful in asking clients about symptoms of anxiety disorders. You may find that you prefer to word these questions somewhat differently, but the important thing is to ask them. Many clients experience anxiety symptoms for years before a doctor, nurse, or psychologist takes the time to ask about these symptoms.

Generalized Anxiety Disorder

Do you find yourself worrying frequently about a number of different things, such as the way things are going for you at home, work, or school?

Do you find yourself feeling anxious or tense much of the time without any obvious reason?

Panic Disorder

Have you ever experienced sudden, intense fear for no reason?

Have you found yourself experiencing intense physical symptoms of chest pain, shortness of breath, dizziness, or sweating, along with a sense that something terrible or life-threatening was happening to you?

Agoraphobia

Do you find yourself uncomfortable in places where you can't get help or escape, such as walking alone, or on a bridge, or in a crowded area?

Are you uncomfortable leaving your home or going traveling without a friend or companion?

Specific Phobia

Are there certain things, places, or activities that you usually or always find fearful—such as spiders, high places, or flying in an airplane?

If you do have fears about specific things, places, or activities, do these fears affect any of your activities at work, home, or school?

Obsessive-Compulsive Disorder

Do you find yourself troubled by persistent or recurrent thoughts that you can't easily get out of your mind—such as thoughts of death, illness, or doing something socially embarrassing (for example, saying something inappropriate, rude, or indecent)?

Do you find yourself unable to easily stop doing certain activities over and over again: activities such as checking that doors are locked, washing your hands, or counting objects?

Post-Traumatic Stress Disorder

Have you ever had a particularly traumatic experience such as witnessing or experiencing violence or a catastrophic event (such as a flood or fire)?

Have you ever found yourself re-experiencing a violent or catastrophic event through dreams or waking "flashbacks"?

---

may frequently fill the role of coordinating various community resources, such as visits to mental health clinics, participation in support groups, and follow-up home visiting services evaluating the effects of medication.

Nurses can be involved in a collaborative role in all treatments previously described, including cognitive-behavioral training, supportive group therapy, insight-based psychotherapy, and use of medications. Further, the nurse will frequently be in a position to provide support and guidance to family members who are attempting to live their own lives while accommodating the special needs of the client. Family members will need information, suggestions for reasonable accommodation of family processes, and emotional support.

▽ EVALUATION

Nursing care should be evaluated in terms of whether or not the expected outcomes were achieved. In anxiety disorders, one cannot expect the client to experience a complete "cure" or remission of the disorder. However, the therapeutic goal should be that the client achieve a level of control over his anxieties and be able to experience life in a personally satisfying manner. There is obviously a need for the nurse and client to discuss realistic expectations and to determine the client's needs and wants in relation to his own illness.

The following three case studies illustrate the application of the nursing process to clients having different anxiety disorders.

CASE STUDY/CARE PLAN

MENTAL HEALTH CLINIC

Earlier in the chapter, Professor Leonard explained his own experience with Panic Disorder. He made clear that he was writing for the reader who understood his "fear of Fear," not for the reader who minimalized his overpowering emotions. The nurse will understand that, even though there is no rational basis for the panic, the panic is real and that one attack will leave the professor vulnerable to repeated attacks.

When a client comes to a mental health clinic seeking help for her panic attacks, the psychiatric nurse could assist her, providing support and assurance that others have presented with the same symptoms. One fear of many clients with panic attacks is that they are alone in their symptoms. It is reassuring to the client if the nurse can relay that he has seen others in similar situations and understands both the severity of and the inability to control the symptoms. The nurse would support the treatment plan offered by mental health workers as a team and accepted by the client. Behaviorally based treatment for the purpose of helping the client identify stimuli that precipitate panic would be helpful. Further, since some clients find comfort through the use of transitional objects (for example, carrying an umbrella), this approach could be explored with him.

Imagine that nurses are giving care to Professor Jones, a college professor who experiences panic attacks. The nurses encounter Professor Jones in two settings, an emergency department where he comes for treatment of symptoms, and in the mental health clinic, where he has been referred for follow-up care. A fictionalized nursing care plan follows.

EMERGENCY ROOM

It is highly likely that Professor Jones would, at some point in his illness, appear in an emergency room in the midst of one of his panic attacks. At this point, he would present with symptoms of palpitations, sweating, trembling, shortness of breath, a sensation of choking, chest pain, nausea, and dizziness. Emergency room staff would immediately initiate treatment to rule out physical causes for his symptoms (cardiac arrythmias). By the time such assessments had been completed, the panic attack would be subsiding, and the professor would have diminished symptoms.

Nursing care in this situation first requires an immediate assessment of the potential dangerous physical causes of the symptoms, so that treatment can be provided. Second, the nurse must have a professional understanding of the condition of Panic Disorder to provide compassionate and appropriate care to a client with a psychiatric condition. Because many clients with panic attacks do not seek help for their condition but, rather, live in fear and distress, it is those times when the client is brought into emergency settings that the nurse can provide support and make appropriate referral.

ASSESSMENT

Professor Jones's panic attacks are unpredictable and intense. He has the classic symptoms of breathing abnormalities, chest pain, and a paralyzing fear that led to more frequent attacks over time. He is becoming increasingly debilitated by these attacks and is seeking professional assistance.

Continued

NURSING DIAGNOSIS *Anxiety, severe,* related to increasingly frequent panic attacks and previous experience of panic attacks, as evidenced by tension, apprehension, and uncertainty

Outcomes	Planning/Interventions	Evaluation
◆ Within 1 month Professor Jones will develop an awareness of his own anxiety by becoming aware of the antecedents to his panic attacks. ◆ Within 1 month, the client will practice anxiety control techniques: use of medication, use of transitional object, and use of support system.	◆ Assist the client in evaluating patterns of lifestyle and stress and the number of panic attacks he suffers. ◆ Offer reassurance and support. ◆ Establish a therapeutic relationship with the client. ◆ Engage the client in self-reflective discussions. ◆ Educate the client about prescribed medications and their uses in controlling anxiety. ◆ Explore other approaches, such as use of transitional objects (umbrella), that some find make them feel more secure. ◆ Provide assistance over the phone: Professor Jones may call in if he is afraid he may be developing an attack. He can then talk to someone rather than feel alone.	Professor Jones found that he had many stressors in his life: high work demands, large number of students, and poor time management. He discovered through self-reflection that his number of panic attacks increased when he felt "too much was going on." Professor Jones took prescribed medication and reported feeling less "worried." He disclosed that carrying books made him "feel better." He thought this was silly, but, given that the nurse explained that others with his condition sometimes felt less anxious with an object, he decided he would carry his books when walking to and from work. Professor Jones did call into the clinic—2 or 3 times the first few weeks. The nurse now is helping him to establish and use a support system.

NURSING DIAGNOSIS *Social isolation,* related to alterations in mental status, as evidenced by insecurity in public.

Outcomes	Planning/Interventions	Evaluation
Professor Jones will maintain social contact with at least one personal friend over the next 2 months.	◆ Assist Professor Jones to reflect on the purpose and role social withdrawal served for him right now.	Within 2 weeks, Professor Jones reestablished contact with a trusted friend.

Continued

Outcomes	Planning/Interventions	Evaluation
	◆ Help Professor Jones to establish social contacts lost during his recent experiences with increased panic attacks; encourage him to invite a colleague to lunch, write a note to a friend, and use the phone to talk to others.	Professor Jones attended two campus social events and interacted with other faculty there.
	◆ Invite Professor Jones to attend supportive group therapy/social therapy meetings.	Professor Jones declined the groups at this time, wishing to try other approaches.

NURSING DIAGNOSIS *Risk for injury*, related to the diagnosis of Panic Disorder, as evidenced by psychological alterations.

Outcomes	Planning/Interventions	Evaluation
Professor Jones will make a plan to obtain immediate help should he feel he is going out of control.	◆ Discuss the risks with him. ◆ Identify supports available in his community: emergency department, 911 for ambulance.	Professor Jones never attempted to injure himself. He did not use either the emergency room or the 911 emergency number during the time of treatment.

CRITICAL THINKING BAND

ASSESSMENT
What other aspects of Professor Jones's life should be evaluated as possibly influencing his mental health?

NURSING DIAGNOSIS
What other diagnoses might apply with this client? Could he be having a heart attack? How do we discriminate between extreme anxiety and a physiological emergency?

Outcomes	Planning/Interventions	Evaluation
What other mutual goals would be reasonable? How would goals change if Professor Jones had always been reclusive?	What other strategies might we try? If we found out that he was an academic genius who relied on scientific reports for personal and professional decision making, how might we modify our interventions?	If Professor Jones had more panic attacks rather than fewer, what then?

CASE STUDY/CARE PLAN

Obsessive-Compulsive Disorder is relatively common, and the average person experiencing the disorder is unable to make the world adjust to the obsessions and compulsions in the manner used by Howard Hughes, described earlier in the chapter. Few have the resources to demand so much of others, and accommodation of the individual and his family will require much patience, understanding, and professional support. Consider the following example of Mrs. Vail, who was diagnosed with the same condition.

Mrs. Vail is a 47-year-old woman who lives with her husband, Fred, in a three-bedroom home in a small city. Fred is employed as an accountant.

Continued

The Vails have a number of longtime friends in their community, and they frequently enjoy playing bridge, going to the movies, and participating in social events at their church. The Vails have two children, both grown—a son 23 years old, working in an urban center 50 miles away, and a daughter, 20 years old, who is newly married and living in the same community as her parents. Mrs. Vail has always been a homemaker and takes pride in her ability to organize a household and provide service to community and church groups. For the past 2 years, Mrs. Vail has become increasingly nervous and has become progressively more concerned about the cleanliness of her home.

Over the past three months, she has become excessively concerned with contamination of her household by germs from the outside. She has insisted that family members and guests remove their shoes before entering the house. She washes the floors every day and sometimes two or three times a day. She is uncomfortable with anyone bringing things into the house from outside; for example, she does not want her husband to bring papers home from work. She will wear only one coat when going outside, and she will leave the coat and her shoes on her back porch, never bringing them in. She has become overly concerned with her food as well, and over the past few days, she will not eat food anyone else has purchased or prepared. She has established elaborate rituals of washing vegetables, boiling meat,

and preparing food in a manner that releases her from anxiety over eating contaminated food.

Her husband has attempted to understand her concerns and is willing to "humor" her by removing his shoes and eating foods she has prepared in her "new way." But, he is losing his patience; he wants to go out to eat with friends, and she will go but refuses to eat. Their daughter thinks her mother is "weird" and finally convinced her mother to discuss her feelings with the family doctor. Mrs. Vail readily agreed that her feelings and behaviors are different and changed and describes herself as increasingly lonely, anxious, and afraid of others.

The physician has diagnosed Mrs. Vail as having Obsessive-Compulsive Disorder, prescribed clomipramine, and recommended follow-up care and treatment through the county mental health clinic.

ASSESSMENT

Mrs. Vail is a 47-year-old homemaker who has had difficulty with increasing anxiety over the past 2 years. During the past 2 months, she has become completely focused on the cleanliness of her home and the purity of her food. She has developed and uses to excess elaborate systems for "keeping the germs away," systems that have interrupted and changed every aspect of daily living for the Vail family. Mr. Vail does not understand his wife's unusual behaviors; Mrs. Vail realizes she has a serious problem and is very unhappy.

NURSING DIAGNOSIS *Anxiety*, related to unexplained fears of contamination in the home

Outcomes

♦ The client will acknowledge and discuss her anxiety and preoccupation with home cleanliness, she will recognize her inflexibility and rigidity in her current day-to-day living processes, and she will identify the need for behavioral change.

♦ Mrs. Vail will demonstrate a decrease in repetitive cleaning behaviors in the home within 8 weeks.

Planning/Interventions

♦ Assist the client in recognizing her fears and behaviors.

♦ Communicate to Mrs. Vail unconditional acceptance of her and her problems.

♦ Use active and empathetic listening techniques. Recognize Mrs. Vail's strengths in these situations: her clear role with the family, her protection of the family, and her concern for her family.

♦ Collect data with Mrs. Vail and set mutual goals for decreasing redundant cleaning behaviors over the next 8 weeks (i.e., wash floor six rather than eight times a day the first week; clean vegetables three times rather than four).

Evaluation

Within 8 weeks, Mrs. Vail was able to discuss her anxieties and behaviors. She identified the behaviors she most wanted to change—the redundant cleaning behaviors involved with food preparation.

Mrs. Vail was able to see her desire to change the behavior as a strength.

Continued

Outcomes	Planning/Interventions	Evaluation
◆ Mrs. Vail will demonstrate at least one problem-solving skill that can be used to decrease her feelings of anxiety.	◆ Encourage Mrs. Vail to become involved in other activities, to redirect her focus to other events.	The data collection was useful. Mrs. Vail was unaware of how many times she had performed the same activities. Mrs. Vail explored different activities she could pursue when she thought she was becoming anxious, like taking a walk. Medication also decreased both her anxiety and her repetitive actions in the home.

NURSING DIAGNOSIS *Powerlessness*, related to her lifestyle and feeling of helplessness, as evidenced by inability to control her repetitive cleaning behaviors.

Outcomes	Planning/Interventions	Evaluation
Mrs. Vail will verbalize feeling in control of her actions in the home within 8 weeks.	◆ Provide expert assistance to Mrs. Vail by encouraging her to discuss and learn about Obsessive-Compulsive Disorder. ◆ Help Mrs. Vail construct a reasonable work schedule at home that builds in time for cleaning, food preparation, and other home activities not currently part of the obsessive-compulsive behaviors.	Mrs. Vail maintained schedule.

NURSING DIAGNOSIS *Social isolation*, related to absence of satisfying personal relationships, as evidenced by repetitive meaningless actions (preoccupation with repetitive cleaning behaviors) and values (excessive cleanliness) unacceptable to family.

Outcomes	Planning/Interventions	Evaluation
◆ Mrs. Vail will identify previous social activities that she enjoyed before becoming so anxious. ◆ Mrs. Vail will leave the home at least twice a week for activities unrelated to homemaking activities.	◆ Discuss with the family unit Mrs. Vail's need for support in making gradual changes. ◆ Identify social activities and networks Mrs. Vail had before her Obsessive-Compulsive Disorder became problematic.	Mrs. Vail began to identify social activities. She left the home once during the past two weeks.

Continued

NURSING DIAGNOSIS *Altered family processes*, related to situation transition (the need of the family to accommodate Mrs. Vail's behaviors), as evidenced by inability to accept Mrs. Vail's behavior.

Outcomes	Planning/Interventions	Evaluation
◆ The family will gain knowledge about Obsessive-Compulsive Disorder. ◆ The family will express concern about Mrs. Vail's condition and support her in obtaining professional help. ◆ The family will distinguish between supportive and nonsupportive behaviors for both Mrs. Vail and each other.	◆ Educate and provide materials to the family about Obsessive-Compulsive Disorder, its course, and its treatment. ◆ Supervise Mrs. Vail's medication regimen. ◆ Support Mr. Vail by encouraging his questions, concerns, and expressions of feeling. ◆ Encourage Mrs. Vail's children to become more involved in Mrs. Vail's progress and to provide respite to Mr. Vail.	Within 6 weeks, the Vail family had a better understanding of the behaviors Mrs. Vail has been demonstrating. They were relieved to have a supportive nurse of whom they could ask a myriad of questions. They had initially thought that Mrs. Vail was "beyond help" and were encouraged to see early progress. Mr. Vail was especially glad to have help with his wife's problems; he said, "You know I love her. I just didn't know what to do."

CRITICAL THINKING BAND

ASSESSMENT
What other environmental factors should be considered concerning Mrs. Vail and her family?

NURSING DIAGNOSIS
What other diagnoses might apply to this client's situation?

Outcomes
Were mutual goals with Mrs. Vail possible during the initial phases of contact? How might those goals change once Mrs. Vail was beginning to improve?

Planning/Interventions
What nursing interventions were used to engender trust with Mrs. Vail? How could you move beyond her anxiety without adding to that anxiety?

Evaluation
In what other ways might this scenario have gone? If Mrs. Vail's behaviors had actually escalated with this plan?

CASE STUDY/CARE PLAN

Returning to the literary excerpt presented in Chapter 9—the story of Wilbur, the man who experienced the crisis of the West Virginia flood—one can recognize the tragedy of significant disaster. Wilbur is experiencing Post-Traumatic Stress Disorder. One year after the flood experience, he describes guilt, anxiety, sleeplessness, and fear of water/rain. A nurse involved in his care recognizes that the anxiety is recurrent and,

after 1 year, becoming a pattern that Wilbur cannot control. Upon evaluation of those losses in his life that are associated with the flood, the nurse uncovers that the grief is prolonged; that is, he has not worked through the grief he is holding.

Imagine that nurses are giving care to Wilbur, who has come to the facility for treatment. A fictionalized nursing care plan follows.

Continued

NURSING DIAGNOSIS   *Post-trauma response*, related to disaster (flood), as evidenced by flashbacks and nightmares and verbalization of guilt.

Outcomes

◆ Wilbur will verbalize an understanding of Post-Traumatic Stress Disorder (PTSD).

◆ Wilbur will begin to be more involved with his family and community; his anxiety will decrease over the next 6 months as his interest in others increases.

Planning/Interventions

◆ Provide information to Wilbur regarding post-traumatic response: the relationship among his fear of rain, sleeplessness, and anxiety.

◆ Assist Wilbur to identify activities he might enjoy to redirect his attention to the present.

◆ Identify support groups that might be available in Wilbur's local area.

Evaluation

Within 1 month, Wilbur had a good understanding of PTSD and could relate the information to his own experience.

Wilbur began to enjoy and engage in outdoor activities with old friends, for example, hiking.

NURSING DIAGNOSIS   *Dysfunctional grieving*, related to actual losses, as evidenced by reliving of past experiences, interference with life functioning, and alterations in sleep habits.

Outcomes

Wilbur will begin the grieving process to identify his losses and work through the emotions of anger and depression.

Planning/Interventions

◆ Encourage Wilbur to slowly and gradually discuss his experiences in a safe and secure setting.

◆ Assess Wilbur for depression, anxiety, and the potential for self-harm or neglect.

◆ Support Wilbur through the grieving process.

◆ Facilitate creating an environment that would most enable Wilbur to heal based on his perspective.

◆ Provide positive feedback for Wilbur's growth and improvement.

Evaluation

Over time, Wilbur dealt with the severe losses from the flood. He realized the normalcy of grieving and how one "sometimes cannot make sense of these things." He kept thinking that he and his whole family would have died had he not gotten up to smoke. When the most intense grieving period had passed, he grinned and commented that everybody thinks smoking is so bad. He believes it saved his life.

CRITICAL THINKING BAND

ASSESSMENT
How could you assess the impact of Wilbur's relationship with his family members over the past year on his current state of mental health?

NURSING DIAGNOSIS
Are there other diagnoses that might better manage Wilbur's issues?

Outcomes
What do you think Wilbur thought about these goals? Would they have to be mutual to work?

Planning/Interventions
Could the same strategies used with Wilbur work for other flood victims? Where does care need to be personalized?

Evaluation
Do plans always work? How would we know with Wilbur? With other clients?

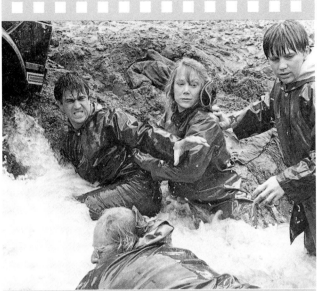

The River. Source: Universal/Courtesy Kobal.

The trauma of a flood, causing loss of life and property, leave many in a state of shock and grief. In the example of our case study, Wilbur is left with Post-Traumatic Stress Disorder after the experience of a devastating flood.

KEY CONCEPTS

◆ Anxiety is a subjective feeling of uneasiness associated with the autonomic nervous system.

◆ Anxiety and fear have much in common; however, anxiety is a generalized response, and fear is a response to a specific, identified object or situation.

◆ While there is some disagreement among psychiatrists, most believe that anxiety is a part of the human condition. In its extremes, however, anxiety results in serious limitations.

◆ Stages of anxiety have been described to identify the emotions and responses on a continuum of severity.

◆ There are six major anxiety disorders (summarized in Table 10-2).

◆ Treatment for anxiety disorders includes psychotherapy, which can be insight based or behaviorally based, as well as medication. Therapy and drugs are frequently used in combination.

◆ Nursing theory, particularly the Modeling and Role-Modeling Theory, provides direction for nursing care, beginning with the need to establish trust and understand the client's subjective experience of emotion.

REVIEW QUESTIONS AND ACTIVITIES

1. Define anxiety and fear and differentiate between the two.

2. Describe what is meant by calling modern times the "age of anxiety." Describe when anxiety becomes a psychiatric concern.

3. List the six major anxiety disorders and describe their symptoms.

4. Select one client you have cared for in the general hospital who exhibited anxiety. Describe the presenting symptoms of the anxiety, the client's need for support, and the response of the nursing staff.

5. Select one client you have cared for in the psychiatric setting who exhibited a phobia. Describe the presenting symptoms of the anxiety, the client's need for support, and the response of the nursing staff.

6. Plan out an information session you would have with a family who had a son with Obsessive-Compulsive Disorder. What does this family need to know and how will you teach it?

7. Do the same exercise in question 6 for a woman who has a husband with Post-Traumatic Stress Disorder.

EXPLORING THE WEB

◆ Visit this text's "Online Companion™" on the Internet at **http://www.DelmarNursing.com** for further information on anxiety and anxiety disorders.

◆ What sites could you recommend to clients and families experiencing anxiety who are looking for self-help, chat rooms, or other electronic information sources?

◆ What resources are listed for caregivers and health care professionals?

◆ Is there a listing on the Internet of books, videos, or other media on anxiety and anxiety disorders? Are these resources available in your local library or through purchase over the Web?

◆ What other key terms might you search (e.g., phobia, Panic Disorder, Obsessive-Compulsive Disorder, Post-Traumatic Stress Disorder)?

◆ What organizations or professional journals could you search for information on anxiety?

REFERENCES

American Psychiatric Association *Diagnostic and Statistical Manual of Mental Disorders*, Fourth Edition. Washington, DC: American Psychiatric Association, 1994.

Andrews, G. (1993). The benefits of psychotherapy. In N. Sartorius, G. Girolamo, G. Andrews, G. A. German, & L. Eisenberg (Eds.), *Treatment of mental disorders*, (pp. 235–247). Washington, DC: American Psychiatric Press.

Blacher, R. S. (1975). On awakening paralyzed during surgery. *Journal of the American Medical Association, 234*, 67–68.

Blazer, B. G., Hughes, D., George, L. K., Swartz, M., & Boyer, R. (1991). Generalized anxiety disorder. In L. Robins & D. Regier (Eds.), *Psychiatric disorders in America* (p. 192). New York: Free Press.

Busch, P. E. (1996). Panic disorder. *Home Healthcare Nurse, 14*, 111–116.

Bystritsky, A., Munford, P., Rosen, R., Martin, K., Vapnik, T., Gorbis, E., & Wolson, R. (1996). A preliminary study of partial hospital management of severe Obsessive-Compulsive Disorder. *Psychiatric Services, 47*, 170–174.

Cohen, J., & Stewart, I. (1995). Beyond all reasonable DNA. *Lancet, 345*, 1586–1587.

Cottraux, J. (1993). Behavior therapy. In N. Sartorius, G. Girolamo, G. Andrews, G. A. German, & L. Eisenberg (Eds.), *Treatment of mental disorders* (p. 199–233). Washington, DC: American Psychiatric Press.

Crews, F. (1994). The revenge of the repressed. *New York Review of Books, 41*, 54–60.

Eaton, W., Dyman, A., & Weissman, W. W. (1991). Panic and phobia. In L. N. Robins & D. A. Regier (Eds.), *Psychiatric disorders in America: The epidemiologic catchment area study.* New York: Free Press.

Estrum, M. (1996). Generalized anxiety disorder in stroke patients: A 3 year longitudinal study. *Stroke, 27*, 270–275.

Fryer, A. (1992). *National anxiety disorders screening day screening questionnaire.* New York: Anxiety Disorders Clinic, New York State Psychiatric Institute.

Garbowsky, M. (1989). *The house without the door: A study of Emily Dickinson and the illness of agoraphobia.* Cranbury, NJ: Associated University Presses.

Goldfried, M. R., Greenberg, L. S, & Marmar, C. (1990). Individual psychotherapy: Process and outcome. *Annual Review of Psychology, 41*, 659–688.

Goodwin, D. W. (1986). *Anxiety.* New York: Oxford University Press.

Griest, J. H. (1990). Treatment of obsessive compulsive disorder: Psychotherapies, drugs and other somatic treatments. *Journal of Clinical Psychiatry, 51*(8, Suppl.), 44–50.

Kanton, W. (1989). *Panic disorder in the medical setting* (DHHS Pub. No. ADM 89-1629). Washington, DC: U.S. Government Printing Office.

Kupfermann, I. (1985). Hypothalamus and limbic system I: Peptidergic neurons, homeostasis, and emotional behavior. In E. R. Kandel & J. H. Schwartz (Eds.), *Principles of neural science* (2nd ed., pp. 623–624). New York: Elsevier.

Marks, I. (1987). *Fears, phobias, and rituals: Panic, anxiety, and their disorders.* New York: Oxford University Press.

Mavissakalian, M. R., & Jones, B. A. (1989). Antidepressant drugs plus exposure treatment of agoraphobia/panic and OCD. *International Review of Psychiatry, 1*, 275–282.

Nagel, T. (1994a). Freud's permanent revolution. *New York Review of Books, 41*, 34–38.

Nagel, T. (1994b). Letter to editor. *New York Review of Books, 41*, 56.

North American Nursing Diagnosis Association. (1996). NANDA nursing diagnoses: Definitions and classification 1997–1998. Philadelphia: NANDA.

Nymberg, J. H., & Van Noppen, B. (1994). Obsessive-compulsive disorder: A concealed diagnosis. *American Family Physician, 49*, 1129–1137.

Power, K. G., Simpson, R. J., Swanswon, V., & Wallace, L. A. (1990). A controlled comparison of cognitive-behavior therapy, diazepam, and placebo, alone and in combination, for the treatment of generalized anxiety disorder. *Journal of Anxiety Disorders, 4,* 267–292.

Rauch, S. L., Jenike, M. A., Alpert, N. M., Baer, L., Breiten, H. C., Savage, C. R., & Fischman, A. J. (1994). Regional cerebral blood flow measured during symptom provocation in obsessive compulsive disorder using oxygen-15 labeled carbon dioxide and positron emission tomography. *Archives of General Psychiatry, 51,* 66.

Rauch, S. L., Baer, L., Breiten, H. C., Fischman, A. J., Manzo, P. A., Moretti, C., & Jenike, M. A. (1995). A positron emission tomographic study of simple phobic symptom provocation. *Archives of General Psychiatry, 52,* 20–28.

Rauch, S. L., Vanderkolk, B. A., Fisher, R. E., Alpert, N. M., Orr, S. P., Savage, C. R., Fischman, A. J., Jenike, M. A., & Pitman, R. K. (1996). Symptom provocation study of post-traumatic stress disorders using positron emission tomography and sight-driven imagery. *Archives of General Psychiatry, 53,* 385. New York: American Medical Association.

Rickelsk, P., & Schweizer, E. (1990). The clinical course and long term management of generalized anxiety disorder. *Journal of Clinical Psychopharmacology, 10*(Suppl.), 101S–110S.

Robins, L. N., & Regier, D. A. (1991). *Psychiatric disorders in America: The epidemiologic catchment area study.* New York: Free Press.

Saraceno, B., Tognoni, G., & Garattini, S. (1993). Critical questions in clinical psychopharmacology. In N. Sartorius, G. Girolamo, G. Andrews, G. A. German, & L. Eisenberg (Eds.), *Treatment of mental disorders* (pp. 63–87). Washington, DC: American Psychiatric Press.

Spear, H. L. (1996). Anxiety: When to worry, what to do. *RN, 59*(7), 40–45.

Verkuyl, D. A. A. (1995). Practising obstetrics and gynecology in areas with a high prevalence of HIV infection. *Lancet, 346,* 293–296.

Weissman, M., Klerman, G., Markowitz, J., & Ouelette, R. (1989). Suicidal ideation and suicide attempts in panic disorder and attacks. *New England Journal of Medicine, 321,* 1209–1214.

LITERARY REFERENCES

Auden, W. H. (1948). *Age of anxiety.* London: Faber and Faber.

Bartlett, D. L., & Steele, J. B. (1979). *Empire: The life, legend, and madness of Howard Hughes.* New York: W.W. Norton.

Blacher, R. S. (1975). On awakening paralyzed during surgery. *Journal of the American Medical Association, 234,* 67–68.

Brookner, A. (1984). *Hotel du Lac.* New York: EP Dutton/Obelisk.

Darwin, C. (1965/1872). In K. Lorenz *The expression of the emotions in man and animals.* Chicago: University of Chicago Press.

de Maupassant, G. (1989). He? In *The dark side: Tales of terror and the supernatural* (A. Kellett, Trans.). New York: Carol & Graf.

Dickinson, E. (1955). In T. H. Johnson (Ed.), *The poems of Emily Dickinson.* Cambridge: Belknap Press of Harvard University.

Eliot, T. S. (1970). The love song of J. Alfred Prufrock. In *Collected poems 1919–1962.* New York: Harcourt, Brace, and World.

Jong, E. (1973). *Fear of flying.* New York: Holt Rinehart and Winston.

Leonard, W. (1927). *The locomotive-god.* New York: Century. As quoted in L. Y. Rabkin (Eds.), *Psychopathology and literature* (pp. 66–71). San Francisco: Chandler.

White, E. B. (1954). *The second tree from the corner.* New York: Harper and Brothers.

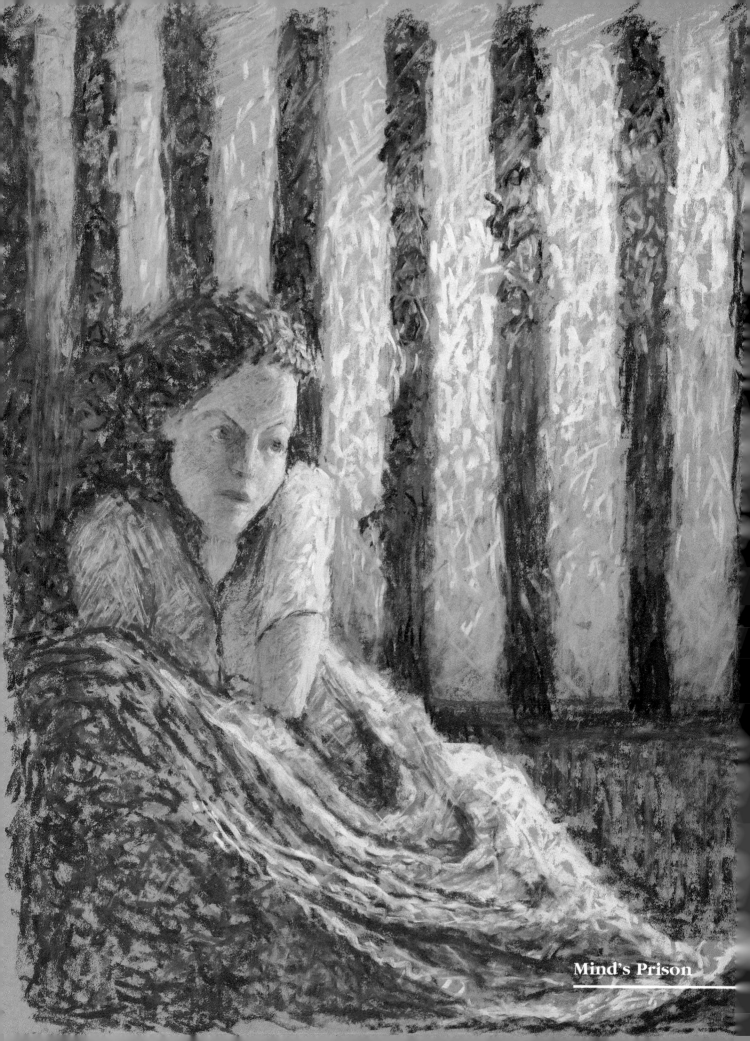

Mind's Prison

Chapter

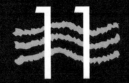

11

THE CLIENT
EXPERIENCING SCHIZOPHRENIA

Noreen Cavan Frisch

Lawrence E. Frisch

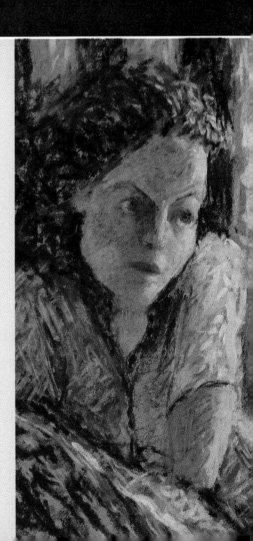

In Touch with Reality

Nurses may become apprehensive when they begin working with clients who are out of touch with reality. Consider the following:

◆ Think of the last time you tried to talk to someone who, no matter how hard you tried to explain, just could not understand you or your perspective?

◆ When falling asleep at night in a darkened room, have you ever thought someone was present, only to alert yourself and see that there was just a pile of clothes on a chair that gave you the illusion that a person was in the room?

◆ Have you ever been certain you heard something (the door bell, for example) when no one else in the room heard the sound?

◆ Have you ever experienced a life event that seemed overwhelming and incomprehensible and learned you still had to go on with life even if you couldn't explain all that had happened to you?

Most persons have experienced at least one of the above. These represent relatively common and completely normal experiences. As you begin to study those conditions that cause altered thought processes, remember that altered thought processes and the other accompanying human responses are part of the human condition. What one sees in mental illness is an exaggeration of the normal human response, not something totally different but, rather, something different only in degree. It is the degree that makes the condition a mental illness.

≋ CHAPTER OUTLINE

THE EXPERIENCE OF SCHIZOPHRENIA
Disordered Thoughts

Incomprehensible Language

Loss of Function

Delusions

Hallucinations

SYMPTOMS

CLINICAL COURSE

EPIDEMIOLOGY
Social Costs

ETIOLOGY
Psychoanalytic Theory

Genetics

Current Views
    Dopamine Hypothesis
    Etiology Unknown

TREATMENT
Psychosocial Treatment
    Clinical and Family Support Services
    Rehabilitation
    Humanitarian Aid/Public Safety

Pharmacological and Physical Treatments
    Neuroleptic Medications
    Other Physical Treatments

NURSING PERSPECTIVES

NURSING THEORY

▽ NURSING PROCESS

▽ CASE STUDY/CARE PLAN

≋ COMPETENCIES

Upon completion of this chapter, the reader should be able to:

1. Contrast altered thought processes as normal human responses with the psychiatric conditions schizophrenia and psychosis.
2. Empathize with the lived experiences of those who have schizophrenia and those who have a family member with the condition.
3. Recognize the presenting symptoms of schizophrenia.
4. Discuss the epidemiology of schizophrenia.
5. Explain the etiology of schizophrenia as an organic disease.
6. Discuss the genetic factors known with regard to the transition of schizophrenia.
7. Engage in psychosocial therapeutic treatments for individuals and their families.
8. Explain the role of neuroleptic drugs in management of schizophrenia.
9. Provide nursing care to persons suffering from schizophrenia, based on nursing theory and the nursing process.
10. Develop a personal perspective on the social policies that guide treatment and care of chronically mentally ill persons in the United States.

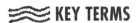 **KEY TERMS**

Akathisia   Reaction involving physical restlessness and inability to sit still.

Akinesia   Reaction involving loss of movement.

Alogia   Tendency to speak very little and use brief and seemingly empty phrases.

Anhedonia   Inability to find enjoyment in daily activities.

Avolition   Lack of motivation for work or other goal-oriented activities.

Catatonia   Behavior disorder marked by a decrease in reactivity to the environment, sometimes reaching an extreme degree of complete unawareness.

Delusion   False belief that misrepresents either perceptions or experiences.

Derailment   Speech that gets off the point or subject.

Dystonia   Reaction manifested by painful muscle spasms lasting from a few seconds to several days.

Flattened Affect   Loss of expressiveness.

Grandiose Delusion   Perception of importance, special powers, or religious significance that is not in line with reality.

Hallucination   Sensory experiences not perceptible to other nonpsychotic individuals.

Incoherence   Speech that is not logically connected.

Neologistic Word   Invented word, often used by persons suffering from schizophrenia.

Persecutory Delusion   Paranoid perception that others are "out to get me."

Psychotic   Mental state involving the loss of rational thought and/or loss of ability to accurately interpret the environment.

Referential Delusion   Perception that common events refer specifically to the individual.

Schizophrenia   Mental disorder characterized by disordered thoughts, hallucinations, and delusions.

Tangentiality   Speech marked by failure to reach a goal or stick to the original point.

Tardive Dyskinesia   Movement disorder characterized by repetitive motions such as chewing or grimacing.

Word Salad   Speech marked by a group of disconnected words.

The *Diagnostic and Statistical Manual*, 4th ed. (DSM-IV) describes psychotic symptoms as the defining feature of several disorders, schizophrenia being the one most commonly seen by nurses. While the term **psychotic** has had many interpretations, all include the loss of rational thought and/or loss of ability to accurately interpret the environment. **Schizophrenia** is defined as a mental disorder characterized by disordered thoughts, hallucinations, and delusions.

Many persons have heard a lot about the word *schizophrenia*, and many believe that the term means split or dual personality; this, however, is not the case. Another common misconception is that schizophrenia is caused by factors such as family dysfunction or drug and alcohol abuse. The accompanying display lists these and other myths about the disease.

DISPELLING COMMON MYTHS ABOUT SCHIZOPHRENIA

◆ Schizophrenia does not mean split personality as in Dr. Jekyll and Mr. Hyde. There *are* psychiatric disorders of multiple personalities, but they are very different from schizophrenia. The word *schizophrenia* does mean *splitting of the mind*, but this name was chosen to reflect the effects of schizophrenia on thought and language, not personality.

◆ Schizophrenic individuals are *not* unusually prone to violence. While schizophrenic persons do commit crimes and some are very dangerous, the majority of schizophrenic individuals are not violent. Although schizophrenic persons are rarely dangerous to others, their risk of suicide is very high, approaching 10%.

◆ Schizophrenia is not caused by family dysfunction. Psychological factors influence the way individuals and families cope with schizophrenia, but families do not cause schizophrenia any more than they cause multiple sclerosis or cancer. While the biological factors leading to schizophrenia remain unknown, schizophrenia is clearly a disease of the brain, not a primary psychological disorder.

The reader needs to leave the myths and preconceptions behind and consider the following excerpt as the actual, real-life experience of one person:

Anonymous Autobiography

On my first day of externship at a hospital
I was waiting for the pharmacy to open since I was

early by an hour. I was sitting in a lobby wearing a white lab coat and required name tag and catching a catnap. A young male patient approached me.

"Excuse me, miss. Do you know that every morning when I get out of bed I feel there is danger everywhere?"

Because I had a white coat he assumed I had an answer to this problem, or at least that I was not in his situation and could offer some assistance. I was taken off guard by this psychiatric patient but said, "You sound very frightened." He said, "Yes. Are you sad or just resting?" I felt he was seeing right through me. "No," I replied, "I'm not sad; I'm just very tired." "Oh," he said, "then I'll leave you alone," and he walked away.

My white coat and name tag offered me no immunity from schizophrenia. Pharmacy students are vulnerable just as everyone else is, in spite of the fact that we are taught about all diseases as if we were an immune group.

Inside, while I spoke to this patient I wanted to say: "Yes, I too sense danger everywhere, each morning and all day. It's hard for me to get out of bed, to go out of the house, to talk to people; it's hard just to get dressed and get outside and function. I'm afraid of people, of change. I'm sensitive to sunlight and noise. I never watch the news or read a newspaper because it frightens me."

Talking to this patient had made the conflict within me very obvious. This young man and I are related in a way I cannot share with him, with my fellow students, or with faculty. Yes, I am a pharmacy student. But yes, I have been diagnosed as schizophrenic and have been hospitalized on three occasions when I could not function. Yes, I am on neuroleptics and must see a psychologist at least once a week, and sometimes more often, in order to function.

I wanted to tell him, "Yes, I know how it feels, and isn't it terrible?" . . . Even now . . . in a professional pharmacy school, it would probably shock many people to know a schizophrenic was in their class, would be a pharmacist, and could do a good job . . . So even now I must write this article anonymously. But I want people to know I have schizophrenia, that I need medicine and psychotherapy, and at some times I have required hospitalization. But I also want them to know that

I have been on the dean's list, and have friends, and expect to receive my pharmacy degree from a major university.

When you think about schizophrenia next time, try to remember me; there are more people like me out there trying to overcome a poorly understood disease and doing the best they can with what medicine and psychotherapy have to offer them. And some of them are making it.

(Anonymous, 1983, pp. 152–155)

Disordered thought is a major characteristic of schizophrenia, and while all persons with this diagnosis have had disordered thought at some time in their lives, they do not have disordered thoughts all of the time, as the excerpt from a pharmacy student makes clear. However, disordered thoughts occur in schizophrenia and often present along with hallucinations and delusions. These three phenomena—disordered thought, delusions, and hallucinations—are the characteristics of psychosis. While not all three are present in every psychotic client, most schizophrenic individuals manifest a complex mixture of all three. Along with manic-depressive disorder, schizophrenia is the major cause of prolonged psychosis seen in psychiatric practice. Distinguishing between these two major causes of psychosis may be difficult, and reflecting this difficulty, some clients who manifest characteristics of both manic-depressive disorder and schizophrenia are given the DSM-IV diagnosis of Schizoaffective Disorder. Schizoaffective Disorder is discussed briefly in Chapter 16; this chapter focuses on schizophrenia.

THE EXPERIENCE OF SCHIZOPHRENIA

A nursing perspective on disordered thought requires consideration of the subjective human experience of the disease. Because rational cognitive ability is so important for functioning, there are human responses that pervade every aspect of a person's living when one is unable to think. Several nursing diagnoses apply when caring for such a person. These will be discussed as the reader examines the presenting symptoms and current definitions of schizophrenia.

Disordered Thoughts

Altered, or disordered, thoughts are a major characteristic of schizophrenia. When schizophrenic individuals talk, they demonstrate a flow of thought that can be described as "loose"; that is, topics and ideas follow one another with far less order than one expects in everyday speech. Often one idea or thought is followed by a seemingly unrelated one; either topic might make good conversational sense, but when put together, the ideas do not quite seem to mesh. Here is an example of fairly disordered thinking from a published study of schizophrenic language:

[You ask me to define] contentment? Well uh, contentment, well the word contentment, having a book perhaps, perhaps your having a subject, perhaps you have a chapter of reading, but when you come to the word "men" you wonder if you should be content with men in your life and then you get to the letter "I" and you wonder if you should be content having tea by yourself or be content with having it with a group and so forth.*

(Lorenz, 1961, p. 604)

In this passage, the speaker at times seems to make quite good sense (it is perfectly reasonable to wonder if it is better to have tea by oneself or in a group), but the rapid shift of ideas (here around the focus of a single word—*contentment*) is characteristic of disordered thought. The confusion is not in speech alone, but in the thinking process itself. One schizophrenic individual reported: "I try to read even a paragraph in a book, but it takes me ages because each bit I read starts me thinking in ten different directions at once" (Sass, 1992, p. 178). More extreme examples of schizophrenic thought may be completely devoid of any obvious sense:

Chirps in a box. If you abstract yourself far enough from a given context you seem somehow to create a new kind of concretion . . . You explode like when stars explode. In the sky a plate which burned bright. Symbol of all light and energy with me contracted into this plate.

(Lorenz, 1961, p. 604)

Schizophrenia often evolves slowly over years. In the early stages of schizophrenia, formal thought disorder may be very subtle and hard to recognize (Harrow & Quinlan, 1985). As the condition evolves, language becomes even more bizarre than the examples preceding. The person loses ability to communicate.

Incomprehensible Language

The following example illustrates a further degree of disordered communication in schizophrenia:

That's wish-bell double vision. Like walking across a person's eye and reflecting personality. It works on you like dying and going into the spiritual world but landing in the vella world.

(Harrow & Quinlan, 1985, p. 423)

In this last passage, the word *vella* is an invented or **neologistic word**. Schizophrenic individuals frequently invent their own vocabularies and may sometimes offer definitions so that others can better understand their worlds:

Snortie—to talk through walls.

Trominoes—tiny people who live in one's body.

Split-kippered—to be simultaneously alive in Lancashire and dead in Yorkshire.*

(McKenna, 1994, p. 14)

There have been a number of studies of schizophrenic language, and many aspects of thought disorder have been formally categorized (Andreasen, 1979). There are specific terms used to describe schizophrenic speech: **derailment**, going off the point or subject; **tangentiality**, failure to reach a goal or stick to the original point; **incoherence**, speech that is not logically connected; and **word salad**, a group of disconnected words. These characteristics of speech are part of DSM-IV diagnostic criteria for schizophrenia (American Psychiatric Association, 1994).

Without coherent language, the individual loses ability to communicate verbally. When trying to communicate, it becomes very difficult for the client and his family/friends and others because, as hard as they try, they cannot connect with and understand each other. The client sometimes recognizes his communication deficits, but is unable to express his needs, ideas, and intentions to others. Not surprisingly, the progressive loss of language leads to social failure.

Loss of Function

A person without ability to think and communicate cannot maintain social norms. Behavior in schizophrenia is often as disordered as thought. Appearance and dress may range from sloppy to eccentric or even bizarre. Social and verbal behavior are also often affected:

The person may appear markedly disheveled, may dress in an unusual manner (e.g., wearing multiple overcoats, scarves, and gloves on a hot day), or may display clearly inappropriate sexual behavior (e.g., public masturbation) or unpredictable and untriggered agitation (e.g., shouting or swearing).

(American Psychiatric Association, 1994, p. 276)

The extreme of disordered behavior is **catatonia**: "a marked decrease in reactivity to the environment, sometimes

*From "Problems Posed by Schizophrenic Language," by M. Lorenz, 1961, *Archives of General Psychiatry, 4,* pp. 603–610 Copyright 1961, American Medical Association.

*From *Schizophrenia and Related Syndromes*, by P. J. McKenna, 1994, New York: Oxford University Press. By permission of Oxford University Press.

reaching an extreme degree of complete unawareness . . . maintaining a rigid posture and resisting efforts to be moved . . . the assumption of bizarre postures" (American Psychiatric Association, 1994, p. 276). Catatonia is among the most striking psychotic manifestations. The following reflections of one psychotic young woman, edited and published by her therapist, may give some insight into the perceived world that holds a catatonic individual in such rigidity:

Autobiography

For me, madness was definitely not a condition of illness; I did not believe that I was ill. It was rather a country, opposed to Reality, where reigned an implacable light, blinding, leaving no place for shadow; an immense space without boundary, limitless, flat; a mineral, lunar country, cold as the wastes of the North Pole. In this stretching emptiness, all is unchangeable, immobile, congealed, crystallized. Objects are stage trappings, placed here and there, geometric cubes without meaning.

People turn weirdly about, they make gestures, movements without sense; they are phantoms whirling on an infinite plain, crushed by the pitiless electric light. And I—I am lost in it, isolated, cold, stripped, purposeless under the light . . . This was it; this was madness . . . I called it the "Land of Light" because of the brilliant illumination, dazzling, astral, cold, and the state of extreme tension in which everything was, including myself.

(Sechehaye, 1970, p. 24)

Delusions

Many schizophrenic persons express **delusions**, false beliefs that misrepresent either perceptions or experiences. Delusions are a major defining characteristic of psychosis. Delusions are commonly characterized as grandiose, persecutory, or referential. **Grandiose delusions** involve perceptions of importance; delusional persons often believe themselves to have special powers and may claim to be religious Messiahs. Persons with **persecutory delusions** are paranoid; they believe that others intend to do them harm. Persons with **referential delusions** believe that common events—passages in songs, patterns of clouds in the sky, comments of passersby—refer specifically to them. In the following passage, written about himself in the third person, a young schizophrenic man describes grandiose delusions and multiple ideas of reference developing after he presented a paper at a psychology conference:

Grandiose Delusions

David's paper was viewed as a monumental contribution to the conference and potentially to psychology in general. If scientifically verified, his concept of telepathy, universally present at birth and measurable, might have as much influence as the basic ideas of Darwin and Freud.

Each speaker focused on David. By using allusions and nonverbal communications that included pointing and glancing, each illuminated different aspects of David's contribution. Although his name was never mentioned, the speakers enticed David into feeling that he had accomplished something supernatural in writing the paper. . . .

David was described as having a halo around his head, and the Second Coming was announced as forthcoming. Messianic feelings took hold of him. His mission would be to aid the poor and needy. . . .

David's sensitivity to nonverbal communication was extreme; he was adept at reading people's minds. His perceptual powers were so developed that he could not discriminate between telepathic reception and spoken language by others. He was distracted by others in a way that he had never been before . . . Several hundred people at the conference were talking about David. He was the subject of enormous mystery, profound in his silence. Criticism, though, was often expressed by skeptics of the anticipated Second Coming. David felt the intense communication about him as torturous. He wished the talking, nonverbal behavior, and pervasive train of thoughts about him would stop. . . .

Everyday, David studied the patterns in the sky formed from clouds of airplane exhaust. These patterns, always vivid, typically expressed a favorable view of David.

(Zelt, 1981, pp. 527–531)

Delusions are described as bizarre if they bear no understandable relationship to ordinary life experiences. David's paranoid and grandiose delusions are relatively nonbizarre: People could be talking about him, in accord with accepted Christian belief that the Second Coming could be imminent. His referential delusions vary from personal hypersensitivity to bizarre delusions of personal messages seen in airplane vapor trails. Particularly bizarre schizophrenic delusions involve the perception that one's body has been physically changed:

Out of the Depths

I was told [by a hallucinatory voice] to feel on the back of my neck and I would find there a sign of my new mission. I therefore examined and found a shuttle-like affair about three-fourths of an inch long.*

(Boisen, 1960, p. 91)

Bizarre delusions may be much more severe, as when a client believes "a stranger has removed his or her internal organs and has replaced them with someone else's organs without leaving any wounds or scars" (American Psychiatric Association, 1994, p. 275).

Delusions of persecution are among those most commonly seen in schizophrenia. David Zelt, in the article previously quoted, goes on to describe elaborate persecutory delusions involving the CIA and thought control. Another first-person account of schizophrenic experience describes vaguely persecutory delusions about the nursing staff of a mental hospital:

Persecutory Delusions

My feelings about the nursing staff during the first episode were rather complicated. I tried to get as much as I could out of contact with the young student nurses in the ward, but I felt that none of them was in a position to take care of me. On the contrary, they were much younger than myself, and I felt protective of them at times when I did not regard them as making active attempts to harm me. In such instances, I was on the defensive and felt some antagonism. It seemed to me that most of the nurses were like marionettes on a string, with no personalities of their own, being manipulated by powerful forces outside themselves. I saw them as under the influence of hypnotic suggestion. They were, I thought, in the control of others whose minds were more powerful than theirs. . . .

Ordinary simple people like these nurses were, I had felt, being educated to hateful, intolerant, and prejudiced attitudes toward others by the dominant forces in the society around them . . . [I] developed a strong attachment to one of the nurses—a head nurse—who seemed to me particularly kind, understanding, and sensitive. There were times when only her presence could reassure

me. In spite of this I began to develop the idea that it would be dangerous for her to have too much to do with me. She could not really help me because she too was subject to influence from my enemies even though her intentions were good.

(Anonymous, 1955, pp. 678–679)

Hallucinations

Hallucinations are another major part of the psychotic experience and are also very common in schizophrenia. **Hallucinations** are sensory experiences not perceptible to other nonpsychotic individuals. While hallucinations can involve virtually any sensory modality, they are most commonly auditory. Psychotic individuals typically describe "hearing voices," and these voices are perceived as quite distinct from the individual's own thoughts. The voices generally have specific content, and this is most frequently of a threatening or negative nature: "The voices schizophrenics hear tend to emanate not from any particular person or object in external space but from inside the body or from the sky, as if permeating the entire universe" (Sass, 1992, p. 233). Schizophrenic hallucinations occur while fully awake, and are thought not to be different from experiences considered normal in some cultures (American Psychiatric Association, 1994). It is not unusual for schizophrenic persons to hear two or more voices talking with each other or actually commenting on the individual's stream of thought. This type of multi-voice auditory hallucination is highly characteristic of schizophrenia:

A twenty-four year old man repeatedly heard a couple of voices discussing him. A deep, rough voice would say, "G.T. is a bloody paradox"; then a higher-pitched one would chime in, "He is that, he should be locked up"; and a female voice would occasionally interrupt, saying, "He is not, he is a lovely man."

(C. S. Mellor, 1970, p. 16)

SYMPTOMS

These features of schizophrenia—disordered thought and behavior, delusions, hallucinations—are often referred to as "positive symptoms." Positive symptoms typically manifest themselves as behaviors that seem clearly bizarre even to persons with no special training in psychology, such as schizophrenic persons displaying eccentricities of language, appearance, and behavior that cause them to seem highly unusual. In fact, some writers and psychiatrists have portrayed persons with schizophrenia as individualistic heroes in a society that celebrates conformity and materialistic values:

**Out of the Depths*, A. Boisen, Copyright 1960. Reprinted with permission of HarperCollins Publishers.

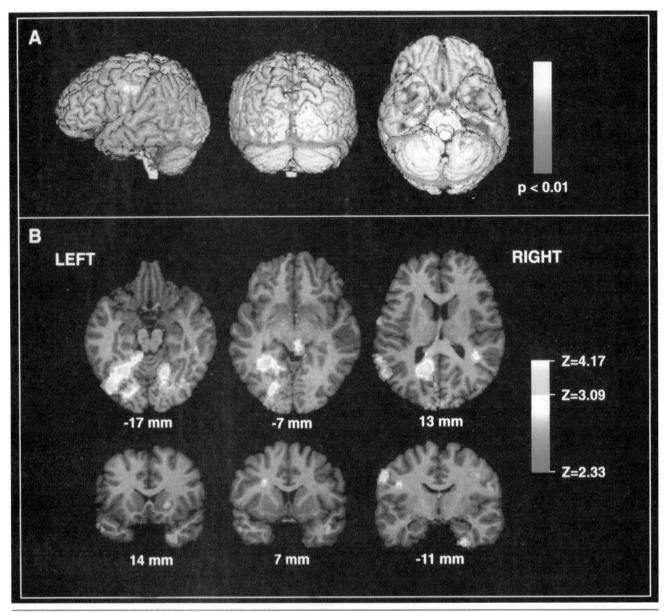

Surface and slice images of the brain of a client with schizophrenia, showing areas of increased activity (in color) while he was having hallucinations—hearing voices and seeing visions that weren't there. These activated brain regions, detected with specifically designed PET imaging techniques, are involved in complex auditory-linguistic, visual, and emotional processing. *Courtesy of D. Silbersweig, M.D. and E. Stern, M.D. Functional Neuroimaging Laboratory, The New York Hospital-Cornell Medical Center. Appeared in: A Functional Neuroanatomy of Hallucinations in Schizophrenia, D. Silbersweig, E. Stern et al. Nature 378: 176–179, 1995.*

In *The Politics of Experience*, R. D. Laing describes madness as a release from constraint and a return to "primal man" that may even have the power to heal "our own appalling state of alienation called normality."

(Sass, 1992, p. 22)

This romantic view of madness has little practical relevance to the very real difficulties that most schizophrenic individuals encounter in finding a satisfactory way to live in modern society. For most schizophrenics, the greatest impediments to social integration come not from their madness—the delusions, hallucinations, and disordered thought—but from what are commonly termed negative symptoms.

Negative symptoms of schizophrenia are both more difficult to describe and, in their subtlest forms, more difficult to detect than are the positive symptoms. In many ways, however, the negative symptoms—flattened affect, alogia, avolition, and anhedonia—are far more debilitating.

◆ **Flattened affect** describes the loss of expressiveness that most schizophrenic persons develop during their illness. While schizophrenic individu-

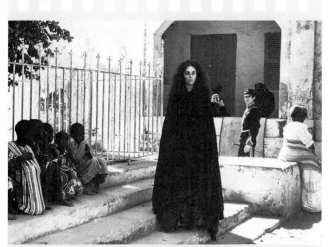

The Story of Adele H.
Source: Films du Carosse/Artistes Associes/Courtesy Kobal.

Once a lively and sociable young woman, Adele becomes obsessed with her love for a young man, and she loses her sanity. She exhibits many characteristics of schizophrenia, including delusions, hallucinations, and psychosis. She is seen above pacing the streets, unable to recognize those whom she once knew well.

als may sometimes smile or seem to develop some human warmth, the overall impression of schizophrenia is that of extreme emotional distance and lack of human response.

◆ **Alogia** refers to the tendency of schizophrenic individuals to speak very little and, even when speaking openly, to use brief and often seemingly empty phrases.

◆ **Avolition** is the tendency for those with schizophrenia to lack motivation for work or other goal-directed activities.

◆ **Anhedonia** is the seeming inability to find enjoyment in activities that would be pleasurable to unaffected individuals. While by no means unique to schizophrenia—indeed, anhedonia is a major part of the experience of depression—most schizophrenic individuals do display a significant degree of loss of pleasure in daily activities.

Unlike the positive symptoms of schizophrenia, negative symptoms do not differ fundamentally from behaviors displayed by many persons. Negative symptoms are more common and more severe in persons with schizophrenia and are most striking when a schizophrenic individual is contrasted with the person he or she was before the illness began. The following passage is an extraordinary description of one family's experience of schizophrenia, seen primarily from the perspective of negative symptoms:

Mourning without End

[Gary's] childhood up to his teenage years was, as we say in medicine, "unremarkable." There was, however, something remarkable for us: Gary was a terrific kid, the kind of appealing child that parents feel lucky to have. If you had been gathering data about him during his senior year of high school, this is what you would have learned: academically, he was ranked first in his class, with a combined score of 1500 on his SATs, and had been accepted to Harvard early decision; he had a close relationship with a girlfriend for 2 years; he was the leader of a jazz group and acknowledged as an outstanding jazz drummer. It is no wonder, then, that he did not go to the 10th reunion of his high school class, because his life has not been the same since his senior year.

I have often been asked, "when did Gary's illness begin?" If I were his psychiatrist writing up the case history, I would say, "when he dropped out of Harvard during his sophomore year" or "at the time of his first hospitalization 2 years later." But when the onset of the illness is so insidious, as it was in Gary's case, and as it is in so many of these young people, it is an impossible question to answer. In retrospect, we have reason to believe that his illness started much earlier . . . During high school Gary quit the tennis team, saying that he wanted to concentrate on his drumming and band work. At the time it seemed reasonable, but in retrospect it was the beginning of a tendency toward isolation. . . .

Since that time there have been three relatively short hospitalizations, the first of which was necessary because he was suicidal . . . What has it been like for us these past 10 years? I will begin with what has always been most painful for me . . . feelings of loss, grief, and mourning . . . I feel the loss of the son that I once had because in many ways he is quite different. Struggling as he does with many of what we now call the "negative symptoms," he has lost that gleam in his eye, that joyous good humor, that zest for life which he once showed. Today, it is hard for him to feel things strongly, or to enjoy his music, sports, or being with the family.

For a long time, when I looked into his eyes I felt that there was no one there. This is one of those manifestations that are difficult for the observer, let alone the person with the illness, to put into words. Some of the expressions that came into my mind were these: "He has become a shell of a person, there is no one there, he has lost his self, he looks different, his face has changed, he's a lost soul" . . . These symptoms and the cognitive impairment disturb me much more than they do my wife, who gets more distressed over his delusional thinking. For me, the delusional thinking, as upsetting as it is, is still a sign of lively mental activity . . . I am more hopeful that the delusions can be altered by medication: I worry that the cognitive impairment cannot be reversed. . . .

I know that I should be most proud of Gary, and I can often feel that. The problem is that it is not easy to see that he is displaying great courage in coping with what has happened to him. The symptoms of the illness make him appear lacking in motivation, initiative, and will, and even he accuses himself of not trying hard enough. It is hard for an observer to see how difficult it must be for him to get up every day, hoping to feel different, only to awake with the same feeling of anhedonia*

(Willick, 1994, pp. 5–19)

As Gary's father observes, cognitive impairment is yet another aspect of schizophrenia, in some ways the most disabling. While not part of the diagnostic criteria for schizophrenia, cognitive impairment has a major influence on functional outcome.

The diagnosis of schizophrenia in DSM-IV (American Psychiatric Association, 1994) requires the presence of two positive or negative symptoms for a significant portion of time during a 1-month period, with some associated social or occupational dysfunction. Even in the absence of symptoms, there must also be a 6-month period of some detectable prodromal or residual symptoms.

CLINICAL COURSE

As in Gary's case, schizophrenia most commonly manifests itself in the early to mid-twenties in men. The disorder often begins somewhat later in women, typically in the late twenties. Gary's case was once again typical in that he had at least 2 years of steadily progressing symptoms before hospitalization was required, and, in retrospect, mild symptoms could be traced back to early

adolescence. The long-term course of schizophrenia is somewhat different in men and women. Overall, women tend to have a somewhat more benign course with fewer negative symptoms and less long-term cognitive impairment. This may be a function of the later onset of the disorder, since the same relatively more benign course is also seen in men whose symptoms start later in life. Other factors associated with relatively better prognosis include a psychologically sound personality prior to developing schizophrenia, good functioning between relatively short episodes of decompensation, the presence of significant depressive symptoms especially in association with a family history of mood disorder, no family history of schizophrenia, and normal neurological status with no signs of structural brain damage on computed tomography (CT) or magnetic resonance imaging (MRI) (American Psychiatric Association, 1994).

Much of the current understanding about the natural course of schizophrenia comes from a landmark 20-year study done by Manfred Bleuler (1974). Bleuler found that schizophrenia most commonly evolved over approximately 5 years, after which time it tended to stabilize with little subsequent deterioration and, in about a third of clients, showed a tendency for some improvement. Unfortunately, another third of clients continued to worsen after 5 years, and a significant proportion of these clients tended to develop very severe intellectual and functional deficits. While negative symptoms surely compounded difficulties of social adjustment, severe cognitive deficits were associated with the worst outcomes.

Numerous other studies have examined cohorts of schizophrenic persons in a variety of settings and countries. The most recent of these studies suggest several interesting findings (McKenna, 1994). First, the outcome for schizophrenia seems to have improved somewhat in the past 20 years, presumably as a result of treatment. Second, despite such improvement, schizophrenia is still a socially devastating disorder: In one recent study, less than 20% of clients were fully employed, and less than 50% were fully independent (Johnstone, 1991). Some clients may be free of positive symptoms and therefore be considered to have a "good outcome," but a good functional outcome may not follow directly from the relative absence of positive symptoms. Finally, it has become evident that the long-term functional outcome of schizophrenia is very difficult to predict for any individual client and may range from near-normal functioning to total dependence. One writer states, "so far as its course is concerned, schizophrenia follows no rules but its own" (McKenna, 1994, p. 72).

No discussion of outcome in schizophrenia would be complete without some discussion of the risk of suicide in this disorder. Suicide is discussed in more detail in Chapter 16, but it is worth emphasizing here that schizophrenia carries a very high suicide risk, possibly the highest of any psychiatric diagnosis (including Major Depressive Disorder). Overall, at least 10% of schizophrenic individuals eventually commit suicide (Gottesman, 1991).

---

*From A Parent's Perspective: Mourning Without End by Martin Willick. (1994). In N. C. Andreasen, *Schizophrenia: From Mind to Molecule* (pp. 5–19). Washington, DC: American Psychiatric Press.

Suicide may occur at any time in the course of the disorder and occurs with equal frequency in men and women, in contrast to suicide in the general population, which is much more common in men. Retrospective studies have not been able identify unusual risk factors in individuals who have killed themselves (Allenbeck, 1989), and the pervasive negative symptoms of schizophrenia make any prediction based on assessing degree of depression exceedingly difficult.

EPIDEMIOLOGY

The major challenge in much of psychiatric epidemiology is case definition: determining who actually has a given diagnosis. While this is of great importance in virtually all psychiatric conditions, nowhere is it more important or difficult than with schizophrenia, for which widely accepted definitions have emerged only recently. Mentally ill individuals frequently tend to have several seemingly different overlapping diagnoses, the border between diagnoses is often obscure, and social and economic factors may play a major role both in cause and in outcome of psychiatric disorders. The *Diagnostic and Statistical Manual* has been of value in standardizing case definitions, but as DSM evolves through DSM-III, IIIR, and now IV, criteria continue to change, potentially affecting conclusions of earlier studies.

Despite these limitations, there is actually much known about the epidemiology of schizophrenia (Gottesman, 1991). One highly regarded study using a cross-sectional methodology was a Swedish door-to-door survey of all 2,550 individuals in a rural community. Careful psychiatric interviews were conducted, and to these were added data from hospital and other community health records. There is reason to believe that the case definitions used for schizophrenia were similar to those in use today. Twenty-one schizophrenic persons were found, for a prevalence of 8.2 per 1,000 persons in the community. It is important to recognize that a number of the schizophrenic community members interviewed in this study had neither been previously diagnosed with schizophrenia nor received any mental health treatment (in several cases despite obvious psychosis). Based on a set of plausible assumptions, the lifetime risk for schizophrenia in this part of Sweden was estimated to be 1.39%. This study established that at any point in time, 8.2 persons with schizophrenia would likely be found for every 1,000 residents of a particular community. If the entire population were followed for a lifetime, it is probable that 1.39% would develop sufficient symptoms to result in a diagnosis of schizophrenia.

An even more ambitious Danish study followed a cohort of persons born during a 4-year period on a small Danish island. Those who lived to age 11 years (N=4,130) were entered in the study and followed for the next 55 years. Over this period, 38 developed schizophrenia,

for a lifetime risk of just under 1%, reasonably close to the 1.39% figure in the Swedish cross-sectional study.

Yet other studies report an incidence rate of 1 new case per 10,000 individuals yearly (American Psychiatric Association, 1994).

Social Costs

Epidemiological studies can help understand how common schizophrenia is, but a broader viewpoint is required to understand the very high social and financial costs of this relatively uncommon disorder (Flynn, 1994). In a recent year, it is estimated that mental illness cost Americans $129.7 billion. About half this amount was attributed to lost productivity and the other half to actual medical care. While schizophrenic persons represent only 10% of the outpatient mental health case load in the United States and only 15% of the overall inpatient case load (36% in state and county mental hospitals), their care accounts for 75% of all mental health direct costs and 90% of all costs due to loss of productivity (Flynn, 1994). While it would appear that by far the majority of United States mental health care expenditures are devoted to persons with schizophrenia, these expenditures by no means benefit all schizophrenic individuals. Many, if not most, schizophrenic persons live without any ongoing contact with the formal mental health system:

> A rising tide of schizophrenic and other severely disordered individuals are now being seen in American jails . . . Jails have, in fact become the new asylums as many police departments feel that it is more humane to arrest severely mentally ill people than to leave them outdoors where they risk freezing to death under bridges or in city parks. Today, we have more seriously mentally ill individuals in the Los Angeles County Jail than in all five California mental hospitals combined. In fact, the Los Angeles County Jail has more mentally ill individuals than the nation's largest state hospital.[*]
>
> (Flynn, 1994, p. 21)

ETIOLOGY

The 19th-century search for etiology was based on the widely held conviction that schizophrenia is a disorder of the brain and not primarily a psychological condition. This view that organic or biological factors are more important than psychological factors in causing schizophrenia has emerged more clearly in recent years. When schizophrenia made its appearance at the end of

[*]From *Schizophrenia From a Family Point of View* by L. Flynn (1994). In N. C. Andreasen, *Schizophrenia: From Mind to Molecule* (pp. 21–30). Washington, DC: American Psychiatric Press.

the 18th century, there were several theories about its cause. Given that its discovery coincided with the European Industrial Revolution, schizophrenia was initially thought to be a direct consequence of stress and urbanization (Gottesman, 1991).

Psychoanalytic Theory

While Freud did not believe that psychotherapy could cure psychosis, he did offer a range of potential psychoanalytic explanations for the symptoms of schizophrenia. Spurred by some apparent therapeutic successes, some of his followers eventually proposed psychoanalytical theories of the etiology of schizophrenia. These included a view that childhood temper tantrums and other unneutralized aggressions might ultimately lead to psychosis. At about the same time, a psychoanalytic theory emerged that portrayed schizophrenia arising out of inadequate maternal nurturance in early infancy (Fine, 1979). Gottesman, a psychologist, makes the following observations about psychological theories of schizophrenia:

> It must be said that much of Freud's doctrine has been overly generalized by his disciples and followers beyond the conditions for which it may be of use. This has confused the study and understanding of schizophrenia by delaying biological and genetic research, and we have lived with that confusion for much of the twentieth century. Mental health professionals believe that environmental, interpersonal, and intrapsychic stressors are contributing factors; we do not believe, however, that a bad mother or father, bad mothering, or any other environmental factor alone can cause someone to become schizophrenic.*
>
> (Gottesman, 1991, p. 15)

In actuality, multiple research studies have evaluated a wide range of developmental, environmental, and psychological factors and have failed to find any suggestion that such factors are in any way direct causes of schizophrenia (McKenna, 1994).

Genetics

For individuals of certain genetic background the incidence of schizophrenia may be very much higher than average. For example, while the overall risk of schizophrenia developing in a lifetime is about 1%, an individual with two schizophrenic parents has nearly a 50% chance of becoming schizophrenic. Schizophrenia is clearly a disorder with a major genetic component. This component has been investigated most dramatically

---

*From *Schizophrenia Genesis* by Gottesman, Copyright ©1991 by Irving I. Gottesman. Used with permission of W. H. Freeman and Company.

RESEARCH HIGHLIGHT

Twin Studies in Schizophrenia

There are three types of twin studies that have been conducted, and the major findings are the following (McKenna, 1994; Gottesman, 1991; Reveley, 1994):

1. Studies have examined hospitalized clients and compared the frequency of similarly affected twins for both identical (monozygotic) and fraternal (dizygotic) twins. In four studies, 60% to 70% of hospitalized identical twins had a monozygotic sibling who also had the disease; for fraternal twins, only 0% to 15% had a dizygotic sibling with the disease (McKenna 1994).

2. Other studies have focused on cross-sectional population samples rather than on hospitalized individuals. For identical twins, if one twin had schizophrenia, his co-twin was 2 to 3 times more likely to have schizophrenia than were co-twins of fraternal twins who had the disease (Gottesman, 1991).

3. In studies that evaluated identical twins reared apart, although the number is small and cannot permit generalizations, if one twin had schizophrenia, the co-twin also had schizophrenia in 64% of the pairs (Reveley, 1994).

---

through studies of twins. These studies are summarized in the accompanying Research Highlight, and the results of twin studies argue convincingly that there is a genetic component to the disease (McKenna, 1994; Gottesman, 1991; Reveley, 1994).

The inheritance of schizophrenia, however, is very complex and still incompletely understood. As can be seen from Figure 11-1, there is a clear genetic risk for developing schizophrenia, with the highest risk occurring for identical twins and for children whose parents both have schizophrenia. Intermediate (10% to 15%) risk occurs for non-identical-twin siblings of schizophrenic individuals and for children of schizophrenics. Risk for other genetic relationships, while higher than the general population's baseline of 1%, are under 10%.

Despite the well-demonstrated contribution of genetics to the development of schizophrenia, the majority of schizophrenics (63%) have absolutely no family history of the disease. Even monozygotic twins (who have virtually all of their genes in common) have less than 100% likelihood of one developing schizophrenia when the other is afflicted. Genetics clearly plays a role but by no means a decisive one. Scientists have so far sought the actual cause of schizophrenia with great effort, but to date, no certain answer has emerged.

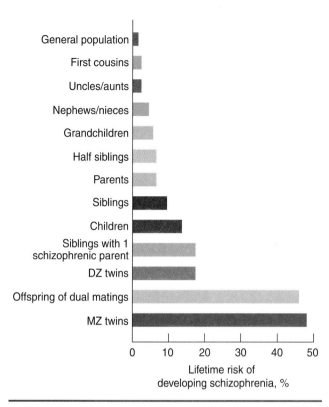

Figure 11-1   **Genetic risk for developing schizophrenia.** *Adapted from* Schizophrenia Genesis *by Gottesman. Copyright © 1991 by Irving I. Gottesman. Used with permission of W. H. Freeman and Company.*

⟲ *REFLECTIVE THINKING*

Schizophrenia and Genetic Tendency

If a family had one child with schizophrenia and asked you about the genetic tendencies of the disease, what would you tell them?

Current Views

If psychological factors are not fundamental causes and genetic factors only play a partial role, what *does* cause schizophrenia? By the end of the 19th century some leading psychiatrists felt strongly that schizophrenia was due to "organic causes"; that is, there was something physically and structurally wrong with the brains of schizophrenic individuals. The trouble with this theory was that no one could find any structural abnormalities in brains examined at autopsy. Dr. Alzheimer (who was able to show a definitive link between senile dementia and brain structure) was able to show only mild generalized cell loss and scarring (gliosis) in schizophrenia, findings too nonspecific to offer clues to causation (Johnstone, 1991).

There was little progress in the search for organic causes of schizophrenia until the mid-1970s, when the

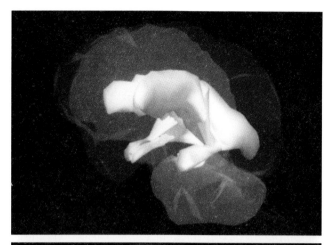

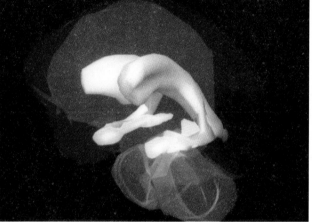

MRI images in schizophrenia. These two MRI images depict a person with schizophrenia (top) and a normal control (bottom). The brain is seen from the side. The most striking difference is in the hippocampus (yellow), which is much smaller in the schizophrenic individual. The ventricles (grey) are larger in the person with schizophrenia. *Permission granted by Nancy C. Andreasen of the University of Iowa.*

newly developed CT scanner was used to evaluate brain structure in schizophrenic individuals. This powerful tool was able to show that schizophrenic males (but not females) have larger lateral ventricles than do nonschizophrenic persons. It appears that this finding has been established beyond any reasonable doubt, but its meaning is unclear. No one knows if the ventricular enlargement is a cause or a consequence of schizophrenia, and the degree of enlargement seems to have no consistent relationship to the degree or nature of illness.

Soon after the development of CT scanning, various techniques became available to study regional brain blood flow and metabolic activity, and these techniques were soon used to study clients with schizophrenia. Despite early suggestions of regional blood flow abnormalities, two decades of research has produced many interesting findings in different forms of schizophrenia

(Liddle et al., 1992) but little insight into the cause of the disorder.

Dopamine Hypothesis

While the cause of schizophrenia remains unknown, the brain in this disorder has been examined in remarkable detail. It seems extraordinary that such profound disruption of function can result with such little anatomic change. Many scientists feel that the pathological explanation for such profound but as yet invisible abnormalities can only be found at the molecular level: in specific enzymes and neurotransmitters. This view has given rise since the 1960s to what is termed the *dopamine hypothesis* (McKenna, 1994). This hypothesis states that the functional abnormalities in schizophrenia are due to excessive activity of brain dopamine. Dopamine is normally produced in the brain, and it serves as a signaling molecule or neurotransmitter. Dopamine seems to have its most important effects in the basal ganglia of the brain; reduction of dopamine in these structures leads to Parkinson's disease (a movement disorder most commonly seen in the elderly). Several pieces of evidence provide support for this hypothesis. First, drugs effective in the control of positive symptoms of schizophrenia all seem to have significant dopamine receptor blocking activity; that is, these drugs seem to work because they reduce the effect of an individual's own dopamine on his or her brain. Secondly, drugs like amphetamines, which have the ability to cause strikingly schizophrenic-like psychoses, act by increasing brain dopamine concentrations (McKenna, 1994). Finally, of all the neuropathological findings from multiple autopsies of persons dying with schizophrenia, the most reproducible is an increase in dopamine receptors in the brain's basal ganglia. If receptors are increased in number, then any given amount of brain dopamine can exert a stronger biological effect (Clardy, Hyde, & Kleinman, 1994).

Etiology Unknown

Despite the intriguing evidence supporting the finding of increased dopamine and dopamine receptors in schizophrenia, there is also some strong evidence against the hypothesis, and the hypothesis remains highly controversial. The 1990s—at one time optimistically proclaimed to be the "decade of the brain"—currently seem likely to pass without the emergence of a definitive understanding of schizophrenia.

TREATMENT

There are two main approaches to the treatment of schizophrenia: the psychosocial approach and the pharmacological approach. The nurse has a role in each.

There is certainly an autonomous nursing role in directing and managing the psychosocial treatment as well as an obvious collaborative role in working with other professionals to provide for the psychosocial therapies and to monitor the pharmacological treatment. Each will be discussed next, with specific attention paid to nursing perspectives on care in the section that follows.

Psychosocial Treatment

The goals of psychosocial treatment interventions can be conceived in a number of different ways, but one useful approach has been to divide interventions into three categories: clinical and family support services, rehabilitative services, and humanitarian aid/public safety (Hargreaves & Shumway, 1989). The goal of clinical interventions is to reduce both positive and negative symptoms and to maximize functional outcome. Clinical support involves outpatient management and family/community services. Rehabilitation involves increasing clients' capacities, both for social interactions and for productive activity (including gainful employment when feasible). Humanitarian interventions are those efforts that maximize an individual's independence and quality of life within the bounds of his or her mental disability. Public safety involves balancing personal liberty with the recognition that some social control may be needed to prevent harm, both to the individual and to society.

Clinical and Family Support Services

Clinical and family support services include educating family members about the nature and meaning of schizophrenia as well as providing specific skills training for both client and family. Stress management skills and functional coping responses are of high priority.

Assisting family members is a priority of nursing care. One study of mothers of schizophrenic young men revealed that the mothers felt fear, distress, uncertainty, and powerlessness (Wheeler, 1994). Another evaluation of parents' experiences of caring for chronically mentally ill children revealed that sorrow is often triggered by the unending caregiving responsibilities (Eakes, 1995). Families can be supported through education, group activities, and community involvement/advocacy. Internet bulletin boards and discussion groups provide new methods of linking individuals and family members with others around the world in electronic support groups. For example, over a three-month time period, one discussion group on the general topic of schizophrenia had 54 named participants from 10 countries with over 1,000 entries (Schizophrenia Discussion Group, 1997).

In addition, educating families to understand the purpose and side effects of medication can help them work to ensure compliance. Multiple studies have shown that adding these kinds of psychosocial interventions to drug

NURSING TIP

Family Management of Members with Schizophrenia

Three underlying concepts of programs directed to families have been summarized as follows (Barrowclough & Tarrier, 1992):

1. Living with a person who suffers from schizophrenia can be very difficult; most relatives feel stressed and upset, at least some of the time.

2. When the client with schizophrenia lives with his family, a lot of the day-to-day help and rehabilitation is carried out by family members. Thus, if they are to effectively help the client, family members must have help in managing their stress and coping with difficult situations.

3. Additionally, people who suffer from schizophrenia are unusually sensitive to stress in others, so by feeling more in control oneself, a family member may indirectly help the client.

treatment significantly reduces the frequency of relapses (McGlashan, 1994).

Rehabilitation

Rehabilitation efforts for persons with schizophrenia may be directed toward vocational goals for some individuals, but for a majority, the presence of negative symptoms makes any kind of social functioning so problematic that the primary focus has to be on enhancing social skills. Training in social functioning can potentially increase clients' knowledge and skill levels; it may also sometimes reduce rates of psychotic relapse (Hogarty et al., 1986). Programs can address emotional insight and family problem solving skills and both verbal and nonverbal communication, including the importance of eye contact and facial expressions. As two authorities observe:

The most effective psychosocial treatment— whether provided in individual, group, or family therapy, inpatient ward or community program— contains elements of practicality, problem-solving of everyday challenges, socialization and vocational activities, and specific goal orientation . . . It is likely that future research will establish the benefit of indefinite psychosocial support and training in the long-term management of schizophrenia. Just as neuroleptic drugs are most effective in maintaining

symptomatic improvement when continued indefinitely, it is not surprising that psychosocial treatments are similarly optimized by continuity.*

(Vaccaro & Roberts, 1992, p. 114)

Individual and family stress is clearly associated with both onset and exacerbation of schizophrenic symptoms. Failure to take medication is a major cause of symptoms worsening. Enhancing family functioning, decreasing measures of interpersonal stress, and maximizing medication compliance are among the important areas for psychosocial intervention. This intervention may be effected by a nurse, a social worker, a psychologist, or a multidisciplinary team involving all three professions.

Humanitarian Aid/Public Safety

In recent years mental health workers have used the term *challenging behavior* to describe the most difficult positive symptoms of schizophrenia: bizarre, socially disruptive, and perhaps potentially dangerous behavior. Prior to deinstitutionalization, many such clients would have been hospitalized in an effort to enhance their own safety as well as that of the public. Today the options for managing and treating such challenging behavior are probably more limited.

Beginning in the mid-1960s, the United States embarked on an extraordinary program to remove the severely mentally ill from mental hospitals. Many hospitals were indeed uncaring, filthy, and brutal; from a human perspective, "deinstitutionalized" care seemed to offer the severely mentally ill potential for far more normal lives. As a result, between 1965 and 1975 the population of United States mental institutions was purposefully reduced by 60%; and it had actually declined even more dramatically between 1955 and 1965. Experts have observed that the results were not quite as intended: "With help from improvements in antipsychotic drugs, many schizophrenics have returned to the community. Some are in supervised public settings, and we are still able to count those, but some are in jails and prisons, others are lost among the hordes of homeless, and a few are in private treatment" (Gottesman, 1991, p. 64).

While this revolutionary program of deinstitutionalization is not fully responsible for the current American epidemic of homelessness, many feel it has contributed significantly. About a third of the homeless are estimated to be seriously mentally ill, as are up to 20% of the nearly 1 million individuals in United States jails and prisons (Gottesman, 1991).

While numerous problems were documented and care in some hospitals was inappropriate, the best psychiatric facilities of the 1960s provided clients with a

---

*"Teaching Social and Coping Skills," J. V. Vacarro & L. Roberts, ©1992. Reprinted by permission of John Wiley & Sons Ltd.

ஒ *REFLECTIVE THINKING*

Schizophrenia and the Homeless

Clinicians who examine the homeless consistently conclude that about a third of them have severe mental disorders, and in direct surveys of the homeless, the homeless themselves report clear symptoms of psychosis.

In the 1950s and 1960s, most of these persons would have been placed in hospitals on the basis of their mental illnesses. Deinstitutionalization moved these persons to the least restrictive environment, and in the 1980s and 1990s, social policies are such that these persons have the right to be on their own but with little support and no money with which to manage other than on the street. Courts have ruled that mental illness is not sufficient justification for involuntary commitment to a hospital. And hospitals are not allowed (or, at least, are not reimbursed) for keeping clients longer than a specified number of days.

◆ How would you create social policy to maintain the individual rights of mentally ill persons and at the same time provide them with care and treatment?

◆ Who would agree with your position and who would not?

◆ What role does the professional nurse have in advocacy for clients' rights? How can the nurse best implement this role?

protective and supportive environment that cannot be duplicated today. As the distinguished Yale University psychiatrist Thomas McGlashan observes:

> We must tell the accountants that the alternatives to institutionalization are equally if not more expensive . . . We have thrust the severely mentally ill out of the institutions [onto the sidewalks] only to forget that . . . they are disabled and they need asylum, in the sense of support and protection from stress . . . I am not sure what will be our next great leap forward, but I do know one thing—we sure are ready for something because it sure is bad out there.*

(McGlashan, 1994, p. 213)

Many mental health workers define humane care as the least restrictive care needed to provide psychosocial and rehabilitative services to the client. While deinstitutionalization ensured that persons live in environments with fewer restrictions, one knows from a social perspective that the settings in which many schizophrenic persons currently live are neither caring nor therapeutic. The individual's right to the least restrictive environment has all too often meant the right to be homeless, starving, and without treatment.

Pharmacological and Physical Treatments

Neuroleptic Medications

For centuries, rauwolfia root had been used in India to sedate persons with severe psychiatric disorders. In 1952, the active ingredient of rauwolfia, reserpine, was found to have useful properties in the management of schizophrenia. At virtually the same time, two newly synthesized antihistamine-like drugs, promethazine and chlorpromazine, were found to have very similar effects in clients. By the mid-1960s, multiple placebo-controlled double-blind trials had established beyond any doubt the effectiveness of chlorpromazine in controlling both negative and positive symptoms of schizophrenia, although the effect on negative symptoms was far less than that on positive symptoms. Not only was the effectiveness of chlorpromazine proven by these careful studies, but the improvement—especially in positive symptoms of paranoia, hallucinations, and agitation—was quite remarkable for some clients. While reserpine soon fell out of favor as a psychiatric drug, numerous other "antipsychotic" medications became available over the next few years; collectively, these drugs have become known as "neuroleptics."

Several decades of neuroleptic usage have led clinicians to a variety of conclusions about these drugs,

*From Psychosocial Treatments of Schizophrenia by T. H. McGlashan. (1994). In N. C. Andreasen, *Schizophrenia: From Mind to Molecule* (p. 213). Washington, DC: American Psychiatric Press.

NEUROLEPTIC DRUGS

◆ Neuroleptics are valuable medications, but they do not cure schizophrenia.

◆ In about a quarter of clients, even positive symptoms remain highly resistant to neuroleptic drugs.

◆ While the neuroleptic drugs do have an effect on negative symptoms, these symptoms frequently remain socially incapacitating.

◆ These medications have a range of significant adverse side effects.

◆ With the exception of clozapine, there is little evidence that any one neuroleptic is more effective than the others.

◆ All the neuroleptics seem to share the ability to block dopamine from interacting with brain dopamine receptors.

summarized in the accompanying display. These drugs are helpful, but they do not cure schizophrenia, and they have some significant adverse side effects, which are discussed following.

Side effects of neuroleptics. Most of the neuroleptics share similar therapeutic properties and side effects. Sudden death has occasionally been reported after neuroleptic administration, especially by injection, but experts are not yet sure whether medication has caused these deaths (Editors, 1995). Other than this still unresolved concern, the most serious neuroleptic side effects involve the nervous system and appear to result from the very dopamine receptor blockade that makes these drugs so useful.

The most readily treated side effect is called **dystonia**. Dystonic reactions usually manifest as painful muscle spasms lasting anywhere from a few seconds to days. These may involve any muscle group and are most often localized to just a few muscles at a time. Contractions of the neck, known as torticollis, and of the facial muscles are probably most common. Clients may present with the head drawn forcefully to one side, with spasms of the mouth muscles, or with fixed tongue protrusion. These spasms are rarely dangerous unless the laryngeal muscles are involved, in which case the airway is at risk of obstruction. Dystonic reactions typically occur within a few hours or days of starting a neuroleptic, stop fairly quickly when medication is discontinued, and respond almost instantaneously to intravenous diphenhydramine (benadryl) or to other anticholinergic medications. Benzodiazepines (diazepam or clonazepam) are also effective. Acute dystonia is fairly rare but occurs in 2% to 3% of clients given chlorpromazine and rather more commonly in clients given haloperidol (haldol) and a long-acting injectable neuroleptic such as fluphenazine.

Akathisia is a somewhat more common side effect that affects both motor function and behavior. Clients with akathisia become physically restless and unable to sit still: they pace, shift their weight from foot to foot, and tap their feet. The upper extremities or face is rarely involved, but many clients develop emotional changes: at times, decreased ability to concentrate along with euphoria but sometimes malaise, depression, and worsening psychosis. Compared to acute dystonia, akathisia begins somewhat later in the course of treatment, but rarely after 6 months. It sometimes diminishes or disappears without stopping treatment, but virtually always goes away when the neuroleptic medication is stopped.

Symptoms of parkinsonism may be induced by neuroleptic drugs and occur in up to 40% of clients treated with these medications. Older clients are affected more than younger, and, like akathisia, parkinsonism tends to occur within the first months of treatment. The primary finding is **akinesia**, or poverty of movement. This is different from the usual avolition of schizophrenia; clients with parkinsonian akinesia initiate very slowly any movement (seen commonly in getting out of a chair) and

show reduced arm swinging when walking. In most cases, symptoms resolve even without stopping medication, but about 1% of individuals continue to have parkinsonism despite drug withdrawal. It is felt by many that these individuals had underlying "idiopathic" parkinsonism that was unmasked by neuroleptic treatment. Clients with drug-induced parkinsonism are thought to respond particularly well to anticholinergic medication treatment.

Tardive dyskinesia is a troublesome movement disorder that is commonly found in schizophrenic clients maintained on neuroleptics for long periods of time. The incidence is said to be up to 4% per year but is clearly highest in older clients, especially women. The movements of tardive dyskinesia are typically repetitive and most commonly involve the face. Common findings are repetitive smacking, chewing, grimacing, cheek puffing, and tongue protrusion. Similar movements can involve the hands, and on occasion, ticlike movements occur, including grunts or other vocal utterances.

> ⚡ **NURSING ALERT!**
>
> **Tardive Dyskinesia**
>
> Unlike the other neuroleptic-induced movement disorders, tardive dyskinesia frequently cannot be reversed by withdrawing medication.

Curiously, increasing the dose of medication sometimes significantly suppresses tardive dyskinesia. However, tardive dyskinesia is often very resistant to any treatment and permanently stigmatizes clients who have the misfortune to develop symptoms unresponsive to treatment. Early diagnosis and treatment, including drug holidays and decreased dosages, are the best courses of action.

The most serious neuroleptic side effect, the neuroleptic malignant syndrome, is also the rarest, but nurses must be familiar with it because if left untreated, it may rapidly lead to death. Most clients develop this syndrome only when on high or increasing doses of medication and often after a dosage increase. The most striking features are confusion or decreased level of consciousness and high fever. Clients also acutely develop parkinsonian symptoms of rigidity and akinesia, but the significance of these is sometimes overlooked in the erroneous search for an infectious cause of fever. Fever is most often very high in neuroleptic malignant syndrome, not infrequently rising to dangerous levels (above 106° F); but in rare cases, it may be absent, and high fever is not required to make the diagnosis. Serum creatine kinase (CK) is the definitive diagnostic test; because of muscle damage, presumably due to extreme rigidity, CK reaches very high levels, often associated with myoglobinuria. Treatment is largely symptomatic, and both vigorous hydration and cooling are often required to ensure survival. Neuroleptic medication is stopped, and various medications to increase central nervous system (CNS) dopamine levels may be given.

Atypical neuroleptics. Thioridizine and clozapine are regarded as atypical neuroleptics partly because they do not seem to cause movement disorders. While thioridizine is clearly *less* effective than the other neuroleptics, clozapine has been shown in controlled trials to be more effective and often to produce improvement in clients resistant to the classical neuroleptics. Unfortunately, this improvement sometimes comes at a price: Clozapine occasionally and unpredictably causes severe agranulocytosis (reduction in numbers of white blood cells). This complication has proven fatal for some clients, and in some states, mental health client advocacy groups have forced tight regulation in the use of clozapine. With careful monitoring of white blood cell counts, clozapine can be used with relative safety, but this requirement for monitoring makes it very difficult to employ in community outpatient settings unless compliance can be ensured. There is currently much interest in developing new drugs that have clozapine's effectiveness without its effect on white blood cells.

Other Physical Treatments

Medication is not the only treatment employed for schizophrenia. Electroconvulsive therapy (shock therapy) has been used, especially for individuals in catatonic states, and is felt by many psychiatrists to be valuable (see Chapter 30 for further discussion of electroconvulsive therapy). However, no scientific basis for its use has yet been established; the best and safest use is in conjunction with an affective component.

NURSING PERSPECTIVES

The nurse is a major participant in the care of schizophrenic persons.

Nurses will work with other mental health care workers and be part of a collaborative team providing service to and advocacy for clients. A nursing perspective, however, is unique because the nursing focus is on the human response to the condition. As demonstrated in the discussions preceding, the human responses to living with schizophrenia are directly related to the individual's experience and symptoms. Applicable nursing diagnoses parallel these symptoms, as illustrated in Table 11-1.

What approach to care should the nurse use? There are basic guidelines for each nursing diagnosis. To address the diagnosis of *altered thought processes*, the nurse must first recognize that the client is unable to easily follow verbal speech. The nurse must speak clearly, making only one point at a time or giving clear and simple directions. When a client is delusional, the nurse should not enter into the delusion, that is, should not ask the client to "tell me more" and/or engage the client in conversation about

Table 11-1   Symptoms Experienced with Schizophrenia and Associated Nursing Diagnoses

SYMPTOMS	NURSING DIAGNOSES
Disordered thought	*Altered thought processes*
Incomprehensible language	*Impaired verbal communication*
Loss of function	*Altered role performance*
Delusions	*Altered thought processes*
Hallucinations	*Impaired sensory perception*

the delusional ideas. Rather, the nurse should attempt to learn the meaning of the delusion to the client. Also, the nurse can and should express doubt over the reality of delusional thoughts; for example, the nurse could say, "I don't see how you can be receiving messages from outer space," but must avoid entering into an argument with the client over the validity of his thoughts. The nurse should redirect the conversation away from the delusions and back to reality by introducing another topic. When a client has been diagnosed with *impaired verbal communication* because of disordered speech, the nurse can assist by taking time to understand the client's needs, maintaining a calm and peaceful environment to help the client center and express himself, and communicating to the client in clear, short phrases. Interventions aimed at developing and maintaining social skills (to be discussed later) will also apply.

The diagnosis of *altered role performance* will cause great difficulty for the client in society. Loss of job, friends, and support may be results of the client's inability to perform in socially acceptable ways. The client may lose the ability to care for himself. Such situations lead to dependence on others to the degree where hospital care or care through structured settings like board-and-care homes is necessary. The community nurse will frequently have a role in evaluating the living and care environments for clients and assisting in procuring appropriate and safe arrangements. Further, the nurse should assist the client in activities that foster socially acceptable interactions with others.

The diagnosis of *altered sensory perceptions* due to hallucinations can be frightening to the client, his family and friends, other clients on a hospital unit, and the nurse herself. The nurse must understand that the hallucinations are very real to the client and that clients will respond to their hallucinatory experiences. In an acute setting, the nurse should provide a quiet and nonstimulating environment and talk to the client, letting him know that she is present and will maintain safety for the client. It is appropriate for the nurse to tell the client that she does not see or hear the client's hallucination. For example, the nurse might say, "I know it is very real to you, but I do not hear the voice." Because medications can control hallucinations, the nurse can administer medication as prescribed by the physician. The nurse must remember that clients

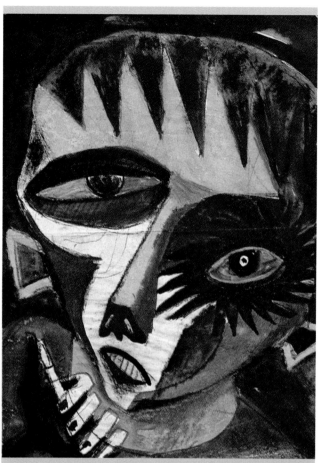

From *Art as Healing* by Edward Adamson and John Timlin.
Reprinted with permission of Adamson Collection Charity.

While the influences of Cubism may be apparent, this painting is not by a follower of Picasso or Braque but was painted by an individual suffering from schizophrenia. The intensity of schizophrenic experience is evident in the frenzied shapes and colors.

may respond to hallucinations in unpredictable ways and that there is always a potential for violent outbursts. For example, a client may hear voices telling him to harm someone else. The goals of the nursing interventions are to establish safety and to help attune the client to reality.

Impaired social interactions result from the negative symptoms of the disease. Social support and social training groups can be important interventions. The nurse must begin by establishing a one-on-one, supportive, therapeutic relationship and build from that relationship to assist the client to interact with others. On an interdisciplinary team, recreational and occupational therapists can make important contributions to meeting the client's needs for socialization through planned therapeutic activities.

NURSING THEORY

The overriding need of a long-term schizophrenic client is to be supported so that he can maintain ability to function as independently as possible. Frequently, the client's inability to interact with others and meet expected social norms prevents independent functioning. Nursing theories grounded in establishing a trusting nurse-client relationship help provide the framework to serve as a basis for all therapeutic interaction.

The Modeling and Role-Modeling Theory (Erickson, Tomlin, & Swain, 1983; Frisch & Bowman, 1995) assists by providing the nurse with the five aims of intervention that can become the foundation for all work with the schizophrenic client:

1. Build trust.
2. Promote positive orientation.
3. Promote perceived control.
4. Promote strengths.
5. Set mutual goals that are health directed.

The nurse can begin with building trust and work from an established nurse-client relationship to design care aimed at realistic and appropriate goals.

N U R S I N G   P R O C E S S

▽ ASSESSMENT

An important consideration in assessing a client with schizophrenia is the degree to which symptoms of the disease are currently affecting the client's functioning. The display on the following page lists important parameters of assessment. The nurse will need to obtain information from the client and, often, from other sources. For example, a schizophrenic individual may not be able to communicate regarding negative symptoms, such as lack of

motivation or poverty of speech, and will not be able to tell the nurse if current behavior is a change from previous functioning. Such information is appropriately obtained from family members or others who may relate observations over a period of time.

In assessment, the nurse is not just looking for evidence that symptoms of schizophrenia exist; she is also looking for clues as to the immediate concerns of and the kind of assistance desired by the client or family members/caretakers.

ASSESSMENT PARAMETERS FOR SCHIZOPHRENIC CLIENTS

Observe for:

1. Presence of delusions
   - Does the client have ideas or beliefs that others say are untrue?
   - Does the client have the belief that neutral cues in the environment refer to him?
   - Does the client believe he has special talents and extraordinary powers?
2. Presence of hallucinations
   - Does the client see, hear, or smell things others do not?
3. Disorganized speech
   - Can the client communicate logically and rationally?
4. Problems in basic grooming
5. Negative symptoms of schizophrenia, including:
   - Flat affect (dampening of emotions)
   - Poverty of speech
   - Lack of motivation
   - Symptoms of depression
6. Level of independence and functioning

▽ NURSING DIAGNOSIS

Nursing diagnoses are made based on priority needs. For example, in an acute episode where the client is being admitted to hospital for symptoms of disordered thoughts, hallucinations, delusions, and loss of function, control and management of the symptoms are the highest priority. Once symptoms are brought under control, the concerns of loss of function, social isolation, and role performance can be addressed over a rehabilitative plan of care.

Nursing diagnoses made during the acute episode may be:

- *Altered thought processes,* related to inability to think rationally, complete a sentence, or communicate coherently
- *Altered thought processes,* related to persecutory delusions
- *Altered sensory perceptions,* related to auditory hallucinations
- *Self-care deficit (specify),* related to inability to maintain personal hygiene

- *Sleep pattern disturbance,* related to fear of falling asleep

In contrast, in a rehabilitative phase of treatment, the nursing diagnoses may be:

- *Altered role performance,* related to change in self-perception of role
- *Social isolation,* related to absence of or inability to engage in satisfying personal relationships
- *Ineffective management of therapeutic regimen,* related to knowledge deficit and complexity of therapeutic regimen

▽ OUTCOME IDENTIFICATION

For each diagnosis, the nurse must establish appropriate and expected outcomes and goals. Again, the expected outcomes will be different depending on whether the client is being treated in an acute or rehabilitative phase.

Acute Phase

In the acute phase, the immediate goal of treatment is to bring symptoms under control. For example, for the diagnosis of *altered thought processes,* a stated outcome might be "within 3 days of initiating treatment, the client will be able to answer simple direct questions." For the diagnosis of *altered sensory perception,* related to hallucinations, the outcome might be "within 3 days of initiating medication, the client will experience a decline in number of hallucinations." For the diagnosis of *sleep pattern disturbance,* the stated outcome might be "within 3 days of hospital admission, the client will sleep through the night."

Rehabilitative Phase

Clearly, the nurse providing care in the rehabilitative phase will establish goals aimed at helping the client and his family to make the best adjustment possible to a chronic illness and will take any measures possible to maintain the client's independence to whatever degree possible. Outcomes should be identified for every nursing diagnosis. Examples are: for the diagnosis of *altered role performance,* related to inability to keep a job, the nurse and client together might determine that the problem is getting up to go to work and might establish a goal that the client will attend work regularly by going to work with his neighbor; for the diagnosis of *ineffective management of the therapeutic regimen,* related to forgetting to take needed medications, the nurse and client might come up with an outcome that the client will take medications regularly and that his sister will visit daily to inquire about medication.

CARING FOR SCHIZOPHRENIC CLIENTS: ACUTE PHASE

The following principles are helpful in planning interventions for schizophrenic clients in the acute phase:

- The symptoms of disordered thoughts, hallucinations, and loss of function are often frightening to the client. Nursing actions to promote a calm, peaceful, trusting atmosphere are essential in alleviating fear and establishing a nurse-client relationship.

- The nurse should express reality regarding client reports of hallucinations and delusions but should not enter into arguments regarding whether or not the delusions are true or the hallucinations are real. For example, the nurse should say, "I don't understand how you could be getting secret messages from the President of Poland while you are here in our hospital," and then should redirect the conversation to another topic. Regarding hallucinations, the nurse should say, "I don't hear the voices you are talking about, but I understand they are real to you."

- The nurse should work collaboratively with the treatment team to initiate a plan to control the acute symptoms and move the client into rehabilitative care.

CARING FOR SCHIZOPHRENIC CLIENTS: REHABILITATIVE PHASE

The following principles are helpful in planning interventions for schizophrenic clients in the rehabilitative phase:

- Schizophrenic clients tend to do better with a structured daily schedule and a daily plan of activities. Therefore it is helpful for the client to have a written schedule to follow.

- Social isolation is common, and activities that promote supportive contacts with others help to meet social needs and to boost self-esteem.

- *Risk for ineffective management of therapeutic regimen* is high, such that frequent home visits from the nurse coupled with assistance from family or significant others may be essential for success.

- Factors such as lack of transportation to follow-up visits, lack of supportive and affordable housing, and difficulty in obtaining health care insurance or social assistance usually require that the nurse work closely with social workers and community agencies to meet client needs.

- Family members and/or significant others are frequently involved in client care; nurse's care to the caregiver and elimination of caregiver role strain are always important considerations.

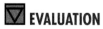 PLANNING/INTERVENTIONS

Acute Phase

In the acute phase of schizophrenia, the assessment, plan, and outcomes are all based on alleviating acute symptoms. Thus, much of the nursing care will be collaborative and involve use of medications to bring symptoms under control. Independent nursing care—for example, care directed at assisting a client to sleep—will be done through interventions that establish a safe and trusting environment and provide an acutely ill client a space for sleep without interference from others.

Rehabilitative Phase

In the rehabilitative phase, the interventions must be planned by the nurse and client together, not by the nurse alone. The most successful interventions will be creative, as the nurse and client attempt to identify the reasons that impede successful meeting of client goals and to come up with plans that work for the client. For example, the nurse helps her client find volunteer work in his community, assists the client to interact with others, and helps him maintain a socially acceptable role within the community. The nurse also works with her client and his family members to monitor daily medication intake and assists the client to keep acute symptoms under control.

EVALUATION

Evaluation of nursing care is always based on whether or not the identified outcomes have been met. When the outcomes are written in behavioral and measurable terms, the nurse can readily evaluate if the outcome has been met.

CASE STUDY/CARE PLAN

Refer to the literary excerpt "Mourning without End." Imagine that nurses are giving care to Gary as if he were coming to the hospital for an acute admission. His symptoms and behaviors are expected to be similar to those of other schizophrenic clients. This is a fictionalized nursing care plan.

ASSESSMENT

Gary is a highly intelligent college student who has first-hand experience with schizophrenia. He is currently in school, and until recently has adequately managed his academic work. Gary has been hospitalized three times in the past for acute schizophrenic episodes that included delusions and suicidal ideation. He has been well maintained for several months on medications and weekly psychotherapy. Gary has noticed an increase in problems over the past 3 weeks. He is having difficulty concentrating, is increasingly afraid of people, and senses danger is everywhere. Gary has cut the cable of his television because he believes it has the power to hurt him and refuses to deal with answering the phone or checking his messages. He recognizes he is increasingly isolating himself from his friends, his peers, his family, and his work. It is very hard to even get up in the morning. He forgets to take his prescribed medications. Gary is very close to his father, who has stood by him since his illness began. Gary decides to drive to his father's private office to talk to him about getting help. He is very fearful.

Gary and his father decide that he needs some intensive intervention. The psychotherapist is called and Gary is admitted to a private mental health clinic. Gary's dad arranges for a short-term leave of absence from the college for Gary.

NURSING DIAGNOSIS *Ineffective individual coping*, related to situational crises, as evidenced by inability to cope, meet role expectations, or meet basic needs

Outcomes	Planning/Interventions	Evaluation
◆ Within 4 days, Gary will identify those factors he believes may have precipitated the need for this hospitalization.	◆ Assist Gary in verbally exploring the source of his stress over the past 3 weeks by asking about life events prior to hospitalization.	Gary's stress was primarily in response to his classes, where he has had stress related to performance.
◆ Within 4 days, Gary will reestablish the effective coping strategies he has used in the past (physical exercise in the form of two 30-minute walks a day).	◆ Encourage Gary to use strategies that have worked well in the past, such as taking supervised walks or setting up a structured daily schedule.	Gary's greatest fear was of slipping back into a delusional state and "losing all the progress I had made."
◆ Within 7 days, Gary will demonstrate an ability to manage his medications and daily activities in a supervised home setting.	◆ Work with Gary to achieve understanding of the importance of establishing a schedule as a means of maintaining control of his life and a link to reality.	Gary did not initially make the connection, but as his fear escalated, he stopped walking each day, missed two appointments with his therapist, and forgot to take his medications. His symptoms increased. Once hospitalized, he realized he was perfectly capable of staying well enough to manage his daily affairs.
◆ Within 2 weeks, Gary will return to his apartment, demonstrating prehospital behavior, as evidenced by pre-illness stable eating, sleeping, and activity patterns.	◆ Help Gary to reestablish normal perspectives about his behavior, his medications, his stress level, and his environment.	

Continued

NURSING DIAGNOSIS *Impaired social interaction*, related to social withdrawal, as evidenced by verbalization of discomfort in social situations and dysfunctional interactions with peers

Outcomes	Planning/Interventions	Evaluation
◆ Within 24 hours of hospitalization, Gary will establish a beginning relationship with a nurse.	◆ Assist Gary in his socialization, starting with one-on-one interactions. ◆ Encourage Gary to expand his world by initiating conversation with one staff person and one client per day.	In the hospital, Gary was open to discussing his problems. He felt particularly comfortable with Ben, a nurse who expressed how much he respected Gary for work-ing toward a college degree. Ben liked to walk and talk, so he and Gary were able to do a lot of reflection about what had gone on the past few weeks. With Ben's encouragement, Gary did get involved in inpatient and outpatient counseling sessions. Gary also asked his psychotherapist to let Ben know he was "back on track with school."
◆ Within 4 days, Gary will attend a small in-patient group session.	◆ Attend a small inpatient counseling session with Gary.	
◆ Within 2 weeks, Gary will attend an out-patient group meeting (with his father, if he so chooses).	◆ Include outpatient meetings in the discharge plan for Gary.	
◆ Within 1 month, Gary will reconnect with at least two friends and regularly attend his therapy sessions.	◆ Help Gary locate and reestablish contact with one or two friends of his choice. ◆ Follow up with telephone calls first to Gary's dad (with Gary's permission) and then to Gary to encourage his continued participation in group and other interactions.	

CRITICAL THINKING BAND

ASSESSMENT

What additional personal or environmental factors should be evaluated as possible stressors for Gary?

NURSING DIAGNOSIS

What is the role of family in mental health prob-lems such as Gary's? What additional nursing diag-noses, including family-oriented diagnoses, might be appropriate in Gary's case?

Outcomes

Where do regular life challenges fit in the lives of persons with schizophrenia?

Do you think the out-comes identified for Gary would be typical or expected for other individuals with schizophrenia?

Planning/Interventions

What are the best ways to instill "hope" in the lives of clients? Where did hope fit for Gary?

What additional interventions would you recom-mend to get Gary back to his prehospital level of functioning?

Evaluation

Does successful manage-ment of acute mental ill-nesses engender success in future potential episodes? Why or why not? Do you think that Gary's initial progress promises con-tinued improvement?

KEY CONCEPTS

◆ *Altered thought processes* is a nursing diagnosis representing the human response to situations where a person has lost ability to use rational mental processes.

◆ Schizophrenia is a major debilitating disease where the client loses rational thought and/or ability to interpret the environment.

◆ An individual experiencing schizophrenia may present with disordered thoughts, incomprehensible language, loss of function, delusions, and hallucinations.

◆ Positive symptoms of schizophrenia include outward behaviors that clearly display pathology.

◆ Negative symptoms of schizophrenia include behaviors that represent a change from the individual's prior personality and lead to social isolation and anhedonia.

◆ There is no predictable clinical course for any individual person diagnosed with schizophrenia.

◆ With about one new case of schizophrenia per 10,000 persons, the social costs are exceedingly high.

◆ Schizophrenia is an organic disease with a strong genetic component.

◆ Psychosocial treatment includes individual and family support services as well as socially directed rehabilitation.

◆ Pharmacological treatment is primarily through neuroleptic drugs.

◆ Nursing theory focusing on the nurse-client interactions are most helpful.

◆ The five aims of intervention provide a framework for nursing care.

REVIEW QUESTIONS AND ACTIVITIES

1. How would you identify that a client brought to your emergency room had had an altered thought process?

2. How would you tell the difference between a drug-induced condition and schizophrenia?

3. Describe the clinical course of schizophrenia.

4. Explain the difference between positive and negative symptoms of the disease.

5. How would you design social supports for schizophrenic persons in your community?

6. What is your opinion of the current supports and services in your community?

7. Explain the major neuroleptic drugs and their side effects.

8. How does the nurse-client relationship impact care of the schizophrenic person?

9. Explain how the five aims of intervention assist in planning nursing care.

EXPLORING THE WEB

◆ Visit this text's "Online Companion™" on the Internet at **http://www.DelmarNursing.com** for further information on schizophrenia.

◆ What resources are listed for caregivers and health care professionals on the Web?

◆ Explore the Web to locate various discussion areas and conferences that link clients, families, and caregivers involved with schizophrenia.

REFERENCES

Allenbeck, P. (1989). Schizophrenia: A life-shortening disease. *Schizophrenia Bulletin, 15,* 81–89.

American Psychiatric Association. *Diagnostic and Statistical Manual of Mental Disorders*, Fourth Edition. Washington DC: American Psychiatric Association, 1994.

Andreasen, N. C. (1979). Thought, language and communication disorders: Clinical assessment, definition of terms and evaluation of their reliability. *Archives of General Psychiatry, 36,* 1315–1321.

Barrowclough, C. B., & Tarrier, N. T. (1992). Interventions with families. In M. Birchwood & N. Tarrier (Eds.), *Innovations in the psychological management of schizophrenia*. Chichester: Wiley.

Bleuler, M. (1974). The long term course of the schizophrenic psychoses. *Psychological Medicine, 4,* 244–254.

Byrne, C. M., Woodside, H., Landeen, J., & Kirkpatrick, H. (1994). The importance of relationships in fostering hope. *Journal of Psychosocial Nursing and Mental Health Services, 32,* 31–34.

Clardy, J. C., Hyde, T. M., & Kleinman, J. E. (1994). Postmortem neurochemical and neuropathological studies in schizophrenia. In N. C. Andreasen (Ed.), *Schizophrenia, from mind to molecule*. Washington, DC: American Psychiatric Press.

Eakes, G. G. (1995). *Archives of Psychiatric Nursing, 9,* 77–84.

Editors. (1995). Anti-drug counterblast in mental health [Editorial]. *Lancet, 346,* 323.

Erickson, H., Tomlin, E., & Swain, M. A. (1983). *Modeling and role-modeling: A theory and paradigm for nursing*. Lexington, KY: Pine.

Fine, R. (1979). *A history of psychoanalysis*. New York: Columbia University Press.

Flynn, L. (1994). Schizophrenia from a family point of view. In N. C. Andreasen (Ed.), *Schizophrenia, from mind to molecule* (pp. 21–30). Washington, DC: American Psychiatric Press.

Frisch, N., & Bowman, S. (1995). The modeling and role-modeling theory. In J. George (Ed.), *Nursing theories: The base for professional practice* (4th ed., pp. 355–372). Norwalk, CT: Appleton and Lange.

Gottesman, I. I. (1991). *Schizophrenia genesis.* New York: Freeman.

Hargreaves, W. A., & Shumway, M. (1989). Effectiveness of mental health services for the severely mental ill. In C. A. Taube & A. Hohmann (Eds.), *The future of mental health services research.* Washington, DC: NIMH, U.S. Government Printing Office.

Harrow, M., & Quinlan, D. M. (1985). *Disordered thinking and schizophrenic psychopathology.* New York: Gardner.

Hogarty, G. E., Anderson, C. M., Reiss, D. J., Kornblith, S. J., Greenwald, D. P., Javna, C. D., & Madonia, M. J. (1986). Family psychoeducation, social skills training and maintenance chemotherapy. *Archives of General Psychiatry, 43,* 633–642.

Jablensky, A., Sartorius, N., Ernberg, G., Anker, M., Korten, A., Cooper, J. E., Day, R., & Bertelsen, A. (1992). *Psychological medicine monograph* (Suppl. 20). Cambridge: Cambridge University Press.

Johnstone, E. C. (1991). Disabilities and circumstances of schizophrenic patients: A follow-up study. *British Journal of Psychiatry, 159* (Suppl.) pp. 4–46.

Liddle, P. F., Friston, K. J., Frith, C. D., Hirsch, S. R., Jones, T., & Frackowisk, R. S. J. (1992). Patterns of cerebral blood flow in schizophrenia. *British Journal of Psychiatry, 160,* 179–186.

Lorenz, M. (1961). Problems posed by schizophrenic language. *Archives of General Psychiatry, 4,* 604.

McGlashan, T. H. (1994). Psychosocial treatments of schizophrenia. In N. C. Andreasen (Ed.), *Schizophrenia, from mind to molecule* (pp. 189–215). Washington, DC: American Psychiatric Press.

McKenna, P. J. (1994). *Schizophrenia and related syndromes.* New York: Oxford University Press.

Mellor, C. S. (1970). Firsthand symptoms in schizophrenia. *British Journal of Psychiatry, 117,* 16–18.

Mueser, K. T., & Gingerich, S. (1994). *Coping with schizophrenia: A guide for families.* Oakland: New Harbinger.

North American Nursing Diagnosis Association. (1996). *NANDA nursing diagnoses: Definitions and classification: 1997–1998.* Philadelphia: Author.

Reveley, A. M. (1994). Phenomenology, environmental risk, and genetics: Twin studies of schizophrenia. In N. C. Andreasen (Ed.), *Schizophrenia, from mind to molecule* (pp. 105–118). Washington, DC: American Psychiatric Press.

Sass, L. (1992). *Madness and modernism.* New York: Basic Books.

Schizophrenia Discussion Group. (1997). homepage, www.araby-station.com/webboard/guest2.exe.list.

Vaccaro, J. V., & Roberts, L. (1992). Teaching social coping skills. In M. Birchwood & N. Tarrier (Eds.), *Innovations in the psychological management of schizophrenia.* Chichester: Wiley.

Wheeler, C. (1994). The diagnosis of schizophrenia and its impact on the primary caregiver. *Nursing Practice in New Zealand, 9,* 15–23.

≋ LITERARY REFERENCES

Anonymous. (1955). An autobiography of a schizophrenic experience. *Journal of Abnormal and Social Psychology, 51,* 677–689.

Anonymous. (1983). *Schizophrenic Bulletin, 9,* 152–155.

Boisen, A. (1960). *Out of the depths.* New York: HarperCollins.

Sechehaye, M. (Ed.). (1970). *Autobiography of a schizophrenic girl.* New York: New American Library.

Willick, M. S. (1994). A parent's perspective: Mourning without end. In N. C. Andreasen (Ed.), *Schizophrenia: From mind to molecule* (pp. 5–19). Washington, DC: American Psychiatric Press.

Zelt, D. (pseudonym). (1981). *Schizophrenic Bulletin, 7,* 527–531.

≋ SUGGESTED READINGS

Chouvardas, J. (1996). The symbolic and literal in schizophrenic language. *Perspectives in Psychiatric Nursing, 32,* 20–22.

Keltner, N. (1996). Brain update: Pathoanatomy of schizophrenia. *Perspectives in Psychiatric Care, 32,* 32–35.

McKenna, P. J. (1995). *Schizophrenia and related syndromes.* Oxford: Oxford University Press.

Mueser, K. T., & Gingerich, S. (1994). *Coping with schizophrenia: A guide for families.* Oakland, CA: New Hudinger.

Shriqu, C. L., & Nasrallah, H. A. (1995). *Contemporary issues in the treatment of schizophrenia.* Washington, DC: American Psychiatric Press.

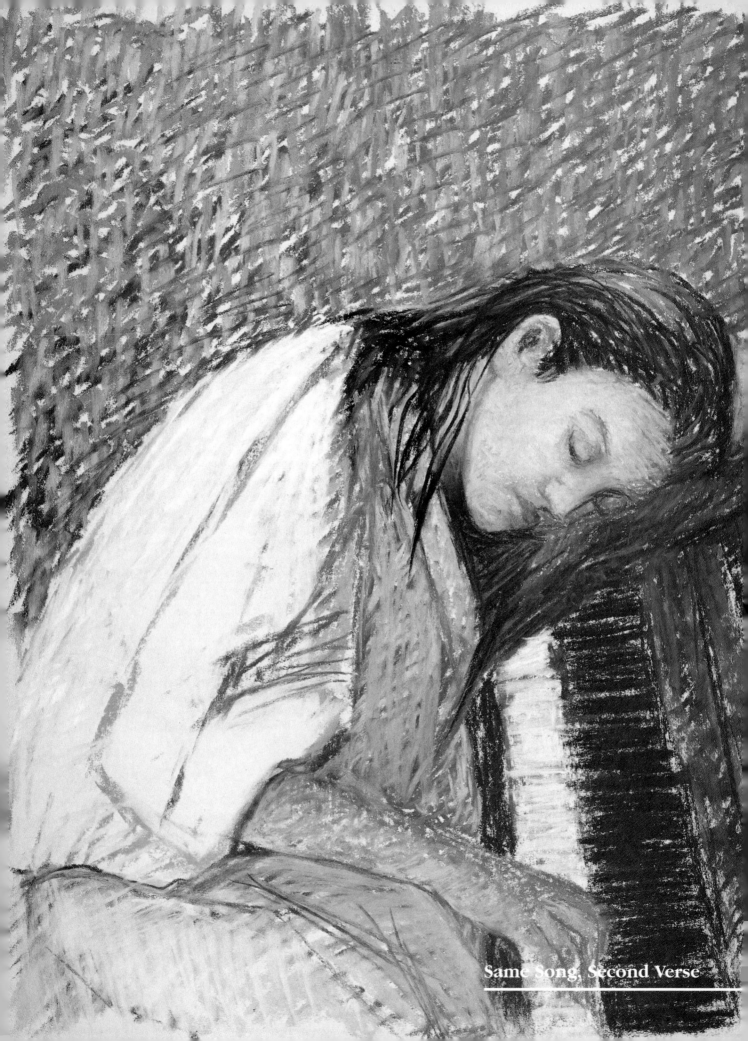

Same Song, Second Verse

Chapter

12

THE CLIENT
EXPERIENCING DEPRESSION

Noreen Cavan Frisch
Lawrence E. Frisch

Mood Swings and You

Consider your life over the past few months:

♦ What were the "ups" and "downs" for you?
♦ Do you notice changes in emotions or energy over time?
♦ Are there days (or times) when you feel closer to people around you and other times when you feel isolated?
♦ Can you identify patterns in the moods of your life?
♦ Do you notice patterns in mood in persons close to you?

Everyone has mood swings. Life events affect each of us such that some days are happier ("better") than others. In this chapter, we will begin to explore the range of moods that people experience.

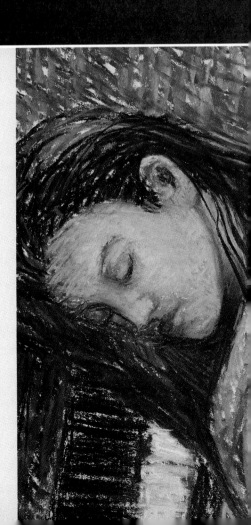

≋ CHAPTER OUTLINE

WHAT IS DEPRESSION?

Major Depressive Disorder

Minor Depressive Disorder

Dysthymic Disorder

Bereavement Versus Depressive Disease
    Stage 1: The Period of Shock
    Stage 2: The Reality Stage
    Stage 3: The Recovery Stage

THEORIES OF DEPRESSION

Psychoanalysis

Object Loss Theory

Learned Helplessness Theory

Cognitive Theory

Physical/Biological Models

TREATMENT

Psychotherapy
    Effect of Psychotherapy

Physical Therapies
    Electroconvulsive Therapy
    Light Therapy

Medications
    Tricyclic and Related Antidepressants
    Selective Serotonin Reuptake Inhibitors
    Monoamine Oxidase Inhibitors
    Effect of Medications

NURSING PERSPECTIVES

Caring Theories

Self-Care Deficit Theory

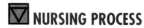 **NURSING PROCESS**

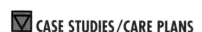 **CASE STUDIES/CARE PLANS**

FUTURE DIRECTIONS

≋ COMPETENCIES

Upon completion of this chapter, the reader should be able to:

1. Identify mood swings as a normal part of the human emotional experience.

2. Employ empathy to understand one's own experience of depression and to understand the depressive feelings of others.

3. Define depression and differentiate between major and minor depressive disorders.

4. Describe the concepts of grief and bereavement.

5. Analyze predisposing factors to grief and depression.

6. Identify major psychological theories that explain depression.

7. Integrate a nursing theory base into care for depressed clients.

8. Apply the nursing process to clients who are depressed by:

    ♦ Performing nursing assessments for depression

    ♦ Analyzing data in terms of nursing and psychological theories

    ♦ Formulating individualized nursing diagnoses

    ♦ Suggesting appropriate outcomes

    ♦ Deriving a plan of care

    ♦ Evaluating nursing care based on outcomes

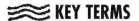

KEY TERMS

Bipolar Depression   Mood disorder characterized by up and down swings.

Brief Dynamic Therapy   Short-term psychotherapy that focuses on resolving core conflicts that derive from personality and living situations.

Chronic Grief   Unresolved bereavement.

Cognitive Therapy   Short-term psychotherapy that focuses on removing symptoms by identifying and correcting perceptual biases in client's thinking and correcting unrecognized assumptions.

Delayed Grief   Bereavement that is not accomplished at the time of the loss and remains with the individual.

Depression   State wherein an individual experiences a profound sadness.

Ego   Conscious self.

Exaggerated Grief   Bereavement that is overwhelming.

Grief   Healthy expression of bereavement.

Marital Therapy   Short-term psychotherapy that attempts to resolve problems that occur within a marriage.

Masked Grief   Bereavement that is hidden by either a physical symptom or a maladaptive behavior; the individual is unaware of the connection to the grief or loss.

Mood Disorder   Pattern of mood episodes that results in difficulty functioning in family, work, and social affairs.

Mood Episode   Experience of a strong emotion of depression, mania, or a mixture of both for a period of at least 2 weeks.

Nurse Agency   Nursing activities required to compensate for the client's inability to meet his own self-care needs (Orem's Theory).

Self-Care Agency   Client's ability to provide for own needs (Orem's Theory).

Superego   Inner voice.

Supportive-Educative Role   Nursing activities that focus on enhancing the client's ability both to carry on effectively without nursing support and to rise above the feelings of depression (Orem's Theory).

Unipolar Depression   Disorder in which mood swings are always in one direction, toward depression.

Mood swings are a part of everyone's life. There are days when each of us feels up, and days when we feel down. To live and understand our emotions means to experience a range of feelings. While most people are happy when they feel cheerful and energetic, they often forget that it is not always healthy or appropriate to feel this way. Loss is one of the inevitable human experiences. Here are some lines written 650 years ago by a Chinese mother whose young child has recently died:

Written on Seeing the Flowers, and Remembering my Daughter

I grieve for my second daughter.
Six years I carried her about,
Held her against my breast and helped her eat,
Taught her rhymes as she sat on my knee.
She would arise early and copy her elder
sister's dress,
Struggling to see herself in the dressing table
mirror.
She had begun to delight in pretty silks and lace
But in a poor family she could have none of
these.
I would sigh over my own recurring frustrations,
Treading the byways through the rain and
snow.
But evenings when I returned to receive her
greeting
My sad cares could be transformed into
contentment.
What were we to do, that day when illness
struck?
The worse because it was during the crisis of
war;
Frightened by the alarming sounds, she sank
quickly into death.
There was no time even to fix medicines for her.
Distraught, I prepared her poor little coffin;
Weeping, accompanied it to that distant
hillside.
It is already lost in the vast void.
Disconsolate, I still grieve deeply for her.
I think how last year, in the spring,
When the flowers bloomed by the pond in our
old garden
She led me by the hand along under the trees
And asked me to break off a pretty branch for
her.

This year again the flowers bloom;
Now I live far from home, here by this river's edge.
All the household are here, only she is gone.
I look at the flowers, and my tears fall in vain.
A cup of wine brings me no comfort.
The wind makes desolate sounds in the night
curtains.*

(Ch'i K. in Weir, 1980, p. 156)

The loss of a child is such an overwhelming experience that even this beautiful poem can only hint at a mother's grief. What would we think if, instead of telling us that "I still grieve deeply for her," Kao Ch'i described how cheerful and happy she was? When the French writer Camus opens his famous novel *The Stranger* with the lines "Mother died today, or maybe yesterday. I can't be sure," the reader knows something is profoundly wrong. Death and loss call for grief and sadness. These are the *normal* human responses; anything less is a sign of poor mental health, of blocked emotions, of crisis.

So, it is clear that feelings of sadness are normal for each of us at some times. Losses and stresses far less profound than death can make us sad, but the feelings are usually fleeting, perhaps lasting a few hours or days. These fluctuations in mood are so much a part of life that the thought of life with all ups and no downs seems to be completely outside of normal human experience. And yet, there are people for whom the downs or the ups become too extreme and last too long. Because of their moods, these people may find it hard or impossible to function in their families, in their work, or in social affairs. They may behave bizarrely, hold unreasonable beliefs, and in their extremes of mood, bring harm to themselves or to others. These people have what we term a **mood disorder**. In his book *As a Man Grows Older*, the Italian novelist Italo Svevo describes an extreme example of such a mood disorder:

Amalia

He had just shut the door of his flat behind him and was standing hat in hand in the dining room, uncertain what to do next, and wondering whether he could after all face an hour of boredom in his sister's mute society. Suddenly there came from Amalia's room the sound of two or three unintelligible words, and finally a whole phrase: "Get away, you ugly brute!" He shuddered. Her voice was so changed by fatigue or emotion that it resembled his sister's only as an inarticulate shout proceeding from the throat can resemble the

modulated speaking voice. Was she asleep at this hour and dreaming by day?

He opened the door noiselessly, and a sight presented itself to his eyes which till his dying day he could never forget. For ever afterwards one or other of the details of that scene had only to strike his senses for him to recall the whole of it immediately and to feel again the appalling horror of it. . . .

Amalia's clothes lay scattered all over the floor and a skirt prevented him from opening the door completely; there were a few garments under the bed . . . her boots had been arranged with evident care in the middle of the table.

Amalia was sitting on the edge of the bed, clothed only in a short chemise. She had not noticed her brother's entry, and continued gently to pass her hands up and down her legs, which were as thin as spindles. Emilio was surprised and shocked to see that her naked body resembled that of an ill-nourished child. . . .

"Amalia! What are you doing?" he said reprovingly. She did not hear him, though she seemed to be conscious. . . .

"Amalia!" he repeated in a faint voice, overwhelmed by this obvious proof that she was delirious. He put his hand on her shoulder. Then she turned. She looked first at the hand whose touch she had felt, then she looked him in the face. . . . It was a slight relief to him to notice that she had heard him. She looked at him again, thoughtfully, as if she were trying to understand the meaning of those cries and of the repeated pressure on her shoulder. She touched her chest as if she had suddenly become conscious of the weight upon it which tormented her. Then forgetting Emilio and her own exhaustion, she shouted again: "Oh, still those horrible creatures!" and there was a break in her voice as if she were going to burst out crying. She rubbed her legs vigorously with both her hands; then bent down with a swift movement as if she were about to surprise an animal in the act of escaping. She seized one of her toes in her right hand and covered it over with her left, then carefully raised both her closed hands as if she were holding something in them. When she saw they were empty she examined them several times, then returned to her foot, ready to stoop down again and renew her strange chase.

---

*From *Death in Literature*, by Robert F. Weir. Copyright © 1980 by Columbia University Press. Reprinted with permission of the publisher.

A shivering attack reminded Emilio that he ought to induce her to get into bed. He approached her. . . . His task was however quite easy, for she obeyed the first firm pressure of his hand; she lifted one leg after the other on to the bed, without any shame, and allowed him to pull the bedclothes over her. But she showed an inexplicable reluctance to lie down altogether, and remained leaning on one elbow. Very soon, however, she could no longer hold out in that position, and abandoned herself on the pillow, uttering for the first time an intelligible sound of grief. "Oh, my God! my God!"

"But what has happened to you?" asked Emilio who, at the sound of that one sensible cry, thought that he could talk to her like a reasonable person. She made no reply, for she was intent on discovering what it was that still went on tormenting her. . . . She hunched herself all up together, sought out her legs with her hands, and in the deep plot she was evidently meditating against the things or creatures which tormented her, she even contrived to make her breathing less noisy. Then she drew up her hands again and gazed at them in incredulous surprise when she found them empty. She lay for a while beneath the sheets in a state of such distress that she seemed even to forget her terrible bodily fatigue.

"Are you better?" Emilio asked, in a tone of entreaty. He wanted to console himself by the sound of his own voice. . . . He bent over her, so that she might hear him better.

She lay looking at him for a long time, while her quick feeble breath rose towards him. She recognised him; the warmth of the bed seemed to have revived her senses. However far she wandered afterwards in her delirium, he never forgot that she had recognised him. . . .

Amalia listened to all he had to say, but she seemed also to be listening inwardly to other words beside his; then she said "If you want it I must do it. We will stay here then, but . . . so much dirt. . . ." Two tears flowed down her cheeks which had been dry till that moment; they rolled like two pearls down her flaming cheeks. . . .

Soon after she forgot that grievance, but her delirium soon produced another source of distress. She had been out fishing and could not catch any fish: "I can't understand! What is the good of going out fishing if there are not any fish? One has to go

such a long, long way and it is so cold." The others had taken all the fish and there were none left for them. All her grief and fatigue now seemed to be due to that fact. Her fevered words, to which her exhaustion gave a kind of tired rhythm, were continually interrupted by some sound of distress.

He had ceased to pay any attention to her; he must find some way out of the situation, he must devise some means of fetching a doctor. . . . He had not made up his mind yet what he should do, but he must make haste and get some help for his unfortunate sister.[*]

(Svevo, 1949, pp. 193–199)

Amalia's mood disorder of **depression**, the state wherein an individual experiences a profound sadness, has become so severe that she has become psychotic; she has almost completely lost touch with reality. She very likely needs psychiatric hospitalization to recover, as she has a profound depressive disorder. This chapter will discuss depressive disorders, those mood disorders where mood swings are always down (or **unipolar depression**). The next chapter will discuss mood disorders in which, at least some of the time, persons experience up swings to a manic or hypomanic level (referred to as **bipolar depression**, even in those rare instances where the swings are only up). The reader cannot tell from the preceding excerpt whether Amalia's depression is unipolar or bipolar: The symptoms and severity of depression may be identical in both conditions.

WHAT IS DEPRESSION?

Sadness and loss are universal, but symptoms severe enough or long-lasting enough to justify a diagnosis of depression are much rarer. Epidemiological studies suggest that 7% to 12% of men and 20% to 25% of women are likely to become significantly depressed at some time in their lives. The definition of "significantly depressed" is clearly arbitrary, but the fourth edition of the *Diagnostic and Statistical Manual* (DSM-IV) is currently the best guide to definition. DSM-IV presents definitions and criteria for mood disorders so that there can be definitional consistency in mental health care.

DSM-IV makes a fundamental distinction between a mood episode and a mood disorder. A **mood episode** is the experience of a strong emotion of depression, mania, or a mixture of both for a period of at least 2 weeks. To be diagnosed as an episode, the symptom must be newly

---

*By Italo Svevo from *As a Man Grows Older* Copyright © 1949 by Italo Svevo and Beryl de Zoete. Reprinted by permission of New Directions Publishing Corp.

present or have clearly worsened over the preepisode state and must be present nearly every day for most of the day for 2 consecutive weeks. A mood disorder is diagnosed based on the pattern of mood episodes.

Depression is the intense feeling of a depressed, down mood. However, not everyone who feels depressed meets DSM-IV criteria for depression and it is *possible* (but *unusual*) to meet those criteria *without feeling depressed*. DSM-IV defines a range of depressive mood disorders, the most important of which are Major Depressive Disorder, Minor Depressive Disorder, Dysthymic Disorder, and Bereavement. These are common and important clinical conditions with which the nurse should be thoroughly familiar.

Major Depressive Disorder

To qualify for this diagnosis, DSM-IV requires the presence of at least one Major Depressive Episode. This episode must (1) last at least 2 weeks, (2) represent a change from previous functioning, and (3) cause some impairment in a person's social or occupational functioning. During an episode, it is also required that five or more symptoms be present. One of these symptoms *must* be either depressed mood or loss of interest in previously enjoyable activities. The individual must also experience at least four additional symptoms, which may include changes in appetite or weight; sleep disturbance (usually trouble staying asleep); fatigue or loss of energy; feelings of worthlessness or guilt; difficulty concentrating, thinking, or making decisions; or recurrent thoughts of death or suicide.

A person experiencing a depressive episode may express feelings of sadness and hopelessness or may express the sense of feeling empty or having no feelings. Some persons express somatic symptoms such as bodily aches and pains rather than sadness. Also, some individuals, particularly adolescents, will exhibit irritability or crankiness rather than sadness. Family members or close friends will notice a change in the individual, most commonly a social withdrawal and a neglect of activities that previously brought the person pleasure. Nearly 100 years ago, the great Russian writer Leo Tolstoy eloquently described the onset of his own recurrent major depressive episodes:

My Confessions

But five years ago something very strange began to happen to me. At first I experienced moments of perplexity and arrest of life, as though I did not know how to live or what to do; and I felt lost and became dejected. But this passed, and I went on living as before. Then these moments of perplexity began to recur oftener and oftener, and always in

the same form. They were always expressed by the questions: What's it for? What does it lead to? . . .

My life had come to a standstill. I could breathe, eat, drink, and sleep, and I could not help doing these things; but there was no life, for there were no wishes the fulfillment of which I could consider reasonable. If I desired anything, I knew in advance that whether I satisfied my desire or not, nothing would come of it. Had a fairy come and offered to fulfill my desires I should not have known what to ask. If in moments of intoxication I felt something which, though not a wish, was a habit left by former wishes, in sober moments I knew this to be a delusion, and that there was really nothing to wish for. I could not even wish to know the truth, for I guessed of what it consisted. The truth was that life is meaningless. I had, as it were, lived, lived and walked, walked, till I had come to a precipice and saw clearly that there was nothing ahead of me but destruction. . . .

It had come to this, that I, a healthy, fortunate man, felt I could no longer live; some irresistible power impelled me to rid myself one way or other of life. I cannot say I wished to kill myself. The power which drew me away from life was stronger, fuller, and more widespread than any mere wish. It was a force similar to the former striving to live, only in the opposite direction. . . .

And all this befell me at a time when all around me I had what is considered complete good fortune. I was not yet fifty; I had a good wife who loved me and whom I loved, good children, and a large estate which without much effort on my part improved and increased. I was respected by my relations and acquaintances more than at any previous time. I was praised by others, and without much self-deception could consider that my name was famous. And far from being insane or mentally diseased, I enjoyed on the contrary a strength of mind and body such as I have seldom met with among men of my kind; physically, I could keep up with the peasants at mowing, and mentally I could work for eight and ten hours at a stretch without experiencing any ill results from such exertion. . . .

But life had lost its attraction for me; so how could I attract others? . . . I was like one lost in a wood who, horrified at having lost his way, rushes about, wishing to find the road. He knows that

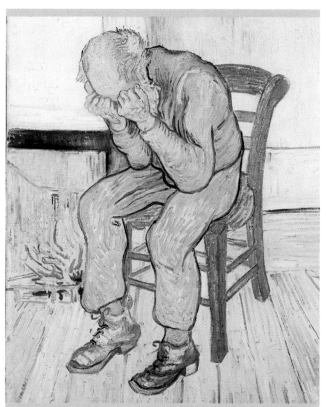

Old Man in Sorrow by Van Gogh.
Source: Collection Kröller-Müller Museum, Otterlo, The Netherlands.

Van Gogh painted this relatively unknown picture not long before he killed himself, a few months after his release from the asylum at Arles (see Van Gogh painting in Chapter 2). Although the chair recalls several famous paintings from somewhat happier days (*The Rocking Chair, Gauguin's Armchair*), the figure is an extraordinary evocation of despair.

each step he takes confuses him more and more; but still he cannot help rushing about.

. . . The horror of darkness was too great.
*. . . That was the feeling which drew me most strongly towards suicide.**

(Tolstoy, 1932, pp. 201–207)

Major depressive episodes frequently develop over a few days or weeks, and without treatment they most commonly last for longer than 6 months. Up to 10% of persons with Major Depressive Disorder have, as did Tolstoy, symptoms that persist for 2 or more years. Major Depressive Disorder is quite common in clients visiting general medical outpatient facilities: It appears to occur in up to 9% of clients.

---

*From *A Confession and What I Believe*, by L. Tolstoy, Translated by A. Maude, 1932, London: Oxford University Press. Reprinted with permission.

Minor Depressive Disorder

An additional 10% of clients may suffer from less severe symptoms that may interfere with their functioning but may not qualify for a diagnosis of Major Depressive Disorder. The diagnosis Minor Depressive Disorder has been proposed for these individuals but has not yet been validated within DSM. Clearly, many persons can be greatly troubled by depression without having enough symptoms to qualify for a major psychiatric diagnosis. The American novelist F. Scott Fitzgerald described his own struggles with depression, which are consistent with the minor category, in an essay that he called "The Crack-Up":

The Crack-Up

Of course all life is a process of breaking down, but the blows that do the dramatic side of the work—the big sudden blows that come, or seem to come, from outside—the ones you remember and blame things on and, in moments of weakness, tell your friends about, don't show their effect all at once. There is another sort of blow that comes from within—that you don't feel until it's too late to do anything about it, until you realize with finality that in some regard you will never be as good a man again. The first sort of breakage seems to happen quick—the second kind happens almost without your knowing it but is realized suddenly indeed.

Before I go on with this short history, let me make a general observation—the test of a first-rate intelligence is the ability to hold two opposed ideas in the mind at the same time and still retain the ability to function. One should, for example, be able to see that things are hopeless and yet be determined to make them otherwise. This philosophy fitted on to my early adult life, when I saw the improbable, the implausible, often the "impossible," come true. . . .

For seventeen years, with a year of deliberate loafing and resting out in the center—things went on like that, with a new chore only a nice prospect for the next day. I was living hard, too, but: "Up to forty-nine it'll be all right," I said. "I can count on that. For a man who's lived as I have, that's all you could ask."

—And then, ten years this side of forty-nine, I suddenly realized that I had prematurely cracked.

Now a man can crack in many ways—can

crack in the head—in which case the power of decision is taken from you by others! or in the body, when one can but submit to the white hospital world; or (like the present writer) in the nerves . . . *too much anger and too many tears*. . . .

Suffice it to say that after about an hour of solitary pillow-hugging, I began to realize that for two years my life had been a drawing on resources that I did not possess, that I had been mortgaging myself physically and spiritually up to the hilt. . . .

I realized that in those two years, in order to preserve something—an inner hush maybe, maybe not—I had weaned myself from all the things I used to love—that every act of life from the morning tooth-brush to the friend at dinner had become an effort. I saw that for a long time I had not liked people and things, but only followed the rickety old pretense of liking. I saw that even my love for those closest to me has become only an attempt to love, that my casual relations—with an editor, a tobacco seller, the child of a friend, were only what I remembered I should do, from other days. All in the same month I became bitter about such things as the sound of the radio, the advertisements in the magazines, the screech of tracks, the dead silence of the country—contemptuous at human softness, immediately (if secretly) quarrelsome toward hardness—hating the night when I couldn't sleep and hating the day because it went toward night. I slept on the heart side now because I knew that the sooner I could tire that out, even a little, the sooner would come that blessed hour of nightmare which, like a catharsis, would enable me to better meet the new day. . . .

Trying to cling to something, I liked doctors and girl children up to the age of about thirteen and well-brought-up boy children from about eight years old on. I could have peace and happiness with these few categories of people. I forgot to add that I liked older men—men over seventy, sometimes over sixty if their faces looked seasoned. I liked Katharine Hepburn's face on the screen, no matter what was said about her pretentiousness, and Miriam Hopkins' face, and old friends if I only saw them once a year and could remember their ghosts.

All rather inhuman and undernourished,

isn't it? Well, that, children, is the true sign of cracking up.

It is not a pretty picture. Inevitably it was carted here and there within its frame and exposed to various critics.

"Instead of being so sorry for yourself, listen—"(one of the critics) said. (She always says "Listen," because she thinks while she talks—really thinks.) So she said: "Listen. Suppose this wasn't a crack in you—suppose it was a crack in the Grand Canyon."

"The crack's in me," I said heroically.

"Listen! The world only exists in your eyes—your conception of it. You can make it as big or as small as you want to. And you're trying to be a little puny individual. By God, if I ever cracked, I'd try to make the world crack with me. Listen! The world only exists through your apprehension of it, and so it's much better to say that it's not you that's cracked—it's the Grand Canyon."

. . . She spoke, then, of old woes of her own, that seemed, in the telling, to have been more dolorous than mine, and how she had met them, over-ridden them, beaten them.

I felt a certain reaction to what she said, but I am a slow-thinking man, and it occurred to me simultaneously that of all the natural forces, vitality is the incommunicable one. . . . You have it or you haven't it, like health or brown eyes or honor or a baritone voice. I might have asked some of it from her . . . but I could never have got it—not even if I'd waited around for a thousand hours with the tin cup of self-pity. I could walk from her door, holding myself very carefully like cracked crockery, and go away into the world of bitterness, where I was making a home.*

(Fitzgerald, 1945, pp. 520–524)

Dysthymic Disorder

Whereas the essence of Major Depressive Disorder is discrete episodes of depression, persons with Dysthymic Disorder feel depressed nearly all of the time. DSM-IV criteria for Dysthymic Disorder include "depressed mood for most of the day, for more days than not . . . for at least

---

*By F. Scott Fitzgerald from *The Crack-Up* Copyright © 1945 by New Directions Publishing Corp. Reprinted with permission of New Directions Publishing Corp.

2 years." A person with Dysthymic Disorder must also have at least two of the following symptoms: appetite disturbance, sleep disturbance, fatigue, low self-esteem, poor concentration or difficulty making decisions, and feelings of hopelessness. As with Major Depressive Disorder, the symptoms must cause clinically significant distress or impairment in social or occupational functioning. Dysthymic Disorder is somewhat rarer than Major Depressive Disorder, occurring during a lifetime in about 6% of persons. At any time, between 2% and 4% of persons visiting outpatient medical facilities have Dysthymic Disorder. Like Major Depressive Disorder, Dysthymic Disorder often begins in childhood or adolescence. In his play *Uncle Vanya*, the great writer Chekhov would seem to be convincingly describing Dysthymic Disorder. Here, the middle-aged country doctor Astrov is visiting in the home of Sonia, a young woman who is in love with him:

Uncle Vanya

SONIA: You're dissatisfied with life then?

ASTROV: I love life as such—but our life, our everyday provincial life in Russia, I just can't endure. I despise it with all my soul. As for my own life, God knows I can find nothing good in it at all. You know, when you walk through a forest on a dark night and you see a small light gleaming in the distance, you don't notice your tiredness, not the darkness, nor the prickly branches lashing you in the face. . . . I work harder than anyone in the district—you know that—fate batters me continuously, at times I suffer unbearably—but there's no small light in the distance. I'm not expecting anything for myself any longer, I don't love human beings . . . I haven't cared for anyone for years.

SONIA: Not for anyone?

ASTROV: No one. I feel a sort of fondness for your old nurse—for the sake of old times. The peasants are all too much alike, undeveloped, living in squalor. As for the educated people—it's hard to get on with them. They tire me so. All of them, all our good friends here are shallow in thought, shallow in feeling, unable to see further than their noses— or to put it quite bluntly, stupid. And the ones who are a bit more intelligent, of a higher mental calibre, are hysterical, positively rotten with intro- spection and futile cerebration. They whine, they are full of hatreds and morbidly malicious, they sidle up to a man, look at him out of the corner

of their eyes, and pronounce their judgement: 'Oh, he's a psychopath!,' or 'Just a phrase-monger.' And when they don't know how to label me, they say: 'He's a queer fellow, very queer!' I love forests— that's queer, I don't eat meat—that's queer too. There isn't any direct objective, unprejudiced attitude to people or nature left. . . . No, there isn't! [About to drink.]

SONIA: [Prevents him.] No, I beg you, I implore you, don't drink any more.

ASTROV: Why not?

SONIA: It's so unlike you! You have such poise, your voice is so soft. . . . More than that, you are beautiful as no one else I know is beautiful. So why do you want to be like ordinary men, the kind who drink and play cards? Don't do it, I implore you. You always say that people don't create anything, but merely destroy what has been given them from above. Then why, why are you destroying yourself? You mustn't, you mustn't, I beseech you, I implore you!

ASTROV: [Holds out his hand to her.] I won't drink any more!

SONIA: Give me your word.

ASTROV: My word of honour.

SONIA: [Presses his hand warmly.] Thank you!

ASTROV: Enough! My head's clear now. You see I'm quite sober—and I'll stay sober to the end of my days. [Looks at his watch.] Well, to continue. As I said, my time's over, it's too late for me now . . . I've aged too much, I've worked myself to a standstill, I've grown coarse and insensitive . . . I believe I could never really become fond of another human being. I don't love anybody and never shall now. What still does affect me is beauty. I can't remain indifferent to that. I believe that if Yeliena Andryeevna wanted to, for instance, she could turn my head in a day. . . . But that's not love, of course, that's not affection. . . . [Covers his eyes with his hands and shudders.]

SONIA: What is it?

ASTROV: Nothing. . . . In Lent one of my patients died under chloroform.

SONIA: It's time to forget about that. [A pause.] Tell me, Mihail Lvovich. . . . If I had a girl friend, or a young sister and if you got to know that she . . . well, suppose that she loved you, what would you do?

ASTROV: [Shrugging his shoulders.] I don't know. Probably nothing. I should let her know that I couldn't love her . . . besides I've got too many other things on my mind. However, if I'm going, I'd better start now. I'll say goodbye, my dear girl, or we'll not finish till morning. [Shakes hands with her.] *

(Chekhov, 1954, pp. 210–212)

Nurses must be aware of the fact that nearly 15% of hospitalized clients may meet criteria for Major Depressive Disorder. This is a complex issue however, because neither Dysthymic Disorder nor Major Depressive Disorder should be diagnosed when depressive symptoms are thought to be due to physical illness. Some additional material on depressive illness in persons with physical illness is found in Chapter 19 (on care of the physically ill) and in Chapter 23 (on care of the elderly client).

⚙ NURSING ALERT!

Risk Factors for Depression

- ◆ Family history of depression
- ◆ Having experienced recent negative stressors
- ◆ Having childhood experiences in a negative home environment
- ◆ Lacking a social support system
- ◆ Having significant, physical disease

Bereavement Versus Depressive Disease

It is important that the nurse understand and recognize the difference between bereavement or **grief**, a normal and healthy condition, and depressive disease. While DSM-IV recognizes the diagnosis of Bereavement (loss), no diagnostic criteria are given because this is assumed to be a normal human condition. However, the nurse will recognize grieving—anticipatory or dysfunctional as nursing diagnoses recognized by NANDA (1996)

---

*From Uncle Vanya, in *Plays*, by Anton Chekhov, pp. 210–212, translated by Elisaveta Fen (Penguin Classics, 1954) Copyright © Elisaveta Fen, 1954. Reproduced by permission of Penguin Books, Ltd.

and calling for a nursing response. A person experiencing grief will have many of the same symptoms as one who is depressed. That is, a grieving person will feel sad and hopeless and express feelings of depression. A grieving person may also exhibit loss of appetite, weight loss, sleep disturbances, and inability to concentrate, make decisions, and carry out daily activities. The difference is that the grieving person has experienced a recent loss, acknowledges that loss, and experiences great pain in giving up attachment to that which was lost. Bereavement may last for days or months, depending on the degree of attachment involved. The level of severity can only be determined by the individual grieving, not the particular circumstances that provoked the grief. A person will respond to the emotions of grief using the same coping strategies that he has used to deal with other, powerful emotions in the past. One learns how to grieve by learning how to understand and accept emotions, how to feel emotions, and how to use supportive persons to talk about feelings. Successful resolution of normal grief requires that a person accept, understand, and deal with painful emotions.

Manning (1984) described stages of the normal grieving process, discussed following.

Stage 1: The Period of Shock

The person describes feeling "numb." This stage lasts from days to a month or more. The following poignant poem was written by 12-year-old Jeff Irish a few days after his brother had died of bacterial meningitis. It captures with great feeling the sense of shock and disbelief that accompanies unexpected loss:

A Boy Thirteen

He had red hair,
Was thin and tall,
One could never eat as much as he,
He hiked in the sierras,
Went back-packing and even planned a trip
for the family
Even got me to join Boy Scouts,
Always wanted me to backpack with him,
We went to Germany,
He and I went to German schools and learned
German
Then it came time for our trip to Rome,
By train,
He and I couldn't wait to come back to
Germany and go sledding,
We passed through the Alps on the way
to Rome,

I looked up to him,
I twelve and HE "A BOY THIRTEEN,"
He was five feet and nine inches tall,
I remember very well looking up and there
He was with the train window down, His head
a little ways out with the wind blowing
his red hair as he watched the Alps
passing by,
He was my brother,
My only brother,

. . .

One I could play Baseball with,
Someone I could talk to,
In Germany he had bought a camera,
A single lense reflex,
HE had alot of new things going on,
Then on Feb. 6 He died.
He my only brother the one I planned to
backpack with, the guy I wanted to sled with,
the person I looked up to, the boy that
played baseball with me, the guy with a
new camera, my brother who I could talk to, the
one who could eat as no one else, my brother
that
     was five feet and nine inches tall, tall and thin
with red hair "THE BOY THAT WAS THIRTEEN"
He died because he happened to breathe in
some bacteria that probably can only be seen
under some special microscope,
     I guess all I can say is I loved him and needed
him and that
     *I don't understand.**

(Irish, 1980, pp. 180–181)

Stage 2: The Reality Stage

Most of the painful experience begins here, when the individual consciously realizes the meaning of the loss to her life. Reactions may include anger, guilt, hurt, frustration, helplessness, or fear. The following selection is from Julian Barnes's novel *Flaubert's Parrot*. The narrator is an English doctor, Geoffrey, whose wife has recently committed suicide. Geoffrey is obsessed by the life and writings of Gustave Flaubert, who wrote *Madame Bovary*, a 19th-century novel about the adultery and suicide of a country doctor's wife.

---

*From *Death in Literature*, by Robert F. Weir, Copyright © 1980 by Columbia University Press. Reprinted with permission of the publisher.

Flaubert's Parrot

This is a pure story, whatever you may think. When she dies, you are not at first surprised. Part of love is preparing for death. You feel confirmed in your love when she dies. You got it right. This is part of it all.

Afterwards comes the madness. And then the loneliness: not the spectacular solitude you had anticipated, not the interesting martyrdom of widowhood, but just loneliness. You expect something almost geological—vertigo in a shelving canyon—but it's not like that; it's just misery as regular as a job. What do we doctors say? I'm deeply sorry, Mrs Blank . . . rest assured you will come out of it; . . . I would suggest; perhaps a new interest, Mrs Blank; car maintenance, formation dancing?; don't worry, six months will see you back on the roundabout; come and see me again any time; oh nurse, when she calls, just give her this repeat prescription will you, no I don't need to see her, well it's not her that's dead is it, look on the bright side. What did she say her name was?

And then it happens to you. There's no glory in it. Mourning is full of time; nothing but time . . . I've tried drink, but what does that do? Drink makes you drunk, that's all it's ever been able to do. Work, they say, cures everything. It doesn't; often, it doesn't even induce tiredness; the nearest you get to it is a neurotic lethargy. And there is always extra time. Have some more time. Take your time. Extra time. Time on your hands.

Other people think you want to talk. "Do you want to talk about Ellen?" they ask, hinting that they won't be embarrassed if you break down. Sometimes you talk, sometimes you don't; it makes little difference. The words aren't the right ones; or rather, the right words don't exist. "Language is like the cracked kettle on which we beat out tunes for bears to dance to, while all the time we long to move the stars to pity." You talk, and you find the language of bereavement foolishly inadequate. You seem to be talking about other people's griefs. I loved her; we were unhappy; I miss her. . . . There is a limited choice of prayers on offer: gabble the syllables.

"It may seem bad, Geoffrey, but you'll come out of it. I'm not taking your grief lightly; it's just

that I've seen enough of life to know that you'll come out of it." The words you've said yourself while scribbling a prescription. . . . And you do come out of it, that's true. After a year, after five. But you don't come out of it like a train coming out of a tunnel, bursting through the Downs into sunshine and that swift, rattling descent to the Channel; you come out of it as a gull comes out of an oil slick. You are tarred and feathered for life.

And still you think about her every day . . .

I sometimes feel embarrassed by people's sympathy.*

(Barnes, 1985, p. 190)

Stage 3: The Recovery Stage

During the final, recovery phase, the person integrates the loss into the reality of her life and begins to live again. From Flaubert's *Madame Bovary*, a friend tries to console Dr. Bovary after his wife's suicide:

Madame Bovary

I know what it's like, he said, slapping him on the shoulder. I was like you, I was! After I lost my poor departed wife, I used to go off into the fields, to be on my own. I'd drop down at the foot of a tree, crying, calling on the good Lord, telling him off. I wanted to be like the moles, hung up on the branches, their bellies crawling with maggots—dead, I mean. And when I thought of the others, at that very moment, hugging their bonny little wives close to them, I'd strike the ground with my stick, hard. I was crazy, like, didn't even eat, the thought of going to the inn sickened me, you wouldn't believe it. Ah well, slowly but surely, one day chasing another, spring on top of winter, autumn on top of summer, it leaked away, drop by drop, little by little; it left, it went away—it sank down, I should say, because there's always something stays, at the bottom, so to speak . . . a weight there, on the chest! But it's the same for all of us, we mustn't let ourselves go, and want to die just because others are dead. . . . You must pull yourself together Monsieur Bovary—it will pass! Come

and see us. My daughter thinks of you from time to time, you know, and you are forgetting her, so she says. It'll be spring soon; we'll get you to shoot a rabbit in the woods, to help take your mind off things.

(Flaubert, 1983, pp. 113–114)

Grief experienced after the death of a loved one was once thought to take about 1 year to reach resolution. Now it is clear that normal grieving may take 2 or even 3 years, depending on many factors surrounding the attachment and loss (Bower, 1987). During normal grieving, however, the person is progressing through the stages described above and exhibiting adaptive behaviors.

Even when depressive symptoms are severe, unless a grieving individual is suicidal, Major Depressive Disorder is not diagnosed within the first two months after the loss of a loved one. Abnormal grief reactions do occur, particularly in situations where the individual had ambivalent feelings toward the person lost and/or unresolved emotional work within that relationship.

In abnormal grieving, the individual experiences grief as overwhelming and resorts to maladaptive behaviors. The literature describes four types of abnormal grief reactions (Worden, 1991): **chronic grief**, where the grief never reaches conclusions; **delayed grief**, where the grief work is not accomplished at the time of loss and remains with the individual; **exaggerated grief**, where the grief is experienced as overwhelming; and **masked grief**, where the grief is masked by either a physical symptom or a maladaptive behavior and the person is unaware of the connections to grief and loss.

A nurse will need to support and care for persons undergoing grief, and some of the nursing interventions will be similar to those used when caring for one who is depressed. It is important, though, that the nurse have

---

*From FLAUBERT'S PARROT, by Julian Barnes, Copyright © 1984 by Julian Barnes. Reprinted by permission of Alfred A. Knopf, Inc.

> ✳ **NURSING TIP**
>
> **Identifying Successful Grieving**
>
> A person moving successfully through normal grieving will:
>
> ◆ Consciously recognize she has experienced a significant loss
>
> ◆ Progress through the stages of shock (emotional numbness), reality (deep pain), and recovery (beginning to live again)
>
> ◆ Use adaptive coping behaviors such as action strategies (keeping busy), cognitive coping ("can do" attitude), and interpersonal coping (talking with others, joining a support group)

basic underlying knowledge of the course and dynamics of both grief and depression so that specialist care can be sought for grieving complicated by a mood disorder.

THEORIES OF DEPRESSION

Depression is such a profound and devastating human experience that it seems to demand an explanation. As in the story of Amalia, depression can rapidly transform a person from relatively normal functioning to psychosis. F. Scott Fitzgerald describes his own "cracking up" as occurring both more slowly and less profoundly, but neither he nor his friend nor his readers have a clear understanding of why this has happened to him. There are numerous psychological theories that try to explain the cause of mood disorders. The nurse should have at least some acquaintance with a few of the major theories of depression.

Psychoanalysis

Psychoanalysis derives from Sigmund Freud's studies of dreaming as a window into the unconscious mind (Fine, 1979). Since there are currently many schools of psychoanalysis, not all strictly adhering to Freud's theories, it is not possible to define a single psychoanalytic perspective on depression. In fact, while Freud himself suffered from symptoms of depression, neither the diagnosis nor the explanation of depressive symptoms plays a large part in his work. In 1917 Freud published "Mourning and Melancholia," a paper that described mourning as the "psychically prolonged . . . existence of the lost object (of love)." By this he meant that the mourner feels as if somehow the lost person is still emotionally present until "the work of mourning is completed." In this paper, Freud described depression (melancholia) as loss of an *internal* quality such as self-esteem during the crisis deriving from a child's discovery of his inability to assume the social and sexual role of the same-sex parent. Freud later viewed depression as a conflict between the **ego** (the conscious self) and the **superego** (an inner voice, something like an internalized parent). In depression, the superego punishes the ego for having forbidden wishes or for not living up to the superego's expectations (usually similar to those of one's actual parents). The result of that conflict was guilt, self-hate, and anger turned inward; these processes in turn led to depression.

While perhaps somewhat out of favor presently, psychoanalysis offers at least two important insights into the understanding of depression. First, the concept that depression may derive from the superego allows the nurse or other therapist to explore with a client how childhood experiences and parental expectations may influence present feelings. Second, since psychoanalysis traces the roots of depression into childhood, it supports

the understanding that children may be significantly depressed. Depression *does* occur in children, and the nurse who works with children and their families should be alert to its detection and treatment.

Object Loss Theory

Object loss theory is also based in psychoanalysis but derives from a specific historical event. After World War II, millions of children were orphaned and left homeless and grew up in abject poverty. John Bowlby's psychoanalytic study of these children concluded that adult mental health required a young child to experience a close and loving relationship with its mother (or an appropriate mother substitute) (Fine, 1979). Two ideas are important in the theory that derived from Bowlby's observations: (1) a traumatic loss early in life may predispose one to depression and (2) a subsequent loss or separation in adulthood may serve as a stimulus to depression. These ideas have been strongly attacked by other psychoanalysts, particularly Freud's daughter, Anna. Anna Freud believed that many factors other than maternal separation influence the development of a child's personality (more precisely, *ego*) and that a strong ego can resist the crisis of maternal loss. This disagreement over the role that object loss plays in depression was once known as the Bowlby controversy. Object loss theory may be important in understanding the personal histories of depressed individuals whose childhoods were particularly traumatic and loss filled.

Learned Helplessness Theory

The learned helplessness theory of depression is based on the work of Seligman (1974). He defines helplessness as the sense that one has no control over life events and defines hopelessness as the sense that no one can do anything about life's events. This theory suggests that it is not any specific situation that causes depression, but, rather, it is the individual's belief that there is nothing either he or anyone else can do to make things better. Learned helplessness is caused by a series of reinforcers in one's environment that serve to take control away from the individual, thus producing a personality trait of "giving up." A person who has learned helplessness in growing up has no sense of herself as master of her own destiny and will lack the skills and incentive to try.

Cognitive Theory

Cognitive theory emerged in contrast to psychoanalysis. Psychoanalysis emphasizes the unconscious childhood origins of adult emotional experiences. While clients may be very aware of their feelings, they rarely, according to psychoanalysts, can understand the origin of those feelings without extensive psychotherapy. Psychoanalysts believe that only through that lengthy process of understanding can uncomfortable feelings of anxiety and depression be set aside. Psychoanalysts Albert Ellis and Aaron Beck initiated something of a revolution when they came to believe that how clients *think about their feelings* may be more important for their recovery than *deep understanding of the origins of those feelings.* Beck views depression as a condition in which the individual has come to accept faulty thoughts and to hold dysfunctional assumptions. Ellis termed these thoughts "irrational beliefs" (Beck, 1967). Cognitive theory itself is a little more complicated than this: The client is depressed because he accepts a view of himself and the world that allows for dysfunctional thoughts, painful emotions, and maladaptive behaviors (Perris & Herlofson, 1993). By learning to see the world differently, the client comes to adopt a healthier and more functional self-image. Cognitive therapy relies on individual learning and teaching from a skilled therapist. Psychologists refer to the recent developments leading to cognitive therapy as the "cognitive revolution," in part because supporters of cognitive approaches have consistently demanded that their theories be judged on whether they make clients better. Cognitive treatments *do* work, and it has been difficult to demonstrate such consistent effectiveness for any other type of psychotherapy. In this successful insistence on demonstrable effectiveness, cognitive therapy truly *is* revolutionary.

Physical/Biological Models

With recent advances in biochemical studies, explicitly biological and biochemical models of depression have been proposed. It has long been known that some drugs make depression worse, while others clearly improve depressive symptoms. While their effects may be different, such drugs seem to have in common that they affect concentrations of monoamines (especially norepinephrine and serotonin) in the brain. This effect on monoamines has been of interest to physiologists because norepinephrine and serotonin are produced in only very localized areas of the brainstem. This localized production might imply that depression is a disease that could be shown to have its origins in a very specific area of brain. So far these ideas remain theoretical only. Many researchers believe that monoamines do play a role in producing depressive symptoms, but no biochemical theory can yet account for the causes of depression in individual humans.

Recently, the very powerful tools of single-photon emission computed tomography (SPECT) and positron emission tomography (PET) have allowed measurements to be made of metabolism and blood flow in different parts of the brain in depressed and nondepressed persons (George, Ketter, & Post, 1993). These scanning techniques can measure both blood flow and glucose utilization in different very highly localized brain areas. Emerging

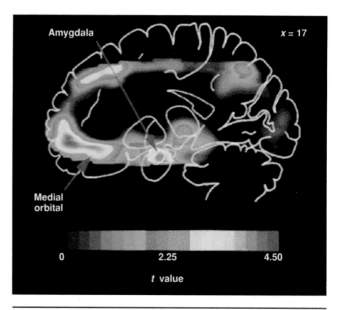

PET scanning in depression. This PET image shows that depressed persons commonly have increased blood flow in specific brain areas as compared to nondepressed persons. This image depicts a parasaggital "slice" as if the image were seen from the left side of a transparent head. Areas depicted in yellow, orange, or red have more blood flow than do comparable anatomic areas in persons without depression. This scan provides evidence for increased metabolic activity in the amygdala (and other brain areas) in persons with familial major depression. *From J. L. Price, S. T. Carmichael, & W. C. Drevets,* Progr. Brain Research, 107 *523, (1996) with kind permission of Elsevier Science—NL—Sara Burgerharstraat 25, 1055 KV, Amsterdam, The Netherlands.*

studies seem to show that depression is associated with consistent changes in the temporal and especially the frontal lobes: Depressed persons do not metabolize glucose well in these areas, but when their depression resolves, metabolism returns to normal (Bench, Friston, Brown, Frackowial, & Dolan, 1993). There is increased metabolic activity within the amygdala in persons with familial major depression as compared to a control group.

These findings are both interesting and important, and they suggest that depression is truly, at some level, a disease of the brain. The findings do not explain *why* glucose uptake is abnormal, and they do not explain how (or whether) psychological factors such as grieving can affect brain function measured by PET scanning. As a result, it still remains unknown whether the observed PET findings are a *cause* or an *effect* of depression. While PET and SPECT findings do not yet hold clinical importance for the nurse, it is likely that evolving highly technical studies will cast new light and understanding on both the causes and treatments of depression.

TREATMENT

Current treatments for depression include psychotherapy, somatic or physical therapies, and medications.

Psychotherapy

Psychotherapy refers to any of over 250 types of largely verbal techniques designed to help individuals surmount psychological stresses including depression. Psychotherapy based on psychoanalytic interventions emphasize helping clients gain insight into the causes of their depression. This approach is long term and requires much motivation on the part of the client to invest considerable time, effort, and money. While psychoanalytic interventions have long been used in treating depression, several newer approaches have gained favor in recent years. The discussion that follows will cover three types of short-term psychotherapy: brief dynamic therapy, marital therapy, and cognitive therapy. Nurses will have many clients who receive other types of therapeutic interventions, but these three therapies are among the most carefully studied in mood disorders.

Brief dynamic therapy focuses on core conflicts that derive from personality and living situations. The goal is to resolve depressive symptoms by improving these conflicts and resolving stresses. The therapist in this approach takes an active role to direct sessions toward resolution of conflicts. Techniques of confrontation and interpretation of behaviors and events are frequently used. Conflicts, their meanings, and individuals' choices are emphasized. This type of therapy can be done either with individuals or in a group format.

Marital therapy attempts to resolve problems that occur with a marriage. Marital therapy is relevant to the treatment of depression because marital distress is common and often includes at least one depressed spouse. Studies suggest that relapses of depression are often preceded by marital discord. Behavioral marital therapy focuses on enhancing behaviors that are supportive of healthy marital relationships. Through therapy sessions, each partner comes to understand the feelings and experiences of the other. Building a stronger marital bond helps to ward off future depressive episodes. The therapist here takes an active role as well and uses techniques similar to those in brief, dynamic therapy.

Cognitive therapy has already been discussed as it derives from a theoretical perspective about the management of depression. Cognitive therapy focuses on removing symptoms by identifying and correcting perceptual biases in clients' thinking and correcting unrecognized assumptions. The therapy concentrates on changing negative thoughts and behaviors into alternatives that do not sustain depression (Abraham, Neese, & Westerman, 1991).

Most psychotherapists currently endorse brief treatment approaches. Significant improvement should be seen by 6 to 12 weeks. In contrast to long-term psychotherapy, which may extend over years, brief treatment does not generally exceed 40 sessions (see also Chapter 26).

Effect of Psychotherapy

Studies of psychotherapy have shown fairly consistent benefit for depression. Brief dynamic psychotherapy has not been compared to placebo, but overall efficacy in six studies appeared to be about 35%. Marital therapy has been shown to effectively alleviate depressive symptoms especially and, not surprisingly, in clients who report marital discord. Cognitive therapy has been extensively studied and compared to both placebo and drug treatment. No studies show that cognitive therapy differs in effectiveness from any other psychotherapeutic technique *or* that medication treatment is more effective than cognitive therapy. In some studies, cognitive therapy seems to be more effective than medication. One study has shown the effectiveness of computer-assisted cognitive therapy. This may be an important advance since one of the strongest criticisms of psychotherapy is its cost in comparison to treatment with medications.

Physical Therapies

While many physical therapies have been in use for depressed clients, this discussion will be limited to two: electroconvulsive therapy and light therapy.

Electroconvulsive Therapy

Electroconvulsive therapy (ECT) is a procedure in which clients are treated with pulses of electrical energy sufficient to cause a brief convulsion or seizure (Bolwig, 1993). Electroconvulsive therapy is carried out under anesthesia. Muscle-depolarizing agents are also given so that no actual convulsive movements occur; the primary effect of ECT is on the brain itself. Studies show that clients do not find the actual ECT treatment frightening, painful, or unpleasant. Although deaths have occurred from ECT, particularly in elderly clients or those with heart disease, the risk is quite low. Side effects depend on the specific technique used but are mostly limited to memory deficits. These are typically mild but may be permanent (see also Chapter 30).

Effect of ECT. Electroconvulsive therapy is utilized in depression because multiple studies have shown it to be highly effective in helping severe depression resistant to all other treatments. Many studies on ECT and depression produce response rates as high as 90%. In comparison to medications [tricyclic antidepressants and monoamine oxidase (MAO) inhibitors], ECT has been clearly shown to be the superior treatment (Abraham, Neese, & Westerman, 1991). Studies using "sham ECT" have demonstrated that ECT effectiveness is not solely due to a placebo effect. Despite its proven effectiveness, ECT is usually reserved only for the most severely depressed clients who have failed to respond to one or more medication trials.

Light Therapy

Light therapy is a new form of treatment, the indications for which have yet to be completely established (Depression Guideline Panel, 1993; Ford, 1992). It is most commonly indicated for clients who have Seasonal Affective Disorder (SAD), a nonpsychotic depression that occurs repeatedly during the winter months and is usually seen in areas of high latitude where daylight time during the winter is limited. By exposing clients to bright lights for a period of time each day, light therapy simulates summer light conditions (Figure 12-1).

Effect of Light Therapy. When used for SAD, light therapy relieves symptoms in about 75% of persons. Response should occur within 2 weeks, and neither safety nor efficacy has been established for treatment lasting longer than this (see also Chapter 30).

Medications

Four types of medications are commonly used to treat depression. Lithium and some anticonvulsants (especially carbamazepine) are most commonly, but not exclusively, used for clients with bipolar disorder. They will be discussed in Chapter 13. The other three categories are

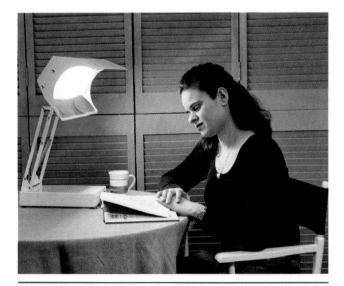

Figure 12-1   Many clients with seasonal affective disorder will find their spirits lifted when using light therapy. *Courtesy Northern Light, Montreal, Canada.*

tricyclic and related antidepressants, selective serotonin reuptake inhibitors (SSRIs), and MAO inhibitors.

Drugs are chosen based on client characteristics, prior response to medications, family history of response to medication, concurrent illnesses and medications, and the provider's preferences. Since most medications take a month or more to be effective, dose increases or changes in medication should generally be made only after several weeks. Some clinicians begin tricyclic antidepressants at low doses and increase at 1- to 3-day intervals in an effort to accommodate clients to medication side effects.

Antidepressant medications are generally prescribed for 4 to 9 months and may then be discontinued. Many clients, however, should remain on antidepressants indefinitely. Indications for continuing antidepressant treatment include three or more episodes of Major Depressive Disorder, history of recurrence within 1 year of discontinuing previous antidepressants, family history of recurrent depression or bipolar depression, onset of depression before age 20, and sudden onset of past depressions.

Psychotically depressed clients like Amalia are likely to receive antipsychotic medications such as phenothiazines. Since psychosis is such an important part of the psychiatric disorder schizophrenia, these medications are discussed at length in Chapters 11 and 25. When indicated by psychotic symptoms, they are used comparably in depressed and schizophrenic clients.

Because symptoms of anxiety are typically prominent in depressed clients seen in primary care, these clients are often treated with antianxiety medications. The excerpt "The Crack-Up," presented earlier, offers a good example of depression in which anxiety is a major symptom: The very idea of "cracking" is an anxiety-related symptom. While it may seem logical to use antianxiety medications when treating individuals like the narrator in Fitzgerald's essay, experts strongly oppose such treatment except in highly unusual cases (Wells, Katon, Rogers, & Camp, 1994). Anxiolytics (antianxiety medications) should be avoided for at least three reasons: (1) symptoms of anxiety in depressed clients almost always respond to antidepressant medications; (2) controlled studies show no benefit from adding anxiolytics to antidepressants; and (3) most anxiolytic medications have a strong tendency to produce dependency.

The following is a discussion of the commonly used medications.

Tricyclic and Related Antidepressants

Tricyclics and related antidepressants were the first medications to prove effective in the management of depression. They are still the standard against which newer drugs are measured. While called *antidepressants*, these medications do have other uses in client care. For example, they are used to treat enuresis (bed wetting in children), chronic pain, Panic Disorder, Obsessive-

Table 12-1   Common Antidepressants

GENERIC NAME	PROPRIETARY NAME	DOSE RANGE (mg)	SEDATION	ANTICHOLINERGIC EFFECTS	ORTHOSTATIC EFFECTS
Amitryptyline	Elavil	150–200	High	High	High
Amoxepine	Ascendin	150–200	Low	Low	Moderate
Clomipramine	Anafranil	150–200	High	High	High
Desipramine	Norpramin	150–200	Low	Low	Moderate
Doxepin	Sinequan/Adapin	150–200	High	Moderate	Moderate
Imipramine	Tofranil	150–200	Moderate	Moderate	High
Maprotiline	Ludiomil	150–200	Moderate	Low	Moderate
Nortriptyline	Pamelor	75–100	Low	Low	Lowest
Protriptyline	Vivactil	30	Low	High	Low
Trimipramine	Surmontil	150–200	High	Moderate	Moderate
Bupropion	Wellbutrin	300	Low	Very low	Very low
Trazodone	Desyrel	150–400	High	Very low	High

Notes: Bupropion and trazodone are pharmacologically not tricyclic antidepressants. Bupropion may cause seizures, especially in doses above 300 mg daily.

Compulsive Disorder, migraine headaches, and bulimia as well as depression. Table 12-1 lists tricyclic and related antidepressants, daily dosage ranges, and common side effects. Clients with sleep disturbances are often given a drug with high to moderate sedative effects. Anticholinergic effects (dry mouth, constipation, inability to pass urine) are often the side effects that clients find most unacceptable and lead to discontinuation of medication. Orthostatic effects result in dizziness or fainting on changing position and are especially troublesome for elderly clients and those with relatively low blood pressure. Moderate weight gain is another common side effect of many of these medications, and most can cause sexual dysfunction in both men and women. All of the medications in Table 12-1 except trazodone and bupropion are very dangerous and often fatal if taken in overdose. For

this reason, great caution is used in prescribing these medications to potentially suicidal clients. Trazadone and the SSRI medications may be much safer and rarely result in death if taken in large quantities.

Tricyclic antidepressants are usually given as a single dose at bedtime. Sleep may improve almost immediately (though some clients are troubled by vivid dreams), but any improvement in depressive symptoms takes at least 2 to 3 weeks. Full response typically requires 4 to 6 weeks. Blood testing to determine plasma levels of antidepressant drugs is often used for amitryptiline (Elavil), imipramine (Tofranil), desipramine (Norpramin), and nortriptyline (Pamelor). If medication is stopped, it should be tapered rather than withdrawn abruptly.

Selective Serotonin Reuptake Inhibitors

The SSRIs have become increasingly popular in recent years. They have not yet been clearly demonstrated to be effective in treating severely depressed individuals but are widely used among outpatients. There are currently four SSRIs available: fluoxetine (Prozac), sertraline (Zoloft), paroxetine (Paxil), and fluvoxamine (Luvox). They differ in recommended dose but otherwise seem to have relatively few differences between them. Fluoxetine (Prozac) seems to have the highest incidence of interactions with other drugs, and paroxetine (Paxil) is excreted at high levels in breast milk, making it perhaps less desirable for treating women of reproductive age.

The SSRIs work by inhibiting the reuptake of serotonin at brain synapses and hence increasing the available serotonin at serotonin-sensitive receptors. Some newer SSRIs under development also stimulate the serotonin receptors. Like tricyclics, the SSRIs take several weeks to

⚡ NURSING ALERT!

Bupropion

Bupropion may cause seizures, especially in doses above 300 mg daily.

⚡ NURSING ALERT!

Tricyclic Antidepressants

Tricyclic antidepressants are very dangerous in overdose; administration must be carefully monitored, especially in clients at risk for suicide.

have an effect and may not achieve maximum effectiveness for 4 to 6 weeks.

These medications have achieved their current popularity not because they are more effective than tricyclic antidepressants, but, in large part, because their side effects are less troublesome. The SSRIs lack the anticholinergic and orthostatic side effects of tricyclic antidepressants. The SSRI side effects may include agitation, restlessness, insomnia, weight loss, headache, nausea, and diarrhea. Sexual dysfunction may also occur, especially in men. The SSRIs are generally safe if taken in overdose, a major advantage for treating potentially suicidal clients. While SSRIs still cost a great deal more than generic tricyclic drugs, many clients prefer more expensive SSRI treatment because of fewer significant side effects.

Monoamine Oxidase Inhibitors

Monoamine oxidase (MAO) inhibitors increase the availability of brain neurotransmitters by interfering with their metabolism. These drugs act to increase the concentrations of serotonin, epinephrine, and norepinephrine in brain tissue. This metabolic effect seems to be responsible for their usefulness as antidepressants. The MAO inhibitors are not used frequently because they require clients to use great care in choosing foods and over-the-counter medications. Since these inhibitors act both on the brain and in the gut, they also prevent the gastrointestinal tract from breaking down ingested catecholamines, which are found in large quantities in some foods and medications. Clients taking MAO inhibitors who consume substances listed in the accompanying display typically experience a dangerous rise in blood pressure. This may result in stroke or other cardiovascular catastrophe.

New MAO inhibitors whose effects can be rapidly reversed have recently been marketed. These drugs may increase the safety and popularity of the MAO group of medications. Drugs that have no gut effects and are active *only* in the brain are also being developed. Whether safer MAO inhibitors will have therapeutic advantages over SSRIs remains to be seen. Currently available MAO inhibitors include tranylcypromine (Parnate), phenelzine (Nardil), and isocarboxazid (Marplan). Moclobemide is a reversible MAO inhibitor that may be released soon (see also Chapter 25).

Effect of Medications

Multiple studies have shown that antidepressant medications are more effective than placebo in resolving symptoms of depression. Effectiveness persists for at least 1 to 2 years in follow-up studies. Few studies suggest any major difference in effectiveness among any of the available drugs. In general, if clients can tolerate medication

---

FOODS AND MEDICATIONS THAT MUST BE AVOIDED BY CLIENTS TAKING MAO INHIBITORS

FOODS TO BE COMPLETELY AVOIDED

- ◆ Cheese: except for cottage and cream cheese
- ◆ Smoked, dried, pickled, cured, or preserved meats and fishes
- ◆ Caviar
- ◆ Fava beans
- ◆ Avocados (probably only if overripe)
- ◆ Yeast extracts
- ◆ Chianti wine
- ◆ Beer containing yeast

FOODS WITH SOME RISK UNLESS USED IN MODERATION

- ◆ Chocolate
- ◆ Coffee

MEDICATIONS TO BE AVOIDED

- ◆ Prescription medications: tricyclic antidepressants, Prozac, Demerol, amphetamines and amphetamine-like medications including all sympathomimetics
- ◆ Nonprescription medications: cold or allergy medications, nasal decongestants and inhalers, cough medications except for plain guaifenesin, stimulants and diet pills, pain medications except for aspirin, acetaminophen, and ibuprofen

---

side effects, a response occurs in 60% to 70% of both inpatients and outpatients. Most studies show a placebo improvement in depression of about 18% to 30%.

NURSING PERSPECTIVES

Nursing theories assist nurses in planning care for a client who is depressed, but the particular theory a nurse selects will depend on many factors. Although the authors believe that caring theories and Self-Care Deficit Theory are especially helpful in approaching and planning nursing care for depressed clients, other practitioners may choose different theories with equally good results. The principles of theory application highlighted in the following discussion should be applicable to many alternative theoretical frameworks.

Caring Theories

Isolation and loneliness are among the most prominent personal characteristics of persons who are depressed. For example, earlier in this chapter, Tolstoy describes his depression as a *force* drawing him away from life, work, and family. Comparable feelings of detachment are expressed in many of the other excerpts quoted and by almost all depressed persons. In some cases social isolation is a major *cause* of an individual's depression: A person who has no important others in his life may become depressed as a consequence of isolation. This is often the case for the elderly. In contrast, other depressed people have opportunities for social interaction that they actively reject: Their depression results in social isolation. For example, Tolstoy was a father, a world-famous author, and a large landowner at the time of his depression. He had friends, family, colleagues, and numerous admirers; for him, social isolation was entirely self-imposed. Whether the client chooses isolation or has it thrust on him by depression, an interpersonal, caring approach will provide the basis for a helping relationship. Although Wiedenbach (1964) and Leininger (1978) have also developed important theories based on caring, this discussion will focus on Watson's (1988) theory of human care.

Watson's theory calls for each individual to be "valued in and of him- or herself to be cared for, respected, nurtured, understood and assisted" (p. 14). In caring for a depressed person, the nurse would value the individual, seek to understand him, and provide respect, nurturing, and support. The nurse will initiate a nurse-client relationship that is based on mutuality and affirmation. The nurse should approach the depressed client with an attitude of sincere caring and strive to build a relationship with the client that demonstrates the nurse's respect for the person.

Watson (1988) believes that nursing is a transpersonal value. She writes that "the transpersonal nature and presence of the union of two persons' souls allow for some unknowns to emerge from the caring itself" (p. 71). The "unknowns" that can emerge from human caring may create a bridge for the depressed person to reach out, to feel and experience human interaction once again.

A caring approach could serve to provide the client with a sense of belonging as well as a sense that he is "likeable." The nurse would strive to understand the world from the client's perspective and be willing to listen to the client's subjective experiences. Through a positive nurse-client relationship, the nurse could aid the client in experiencing a positive view of self and a positive sense of future hope.

It is important to recognize that Watson's theory requires mutuality, that is, that the client respond with some kind of involvement in the therapeutic relationship. The withdrawn, angry, suspicious, and depressed person may be very slow to enter into this kind of mutuality. Despite the strong therapeutic potential of nursing intervention based on caring, some depressed individuals may respond slowly or not at all. The nurse faced with such a client must be willing to persevere, to consult with colleagues and mentors who have extensive experience in reaching the depressed, to carefully examine her own feelings and responses, and perhaps at some point to consider a switch in theory and approach.

Self-Care Deficit Theory

Although diagnosis often focuses on how a depressed person feels, for many depressed individuals the biggest problems are not those of affect (feeling) but of self-care. For example, weight loss is a cardinal symptom of depression, and it frequently results from failure to eat. The depressed may lose interest in their appearance, in hygiene, and in their surroundings. In the excerpt from Italo Svevo's writing quoted earlier, both Amalia's personal appearance (especially her weight loss) and the dishevelment of her dressing and room emphasize her profound self-care deficit.

Orem's (1985) self-care deficit theory views nurses' work to be doing for the client that which he cannot do for himself. In this theory, the concept of **nurse agency** refers to nursing activities required to compensate for the client's inability to meet his own self-care needs. Since a depressed client is often neglectful of basic health and personal requirements, the nurse should direct the client's activities toward correcting any apparent care deficit. The nurse may do this both by directly assisting the client to meet health needs and by demonstrating to the client that the nurse believes he is sufficiently important and worthy of his needs being met.

In using this approach with a depressed client, the nurse must take care not to do for the client anything he is truly capable of doing for himself. In Orem's theory, the concept of **self-care agency** refers to the client's ability to provide for his own needs. Whenever possible, the nurse should encourage the client to meet his own health requirements, thus increasing self-care agency. The nurse will approach the client with an attitude of kindness and understanding and demonstrate via behaviors that the client is valued as a person. When the client begins to be able to care for his basic physical and personal needs, the nurse will move to a **supportive-educative role**, which focuses on enhancing the client's ability both to carry on effectively without nursing support and to rise above the feelings of depression that brought on the initial deficit in self-care.

NURSING PROCESS

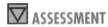 ASSESSMENT

The majority of depressed persons are seen in general medical settings, not in psychiatric clinics and wards. The nurse will come in contact with depressed persons in all areas of practice and on virtually every working day. Thus, all nurses should have basic skills in the assessment and management of depression. While for many nurses that management may be referral to a mental health professional, initial assessment is a fundamental nursing skill. The recognition of depression is an important collaborative issue as well: The Medical Outcomes Study clearly showed that primary care practitioners do not do a good job of recognizing or treating depression (Wells et al., 1989). This failure is important because depression itself, far from being a minor problem, causes more functional impairment than do many chronic medical disorders, such as diabetes. Recognizing and treating depression are not only of critical importance in primary care but also equally necessary for hospitalized medical clients, the elderly, new mothers, children, and adolescents.

How, then, does one know that an individual is depressed? The answer is simple: by observing and talking to him. However, even if the answer is simple, the process of discovering depression is often far from easy. Relatively few individuals present to the nurse with a ready-made diagnosis of depression, and even fewer seek care complaining primarily of depression. From past

---

⁂ NURSING TIP

Recognizing Depression

Persons who are depressed often have the following characteristics:

♦ Find that previously enjoyable activities no longer produce joy

♦ Loss of interest in friends; isolation from others

♦ Difficulty concentrating

♦ A history of significant loss or trauma

♦ A sense of powerlessness and hopelessness

♦ Loss of appetite and weight

♦ Sleep disturbances, particularly early morning awakening with inability to fall back asleep

♦ Make few demands on nursing staff

---

experience, persons may feel that doctors and nurses want to hear only about physical symptoms; so depressed persons are far more likely to volunteer information about their physical symptoms than about their feelings. In addition, many people just do not talk well about feelings, or they may come from a culture in which admitting depression results in loss of face or status. Even a person who knows his symptoms are due to depression is likely to share information about his feelings only with an interviewer he feels to be sympathetic and unhurried. Open-ended questions are best for eliciting feelings, questions like "So how would you say your life has been going?" or "How does this illness make you feel?" More direct questioning may also be helpful and sometimes necessary: "Do you ever feel down-in-the-dumps or sad?"

The nurse should ask most, if not all, clients about their feelings. However, certain individuals should be interviewed more intensively. These include persons with prior episodes of depression or suicide attempts, persons under age 40 or over 70, postpartum mothers, persons with significant medical illness, persons who have limited social support or stressful life circumstances, and persons who abuse alcohol or other substances. Each of these groups is at higher than average risk for significant depression (Depression Guideline Panel, 1993). Women seem to suffer more commonly from depression than do men, so some experts recommend that women be interviewed about depressive symptoms somewhat more intensively than men. A family history of depression should probably also prompt more detailed questioning, although unipolar Major Depressive Disorder only sometimes runs in families. People who present with or admit to problems with sleep, appetite, sexual functioning, chronic pain, or weight change may have depression even if they deny depressed mood. They may instead have fatigue, trouble concentrating, anxiety, or guilt as important alternate symptoms of depression (Depression Guideline Panel, 1993).

The effectiveness of a nurse's interview can be enhanced by questionnaires designed to assist in the detection of depression. These are of two general types: those intended to be completed by the client (self-rating scales) and those intended to be completed by the nurse during an interview. Common self-rating scales are the Beck Depression Inventory and the Zung Self-Rating Depression Scale. These scales are valuable instruments for nursing practice because they rarely miss persons who are significantly depressed. However, they *do not diagnose depression*. A skilled interviewer familiar with DSM-IV should evaluate any client who has an abnormal result on

CULTURAL ASPECTS OF DEPRESSION: REPORT OF A CHINESE AMERICAN POPULATION

In reviewing available literature on the topic, the authors remind the reader that for most of the world's population, psychobiological affect is presented through physical complaints. In Confucian tradition, there is emphasis on inhibiting emotions. Emotions are understood as pathogenic factors that can cause bodily disturbances. Therefore, emotions will frequently be expressed through somatic metaphors.

Investigators of Chinese American populations have documented that somatic complaints are intermixed with affective complaints. Health is seen as a balance between positive and negative forces; illness and emotional states are attributed to imbalances. While available studies are limited to college student populations, data suggest that depressive symptomatology combines with somatic complaints such as poor appetite and disturbed sleep. The somatic complaints become the presenting symptoms. Stress of acculturation may also result in self-rejection, and this aspect of depression has not been fully explored in Chinese Americans.

Nurses caring for certain Chinese Americans must seek to interpret symptoms and behaviors from a Chinese worldview and to understand the client's presenting complaints as reflective of specific cultural ideals and adaptations.

Nurses are cautioned that depression in any client cannot be fully understood without entering into the client's culture. These issues are thoroughly discussed in Chapter 6

Reprinted with permission, "Depression among Chinese Americans: A Review of the Literature," by B. Tabna and J. N. Flaskerud, 1994, *Issues in Mental Health Nursing,* 15(6), pp. 569–584. Copyright 1994 American Association for the Advancement of Science.

SAMPLE ITEMS FROM THE BECK DEPRESSION INVENTORY

Name _____ Date _____

The questionnaire provides groups of statements. Clients are asked to read all statements in the group and to circle the number that best describes their feelings. The following are two samples:

1. 0 I get as much satisfaction out of things as I used to.
1 I don't enjoy things the way I used to.
2 I don't get real satisfaction out of anything anymore.
3 I am dissatisfied or bored with everything.

2. 0 I have not lost interest in other people.
1 I am less interested in other people than I used to be.
2 I have lost most of my interest in other people.
3 I have lost all of my interest in other people.

Beck Depression Inventory. Copyright © 1987, 1993 by Aaron T. Beck. Adapted and reproduced by permission of the publisher, The Psychological Corporation. All rights reserved. "Beck Depression Inventory" and "BDI" are registered trademarks of The Psychological Corporation.

✿✿ REFLECTIVE THINKING

How Do You Feel When Interviewing a Depressed Client?

Think about a depressed individual you have worked with and reflect on the following:

◆ Do depressed clients raise feelings of depression or grief in you? If yes, how do you know this has happened?
◆ Do you believe that depression is justified in some persons and situations and not in others? If yes, what is the difference?
◆ Is it hard to empathize with one who is depressed, particularly if you do not believe he has the "right" to feel so down?
◆ Do some clients leave you feeling drained and fatigued? Which ones? In what settings?
◆ Do some clients leave you feeling angry? Which ones? In what settings?

one of the depression questionnaires; while only 60% to 75% of these people have a final diagnosis of depression, many of the remainder who score "falsely positive" can benefit from supportive nursing interventions.

The nurse should also remember that intuition can be one of the most powerful tools for detecting depression. The appearance of a depressed person can often be a strong clue to feelings and diagnosis. In general, a depressed person presents with little affect or (even if they deny feeling sad) with visible sadness. The individual may look tired, appear withdrawn, and have less facial and bodily expression than is normal. Of course, many medical conditions (hypothyroidism is an excellent example) can produce such an appearance, but the person's appearance is often an important clue for recognition of depression. Another very important diagnostic clue is much harder to describe and learn: Many skilled nurses report that depressed people make them (the nurses) feel a certain way. After talking for a few minutes to a depressed client, many sensitive persons find themselves fatigued and a little depressed. By listening to her own feelings, the nurse can greatly enhance her ability to recognize depression and so provide caring help to clients in need. Many nurses are attracted to psychiatric care precisely because it gives them an opportunity to develop and use their highest intuitive skills.

▽ NURSING DIAGNOSIS

By listening and hearing the experience of a depressed person, the nurse will be able to assess that individual's response to the emotion. Some persons will feel lonely; others guilty. Some will describe not having feelings. Some will lose all connection to others and to a meaning and purpose in their lives. Some, as in F. Scott Fitzgerald's writing, will be personally and spiritually bankrupt. The following is a list of nursing diagnoses (NANDA, 1996) that are common in depressed persons:

- *Hopelessness*, related to long-term stress; abandonment; lost belief in transcendent values
- *Powerlessness*, related to lack of ability to exert control
- *Spiritual distress*, related to challenged belief and value system
- *Self-esteem disturbance*, related to lack of positive reinforcement of one's value and worth
- *Social isolation*, related to inability to engage in satisfying personal relationships
- *Self-care deficit*, related to lack of concern or regard toward self
- *Sleep pattern disturbance*, related to internal stress

The first five of these diagnoses can be made only when the nurse has sufficient interactions with the client to be able to validate that the defining characteristics of the diagnosis are present. The definition of the diagnosis of *hopelessness* states that it is a "subjective state," and the major defining characteristics include both physical observations and verbal cues (NANDA, 1996, p. 71). A nurse must validate that the client's subjective feelings are those of seeing limited or no alternatives or choice, and having no energy to mobilize resources, in order to make the diagnosis of *hopelessness*. *Powerlessness* is diagnosed when an individual feels that his own action cannot affect an outcome; the person has a perceived lack of control over his current situation. *Spiritual distress* is used as a

nursing diagnosis when there is a disruption in a person's life principles such that he questions the meaning of life and of his own existence and lacks a sense of future and of belonging. *Self-esteem disturbance* refers to negative evaluations of self or of self-capabilities. *Social isolation* is diagnosed when a client expresses the desire to be more involved with others than he is currently able to be. Clearly, formulating and validating these diagnoses require considerable nursing skill and effort toward establishing therapeutic communication and rapport with the client.

The diagnoses of *self-care deficit* and *sleep pattern disturbance* can be made through objective observation and the client's subjective feelings. *Self-care deficit* is diagnosed when the client is unable to perform basic activities of daily living and hygiene. *Sleep pattern disturbance* can be used as a diagnosis when the client's sleep cycle causes discomfort. For many depressed individuals, early morning awakening with inability to fall back asleep and feelings of never being rested would lead to this diagnosis. Accuracy in diagnoses is important in guiding nursing staff to individualize care. In each case, nursing staff will address the client's human response to the depression.

▽ OUTCOME IDENTIFICATION

Expected outcomes of nursing care will be as varied as the individual clients and the circumstances surrounding their needs for care. For a client hospitalized with psychotic depression, the nurse may focus on risk for injury related to loss of touch with reality. A reasonable expected outcome would be that the client remain free of injury during the hospitalization. When the focus of care is self-care deficit, an expected outcome could be that within 1 week the client will initiate activities of grooming and daily living. In contrast, when the client is being followed as an outpatient and the depression is of long-term duration, the expected outcomes of care will take longer to achieve. For example, for a client experiencing social isolation and feelings of loneliness, the expected outcome of therapy combined with a socialization group could be that within 1 month the client will initiate a social contact with one person. The three care plans presented at this chapter's end illustrate differing care situations and a range of expected outcomes of care.

▽ PLANNING/INTERVENTIONS

There are several interventions for the depressed client. These include (1) independent nursing actions based on nursing diagnoses and (2) collaborative interventions associated with treatment plans made by a multidisciplinary psychiatric team. Major approaches are discussed following.

NURSING LITERATURE ON DEPRESSION: FINDINGS AND REPORTS

◆ In a study designed to evaluate the effectiveness of a structured cognitive-behavioral group intervention, researchers found that depressed women who participated in a structured group intervention were significantly improved when compared to women who attended a support group or women who served as controls (Maynard, 1993).

◆ The major social factors contributing to depression among the elderly are widowhood or divorce, low socioeconomic status, stressful life events such as personal illness/disability, illness of family members, problems with interpersonal relationships, accidents, a move within the past year, and lack of community networks (Kurlowicz, 1993).

◆ In a study of 12 inpatients diagnosed with Major Unipolar Depression, researchers evaluated effects of movement therapy on mood. Results show that movement therapy has a positive impact on mood and suggest that a movement therapy program could be instituted and evaluated as a nursing intervention for depression (Steward, McMullen, & Rubin, 1994).

◆ In a sample of elderly residents of urban housing units, researchers evaluated effects of a cognitive therapy group, a crafts group, and a control group. Data indicated that subjects in the cognitive therapy group showed significant lessening of depression, those in the craft group showed some lessening of depression, and controls remained unchanged. Researchers reported that the use of diaries was helpful in clarifying thoughts and experiences in the cognitive therapy group (Campbell, 1992).

◆ In a study of myocardial infarction (MI) survivors, researchers found that mood was related to performance of self-care behaviors. Depression was an important predictor of post-MI quality of life. Nursing interventions aimed at assessing for depression and minimizing depression, when present, are needed in this population (Conn, Taylor, & Wiman, 1991).

◆ Exercise was found to be an effective antidepressant in a meta-analysis of 77 studies on exercise and depression (North, 1989).

The nurse would identify the priority diagnoses for each client and establish a plan of care directed toward the circumstances that contributed to the condition. A depressed person will not take initiative to solve problems and find solutions to uncomfortable conditions. A nurse must take care to use a nursing perspective/theory to build a relationship with the client and suggest options for care that serve to keep the client in control of his own treatment and that move the client and nurse to mutually agreed-upon interventions.

Nursing interventions include establishing a one-on-one relationship to provide human contact and relief from the loneliness often described by clients who are depressed; providing positive regard and unconditional acceptance to enhance client self-esteem and feelings of worthiness; engaging the client in activities, often beginning with activities of daily living and moving to social activities, to provide a pattern of functional living and recreation; listening to the client, providing time to understand the client's subjective experience of depression and pain; educating the client (and client's family/significant others) about the prevalence of depression and the use of antidepressive medications; assisting the client to establish a true sense of his own strengths and weaknesses; and addressing the feelings of hopelessness and lack of future by permitting the client to talk through his feelings. The accompanying display discusses other techniques found useful, including group therapy (Chapter 28), movement therapy, and exercise (Chapter 30) (Figure 12-2).

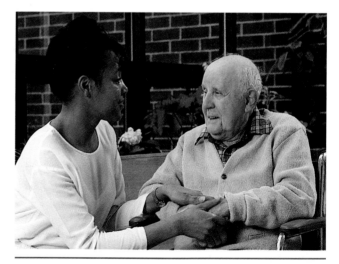

Figure 12-2   Supportive nursing care for depressed clients can include one-on-one interactions, caring touch, listening with empathy, and helping the client to identify personal strengths.

▽ **EVALUATION**

When evaluating a client's progress in managing depression, the nurse should first ask the client's view of changes that have occurred since therapy began. Specific indicators such as stronger sleep patterns, return of appetite, renewed or increasing sense of control and self-worth, and renewed interest in previous or new activities are all good signs of progress. Depressed individuals may experience progress in some areas (return to normal weight) but not in others (continued lack of ability to concentrate). The nurse needs to keep in mind and to remind the client that managing depression often requires significant energy and a conscious effort on the client's part to balance emotions and maintain perspective. It is also important to remember that depression resulting from a significant loss, such as loss of a loved one, may take many weeks or months to overcome and that the client will need sensitive nursing care to adapt to the new situations and roles that accompany such a loss.

CASE STUDY/CARE PLAN

The description of Amalia is presented in the introductory section of this chapter.

Amalia is experiencing a major depressive disorder. She has lost touch with reality; she does not respond to her brother as he enters her room and calls to her; she is uttering words that are unintelligible; she responds to unknown images as she talks about horrible creatures; she cries; and she is in obvious distress and fatigue. While her brother refers to her condition as *delirium*, it is really *psychosis*, the difference being that a person in a psychotic state can be brought back to reality and can acknowledge others in the real world, whereas the person in a delirious state cannot recognize reality. Amalia can recognize and interact with her brother, and she does so when he puts his hand on her shoulder and speaks to her firmly; thus she is psychotic. Imagine that nurses are giving care to Amalia. A fictionalized nursing care plan follows.

ASSESSMENT

Amalia's psychotic depression has incapacitated her. She is nonverbal, minimally responsive, fearful of unknown images, and unable to meet the most basic of needs. She is admitted to an inpatient unit by her brother, who is absolutely shocked by what he has seen.

NURSING DIAGNOSIS *Risk for injury*, related to loss of touch with reality

Outcomes	Planning/Interventions	Evaluation
◆ Amalia will remain free of injury during the inpatient period	◆ Monitor Amalia's condition and location frequently to ensure her safety. ◆ Assign a one-to-one nurse-client ratio. ◆ Provide a private room and remove any object that could potentially be used for self-harm.	Amalia was admitted without any sense of reality. She was tormented by creatures and was extremely fearful. She was put into a protected environment with frequent monitoring. She remained free of injury during the inpatient period.

Continued

NURSING DIAGNOSIS *Altered thought processes*, related to loss of touch with reality and lack of sleep, as evidenced by inaccurate interpretation of environment and distractibility

Outcomes	Planning/Interventions	Evaluation
◆ Amalia will experience fewer psychotic symptoms within 48 hours and remain oriented to person, time, and place.	◆ Engage Amalia in brief conversations so that Amalia may learn to trust the nurse. Communicate using simple sentences. ◆ Reorient Amalia as necessary. ◆ Ensure adequate rest periods. ◆ Monitor sleep, food consumption, and affect, closely watching for psychotic tendencies and depression.	Amalia was gradually oriented to person, time, and place. Within 72 hours, Amalia was calmer, was able to interact with her primary caregiver, and finally slept.

NURSING DIAGNOSIS *Self-care deficit*, related to perceptual and cognitive impairment

Outcomes	Planning/Interventions	Evaluation
◆ Amalia will demonstrate functional behaviors with activities of daily living within 48 hours.	◆ Gently guide Amalia through self-care activities, gradually shifting responsibilities for activities of daily living (ADL) to Amalia. ◆ Initially focus on safety, dressing, and eating. ◆ Give progressive activities associated with ADL. ◆ Provide positive feedback for Amalia's increasing assumption of ADL.	Initially, Amalia was minimally responsive, required complete physical care and protection, and was fed. As her condition improved, however, she was able to assume increasing responsibility for her physical care. She remained extremely fatigued and lethargic, so activities were clustered. Rest periods were built into Amalia's day. By day 4, she was able to bathe and dress herself and began to discuss her problems with the nurse.

CRITICAL THINKING BAND

ASSESSMENT
Would it be valuable to also interview Amalia's brother and/or friends?

NURSING DIAGNOSIS
What other diagnoses are especially important with Amalia?

Continued

Outcomes	Planning/Interventions	Evaluation
How dependent can the nurse allow Amalia to be? Is it necessary to get Amalia focused on self-care?	What differences in Amalia's care would there be if she were in an active-destructive state rather than a neglectful one?	Do plans always work? How does the nurse maintain her own positive attitude?

CASE STUDY/CARE PLAN

The description of F. Scott Fitzgerald's feelings of depression are presented within the discussion of Minor Depressive Disorder earlier in this chapter.

Fitzgerald is describing depression in terms of emptiness (drawing on resources he did not possess), being physically and spiritually drained, and feeling anger and annoyance at the world going on around him (being bitter at the sound of the radio). His life has become an extreme effort, and he is worried about his own ability to cope any longer.

Based on this brief description, one could assume that Fitzgerald has a level of depression that could benefit from treatment, medication, and therapy.

Imagine that nurses are giving care to Mr. Curpin, a man expressing his depression in a manner similar to Fitzgerald.

ASSESSMENT

Mr. Curpin is depressed to the point of admitting "I have no real life in me." He has isolated himself from family and friends, sees no purpose in his life, and forces himself to "appear normal." He is reliant on old patterns of behavior to get him through the long days and longer nights. He is restless, fatigued, unhappy, and discouraged.

NURSING DIAGNOSIS *Ineffective individual coping*, related to depression, as evidenced by verbalization of inability to cope and expression of discouragement

Outcomes	Planning/Interventions	Evaluation
◆ Within 6 weeks, Mr. Curpin will demonstrate an increased use of coping mechanisms.	◆ Encourage Mr. Curpin to discuss the loss of life's purpose through use of communication techniques and open-ended questions and by spending time with Mr. Curpin.	Mr. Curpin revealed that part of his life's concerns related to a sense of fatigue and depression over "getting older" and "not feeling well."
◆ Within 1 month, Mr. Curpin will reconnect with family or friends.	◆ Establish a relationship with Mr. Curpin based on trust: set aside time to talk with him; keep promises; initiate interactions; and keep an atmosphere of positive regard.	His coping mechanism was to withdraw and become uninvolved, yet he felt lonely and isolated.
◆ Within 2 months, Mr. Curpin will verbalize feeling a greater sense of control over his life.	◆ Explore the coping mechanisms Mr. Curpin used before to manage difficult times. ◆ Assess the personal meaning of his social isolation; explore means to reach out to others. ◆ Facilitate discussion about his illness, treatment plan, and personal goals. ◆ Emphasize Mr. Curpin's strengths and progress in gaining control over his life. ◆ Clarify Mr. Curpin's understanding of his treatment.	He was willing to try to reach out to others; he willingly agreed to enter therapy and to explore his means of coping.

Continued

NURSING DIAGNOSIS *Spiritual distress*, related to intense suffering, as evidenced by apathy and questioning own existence

Outcomes	Planning/Interventions	Evaluation
◆ Within 4 weeks Mr. Curpin will verbalize a mood change consistent with hope	◆ Encourage Mr. Curpin to discuss his feelings of hopelessness and distress through the use of therapeutic communication and active listening. ◆ Assess and monitor Mr. Curpin's ability to meet his physical needs. ◆ Assess the meaning and purpose of life for Mr. Curpin, to guide future activities.	Mr. Curpin began to explore his life and what a positive future would mean to him. Over time, he was able to identify future-oriented goals.

CRITICAL THINKING BAND

ASSESSMENT

What physical clues might you look for when interviewing someone whom you suspect is suffering from depression?

NURSING DIAGNOSIS

What means do you really have to help someone adopt new coping patterns?

Outcomes

How can you predict outcomes for another's feelings?

Planning/Interventions

What does it mean when someone has truly lost the meaning and purpose of life? What do you think is a nurse's role in relieving the distress of the human spirit?

Evaluation

Have you accomplished your goal as a nurse when this client sees a future and describes a sense of hope? What other role would you have?

CASE STUDY/CARE PLAN

The description of Geoffrey is presented within the discussion of bereavement earlier in this chapter.

Geoffrey is undergoing acute grieving due to the death of his wife through suicide. He is describing the reality stage of grieving, coming to terms with the pain, the emptiness, and the extreme sadness that he feels. He relates that others offer themselves to him should he want to talk but that talking about his grief makes little difference. He implies that others who are concerned for him enter his world, talk, take him out, let him know that he will "get over it," and finally leave him to himself, where he can feel his grief once again.

Normal grieving is one of the most painful events in a person's life. The nurse recognizes that this is so and also is aware of the fact that the pain is a healthy human response to loss. The nurse cannot make the pain go away. Persons who undergo grief do not always want distractions, medications, and the like. They *need* to feel their sorrow.

Imagine that nurses are caring for Harold, a man who has experienced similar circumstances to Geoffrey.

ASSESSMENT

Harold's wife committed suicide three weeks ago. He knew she was depressed but had no idea she would take her own life. He feels detached, lost, depressed, and overwhelmed. He does not feel like eating, has nightmares when he sleeps, and is unable to respond to the many friends and family offering support. He is secluded and withdrawn.

Continued

NURSING DIAGNOSIS *Normal grieving*, related to death of spouse, as evidenced by self-care deficits, social seclusion, withdrawal, and sense of depression and emotional pain

Outcomes	Planning/Interventions	Evaluation
• Within 2 weeks, Harold will begin to express his feelings associated with his wife's death.	• Facilitate Harold's involvement with a therapist or group so he can explore the loss of his wife to suicide.	Harold went to one bereavement group meeting but found it too painful to return.
• Within 2 months, Harold will establish an adequate balance of sleep, rest, activity, and eating.	• Monitor Harold's grief reactions, watching for statements of hopelessness, self-blame, agitation, or threats of suicide. • Encourage and support Harold in completing normal daily activities and contacts by helping him to plan a schedule and carry through with plans.	Harold did agree to meet with a counselor. He needed time to talk, to cry, and to feel the pain of grief. He did so with the counselor.
• Within 3 months, Harold will show evidence of reengaging in life's activities, including work and social interactions.	• Monitor Harold's physical condition. • Teach about grief work, normal responses, and strategies for dealing with grief reactions. • Underscore that grieving is real, it is painful, and it takes time to resolve.	Within 6 weeks, Harold was able to function adequately in the world. He went back to work and continued therapy. Harold understands grief and grief work intellectually. Harold is beginning to see a future for himself. Harold continues in counseling.

CRITICAL THINKING BAND

ASSESSMENT
What characteristics would you look for to distinguish normal grief from dysfunctional grief or depression?

NURSING DIAGNOSIS
How do you think grief is complicated by death through suicide? How can you differentiate normal grief from depression?

Outcomes
The time frame of grief resolution is highly individualized. How does a nurse establish outcomes? What do you do when your outcomes prove unrealistic?

Planning/Interventions
What nursing theory or theories do you think support your work in bereavement? Why?

Evaluation
How would you know if Harold's grief became a dysfunctional grief reaction? What would you look for?

FUTURE DIRECTIONS

The past 30 years have resulted in important advances in our ability to treat depression. New antidepressant medications will likely emerge at an ever-accelerating rate. Whether any of these will prove decisively superior to medications currently available remains to be seen.

One of the most important controversies in psychiatric care today is the role of antidepressant medications in treating persons who do not have Major Depressive Disorder. While the concept of Minor Depressive Disorder remains invalidated, studies suggest that antidepressants and cognitive and marital therapies may benefit persons with less profound depression. In recent years, clinicians have been willing to prescribe Prozac and other SSRIs to individuals who have few (or occasionally no) psychiatric symptoms. Many of these persons report feeling better and functioning more effectively in their jobs and personal lives (Kramer, 1993). Much concern has been expressed about the medical justification for prescribing medications whose primary purpose is to make individuals "feel and perform better." Some see this as a form of medicalized drug abuse, others as a legitimate medical practice (Nuland, 1994). Surely, these issues will continue to be major social and even political concerns in the coming years.

KEY CONCEPTS

◆ Mood swings are part of everyone's life; however, there are people for whom typical ups and downs become too extreme and too long.

◆ Depression is the intense feeling of a depressed, down mood.

◆ DSM-IV lists specific criteria for the depressive conditions of Major Depressive Disorder, Dysthymic Disorder, and Bereavement. Minor Depressive Disorder has not been validated by DSM but exists as a category for many who do not meet the exact criteria of other depressive disorders.

◆ A depressed person loses interest in activities that were previously enjoyable and often experiences loss of appetite or weight; sleep disturbance; fatigue; feelings of worthlessness; trouble with concentration; and recurrent thoughts of death or suicide.

◆ Persons who are grieving experience the same feelings as those who are depressed.

◆ Grief is a normal, albeit painful, human experience.

◆ Major theories that explain depression include psychoanalytic theory, object loss theory, learned helplessness theory, cognitive theory, and physical/biological theories.

◆ The nursing theories of Watson and Orem are particularly helpful in working with depressed clients.

◆ Caring nursing theories emphasize the need for the nurse to establish a trusting relationship with the client.

◆ The self-care deficit nursing theory addresses the need for the nurse to provide care to meet the client's needs that he is not able to meet on his own.

◆ Medications are frequently used in alleviating depressive symptoms. Tricyclic and related antidepressants, SSRIs, and MAO inhibitors are the most frequently used.

REVIEW QUESTIONS AND ACTIVITIES

1. Differentiate between unipolar and bipolar depression.

2. Identify those who are at risk for developing depression.

3. Describe the characteristics of major depression, minor depression, and dysthymia.

4. Describe bereavement or grief; identify the stages of normal grieving.

5. Consider a client diagnosed with major depression. Explain the depression from the perspective of each of the following theories: psychoanalytic, object loss, learned helplessness, cognitive, and physical/biological.

6. Watson's nursing theory guides practice with depressed persons. How would her theory suggest you initiate interaction with a client?

7. What nursing interventions for a depressed person are consistent with Orem's theory?

8. List assessment parameters for nursing care of one who is at risk for depression.

9. What are the cultural considerations related to nursing care of one who is depressed?

10. Suggest the process needed to validate nursing diagnoses associated with depression.

11. Describe independent nursing interventions for depression. How are these interventions evaluated in practice?

12. Describe the nurse's role in monitoring clients on tricyclic antidepressants and other drugs.

EXPLORING THE WEB

◆ Visit this text's "Online Companion™" on the Internet at **http://www.DelmarNursing.com** for further information on depression.

◆ What key terms might you search for on the Internet (for instance, psychosis, grief, bereavement)?

◆ What sites on the Internet could you recommend to families dealing with depression who are looking for self-help, chat rooms, or other electronic information sources?

REFERENCES

Abraham, I. L., Neese, J. B., & Westerman, P. S. (1991). Depression: Nursing implications of a clinical and social problem. *Nursing Clinics of North America, 26*(3), 527–544.

American Psychiatric Association *Diagnostic and Statistical Manual of Mental Disorders*, Fourth Edition. Washington, DC: American Psychiatric Association, 1994.

Beck, A. (1967). Depression: Causes and treatment. Philadelphia: University of Pennsylvania Press.

Bench, C. J., Friston, K. J., Brown, R. G., Frackowiak, R. S., & Dolan, R. J. (1993). Regional cerebral blood flow in depression measured by positron emission tomography: The relationship with clinical dimensions. *Psychological Medicine, 23*(3), 579–590.

Bolwig, T. (1993). Biological treatment other than drugs. In N. Sartorius, G. DeGirdano, G. Andrews, G. A. German, & L. Eisenberg (Eds.), *Treatment of mental disorders* (pp. 92–111). Washington, DC: American Psychiatric Press.

Bower, B. (1987). Bereavement: Reeling in the years. *Science News, 131*(6), 84.

Campbell, J. (1992). Treatment of depression in well older adults: Use of diaries in cognitive therapy. *Issues in Mental Health Nursing, 13*(1), 19–20.

Conn, V., Taylor, S., & Wiman, P. (1991). Anxiety, depression quality of life, and self-care among survivors of myocardial infarction. *Issues in Mental Health Nursing, 12*(4), 321–332.

Depression Guideline Panel. (1993). *Depression in primary care: Detection and diagnosis.* Rockville, MD: Agency of Health Care Policy and Research.

Fine, R. (1979). *A history of psychoanalysis.* New York: Columbia University Press.

Ford, K. (1992). Seasonal depression: Management of seasonal affective disorder. *Professional Nurse, 8,* 94–98.

George, M. S., Ketter, T. A., & Post, R. M. (1993). SPECT and PET imaging in mood disorders. *Journal of Clinical Psychiatry, 54,* 6–13.

Kramer, P. D. (1993). *Listening to Prozac.* New York: Viking Press.

Kurlowicz, L. H. (1993). Social factors and depression in late life. *Archives of Psychiatric Nursing, 7*(1), 30–36.

Leininger, M. M. (1978). *Transcultural nursing: Concepts, theories, and practices.* New York: John Wiley and Sons, Inc.

Manning, D. (1984). *Don't take my grief away.* San Francisco: Harper & Row.

Maynard, A. (1993). Comparisons of effectiveness of group interventions for depression in women. *Archives of Psychiatric Nursing, 7*(5), 277–283.

North, N. (1989). The effect of exercise on depression: A meta analysis. *Dissertation Abstracts International, 49*(11-B), 5027–5028.

North American Nursing Diagnosis Association (NANDA). (1996). *NANDA Nursing diagnosis: Definitions and classification: 1997–1998*. Philadelphia: Author.

Nuland, S. B. (1994). The pill of pills. *The New York Review of Books, XLI*(11), 48.

Orem, D. E. (1985). *Nursing: Concepts of practice* (3rd ed.). New York: McGraw-Hill.

Perris, C., & Herlofson, J. (1993). Cognitive therapy. In G. Andrews, G. A. German, & L. Eisenberg (Eds.), *Treatment of mental disorders* (pp. 151–153). Washington, DC: American Psychiatric Press.

Seligman, M. (1974). Depression and learned helplessness. In R. Friedman & M. Katz (Eds.), *The psychology of depression: Contemporary research and theory*. Washington, DC: Winson & Sons.

Steward, N., McMullen, L. M., & Rubin, L. D. (1994). Movement therapy with depressed inpatients: A randomized multiple single case study design. *Archives of Psychiatric Nursing, 8*(1), 22–29.

Watson, J. (1988). *Nursing: Human science and human care*. New York: National League of Nurses.

Wells, K. B., Katon, W., Rogers, B., & Camp, P. (1994). Use of minor tranquilizers and antidepressant medications by depressed outpatients: Results from the medical outcomes study. *American Journal of Psychiatry, 151*, 694–700.

Wells, K. B., Stewart, A., Hays, R. D., Burnam, M. A., Rogers, W., Daniels, M., Berry, S., Greenfield, S., & Ware, J. (1989). The functioning and well-being of depressed patients: Results from the medical outcomes study. *JAMA, 272*(7), 914–919.

Wiedenbach, E. (1964). *Clinical nursing: A helping art*. New York: Springer.

Worden, J. W. (1991). *Grief counseling and grief therapy* (2nd ed.). New York: Springer.

≋ LITERARY REFERENCES

Barnes, J. (1985). *Flaubert's parrot*. New York: Knopf.

Chekhov, A. (1954). Uncle Vanya. In *Plays* (E. Fen, Trans., pp. 185–247). New York: Viking.

Ch'i, K. (1966). Written on seeing the flowers and remembering my daughter. In R. F. Weir (Ed.), *Death in literature* (p. 156). New York: Columbia University Press.

Fitzgerald, F. S. (1945). *The crack-up*. New York: New Directions.

Flaubert, G. (1983). *Madame Bovary*. In D. J. Enright (Ed.), *The Oxford book of death* (pp. 113–114). Oxford: Oxford University Press.

Irish, J. (1980). A boy thirteen. In R. F. Weir (Ed.), *Death in literature* (pp. 180–181). New York: Columbia University Press.

Svevo, I. (1949). *As a man grows older*. New York: New Directions.

Tolstoy, L. (1932/1882). *A confession and what I believe* (A. Maude, Trans.). London: Oxford University Press.

≋ SUGGESTED READINGS

Cohen, D. B. (1994). *Out of the blue: Depression and human nature*. New York: Norton.

Goodwin, F., & Redfield, K. *Manic-depressive illness*. New York: Oxford University Press.

Jamison, K. R. (1993). *Touched with fire*. New York: Free Press.

Williams, J. M. G. (1995). *The psychological treatment of depression: A guide to the theory and practice of congitive behavioral therapy*. New York: Routledge.

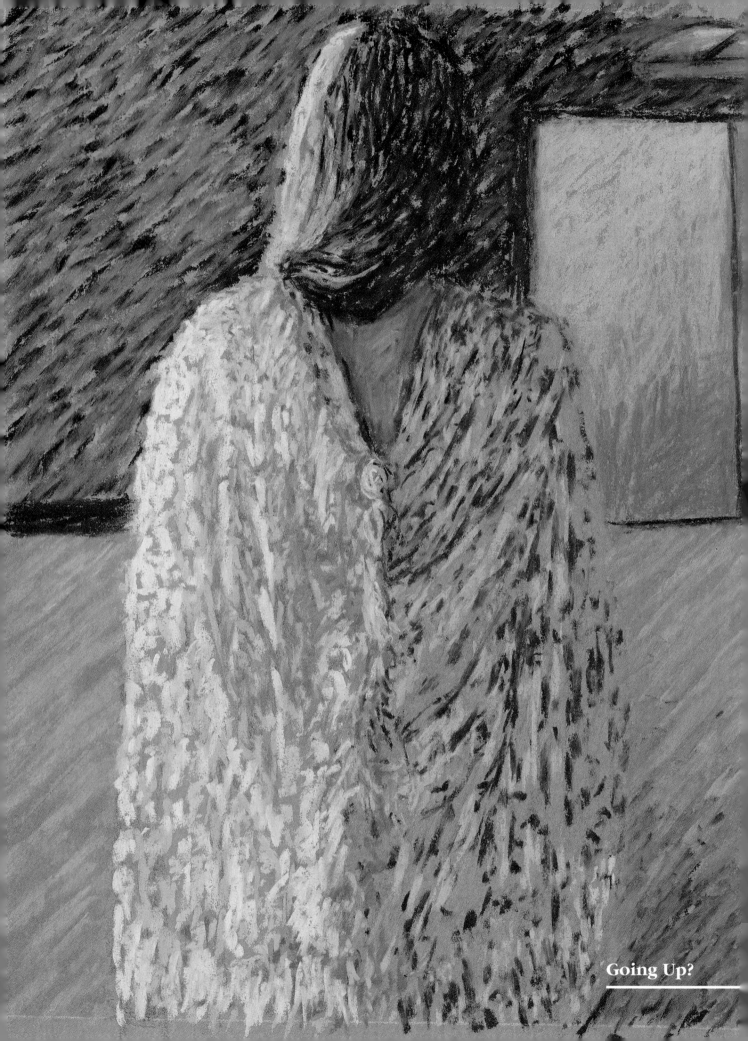

Going Up?

THE CLIENT EXPERIENCING MANIA

Noreen Cavan Frisch
Lawrence E. Frisch

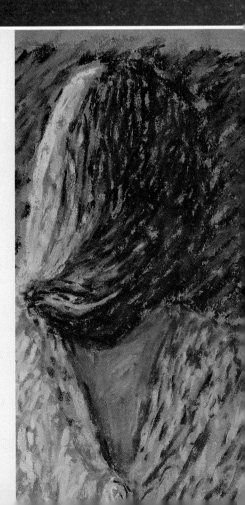

Life in the Fast Lane

Have you ever done any of the following?
- Neglected your physiological need for sleep because you were just too busy to rest?
- Found yourself driving on a freeway late at night with the radio on and the windows open to keep yourself awake when you knew you should be in bed rather than driving?
- Missed meals because work took precedence? Or eaten meals standing up, on the run, or in your car?
- Been completely involved in your own projects, such that you could not really explain to other people what you were doing and why?
- Neglected medical or dental appointments because you were just too busy?
- Became upset with others who told you they just could not understand what you were up to?

If you have experienced any of these situations, you have some notion of that part of life called "the fast lane." As you begin to learn about the mood disorder called mania, think of the disorder as an extension and exaggeration of the situations in which many of us find ourselves.

〰 CHAPTER OUTLINE

MANIA

Manic Episode

Hypomania

Bipolar Disorders

EPIDEMIOLOGY

ETIOLOGY

Molecular Basis

Other Causes
  Drugs
  Physical Disease

CLINICAL COURSE

Social Prognosis

Life Stress

ASSOCIATED DISORDERS/DUAL DIAGNOSES

Substance Abuse

Schizoaffective Disorder

Borderline Personality

BIPOLAR DISORDER AND CREATIVITY

TREATMENT AND CLINICAL MANAGEMENT

Pharmacological Treatment
  Acute Mania
  Maintenance Treatment
  Lithium
  Anticonvulsants

Psychotherapy

Other Treatments

NURSING PERSPECTIVES

NURSING THEORY

  Theory of Human Becoming
  Self-Care Deficit Theory

SUPPORT FOR THE CLIENT'S FAMILY

THE WARD MILIEU AND THE MANIC CLIENT

▽ NURSING PROCESS

▽ CASE STUDY/CARE PLAN

〰 COMPETENCIES

Upon completion of this chapter, the reader should be able to:

1. Define mania and state the behaviors associated with the condition.

2. Describe the cyclical relationship of mania and depression.

3. Explain the genetic and inherited nature of manic disease.

4. Describe the clinical course of mania.

5. Safely administer drugs in the treatment of mania.

6. Integrate nursing theory in assessing and understanding clients with mania.

7. Employ empathy in interactions with manic persons.

8. Use the nursing process and nursing diagnoses to plan and evaluate nursing care.

≋ KEY TERMS

Bipolar Disorder Mood disorder characterized by cyclic experiences with both mania and depression.

Borderline Personality A personality disorder characterized by a pervasive pattern of instability of interpersonal relationships, self-image, and objects, and marked impulsivity.

Continuous Cycling Recurrent movement from mania to depression without an intervening normal period.

Cyclothymic Pattern Cycle of an individual's mood changing back and forth between hypomanic and melancholic states.

Hypomania Mild form of mania (elevated mood) that lasts for only 4 days.

Mania Mood disorder characterized by an elevated, expansive, or irritable mood.

Manic Episode Distinct period of abnormally and persistently elevated, expansive, or irritable mood lasting at least 1 week.

Rapid Cycling Four or more episodes of mania in a year.

Schizoaffective Disorder Condition characterized by elements of schizophrenia and manic-depressive disorder.

Switch Process Mood changes between mania and depression.

Mania is a term used to describe a common disorder associated with an elevated, expansive, or irritable mood. Although many individuals suffer from both mania and depression at times in their lives, mania is in many ways the exact opposite of depression. For example, individuals with depression have a depressed and slowed mood, whereas individuals experiencing mania generally have a markedly elevated mood. Manic individuals are talkative, excitable, and energetic, and their words and ideas often move rapidly from topic to topic. Self-esteem and libido are usually decreased in depression. By contrast, in mania, self-esteem is inflated, often to the point of grandiosity, and sexual behavior may be indiscriminately impulsive. Manic individuals often go for days without sleep, and they may indulge in buying sprees and other impulsive activities with potentially destructive consequences. Many manic individuals lose touch with reality and become psychotic. They may be paranoid, agitated, or delusional, and they may suffer from hallucinations. Manic clients may span the spectrum from fascinating, creative company to violent, out-of-control individuals, highly dangerous to themselves and others. For the manic client, "life is 'effortless,' 'charged with intensity,' and 'filled with special meaning.' [The person] is 'racing,' 'speeded up,' 'wired,' 'hyper,' 'high as a kite,' 'moving in the fast lane,' 'ecstatic,' 'full of energy,' 'flying.' Other people are described as 'too slow' and 'can't keep up.'" (Goodwin & Jamison, 1990, p. 16).

Some psychiatrists have suggested that there are stages of mania, as illustrated in Table 13-1. As an individual moves between these stages, his mood, thinking, and behavior may all change. Like depression, mania is typically a cyclical disorder: Affected individuals go into and out of episodes of mania that may last a few days to many weeks. In between manic episodes, most of these individuals are unaffected and may lead highly productive lives. In fact, as will be discussed later in this chapter, many individuals who suffer from mania seem to be unusually creative, and when well, they may be successful professionals and leaders.

In the early stages of mania, an individual may recognize that his behavior is manic, as in this writing of the poet Theodore Roethke about his own manic episode:

For No Reason

For no reason I started to feel very good.
Suddenly I knew how to enter into the life of every-
thing around me. I knew how it felt to be a tree,
a blade of grass, even a rabbit. I didn't sleep much.
I just walked around with this wonderful feeling.
One day I was passing a diner and all of a sudden
I knew what it felt like to be a lion. I went into the
diner and said to the counter-man, "Bring me a
steak. Don't cook it. Just bring it." So he brought

Table 13-1 Stages of Mania

	STAGE I	STAGE II	STAGE III
Mood	Lability of affect; euphoria predominates; irritability if demands not satisfied	Increased dysphoria and depression, open hostility and anger	Clearly dysphoric; panic stricken; hopeless
Cognition	Expansivity, grandiosity, overconfidence; thoughts coherent but occasionally tangential; sexual and religious preoccupation; racing thoughts	Flight of ideas; disorganization of cognitive state; delusions	Incoherent, definite loosening of associations; bizarre and idiosyncratic delusions; hallucinations in one-third of patients; disorientation to time and place; occasional ideas of reference
Behavior	Increased psychomotor activity; increased initiation and rate of speech; increased spending, smoking, telephone use	Continued increased psychomotor acceleration; increased pressured speech; occasional assaultive behavior	Frenzied and frequently bizarre psychomotor activity

From "The Stages of Mania: A Longitudinal Analysis of the Manic Episode," by G. A. Carlson and F. K. Goodwin, 1973, *Archives of General Psychiatry*, *28*, 221–228.

me this raw steak and I started eating it. The other customers made like they were revolted, watching me. And I began to see that maybe it was a little strange.*

(Seager, 1991, p. 101)

In an excerpt from *Outside the Dog Museum*, the novelist Jonathan Carroll also captures some of the strange behavior seen in Stage I mania:

Going Insane

There was no screech of tires, screams, or thunderous crash when my mind went flying over the cliff into madness, as I gather is true in many cases. Besides, we've all seen too many bad movies where characters scratch their faces or make hyena sounds to indicate they've gone nuts.

Not me. One minute I was famous, successful, self-assured Harry Radcliffe in the trick store, looking for inspiration in a favorite spot. The next, I was quietly but very seriously mad, walking out of that shop with two hundred and fifty yellow pencil sharpeners. I don't know how other people go insane, but my way was at least novel.

Melrose Avenue is not a good place to lose your mind. The stores on the street are full of lunatic desires and are only too happy to let you have them if you can pay. I could.

Anyone want an African gray parrot named Noodle Koofty? I named him in the ride back to Santa Barbara. He sat silently in a giant black cage in the back of my Mercedes station wagon, surrounded by objects I can only cringe at when I think of them now: three colorful garden dwarves about three feet high, each holding a gold hitching ring; five Conway Twitty albums that cost twenty dollars each because they were "classics"; three identical Sam the Sham and the Pharaohs albums, "classics" as well, twenty-five dollars a piece; a box of bathroom tiles with a revolting peach motif; a wall-size poster of a chacma baboon in the same pose as Rodin's The Thinker . . . other things too, but you get the drift.

(Carroll, 1992, pp. 16–17)

Although this last excerpt is from a novel, an almost identical story comes from the real-life descriptions of a manic individual:

Mania

Unfortunately, for manics anyway, mania is a natural (if unnatural) extension of the economy. What with credit cards and bank accounts there is little beyond reach. So, I bought twelve snake bite kits, with a sense of urgency and importance. I bought precious stones, elegant and unnecessary

---

The Glass House: The Life of Theodore Roethke by Allan Seager [Ann Arbor: The University of Michigan Press (1991)].

*From *Outside the Dog Museum*, by J. Carroll, 1992, New York: Doubleday. Reprinted with permission.

furniture, three watches within an hour of one another (in the Rolex rather than Timex class) . . . and totally inappropriate siren-like clothes. During one spree I spent several hundreds on books having titles or covers that somehow caught my fancy: . . . twenty sundry Penguin books because I thought it could be nice if the penguins could form a colony, five Puffin books for a similar reason . . . I imagine I must have spent far more than $30,000 during my two manic episodes.

(Goodwin & Jamison, 1990, p. 29)

Although the experience of Stage I mania is often described as highly pleasant with "great joy and elation" (Goodwin & Jamison, 1990, p. 26), as mania persists and progresses, it takes on more frightening, or ego-dystonic, aspects:

The First Time I Was Manic

In fact, the most awful I have ever felt in my entire life . . . was the first time I was manic. I had been high many times before, but they had never been frightening experiences—ecstatic at best, confusing at worst. In fact, I had learned to accommodate quite well to them. I developed mechanisms of self-control to keep down the peals of otherwise singularly inappropriate laughter, and rigid limits on my irritability. I learned to avoid situations that might otherwise trip or jangle my hypersensitive wiring, and I learned to pretend I was paying attention or following a logical point when my mind was off chasing rabbits in a thousand directions. My work and professional life flowed. But nowhere did this, or my upbringing, or my intellect, or my character, prepare me for insanity. Although I had been building up to this for weeks, and certainly knew something was seriously wrong, there still was a definite point when I knew I was insane. My thoughts were so fast that I couldn't remember the beginning of a sentence halfway through. Fragments of ideas, images, sentences raced around and around. . . . Finally . . . they became meaningless melted pools. Nothing once familiar to me was familiar. I wanted desperately to slow down but could not. Nothing

---

*Excerpted from Manic Depressive Illness by Frederick K. Goodwin and Kay Redfield Jamison. Copyright © 1990 by Oxford University Press, Inc. Reprinted by permission.

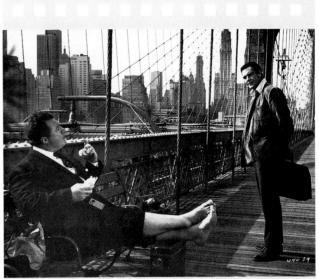

A Fine Madness. Source: Warner Brothers/Courtesy Kobal.

A manic episode was portrayed in *A Fine Madness*—a 1966 movie classic. The main character experiences an expansive, "up" mood, has lots of energy, is impulsive and talkative, and engages strangers in lengthy conversations.

helped—not running around a parking lot for hours on end or swimming for miles. My energy level was untouched by anything I did.

(Goodwin & Jamison, 1990, p. 27)

MANIA

While the excerpts provide an intuitive idea of which behaviors are considered manic, there are specific definitions of the mania. These are divided into categories, based on the severity of the symptoms.

Manic Episode

A **manic episode** is defined as follows:

◆ A distinct period of abnormally and persistently elevated, expansive, or irritable mood lasting at least 1 week (or any duration if hospitalization is necessary).

◆ During the period of mood disturbance, three (or more) of the specific symptoms listed in the display on the next page have persisted to a significant degree.

For a diagnosis of manic episode, symptoms causing marked impairment in job or personal functioning that are not due to illness, drugs, or medications must be present.

MANIC BEHAVIORS

◆ Inflated self-esteem or grandiosity

◆ Decreased need for sleep (e.g., feels rested after only 3 hours of sleep)

◆ More talkative than usual or pressure to keep talking

◆ Flight of ideas or subjective experience that thoughts are racing

◆ Distractibility (i.e., attention too easily drawn to unimportant or irrelevant external stimuli)

◆ Increase in goal-directed activity (either socially, at work or school, or sexually) or psychomotor agitation

◆ Excessive involvement in pleasurable activities that have a high potential for painful consequences (e.g., engaging in unrestrained buying sprees, sexual indiscretions, or foolish business investments)

Reprinted with permission from *Diagnostic and Statistical Manual of Mental Disorders* (4th ed.). American Psychiatric Association, Copyright 1994, Washington, DC: Author.

Hypomania

While extreme mania is clearly abnormal, some experts believe that there is no fine line dividing normal happiness and mild mania: Indeed most of us probably have some maniclike experiences at times in our lives (Klerman, 1981). Mild manic states may become abnormal when they are recurrent, lengthy, and associated with "an unequivocal change in functioning that is uncharacteristic of the person when not symptomatic" (American Psychiatric Association, 1994, p. 338). In an effort to capture this difference between normal happiness and mild mania, the fourth edition of the *Diagnostic and Statistical Manual* (DSM-IV) also defines **Hypomania**. The defining characteristics of hypomania include the same seven criteria for mania, but to diagnose hypomania, only three symptoms need be present, and these need only have lasted 4 days. In contrast to mania, hypomanic symptoms need not cause any disturbance in functioning but must be observable by others.

Bipolar Disorders

While mania is an important psychiatric condition and requires unique nursing and medical interventions, it is most commonly seen along with Major Depressive Disorder (MDD). The combination of mania and depression is typically referred to as **Bipolar Disorder** (**BPD**). Although clients may be depressed and manic at the same

time, the two conditions most commonly occur sequentially: Most often the mania comes first, followed soon after by depression. Psychiatrists refer to the mood change from mania to depression or depression to mania as the **switch process**. The association between depression and mania has been recognized for more than 2,000 years:

Aretaeus

According to Aretaeus (100 AD), the classical form of mania was the bipolar one: the patient who previously was gay, euphoric, and hyperactive suddenly "has a tendency to melancholy; he becomes, at the end of the attack, languid, sad, taciturn, he complains that he is worried about his future, he feels ashamed."

"Melancholia is without any doubt the beginning and even part of the disorder called mania."*

(Roccataggliata, 1986, pp. 230–231)

This linkage between mania and depression had not been forgotten when in 1679 Brouchier wrote about a client: "There are twin symptoms, which are her constant companions, Mania and Melancholy, and they succeed each other in a double and alternate act" (Goodwin & Jamison, 1990, p. 45). While the association between these disorders has been long and consistently recognized, modern clinicians now regard mania and depression (when they occur together in the same client) as a single disorder with two manifestations. This synthesis into the term *bipolar* or *manic-depressive illness* was most decisively made in the early years of this century by the German psychiatrist Kraepelin. In recent years, Post and coworkers at the National Institute of Mental Health have tried to summarize Bipolar Disorder graphically. Figure 13-1 presents a summary of the clinical course of 82 bipolar persons (Post, Roy-Byrne, & Uhde, 1988). From this representation, it can be seen that depression and mania may occur either separately or in close proximity to each other. Except when due to organic causes, mania almost never occurs without depression: Nearly all persons with mania have a form of Bipolar Disorder.

DSM-IV defines two types of bipolar major depressive disorders: Bipolar I and Bipolar II. Bipolar I is classic manic-depressive disease, with the combination of depression and at least one episode of mania. Bipolar II is diagnosed when one hypomanic episode has accompanied major depression but there has been no mania. DSM-IV also describes **cyclothymic patterns** in which individuals cycle between hypomanic and melancholic states but do not qualify for a diagnosis of Major Depressive Disorder (and hence Bipolar II).

---

*From A HISTORY OF ANCIENT PSYCHIATRY, G. Roccataggliata. Copyright 1986 by Greenwood Publishing Group Inc., Westport, CT.

Median Course of Affective Illness in 82 Manic-Depressive Patients

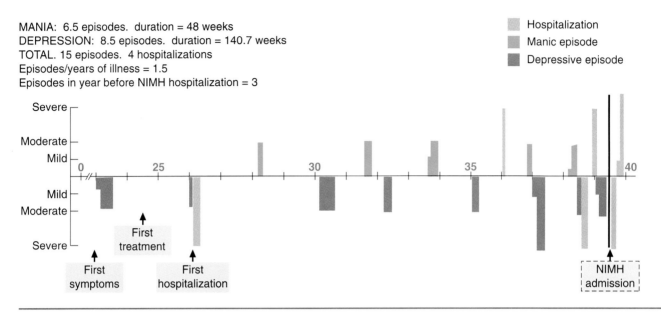

MANIA: 6.5 episodes. duration = 48 weeks
DEPRESSION: 8.5 episodes. duration = 140.7 weeks
TOTAL. 15 episodes. 4 hospitalizations
Episodes/years of illness = 1.5
Episodes in year before NIMH hospitalization = 3

Figure 13-1   Clinical course of mania. *From "Graphic Representation of the Life Course of Illness in Patients with Affective Disorder," by R. M. Post, P. P. Roy-Byrne, and T. W. Uhde, 1988,* American Journal of Psychiatry, 145, *p. 847. Copyright 1988 by the American Psychiatric Association. Reprinted by permission.*

EPIDEMIOLOGY

Epidemiological surveys are consistent in showing that neither mania nor bipolar disorder are particularly common in the population as a whole. Leff, Fischer, and Bertelson (1976) found that in 1976 only 2.6 persons per 100,000 were newly hospitalized for mania each year. Others have confirmed similar values and suggested that mania (of a degree requiring hospitalization) is the rarest of all the major psychoses (Krauthammer & Klerman, 1979). While severe mania may be relatively rare, the nurse working at a community mental health facility is certain to see this condition regularly, in part because individuals with severe mania often experience recurrent manic episodes. For example, in a random community-based household survey, Fogarty, Russell, Newman, and Bland (1994) found a lifetime prevalence of mania of 0.6%, but in those who reported mania, the mean number of manic episodes was 23.

While severe mania is relatively rare, the milder forms, for which clients may often not seek hospitalization—or even treatment—are not uncommon. The Epidemiologic Catchment Area Study (discussed in more detail in Chapter 7) found lifetime prevalence rates for Bipolar I disorder of 4.4% (Weissman, Bruce, Leaf, Florio, & Holzer, 1991). This means that over a lifetime, about 4% of individuals are likely to experience at least one manic episode. Unipolar depressive disorder is about two to four times more common than is bipolar disease, but the difference in rate of occurrence is obscured somewhat by the way in which the two conditions affect men and women differ-

ently. Since women are about twice as likely to be affected by unipolar depression as are men but women are no more likely than are men to have Bipolar Disorder, some of the difference in rate between the two conditions is due to the increased frequency of unipolar disorder in women. Depressive disease in men is about evenly divided between unipolar and Bipolar Disorder.

While women may not have a higher overall incidence of bipolar depression than do men, the length of their symptom cycles can be different in important ways from those of men. One of the major characteristics of Bipolar Disorder is cycle length: the time between episodes. While cycle length may vary from weeks to years and may gradually accelerate over time (with episodes eventually coming more frequently; see Figure 13-1), psychiatric epidemiologists have arbitrarily divided persons with manic-depressive disorder into those with long and those with short cycle lengths, the latter being called rapid cyclers. Rapid cyclers are defined as individuals who have four or more episodes in a year. While the overall incidence of Bipolar Disorder does not differ much between men and women, nearly all rapid cyclers are women (Pariser, 1993). Rapid cyclers may be particularly difficult to treat, so that, while rapid cyclers constitute only 13% to 20% of persons with manic-depressive disorder (Calabrese & Woyshville, 1994), these persons may seek care more frequently than would be predicted from their absolute numbers.

While the onset of bipolar disease can occur from childhood to old age, on the average, persons with Bipolar Disorder tend to become ill in their 30s or before, a decade earlier than do those with unipolar disease (Goodwin & Jamison, 1990). Bipolar Disorder seems to occur with fairly comparable incidence among persons of widely differing ethnicity and race. Carefully controlled studies in China suggest few differences from manic-depressive disorder seen in the United States (Dunner, Jie, Ping, & Dunner, 1984) Although most mental illness seems to disproportionately affect the poor, at least some forms of bipolar disease occur more often among the well-off, particularly affecting men with professional or managerial jobs (Coryell et al., 1989).

ETIOLOGY

A very striking finding about bipolar depressive disorder is its tendency to be inherited. Some of the best data on the inheritance of manic-depressive illness come from studies of twins (Goodwin & Jamison, 1990). If one of two identical twins is manic-depressive, the other is almost certain to develop the disease. For fraternal twins (who share much less of their genetic makeup), the risk is much lower, about 20%. While social and environmental factors surely play a role in how (and perhaps whether) some mental illness develops, genetics seems to be the strongest influence for manic-depressive disorder. Even when identical twins are separated early in life and brought up in completely different adoptive families, when one has manic-depressive disorder, the risk for the second twin seems to be at least 70%. Manic-depressive disorder is not only shared between twins, it is also often passed from parents to their children.

Mariana

With blackest moss the flower-plots
Were thickly crusted, one and all:
The rusted nails fell from the knots
That held the pear to the gable-wall.
The broken sheds looked sad and strange:
Unlifted was the clinking latch;
Weeded and worn the ancient thatch
Upon the lonely moated grange.
She only said, 'My life is dreary,
He cometh not,' she said;
She said, 'I am aweary, aweary,
I would that I were dead!'

(Tennyson, 1830)

Here is Tennyson at his poetic gloomiest and seemingly a match for the tragic story told by Jamison's psychological genealogy of the Tennyson family (Figure 13–2). While the Tennyson family tree illustrates a remarkable inheritance of mental illness, including manic-depressive disease, it also illustrates the inheritance of both unipolar and bipolar depression within manic-depressive families. The finding that unipolar depression is common in relatives of clients with Bipolar Disorder has been shown in more formal studies as well: Clients with manic-depressive disorder are two to three times more likely to have relatives with unipolar or bipolar disorder than are controls (Gershon et al., 1982).

While twin studies and case-control studies provide strong evidence that manic-depressive disorder is often inherited, in recent years geneticists have sought stronger confirmation of the way in which Bipolar Disorder is transmitted. There are potentially two approaches to obtaining this confirmation. The first is to define a defective gene product (typically a protein) thought to cause manic-depressive illness and then look for its presence in affected persons and their relatives. This approach has not yet proved possible. The second approach is to seek other well-defined genetic conditions that are inherited along with Bipolar Disorder. Often, the conditions sought produce no symptoms but are only detected by chemical analysis of protein or DNA. These kinds of studies, known as linkage studies, can be powerful genetic tools and have been remarkably productive in studying other psychiatric/neurological conditions (Gusella et al., 1983). Studies to date have suggested some linkage between Bipolar Disorder and several chromosome sites—most recently on chromosome 18—but have not produced any breakthroughs in our understanding of the genetics of manic-depressive disease. It is highly probable that the next decade will see major advances in this field.

Most of the previous observations apply largely to Bipolar I disorder. The frequency of Bipolar II disorder is less well understood. One study suggested a community prevalence of between 8% and 12% percent (double that for Bipolar I), but this finding has not been confirmed, in part because questionnaire survey instruments may be less reliable for manic symptoms than they are for depression (Goodwin & Jamison, 1990).

The cause of manic-depressive illness is not known. There have been numerous theories about the factors causing the disorder, but none yet seems remotely adequate to explain the clinical findings. It is widely believed that manic-depressive disease is due to some genetically determined biochemical abnormality of the brain. Support for this view comes from the technique of positron emission tomography (PET) scanning. The PET scan is somewhat similar to the computed tomography (CT) scan, but instead of viewing brain structure, it detects areas of metabolic activity. While the significance of findings remains unknown, there do appear to be recognizable differences between brain metabolism in normal persons and in persons suffering from mania. As noted in Chapter 12 on depression, many experts believe that abnormalities of brain neurotransmitters such as serotonin and dopamine

Alfred, Lord Tennyson Partial Family History

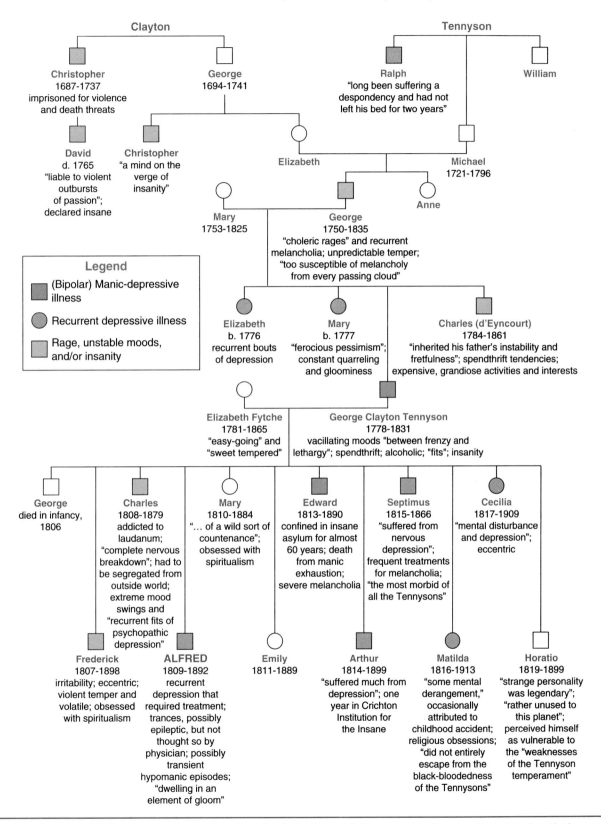

Figure 13-2 Psychologic genealogy: family with bipolar and depressive disease. *Reprinted with the permission of the Free Press, a division of Simon & Schuster from TOUCHED WITH FIRE: Manic Depressive Illness and the Artistic Temperament by Kay Redfield Jamison. Copyright © 1993 by Kay Redfield Jamison.*

play a major role in affective disorder. Bipolar clients have different patterns of urinary and plasma catecholamines than do unipolar depressed patients. Although these findings are interesting and fairly consistent (Goodwin & Jamison, 1990), they do not yet offer any clear causal information about bipolar depression. Recently, scientists have sought an explanation for Bipolar Disorder in brain serotonin's transporting protein, but while serotonin surely plays a role in depressive symptoms, its transporting protein may not be involved.

Molecular Basis

One of the interesting goals of research on Bipolar Disorder has been to define the molecular basis for the switch process—the change, often very sudden, between depressive and manic states. Work on switching has been limited by the great difficulty in distinguishing between cause and effect: Although a given measurement—typically an increase in a chemical substance in blood, urine, or spinal fluid—may cause switching, it may also be, like the observed change in mood, merely the result of switch.

Other Causes

Drugs

A diagnosis of a manic episode can be made only when symptoms have no definable organic cause. Some illnesses and many drugs can precipitate mania. It is important that these factors be considered before a client is labeled with a psychiatric diagnosis or potentially treated inappropriately. While persons of any age may have organic causes of mania, since most manic episodes present for the first time before the age of 40, organic causes should always be sought in older adults presenting with a first episode of mania (Young & Klerman, 1992).

Alcohol and drug withdrawal (particularly from benzodiazepines) are among the most common extrinsic factors leading to agitated states and may be particularly hard to diagnose if, as is often the case, clients do not admit to drug use. The administration of antidepressants [including selective serotonin reuptake inhibitors (SSRIs) like Prozac (see Chapter 12)] may precipitate mania in some individuals. Although these individuals probably do have Bipolar Disorder, control of manic symptoms usually requires stopping antidepressant medication. The elderly are particularly sensitive to drug effects and may develop either mania or delirium in response either to single drugs or to polypharmacy (the administration of multiple drugs, often for multiple medical indications). Common drugs that may induce mania in clients of any age include oral corticosteroids and levodopa. Clients taking anabolic steroids may be at particular risk for mania and may not admit to steroid use even if asked (Pope & Katz, 1994). Other medications that may occasionally cause mania

include baclofen, bromocriptine, captopril, chloroquine, and thyroxine (Peet & Peters, 1995). Intoxicated persons (particularly with stimulant drugs such as cocaine, PCP, or amphetamines) frequently present with mania.

Physical Disease

A wide range of diseases can also produce mania. Among infectious diseases, syphilis, human immunodeficiency virus (HIV), and Lyme disease should always be considered (Fallon, Nields, Parsons, Liebowitz, & Klein, 1993). Thyroid and other endocrine abnormalities (particularly Cushing's disease or syndrome) can cause manic symptoms. Many neurological conditions, including brain tumors and the aftermath of brain injury from trauma or stroke, can precipitate mania (Strakowski, McElroy, Keck, & West, 1994).

CLINICAL COURSE

As emphasized in Figure 13-1, the spectrum of Bipolar I disorder includes recurrent episodes of both mania and depression. Episodes may last several months to a year or more and are often shortened by effective treatment. For any given person, the length of episodes is fairly constant, with manic episodes typically somewhat shorter than depressive episodes (Goodwin & Jamison, 1990). As implied in the passage from Theodore Roethke quoted earlier in this chapter, the following excerpt relates how suddenly manic episodes can appear:

In the Summer of 1955

In the summer of 1955 when I was 33, the thousand unacknowledged human . . . pressures in my being exploded. I ran barefooted in the streets, spat at members of my own family, exposed myself, was almost bodily thrown out of the house of a Nobel Prize-winning author, and believed God had ordained me to act out every conceivable human impulse without an ounce of hypocritical caution.

(Krim, 1961, p. 64)

Depressive symptoms are generally thought more likely to develop over days or weeks, although, as in the following personal description by the famous psychologist William James, they can also occur with striking rapidity:

Suddenly

Suddenly there fell upon me without any warning, just as if it came out of the darkness, a horrible fear of my own existence. Simultaneously *there arose in my mind the image of an epileptic patient whom I had seen in the asylum, a black-haired youth with greenish skin, entirely idiotic, who used to sit all day on one of the benches . . . with his knees drawn up against his chin. . . . This image and my fear entered into a species of combination with the other. . . . It was as if something hitherto solid within my breast gave way entirely, and I became a mass of quivering fear. After this the universe was changed for me altogether. . . . (My fear) gradually faded, but for months I was unable to go out into the dark alone.**

(James, 1961, pp. 160–161)

Individual episodes in clients with manic-depressive disease may be either manic or depressive. Manic and depressive phases may follow each other rapidly (Winokur, Clayton, & Reich, 1969), or clients may have only a single episode of either mania or depression. About half of persons with Bipolar Disorder begin their illnesses each with a single depressive episode and no history of mania. Individuals differ widely in cycle length, with more than four episodes per year defined as **rapid cycling**; occasional clients exhibit **continuous cycling**, which is defined as recurrent movement from mania to depression without an intervening normal period.

Social Prognosis

Although continuous cyclers do not have normal intercycle periods, the remainder of bipolar individuals seem quite unaffected between episodes. On recovery, many return successfully to their families and jobs; however, the social prognosis of bipolar disorder is not uniformly good. In one study where clients were followed up 6 months after hospital admission for mania, 80% were free of symptoms, but only 21% were fully employed (Dion, Tohen, Anthony, & Watermaux, 1988). In a longer follow-up study, significant psychosocial and occupational impairments were documented in clients, despite remissions of up to 2 years (Coryell et al., 1993).

Clients with manic-depressive disorder not only have psychosocial difficulties as a result of their illness, they are also at risk of dying from it. All-cause mortality is approximately twice as high for manic-depressive clients as for age-matched controls, but coexisting medical conditions seem to account for most natural causes of death (Black, Winokur, & Nasrallah, 1987). Suicide, discussed at more length in Chapter 14, is a major risk for clients with

---

*From THE VARIETIES OF RELIGIOUS EXPERIENCE, by William James (New York: Macmillan, 1961).

> ### ⚡ NURSING ALERT!
> #### Risk for Suicide in Mania
> The risk of successful suicide in persons with mania increases in the presence of substance abuse or prior suicide attempt (Goodwin & Jamison, 1990).

Bipolar Disorder. Although one older study suggested that 46% of all suicides occur in persons with manic-depressive illness, this finding has not been corroborated by other studies. More consistently, researchers have found a high suicide rate among persons with Bipolar Disorder: as high as 60% in some studies, but with a mean of 19% (Goodwin & Jamison, 1990).

There is some evidence that persons who are appropriately treated and intensively followed have diminished likelihood of suicide. Nonetheless, a retrospective review of 92 suicides by manic-depressive individuals found that 70% of these occurred despite high-quality medical and psychiatric care (Schou & Weeke, 1988).

Life Stress

Life stresses may precipitate manic-depressive illness, particularly the first-ever episode, but the majority of recurrent episodes seem to occur without external stimuli (Goodwin & Jamison, 1990). Sleep deprivation may sometimes trigger mania, and in some persons, symptoms seem to respond to restorative sleep (Nowlin-Finch, Altshuler, Szuba, & Mintz, 1994).

One of the curious, and not absolutely consistent, aspects of mania is its seasonal tendency. Numerous studies suggest that mania is more likely to present in the summer than at other times of the year (Takei et al., 1992).

ASSOCIATED DISORDERS/DUAL DIAGNOSES
Substance Abuse

One of the factors that complicates both the understanding and the treatment of manic-depressive disorder is that many persons with this diagnosis have other complicating psychiatric diagnoses. Among such dual diagnoses, alcohol abuse plays a particularly important role since there are strong associations between Bipolar Disorder and alcohol abuse, especially in men. Although there are problems with consistent definition of alcohol abuse among different studies, about 35% of persons with manic-depressive disorder is said to abuse alcohol. The corresponding rate for the population as a whole is probably one-third to one-half of this (Goodwin & Jamison, 1990). At least one study suggested a much stronger relationship between alcoholism and mania than between alcohol and depression (Helzer & Prybeck, 1988). While studies have not consistently shown higher alcohol intake during manic as compared to depressive phases, some observers have suggested steady and frequent drinking during mania contrasted with more binge drinking during depressive phases. There have been few studies comparing individuals with Bipolar I and Bipolar II disorders, but where this question has been examined, alcohol abuse does seem to be associated with both diagnoses (Goodwin & Jamison, 1990). Non-alcoholic-substance abuse is similarly associated with Bipolar Disorder, cocaine being a particularly commonly used substance during manic episodes. Whether the high frequency of cocaine use reflects specific efforts to replicate or prolong manic euphoria or merely reflects community drug usage patterns is unknown. Persons with bipolar disorders are also said to engage in excessive use of narcotics, marijuana, and hallucinogens.

Schizoaffective Disorder

A second very important dual diagnosis is **schizoaffective disorder**, bipolar type, a condition in which elements of schizophrenia combine with manic-depressive disorder. Schizoaffective persons have prolonged delusions and/or hallucinations, typically at times when their mood disorders (either mania or depression or both) are in remission. It is often difficult to determine whether persons have pure manic-depressive illness or are schizoaffective, but long-term prognosis may be worse for individuals in the latter category (Goodwin & Jamison, 1990). Since they are by definition psychotic, schizoaffective clients are more difficult to treat successfully than are purely manic-depressive individuals, and, like schizophrenics whom they resemble, they often have major difficulties holding jobs and maintaining personal relationships.

Borderline Personality

Clients with **borderline personality** often overlap diagnostically with Bipolar II disorder. As discussed in Chapter 16, these individuals have very rapid mood swings that tend to react much more to their environment than do the moods of purely hypomanic clients. Recognizing subtle bipolar features is important in the assessment of borderline personality. If Bipolar II is present and not diagnosed, a manic attack may result from administering antidepressant medication to one who is bipolar but thought to be borderline.

BIPOLAR DISORDER AND CREATIVITY

Madness

The greatest of goods comes to us through madness. . . . The prophetess at Delphi and the priestesses at Dodona achieve much that is good for Greece when mad, both on a private and on a public level, whereas when sane they achieve little or nothing; . . . Among the ancients too those who gave things their names did not regard madness as shameful or a matter of reproach; otherwise they would not have connected the very word with the finest of the sciences, that by which the future is judged, and named it "manic." No, they gave it the name thinking madness a fine thing. . . . The man who arrives at the doors of poetry without madness from the muses, persuaded that expertise will make him a good poet, both he and his poetry, the poetry of the sane, are eclipsed by that of the mad.

(Plato in Rowe, 1974)

Thus, the ancient Greeks appreciated that madness and mania could form the basis for poetic inspiration. A remarkable number of modern poets, writers, artists, and musicians have suffered from manic-depressive disorder, and many psychologists and artistic critics have felt that this illness contributed significantly to their artistic greatness. Experts may not agree that the manic state truly facilitates artistic creativity—surely few individuals in Stage 2 or 3 mania are sufficiently in touch with reality to produce creatively—but there is little doubt that the unusual psychic energy and decreased needs for sleep associated with hypomania make for enhanced productivity. Perhaps the willingness to take risks seen in mania also has a counterpart in productive creative work, where risk taking may lead to unanticipated accomplishment.

Not only is manic-depressive illness frequently seen among creative artists, but striking mood swings also appear with some frequency among political and military leaders. When writing of historical figures or creative artists, it is of course highly risky to try to make psychological diagnoses from fragmentary sources. Despite this problem, Goodwin and Jamison (1990) suggest after careful consideration that a surprising array of famous historical figures may have suffered from elements of manic-depressive illness. Individuals considered by Goodwin and Jamison to have been influenced by cyclothymia or hypomania include Oliver Cromwell, Alexander Hamilton, Napoleon Bonaparte, Robert E. Lee, Theodore Roosevelt, Winston Churchill, and Benito Mussolini. Goodwin and Jamison note that biographies of notable poets, composers, and artists document a prevalence of extremes in mood; however, it is important to recognize that many creative persons have no psychopathology: "that the illness and its related temperaments are associated with creativity seems clear. The clinical, ethical, and social implications of this association are less so" (p. 367).

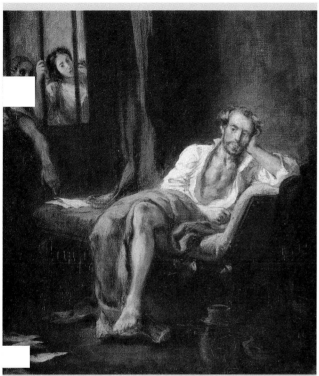

Tasso in the Asylum by Eugene Delacroix.
Courtesy of Oskar Reinhart Collection. "Am Römerholz," Winterthur.

The English Romantic poet Lord Byron was one of the 19th century's best documented manic-depressives. Not surprisingly, he wrote a number of long poems whose narrators or subjects were either frankly manic or had manic characteristics: His widely read "Lament of Tasso" romanticized the life of 16th-century Italian poet Torquato Tasso, who was confined seven years for what seems to have been a combination of psychosis (probably manic) and political imprudence. The painting (by another great Romantic artist) contrasts the poet's repose with the manic intensity of the arm forced between the bars of his cell. The woman at the bars is also striking, perhaps an inmate, perhaps a lover or wife.

The Lament of Tasso

When the impatient thirst of light and air
Parches the heart: and abhorred grate,
Marring the sunbeams with its hideous shade,
Works through the throbbing eyeball to the brain
With a hot sense of heaviness and pain.

(Byron, 1905)

TREATMENT AND CLINICAL MANAGEMENT

Pharmacological Treatment

Acute Mania

The acute condition is most effectively treated with either benzodiazepines or neuroleptic (antipsychotic) agents (see also Chapter 25). Benzodiazepines [clonazepam (Klonopin) is frequently used] are helpful in controlling nonpsychotic symptoms of pressured speech, hyperactivity, agitation, and anxiety. Delusions, flight of ideas, and extreme combativeness may require an antipsychotic such as haldol. Neither antipsychotic medications nor benzodiazepines have any direct effect on the manic process. Valproic acid (Depakene) does have a direct mood-stabilizing effect, and it may begin to work within 24 to 72 hours. Consequently, it is sometimes administered as part of the initial pharmacological treatment of acute mania. One report documents the effectiveness of a lengthy first night of sleep in some patients presenting with acute mania to an inpatient facility (Nolan-Finch et al., 1994). While such sleep therapy may be potentially dangerous if it is achieved only with high doses of medication, it certainly has much to commend it for simplicity and the client's need for rest.

Maintenance Treatment

The 1993 AHCPR Clinical Practice Guidelines for depression do not treat bipolar depression separately from unipolar depression. These guidelines recommend maintenance pharmacological treatment for all persons who have had three or more episodes of major depressive disorder or for those with two episodes of major depression and one of the following:

1. Family history of bipolar disorder or recurrent major depression (parent or sibling)
2. History of recurrence within 1 year after medication being discontinued
3. First episode occurring before age 20
4. Both episodes that were severe, sudden, or life-threatening and occurred within 3 years

Analysis of published data suggests that for Bipolar Disorder, only two relapses might justify maintenance without any of the additional preceding criteria. Goodwin and Jamison (1990) suggest that even a single episode justifies long-term prophylaxis if the first episode is manic, the client is male, onset is sudden or later than age 30, the episode is severe or suicidal, no external precipitants were involved, and/or the client is an adolescent.

Lithium

Clients with mania are often treated with lithium, a widely used medication for manic-depressive disorder. Discovered to be effective in 1949 and used in this country since the late 1960s, lithium has been shown to have beneficial effects in the great majority of people treated. Lithium is used both to treat individual episodes of mania and to prevent recurrences of both mania and depression. Multiple studies have established the efficacy of lithium in both treatment and prevention of symptom recurrence. Lithium is most effective in persons whose symptoms began after puberty (Goodwin & Jamison, 1990) and who are not short cyclers (have fewer than four episodes yearly). Other than a therapeutic trial, there is no satisfactory way to predict which individuals will or will not respond to lithium.

Lithium is given orally in one to three 300-mg doses. Lithium affects all parts of the body; however, three organs are most important to evaluate for potential adverse effects: the thyroid gland, for possible hypothyroidism, which occurs in 5% to 35% of cases; the kidneys, since lithium is excreted through the kidneys and it has been established that lithium decreases renal concentrating ability; and the nervous system, since tremor and decreased motor coordination occur in some individuals. Before initiating treatment, blood counts, electrolyte and other chemistry determinations, urinalysis and creatinine clearance, and thyroid studies should be done; these should be repeated at 6-month to yearly intervals during maintenance treatment. After an acute episode of mania, lithium is typically continued for at least 6 to 12 months (Goodwin & Jamison, 1990) and then consideration is given to long-term maintenance treatment. Lithium levels must be carefully monitored to prevent toxicity associated with overdose. Potentially interfering drugs must be avoided. These include certain antibiotics, many antihypertensive drugs, and anticonvulsants. Lithium takes up to 2 weeks to have any effect on mood. Side effects include increased thirst and appetite, weight gain, memory problems, and impaired motor coordination. While lithium may cause cardiac arrhythmias, there is no evidence that this is dangerous in persons without heart disease (Albrecht & Muller-Oerlinghausen, 1980). Thyroid replacement treatment is occasionally required in clients on long-term lithium treatment. Lithium is embryotoxic, particularly in the first trimester, so women taking lithium need to avoid pregnancy or at least understand the risks of fetal anomaly (see also Chapter 25).

Lithium's major side effects concern neurological and cognitive functioning. While some psychiatrists believe that these effects may be lessened by keeping lithium blood levels at the lowest consistent with effectiveness, there is little scientific data to support this view. Clients may need to accept slowed mental functioning in trade for the "leveling off" of emotions that typically results from lithium use. This is not a trade-off that will be acceptable to all clients.

Compliance is a problem for many clients. Kate Millett, author and painter, has described her own ambivalence about restarting lithium in the face of recurrent symptoms of mania:

⚡ NURSING ALERT!

Lithium Toxicity

Warning Signs of Lithium Toxicity

- ◆ Anorexia
- ◆ Nausea and vomiting
- ◆ Hand tremor
- ◆ Muscle twitching
- ◆ Hyperactive deep tendon reflexes
- ◆ Ataxia
- ◆ Tinnitus
- ◆ Vertigo
- ◆ Weakness, drowsiness

Signs of Lithium Intoxication

- ◆ Fever
- ◆ Decreased urine output
- ◆ Decreased blood pressure
- ◆ Irregular pulse
- ◆ Electrocardiographic changes
- ◆ Altered level of consciousness
- ◆ Seizures
- ◆ Coma
- ◆ Death

✳ NURSING TIP

Managing Lithium Toxicity

- ◆ Obtain history.
- ◆ Discontinue lithium doses.
- ◆ Evaluate vital signs.
- ◆ Obtain blood lithium level.
- ◆ Obtain other blood work: electrolytes, blood urea nitrogen, creatinine, urinalysis, and complete blood count.
- ◆ Evaluate cardiac status through electrocardiography.
- ◆ If acute overdose, provide emetic.
- ◆ Provide hydration.
- ◆ In severe cases, implement osmotic diuresis (with urea or mannitol), increase lithium clearance (with aminophylline), provide intake of NaCl to promote lithium excretion, and implement dialysis.

Lithium

I maintain that . . . the issue is my own free-dom: to take lithium or not to as I choose. It's a voluntary program I was in. Even my shrink doesn't capture people and put them away; he has given me his word on this a number of times. I am free to go off lithium, then if I so choose, though the results of doing so are in his opinion dire. And the experience of my friend Martha Ravich is dire too . . . a professional photographer. She was manic as a monkey, they say. I'd like to know what she says. But I know she's back on lithium. Humiliation, capitulation, cure? That was her attempt to throw the drug; the shaky hands (lithium's side effect), which she hated just as I do, needing steady hands for the camera as I do for the brush. The fear in the trembling hands that hold a 16mm movie camera. I always thought her hands were unsteady because they had scared her, broken her confidence. Thereafter you are afraid, unsound; they have said so, proved it with incarceration with the parole of medication, the continual and eternal doses of lithium—without which you will always be crazy, will lapse into it again in weeks. Look at me—it is six weeks, and I do not feel crazy even though now they say I am. Because I stopped lithium? . . . If I had never told would they know?*

(Millett, 1990, pp. 65–66)

The use of lithium in writers and creative artists has been studied, and there is a suggestion that lithium does have negative effects on some aspects of creativity (Shaw, Mann, Stokes, & Manevitz, 1987). In studies reported by Goodwin and Jamison (1990), 4 of 24 artists and writers refused to continue taking lithium because of side effects of loss of work effectiveness. Two other subjects reported that their productivity was decreased but agreed to continue medication at least for the study's duration.

One client with manic-depressive illness came to terms with the meaning of lithium in his life. He wrote the "Rules for the Gracious Acceptance of Lithium into Your Life," presented in the accompanying display as a guide for all.

Clearly, with a medication that has so many actual and potential physical and psychological side effects, it is important for clients to clearly understand the risks and benefits of taking lithium, particularly when it is given for long-term prophylaxis of mood symptoms. The nurse has

---

*Copyright © 1990 by Kate Millett. Reprinted by permission of Georges Borchardt, Inc. for the author.

RULES FOR THE GRACIOUS ACCEPTANCE OF LITHIUM INTO YOUR LIFE

1. Clear out the medicine cabinet before guests arrive for dinner or new lovers stay the night.
2. Remember to put the lithium back into the cabinet the next day.
3. Don't be too embarrassed by your lack of coordination or your inability to do well the sports you once did with ease.
4. Learn to laugh about spilling coffee, having the palsied signature of an eighty year old, and being unable to put on cufflinks in less than 10 minutes.
5. Smile when people joke about how they think they "need to be on lithium."
6. Nod intelligently, and with conviction, when your physician explains to you the many advantages of lithium in leveling out the chaos in your life.
7. Be patient when waiting for this leveling off. Very patient. Re-read the Book of Job. Continue being patient. Contemplate the similarity between the phrases "being patient" and "being a patient."
8. Try not to let the fact that you can't read without effort annoy you. Be philosophical. Even if you could read, you probably wouldn't remember most of it anyway.
9. Accommodate to a certain lack of enthusiasm and bounce which you once had. Try not to think about all the wild nights you once had. Probably best not to have had those nights anyway.
10. Always keep in perspective how much better you are. Everyone else certainly points it out often enough and, annoyingly enough, it's probably true.
11. Be appreciative. Don't even consider stopping your lithium.
12. When you do stop, get manic, get depressed, expect to hear two basic themes from your family, friends, and healers:
    ◆ But you were doing so much better, I just don't understand it.
    ◆ I told you this would happen.
13. Restock your medicine cabinet.

From MANIC-DEPRESSIVE ILLNESS by Frederick K. Goodwin and Kay R. Jamison. Copyright © 1990 by Oxford University Press, Inc. Used by permission of Oxford University Press, Inc.

a major role in assisting clients to understand the known effects of lithium and the reasons why it is recommended. Unfortunately, because of the variable and highly individual course of bipolar disorder, it is hard to assess any individual's outcome with certainty. Still, several studies (Page, Benaim, & Lappin, 1987; Coppen & Abou-Saleh, 1988) show excellent long-term prevention of both mania and depression with the use of lithium.

Anticonvulsants

Anticonvulsants, particularly carbamazepine (Tegretol) and valproic acid, have been used with some frequency in treating manic-depressive disorder. Their quicker action may make them of value in acute mania, and their different profile of side effects may offer advantages when, for example, renal dysfunction makes the use of lithium difficult or dangerous. These medications, particularly carbamazepine, seem to have their most important use in clients who do not respond to a therapeutic trial of lithium. Because of the high incidence of nonresponse among rapid-cycling bipolar clients, some psychiatrists will begin them directly on an anticonvulsant. The indications for acute and maintenance use of anticonvulsants are probably the same as those for lithium. Carbamazepine is begun at low dose (typically 100 mg in a single dose) and increased as tolerated, usually to 600 to 1,000 mg/day in divided doses, until blood levels reach a therapeutic level of 6 to 10 µg/ml. Valproic acid (most commonly, Depakene) is typically given in a dose of 500 to 1,000 mg daily with blood levels of 50–100 micrograms per ml.

Lithium and carbamazepine can be used together, particularly for rapid cyclers or for those who have dose-dependent lithium side effects such as excessive urination or memory difficulties. While the antimanic effectiveness of carbamazepine has been well established, there is somewhat less evidence demonstrating its antidepressant effect in bipolar disorder.

Side effects of carbamazepine include drowsiness, ataxia, dizziness, visual difficulties, tremor, nausea, rash, liver test abnormalities, and changes in white blood count. Carbamazepine is related to tricyclic antidepressants, so persons sensitive to these drugs should not use carbamazepine. Periodic blood testing and serum levels are required for safe and effective use. Valproic acid side effects are usually minimal but include sedation, tremor, headache, and visual disturbance. A small percentage of clients develop massive liver damage while on valproic acid. This typically occurs without warning, is independent of dosage, and to date has not affected persons over 12 years of age (Werder, 1995).

Psychotherapy

It is uniformly accepted that the primary treatment for Bipolar Disorder is medication. Treating bipolar

---

⚙ RESEARCH HIGHLIGHT

Incorporating Research into Practice

PURPOSE

A nurse researcher reports on the development, initial use, and evaluation of self-management groups for inpatients with bipolar disorder.

METHODS

Using research as a basis for designing the groups, the nurse changed the emphasis of inpatient groups from an interactional to a self-management model. The primary difference between the two is in the degree of structure for setting an agenda for the group sessions. In the interactional model, the session topics are identified by the participants at the beginning of each session. In the self-management groups, a structure is provided by having the therapist set a theme for each meeting. The topics for the self-management group sessions were taken from data obtained from a group of prior patients.

FINDINGS

An evaluation of the sessions was completed by surveying participating patients at discharge. Inpatients reported value in the educational aspects of the groups. The researcher reports plans to further compare the interactional approach to the self-management approach.

IMPLICATIONS

The study demonstrates a direct link of research to practice back to research. Thus, nursing interventions can be grounded in knowledge of what is most beneficial to clients.

From "Treatment of Inpatients with Bipolar Disorders: A Role for Self-Management Groups," by L. E. Pollack, 1995, *Journal of Psychosocial Nursing, 33*(1), pp. 13–16.

---

clients with psychotherapy alone is thought by some to be at least ethically dubious (Goodwin & Jamison, 1990) if not negligent. Nonetheless, there is much support in the literature for the combined use of medication and psychotherapy in the management of manic-depressive illness. There have been few if any good clinical trials showing that psychotherapy adds to the effectiveness of treatment, and it is likely that not all clients require psychotherapeutic interventions. At least two studies (Cochran, 1984; Glick et al., 1985) do suggest better outcome for clients receiving individual and family psychotherapy. One of the major goals in psychotherapy is to increase compliance in taking lithium, and there is evidence that psychotherapy does enhance that compliance (Paykel, 1995). From a nursing perspective, Pollack (1994) has conducted self-management groups for clients with Bipolar Disorder (see Research Highlight). In addition to compliance, issues addressed by nurse-led psychotherapy can include dealing with vocational and interpersonal issues, helping clients come to terms with their feelings about past manic and depressive episodes, and assisting clients in dealing with fear about the potential recurrence of symptoms. For some clients, there is real concern about the risk of passing manic-depressive disorder on to children, and this concern can be addressed in a group setting. For many clients, group therapy can be guided to help persons deal with common problems affecting those with bipolar disorder (Goodwin & Jamison, 1990).

Other Treatments

There are some situations where treatments other than medications and psychotherapy will be used, and the following merit mention. Although rarely used, electroconvulsive therapy is effective in treating mania (Small, Milstein, & Small, 1991) (see Chapter 30). It may have a role in situations where lithium is contraindicated, particularly during early pregnancy. Some evidence supports the usefulness of calcium channel blockers in mania unresponsive to either lithium or anticonvulsants (Cook & Winokur, 1990).

NURSING PERSPECTIVES

The nurse caring for a manic client must begin with an understanding of the disorder and a recognition that the experience of the condition is unique to each individual. To be effective, the nurse will need to handle three major components of care:

1. Use nursing theory to assess how to best assist the client in dealing with a chronic condition.

2. Determine how to support the client's family in adapting to having a family member with Bipolar Disorder.

3. In cases where the nurse works on an inpatient unit, establish a supportive ward milieu for the manic client and the other clients on the unit.

Each of these will be addressed in the following discussion.

NURSING THEORY

It often is difficult for nurses to understand the experiences and the point of view of a manic client. In a manic state, the client appears out of control or on the verge of being so. The client does not have the time or interest to sit and talk with the nurse and frequently does not see any way that a nurse can assist him and/or does not understand why others view him as confused. In between manic episodes, the client must come to terms with the knowledge that he has a chronic illness and that professionals are recommending a continuous dose of medications for management of the condition. Further, the client experiences a range of emotions—ecstasy, joy, fear, depression, embarrassment, guilt—when going through life and reflecting on his past behaviors.

Theory of Human Becoming

Parse's theory (Hickman, 1995) is a very useful perspective in a situation where the nurse must build rapport and a beginning level of trust with a client too busy to be bothered with establishing a nurse-client relationship and in a situation where the client seeks ongoing support in coming to terms with illness. The theory suggests that individuals find personal meaning in the process of living. Further, the theory states that each person establishes his own value priorities, making sense out of his existence. Thus, the nurse does not need to focus on the nurse's reality or bring control to her interactions with the client (neither of which the client would easily accept). Rather, the nurse brings presence and unconditional support. The nurse seeks to understand the client's interpretation of his lived experiences. Nursing interventions begin with being fully present for the person and making no demands.

⊗⊘ *REFLECTIVE THINKING*

The Decision To Use Lithium

Consider Kate Millet's discussion on her own, very personal decision to use or not to use lithium. (Excerpt can be found in lithium discussion found earlier in this chapter.)

Understanding that each individual makes personal choices and understands his condition based on his own interpretation of life, his own values, and his own lived experiences, consider the following:

◆ Can a nurse or psychiatrist ever really know what is best for another?

◆ Under what conditions can mental health professionals force an individual to receive treatments or medications he does not choose to take?

◆ Describe a collaborative (rather than paternalistic) model of psychiatric care.

Next, in the context of caring and support, the nurse will tease out multiple complex realities of the client's experiences. Understanding the client's world will form the basis for nursing care. Nursing interventions must be planned, then, within the context of the client's meaning in life, his goals, and his illness. Consider the exercise in the Reflective Thinking display on previous page from the perspective of Parse's theory.

Self-Care Deficit Theory

When a client is clearly out of control and unable to meet even his own basic needs, the nurse may use Orem's Self-Care Deficit theory to guide the nursing role. According to Orem's theory, in situations where patient agency is limited and the client is unable to care for his own health needs, the nurse must ensure that those needs are met. Thus, in situations where the client is potentially dangerous to self or others, the nurse has a role to intervene and provide for safety. For example, when a manic client is on the verge of physical exhaustion and yet does not see the need to stop physical exercise, the nurse may have to establish her ability and authority to see that the client stops, rests, and takes fluids as the nurse cares for the client's physical needs.

In other situations, particularly when the nurse and client have an ongoing therapeutic relationship, the client may ask the nurse to intervene in his manic behaviors before he engages in behaviors that will be hurtful and/or embarrassing to him later. In such cases, the client will tell the nurse or his psychiatrist or mental health workers that he wants to be stopped if he stops sleeping, becomes agitated, spends large sums of money, and the like. In such a case, the client tells the nurse in advance which behaviors he believes indicate he has lost ability to care for himself, and the nurse knows when interventions (such as hospital admission) are indicated.

SUPPORT FOR THE CLIENT'S FAMILY

Family members and close friends/significant others are often involved in the client's care and frequently seek support and education from nurses. Because of the inherited nature of the disorder, family members may request genetic counseling and may report others in the family who are either depressed or manic. These family members may seek education about the disease, and most will benefit from having someone listen to their feelings and responses to the information that a family member has

bipolar disease. Worry of becoming ill, fear of not being able to handle the client, and guilt over the genetic aspects of passing a disease on to offspring are common themes expressed by families. The nurse's role is one of both support and listening as well as one of educating the family and friends about the disease and what to expect. Because manic individuals may rapidly cycle into depression, the risk of self-injury and suicide must be discussed with family and friends.

THE WARD MILIEU AND THE MANIC CLIENT

One aspect of caring for the manic individual that challenges every psychiatric nurse is the overall management of a hospital inpatient unit when one (or two or three) manic individual(s) arrive on the floor. Taking a perspective from systems theory, consider that a ward may be in equilibrium. Clients and staff have their personalities, activity levels, patterns for day-to-day activities, and unwritten rules of how interactions take place. Once an individual arrives in a state of mania, the equilibrium is upset, and all of the old, predictable patterns of activity and interactions change. The manic client is hospitalized because he is unable to control racing thoughts, feels full of energy, and knows that his life is filled with special meaning. Feelings of grandiosity are a common part of the presenting symptoms, as are feelings of paranoia. Thus, the manic client has more energy and stamina than anyone else present, more ideas of what should be done on the unit, and more confidence than others in his abilities to fix any perceived problem. In addition, the manic client has less ability to use social conventions when approaching others and will not pick up on other's nonverbal indicators that they want to be alone. Experienced nurses offer the following suggestions for coping with this situation:

1. Take a deep breath and relax.
2. Remember that just as anxiety is contagious, so are feelings of calm and peace.
3. Work together with all unit staff to project an image of patience and confidence.
4. Treat all persons with respect and dignity.
5. Provide the manic client with enough personal space so that he does not disturb others with behaviors he cannot control. Often a private room is indicated.

Take these suggestions and ask other psychiatric nurses for additional ideas.

NURSING PROCESS

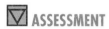 ASSESSMENT

Nursing assessment should begin with presenting symptoms, past history of manic and depressive cycles, evaluation of compliance with prescribed medications, and supporting data. Assessment for a newly hospitalized client should include the current status of the client, including information on the following:

♦ How long has this manic episode lasted?

♦ When was the last time the client slept or ate?

♦ What is the degree of irritability?

♦ What is the potential for violent outbursts?

♦ Is the client oriented and in touch with reality?

♦ Is the client exhibiting delusions?

♦ What event precipitated the client's coming in for care?

Further, assessment should include observations for data that support the diagnosis of mania. The accompanying displays present such supporting data and present questions the nurse might ask when completing the initial assessment interview.

NURSING DIAGNOSIS

Nursing diagnoses most commonly assigned manic individuals are listed in Table 13-2 on the following page. These nursing diagnoses are grouped into categories: safety needs, physical needs, social needs, cognitive needs, and family needs.

OUTCOME IDENTIFICATION

First, outcomes will be based on meeting immediate needs of safety and physical supports. The nursing care plan should reflect these as priorities and establish that these basic needs must be met. Second, the nurse will initiate care directed at meeting the client's needs and desires for appropriate social contacts with others; the expected outcome will be that client will interact within socially acceptable boundaries. Lastly, the nurse will provide care related to cognitive aspects of the disease, with a focus on assisting the client to manage his illness. Outcomes such as "the client will recognize own behaviors that place him at risk for manic episodes" or "the client will seek help to prevent the exacerbation of symptoms" are examples of outcome statements that may be appropriate.

SUPPORTING ASSESSMENT DATA FOR THE CLIENT WITH MANIA

Evaluate for the presence of the following:

♦ Euphoric, expansive, or irritable mood

♦ Excessive use of make-up, jewelry, and brightly colored clothing, which the person may change several times a day

♦ Hyperverbal speech, including slurred speech, flight of ideas, loose associations, and racing thoughts

♦ Irritability when ideas and plans are thwarted

♦ Intrusiveness and poor sense of boundaries

♦ Inability to sit still or join an activity that requires participation

♦ Expansiveness, with indiscriminate enthusiasm for interpersonal, sexual, or occupational interests

♦ Inflated self-esteem or grandiosity

Adapted from *Instant Nursing Assessment: Mental Health*, by P. D. Mabbett, 1996, Albany, NY: Delmar.

SEVEN QUESTIONS TO ASK WHEN ASSESSING A MANIC CLIENT

1. Do you experience ups and downs in your moods?

2. Do you have difficulty focusing your thoughts or conversation?

3. Have you spent more money than usual recently?

4. When is the last time you slept, and how long did you sleep?

5. Have you noticed a change in your sexual interest or sexual activity recently?

6. Do you feel irritated when other people tell you to slow down or when they do not seem to follow your thoughts?

7. Do you believe you have extraordinary abilities or powers?

Adapted from *Instant Nursing Assessment: Mental Health*, by P. D. Mabbett, 1996, Albany, NY: Delmar.

Table 13-2 Common Nursing Diagnoses for a Manic Client

AREA OF NEED	NURSING DIAGNOSIS
Safety needs	*Risk for violence*
	Risk for suicide
Physical needs	*Sleep pattern disturbance*
	Altered nutrition: less than body requirements
	Risk for exhaustion
Social needs	*Impaired social interaction*
Cognitive needs	*Altered thought processes*
	Impaired individual coping
	Ineffective management of the therapeutic regimen
Family needs	*Altered family processes*
	Risk for caregiver role strain

▽ PLANNING/INTERVENTIONS

Interventions include providing a safe and structured environment for the manic client, free of objects that could be used to harm self or others and free of extraneous noise or stimulation. All verbal communication from the nurse should be short, concise, and clear. With regard to client socialization, the nurse should provide an environment with minimal social contacts until the client is able to interact and must always ensure that the client is redirected away from situations that could be embarrassing upon recovery. Nursing interventions focus on the client's need to learn to manage his own condition. It is important to provide information about the disease, its treatment and progression, and sources of help. Lastly, assistance to the client's family/significant others is almost always required, as these persons need to become partners in the management of the condition.

▽ EVALUATION

When evaluating client progress, the nurse can first look at the client's surrounding environment to see that potential hazards have been removed and that excessive stimuli have been reduced or eliminated. Once immediate dangers to the client's physical well-being have been controlled, the nurse should consider the client's level of functioning and social interactions as compared to those at the beginning of treatment. The level of social interaction, for example, must take into account the client's cognitive abilities, desires, and initial level of functioning. The nurse must be careful to view progress in terms of degree and to view the actions of a client who has not inflicted physical harm to self or others during treatment as the first positive steps in a potentially long road to recovery.

CASE STUDY/CARE PLAN

Refer to the excerpt "The First Time I Was Manic," found in the introductory section of this chapter. Consider a client, whom we shall call Joe, who is describing his feelings that he knew he was going insane. He states, "My thoughts were so fast that I couldn't remember the beginning of a sentence halfway through." Further, he relates, "I wanted desperately to slow down but could not. Nothing helped—not running around a parking lot for hours on end or swimming for miles."

Imagine that Joe is our client.

ASSESSMENT

Joe has been admitted to the psychiatric hospital in an acute manic episode, referred from the emergency department. His three friends brought him to the hospital; they know him well and know that he has had two manic episodes before. His friend Tom states that Joe (34 years old) has been prescribed lithium, but that no one really knows if Joe has been taking it. Tom says that Joe has not slept in days and that he has been out running today for approximately 3 hours. No one knows the last time Joe had anything to eat. Joe agreed to come to the hospital with his friends, evidently willing to accept that he "needed a rest." Upon admission, Joe could not communicate well and exhibited flight of ideas. Although he was oriented to person and place, Joe did not know the date. Joe has agreed to get a rest; however, he is pacing the floor when the psychiatric nurse arrives and states he is "ready to rest, but there are a lot of things that need help around this place, and it took forever to get the doc to bring me here, and I ran across the marsh today and saw the gulls, and it's time for spring and when will school be out?"

ACUTE PHASE

NURSING DIAGNOSIS *Sleep pattern disturbance*, related to sensory alterations (psychological stress), as evidenced by verbal complaint of difficulty sleeping

Outcomes	Planning/Interventions	Evaluation
◆ Within the first 24 hours on the unit, Joe will sleep 4 hours and obtain rest.	◆ Provide Joe a private room. ◆ Keep stimulation to a minimum. ◆ Orient Joe to his room, letting him know that you are present and willing to assist him. ◆ Keep all conversation to a minimum. ◆ Establish trust by letting Joe know you are there to help meet his needs. Speak clearly, letting him know that you agree he does need rest. ◆ Administer medications as prescribed (Divalproex/valproic acid). ◆ Talk with Joe about the need for rest.	Joe says he isn't tired at all; he wants to know what is going on around the unit. Joe decides to take a shower; only after the shower does he agree to try to sleep; he goes to bed at 1:00 AM and does sleep until 7:00 AM.

NURSING DIAGNOSIS *Altered nutrition: less than body requirements*, as evidenced by reported inadequate food intake

Outcomes	Planning/Interventions	Evaluation
◆ Within 2 hours after admission, Joe will be adequately hydrated and will have eaten some food.	◆ Bring water, juice, cold beverages to Joe's room. ◆ Arrange for "finger foods" (sandwiches, crackers, and fruit) to be brought to Joe's room. For the first hour on the unit, offer food every 15 minutes.	At the nurse's direction, Joe consumed four glasses of water and two glasses of juice during the first 2 hours in the hospital. He also consumed one sandwich and three pieces of fruit over the next 24 hours.

NURSING DIAGNOSIS *Altered thought processes*, related to distractibility, racing thoughts, and inability to concentrate

Outcomes	Planning/Interventions	Evaluation
◆ Within 48 hours of admission, Joe will be able to concentrate on the immediate task at hand; he will be able to complete a sentence and carry on a simple conversation.	◆ Administer medications as prescribed; talk to Joe in simple, clear language; direct Joe to unit activities. ◆ Invite Joe to participate in a volley ball game. ◆ By late afternoon, communicate with Joe regarding his feelings of "things moving too fast."	Joe takes his medications; he states that the unit needs help in decorating and in making the environment "fun." He asks why there isn't more going on. Joe played the volleyball game, although he did not follow the rules of keeping score.

Continued

Outcomes	Planning/Interventions	Evaluation
		Joe states he understands he can't keep up with his thoughts; he has felt this way before.

RECOVERY PHASE

After 3 days in the hospital, Joe enters the recovery phase. He has slept well for two nights; he describes a basic understanding that he has missed medications and has entered a manic state again. The nursing care is now focused on helping Joe recognize risks for exacerbation of his symptoms and learn how to manage his own care at home. His friends have come to visit and have all told him he is doing much better. He is able to communicate with his friends.

NURSING DIAGNOSIS *Ineffective management of therapeutic regimen,* related to inability to report or recall prior compliance to medication regimen

Outcomes	Planning/Interventions	Evaluation
◆ By the time of hospital discharge, Joe will have a plan for compliance with his prescribed medication regimen and will understand the reasons for taking his medication.	◆ Refer Joe to a cognitive-therapy group for persons with bipolar disorder who have similar challenges and needs to Joe's. ◆ Instruct Joe about medications, diet, and side effects and provide information in writing. ◆ Arrange for the community mental health nurse to visit Joe's home for follow-up.	Joe attends the first group meeting his fourth day in the hospital (other clients in the group are outpatients); Joe indicates an understanding of his medications. Joe is willing to have the community nurse visit; the hospital nurse arranges for Joe to meet this nurse before discharge.

CRITICAL THINKING BAND

ASSESSMENT
How would you assess the safety of Joe's environment? What other questions could you ask Joe's friends to gain insight into the course of his illness?

NURSING DIAGNOSIS
What other nursing diagnoses would you develop for Joe? How do you assess for his safety? Do you have a concern regarding self-esteem and socialization?

Outcomes	Planning/Interventions	Evaluation
What outcomes are realistic for Joe? Can he return home to his own care? How will you know what is safe for him?	Are there other approaches to the care plan? Why does the nurse ask him to participate in a volleyball game? What activities are appropriate for a manic client on the unit where you work?	The nurse did not encounter escalating mania or violence with Joe. Have you seen risk for violence in a manic client? What did the nurse do? What are your feelings regarding the role of medication in the treatment of bipolar disorder?

⟪ KEY CONCEPTS

- ◆ The term *mania* is used to describe a disorder associated with an elevated, expansive, and/or irritable mood.

- ◆ Manic individuals frequently have grandiose thoughts and may become psychotic.

- ◆ There is a cyclical nature to the condition such that persons move between mania and depression.

- ◆ There are categories of mania, depending on severity. These include manic episode, hypomania, and bipolar disorder.

- ◆ Prevalence of mania is low; however, individuals with severe mania experience recurrent episodes and are frequently seen in psychiatric facilities.

- ◆ There is a tendency for Bipolar Disorder to be inherited.

- ◆ Current belief is that bipolar disease is due to some genetically determined abnormality.

- ◆ Certain drugs and physical diseases may produce symptoms of mania.

- ◆ Many persons with manic disease exhibit significant psychosocial and occupational impairments over time.

- ◆ There is a link between mania and mood disorders and persons with artistic and creative abilities.

- ◆ The primary treatment for mania is pharmacological.

- ◆ Due to unwanted side effects, lithium is a difficult drug for many to take over time.

- ◆ Nursing theory suggests means for the nurse to establish trust with manic clients.

- ◆ Specific nursing diagnoses can be used to describe and plan nursing care.

⟪ REVIEW QUESTIONS AND ACTIVITIES

Consider the following case: Mari, a 20-year-old college student, has been up for five nights in a row working on a project for her design class. She has not had time to sleep, eat, or bathe. She has plans to win a prize at an international exhibit, although this is her first attempt at design. She is enthusiastic and seems capable. When her roommates suggest that she take a break, she becomes angry and verbally abusive to them, stating she has to continue with her work. Her closest friend has just discovered that Mari has spent over $5,000 on this project and has neglected all of her other classes for the past week. Because you are a nursing student, her roommates come to you for advice.

1. What evidence do you have that Mari is exhibiting mania?

2. Does Mari fit into a risk category? How would you know?

3. What else would you want to know about Mari?

4. How could you tell if there were a potential for violence?

5. Where on your campus could you refer Mari for help?

6. At what point would you notify an authority on your campus about Mari's condition?

⚛ EXPLORING THE WEB

- ◆ Visit this text's "Online Companion™" on the Internet at **http://www.DelmarNursing.com** for further information on mania.

- ◆ What resources are listed for caregivers and health care professionals?

- ◆ Explore the various discussion areas and conferences that link clients, families, and caregivers involved with manic-depressive disease.

- ◆ What other key terms might you search (for instance, bipolar disorder, hypomania)?

⟪ REFERENCES

Albrecht, J., & Muller-Oerlinghausen, B. (1980). [Cardiovascular side effects of lithium]. *Dtsch Med Wochenschr, 105*, 651–655.

American Psychiatric Association. *Diagnostic and Statistical Manual of Mental Disorders* Fourth Edition. Washington, DC, American Psychiatric Association, 1994.

Bakker, R. H., Kastermans, M. C., & Dassen, T. W. N. (1995). An analysis of the nursing diagnosis *ineffective management of therapeutic regimen* compared to *noncompliance* and Orem's self care deficit theory. *Nursing Diagnosis, 7*, 161–166.

Black, D. W., Winokur, G., & Nasrallah, A. (1987). Is death from natural causes still excessive in psychiatric patients? A follow-up of 1593 patients with major affective disorder. *Journal of Nervous and Mental Diseases, 175*, 674–680.

Calabrese, J. R., & Woyshville, M. J. (1994). A medication algorithm for bipolar rapid cycling. *Journal of Clinical Psychiatry, 56* (Suppl. 3), 11–18.

Carlson, G. A., & Goodwin, F. K. (1973). The stages of mania: A longitudinal analysis of the manic episode. *Archives of General Psychiatry, 28*, 221–228.

Cochran, S. D. (1984). Preventing medical noncompliance in the outpatient treatment of bipolar affective disorders. *Consulting Clinical Psychology, 52*, 873–878.

Cook, B. L., & Winokur, G. (1990). Perspective on bipolar illness. *Comprehensive Therapy, 16*, 18–23.

Coppen, A., & Abou-Saleh, M. T. (1988). Lithium therapy, from clinical trials to practical management. *Acta Psychiatrica Scandinavica, 78*, 754–762.

Coryell, W., Endicott, J., Keller, M., Anderson, M., Growe, W., Hirschfield, R. M. A., & Scheftner, W. (1989). Bipolar affective disorder and high achievement: A familial association. *American Journal of Psychiatry, 146*, 983–988.

Coryell, W., Scheftner, W., Keller, M., Endicott, J., Maser, J., & Klerman, G. L. (1993). The enduring psychosocial consequences of mania and depression. *American Journal of Psychiatry, 150*, 720–727.

Depression Guideline Panel. (1993). *Depression in primary care: Detection and diagnosis.* Rockville, MD: Agency of Health Care Policy and Research.

Dion, G. L., Tohen, M., Anthony, W. A., & Watermaux, C. S. (1988). Symptoms and functioning of patients with bipolar disorder six months after hospitalization. *Hospital and Community Psychiatry, 39*, 652–657.

Dunner, D. L., Jie, S. Q., Ping, Z. Y., & Dunner, P. Z. (1984). A study of primary affective disorder in the People's Republic of China. *Biological Psychiatry, 19*, 353–359.

Fallon, B. N., Nields, J. A., Parsons, B., Liebowitz, M. R., & Klein, D. F. (1993). Psychiatric manifestations of lyme borreliosis. *Journal of Clinical Psychiatry, 54*, 263–268.

Fogarty, F., Russell, T. M., Newman, S. C., & Bland, R. C. (1994). Mania. *Acta Psychiatrica Scandinavica, 376* (Suppl.), 16–23.

Gershon, E. S., Hamovil, J., Guroff, J. J., Dibble, E., Leckman, L. R., & Banney, W. E., Jr. (1982). A family study of schizoaffective, bipolar I, bipolar II, unipolar, and normal control probans. *Archives of General Psychiatry, 39*, 1157–1167.

Glick, T. V., Clarkin, J. F., Spencer, J. H., Maas, G. L., Lewis, A. B., Peyser, J., DeMane, N., Good-Ellis, M., Harris, E., & Lestelle, V. (1985). A controlled evaluation of inpatient family intervention: Preliminary results of the six month follow up. *Archives of General Psychiatry, 42*, 882–886.

Goodwin, F. K., & Jamison, K. R. (1990). *Manic-depressive illness.* New York: Oxford University Press.

Gusella, J. F., Wexler, N. S., Conneally, P. M., Naylor, S. L., Anderson, M., Tanzi, R. E., Watkins, P. C., Ottina, K., Bonella, E., & Martin, J. B. (1983). A polymorphic DNA marker genetically linked to Huntington's disease. *Nature, 306*, 234–238.

Helzer, J. E., & Prybeck, T. R. (1988). The co-occurrence of alcoholism with other psychiatric disorders in the general population and its impact on treatment. *Journal on Studies of Alcohol, 49*, 219–224.

Hickman, J. S. (1995). Rosemarie Rizzo Parse. In J. George (Ed.), *Nursing theories: The base for professional nursing practice* (4th ed., pp. 335–354). Norwalk, CT: Appleton & Lange.

Klerman, G. L. (1981). The spectrum of mania. *Comprehensive Psychiatry, 22*, 11–20.

Krauthammer, C., & Klerman, G. L. (1979). The epidemiology of mania. In B. Shopsin (Ed.), *Manic illness* (pp. 11–28). New York: Raven.

Leff, J. P., Fischer, M., & Bertelson, A. C. (1976). A cross-national study of mania. *British Journal of Psychiatry, 129*, 428–442.

Mabbett, P. D. (1996). *Instant nursing assessment: Mental health.* Albany, NY: Delmar.

Nolan-Finch, N. L., Altshuler, L. L., Szuba, M. P., & Mintz, J. (1994). Rapid resolution of first episodes of mania: Sleep related? *Journal of Clinical Psychiatry, 55*, 26–29.

North American Nursing Diagnosis Association (1996). *NANDA nursing diagnoses: Definitions and classifications 1997–1998.* Philadelphia: NANDA.

Page, C., Benaim, S., & Lappin, F. (1987). A long term retrospective follow-up study of patients treated with prophylactic lithium carbonate. *British Journal of Psychiatry, 150*, 175–179.

Pariser, S. F. (1993). Women and mood disorders: Menarche to menopause. *Annals of Clinical Psychiatry, 5*, 249–254.

Paykel, E. S. (1995). Psychotherapy, medication combinations, and compliance. *Journal of Clinical Psychiatry, 56* (Suppl. 1), 24–30.

Peet, M., & Peters, S. (1995). Drug induced mania. *Drug Safety, 12,* 146–153.

Pollack, L. E. (1994). Treatment of inpatients with bipolar disorders: A role for self management groups. *Journal of Psychiatric Nursing and Mental Health Services, 33,* 11–16.

Pope, H. G., Jr., & Katz, D. L. (1994). Psychiatric and medical effects of anabolic-androgenic steroid use: A controlled study of 160 athletes. *Archives of General Psychiatry, 51,* 375–382.

Post, R. M., Roy-Byrne, P. P., & Uhde, T. W. (1988). Graphic representation of the life course of illness in patients with affective disorder. *American Journal of Psychiatry, 145,* 844–848.

Schou, M., & Weeke, A. (1988). Did manic-depressive patients who committed suicide receive prophylactic or continuation treatment at the time? *British Journal of Psychiatry, 153,* 324–327.

Shaw, E. D., Mann, J. J., Stokes, P. E., & Manevitz, A. Z. A. (1987). Effects of lithium carbonate on associative productivity and idiosyncrasy in bipolar outpatients. *American Journal of Psychiatry, 143,* 1166–1169.

Small, J. G., Milstein, J., & Smill, I. F. (1991). Electroconvulsive therapy for mania. *Psychiatric Clinics of North America, 14,* 887–903.

Strakowski, S. M., McElroy, S. L., Keck, P. W., Jr., & West, S. A. (1994). The co-occurrence of mania with medical and other psychiatric disorders. *International Journal of Psychiatry, 24,* 305–328.

Strober, M., & Carlson, G. (1982). Bipolar illness in adolescents with major depression: Clinical, genetic, and psychopharmacologic predictors in a three- to four-year prospective follow-up investigation. *Archives of General Psychiatry, 39,* 549–555.

Takei, N., O'Callaghan, E., Sham, P., Glover, G., Tamura, A., & Murry, R. (1992). Seasonality of admission in the psychoses: Effect of diagnosis, sex, and age at onset. *British Journal of Psychiatry, 161,* 506–511.

Weissman, M. M., Bruce, M. L., Leaf, P. J., Florio, L. P., & Holzer, C., III. (1991). Affective disorders. In L. N. Robins & D. A. Regier (Eds.), *Psychiatric disorders in America: The epidemiologic catchment area study* (pp. 53–80). New York: Free Press.

Werder, S. F. (1995). An update on the diagnosis and treatment of mania in bipolar disorder. *American Family Physician, 51,* 1126–1136.

Winokur, G., Clayton, P. J., & Reich, T. (1969). *Manic depressive illness.* St. Louis: Mosby.

Young, R. C., & Klerman, G. N. (1992). Mania in late life: Focus on age at onset. *American Journal of Psychiatry, 149,* 867–875.

⟿ LITERARY REFERENCES

Byron, Lord. (1905). *The complete poetical works of Lord Byron.* Boston: Houghton, Mifflin Company.

Carroll, J. (1992). *Outside the dog museum.* New York: Doubleday.

James, W. (1961). *The varieties of religious experience.* New York: Macmillan.

Krim, S. (1961). *Views of a nearsighted cannoneer.* New York: Excelsior.

Millett, K. (1990). *The looney-bin trip.* New York: Simon & Schuster.

Plato. (1988, c1986). *Phaedrus and the seventh and eight letters* (2nd ed.). (Trans. C. J. Rowe). Warminster, Wiltshire, England: Aris & Phillips.

Roccataggliata, G. (1986). *A history of ancient psychiatry.* Westport, CT: Greenwood Press.

Seager, A. (1991). *The glass house: The life of Theodore Roethke.* Ann Arbor, MI: University of Michigan Press.

Tennyson, A. (1968). *Poems & plays.* Oxford, England: Oxford University Press.

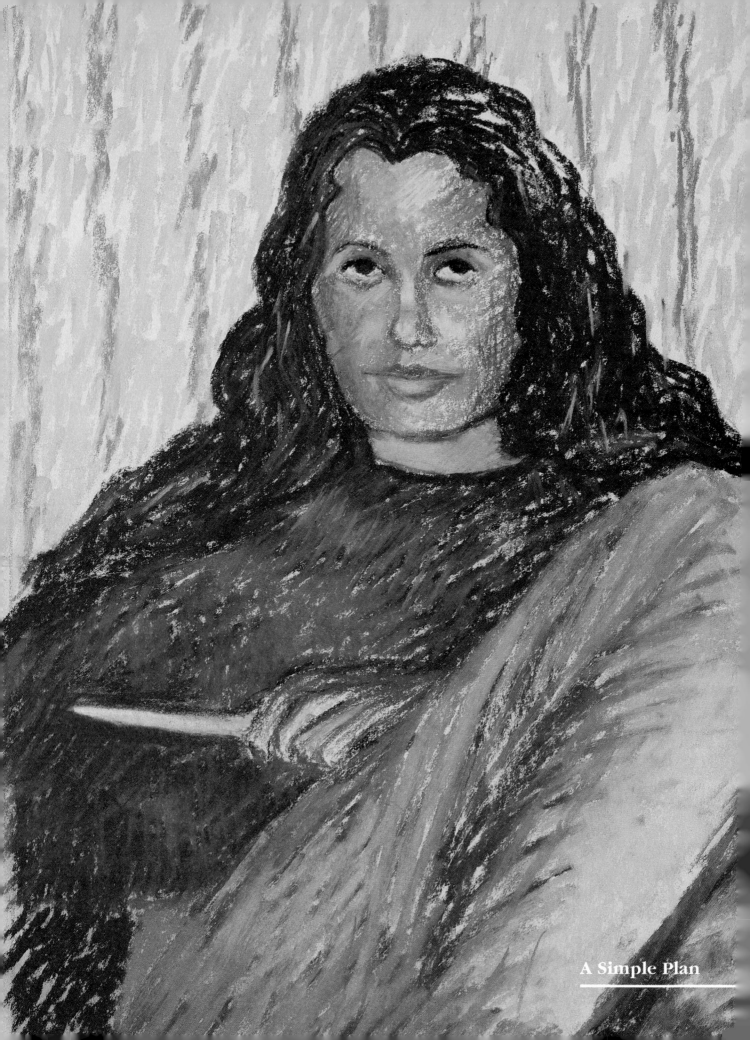

A Simple Plan

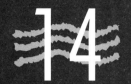

Chapter

14

THE CLIENT
WHO IS SUICIDAL

Noreen Cavan Frisch
Lawrence E. Frisch

Exploration of Hope and Hopelessness

- ◆ What does it mean to you to have meaning and purpose in life?
- ◆ What is your source of inner strength?
- ◆ What in your life helps to make you feel connected to others?
- ◆ Do you believe that those around you can support your needs?
- ◆ Do you have a sense of your own future?

Consider your own very personal answers to these questions. And recognize that hopelessness is a human emotion stemming from a distress of the human spirit.

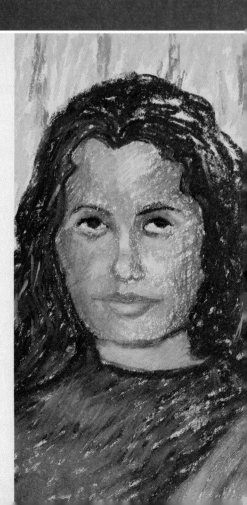

≋ CHAPTER OUTLINE

PREVALENCE OF SUICIDE AND RELATED STATISTICS

Suicide Potential

Suicide or Accident

Suicide Attempts

Suicidal Ideation

Methods

Suicide and Psychiatric Illness
  Bipolar Disorder
  Schizophrenia
  Alcohol and Substance Abuse
  Conduct Disorder
  Mixed Diagnoses

Medical Conditions and Suicide

THEORIES OF SUICIDE

Sociological Theory

Psychological Theory

Biological Explanations

Nursing Theory

SPECIAL POPULATIONS

Adolescents and Young Adults

The Elderly

The Incarcerated

SUICIDE SURVIVORS

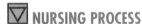 **NURSING PROCESS**

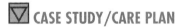 **CASE STUDY/CARE PLAN**

≋ COMPETENCIES

Upon completion of this chapter, the reader should be able to:

1. Explore the significance of hopelessness and loss of meaning and purpose in life.

2. Identify the conditions and circumstances that make an individual at high risk for suicide.

3. Describe a means of assessing suicide potential in a client.

4. Know the means of providing a safe environment for the suicidal client.

5. State the psychiatric and medical conditions that significantly increase a client's risk of suicide.

6. Use theory to understand and interpret suicidal behaviors.

7. Use the nursing assessment to evaluate one's sense of meaning and purpose in life.

8. Use nursing theory to develop a therapeutic nurse-client relationship and as a framework to provide care.

9. Apply the nursing process when providing care to individuals at risk for suicide.

10. Administer care to family members who have experienced the loss of a loved one to suicide.

≋ KEY TERMS

Euthanasia Act of killing or permitting a death for reasons of mercy.

Suicidal Ideation   Thoughts of taking one's life.

Suicide   Purposefully taking one's own life.

Suicide Potential   Person's risk level for completing a suicide.

Suicide Survivors   Friends and family of an individual who dies from suicide.

Purposefully taking one's own life, or **suicide**, is the ultimate form of self-destruction. Clients who are suicidal often feel overwhelmed by life events and decide that the only relief will come from ending their own lives. Intense feelings of fear, loss, anger, or despair can drive individuals to commit suicide, and the effects of an attempted or completed suicide can be devastating and long lasting. Nurses must learn how to recognize the danger signs of clients at risk for suicide and know the appropriate interventions to help clients preserve their health and dignity.

On Death

I am a student nurse. I am dying. I write this to you who are, and will become, nurses in the hope that by my sharing my feelings with you, you may someday be better able to help those who share my experience.

I'm out of the hospital now—perhaps for a month, for six months, perhaps for a year—but no one likes to talk about such things. In fact, no one likes to talk about much at all. Nursing must be advancing, but I wish it would hurry. We're taught not to be overly cheery now, to omit the "Everything's fine" routine, and we have done pretty well. But now one is left in a lonely silent void. With the protective "fine, fine" gone, the staff is left with only their own vulnerability and fear. The dying patient is not yet seen as a person and thus cannot be communicated with as such. He is a symbol of what every human fears and what we each know, at least academically, that we too must someday face. What did they say in psychiatric nursing about meeting pathology with pathology to the detriment of both patient and nurse? And there was a lot about knowing one's own feelings before you could help another with his. How true.

But for me, fear is today and dying is now. You slip in and out of my room, give me medications and check my blood pressure. Is it because I am a student nurse, myself, or just a human being, that I sense your fright? And your fears enhance mine. Why are you afraid? I am the one who is dying!

I know you feel insecure, don't know what to say, don't know what to do. But please believe me, if you care, you can't go wrong. Just admit that you care. That is really for what we search. We may ask for why's and wherefore's, but we

don't really expect answers. Don't run away— wait—all I want to know is that there will be someone to hold my hand when I need it. I am afraid. Death may get to be a routine to you, but it is new to me. You may not see me as unique, but I've never died before. To me, once is pretty unique!

You whisper about my youth, but when one is dying, is he really so young anymore? I have lots I wish we could talk about. It really would not take much more of your time because you are in here quite a bit anyway.

If only we could be honest, both admit of our fears, touch one another. If you really care, would you lose so much of your valuable professionalism if you even cried with me? Just person to person? Then it might not be so hard to die—in a hospital— with friends close by.*

(Anonymous, 1970, p. 336)

Death of the young and suicide have much in common: Each seems particularly tragic, somehow avoidable, in some way incomprehensible. It is rare that the dying can call so eloquently for understanding, comfort, simple touch, and friendship as does this anonymous student nurse. Much is both said and unsaid in this moving essay. As readers, we sense remarkable self-awareness, a resignation coupled with defiance, a strong expression of fear, and anger: "Why are *you* afraid? I am the one who is dying! . . . I write this . . . in the hopes . . . you may someday be *better able* to help. . . . Then, it might not be so hard to die" (italics added). Today it may not be so hard for some to die. The years since 1970 have seen many changes in our understanding of the process of death, in the way we can reach out to the dying of all ages, and in the tools we can offer to ease the pain and fear that so often accompany death. But the mixture of fear, anger, despair (veiled but seemingly just under the surface of this remarkable essay), and the loss both of human touch and of any control over life and death are present, and these experiences are the stuff of which suicide is made.

The purpose of this chapter is to address the topic of suicide from the perspective of psychiatric nursing. Suicide is not inherently a psychiatric problem: By no means do all persons who commit suicide have a psychiatric illness. Indeed, there is growing pressure for medical and nursing involvement in legally assisted suicide of persons thought to be fully mentally competent who decide to end their lives. Nonetheless, suicide currently takes place primarily among the psychiatrically disturbed and in an atmosphere of alienation, disconnectedness, and

---

*From "On Death—I Am a Student Nurse," by Anonymous, 1970, *American Journal of Nursing, 70*, p. 336. Reprinted with permission.

despair. Most who kill themselves are no less in need of solace, touch, and listening than was the student nurse who wrote so eloquently about impending death. Many reach out prior to acting and, like the student nurse, find there is no human response:

On Christmas Eve

On Christmas Eve, the other couple went off on a skiing holiday. My wife and I were left staring at each other. Silently and meticulously, we decorated the Christmas tree and piled the presents, waiting. There was nothing left to say.

Late that afternoon I had sneaked off and phoned the psychotherapist whom I had been seeing, on and off, before I left for the States.

"I'm feeling pretty bad," I said, "Could I possibly see you?"

There was a pause. "It's rather difficult," he said at last. "Are you really desperate, or could you wait till Boxing Day?"

Poor bastard, I thought, he's got his Christmas, too. Let it go. "I can wait."

"Are you sure?" He sounded relieved. "You could come round at 6:30, if it's urgent."

That was the child's bed-time; I wanted to be there. "It's all right," I said, "I'll phone later. Happy Christmas." What did it matter? I went back downstairs.

All my life I have hated Christmas: the unnecessary presents and obligatory cheerfulness, the grinding expense, the anticlimax. It is a day to be negotiated with infinite care, like a minefield. So I fortified myself with a stiff shot of whisky before I got up. It combined with my child's excitement to put a glow of hope on the day. The boy sat among the gaudy wrapping-paper, ribbons and bows, positively crowing with delight. At three years old, Christmas can still be a pleasure. Maybe, I began to feel, this thing could be survived. After all, hadn't I flown all the way from the States to pull my marriage from the fire? Or had I? Perhaps I knew it was unsavable and didn't want it to be otherwise. Perhaps I was merely seeking a plausible excuse for doing myself in. . . .

There was the usual family turkey for the child and my parents-in law. In the evening we went out to a smart and subdued dinner-party, and on from there, I think, to something wilder. But

I'm not sure. . . . After that, I remember nothing at all until I woke up in the hospital and saw my wife's face swimming vaguely towards me through a yellowish fog. She was crying. But that was three days later, three days of oblivion. . . .

It happened ten years ago now, and only gradually have I been able to piece together the facts from hints and snippets, recalled reluctantly and with apologies. Nobody wants to remind an attempted suicide of his folly, or to be reminded of it. Tact and taste forbid. Or is it the failure itself which is embarrassing? Certainly, a successful suicide inspires no delicacy at all; everybody is in on the act at once with his own exclusive inside story. In my own case, my knowledge of what happened is partial and second-hand; the only accurate details are in the gloomy shorthand of the medical reports. Not that it matters, since none of it now means much to me personally. It is as though it had all happened to another person in another world. . . . As for suicide . . . it is not for me. Perhaps I am no longer optimistic enough. I assume now that death, when it finally comes, will probably be nastier than suicide, and certainly a great deal less convenient.[*]

(Alvarez, 1971, pp. 228–237)

This writer gives us a beginning understanding of the feelings and emotions associated with suicide. The nurse must not only understand these and related feelings but also learn to identify those situations when and where suicide might occur. While for some, suicide seems a distant and unusual occurrence, statistics show that hundreds of persons have been touched deeply by the experience of suicide or suicidal thoughts in themselves or someone they know well.

PREVALENCE OF SUICIDE AND RELATED STATISTICS

In the United States, suicide accounts for approximately 13 deaths yearly per 100,000 persons: a total of 30,232 deaths in one recent year (Unnithan, Huff-Corzine, Corzine, & Whitt, 1994). Before 1978, the suicide rate was highest for persons older than 24 years, but between 1955 and 1978, a steady rise in adolescent and young adult suicide brought the rates for this age range from 5 per 100,000 to over 13 per 100,000. In 1987, there were 4,924 suicidal deaths among persons aged 15 to 24, making

---

*From *The Savage God*, by A. Alvarez, 1971, London: Weidenfeld and Nicholson. Reprinted by permission.

suicide the third leading cause of death among young persons (Berman & Jobes, 1991).

Suicide occurs at all ages, however, and males over age 65 have a suicide rate four times higher than the national average. The overall suicide rate for elderly Americans has been increasing steadily for over a decade, although it is still much lower than it was at the height of the Great Depression (Osgood, 1992). Suicide is more common among the divorced and separated (Smith, Mercy, & Conn, 1988). While suicide rates rose in nearly all countries during the Great Depression of the 1930s, there has not been any consistent correlation of current suicide rates with overall rates of unemployment. Nonetheless, individual suicides, especially men, are more frequently unemployed than are controls (Platt, 1984). Among the employed, neither occupation nor income correlate consistently with suicide rates, but high rates have been reported for U.S. physicians (notably women and psychiatrists), though not for nurses (Lester, 1992).

Suicide Potential

The nurse must be able to assess for **suicide potential** and know when a client's risk is severe and chance of completing suicide is imminent. Prevalence data assist in establishing those instances where the risk is high. In general, a client who is rational, has a suicidal plan, and has the means to carry out the plan is at very high risk. For example, a client who expresses suicidal thoughts, has a plan to shoot himself, and has a loaded gun in the closet is at very high risk for completing suicide. Table 14-1 presents a tool for assessing suicide potential. The reader should examine each aspect to become familiar with high-risk behaviors.

Suicide or Accident

It is important to recognize that statistics related to suicide may be subject to underreporting bias because some deaths attributed to accidental causes are likely self inflicted:

The Observer *sent me [Sylvia Plath's] first book of poems to review. It seemed to fit the image I had of her: serious, gifted, withheld, and still partly under the massive shadow of her husband. . . . "Her poems," I wrote, "rest secure in a mass of experience that is never quite brought out into the daylight. . . ."*

When I saw [her husband] later in London, he was tense and preoccupied. Driving on her own, Sylvia had some kind of accident; apparently, she had blacked out and run off the road on to an old airfield, though mercifully without damaging her-

self or their old Morris station-wagon. . . .

After that, Sylvia dropped in fairly often on her visits to London, always with a batch of new poems to read. She talked too about suicide . . . about her attempt ten years before which, I suppose, must have been very much on her mind as she corrected the proofs of her novel [The Bell Jar], and about her recent incident with the car. It had been no accident; she had gone off the road deliberately, seriously, wanting to die.

(Alvarez, 1971, p. 12–16)

While it may sometimes not be possible to identify suicidal intent in accidents, one study found that nearly 25% of actual suicides were misclassified as nonsuicidal in official death reports (Hlady & Middaugh, 1988). Clearly, efforts to understand the phenomenon of suicide are potentially made more complicated by the difficulties of ensuring accurate recording of events.

Suicide Attempts

Suicide attempts appear to be strikingly more common than are completed suicides. Community surveys from Canada document that up to 10% of people report having made a suicide attempt sometime in their lives (Bagley, 1985). Most similar studies have reported rather lower lifetime rates for suicide attempts, ranging from 2.9% in the U.S. Epidemiologic Catchment Area Study (Moscicki et al., 1988) to 7.9% in an Israeli study (Levav, Magnes, Aisenberg, & Rosenblum, 1988). When surveyed, 5% to 6% of college students report having previously made a suicide attempt (Rudd, 1989; Wellman & Wellman, 1988; Westefeld & Furr, 1987). Data consistently show that suicide attempts are more common in women, whereas successful suicide is more common in men (Lester, 1992).

Suicidal Ideation

Suicidal thoughts, called **suicidal ideations**, are even more common than suicidal attempts for persons in all age groups. The Epidemiologic Catchment Area Study (described in Chapter 7) reported a history of suicidal ideation (ever having thought seriously about suicide) in 10.7% of persons surveyed (Robins & Regier, 1991).

Methods

There is an extensive literature on methods chosen by persons attempting and successfully completing suicide (Lester, 1992). Firearms are used by the majority of persons, particularly younger individuals. Medication

Table 14-1 Assessment of Suicide Potential

Name _____ Age _____ Sex _____ Date _____

Rater _____ Evaluation _____

	1 2	3 4 5 6	7 8 9
	Low	Medium	High

Suicide potential

Age and sex	_____	Resources	_____	Total	_____
Symptoms	_____	Prior suicidal behavior	_____		
Stress	_____	Medical status	_____	Number of categories related	_____
Acute vs. chronic	_____	Communication aspects	_____		
Suicidal plan	_____	Reaction of significant other	_____	Average	_____

Rating for category

1. Age and sex (1–9) ☐

    Male
    50 plus (7–9) ☐
    35–49 (4–6) ☐
    15–34 (1–3) ☐

    Female
    50 plus (5–7) ☐
    35–49 (3–5) ☐
    15–34 (1–3) ☐

2. Symptoms (1–9) ☐
    Severe depression: sleep disorder, anorexia, weight loss, withdrawal, despondency, loss of interest, apathy (7–9) ☐
    Feelings of hopelessness, helplessness, exhaustion (7–9) ☐
    Delusions, hallucination, loss of contact, disorientation (6–8) ☐
    Compulsive gambler (6–8) ☐
    Disorganization, confusion, chaos (5–7) ☐
    Alcoholism, drug addiction, homosexuality (4–7) ☐
    Agitation, tension, anxiety (4–6) ☐
    Guilt, shame, embarrassment (4–6) ☐
    Feelings of rage, anger, hostility, revenge (4–6) ☐
    Poor impulse control, poor judgment (4–6) ☐
    Frustrated dependency (4–6) ☐
    Other (describe): ☐

3. Stress (1–9) ☐
    Loss of loved person by death, divorce, separation (5–9) ☐
    Loss of job, money, prestige, status (4–8) ☐
    Sickness, serious illness, surgery, accident, loss of limb (3–7) ☐
    Threat of prosecution, criminal involvement, exposure (4–6) ☐
    Change(s) in life, environment, setting (4–6) ☐
    Success, promotion, increased responsibilities (2–5) ☐
    No significant stress (1–3) ☐
    Other (describe): ☐

4. Acute versus chronic (1–9) ☐
    Sharp, noticeable, and sudden onset of specific symptoms (1–9) ☐
    Recurrent outbreak of similar symptoms (4–9) ☐
    Recent increase in long-standing traits (4–7) ☐
    No specific recent change (1–4) ☐
    Other (describe): ☐

5. Suicidal plan (1–9) ☐
    Lethality of proposed method—gun, jump, hanging, drowning, knife, poison, pills, aspirin (1–9) ☐
    Availability of means in proposed method (1–9) ☐
    Specific detail and clarity in organization of plan (1–9) ☐
    Specificity in time planned (1–9) ☐
    Bizarre plans (4–6) ☐
    Rating of previous suicide attempt(s) (1–9) ☐
    No plans (1–3) ☐
    Other (describe): ☐

Rating for category

6. Resources (1–9) ☐
    No sources of support (family, friends, agencies, employment) (7–9) ☐
    Family and friends available, unwilling to help (4–7) ☐
    Financial problem (4–7) ☐
    Available professional help, agency, or therapist (2–4) ☐
    Family and/or friends willing to help (1–3) ☐
    Stable life history (1–3) ☐
    Physician or clergy available (1–3) ☐
    Employed (1–3) ☐
    Finances no problem (1–3) ☐
    Other (describe): ☐

7. Prior suicidal behavior (1–7) ☐
    One or more prior attempts of high lethality (6–7) ☐
    One or more prior attempts of low lethality (4–5) ☐
    History of repeated threats and depression (3–5) ☐
    No prior suicidal or depressed history (1–3) ☐
    Other (describe): ☐

8. Medical status (1–7) ☐
    Chronic debilitating illness (5–7) ☐
    Pattern of failure in previous therapy (4–6) ☐
    Many repeated unsuccessful experiences with physicians (4–6) ☐
    Psychosomatic illness (asthma, ulcer, etc.) (2–4) ☐
    Chronic minor illness complaints, hypochondria (1–3) ☐
    No medical problems (1–2) ☐
    Other (describe): ☐

9. Communication aspects (1–7) ☐
    Communication broken with rejection of efforts to reestablish by both patient and others (5–7) ☐
    Communications have internalized goal (e.g., declaration of guilt, feelings of worthlessness, blame, shame) (4–7) ☐
    Communications have interpersonalized goal (to cause guilt in others, to force behavior, etc.) (2–4) ☐
    Communications directed toward world and people in general (3–5) ☐
    Communications directed toward one or more specific persons (1–3) ☐
    Other (describe): ☐

10. Reaction of significant other (1–7) ☐
    Defensive, paranoid, rejected, punishing attitude (5–7) ☐
    Denial of own or patient's need for help (5–7) ☐
    No feelings of concern about the patient; does not understand the patient (4–6) ☐
    Indecisiveness, feelings of helplessness (3–5) ☐
    Alternation between feelings of anger and rejection and feelings of responsibility and desire to help (2–4) ☐
    Sympathy and concern plus admission of need for help (1–3) ☐
    Other (describe): ☐

Reprinted with permission from Los Angeles Suicide Prevention Center.

overdose is another commonly chosen method, and most dangerous overdoses involve psychotropic prescription medications. Both of these facts have implications for suicide prevention, and these issues of prevention are discussed later in this chapter.

Suicide and Psychiatric Illness

Suicide is clearly associated with psychiatric illness. Psychiatric conditions that have high incidence of suicide include depression (both unipolar and bipolar), schizophrenia, alcoholism, drug abuse, Panic Disorder, personality disorders, and Obsessive-Compulsive Disorder (Lester, 1992). While it seems likely that clients with each of these disorders have increased suicidal risk, it is far more difficult to assess what percentage of persons who commit suicide have a psychiatric disorder. One major Swedish study (Hagnell & Rorsman, 1979) found that 93% of persons who completed suicide had previously received some kind of psychiatric diagnosis. Not surprisingly, most studies suggest that depression is commonly associated with both completed suicides (Barraclough, 1970) and suicide attempts (Chabrol & Moron, 1988). The Lundby study found that in a small, well-studied Swedish community, the diagnosis of either Unipolar or Bipolar Major Depressive Disorder increased suicide risk by 78 times compared to persons in the population with no psychiatric diagnosis (Hagnell, Lanke, & Rorsman, 1981).

Bipolar Disorder

While data are conflicting on whether suicide risk for bipolar depression is greater than for unipolar depression, clients with Bipolar Disorder have a much higher lifetime suicide risk than does the general population (Guze & Robins, 1970). Early work had suggested manic-depressive illness to be present in 46% of all persons who completed suicide (Robins, Murphy, Wilkinson, Glassner, & Kayes, 1959). More recent studies suggest that between 25% and 50% of clients with manic-depressive illness attempt suicide during their lives, the rates being higher for women than for men (Goodwin & Jamison, 1990). One study has suggested that persons with Bipolar II Disorder (Major Depressive Disorder combined with Hypomania, see Chapter 15) are at higher risk for suicide attempt than are persons with Bipolar I Disorder (Stallone, Dunner, Ahearn, & Fieve, 1980).

Schizophrenia

Persons with schizophrenia are another group with a very high rate of suicide attempts. Two studies have documented an 8% lifetime rate of successful suicide, with an attempt rate over four times higher (Allebeck & Wistedt, 1981; Roy, 1986). Suicide tends to be more common in younger males within the first 10 years of the onset of schizophrenia than in older individuals. In com-

> ### ⟳ NURSING ALERT!
>
> #### Suicide Among Hospitalized Schizophrenic Clients
>
> Schizophrenic persons have a higher than average rate of suicide and suicide attempts. A number of these attempts occur during hospitalization, and the client will rarely tell others of his intent.

parison to persons who do not have the diagnosis of Schizophrenia, schizophrenic individuals are less likely to tell others of their intentions, and, perhaps not surprisingly, they are also depressed, socially isolated, more often college educated, and in significant fear of mental disintegration than are others (Brier & Astrachen, 1984). It is important for nurses to be aware that a number of schizophrenic suicides occur during hospitalization—often not in the hospital itself, but during escapes from involuntary confinement or while out on pass (Wollersdorf et al., 1989).

Alcohol and Substance Abuse

It should not be a surprise that alcohol and substance abuse are strongly related to suicide, but the relationships are difficult to study and to describe. Alcohol probably plays a role in some suicidal decisions: Several studies show that 30% to 40% of suicide victims have significant blood alcohol levels at postmortem examination (Varadaraz & Mendonca, 1987; Welte, Abel, & Wieczorek, 1988). Alcohol may be importantly involved in suicides that are impulsive and violent. One study found that 40% of persons attempting suicide acted within 5 minutes of considering self-harm (Williams, Davidson, & Montgomery, 1980). Such rapid decision making may be highly influenced by alcohol and other substances. Other data on adolescents suggest that acute alcohol and substance use may significantly influence the lethality of the suicidal method chosen (Brent, 1987). Newly admitted psychiatric clients hospitalized for unsuccessful suicide attempts were found in one study to have used alcohol and marijuana more frequently in the preceding 24 hours than were clients admitted for other reasons (Chiles, Strosaht, Cowden, Graham, & Linehan, 1986). Chronic alcohol dependency and abuse are also major risk factors for suicide. Alcoholics are four times more likely to commit suicide than are nonalcoholics and have a lifetime suicide risk that is much higher than that of the general population (Gipps, 1978; Ohara et al., 1989). The combination of alcohol abuse with other psychiatric diagnoses (particularly depression) may be especially lethal (Whitters, Cadoret, & Widmer, 1985). There is strong expert belief that alcohol abuse is associated with suicide among both the elderly (Osgood, 1992) and the very young (Shafii, Corrigan, Whittinghill, & Derrick, 1985). These findings of an association between depression, suicide, and alcoholism seem to hold across cultures as well.

Nonalcohol drug dependency and abuse is also related to suicide, especially in adolescents and young adults (Shafii et al., 1985). Significant percentages of adolescents who commit suicide have a history of substance abuse (Hoberman & Garfinkel, 1988). Suicide attempts occur three times more often in adolescent substance abusers than in the general population, and there is some evidence that suicidal ideation comes on only after drug use begins (Berman & Schwartz, 1990). While this latter finding does not establish that drug use leads to suicide, it does suggest that drug experiences may worsen depressive and other self-destructive feelings. Stimulant drugs may be particularly likely to provoke "post-high depression," and in one study, 7% of cocaine-related deaths were judged suicidal (Tardiff, Gross, Wu, Stajic, & Millman, 1989). Substance abuse may be more common in completed suicides than in suicide attempts among adolescents (Bagley, 1989), and even after unsuccessful attempts, the presence of substance abuse may predict subsequent completed suicide (Cullberg, Wasserman, & Stefanson, 1988).

Conduct Disorder

While depression and substance abuse figure strongly in the phenomenon of adolescent suicide, another DSM-IV diagnosis—Conduct Disorder—may play an even greater role (Apter, Bleich, Plutchik, Mendelsohn, & Tyano, 1988). Conduct Disorder is a repetitive and persistent pattern of behavior in which the basic rights of others or major age-appropriate societal norms or rules are violated. Although Conduct Disorder may be one of the most common psychological findings among adolescent suicide victims, the not-unusual combination of Conduct Disorder, depression, and substance abuse is significantly associated with both the frequency and severity of suicide attempts (Frances & Blumenthal, 1989).

Mixed Diagnoses

While classifications such as DSM-IV and textbooks such as this one require that psychiatric diagnoses be neatly separated into discrete categories, clinicians caring for real-life clients much more commonly find mixtures and combinations of diagnoses present in the same person. Many separate conditions that predispose one to suicide can be found in individual clients. For example, it is not at all uncommon for persons with bipolar disease to abuse alcohol or other substances. This combination of morbidities significantly raises suicide risk (Berglund,

1984). Bipolar Disorder in an individual who also experiences panic attacks constitutes yet another combination posing significant suicide risk (Fawcett, Scheftner, Clark, Gibbons, & Coryell, 1987). Schizoaffective Disorder (see Chapter 15), a psychotic condition combining elements of major depression and schizophrenia, is a highly significant risk factor for suicide, especially in men (Fawcett et al., 1987). Finally, referring particularly to the elderly, Osgood describes the combination of alcoholism, depression, and suicide as "the Deadly Triangle," implying that the combination of depression and alcohol abuse is particularly lethal among older individuals (Osgood, 1992). In general, although depression is certainly present in the vast majority of persons who complete suicide, other comorbidities are almost invariably present as well.

Medical Conditions and Suicide

Although the risk for suicide might be expected to be higher among persons with chronic medical conditions that result in pain, serious risk to life, or severe physical limitations, the literature on this subject, though extensive, is somewhat inconclusive (Barraclough, 1970; Whitlock, 1986). The best evidence supports a link between suicide and the following conditions: epilepsy, cerebrovascular disease, dementia, visual defect, multiple sclerosis, head injury, and brain tumor. With the exception of visual defect, these are all conditions in which brain centers affecting impulse, judgment, or affect might be involved. Two other conditions that appear to have increased suicide rates, lupus and Huntington's disease, may likewise affect both mood and overall cerebral functioning. Several studies have shown that suicide is paradoxically quite rare in Parkinson's disease, a condition characterized by both loss of physical and mental functioning and depressed mood (Whitlock, 1982).

High suicide rates have been reported among persons with duodenal ulcer and liver cirrhosis, but in both cases, suicide may be related to associated alcoholism rather than to the medical condition. There has also been a high incidence of suicide among persons with acquired immunodeficiency syndrome (AIDS) and human immunodeficiency virus (HIV) (Kizer, Green, Perkins, Dobber, & Hughes, 1988).

The suicide rate among clients with cancer is probably elevated, particularly in the first year after diagnosis (Allebeck, Bolund, & Ringback, 1989). Not surprisingly, most studies suggest that a diagnosis of cancer leads to depression, which in turn results in suicide. While other conditions that not infrequently lead to depression—rheumatoid arthritis, chronic low-back pain, cardiovascular disease, asthma, diabetes—might similarly seem candidates for elevated suicide rate, several studies have failed to document any unusual incidence (Stensman &

RESEARCH HIGHLIGHT

Suicide in Cancer Patients: Findings of Three Reports

1. Cancer patients, particularly those with advanced disease, question the point of carrying on. Nurses need to address the potential for suicide by bringing such feelings out into the open.

From "Finding the Means to Carry On. Suicidal Feelings in Cancer Patients," by S. H. Richards, 1994, *Professional Nurse, 9,* pp. 334–336, 338–339.

2. Chemotherapy and other cancer treatments cause emotional distress in 40% to 60% of clients. Major depression developed in 25% of persons with cancer. Detection of suicide risk is essential.

From "Evaluating Depression among Patients with Cancer," by S. M. Valente, J. M. Saunders, and M. Z. Cohen, 1994, *Cancer Practice, 2,* p. 65.

3. In a study of oncology nurses' knowledge of suicide risk, many nurses demonstrated lack of complete knowledge of the risk. Few nurses asked about a suicide plan in an assessment of risk; less than one-third recommended taking suicide precautions. Few knew risk factors of male gender or advanced age. Need for education was demonstrated.

From "Oncology Nurses' Knowledge and Misconceptions about Suicide," by S. M. Valente, J. M. Saunders, and M. Grant, 1994, *Cancer Practice, 2,* p. 209.

Sundqvist-Stensman, 1988; Whitlock, 1982). It is difficult to determine correlations between suicide and relatively infrequent conditions, and negative findings in these studies do not eliminate the possibility of elevated suicide risk among persons with some chronic medical conditions.

THEORIES OF SUICIDE

In general, theories about why people commit suicide fall into three categories: sociological, psychological, and biochemical. Each of these will be discussed separately.

Sociological Theory

In 1897, the French sociologist Emile Durkheim wrote a highly influential book entitled *Suicide* (Durkheim, 1951/1897). In this book, he argued that only social factors could explain suicide, and chief among these was *anomie,* which might be described as the combination of social disconnection and loss of societal control over individuals' impulsive behavior. In Durkheim's view, suicide often occurs because society fails to either control individual impulses or allow individuals a sense of social connectedness and hope.

Psychological Theory

There are numerous psychological models of suicide based on psychological theories as diverse as psychoanalysis and behavioral theories (described in Chapters 3 and 26). One integrative approach to modeling suicide was proposed by Schneidman (1987). His model suggests that three factors affect suicidal ideation: pain, perturbation, and press. In this model, pain is viewed as a psychological phenomenon but is unlikely to exclude physical pain. Perturbation is the degree of emotional distress reflected in the presence or absence of impulse control. Press is a concept describing the various stresses or pressures on an individual; these "presses" can come from inside the individual, from others, or from society as a whole. In Schneidman's view, suicide occurs when psychological pain results from blocked psychological needs in the context of high levels of perturbation (distress) and press (sense of overwhelming internal or external pressures).

Simpler psychological theories have been proposed that focus on depression alone. One major theory posits that depression is a major factor in suicide and that depression results from the belief, typically based on experience, that an individual is helpless to affect the outcome of his or her life events. In addition, it is theorized that depressed individuals tend to take psychological responsibility for their perceived failures. According to this "depression paradox theory" of suicide, the depressed person may be caught between strong feelings of helplessness and equally strong feelings of responsibility. The bind generated by this conflict between feeling both responsible and helpless may lead people to feel that only suicide gives them a way out of their troubles (Lester, 1992).

Biological Explanations

Not content with sociological and psychological theories alone, many investigators have sought more strictly biological explanations of suicide. Since suicide is closely related to depression, both theoretically and empirically, and since depression has in many cases shown a strong relation to neurotransmitter imbalances, it is not surprising that much work has focused on serotonin metabolites in suicide. The literature is complex and unsettled, but the findings do show some striking consistencies. Serotonin is an important monoamine brain neurotransmitter, and it is readily metabolized to 5-hydroxyindoleacetic acid (5-HIAA), which circulates in blood and cerebrospinal fluid. In general, 5-HIAA levels in assayable body fluids are thought to reflect levels of brain serotonin (which cannot be directly measured). Multiple studies suggest that a subset of suicide attempters and completers, perhaps particularly those who use violent means of self-destruction, have very low 5-HIAA levels in the cerebrospinal fluid (Asberg, 1989). While a full-scale biological theory of suicide has yet to emerge from these neurotransmitter observations, scientists continue to be greatly interested in this area of research, and new results should be expected in the future.

Nursing Theory

Of all nursing theories, the work of Peplau speaks directly to the work of nurses in working with the suicidal and potentially suicidal client. Developing her theory of nursing in the 1950s, Peplau (1988) believed that nursing is therapeutic because it is a healing art, because nursing engages two or more people in an interaction with a common goal, and because both nurse and client learn and grow as a result of the nurse-client interaction. Peplau considers nursing to be a significant, interpersonal process; the tools of nursing are communication and interviewing skills, that is, tools of self.

There is strong evidence that one thing the nurse can do for the suicidal client is to form a significant, interpersonal relationship. Studies of persons who were hospitalized because of failed suicide attempts indicate that those clients felt isolated and ignored during their hospital stays (Dunleavey, 1992) and that their major needs were to be loved, to maintain a high level of self-esteem, to begin to have control over their lives, and to be supported (Carrigan, 1994). Another evaluation indicated that nurses consistently found that persons who exhibited self-harm behaviors and persons who did not readily form therapeutic alliances with their nurses were difficult to treat (Gallop, Lancee, & Shuger, 1993). Researchers conclude that the nurse must take time with suicidal clients and engage them in interactions. Further, researchers recommend that there is a need for nurses to have a better understanding of clients who have attempted suicide (Carrigan, 1994).

Peplau (1988) provides direction on how to intervene. First, the nurse and client meet as strangers. The nurse provides time, support, and interactions aimed at assisting the client to identify problems and concerns and what resources can be used to meet the client's needs. The nurse and client clarify each other's perceptions and expectations. The nurse will make clear to the client that she will both protect him from self-harm and continue to provide opportunity for interaction and unconditional support. The nurse will assist the client to take advantage of all available services: hospitalization, if indicated; family supports; group therapy; medications;

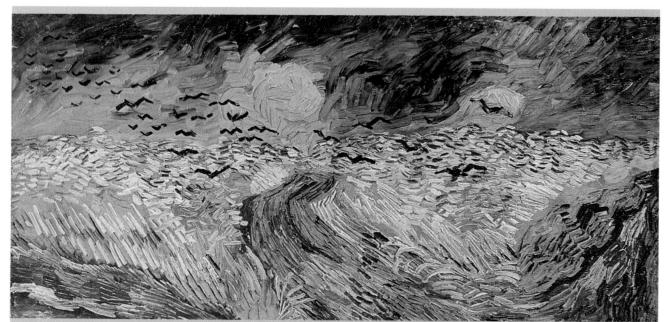

Wheatfield with Crows by Van Gogh. Source: Art Resource, NY. Van Gogh Museum, Amsterdam, The Netherlands.

The last of Van Gogh's paintings, this was painted only a few days before his suicide. It is hard not to see death in this painting. The sky is ominously bearing down on the dry and yellowed wheat; a green road seems to go nowhere; the crows disappear into the sky at the upper right of a picture that has no focus or center. Even the brushstrokes seem undirected and despairing.

and community services. The client may learn a new independence and develop self-care skills. When the client has resolved his initial suicidal crisis, and the underlying depression and distress have been addressed, the nurse can then terminate the relationship, ensuring that the client has a support system and knows where he can call for help and receive help should the need arise again.

The art of nursing, in this case, is the art of being in a relationship with another who is in need. While other nursing theories, most notably Watson's, Parse's, and Erickson's, are grounded in the concepts of caring, presence, and nurturing, respectively, the basic work of Peplau provides a foundation and framework for all nursing care of the suicidal client.

SPECIAL POPULATIONS

There are three populations that merit attention because of their elevated risk for suicide and/or the fact that many overlook their calls for help. These are adolescents/young adults, the elderly, and the incarcerated.

Adolescents and Young Adults

I knew just how to go about it.

The minute the car tires crunched off down the drive and the sound of the motor faded, I jumped out of bed and hurried into my white blouse and green figured skirt and black raincoat. The raincoat felt damp still, from the day before, but that would soon cease to matter.

I went downstairs and picked up a pale blue envelope from the dining room table and scrawled on the back, in large painstaking letters: I am going for a long walk.

I propped the message where my mother would see it the minute she came in.

Then I laughed.

I had forgotten the most important thing.

I ran upstairs and dragged a chair into my mother's closet. Then I climbed up and reached for the small green strongbox on the top shelf. I could have torn the metal cover off with my bare hands, the lock was so feeble, but I wanted to do things in a calm, orderly way.

I pulled out my mother's upper right-hand bureau drawer and slipped the blue jewelry box from its hiding place under the scented Irish linen handkerchiefs. I unpinned the little key from the dark velvet. Then I unlocked the strongbox and took out the bottle of new pills. There were more than I had hoped.

There were at least fifty.

If I had waited until my mother doled them out to me, night by night, it would have taken me fifty nights to save up enough. And in fifty nights, college would have opened, and my brother would have come back from Germany, and it would be too late.

I pinned the key back in the jewelry box among the clutter of inexpensive chains and rings, put the jewelry box back in the drawer under the handkerchiefs, returned the strongbox to the closet shelf and set the chair on the rug in the exact spot I had dragged it from.

Then I went downstairs and into the kitchen. I turned on the tap and poured myself a tall glass of water. Then I took the glass of water and the bottle of pills and went down into the cellar.

A dim, undersea light filtered through the slits of the cellar windows. Behind the oil burner, a dark gap showed in the wall at about shoulder height and ran back under the breezeway, out of sight. The breezeway had been added to the house after the cellar was dug, and built out over this secret earth bottomed crevice.

A few old, rotting fireplace logs blocked the hole mouth. I shoved them back a bit. Then I set the glass of water and the bottle of pills side by side on the flat surface of one of the logs and started to heave myself up.

It took me a good while to heft my body into the gap, but at last, after many tries, I managed it, and crouched at the mouth of the darkness, like a troll.

The earth seemed friendly under my bare feet, but cold. I wondered how long it had been since this particular square of soil had seen the sun.

Then, one after the other, I lugged the heavy, dust-covered logs across the hole mouth. The dark felt thick as velvet. I reached for the glass and bottle, and carefully, on my knees, with bent head, crawled to the farthest wall.

Cobwebs touched my face with the softness of moths. Wrapping my black coat round me like my own sweet shadow, I unscrewed the bottle of pills and started taking them swiftly, between gulps of water, one by one by one.

At first nothing happened, but as I approached the bottom of the bottle, red and blue lights began

⚕ NURSING ALERT!

Adolescent Suicide

Most adolescent suicide completers have never received mental health treatment, although the majority of these adolescents had exhibited psychiatric symptoms prior to their deaths.

to flash before my eyes. The bottle slid from my fingers and I lay down.

The silence drew off, baring the pebbles and shells and all the tatty wreckage of my life. Then, at the rim of vision, it gathered itself, and in one sweeping tide, rushed me to sleep.[*]

(Plath, 1971, 189–190)

In this passage, Sylvia Plath has captured some of the essential elements of adolescent suicide. Drug ingestions are common in suicide attempts among the young, particularly young women, and the home is the most common suicide site. The attempt described here seems particularly serious; adolescent ingestions more typically occur in the presence of others and are of relatively low lethality. Studies suggest that 8% to 9% of high school students have made one or more suicide attempts (Harkavy-Friedman, Asnis, Boeck, & DiFiore, 1987). While most attempts clearly do not result in death, the triad of homicide, accident, and suicide is by far the leading cause of death in adolescents and young adults. Indeed, there is persuasive sociological theory that homicide and suicide are closely related phenomena. This theory is based on observations that suicide rates are often inversely related to homicide rates; that is, geographic regions with low suicide rates tend to have high homicide rates (Unnithan et al., 1994).

The Elderly

A Summer Tragedy

Old Jeff Patton, the black share farmer, fumbled with his bow tie. His fingers trembled and the high stiff collar pinched his throat. A fellow loses his hand for such vanities after thirty or forty years of simple life. Once a year, or maybe twice if there's a wedding among his kinfolks, he may spruce up; but generally fancy clothes do nothing but adorn the wall of the big room and feed the

moths. That had been Jeff Patton's experience. He had not worn his stiff-bosomed shirt more than a dozen times in all his married life. His swallow-tailed coat lay on the bed beside him, freshly brushed and pressed, but it was as full of holes as the overalls in which he worked on weekdays. The moths had used it badly. Jeff twisted his mouth into a hideous toothless grimace as he contended with the obstinate bow. He stamped his good foot and decided to give up the struggle.

"Jennie," he called.

"What's that, Jeff?" His wife's shrunken voice came out of the adjoining room like an echo. It was hardly bigger than a whisper.

"I reckon you'll have to he'p me wid this heah bow tie, baby," he said meekly. "Dog if I can hitch it up."

Her answer was not strong enough to reach him, but presently the old woman came to the door, feeling her way with a stick. She had a wasted, dead-leaf appearance. Her body, as scrawny and gnarled as a string bean, seemed less than nothing in the ocean of frayed and faded petticoats that surrounded her. These hung an inch or two above the tops of her heavy unlaced shoes and showed little grotesque piles where the stockings had fallen down from her negligible legs.

Jennie sat on the side of the bed and old Jeff Patton got down on one knee while she tied the bow knot. It was a slow and painful ordeal for each of them in this position. Jeff's bones cracked, his knee ached, and it was only after a half dozen attempts that Jennie worked a semblance of a bow into the tie. . . .

Jeff opened the door and helped his wife into the car. A quick shudder passed over him. Jesus! . . .

"How come you shaking so?" Jennie whispered.

"I don't know," he said.

"You mus' be scairt, Jeff."

"No, baby, I ain't scairt. . . ."

Jeff's thought halted there. . . . Before he knew it, some remark would slip out of his mouth and that would make Jennie feel blue. Perhaps she would cry. A woman like Jennie could not easily throw off the grief that comes from losing five grown children within two years. Even Jeff was still staggered by the blow. His memory had not

---

been much good recently. He frequently talked to himself. And, although he had kept it a secret, he knew that his courage had left him. . . .

The road became smooth and red, and Jeff could tell by the smell of the air that they were nearing the river. . . . Suddenly Jennie leaned forward, buried her face in the nervous hands and burst into tears. She cried aloud in a dry cracked voice that suggested the rattle of fodder on dead stalks. She cried aloud like a child, for she had never learned to suppress a genuine sob. Her slight old frame shook heavily and seemed hardly able to sustain such violent grief. . . .

"So you the one what's scairt now, hunh?"

"I ain't scairt, Jeff. I's jess thinking' 'bout leavin' eve'thing like this—eve'thing we been used to. It's right sad-like. . . .

"You mustn't cry, baby," he said to his wife. "We gotta be strong. We can't break down. . . ."

Jeff thought of the handicaps, the near impossibility, of making another crop with his leg bothering him more and more each week. Then there was always the chance that he would have another stroke, like the one that had made him lame. Another one might kill him. The least it could do would be to leave him helpless. Jeff gasped—Lord, Jesus! He could not bear to think of being helpless, like a baby, on Jennie's hands. Frail, blind Jennie. . . .

Below, the water of the stream boomed, a soft thunder in the deep channel. Jeff ran the car onto the clay slope, pointed it directly toward the stream and put his foot heavily on the accelerator. The little car leaped furiously down the steep incline toward the water. The movement was nearly as swift and direct as a fall. The two old black folks, sitting quietly side by side, showed no excitement. In another instant the car hit the water and dropped immediately out of sight.

A little later it lodged in the mud of a shallow place. One wheel of the crushed and upturned little Ford became visible above the rushing water.

(Bontemps, 1961, pp. 253–262)

Writing over 30 years ago, Arna Bontemps raised the issue of suicide among the elderly, a problem that has only recently received significant attention. As Frank and Lester observed 17 years after this story was written, suicide in older individuals does tend to be a summer tragedy,

peaking somewhat in May (Lester, 1992). Suicide among the elderly is a much greater problem in the isolated Western states (Arizona, Wyoming, Montana, and Alaska) than it is in the South, which, at least in urban areas, has long had a lower suicide rate than other areas in the country (Osgood, 1992). Couple suicide, as in Bontemps's story, is actually a very rare event. Between 1980 and 1987, Wickett (1989) was able to document only 97 U.S. cases, and the method almost always involved firearms. Rare as they may be, couple suicides typically involve all of the elements of tragedy found in Jeff and Jennie's story: unemployment, physical loss, financial troubles, recent emotional loss, and an event occurring in the morning (Fishbain & Aldrich, 1985). In real-life double suicides, alcohol is commonly involved, but as in Jeff and Jennie's story, depression and guilt are not typically prominent.

Elderly suicide more commonly affects individuals living alone and is an especially serious problem for men over age 75. Individual suicides among the elderly are related to depression as well as to alcohol. The problem of suicide among the elderly is arguably much greater than reflected in statistics if one includes deaths from self-starvation and medication refusal, common self-willed forms of death among older adults. Since the geriatric population is growing steadily, it is likely that the problem of suicide among the elderly will increase in visibility. One authority suggests that at present rates, by the year 2030, an older American will kill him- or herself every 45 minutes (Osgood, 1992).

Conventional preventive efforts seem not to effectively reach the elderly. For example, only 2% of all calls to crisis hotlines are said to be made by persons over the age of 60 years (Osgood, 1992). There is a developing nursing role in activities that serve as preventive efforts for the elderly. These include increasing participation in adult day care and other socialization activities, increasing pet ownership and pet visitation programs, and actively seeking and treating depression in the elderly.

⑨ RESEARCH HIGHLIGHT

Pet Interaction To Decrease Loneliness

A nurse researcher conducted a study of the effects of pet interaction on loneliness by evaluating 65 individuals, some of whom had pets in their homes and some of whom participated in a pet visitation program. Findings indicated that as pet interaction increased, loneliness decreased. Conclusions are that pet interaction is a viable intervention for loneliness and helps prevent depression.

From "Human Pet Interaction and Loneliness," by M. Calvert, 1989, *Nursing Science Quarterly, 2,* 172–182.

The Incarcerated

Behind Bars

In a West Coast community, after smoking "crack," a 34-year old man developed a toxic psychosis that caused hallucinations and paranoid delusions. He heard the voice of his daughter calling. He phoned her but he was so confused he could not recognize her voice. He entered his mother's room at 3:00 AM, holding a knife in one hand and a razor in the other, and threatened to cut his wrists. His mother was able to calm him down and get him to drop his weapons. His sister called the police and stated that her brother and the family wanted him to be admitted to a psychiatric hospital. Sheriff's deputies arrived and obtained his history. When they ran a police check they discovered that he had an outstanding traffic warrant and decided to take him to jail instead of a psychiatric hospital.

The booking officer noted the history and added that he thought the man was a homosexual. He requested a mental health evaluation because he felt that the man was mentally ill and suicidal. A call was made to summon a nurse to evaluate him, but apparently she did not feel that there was any urgency to this request; she made other rounds first and these delayed her for a long time. During this time the man claimed that he was being gassed through the vents in his cell and complained of loud noise when in fact he was in a completely quiet area. . . .

Two hours later when the nurse appeared, she saw the man lying on his cot and because she assumed he was asleep, she did not awaken him or schedule a watch so she could be notified when he awoke. Forty-five minutes later he was found hanging in his cell.

(Lester & Danto, 1993, pp. 9–10)

The suicide rate for incarcerated persons is much higher than for the population as a whole, but, as in the case presented above, suicide events are much more common in local jails and holding facilities than they are in prisons.

*Used with permission from The Charles Press, Publishers, Philadelphia, from D. Lester and B. Danto, *Suicide Behind Bars* (1993).

While there are exceptions—rates may be particularly high in units for psychiatrically disturbed inmates and on "death row"—suicide rates in federal and state prisons are generally not much different than those in the general population. There are also very high reported suicide rates among youthful offenders placed in facilities for adults (Lester & Danto, 1993). As in the case reported preceding, nurses are often major care providers in local jails and so may be the first to recognize the potential for suicide. Failure to recognize risk may result in not only potentially avoidable loss of life, as in this case, but also in serious legal liability.

SUICIDE SURVIVORS

In recent years, more attention has been given to the needs of **suicide survivors**, the friends and family of an individual who dies from suicide. The normal process of bereavement has been discussed elsewhere in this text (Chapter 12), and evidence from a number of studies suggests that the process of grief after suicidal loss is not fundamentally different from that after any other death (Van der Wal, 1990). Nonetheless, the suddenness and, on

---

✳ NURSING TIP

How To Help Survivors of Suicide

◆ Give survivors the opportunity to talk. Allow them to determine how much or how little they wish to share.

◆ Do not intimidate or seek to find blame. Try to see the situation through the survivor's eyes.

◆ Allow the individual the opportunity to express the anger that often accompanies the grieving process. Reassure the survivor that these are normal feelings and emotions.

◆ Offer information and provide practical help. Educate the survivor on literature, community resources, and available support groups.

◆ Provide the survivor with time to heal. Do not suggest "you should be over this by now." Offer unconditional support as they move through the period of bereavement.

◆ Do not abandon the survivor. Send cards, call, or visit. Offer oneself, but allow survivor to refuse invitations. Keep offering oneself over time.

From "Exploring Widows' Experiences After the Suicide of Their Spouse," by B. J. Smith, A. M. Mitchell, A. A. Bruno, and R. E. Constatino, 1995, *Journal of Psychological Nursing, 33*, p. 10. Reprinted with permission.

occasion, the violence of suicide may constitute particular stresses in the grieving process. Over the past two decades, many self-help groups have been formed to assist suicide survivors. These groups may allow survivors to share experiences with others and to channel anger and sadness into socially helpful activities (Billow, 1987). Some survivors have written of their experiences in an effort to assist others with the grieving process.

⊚⊚ *REFLECTIVE THINKING*

A Discussion of Euthanasia

Suicide has long been regarded as a crime, both in Christian doctrine and in English Common Law, and many contemporary authors argue equally eloquently against the moral acceptance of suicide. However, there seems little doubt that academic and public views of suicide have become more liberal during recent past decades: As evidence of this liberalization, psychologists have suggested "rational choice" theories of suicide (Lester, 1988), and, perhaps more importantly, there has been a growing acceptance of the legality and even desirability of **euthanasia**, or the act of killing or permitting a death for reasons of mercy. Since most cases of euthanasia involve the elderly and the terminally ill, many have expressed concerns that euthanasia enthusiasts may have social ends (reducing the number of expensive and dependent individuals) more in view than altruistic ones (reducing individuals' pain and suffering). Nonetheless, even in relatively conservative medical circles there is conditional acceptance of the principles of assisted dying (Lancet editors, 1995b). This willingness to admit "euthanasia openly (and more honestly) into all . . . future discussions of end-of-life decisions affecting competent adults" (Lancet editors, 1995b, p. 259) has already found expression in a number of states. In 1995, Oregon voters narrowly approved a ballot measure authorizing physician-assisted suicide for the terminally ill. Turner (1995) recently reported a euthanasia-related membership poll of the California Academy of Family Physicians. In this poll, 68% of member physicians supported patients' right to euthanasia, but only 37% said they would agree to participate in assisted suicide. Younger physicians, women, and physicians who practiced outside of medical school settings were most likely to support euthanasia and to be willing to participate in suicide. The Netherlands was among the first countries to liberalize laws and practices relating to assisted suicide, but the actual number of patients and physicians involved seems to have remained relatively small. Euthanasia is clearly an issue that deeply divides practitioners of medicine and nursing. The ethical, moral, and religious problems it raises are unlikely to recede.

Each nurse must examine her own views, feelings, and moral convictions in relation to euthanasia.

Refer to the ethical principles described in Chapter 8 of this text to assist you in determining the actions you believe are appropriate for you as a nurse and as a citizen.

NURSING   PROCESS

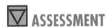 ASSESSMENT

Knowing the prevalence of suicide and the conditions under which it is likely to occur provides the nurse with only beginning information on nursing's unique role and contribution to client care. Because, by definition, nursing is "care of the human response to actual or potential health problems," the nurse must look at suicidal behaviors within the context of the individual's human response to the conditions in which he finds himself.

The nurse must begin her work with the client by making a clear assessment of not just the suicidal risk but also the individual's unique responses in his spiritual domain. The display on the following page provides a series of questions adapted from a nursing spiritual assessment tool that will help the nurse and client evaluate the individual's human response to his present life situations.

▽ NURSING DIAGNOSIS

A common theme in all descriptions of the circumstances of suicide, and in both the sociological and psychological theories, is that the person attempting suicide feels helpless. Nursing literature has addressed these feelings

NURSING ASSESSMENT OF THE HUMAN SPIRIT

- What gives your life meaning?
- Do you have a sense of purpose in life?
- Does your current condition interfere with your life's goals?
- Will you be able to make changes in your life to maintain your health?
- What is the most important or powerful thing in your life?
- What brings you joy and peace in your life?
- What can you do to feel alive and full of spirit?

- What traits do you like about yourself?
- What choices are available to you to enhance your healing?
- How do you feel about yourself right now?
- How do you feel when you have a true sense of yourself?
- What do you do to show love for yourself?
- Is worship important to you?
- Do you have a sense of belonging in this world?
- At some level do you ever feel a connection with the world or universe?

From *Spiritual Assessment Tool, Holistic Nursing: A Handbook for Practice,* by C. Guzzetta and B. Dossey, 1995, Gaithersburg, MD: Aspen Publishers. Adapted with permission.

CLUES TO SUICIDE

SYNDROMATIC CLUES

Depression

- Change in sleep patterns
- Loss of appetite and weight loss
- Complaints about illnesses, real or imaginary, or complaints about body aches and minor or major physical problems, real or imaginary
- Mood changes (sadness, lethargy)
- Loss of interest in usual activities
- Loss of energy and fatigue

Alcoholism

- Increased drinking
- Physical dependence on alcohol
- Loss of control over drinking
- Lying and denial
- Hiding liquor
- Sneaking drinks
- Drinking in spite of medical admonitions against it
- Blackouts
- Hangovers
- Cuts, scratches, bruises, cigarette burns

VERBAL CLUES

- "I am going to kill myself."
- "I am going to commit suicide."
- "I want to end it all."
- "I've had it."

- "I've lived long enough. No more."
- "I'm tired of life."
- "I'm tired of living."
- "My family would be better off without me."
- "Nobody cares about me."
- "Who cares if I'm dead anyway?"
- "I won't be around much longer."
- "Pretty soon you won't have to worry about me anyway."

BEHAVIORAL CLUES

- Previous suicide attempts
- Buying a gun
- Stockpiling pills
- Giving away money or possessions
- Loss of interest in favorite activities, church, or family
- Making or changing a will
- Making funeral plans
- Suspicious behavior

SITUATIONAL CLUES

- Death of spouse, child, or close friend
- Death of a pet
- Major move
- Diagnosis of a terminal illness
- Retirement
- Flare-up with a friend or relative

Reprinted with permission from *Suicide in Later Life,* by N. Osgood, 1992, Copyright © 1992, Jossey-Bass Inc., Publishers. First published by Lexington Books. All rights reserved.

from several perspectives, and a review of the relevant North American Nursing Diagnosis Association (NANDA) diagnoses provides insight. In 1994, introduction of a new diagnosis called *spiritual well-being* provoked an analysis of the then existing diagnoses of *spiritual distress, hopelessness,* and *powerlessness.* Examination of these diagnoses led nurses to identify the linkages among them. *Spiritual distress* is defined as a "disruption in the life principle which pervades a person's entire being and which integrates and transcends one's biological and psychological nature" (NANDA, 1996, p. 47). *Hopelessness* is defined as "a subjective state in which an individual sees limited or no alternatives or personal choices available and is unable to mobilize energy on own behalf" (NANDA, 1996, p. 71). Lastly, *powerlessness* is defined as the "perception that one's own actions will not significantly affect an outcome; a perceived lack of control over a current situation or immediate happening" (NANDA, 1996, p. 72). The common theme underlying these diagnoses is meaning and purpose in life (Dossey, Frisch, Guzetta, & Burkhardt, 1994). Without meaning and purpose, a person may become alienated from others and lose his sense of connectedness—the human response of *powerlessness.* Without meaning and purpose, a person may lose any positive sense of future and give up any belief that the world and those around him will meet his needs—the human response of *hopelessness.* Lastly, without meaning and purpose in life, a person may feel lack of inner strength and lack of his own sense of sacredness or mystery—the human response of *spiritual distress.* Thus, there seems a trio of responses that may even represent a continuum—alienation, despair, and distress of the human spirit. These are the human conditions present in circumstances where a person turns to suicide.

While these three diagnoses have been approved for use for years, nurses have identified that these diagnoses are frequently missed in clients. Case studies presented recently identified two quite separate instances where a client's hopelessness and calls for help were missed by nurses providing care that lacked sensitivity to these issues. One nurse reports a situation where a hospitalized client in critical care presents with the following behaviors: progressive disinterest in her care, sleeping during her daughter's visits, making statements such as "I want to be done with this" and other negative comments, and withdrawing from nursing and medical staff (Perry, 1995). Analysis of the case revealed that the condition of *hopelessness* did exist but that the nurses were too involved with other aspects of this woman's care to make the diagnosis (Perry & Lunney, 1995). In a quite different case, a home care nurse reports on the assessment of an elderly gentleman who was clearly depressed and in need of support. The nurse correctly assessed that the man needed further care, but, despite his comments of "If I can't see, what's the use of living? I wish I had a stroke and finish it off," his potential for suicide was not

addressed (Ryan & Lunney, 1995). These examples underscore the need for nurses to develop sensitivity and to complete assessments when they have ideas that hopelessness may be present. It is imperative that nurses develop an awareness of suicide and risk for suicide in all clients in all clinical settings.

◢ OUTCOME IDENTIFICATION

The immediate outcome for clients at risk for suicide includes preventing harm and ensuring client safety. Establishing a safe or reduced-risk environment is one means of increasing the chances of meeting this goal. An eventual decrease or elimination of the client's desire to commit suicide is an outcome that should also be identified as a goal to work toward.

◢ PLANNING/INTERVENTIONS

While the majority of suicidal or potentially suicidal clients will in all likelihood need to be referred for evaluation, the nurse should nonetheless have a basic understanding of the principles of crisis management as they pertain to suicidal risk.

Tertiary Prevention

One of the best reasons for studying the relationship of suicide to various physical, psychological, and social factors is to seek ways to prevent suicidal behavior. While improved treatment of suicide victims might not seem to really qualify as prevention, the term tertiary prevention is often given to such therapy. Over the past decades there have indeed been advances both in trauma care and in the management of common ingestions. It is certainly likely that some persons who have attempted suicide survive today whereas they would have died in the past. While no one would argue that tertiary prevention is sufficient, no doubt medical advances in the care of the acutely ill and injured will continue to be made.

Secondary Prevention

Secondary prevention focuses on persons who display recognizable risk factors or who have already survived suicide attempts. Some of these latter individuals go on to complete suicide, and they represent a particularly high-risk group for secondary preventive intervention. Other potential risk factors clearly include various psychiatric conditions associated with unusually high rates of suicide, or being in a defined high-risk situation by nature of age or geography. For example, elderly men living in rural areas of the American West have very high suicide risk (Osgood, 1992); these men may therefore be another target for secondary prevention.

For secondary prevention to be effective, mental health workers must have clear data that establish risk factors in the identified population and then develop programs aimed at reducing specific risk factors. Evaluation must be able to show that programs have reduced the suicide risk. Clearly, the more accurately risk can be predicted, the more focused preventive activities can be. Unfortunately, predicting suicide in specific individuals has proven a daunting or even impossible task (Jeanneret, 1992). While previous suicide attempt(s) put an individual at very significantly increased risk for subsequent completed suicide, to date, no criteria have proven effective in identifying suicidal individuals, even among those hospitalized for severe depression (Van Egmond & Diekstra, 1990; Goldstein, Black, Nasrallah, & Winokur, 1991). Consequently, if individuals at highest risk can rarely be identified, secondary prevention must target all patients with known risk factors, particularly Major Depressive Disorder.

Many mental health workers believe that improved detection and effective ongoing treatment of depression offer a real possibility to reduce suicide rates. Current data suggest that primary care providers are increasingly adept at detecting depression (Schwenk, Coyne, & Fechner-Bates, 1996), and well-publicized national guidelines for depression treatment offer some hope of reducing suicide in treated patients. Based on this model of secondary prevention, Osgood offers the "Ten Common Characteristics of Persons Attempting Suicide," which may help guide efforts to detect persons at risk (see accompanying display).

Primary Prevention

Primary prevention describes preventive activities applied to the whole population, regardless of any demonstrable risk factors. While primary prevention might seem futile, given that suicide is a relatively rare occurrence in the general population, a number of primary prevention programs have actually been found effective in reducing suicides.

Access Control

Access control focuses on making it harder for people to gain access to lethal means. For example, over the past 30 years, many countries have greatly reduced carbon monoxide content in cooking gas for the purpose of preventing suicide. As a result, suicides due to oven-related asphyxiation have markedly decreased (Clarke & Mayhew, 1988; Yamasawa, Nishimukai, Ohbora, & Inoue, 1980). The comparable reduction of carbon monoxide in automobile exhaust (this reduction was done for environmental reasons rather than directly for suicide prevention) has also affected use of this suicide method (Lester, 1989). Several "waves" of suicide in specific locations have been stopped by blocking access to well-publicized sites for jumping or self-hanging (Berman, 1990).

Finally, while the data are challenged by some, much evidence supports the concept that reducing access to guns would significantly decrease the prevalence of suicide (Lester, 1984). Guns are commonly available, highly lethal, and frequently used for suicidal purposes. Many feel that further restrictions of gun availability would likely constitute the strongest primary prevention possible (Cantor, 1990). Some critics of this form of primary prevention maintain that decreased lethal access such as might come about through tight gun control would have no overall effect on suicide because alternative methods would be chosen (Lester, 1992). While this is likely true for some highly premeditated suicides, there is mounting evidence that reducing access to lethal means does reduce overall suicide rates, not just those due to the restricted method (Lester & Murrell, 1980). In the United States, gun control has become a highly politicized issue, and it currently seems unlikely that there will be major federal or local efforts to reduce the availability of firearms. This is particularly unfortunate from a public health point of view since data also suggest gun control would reduce homicide rates as well.

Crisis Intervention

Access control is certainly not the only means of primary prevention. Many communities have set up crisis

---

TEN COMMON CHARACTERISTICS OF PERSONS ATTEMPTING SUICIDE

1. Unbearable psychological pain is the common stimulus.
2. Frustrated psychological need is the common stressor.
3. The common purpose is to seek a solution.
4. Cessation of consciousness is the common goal.
5. The common emotion is hopelessness-helplessness.
6. Ambivalence is the common internal attitude.
7. The common cognitive state is constriction.
8. Communication of intention is the common interpersonal act.
9. The common action is escape.
10. The common consistency is difficulty with lifelong coping patterns.

ඟ *REFLECTIVE THINKING*

Gun Control as Primary Prevention of Suicide

In 1992, the Centers for Disease Control and Prevention (CDC) established a Division of Violence Prevention as part of a national effort to view violence as a major U.S. public health problem. The division supports firearms research and has funded research that brought in the following findings: Guns kept in the home nearly triple the risk of homicide; guns in the home increase the risk of death from assault and the risk of suicide nearly fivefold. It has recently been reported (Lancet editors, 1995a) that the CDC's support of firearms research "has the gun lobby up in arms" (p. 563). The National Rifle Association (NRA) and a 500-member physician group called Doctors for Integrity in Research and Public Policy (DIRPP) has been campaigning against politicalization of the injury prevention program. The CDC staff state that it is not possible or creditable to address the problem of violence-related injuries without addressing the role firearms play in such injuries.

As a nurse and as a citizen, what is your view regarding the role of public policy with regard to primary prevention of suicide by limiting access to firearms?

intervention centers and telephone hotline services in an effort to provide resources for individuals in crisis who might otherwise have no nonsuicidal outlet for crises. Not surprisingly perhaps, given the relative rarity of suicide, only 6% to 11% of calls or visits to such centers are suicide related (Franklin, Comstock, Simmons, & Mason, 1989). The evidence that intervention centers and hotline services actually reduce suicide rates is at best equivocal. Data from one study support a significant reduction of suicide among young women (Miller, Coombs, Leeper, & Barton, 1984), but other evaluations have not found any effect on community suicide rates (Dew, Bromet, Brent, & Greenhouse, 1987).

Listening to the Client

While data supporting the effectiveness of crisis intervention and hotlines in suicide prevention may be limited, there is little doubt that many suicides could be prevented if victims' warnings were heeded by friends, relatives, health care providers, and work colleagues. In several studies, up to 94% of persons committing suicide had directly or indirectly communicated their suicidal intent prior to the act (Walk-Wasserman, 1986). While these studies are typically retrospective and subject to

bias, friends and relatives consistently report that individuals committing suicide expressed thoughts of hopelessness, helplessness, suicide, and death. The elderly may be more likely to verbalize suicidal feelings than are the young, but all too often, even the most direct warnings are ignored, as in this example:

The Physics Master

When I was at school there was an unusually sweet-tempered rather disorganized physics master who was continually talking, in a joky way, about suicide. He was a small man with a large red face, a large head covered with woolly grey curls and a permanently worried smile. He was said to have got a First in his subject at Cambridge, unlike most of his colleagues. One day at the end of a lesson, he remarked mildly that anyone cutting his throat should always be careful to put his head in a sack first, otherwise he would leave a terrible mess. Everyone laughed. Then the one o'clock bell rang and the boys all trooped off to lunch. The physics master cycled straight home, put his head in a sack and cut his throat.

(Alvarez, 1971, p. xi)

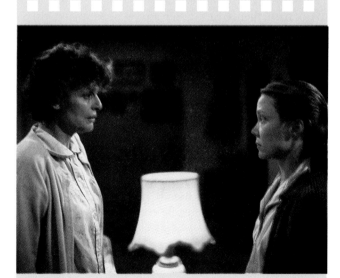

'Night Mother.
Source: Universal/Courtesy Kobal.

A suicidal person feels isolated and lonely. Having someone to stay up all night and listen may assist a suicidal person to avoid an attempt on her own life. This idea is depicted in *'Night Mother*.

Encouraging Hospitalization

Most truly suicidal individuals should be hospitalized for their own protection. Hospitalization affords a safe environment in which subsequent risk can be assessed and ongoing intervention can be planned. Only when risk is judged to be minimal by highly experienced professional personnel should the option of hospitalization not be pursued. Many individuals will recognize that their own interests are best served by protective hospitalization, but for others, short-term involuntary commitment will be necessary.

Restricting Lethal Access

Suicidal individuals should return to environments that have been made as safe as possible. In most cases, firearms should be removed from the access of the suicidal individual. Medication stockpiles should be assessed and placed under others' supervision. Family and household members will likely need education to ensure their willingness to act in a potential victim's interests. While nurses and mental health care workers do everything possible to protect the client and prevent suicidal death, the reader is cautioned that there are times when a person intent on killing himself will do so no matter what is done by professionals and family/friends.

Establishing a "Suicide Contract" or Agreement

Most therapists agree that when clients readily agree to not harm themselves during a prescribed period, risk is decreased. Often such contracts are written and signed, and the client is assured he has someone to call if he cannot bear to be alone.

Decreasing Social Isolation

Even if not hospitalized, suicidal individuals need to have a social network established. Persons in proximity to potentially suicidal clients must be aware of the need to not leave the individual alone. When such supportive networks of family and friends cannot be readily established, hospitalization must be considered.

Decreasing Psychological Symptoms

Medication and psychotherapy should be used to reduce anxiety and stress. Depressive symptoms generally do not respond rapidly to medication, so monitoring is particularly important pending medication effects. Psycho-

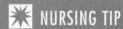 **NURSING TIP**

Suicide Precautions

◆ When a suicidal client is hospitalized, the nurse has a duty to protect the client from self-harm.

◆ The goal of suicide precautions is to create a safe environment.

Precautions usually include:

1. Removing sharp objects, such as knives, scissors, and mirrors, from the client's possession and access

2. Removing toxic substances, such as drugs and alcohol, and ensuring that unit medications are locked

3. Removing clothing that could be used for self-destruction, such as neck ties, belts, stockings, and the like

4. Placing the client under close supervision, including one-to-one supervision with a staff member

therapy is often indicated and initially may focus on personal and social conditions that bring about and/or perpetuate suicidal thoughts. Cognitive-behavioral therapy may be particularly useful, as may techniques to deal with frustration and anger. Substance use and abuse are often involved and may require separate outpatient or inpatient interventions.

▽ EVALUATION

The most obvious measure of success of interventions for suicidal clients is the prevention of suicide attempts or completions. The nurse should also carefully monitor the client's view of self and life situation to assess if the factors contributing to the client's suicidal ideations have changed in any way. The client should also be evaluated for restoration of some sense of hope and life meaning. Plans for ongoing care and evaluation, as well as involvement of family members and significant others, should be implemented for clients at continuing suicide risk.

CASE STUDY/CARE PLAN

Penny is a young woman, 17 years old, who was brought to the emergency department by her mother. Penny had ingested an unknown quantity of medications from the family's medicine cabinet and was found unresponsive by her mother when the mother returned home from work. Penny was treated medically and has been referred to the mental health unit for hospitalization.

ASSESSMENT

Jane is a psychiatric nurse who will be Penny's primary nurse. Jane observes that Penny is withdrawn. Penny's physical appearance is disheveled; her eyes are reddened as if she has been crying recently. Penny avoids eye contact and does not speak much. Penny tells Jane that she is tired, that she has not slept. Penny does not answer the question "Do you feel you could or would harm yourself again tonight?"

NURSING DIAGNOSIS *Risk for injury*, related to psychological dysfunction (suicide attempt)

Outcomes	Planning/Interventions	Evaluation
◆ Penny will not harm herself further while in the hospital.	◆ Initiate suicide precautions to ensure Penny's safety.	Penny did not harm herself during the hospital stay.
◆ Penny will make a verbal contract to not harm herself for the next 4 days.	◆ Begin to establish trust with Penny by approaching her in a nonjudgmental manner. ◆ Establish in each 24-hour period Penny's verbal contract to not harm herself.	Penny did make a verbal contract with the nurse by the second hospital day that she would not harm herself while in the hospital.
◆ Penny will sign a written contract to not hurt herself at any time in the next 4 months.	◆ Offer positive encouragement to Penny for remaining free of injury and/or for taking a positive interest in herself.	Penny did sign a written contract to call a hotline number rather than make another attempt.

NURSING DIAGNOSIS *Ineffective individual coping*, related to situational crisis (suicide attempt), as evidenced by destructive behavior and inability to ask for help

Outcomes	Planning/Interventions	Evaluation
◆ Penny will verbalize one positive statement about herself.	◆ Permit Penny to be herself. ◆ Promote Penny's control by giving her choices of daily activities and of conversation topics.	Penny did respond to the nurse and entered into a relationship with the nurse. Penny began to describe her interests, her feelings.
◆ Penny will begin to examine her coping skills and consider alternatives.	◆ Develop a positive relationship with Penny by remaining caring and truthful in interactions, by actively listening when Penny wants to talk, and by remaining attentive when Penny wishes to be silent.	Penny accepted individual therapy and agreed to weekly sessions.
	◆ Encourage Penny to view others as a source of support and assistance.	
	◆ Encourage Penny to enter therapy on an ongoing basis.	

CRITICAL THINKING BAND

ASSESSMENT
Would you also assess Penny's family situation for possible clues into her present psychological state? What other contacts (friends, school, boyfriend) would you pursue?

NURSING DIAGNOSIS
What family-oriented diagnoses might be uncovered in Penny's case?

Outcomes
What outcomes would you identify for a longer term period (perhaps 2 weeks and beyond)? Are there family-oriented outcomes that you would include?

Planning/Interventions
Identify family interventions that might help in Penny's situation.

Evaluation
How would you plan follow-up care and evaluation for Penny and her family once she is discharged?

≈ KEY CONCEPTS

◆ Suicide is an event rooted in fear, anger, despair, and loss of human touch and solace.

◆ The nurse must understand her own feelings about death, despair, and the human spirit to enter into a therapeutic relationship with a suicidal client.

◆ Suicide accounts for 13 deaths per 100,000 in the United States, with the rates for adolescents and the elderly (particularly elderly men) higher than the national average.

◆ Suicide attempts are much more common than completed suicides, with estimates ranging from 2.9% to as high as 10% of populations studied.

◆ Suicide is clearly associated with other psychiatric illnesses, including depression, bipolar disorders, schizophrenia, and substance abuse.

◆ Some persons with chronic illnesses have an increased risk for suicide; these include persons with epilepsy, cerebrovascular disease, dementia, multiple sclerosis, head injury, and brain tumor.

◆ Theories of suicide include sociological, psychological, and biological perspectives.

◆ The nursing diagnoses of *powerlessness, hopelessness,* and *distress of the human spirit* represent the human conditions of alienation, despair, and spiritual distress, which are linked to suicide.

◆ Preventive services include all levels of prevention: tertiary, secondary, and primary.

◆ Nursing management of clients at risk for suicide centers on protecting from harm and beginning to decrease isolation and psychological symptoms.

◆ Nursing theories that focus on the nurse-client relationship and the need to develop trust are helpful to guide interventions.

◆ Special populations requiring nursing care include adolescents, the elderly, the incarcerated, and family members and friends of those who attempt or complete suicide.

≈ REVIEW QUESTIONS AND ACTIVITIES

1. What is your attitude toward suicide? What do you need to do before you approach a suicidal client?

2. Describe the conditions under which suicide is most likely to occur.

3. What groups in the United States have the highest prevalence of suicide? Suicide attempts?

4. Describe the way a worker on a telephone hotline would assess the suicidal risk in a caller?

5. Use theory to provide an explanation for why a person would choose suicide.

6. Identify the means of validating the presence of the nursing diagnoses of *hopelessness, powerlessness,* and *spiritual distress.*

7. Evaluate how nursing theory helps you in your work to establish a therapeutic relationship with a client.

8. What can be done (and what is being done) to prevent suicide in your community?

9. What are your personal attitudes and beliefs regarding assisted suicide?

⚛ EXPLORING THE WEB

◆ Visit this text's "Online Companion™" on the Internet at **http://www.DelmarNursing.com** for further information on suicide prevention.

◆ Are there separate suicide prevention sources listed for families, caregivers, and health care providers? How does their information differ?

◆ What suicide prevention measures can you find on the Web that differ from those outlined in this chapter?

◆ What resources are available through the Internet for families who have lost a loved one to suicide?

〰 REFERENCES

Allebeck, P., Bolund, C., & Ringback, G. (1989). Increased suicide rate in cancer patients. *Journal of Clinical Epidemiology, 42,* 611–616.

Allebeck, P., & Wistedt, B. (1981). Mortality in schizophrenia. *Archives of General Psychiatry, 43,* 650–653.

Apter, A., Bleich, A., Plutchik, R., Mendelsohn, S., & Tyano, S. (1988). Suicidal behavior, depression, and conduct disorder in hospitalized adolescents. *Journal of the American Academy of Child and Adolescent Psychiatry, 17,* 696–699.

Asberg, M. (1989). Neurotransmitter monoamine metabolites in the cerebrospinal fluid as risk factors for suicidal behavior. In *Alcohol, Drug Abuse and Mental Health Administration, Report of the Secretary's Task Force on Youth Suicide.* Vol. 2: *Risk factors for youth suicide* (DHHA Publication No. ADM 89–1623, pp. 193–212). Washington, DC: U.S. Government Printing Office.

Bagley, C. (1985). Psychosocial correlates of suicide behaviors in an urban population. *Crisis, 6,* 63–67.

Bagley, C. (1989). Profiles of youthful suicide. *Psychiatric Reports, 65,* 234.

Barraclough, B. (1970). The diagnostic classification and psychiatric treatment of 100 suicides. In R. Fox (Ed.), *Proceedings of the fifth international conference for suicide prevention* (pp. 129–132). Vienna: IASP.

Berglund, M. (1984). Suicide in alcoholism: A prospective study of 88 suicides: The multidimensional diagnosis at first admission. *Archives of General Psychiatry, 41,* 888–891.

Berman, A. (Ed). (1990). *Suicide prevention: Case consultation.* New York: Springer.

Berman, A., & Jobes, D. A. (1991). *Adolescent suicide.* Washington, DC: American Psychiatric Press.

Berman, A. N., & Schwartz, R. (1990). Suicide attempts among adolescent drug users. *American Journal of Diseases of Children, 144,* 310–314.

Billow, C. J. (1987). A multiple family support group for survivors of suicide. In E. J. Cunn, J. L. McIntosh, & K. Dunn-Maxim (Eds.), *Suicide and its aftermath* (pp. 208–214). New York: WW North.

Brent, D. A. (1987). Correlates of medical lethality and suicide attempts among children and adolescents. *Journal of the American Academy of Child and Adolescent Psychiatry, 26,* 87–91.

Brier, A., & Astrachen, B. (1984). Characteristics of schizophrenic patients who complete suicide. *American Journal of Psychiatry, 14,* 206–209.

Calvert, M. (1989). Human pet interaction and loneliness. *Nursing Science Quarterly, 2,* 172–182.

Cantor, P. C. (1990). Intervention strategies: Environmental risk reduction for youth suicide. In *Alcohol, Drug Abuse and Mental Health Administration, Report of the Secretary's Task Force on Youth Suicide.* Vol. 3: *Prevention and intervention in youth suicide* (DHHA Publication No. ADM 89–1623, pp. 285–293). Washington, DC: U.S. Government Printing Office.

Carrigan, J. T. (1994). The psychosocial need of patients who have attempted suicide by overdose. *Journal of Advanced Nursing, 20,* 635–742.

Chabrol, H., & Moron, P. (1988). Depressive disorders in 100 adolescents who attempted suicide. *American Journal of Psychiatry, 145,* 379.

Chiles, J., Strosaht, K., Cowden, L., Graham, R., & Linehan, M. (1986). The 24 hours before hospitalization. *Suicide and life-threatening behaviors, 16,* 335–342.

Clarke, R. N., & Mayhew, P. (1988). The British gas suicide stay and its criminological implications. *Crime and Justice, 10,* 79–116.

Cullberg, J., Wasserman, D., & Stefanson, G. G. (1988). Who commits suicide after a suicide attempt? *Acta Psychiatrice Scandinavia, 77,* 598–603.

Dew, M. A., Bromet, E. J., Brent, D., & Greenhouse, J. B. (1987). A qualitative literature review of the effectiveness of suicide prevention centers. *Journal of Consulting and Clinical Psychiatry, 55,* 239–244.

Dossey, B., Frisch, N., Guzetta, C., & Burkhardt, M. (1994). Report of specialty organizations. In R. M. Carroll-Johnson & M. Paquette (Eds.), *Classification of nursing diagnoses: Proceedings of the Tenth conference* (pp. 154–166). Philadelphia: Lippincott.

Dunleavey, R. (1992). An adequate response to a cry for help? Parasuicide patients' perception of their nursing care. *Professional Nurse, 7,* 213–215.

Durkheim, E. (1951). *Suicide, a study in sociology* (J. S. Spaulding & G. Simpson, Trans.; G. Simpson, Ed.). New York: Free Press.

Fawcett, J., Scheftner, W., Clark, D., Gibbons, R., & Coryell, W. (1987). Clinical predictors of suicide in patients with major affective disorders: A controlled prospective study. *American Journal of Psychiatry, 144,* 35–40.

Fishbain, D. A., & Aldrich, T. E. (1985). Suicide pack. *Journal of Clinical Psychiatry, 46,* 11–15.

Frances, A., & Blumenthal, S. J. (1989). Personality as a predictor of youth suicide. In *Alcohol, Drug Abuse, and Mental Health Administration, Report of the Secretary's Task Force on Youth Suicide. Vol. 2: Risk factors for youth suicide* (DHHS Publication No. ADM 89-1622, pp. 160–171). Washington, DC: U.S. Government Printing Office.

Franklin, J. L., Comstock, B. S., Simmons, J. T., & Mason, M. (1989). Characteristics of suicide preventions, intervention programs: Analysis of a survey. In *Alcohol, Drug Abuse, and Mental Health Administration, Report of the Secretary's Task Force on Youth Suicide* (Vol. 3, pp. 93–102). Washington, DC: U.S. Government Printing Office.

Gallop, R., Lancee, W., & Shuger, G. (1993). Residents' and nurses' perceptions of difficult-to-treat short stay patients. *Hospital and Community Psychiatry, 44,* 352–357.

Gipps, C. H. (1978). Alcohol, diseases of alcoholics, and alcoholic liver disease. *Netherlands Journal of Medicine, 21,* 83–90.

Goldstein, R. N., Black, D. W., Nasrallah, A., & Winokur, G. (1991). The predictability of suicide: Sensitivity, specificity and predictive value of a multivariate model applied to suicide among 1906 patients with affective disorders. *Archives of General Psychiatry, 48,* 418–422.

Goodwin, F. K., & Jamison, K. R. (1990). *Manic-depressive illness.* New York: Oxford University Press.

Guze, S. B., & Robin, E. (1970). Suicide and primary affective disorders. *British Journal of Psychiatry, 117,* 437–438.

Hagnell, O., Lanke, J., & Rorsman, B. (1981). Suicide rates in the Lundby study: Mental illness as a risk factor for suicide. *Neuropsychobiology, 7,* 248–253.

Hagnell, O., & Rorsman, B. (1979). Suicide in the Lundby study. *Neuropsychobiology, 5,* 61–73.

Harkavy-Friedman, J., Asnis, G., Boeck, M., & DiFiore, J. (1987). Prevalence of specific suicidal behaviors in a high school sample. *American Journal of Psychiatry, 144,* 1203–1206.

Hlady, W. G., & Middaugh, J. P. (1988). The underrecording of suicides in state and national records, Alaska 1983–1984. *Suicide and Life-Threatening Behavior, 18,* 237–244.

Hoberman, H. M., & Garfinkel, B. D. (1988). Completed suicide in children and adolescents. *Journal of American Academy of Child and Adolescent Psychiatry, 27,* 689–695.

Jeanneret, O. (1992). A tentative epidemiologic approach to suicide prevention in adolescence. *Journal of Adolescent Health, 13,* 409–414.

Kizer, K. W., Green, M., Perkins, C., Dobber, F. G., & Hughes, M. J. (1988). AIDS and suicide in California. *JAMA, 260,* 1881.

Lancet editors. (1995a). US gun lobby takes aim at CDC injury centre. *The Lancet, 346,* 563–564.

Lancet editors. (1995b). The final autonomy. *The Lancet, 346,* 259.

Lester, D. (1984). *Gun control.* Springfield: Charles C. Thomas.

Lester, D. (1988). Rational choice theory and suicide. *Activitas Nervosa Superior, 30,* 309–312.

Lester, D. (1989). Suicide by car exhaust. *Perceptual and Motor Skills, 68,* 442.

Lester, D. (1992). *Why people kill themselves* (3rd. ed.). Springfield, IL: Charles C. Thomas.

Lester, D., & Danto, D. L. (1993). *Suicide behind bars.* Philadelphia: Charles Press.

Lester, D., & Murrell, M. E. (1980). The influence of gun control laws on suicidal behaviors. *American Journal of Psychiatry, 137,* 121–122.

Levav, I., Magnes, J., Aisenberg, E., & Rosenblum, I. (1988). Sociodemographic correlates of suicidal ideation and reported attempts. *Israel Journal of Psychiatry, 25,* 38–45.

Miller, H. L., Coombs, S. W., Leeper, J. D., & Barton, S. N. (1984). An analysis of the effect of suicide prevention facilities on suicide rates in the US. *American Journal of Public Health, 74,* 340–343.

Moscicki, E. K., O'Carrol, P., Rae, D. S., Locke, B. Z., Roy, A., & Regier, D. A. (1988). Suicide attempts in the Epidemiological Catchment Area Study. *Yale Journal of Biology and Medicine, 61,* 259–268.

North American Nursing Diagnosis Association. (NANDA). (1996). *NANDA nursing diagnosis: Definitions and classification, 1997–1998.* Philadelphia: Author.

Ohara, K., Suzuki, Y., Sugita, T., Kobayashi, K., Tamefusa, K., Hattori, S., & Ohara, K. (1989). Mortality among alcoholics discharged from a Japanese hospital. *British Journal of Psychiatry, 84,* 287–291.

Osgood, N. (1992). *Suicide in later life.* Lexington, KY: Lexington Books.

Peplau, H. (1988). The art and science of nursing: Similarities, differences and relations. *Nursing Science Quarterly, 1,* 8–15.

Perry, K. (1995). You make the diagnosis, case study for a patient in respiratory critical care. *Nursing Diagnosis, 6,* 72.

Perry, K., & Lunney, M. (1995). Case study analysis. *Nursing Diagnosis, 6,* 89–90.

Platt, S. D. (1984). Unemployment and suicidal behavior. *Social Science Medicine, 19,* 93–115.

Richards, S. H. (1994). Finding the means to carry on: Suicidal feelings in cancer patients. *Professional Nurse, 9,* 334–336, 338–339.

Robins, E., Murphy, G. E., Wilkinson, R. N., Glassner, S., & Kayes, J. (1959). Some clinical considerations in prevention of suicide based on a study of 134 successful suicides. *American Journal of Public Health, 49,* 888–899.

Robins, L. N., & Regier D. A. (Eds.). (1991). *Psychiatric disorders in America.* New York: Free Press.

Roy, A. (1986). Depression, attempted suicide and suicide in chronic schizophrenia. *Psychiatric Clinics of North America, 9,* 193–206.

Rudd, M. D. (1989). The prevalence of suicidal ideation among college students. *Suicide and Life-Threatening Behaviors, 19,* 173–183.

Ryan, M., & Lunney, M. (1995). You make the diagnosis, case study: Biases that influence the diagnostic process. *Nursing Diagnosis, 6,* 171–172.

Schneidman, E. S. (1987). A psychological approach to suicide. In G.R. Vardenbos & B. K. Bryant (Eds.), *Cataclysms, crises, and catastrophes: Psychology in action.* Washington, DC: American Psychological Association.

Schwenk, T. L., Coyne, J., & Fechner-Bates, S. (1996). Differences between detected and undetected patients in primary care and depressed psychiatric patients. *General Hospital Psychiatry, 18*(6), 407–415.

Shafii, M., Corrigan, S., Whittinghill, J. R., & Derrick, A. (1985). Psychological autopsy of completed suicide in children and adolescents. *American Journal of Psychiatry, 142,* 1061–1064.

Smith, B. J., Mitchell, A., Bruno, A., & Constatino, R. (1995). Exploring widows' experiences after the suicide of their spouse. *Journal of Psychosocial Nursing, 33,* 10–15.

Smith, J. C., Mercy, J. A., & Conn, J. M. (1988). Marital status and the risk of suicide. *American Journal of Public Health, 78,* 78–80.

Stallone, F., Dunner, D., Ahearn, J., & Fieve, R. (1980). Statistical predictions of suicide in depressives. *Comprehensive Psychiatry, 21,* 381–387.

Stensman, R., & Sundqvist-Stensman, U. (1988). Physical disease and disability among 416 suicide cases in Sweden. *Scandinavian Journal of Social Medicine, 16,* 149–153.

Tardiff, K., Gross, E., Wu, J., Stajic, M., & Millman, R. (1989). Analysis of cocaine positive fatalities. *Journal of Forensic Science, 43,* 53–63.

Turner, R. (1995). *California Family Physician, 46,* 6–7.

Unnithan, P. M., Huff-Corzine, L., Corzine, J., & Whitt, H. P. (1994). *The currents of lethal violence.* Albany, NY: SUNY.

Valente, S. M., Saunders, J. M., & Cohen, M. Z. (1994a). Evaluating depression among patients with cancer. *Cancer Practice, 2,* 65–71.

Valente, S. M., Saunders, J. M., & Grant, M. (1994b). Oncology nurses' knowledge and misconceptions about suicide. *Cancer Practice, 2,* 209–216.

Van der Wal, J. (1990). The aftermath of suicide: A review of empirical evidence. *Omega, 20,* 149–171.

Van Egmond, M., & Diekstra, R. F. (1990). The predictability of suicidal behaviors. *Crisis, 11,* 57–84.

Varadaraz, R., & Mendonca, J. (1987). A survey of blood alcohol levels in self-poisoning cases. *Advances in Alcohol and Substance Abuse, 7*(1), 63–69.

Walk-Wasserman, D. (1986). Suicidal communication of persons attempting suicide and response of significant other. *Acta Psychiatrica Scandinavica, 73,* 481–499.

Weissman, M. M., Klerman, G., Markowitz, J., & Ouellette, R. (1989). Suicide ideation and suicide attempts in panic disorder and attacks. *New England Journal of Medicine, 321,* 1209–1211.

Wellman, U., & Wellman, M. M. (1988). Correlates of suicidal ideation in a college population. *Social Psychiatry and Psychiatric Epidemiology, 23,* 90–95.

Welte, J., Abel, E., & Wieczorek, W. (1988). The role of alcohol in suicides in Erie county, NY, 1972–1984. *Public Health Reports, 103,* 648–652.

Westefeld, J., & Furr, S. (1987). Suicide and depression among college students. *Professional Psychology, 18,* 119–127.

Whitlock, F. (1982). The neurology of affective disorder and suicide. *Australian and New Zealand Journal of Psychiatry, 16,* 1–12.

Whitlock, F. (1986). Suicide and physical illness. In A. Roy (Ed.), *Suicide* (pp. 151–170). Baltimore: Williams & Wilkins.

Whitters, A., Cadoret, R., & Widmer, R. (1985). Factors associated with suicide attempts in alcohol abusers. *Journal of Affective Disorders, 9,* 15–23.

Wickett, A. (1989). *Double exit.* Eugene, OR: Hemlock Society.

Williams, C., Davidson, J., & Montgomery, I. (1980). Impulsive suicidal behavior. *Journal of Clinical Psychology, 36,* 90–104.

Wollersdorf, M., Bary, P., Steiner, B., Keller, F., Vogel, R., Hale, G., & Schuttler, R. (1989). Schizophrenia and suicide in psychiatric inpatients. In S. D. Platt & N. Kreitman (Eds.), *Current research on suicide and parasuicide* (pp. 67–77). Edinburgh: University of Edinburgh.

Yamasawa, K., Nishimukai, J., Ohbora, Y., & Inoue, K. (1980). A statistical study of suicide through intoxication. *Acta Medicinae Legalis et Socalis, 30,* 187–192.

〜 LITERARY REFERENCES

Alvarez, A. (1971). *The savage God.* London: Weidenfeld & Nicholson.

Anonymous. (1970). Death in the first person. *American Journal of Nursing, 70,* 336.

Bontemps, A. (1961). *The old south.* Anthologized in R. Weir, *Death in literature* (pp. 253–262). New York: Columbia University Press.

Lester, D., & Danto, B. (1993). *Suicide behind bars.* Philadelphia: Charles Press.

Plath, S. (1971). *The bell jar.* New York: Harper & Row.

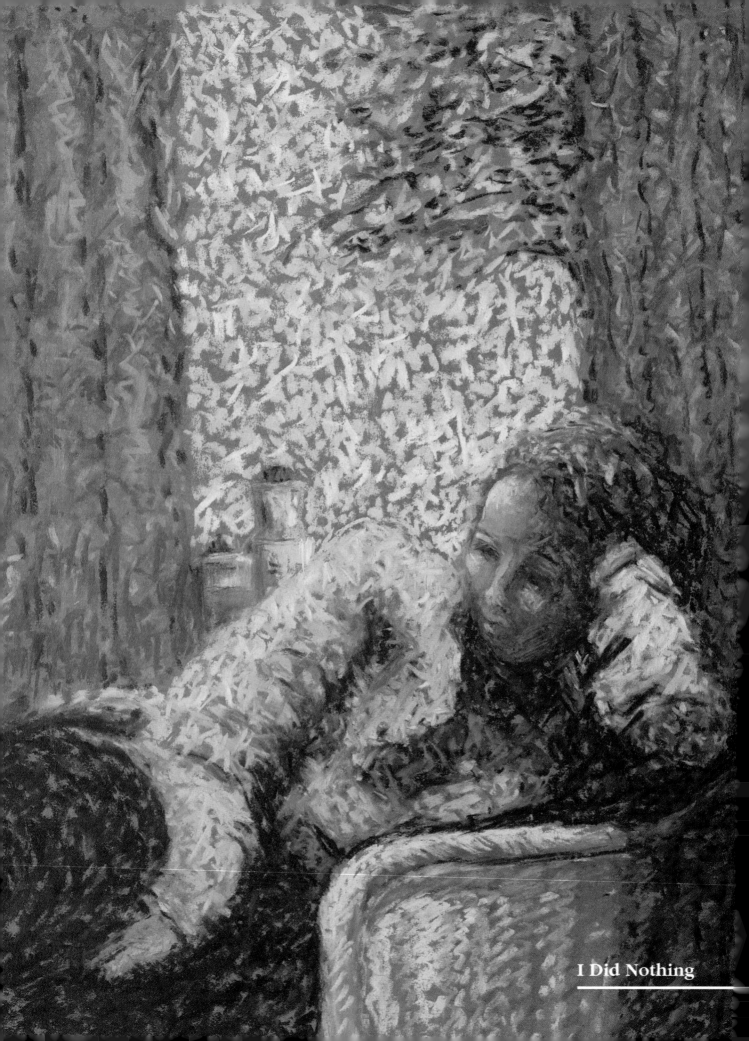

I Did Nothing

Chapter

15

THE CLIENT WHO ABUSES CHEMICAL SUBSTANCES

Noreen Cavan Frisch

Lawrence E. Frisch

Chemical Substances in Your Life

If you are reading this textbook while drinking a cup of coffee or tea, smoking a cigarette, sipping a glass of wine, or drinking a can of beer, you are using the most commonly abused substances in the United States. Chemical substances are a part of our lives. And medications, both over-the-counter and prescription drugs, are a part of our social environment.

Before reading this chapter:

◆ Look in your refrigerator and food cabinets and identify any food or drink that is known to contain habituating substances such as alcohol or caffeine.

◆ Look in your medicine cabinet and identify the number and kind of prescription and over-the-counter drugs.

◆ Take note over the next week of how often you:
  – Use a drug or chemical substance
  – Are offered a drug or chemical substance by another person
  – See an advertisement for a drug or chemical substance

◆ Document for yourself the number and kind of chemical substances in your personal environment.

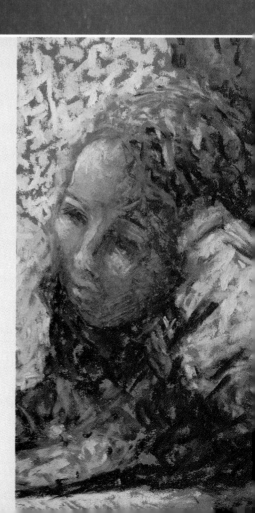

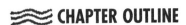 **CHAPTER OUTLINE**

DEFINITIONS RELATED TO SUBSTANCE ABUSE

SUBSTANCE USE AND ABUSE IN SOCIETY

ABUSED SUBSTANCES

EFFORTS TO CONTROL SUBSTANCE ABUSE

Control of Tobacco Use

Control of Alcohol Use

Control of Cocaine and Opiate Use

SPECIFIC ABUSED SUBSTANCES

Nicotine
    Effects
    Dependence and Withdrawal
    Treatment of Dependence
    Nurse's Role in Nicotine Abuse

Alcohol
    Effects
    Dependence and Withdrawal
    Treatment of Dependence
    Nurse's Role in Alcohol Abuse

Cocaine
    Effects
    Dependence and Withdrawal
    Treatment of Dependence
    Nurse's Role in Cocaine Abuse

Opiates
    Effects
    Dependence and Withdrawal
    Treatment of Dependence
    Nurse's Role in Opiate Abuse

Other Commonly Abused Substances
    Hallucinogens
    Inhalants
    Cannabis (Marijuana)

MULTIPLE DRUGS, MULTIPLE DIAGNOSES

SUBSTANCE ABUSE AS A SOCIAL PROBLEM

IMPACT OF DRUG USE/ABUSE ON FAMILIES

Family Dysfunction

Codependence

NURSING THEORY AND PSYCHOLOGICAL THEORY

 NURSING PROCESS

 CASE STUDY/CARE PLAN

COMPETENCIES

Upon completion of this chapter, the reader should be able to:

1. Describe the widespread nature of substance abuse in historical and modern cultures.
2. List the types of substances subject to misuse and abuse.
3. Define and differentiate between the terms *tolerance*, *withdrawal*, *dependence*, *craving*, and *addiction*.
4. Identify the effects, withdrawal symptoms, patterns of abuse, and means of treatment for nicotine, alcohol, cocaine, and opiate abuse.
5. Explain the philosophy and treatment approach of Alcoholics Anonymous and 12-step programs.
6. Explain the relationship between chemical abuse and family dysfunction.
7. Explain the dynamics of codependency.
8. Employ nursing theory and diagnoses to plan care for the individual and family unit affected by chemical abuse.

≋ KEY TERMS

Addiction Inability to abstain from drug use, accompanied by drug tolerance and withdrawal.

Alcoholism Compulsion to drink alcohol.

Codependence Behaviors exhibited by significant others of a substance-abusing individual that serve to enable and protect the abuse at the exclusion of personal fulfillment and self-development.

Craving Strong, overpowering urge for drugs felt by an individual who abuses or is dependent on drugs.

Drug Dependence Condition occurring when individuals exhibit a set of behaviors associated with inability to control use of a drug.

Drug Use Any taking of a drug.

Substance Abuse Maladaptive pattern of use of a drug in situations of real or potential harm.

Tolerance Acquired resistance to the effects of a drug.

Withdrawal Condition occurring when cessation of drug use results in a drug-specific set of symptoms that would be relieved by additional doses of the drug.

While all psychiatric disorders reflect a complex interplay of interpersonal, genetic, and sociocultural factors, perhaps nowhere is this complexity so evident as in the disorders of substance use and dependence. As an introduction to the substance-related disorders, this chapter focuses on some of the most important issues. Four substances are considered in detail: nicotine, alcohol, cocaine, and opiates. This discussion outlines the most common and dangerous substances abused in modern society and provides a broad understanding of the social, psychiatric, and nursing challenges posed by substance use.

The chapter begins with a general discussion of four basic topics: the widespread (if not universal) nature of substance use in human cultures, the very large number of substances subject to misuse and abuse, the varied range of drug effects and dependency symptoms, and the challenges of changing substance-using and substance-abusing behavior.

Following this overview, discussion is devoted to each of four specific substances and to the topic of multiple-drug abuse. Consideration is then given to issues of preventing substance abuse and dependency and the role of families and/or significant others in substance abuse. Independent and collaborative nursing roles of caring for clients and families are examined in the context of nursing theory and diagnosis in planning and evaluating care for individuals and for families.

DEFINITIONS RELATED TO SUBSTANCE ABUSE

One of the difficult problems in coming to an understanding of substance-related disorders is agreeing on definitions of various terms used to describe excessive drug use: These include *use, abuse, tolerance, withdrawal, dependence, craving,* and *addiction.*

Drug use refers to any taking of a drug. **Substance abuse** is quite different from use alone and may be defined in a number of ways. Referring primarily to alcohol, the following definition has been presented in the *Diagnostic and Statistical Manual,* fourth edition (DSM-IV): "A maladaptive pattern of . . . use indicated by one of the following: (1) continued use despite knowledge of having a persistent or recurrent social, occupational, psychological, or physical problem that is caused or exacerbated by . . . use or (2) recurrent use in situations in which . . . use is physically hazardous" (American Psychiatric Association, 1994, pp. 182–183).

In this definition, diagnosing abuse requires that use continue despite real or potential harm. The *Tenth Revision of the International Classification of Diseases* (ICD-10) explicitly incorporates this idea of harm by making reference to "harmful use" of drugs. In ICD-10, harmful use is defined as use causing actual physical or mental damage to the using individual. The ICD-10 definition is somewhat

---

BEHAVIORS ASSOCIATED WITH DRUG DEPENDENCE

◆ Develop tolerance to drug effects

◆ Manifest withdrawal from a drug

◆ Use more drug than intended

◆ Try persistently or unsuccessfully to cut down on use

◆ Spend significant amount of time using or trying to obtain the drug

◆ Give up important activities because of the drug

◆ Continue to use a drug despite knowing it is causing physical or psychological problem(s)

---

more restrictive than the DSM view of abuse. Under the DSM definition, abusers need not actually harm themselves; they only have to use a drug in potentially hazardous ways. For purposes of this text, abuse will be defined in accord with the DSM criteria, so that abuse refers to situations where a drug or substance is used in situations of real or potential harm.

Tolerance is an acquired resistance to the effects of a drug and is defined in DSM-IV as either needing to increase drug dosage to achieve a given effect or finding decreasing effect from a continuing fixed dosage (American Psychiatric Association, 1994). **Withdrawal** is a condition that occurs when stopping a drug results in a drug-specific set of symptoms that are (or would be) relieved by additional doses of the drug. **Drug dependence** occurs when individuals exhibit a set of behaviors associated with inability to control use of the drug. These behaviors are listed in the accompanying display. The DSM-IV definition of dependence requires that three or more of these characteristics occur within one year and be related to one drug.

Craving is a term often used to describe some of the behavior of individuals who abuse or are dependent on drugs. While a totally satisfactory definition of craving has never been offered, it is often taken to describe "the strong, almost overpowering urge for opiates experienced by opiate-dependent clients during acute withdrawal. It has subsequently found favor as a description of the desire to use any abused substance at any time" (Bauer, 1992). Probably because of difficulties with definition, the word *craving* has not found its way into the definition of dependence.

Addiction is an even more difficult term to define. Some have suggested that addiction may be diagnosed when both tolerance and withdrawal are present (Grinspoon & Bakalar, 1992). Others have diagnosed addiction only when an individual demonstrates inability to abstain

from drug use in addition to displaying evidence of both tolerance and withdrawal (Jellinek, 1960). Still others define addiction as the combination of drug craving, compulsive use, and relapse after withdrawal (Rinaldi, Steindler, Wilford, & Goodwin, 1988). Partly because it has proven difficult to define reproducibly, *addiction* is not a term used in DSM-IV. Instead, DSM-IV defines "physiological dependence," in which either tolerance or withdrawal (or both) are included among the three or more criteria used to establish an individual's diagnosis of dependence. In contrast, if neither tolerance nor withdrawal has occurred but criteria for dependence are otherwise met, the condition is described as "without physiological dependence."

SUBSTANCE USE AND ABUSE IN SOCIETY

Since the 1980s there has been such emphasis on controlling drug use in America that it is easy to think drugs are something new and unique. There certainly are importantly unique aspects to drug use in the late 20th century: As with other consumer goods, drugs are currently available in unprecedented variety, potency, and abundance. In 19th-century America, drug users likely had fewer drugs from which to choose, but access was probably easier. In 19th-century America, neither alcohol, nor cocaine, nor opiates were restricted in any effective way, and both adults and children had relatively free access to these substances. Morphine, one of the products of 19th-century chemical technology, was widely used during the Civil War to relieve the pain of battlefield injuries. By the end of the century, 500,000 pounds of opium were imported yearly into the United States and distributed uncontrolled as opium, morphine, or codeine (Musto, 1992). Pure preparations of cocaine became readily available only after the 1880s. Coca-Cola (whose manufacturers voluntarily removed cocaine from the formula in 1903) was only one of many cocaine-containing "tonics" advertised and marketed as stimulants.

The use of drugs seems to have been part of the human condition since earliest human prehistory. The *Old Testament* vividly describes drunkenness and attributes to Noah the discovery of grapes and wine. Indeed, by the time the *Old Testament* was written, the consumption of alcohol had long been a source of both consolation and misery. Beer and wine were produced and consumed by the ancient Egyptians many centuries before the story of Noah was set in writing. Early humans made fermented liquors from algae, tree saps, rice, and numerous fruits, and, in fact, there probably has never been a time since the Bronze Age when humans have not had access to alcohol.

It is harder to trace the past history of other drugs, but archeological evidence suggests coca use in what is now Peru (coca is the leaf from which cocaine is made) for at least the past 5,000 years. However improbable it might seem that early humans would fail to recognize the psychoactive properties of the common hemp plant, Sufi legend claims that marijuana consumption began only 1,000 years ago. Much firmer evidence suggests that tobacco use had its origins at least 7,000 years earlier. Opium use is mentioned in *The Odyssey*, and opium was an important item of commerce throughout the Mediterranean region over 3,500 years ago. The cultivation of opium poppies in Europe can be traced back even further, to Paleolithic and Neolithic times; it is highly likely that Stone Age people had discovered narcotics long before their 20th-century descendants declared war on the drugs (Siegel, 1989).

While use of drugs has been clearly established in the earliest epochs of human history, it is much harder to document drug dependency and abuse. It is difficult to imagine that earlier cultures were more successful in avoiding at least some of the complications of drug use seen today.

ABUSED SUBSTANCES

Psychoactive substances used and abused by humans have their origins either as plant products or as modern laboratory chemicals. Most substances can be classified primarily as stimulant drugs, hallucinogens, or central nervous system (CNS) depressants. Stimulants act on brain neurotransmitter receptors to produce excitation, increased alertness, aggressiveness, and decreased food intake. Hallucinogens produce perceptual and sensory alterations that may involve any sensory modality (vision, hearing, smell, touch, taste) and frequently result in hallucinations. Depressants act to decrease CNS functioning, and as with alcohol, their initial effect may be stimulation if inhibitory brain centers are depressed first. Many drugs have several effects, particularly in higher doses. For example, amphetamines are stimulants that may cause psychosis and hallucinations in high doses; marijuana is both a hallucinogen and a depressant; and nicotine has both stimulant and depressant characteristics. Table 15-1 lists a representative sampling of frequently abused substances.

Table 15-1   Frequently Abused Substances

Depressants	Alcohol, opium, morphine, heroin, barbiturates, benzodiazepines, volatile inhalants
Stimulants	Amphetamines, cocaine, crack, phencyclidine (PCP), nicotine, caffeine
Hallucinogens	LSD, mescaline, psilocybin MDMA (Ecstasy)

Despite concerns over increased use of cocaine and hallucinogens in the United States, the most commonly utilized psychoactive substances are most certainly caffeine, nicotine, alcohol, marijuana, and volatile inhalants. While much evidence suggests that caffeine is habituating and there is a caffeine withdrawal syndrome, psychiatric practice and DSM-IV do not recognize caffeine dependency as a psychiatric condition. Nicotine and alcohol dependence and abuse, however, are clearly defined as disorders and continue to constitute a major health problem. Although experts dispute whether marijuana causes withdrawal symptoms, DSM-IV does define both cannabis (marijuana) dependence and cannabis abuse. Volatile inhalants (paint, glue) are other frequently abused substances whose use may lead not only to intoxication but also occasionally to death.

Individuals become dependent on and abuse substances because these substances act on the brain, most often by producing pleasant sensations or experiences. Not only do wild animals indulge in drug-seeking behavior, but laboratory animals can easily be induced to self-administer drugs in ways that mimic human dependence and abuse. In such laboratory experiments, drugs can be administered directly into specific sites in an animal's brain. Such experiments clearly show that only when a drug is administered into specific brain areas can dependence and abuse be elicited. These experiments suggest that very specific brain centers are involved in dependence. Many psychologists now believe that the brain has built-in "reward centers" that when stimulated electrically or chemically, result in inherently pleasurable stimuli (Pfaffmann, 1960). The best theory of substance dependence is that a variety of abused drugs can stimulate brain reward systems in the process producing a desired "high" (Kornetsky, 1985). Under this hypothesis, pleasurable sensations are actually produced by the brain itself; the drug is only a means to stimulate the necessary brain centers. While most data supporting this hypothesis are based on animal studies, there are also human experiments showing that electrical brain stimulation of discrete "pleasure centers" can produce sensations of intense pleasure (Heath, 1964). In both humans and animals, these centers are widely distributed in the brainstem, midbrain, and forebrain. Scattered and separated from each other as they are, these pleasure centers appear to share neural connections of the so-called dopaminergic brain pathways (Gardner, 1992). This dopaminergic connection means that most of these centers seem to be influenced by the neurotransmitter dopamine.

It is sometimes suggested that humans who abuse drugs may have defective abilities to stimulate their pleasure centers through ordinary daily activities and as a result require the more intense stimulation of drug administration (Weiss, Mirin, Michael, & Sollogrub, 1986). While this idea is far from universally accepted, it offers one attractive explanation for how brain function and psychological behavior might be linked.

EFFORTS TO CONTROL SUBSTANCE ABUSE

Many societies and cultures have made strong efforts to control substance use and abuse. Because of the power that substance dependence can exert over human behavior, it is perhaps not surprising that historical efforts to reduce drug use and abuse have met with at best limited success. Some of these efforts are described in what follows.

Control of Tobacco Use

While efforts to ban smoking in public places seem relatively successful in the 1990s, prior similar rulings failed from the very earliest days of tobacco use. In 1639, the director-general of New Amsterdam (later to become New York City) banned smoking. The city's smokers—most of its male inhabitants—protested by camping outside his office to overturn the edict (Siegel, 1989). By the middle of the 17th century, the addictive nature of tobacco was recognized in Europe, and official edicts banning smoking existed in Bavaria, Saxony, Zurich, and other states. Punishments against smokers were introduced in Russia and Turkey, yet tobacco use continued (Siegel, 1989).

It is probable that no other drug has ever become so widely abused so quickly as did tobacco. Neither King James's condemnation of 1604 nor his heavy taxation stopped the widespread adoption of tobacco use in England. Papal encyclicals in 1642 and 1650 were similarly unsuccessful in changing patterns of increasing use in Catholic countries (Woods, 1993). Recent trends of increasing cigarette use among young persons despite unprecedented educational efforts testify to the immense difficulties of reducing tobacco consumption.

Control of Alcohol Use

Prohibitions have been notably unsuccessful in controlling use of alcohol. While most Americans identify Prohibition with the Eighteenth Amendment of 1920, there was actually a strong prohibition movement in the mid-19th century that led to antiliquor laws in a majority of states. It is likely that prohibition gained popularity because of serious and widespread alcohol abuse: In the early 19th century, Americans were consuming an astonishing yearly average of 7 gallons of 200-proof alcohol (Zimring & Hawkins, 1992). Consumption did significantly decrease over the following century, but only to about 2 gallons per capita on the eve of Prohibition in 1920. Historians dispute the degree to which state and local antiliquor laws were responsible for this decline in use.

The evidence suggests that National Prohibition did result in a further, though temporary, decrease in American per-capita consumption of alcohol (Lender & Martin, 1987). After Prohibition began in 1920, deaths from cirrhosis declined, as did hospital admissions for alcoholic psychosis and arrests for disorderly conduct (Zimring & Hawkins, 1992). Religious use of alcohol was allowed and, interestingly, accounted for almost a million gallons of wine during Prohibition's early years. Ultimately, the voting public found diminishing enthusiasm for restrictions on alcohol use, and the Eighteenth Amendment was repealed in 1933. As one historian has observed, Prohibition proved to Americans that "as bad as a drug might be, there could be laws that were worse" (Zimring & Hawkins, 1992, p. 69).

Control of Cocaine and Opiate Use

The Harrison Act of 1914 prohibited sale of narcotics and cocaine without prescription. Prior to this legislation, both cocaine and opiates could be easily purchased in pharmacies and were widely and legally used by Americans of all social classes. It is thought by some that heroin addiction became less common after the Harrison Act was passed, but many experts believe that formal prohibition of narcotics has had no significant effect on abuse frequency. The cocaine story is similar. The 1914 prohibition of cocaine dramatically increased street prices, and by the 1930s, usage seems to have declined significantly. There was little or no decline in total drug use: Many users switched to less expensive heroin, whereas those whose doctors would supply stimulant needs by prescription began to use amphetamines (synthetic drugs providing much of the high of cocaine but lasting far longer). Widespread marketing and prescription of amphetamines began in the 1920s, and by 1932 these drugs were made available by inhaler for rapid absorption and psychoactive effect. Amphetamine use declined in the 1960s as these drugs became subject to more stringent control. At the same time, cocaine use increased, at first steadily, then at a rapidly accelerating pace, to the very high levels seen in the 1980s and early 1990s. Cocaine use was increasing dramatically when President Nixon first announced and then declared victory in his "War Against Drugs" and increased even more dramatically during First Lady Nancy Reagan's "Just Say No" campaign. If Americans were saying "No" to anything during the 1980s, it was not cocaine (Woods, 1993). Despite major governmental efforts, it seems highly unlikely that prohibition has had a significant effect on the long-term use of either heroin or cocaine in the United States.

SPECIFIC ABUSED SUBSTANCES

In this section, four of the most commonly abused drugs are discussed. The purpose is to provide the reader with background and understanding of the unique properties and difficulties encountered during withdrawal and treatment for nicotine, alcohol, cocaine, and opiates.

Nicotine

On Quitting Smoking

At that time I didn't know whether I liked or hated the taste of cigarettes and the condition produced by nicotine. When I discovered that I really hated it all, it was much worse. That was when I was about twenty. For several weeks I suffered from a violent sore throat accompanied by fever. The doctor ordered me to stay in bed and to give up smoking entirely. I remember being struck by the word entirely, which the fever made more vivid. I saw a great void and no means of resisting the fearful oppression which emptiness always produces.

. . . I was in a state of fearful agitation. I thought: "As it's so bad for me I won't smoke any more, but I must first have just one last smoke." I lit a cigarette and at once all my excitement died down, though the fever seemed to get worse. . . . I smoked my cigarette solemnly to the end as if I were fulfilling a vow. And though it caused me agony I smoked many more during that illness . . . [which] was the direct cause of my second trouble: the trouble I took trying to rid myself of the first. My days became filled with cigarettes and resolutions to give up smoking, and to make a clean sweep of it, that is more or less what they are still. The dance of the last cigarette which began when I was twenty has not reached its last figure yet. . . . I may as well say that for some time past I have been smoking a great many cigarettes and have given up calling them the last.*

(*Svevo, 1958, pp. 5–26*)

Writing of a life lived (or imagined) many years ago, Italo Svevo captures with irony and in remarkably modern terms the smoker's experience: the ambivalence, the multiple broken resolutions to have "just one more," the endless "quit dates." In a similarly ironic vein, Svevo's English contemporary Oscar Wilde wrote that cigarettes are the perfect pleasure: "they are exquisite and they leave one completely unsatisfied." Few drugs have the addictive potential of nicotine. While only a small percentage of persons who have used cocaine or alcohol become addicted, by far the majority of tobacco users are physiologically dependent on this substance (Jarvik, & Schneider, 1992). While nicotine may not be the direct cause of tobacco-

---

*From *CONFESSIONS OF ZENO*, by Italo Svevo, Trans., Beryl deZoete. Copyright 1930 and renewed 1958 by Alfred A. Knopf, Inc. Reprinted by permission of the publisher.

related deaths, tobacco kills 70 times more people every year than do heroin and cocaine combined. The economic and social costs of tobacco dependence are immense.

Even addiction experts have been slow to recognize that nicotine is a powerfully addictive substance capable of producing both tolerance and withdrawal symptoms. Perhaps the widespread social acceptance of smoking has, until recently, made it difficult to acknowledge that nicotine is no less an abused substance than heroin or cocaine. There is little doubt that potent advertising techniques lent a social status to tobacco that continues to make it seem different from street drugs. Such ads proclaim one brand better than another in "taste" or image; the accompanying photographs or, more recently, cartoons are given the nonverbal task of advertising the smoker's high.

Effects

When tolerance limits unpleasant side effects, the "full effect" of nicotine may be surprisingly similar to that of other abused substances. Research indicates that human subjects not only like intravenously administered nicotine as well as morphine or cocaine (Jesinski, Johnson, & Henningfield, 1984) but also sometimes have difficulty in distinguishing which drug they have actually been given because the highs of all three are perceived as similar (Rosencrans & Chance, 1977).

The net result of nicotine intoxication is a peculiar combination of subjective relaxation and excitement. While nicotine users often claim that smoking relieves anxiety, in most cases the perceived anxiety is actually the effect of periodic nicotine withdrawal, an anxiety directly relievable only via nicotine. Users also claim that nicotine alerts them and helps performance, and psychological studies do suggest that nicotine improves performance in some motor tasks (Edwards, Wesnes, Warburton, & Gale, 1985) but not in tasks that are cognitively related. Nicotine does decrease appetite, perhaps more in females than males (Grunberg, 1990).

Dependence and Withdrawal

Nicotine withdrawal was clinically described as early as 1942 (Johnston, 1985). However, for the next 35 years, symptoms of withdrawal were attributed, both by scientists and by the public, purely to psychological distress. More recent investigations have established a wide range of withdrawal symptoms: mood change, exhibited by irritability, frustration, anger, anxiety, and/or depression; physiological symptoms such as drowsiness, fatigue, restlessness, difficulty concentrating, and/or hunger; and measurable physiological changes such as weight gain, decrease in pulse, EEG alterations, performance deficit, and increased sweating (Jarvik & Schneider, 1992). DSM-IV establishes the following criteria for the diagnosis of Nicotine Withdrawal (American Psychiatric Association, 1994):

◆ Daily use of nicotine for at least several weeks

◆ Abrupt cessation or reduction of use followed within 24 hours by four or more of the following symptoms: dysphoria or depression, insomnia, irritability, anxiety, difficulty concentrating, restlessness, decreased heart rate, increased appetite, or weight gain

Since nicotine is too physically and psychologically addicting to be abused without resulting in dependence, there is little distinction between nicotine abuse and dependence. Dependence is defined similarly to that for all other substances and may include tolerance, withdrawal, the use of larger quantities than desired (Svevo's perpetual "last cigarette"), continuing unsuccessful efforts to quit, chain smoking, and continuing use despite widespread knowledge of medical harm. Nicotine tolerance is defined by the absence of common side effects despite high dosage: nausea, dizziness, and rapid heart rate. Withdrawal commonly occurs even with brief abstinence, as in nonsmoking workplaces or airplane rides.

Treatment of Dependence

Curiously, only about 50% of individuals who quit smoking experience physical withdrawal symptoms (American Psychiatric Association, 1994), but the occurrence of withdrawal contributes to the great difficulties many individuals have in discontinuing nicotine use. Failure rates for organized quitting (efforts to bring a cohort of people through cessation efforts together) are very high, frequently 70% to 80%. Specialized modalities such as acupuncture and hypnosis have yet to be shown generally more effective than other techniques (Schwartz, 1987). Most successful ex-smokers have simply stopped on their own. For many others, the use of nicotine replacement (gum, patches, sprays) is an attractive option to help control nicotine withdrawal in the early weeks of quitting. Short-term quit rates are approximately doubled with the use of nicotine replacement, but long-term benefits are less well established. A variety of antidepressant medications have been shown to be of modest value in smoking cessation. For smokers willing to quit, relapse remains the greatest problem. Withdrawal is not the only factor in relapse; many people relapse because they find themselves in situations that they habitually associate with smoking: for example, drinking alcohol or having a morning cup of coffee (Prochaska, Velicer, di Clemente, & Fava, 1988). Behavioral programs have been designed to reduce relapse by recognizing and training for these occurrences, and such programs may prove to have a lasting effect by teaching skills for avoiding relapse in specific high-risk situations (Shiffman, Read, Maltese, Rapkin, & Jarvik, 1985).

Nurse's Role in Nicotine Abuse

Probably the most significant role of nurses in nicotine use and abuse is that of client education and prevention of nicotine use. While virtually all of the American population has heard of the negative health effects caused by smoking, cigarettes and cigars are still quite popular. Nurses are involved in each level of prevention:

◆ Primary prevention: community-wide education efforts to prevent individuals (particularly children) from becoming smokers

◆ Secondary prevention: encouraging smokers to quit smoking through involvement in cessation programs

◆ Tertiary prevention: unbiased treatment for those who have smoking-related disease (i.e., providing quality care to those with emphysema, lung cancer, and heart disease)

Focusing on primary prevention is the activity likely to have the greatest effect on the greatest number of individuals. Antismoking efforts in schools and advocacy for no-smoking legislation in public buildings are examples of wide-reaching primary prevention efforts.

Alcohol

Under the Influence

My father drank. He drank as a gut-punched boxer gasps for breath, as a starving dog gobbles food—compulsively, secretly, in pain and trembling. I use the past tense not because he ever quit drinking but because he quit living. That is how the story ends for my father, age sixty-four, heart bursting, body cooling and forsaken on the linoleum of my brother's trailer. The story continues for my brother, my sister, my mother, and me, and will continue so long as memory holds.

In the perennial present of memory, I slip into the garage or barn to see my father tipping back the flat green bottles of wine, the brown cylinders of whiskey, the cans of beer disguised in paper bags. His Adam's apple bobs, the liquid gurgles, he wipes the sandy-haired back of a hand over his lips, and then, his bloodshot gaze bumping into me, he stashes the bottle or can inside his jacket, under the workbench, between two bales of hay, and we both pretend the moment has not occurred.

"What's up, buddy?" he says, thick-tongued and edgy.

"Sky's up," I answer, playing along.

"And don't forget prices," he grumbles. "Prices are always up. And taxes." . . .

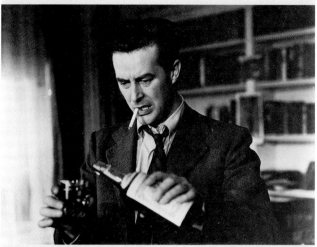

Lost Weekend. Source: Paramount/Courtesy Kobal.

Alcoholism is featured in many movies. The real trauma of the disease and its effects on individuals and families, however, is frequently underplayed by the media.

I still shy away from nightclubs, from bars, from parties where the solvent is alcohol. My friends puzzle over this, but it is no more peculiar than for a man to shy away from the lions' den after seeing his father torn apart. I took my own first drink at the age of twenty-one, half a glass of burgundy. I knew the odds of my becoming an alcoholic were four times higher than for the sons of nonalcoholic fathers. So I sipped warily.

I still do—once a week, perhaps, a glass of wine, a can of beer, nothing stronger, nothing more. I listen for the turning of a key in my brain.*

(Sanders, 1989, pp. 68–75)

Alcohol is such a widely abused substance that there are almost as many "Under the Influence" stories as there are families. Father could have been (and often is) mother, or brother, or sister, or uncle, or grandfather.

Effects

Alcohol is so widely used in American society that virtually all persons are familiar with common effects of acute alcohol intoxication. In most people, alcohol produces varying degrees of talkativeness, disinhibited behavior, uncoordination, irritability and combativeness,

*Copyright © 1989 by *Harper's Magazine*. All rights reserved. Reproduced from the November issue by special permission.

🌀 NURSING ALERT!

Alcohol-Induced Hypoglycemia

A blood sugar determination should always be done on persons brought to medical attention for alcohol-related symptoms because alcohol can significantly lower blood sugar, and symptoms of such hypoglycemia can easily be mistaken for intoxication.

---

slurred speech, and drowsiness, depending on dose and individual susceptibility. Even in fairly small doses, alcohol significantly impedes motor and cognitive function. There is good correlation between measured blood alcohol levels and symptoms, but only in nondependent drinkers. Tolerance to alcohol develops with continued use, and tolerant individuals can perform surprisingly well at blood levels that would produce stupor, if not death, in nontolerant persons (Victor, 1992).

One of the remarkable pharmacological facts about alcohol is its biochemical simplicity: a pair of carbon atoms, a single oxygen atom, and a few hydrogens. Many simple substances have effects on the CNS by dissolving in the lipid layers of brain cells. Indeed, in high doses, ethanol clearly *does* act by dissolving in the lipid membranes that separate cells (Goldstein, Chin, & Lyon, 1982). However, at relatively low doses, other mechanisms are required to explain alcohol's effects. These mechanisms are incompletely understood but do involve a variety of brain neurotransmitter systems (Charness, 1992).

NEUROLOGICAL COMPLICATIONS OF CHRONIC ALCOHOLISM

Korsakoff's Syndrome—Dementia with profound loss of recent memory.

◆ Symptoms: amnesia, dementia, psychosis
◆ Cause: alcoholism, nutritional deficiency
◆ Treatment: supportive care
◆ Prognosis: poor for cognitive recovery

Wernicke's Encephalopathy—Delirium with cranial nerve dysfunction.

◆ Symptoms: mental status changes, paralysis of extraocular eye movements leading to disconjugate gaze
◆ Cause: thiamine deficiency due to poor diet
◆ Treatment: thiamine. Giving glucose without thiamine leads to permanent neurological damage
◆ Prognosis: excellent with early thiamine administration but may also have Korsakoff's Syndrome

The chronic effects of alcohol are also highly complicated. Chronic alcohol abuse may produce serious damage to the bone marrow, heart, liver, pancreas, stomach, intestines, reproductive tract, and developing embryo. Neurological complications of alcoholism are often due to associated nutritional deficiencies and may affect many different parts of the nervous system. Two of these complications are summarized in the display on the preceding page.

Long-term excessive alcohol consumption is associated with an increase in the rates of certain cancers, particularly esophageal and colonic (Korsten & Lieber, 1992). The social and psychological effects of chronic alcohol abuse are widespread and profound. They include job loss, family disintegration, homelessness, depression, ill health, violence, accidents, and multiple concomitant psychiatric disorders. Chronic alcohol use does not cause all of these consequences, but it is strongly associated with a wide range of social dysfunction and pathology.

Dependence and Withdrawal

Alcohol withdrawal is often called delirium tremens (DTs). Because withdrawal from alcohol is so often similar to withdrawal from other substances, terms like DTs are best avoided in favor of the more generic term of withdrawal. Alcohol withdrawal symptoms typically include sweating, rapid pulse, tremor, sleep disorder, nausea and/or vomiting, and agitation. The rarest and most dramatic symptoms of alcohol withdrawal include seizures and hallucinations involving animals, frequently spiders or other insects. In Mark Twain's classic novel *Adventures of Huckleberry Finn*, Huck describes his father's dramatic and frightening alcoholic hallucinations:

Yelling About Snakes

I don't know how long I was asleep, but all of a sudden there was an awful scream and I was up. There was pap looking wild, and skipping around every which way and yelling about snakes. He said they was crawling up his legs; and then he would give a jump and scream, and say one had bit him on the cheek—but I couldn't see no snakes. He started and run round and round the cabin, hollering "Take him off! take him off! he's biting me on the neck!" I never see a man look so wild in the eyes. *

(Twain, 1987, p. 36)

This sort of delirium occurs in only a small proportion of those withdrawing from alcohol, and its occurrence is

---

*From *The Adventures of Huckleberry Finn* by M. Twain. Translated/ Edited by Walter Hunter Blair. Copyright © 1987 The Mark Twain Foundation. Regents of the University of California Press. Reproduced with permission.

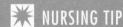

NURSING TIP

The Client in Alcohol Withdrawal
Goals of Care

- Decrease the physical need for alcohol
- Monitor withdrawal
- Prevent alcohol withdrawal delirium
- Control symptoms and prevent injury

Common Sequence of Withdrawal (Untreated)

1. Tremulousness (the shakes)
   - Onset: 3 to 36 hours after last dose (drink)
   - Symptoms: tremors, anorexia, insomnia, tachycardia, agitation, increased blood pressure, anxiety, nausea and vomiting
2. Acute hallucinations
   - Onset: any time after tremors have begun
   - Symptoms: psychomotor agitation; auditory hallucinations
3. Alcohol withdrawal delirium (delirium tremens)
   - Onset: 24 to 72 hours after last drink
   - Symptoms: disorientation, delusions, hallucinations (most often visual but can be tactile), delirium, severe agitation, fever, perspiration, tachycardia, seizures (either petit mal or grand mal)

often a sign of coexisting serious, though often alcohol-related, medical illness. Common underlying conditions predisposing to delirium include liver disease, pneumonia, gastrointestinal (GI) bleeding, hypoglycemia, and electrolyte imbalance. Clients presenting with withdrawal-associated delirium should be carefully monitored for medical problems and treated vigorously. Treatment typically includes medications to suppress agitation (chlordiazepoxide is most commonly used), fluids, and nutritional support including thiamine and other vitamins. Abnormal mental status must not be assumed to be due solely to alcohol withdrawal: Conditions such as head injury, subdural hematoma, and meningitis should be excluded via appropriate testing.

DSM-IV criteria for alcohol abuse and dependence are similar to those for other substances. Abuse is typically diagnosed when alcohol use leads to work problems, hazardous practices (such as driving under the influence), legal difficulties, or continuing use in the face of physical or social problems due to alcohol. Alcohol Dependence is diagnosed on the basis of three or more symptoms from a list that includes withdrawal, tolerance, greater-than-intended use, unsuccessful attempts to control use, and giving up of other activities in favor of alcohol use. Goodwin (1992) offers a simpler definition of **alcoholism**: "a compulsion to drink alcohol, causing harm to self or others" (p. 144).

Dependency on alcohol is more common among men than women and affects up to 14% of the U.S. population at some time in their lives (American Psychiatric Association, 1994). It has been suggested that alcoholism can be classified into two varieties: Type I alcoholism involves men and women equally, is associated with environmental stresses such as poverty, and tends to be relatively mild. Type II alcoholism is well described in the excerpt from Scott Russell Sanders: It affects primarily men, begins in the 20s or earlier, and is associated with binge drinking. Type II alcoholism tends to run in families; genetic predisposition has been suggested (Goodwin, 1992).

Some experts feel that the inclusion of most women alcohol abusers in the Type I classification may underestimate the seriousness of alcohol dependence in women. Women seem to metabolize alcohol differently than do men and attain higher blood levels with lower intake (Frezza, DiPadova, Pozzato, et al., 1990). Although women are proportionately more likely than men to be steady rather than binge drinkers, liver disease and other complications seem to occur at lower drinking intensities in women. While women alcohol abusers do drink less, they are also more likely to start at a later age, to drink privately, and to be socially isolated (Lex, 1992). Some data suggest that these observations apply primarily to older women and that, in recent years, not only has alcohol abuse become more common among women, but also women are beginning to drink at a younger age and

꩜꩜ *REFLECTIVE THINKING*

Acetaldehyde

Alcohol is metabolized in the body to the substance *acetaldehyde*, which in turn is further metabolized and excreted. Acetaldehyde is a toxic substance that in large doses causes flushing, nausea, and sleepiness. Acetaldehyde is a strongly psychoactive substance. Some scientists speculate that it is acetaldehyde formed from alcohol that leads to alcohol dependence, not the alcohol itself. However, alcohol consumption is not the only source of acetaldehyde: Smoking produces significant blood levels of acetaldehyde. Studies in animals suggest that the combination of acetaldehyde and nicotine may have unusually high addictive potential (Raloff, 1994).

As a result of these studies, it has been suggested that acetaldehyde may be a major link between the two most common American addictions: tobacco and alcohol.

Consider what implications this information has for drug prevention and drug treatment.

CAGE QUESTIONNAIRE

C Have you ever felt you should **c**ut down on your drinking?

A Have people **a**nnoyed you by criticizing your drinking?

G Have you ever felt bad or **g**uilty about drinking?

E Have you ever taken a drink the first thing in the morning to steady your nerves or get rid of a hangover (**e**ye opener)?

From "Detecting Alcoholism: The CAGE Questionnaire," by J. A. Ewing, 1984, *Journal of the American Medical Association, 252*, pp. 1905–1907. Copyright 1984, American Medical Association. Reprinted with permission.

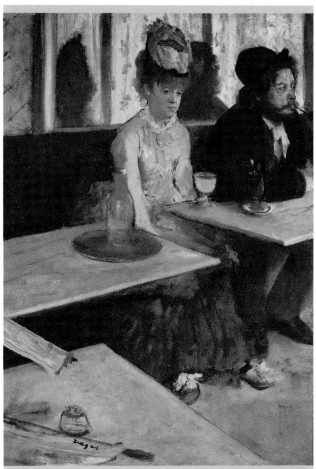

Absinthe (At the Cafe) by Degas. Source: Erich Lessing/Art Resource.

Absinthe (wormwood) was widely used as an intoxicant in 19th-century Europe. This painting hints at withdrawal and social isolation in a young woman who seems well dressed but lost in her (drugged?) thoughts. Absinthe frequently produced permanent brain damage, and not surprisingly, it is rarely used now as a drug of abuse.

drink more heavily than in the past. Any such change in drinking patterns may have a serious long-term impact on the health of alcohol-abusing women (Lex, 1992).

Clients rarely present for health or mental health care complaining of alcohol abuse or dependence. Even clients who present to emergency facilities intoxicated or with high blood alcohol levels often deny that their alcohol use is compulsive or represents a problem. Yet, because of associated medical problems, alcohol abusers commonly seek health care: 90% of alcoholics have significant medical problems in addition to their alcohol dependency (Schuckit, 1992). The four-item CAGE questionnaire (Ewing, 1984), displayed on the previous page, is often used to screen medical clients for alcohol abuse.

"Yes" answers to two or more items on the CAGE constitute a positive response, and in some populations, a positive response is over 90% sensitive in detecting individuals with alcohol problems (Chang & Kosten, 1992). A longer questionnaire, the Michigan Alcohol Screening Test (MAST), is more sensitive but takes more time to administer (Schuckit & Irwin, 1988). Screening tools such as the CAGE or MAST can be used to identify persons at potential risk for alcohol dependence; however, the actual diagnosis should be made by a trained interviewer using accepted criteria such as those in DSM-IV.

Treatment of Dependence

As is demonstrated in the story of Scott Sanders's father, alcohol dependency, or alcoholism, is a condition that persists and develops over many years. There may be a wide array of crises in the life of an alcoholic, but as with many chronic illnesses, the pattern of the disease is to vary in severity over a lifetime. Schuckit (1992) has provided a summary of the typical pattern of Type II alcoholism in men (presented in Table 15-2). In addition, Table 15-3 presents phases of alcoholism, taken from the experiences of many, which document a common evolution in drinking behaviors from moderate drinking to chronic alcoholism.

Any consideration of treatment must take some account of where in the alcoholic "natural history" an individual is, his personal goals for behavioral change, and the likelihood of spontaneous remission. Although studies on remission are difficult to interpret unless criteria for definition are strictly adhered to, a number of studies have shown that 10% to 30% of alcoholics will experience long-term abstention with no formal treatment (Vaillant, 1982). Sanders's father was "dry" for 15 years and only relapsed and died after retirement allowed him to move back to the community in which his drinking had begun five decades before.

Therapy for alcohol abuse and dependency most commonly begins with a 4- to 5-day drug detoxification wherein alcohol is replaced by a benzodiazepine in rapidly decreasing dosages. Detoxification may sometimes take place outside the hospital, but many individu-

Table 15-2 Natural History of Primary Alcoholism in Men

1. Age of first drink	12–14 years
2. Age first intoxicated	14–18 years
3. Age of first minor alcohol problem (missed school or work due to drinking behavior)	18–25 years
4. Usual age of first major problem (lost job because of drinking behavior)	28–30 years
5. Usual age entering treatment	40 years
6. Usual age of death (leading causes: heart disease, cancer, accidents, suicide)	55–60 years
7. Year abstinence alternates with active drinking	Any
8. "Spontaneous remission" rate or response to nonspecific intervention	10%–30%

From *Medical Diagnosis and Treatment of Alcoholism* from Schuckit, M. A. (p. 369), edited by J. H. Mendelson and N. K. Mello, New York: McGraw-Hill. Reprinted with permission.

als require brief hospitalization for either safety or success. Detoxification is followed by a treatment program involving some mixture of counseling, group support, and medication. Schuckit (1992) has summarized six issues that may be useful in forming the basis of alcohol counseling:

- Using free time constructively now that alcohol is no longer available

- Remaining sober while interacting with heavy-drinking friends

- Reestablishing ties with significant others, including the spouse, children, and parents, recognizing that the absence of alcohol will uncover many problems that have built up for years

- Learning how to say no to drinking at a party

- Handling stress

- Coping with general life problems, including the possible need to change jobs (vocational counseling), money management, and learning to deal with the sexual difficulties that often develop in the context of heavy drinking

Alcoholics Anonymous. Alcoholics Anonymous (AA) is a self-help organization of persons who come together to assist each other in dealing with their drinking problems. Alcoholics Anonymous is nonprofessional, self-supporting, nondenominational, apolitical, and multicultural. The AA program is based on 12 steps that offer the individual a way of living without alcohol. Each person considering joining AA is encouraged to seek a sponsor, another AA member willing to offer support to the new member in following the AA treatment program. Alcoholics Anonymous sponsors meetings in nearly every community in the United

Table 15-3 **Phases of Drinking Behavior in Alcoholics**

Phase 1: Prealcoholic	Drinks because of social motivations
	Finds that alcohol relieves stress
	Over time, needs to increase the amount of alcohol needed for relief
	May be told by others that his drinking is too heavy or too frequent
	Can be described as the "nonaddicted heavy drinker"
Phase 2: Early alcoholic	Begins to drink alone
	Becomes preoccupied with the supply of drinks
	Hides bottles of alcohol at work, home, and/or car
	Wakes up in the morning and needs a drink to control tremors (the eye-opener)
	May experience blackouts (memory loss for immediate past events)
	Uses denial as a defense mechanism and does not admit to being dependent on alcohol
Phase 3: True alcoholic	Completely loses control over ability to choose whether or not to drink
	Goes out on binge-drinking episodes; stops drinking only when too sick to take another drink
	Experiences the following: isolation from others, aggression, loss of interest in any activity that once brought pleasure, impotence/frigidity, nutritional impairment
	In this phase, most who were gainfully employed have lost their jobs, many have lost their families, and all have lost their self-esteem
Phase 4: Chronic alcoholic	Over time, the individual's continuous use of alcohol leads to extensive emotional disorganization
	May exhibit impairment of reality testing; regression; and/or loss of a sense of ethics
	Physically the individual exhibits disorders of the CNS (bilateral, progressive neuritis of the lower extremities; temporary nerve palsies) and liver and vascular disease

From "Phases of Alcohol Addiction," by E. M. Jellinek, 1952, *Quarterly Journal of Studies of Alcohol, 13*, pp. 673–684. Reprinted with permission from Quarterly Journal of Studies on Alcohol, Vol. 13, pp. 673–684, 1952 (presently Journal of Studies on Alcohol). Copyright by Journal Studies on Alcohol Inc., Rutgers Center of Alcohol Studies, Piscataway, NJ 08855.

THE TWELVE STEPS OF ALCOHOLICS ANONYMOUS

1. We admitted we were powerless over alcohol —that our lives had become unmanageable.

2. Came to believe that a power greater than ourselves could restore us to sanity.

3. Made a decision to turn our will and our lives over to the care of God as we understood Him.

4. Made a searching and fearless moral inventory of ourselves.

5. Admitted to God, to ourselves, and to another human being the exact nature of our wrongs.

6. Were entirely ready to have God remove all these defects of character.

7. Humbly asked Him to remove our shortcomings.

8. Made a list of all persons we had harmed, and became willing to make amends to them all.

9. Made direct amends to such people wherever possible, except when to do so would injure them or others.

10. Continued to take personal inventory and when we were wrong promptly admitted it.

11. Sought through prayer and meditation to improve our conscious contact with God *as we understood Him*, praying only for knowledge of His will for us and the power to carry that out.

12. Having had a spiritual awakening as the result of these steps, we tried to carry this message to alcoholics and to practice these principles in all our affairs.

The Twelve Steps are reprinted with permission of Alcoholics Anonymous World Services, Inc. Permission to reprint the Twelve Steps does not mean that A.A. has reviewed or approved the contents of this publication, nor that A.A. agrees with the views expressed herein. A.A. is a program of recovery from alcoholism *only*—use of the Twelve Steps in connection with programs and activities which are patterned after A.A. but which address other problems, or in any other non-A.A. context, does not imply otherwise.

States. Meetings may include speakers who tell their personal stories of recovery and may include discussions among several members. The objective is to assist each person by providing a close bond among people. Through AA, the individual accepts that, while he did not choose to become an alcoholic, he has complete responsibility for his own recovery.

Group support for alcoholics, recommended for all persons dealing with alcoholism, almost always includes AA. Available data suggest that alcoholics who become AA members have a 40% to 50% chance of long-term abstention (Emrick, 1987). Some alcohol-dependent individuals, particularly younger men, have difficulty accepting the strongly religious flavor of AA (Boscarino, 1980). However, for those who join, AA offers a strong support program with daily meetings, a remarkably widespread and accepting network, and no-cost treatment.

Medication. Along with formal counseling and AA, medication may sometimes play a role in the management of alcohol dependence. After acute detoxification, there is generally no role for benzodiazepine medications or sleeping pills. Buspirone may be of value when anxiety is a major psychological symptom (Kranzler, Burleson, Del Boca, & Babor, et al., 1994). Antidepressant medications are used for persons who clearly have Major Depressive Disorder, but otherwise are not indicated in treating alcohol abuse or dependence (Kranzler et al., 1995). Disulfiram (Antabuse) remains a frequently prescribed drug for the prevention of relapse in alcohol abuse. The drug inhibits a major enzyme in the pathway that metabolizes alcohol; as a result, toxic metabolites of alcohol accumulate in the body, and a person who drinks while taking disulfiram becomes physically ill, typically with flushing, nausea, and vomiting lasting for up to an hour. The effects of disulfiram persist at least 72 hours after the most recent dose, so disulfiram cannot be conveniently stopped to facilitate an unplanned binge. At one time, the use of disulfiram was common, but its popularity has fallen in recent years for at least three reasons. First, studies have failed to show much benefit in the majority of individuals who receive disulfiram (Fuller, Branchley, & Brightwell, 1986). Second, the side effects of disulfiram toxicity may be serious and may involve rare complications including serious neurological dysfunction and fatal liver disease. Finally, persons who relapse on alcohol, particularly those with significant underlying medical disorders, may become dangerously ill from the combination of disulfiram and alcohol. Despite these problems and concerns, disulfiram remains a useful treatment for some clients and continues to be prescribed for relapse prevention.

Naltrexone is the most widely used of several new drugs that may help prevent relapse in alcohol abusers. Naltrexone is a long-acting, orally administered antagonist of opiate effects that has found a role in preventing relapse among opiate abusers. While the reasons for effectiveness are not yet clear, naltrexone also has some benefit in preventing alcohol craving and relapse (Medical Letter, 1995). Naltrexone seems to work best when combined with supportive psychotherapy (O'Malley et al., 1992). Naltrexone is expensive and carries a risk of producing unanticipated opiate withdrawal in clients who, unknown to their physicians, also abuse these drugs. Newer pharmacological treatments for reducing relapse are based on the theory that dopamine receptors are involved in the high produced by alcohol. Recent studies suggest that some alcohol abusers do have decreased brain dopamine activity and that these individuals may respond to drugs that boost dopamine effect (Bower, 1995). Additionally, studies on nonselected alcohol-dependent individuals have shown some benefit from such dopamine agonists (Hitzig, 1993).

Special treatment issues for women. Most studies on alcohol treatment effectiveness have included few women (Vanicelli & Nash, 1984). Programs targeted to the special problems of alcohol abuse in women can be effective in reducing drinking in this group (Duckert, 1987). Women who abuse alcohol seem to have a very high incidence of past history of physical and sexual abuse. Successful treatment of alcohol dependence in women may require sensitivity to these issues of emotional and physical trauma (Bower, 1994). These issues are addressed more fully in Chapter 24 of this text. Further, use of alcohol during pregnancy has a significant effect on the developing fetus and may lead to Fetal Alcohol Syndrome. Fetal Alcohol Syndrome can result in mental retardation and other developmental disorders.

Nurse's Role in Alcohol Abuse

Nurses are involved in giving care at every phase of alcohol dependence, three of which are discussed here. Two are distinct phases in which the nurse provides in-hospital care: the acute phase, when the client is under care during the period of withdrawal, and the recovery phase, when the client and providers are establishing a treatment plan for immediate follow-up to hospital care. The third phase takes place in the community, when the nurse may follow a client to encourage compliance with a treatment plan and also engage in community-wide alcohol abuse prevention activities. Each of these phases is discussed following.

In the acute phase, the nurse's role is collaborative, monitoring the client's withdrawal from alcohol and taking steps to provide interventions to prevent DTs. Nursing care is provided usually through established protocols, as a physician's order is needed to carry out appropriate treatments. The goals of nursing care are to:

◆ Prevent alcohol withdrawal delirium through administration of drugs that duplicate the depressant action of alcohol on the CNS.

NURSING TIP

Denial: Living with Alcoholism

It is important to remember that many alcohol abusers strongly deny their alcohol-related problems. Consider the following:

Again his hands shook too much for him to run a saw, to make his precious miniature furniture, to drive straight down back roads. Again he wound up in the ditch, in the hospital, in jail, in treatment centers. Again he shouted and wept. Again he lied. "I never touched a drop," he swore. "Your mother's making it up."

(Sanders, 1989, p. 74)

◆ Correct fluid and electrolyte imbalances. Because alcoholics are often overhydrated, electrolytes must be determined by blood chemistries and corrective action must be taken.

◆ Perform diagnostic measures such as evaluating the client for medical conditions associated with alcoholism, such as liver damage, pancreatitis, altered blood glucose levels; evaluating the client for nervous system disorders associated with chronic alcohol use, such as peripheral polyneuritis and temporary nerve palsies; and evaluating nutritional status, particularly vitamin deficiency (B complex).

Further, the nurse must establish rapport with the client and initiate the follow-up plan for recovery from alcoholism. The nurse must recognize that the client will cope according to established patterns. The most frequent defense mechanism used by the alcoholic is denial, and the nurse should expect to encounter it. The client will very likely deny that the alcoholism is a significant problem: He may state that he can handle his condition himself or may flatly deny that there is a condition needing follow-up care. The nursing approach should be firm and based in reality but should also indicate to the client that the nurse cares about his recovery. The alcoholic has lost much or all of his self-esteem; the nurse must provide a balance of reality and caring so that the client has the opportunity to choose recovery.

In the recovery phase, the nurse must work with an interdisciplinary team to develop a discharge plan. Almost always, the client is invited to attend AA or a similar self-help group. The nurse must be aware of the fact that the risk for the alcoholic in the initial stage of recovery is returning to social and work settings where others are drinking. Alcoholics Anonymous attempts to break the cycle by providing the client with an alternative social environment where nondrinking behavior is reinforced.

Initial meetings of AA and treatment with a therapist or counselor should be scheduled while the client is in hospital. The nurse ensures that the client has a plan for where to obtain help before leaving a hospital setting.

In the community setting, the nurse may work to support the client's individual recovery and may also work to support the client's family's needs in dealing with alcohol addiction. An outpatient treatment center may provide a space for AA meetings, individual therapy and counseling, and referral to community services. A nurse working in such a setting will be part of a treatment team and will collaborate with others in the approach used. Issues specifically related to family needs are discussed later in this chapter. Primary prevention programs, those related to community-wide prevention of alcohol abuse, are also important. Projects such as enforcement of drinking laws to prevent underage drinking and programs such as educational activities geared to teach responsible drinking behavior to college students are examples of such preventative activities.

Cocaine

"My Precious Marty"—Sigmund Freud Writes to His Fiancee

I first took 0.05 gram of cocainum muriaticum in a 1% water solution when I was slightly out of sorts due to fatigue. The solution is rather viscous, slightly opalescent, and with an unusual aromatic smell. At first the taste is bitter but this then changes to a series of very nice aromatic flavors. . . . A few minutes after taking the cocaine one suddenly feels light and exhilarated. The lips and palate feel first furry and then warm, and if one drinks cold water it feels warm to the lips but cold to the throat. But on some occasions the main feeling is a rather pleasant coolness in mouth and throat.

(Clark, 1980, p. 59)

April 21, 1884—I am also toying with a project and a hope which I will tell you about; perhaps nothing will come of this, either. It is a therapeutic experiment. I have been reading about cocaine, the effective ingredient of coca leaves, which some Indian tribes chew in order to make themselves resistant to privation and fatigue. A German has tested this stuff on soldiers and reported that it has really rendered them strong and capable of endurance. I have now ordered some of it and for obvious reasons am going to try it out on cases of heart disease, then on nervous exhaustion, particularly in the awful condition following withdrawal of morphine. . . . There may be any number of other people experimenting on it already . . . but . . . as you know an experimenter's temperament requires two basic qualities: optimism in attempt, criticism in work.

(Freud, 1960, pp. 107–108)

June 2, 1884—Woe to you, my Princess, when I come. I will kiss you quite red and feed you till you are plump. And if you are forward, you shall see who is the stronger, a gentle little girl who doesn't eat enough or a big wild man who has cocaine in his body. In my last severe depression I took coca again and a small dose lifted me to the heights in a wonderful fashion. I am just now busy collecting the literature for a song of praise to this magical substance.

(Clark, 1980, p. 59)

June 29, 1884—If you really insist on meeting me at the station, I cannot stop you. . . . I won't be tired because I shall be traveling under the influence of coca, in order to curb my terrible impatience.

(Freud, 1960, p. 115)

May 17, 1885—Yesterday I received from Berlin a very flattering letter. . . . When the letter came I was suffering from migraine. . . . I took some cocaine, watched the migraine vanish at once . . . but I was so wound up that I had to go on working and writing and couldn't get to sleep before four in the morning.

(Freud, 1960, p. 145)

February 2, 1886—The bit of cocaine I have just taken is making me talkative, my little woman. I will go on writing and comment on your criticism of my wretched self. Do you realize how strangely a human being is constructed, that his virtues are often the seed of his downfall and his faults the source of his happiness?

(Freud, 1960, pp. 200–207)

In 1881, Sigmund Freud received his medical degree and almost immediately fell in love with Martha Bernays. Marriage was impossible without a solid career and income, and so Freud sought a subject for scientific study that would potentially bring him both fame and fortune. While the development of psychoanalysis would much later be the real source of Freud's fame, the study of cocaine was his first prominent—and controversial—

accomplishment. He published several scientific papers on cocaine and was among the first to recognize cocaine's potential role as a local anesthetic agent for eye surgery. He also self-administered cocaine in an effort to cure migraine and depression. By 1887 he had come to recognize that the use of cocaine was not without serious risks (Brain & Coward, 1989).

As he himself suggested in his April 21 letter to Martha, Freud was not unique in his pioneering enthusiasm for cocaine. Only a few years later, John Pemberton offered prohibition-minded Americans a new alcohol-free "temperance drink" compounded from caffeine and cocaine. Each 8-ounce glass of Coca-Cola contained 60 mg of cocaine, about the dose Freud recommended for depression (Gold, 1992). Freud could have met his own 200-mg cocaine needs with just under four Coca-Cola bottles a day. For 25 years, until cocaine was removed from the formula, many Americans found Coca-Cola to be very much "the real thing."

Over the next 90 years, the side effects and addictive nature of cocaine seem to have been largely forgotten. The 1980 edition of the *Comprehensive Textbook of Psychiatry* claimed that "used no more than two or three times a week cocaine creates no serious problems. In daily and fairly large amounts, it can produce minor psychological disturbances. Chronic cocaine abuse usually does not appear as a medical problem" (Gold, 1992, p. 206). Only 14 years later, DSM-IV turned these "minor psychological disturbances" into 10 diagnoses: Cocaine Intoxication, Cocaine Withdrawal, Cocaine Intoxication Delirium, Cocaine-Induced Psychotic Disorder (with and without delusions and hallucinations), Cocaine-Induced Mood Disorder, Cocaine-Induced Anxiety Disorder, Cocaine-Induced Sexual Dysfunction, Cocaine-Induced Sleep Disorder, and Cocaine-Related Disorder Not Otherwise Specified. (American Psychiatric Association, 1994). For associated medical problems, DSM-IV details sinusitis, nasal irritation and bleeding, perforated nasal septum, pneumonia, bronchitis, weight loss, chest pain, pneumothorax, myocardial infarction, sudden death, stroke, seizures, cardiac arrhythmias, premature labor and delivery, and acquired immunodeficiency syndrome (AIDS) (American Psychiatric Association). This is a lengthy list for a drug that only a few years before had been authoritatively declared free of adverse medical side effects.

Effects

Cocaine acts in the brain's reward centers to block the reuptake of neurotransmitters, especially norepinephrine and dopamine. This results in excess stimulation of these reward centers by these two excitatory neurotransmitters. In consequence, the brain mediates a release of stress hormones including epinephrine. Psychological effects of cocaine are listed in the accompanying display.

Especially in higher dosages, the effects of cocaine on

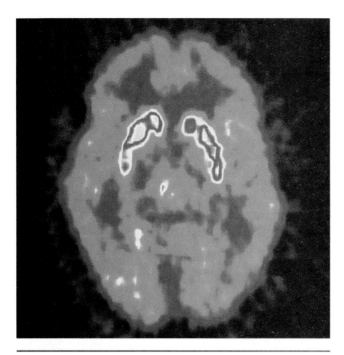

This positron emission tomography (PET) scan shows that cocaine binds to specific brain locations, primarily at dopamine-rich sites in the basal ganglia (white, orange, and yellow areas on the scan). Green areas show lower density binding, and no binding occurs in the ventricles and other blue areas. The maximum binding is in the basal ganglial nuclei, which appear white. *From "Addiction Brain Mechanisms and Their Related Implications," by D. J. Nutt, 1996,* The Lancet, 347, *pp. 33–35.*

PSYCHOLOGICAL EFFECTS OF COCAINE: LOW TO AVERAGE DOSES (25–150 MG)

Generally enjoyable effects with great increase in self-image. Rapid onset of a high with the following components:

◆ Euphoria, seldom dysphoria

◆ Increased sense of energy

◆ Enhanced mental acuity

◆ Increased sensory awareness (sexual, auditory, tactile, visual)

◆ Decreased appetite (anorexia)

◆ Increased anxiety and suspiciousness

◆ Decreased need for sleep

◆ Postponement of fatigue

◆ Increased self-confidence, egocentricity

◆ Delusions—dependence

◆ Physical symptoms of generalized sympathetic discharge

From *Substance Abuse: A Comprehensive Textbook* (2nd ed.), by J. H. Lowinson, 1992, Baltimore: Williams and Wilkins. Reprinted with permission.

Dependence and Withdrawal

Perhaps because some heavy cocaine users do not seem to have withdrawal symptoms, it was once thought that physiological dependence on cocaine was rare. When withdrawal symptoms occur, they include fatigue, vivid or unpleasant dreams, sleep disturbance, increased appetite, and psychomotor changes, either agitation or retardation. Symptoms typically occur a few hours to several days after the prior dose, but with large or repetitive doses may occur almost immediately after a cocaine high. Craving for cocaine is very common but is not included by DSM-IV among symptoms meeting criteria for withdrawal. Two withdrawal symptoms following reduction of cocaine dose are required to make a diagnosis of withdrawal.

The DSM-IV criteria for cocaine dependence and abuse are similar to those for other substances. DSM-IV describes inability to resist cocaine when it is available as an early sign of dependence (American Psychiatric Association, 1994). Tolerance is common, leading to escalating dosage, and larger amounts of money are often required to support a growing cocaine dependence. While the initial experience or experiences with high-dose cocaine may produce highly pleasurable euphoria, subsequent drug use rarely leads to an equally powerful high. Increasing doses or repetitive binging may come closer to

bodily drives are very strong. One authority reports that "so powerful is the direct stimulation provided by cocaine that sleep, safety, money, morality, loved ones, responsibility, even survival become largely irrelevant to the cocaine user" (Gold, 1992, p. 208). In animal studies, given a choice between cocaine and food or sex, rats choose cocaine until they die from overdose or starvation (Siegel, 1989).

Why has medical opinion shifted so strongly between 1980 and 1994 from nonchalance to a view that cocaine is a serious and dangerous drug of abuse? The answer is crack. Crack is a crystallized form of cocaine that can be smoked, gives a brief (5- to 10-min) but almost instantaneous high, and provides cocaine blood levels as high or higher than those that result from intravenous administration. Noncrack cocaine is most commonly inhaled—"snorted"—into the nose, as a (usually impure) powder. Oral administration, as in the original Coca-Cola, has a relatively lower potential for producing dependence than does snorting, in which larger amounts of the drug are carried quickly to the brain. Smoked cocaine—most commonly, crack—has a much higher addictive potential than does any other means of administration.

replicating initial feelings, and this desire for recapturing vivid memories of intoxication may be a strong impetus for compulsive use (Gold, 1992).

Treatment of Dependence

Withdrawal from cocaine is rarely physically dangerous: Cocaine deaths occur from the drug itself, not its absence. The major challenge in treatment is to prevent relapse. Most clients with crack dependency need inpatient care because of both the intensity of drug cravings that crack provokes and the severity of the post-intoxication psychological "crash" that occurs during withdrawal. Day hospitalization is another alternative that offers many of the advantages of inpatient treatment at lower costs (Alterman et al., 1994). Counseling focuses on recognizing and avoiding situations that might lead to renewed use. This often requires changing friends, living situations, and jobs. Depression is often a problem and may benefit from psychological or medical treatment. Cocaine Anonymous programs, self-help groups patterned after AA, are helpful for many in preventing relapse.

Cocaine abuse differs from many other forms of substance abuse in that women are as commonly represented among abusers as are men. Programs specifically designed to address women's needs and concerns may be more attractive to and effective for female abusers (Hughes et al., 1995). Overall, retention is a major problem for all cocaine treatment programs. Effectiveness of treatment is strongly related to motivation and to the level of functioning that the dependent individual had prior to becoming involved with cocaine. With increasing motivation and higher precocaine levels of functioning, treatment outcomes improve.

Nurse's Role in Cocaine Abuse

The nurse working in a chemical dependency unit will provide direct care to clients experiencing intense cravings for the drug and a sometimes overwhelming sense of depression related to the crash of not having another dose. The client may wish to stop his own use of the drug, but such recovery involves changing the client's lifestyle completely. The nurse must work with a treatment team, helping the client to choose recovery and then place himself in settings where recovery is possible. Changing jobs, living situations, and friends is not an easy task. Group support such as that of Cocaine Anonymous is helpful. The nurse is always in a collaborative role, working with other professionals, including addictions counselors, to help the client choose recovery. The nurse also has a role in assessing for depression, as cocaine users frequently experience depression during recovery.

Opiates

I Did Absolutely Nothing

*I lived in one room in the Native Quarter of Tangier. I had not taken a bath in a year nor changed my clothes or removed them except to stick a needle every hour into the fibrous grey wooden flesh of terminal addiction. I never cleaned or dusted the room. Empty ampule boxes and garbage piled to the ceiling. Light and water long since turned off for non payment. I did absolutely nothing. I could look at the end of my shoe for eight hours. I was only roused to action when the hourglass of junk ran out. If a friend came to visit and they rarely did since who or what was left to visit I sat there not caring that he had entered my field of vision a grey screen always blanker and fainter and not caring when he walked out of it. If he had died on the spot I would have sat there looking at my shoe waiting to go through his pockets. Wouldn't you? Because I never had enough junk—no one ever does. Thirty grains of morphine a day and it still was not enough. And long waits in front of the drugstore. Delay is a rule in the junk business. The Man is never on time. This is no accident. There are no accidents in the junk world. The addict is taught again and again exactly what will happen if he does not score for his junk ration. Get up that money or else. And suddenly my habit began to jump and jump. Forty, sixty grains a day. And it still was not enough. And I could not pay.**

(Burroughs, 1960, p. 18)

William Burroughs's testimony is particularly extraordinary because despite living under degrading circumstances in New York and North Africa, he still managed to be a major novelist, writer, and cult figure of the "beat" generation. As an author, Burroughs consciously cultivated the image of an outlaw, a man of evil and degradation. But however much he struck the literary pose of one who has purposefully chosen ugliness and self-destruction, drug dependency governed his life. He had left the protected world of Harvard for a life of filth and poverty, where his only certainty was withdrawal:

---

*From "Deposition: Testimony Concerning a Sickness," by W. Burroughs, 1960, *Evergreen Review*, 4, p. 18. © by Grove Press, Inc. Reprinted with permission.

I was an addict for fifteen years. When I say addict I mean an addict to junk (generic term for opium and/or derivatives including all synthetics from demerol to palfium). I have used junk in many forms: morphine, heroin, dilaudid, eukodal, pantapon, diocodid, diosane, opium, demerol, dolophine, palfium. I have smoked junk, eaten it, sniffed it, injected it in vein-skin-muscle, inserted it in rectal suppositories. The needle is not important . . . the result is the same: addiction.

(Burroughs, 1960, p. 18)

Effects

As Burroughs emphasizes, there are many opiates, all chemical derivatives of opium. Opium is derived from a milky secretion produced by the poppy flower's seed pods as they ripen. Small amounts of opium are found in poppy seeds and in other poppies, but the opium poppy —native to what is now Turkey—has by far the highest concentration. By some extraordinary biological coincidence, opium and its derivatives are a perfect fit for chemical receptor molecules in the nervous system of animals. Animals have a complex neurotransmitter system that regulates pain and activity and is known as the

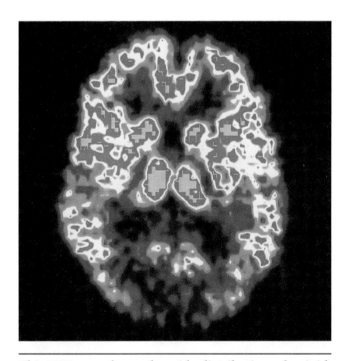

This PET scan shows the wide distribution of opioid binding sites. The highest opioid binding is represented by pink, yellow, and red/orange. Blue and green areas bind the least amount of opioid. *From "Addiction Brain Mechanisms and Their Related Implications," by D. J. Nutt, 1996,* The Lancet, 347, *pp. 33–35.*

endorphin system. Opiates fit into the endorphin receptors as a key fits into a lock, and fitting into that lock, they have profound effects on the brain. Stimulation of endorphin (usually called opiate) receptors produces a wide variety of changes in the nervous system: Perception of pain is diminished, a sense of comfort or pleasure is established, bodily functions slow down, and the brain vomiting center is stimulated. Opiates have important medical use in relieving pain and apprehension. They are also widely abused because of their euphoric properties: They make some users feel contented and free of worry and, depending on the dose and rapidity of administration, may give users a "rush" of intense pleasure. This rush seems to come primarily after intravenous administration and explains the continuing popularity of this exceedingly dangerous means of administering drugs.

Dependence and Withdrawal

As Burroughs implies, withdrawal is a phenomenon well known both to opiate abusers and care providers. Symptoms of withdrawal include depression, restlessness, nausea or vomiting, muscle aches, tearing and/or nasal discharge, dilated pupils, "gooseflesh," sweating, diarrhea, yawning, fever, and insomnia. Perhaps Burroughs was exaggerating when he claimed to need hourly injections: Withdrawal usually occurs 6 to 24 hours after a previous dose and is unlikely to occur at hourly intervals. Still, most addicts make every effort to avoid withdrawal and whenever possible provide themselves with opiates on a schedule that prevents the profoundly uncomfortable symptoms of withdrawal.

Tolerance is highly characteristic of opiate use. Burroughs describes his escalating dose of morphine. Addicts may come to require exceedingly high (and expensive) doses after a relatively brief time. In experimental studies, volunteers can be made tolerant to huge morphine doses (up to 500 mg/day) in only a little more than a week (Jaffe, 1990).

Technically, dependence can be demonstrated even after only one dose of morphine. If a narcotic antagonist (a drug that blocks the effects of opiates) is given soon after a single dose of morphine, mild withdrawal symptoms can be produced. This rapid development of dependence is of no clinical significance, but chronic or dependent users may have very protracted withdrawal that occurs in two phases. The first phase includes the acute symptoms discussed in the previous section and is over in a few days; the second phase may last for 6 months. Symptoms of the second phase include vague malaise, depression, changes in appetite, and measurable differences in temperature and respiration (Jaffe, 1990).

It seems that only some persons become dependent on opiates despite experimentation. There was widespread opiate use among U.S. servicemen in Vietnam, but only about half of those who used heroin became dependent.

Persons who used heroin multiple times were more likely to become dependent while in Vietnam, but many spontaneously stopped use when they returned to the United States (Robins, 1979). DSM-IV defines opiate abuse as occurring in persons who use opiates rarely but find themselves in social or legal difficulties because of that use. The presence of withdrawal or tolerance is far more likely to suggest dependence rather than merely abuse.

Treatment of Dependence

In the second passage from William Burroughs quoted previously, Burroughs claims that "The needle is not important." According to this view, the addict seeks only the chemical reaction of opiates with his or her endorphin receptors. Burroughs reports that addiction follows whatever the form of the substance used. However, while these pharmacological actions of opiates are undoubtedly of very great importance in leading to dependence, opiate addiction is a complex physical, psychological, and social phenomenon in which the *setting*—often including drug injection paraphernalia—is very important. Opiate users constitute a subculture with defined interactions, rituals, and hierarchies. Successful treatment must recognize that opiate abuse is a way of life, that for the addict to say "I did absolutely nothing" really means "I lived for opiates and nothing else." Treatment must not only separate the abuser from his or her junk, but it must also help supply human and spiritual content to a life that would otherwise be spent "looking at the end of a shoe for eight hours."

When opiate-dependent individuals seek treatment, the primary therapeutic decision is whether the goal should be detoxification or substitution of oral methadone for injected opiates. The principles of detoxification are not fundamentally different for opiates than they are for alcohol, tobacco, or cocaine: Drug usage is stopped, and any withdrawal symptoms are managed by medical intervention. Because opiate withdrawal symptoms are common and may be severe, specialized therapeutic and pharmacological approaches have been developed to facilitate detoxification (Vining, Kosten, & Kleber, 1988).

Methadone maintenance is an entirely different concept that bypasses detoxification but substitutes a "more acceptable" substance—medically prescribed methadone —for street opiates. Methadone is a long-acting orally administered opiate that can indefinitely suppress both the symptoms of withdrawal and the craving for intravenous fast-acting opiates such as heroin. At least in dependent individuals, oral methadone seems not to produce euphoria or sedation. It does, however, block opiate receptors so that while on methadone, further doses of intravenous heroin have little psychological or physical effect. In this way, not only does methadone reduce or eliminate opiate craving, but it also makes further administration of the opiate drug less attractive. The experience of 30 years suggests that methadone is safe and does not impair normal client functioning (Lowinson, Marion, Joseph, & Dole, 1992).

One of the strongest arguments in favor of methadone maintenance is that to the extent it is effective, it reduces injection drug use and hence decreases the risk of human immunodeficiency virus (HIV) transmission. Methadone maintenance has been a controversial therapy because it involves the legalized supply of prescription narcotics to clients whose only disease is opiate dependence. There is also little doubt that some of the methadone prescribed in maintenance programs is diverted onto the street, where it becomes part of the fabric of illegal abuse. If the goal is to keep opiate-dependent persons free of injection drugs, functional, and employable, then methadone maintenance has a useful role. The administration of methadone programs is complicated by the realities of current substance abuse. Abuse involving multiple drugs—often mixtures of heroin and cocaine—is very common. Methadone maintenance is, by its nature, focused on opiates alone, but opiate users are also frequently and simultaneously abusing cocaine, amphetamines, marijuana, and alcohol. As will be discussed in the following section, many methadone programs have adapted to the special needs of multidrug abuse (Joseph & Appel, 1985).

While methadone maintenance is strongly advocated by some, many experts equally strongly endorse the alternative goal of detoxification followed by abstinence. The principles of this latter approach are very similar to those employed in alcohol and cocaine treatment. As with these substances, successful treatment seems to require a combination of psychotherapy; attention to social, vocational, and spiritual well-being; and involvement in a 12-step group.

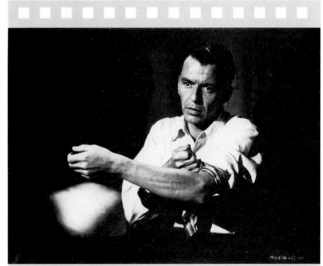

Man with the Golden Arm. Source: United Artists/Courtesy Kobal.

In a movie classic, Frank Sinatra portrays a man addicted to heroin. While the decade has changed, the effects of the drug and addiction remain constant.

Nurse's Role in Opiate Abuse

The nurse has a similar role in treating the opiate addict as in treating the alcoholic. The nurse may be involved with caring for the client in acute withdrawal, initial recovery, and long-term maintenance. In acute recovery, the nurse must monitor the withdrawal and ensure client safety. If methadone is used, the nurse will monitor the dose and effect. The nurse is almost always in a collaborative role, working with addictions counselors and other professionals to assist the client to choose recovery and then find a living situation where recovery is possible.

Other Commonly Abused Substances

Hallucinogens

Hallucinogens are substances such as lysergic acid diethylamide (LSD), mescaline, peyote, psilocybin, and MDMA (Ecstasy) that, when ingested, cause disturbances of perception or frank hallucinations. Hallucinogens were widely used in the 1960s, and reports suggest that they are once again relatively popularly abused substances. While tolerance to hallucinogen use develops quite quickly, dependence is rarely seen. Hallucinogen use is most commonly intermittent, often punctuated by long periods of abstinence. Injury from these drugs typically results from dangerous behaviors that occur when under the immediate influence, for example driving or diving off a building or other high place under the delusion that the individual can fly. Such abuse may result in serious injury or death. In contrast, violent behavior, though reported occasionally, is not frequent.

Inhalants

Inhalants are volatile chemical substances found most often as solvents in common household and industrial products: paints (especially aerosol spray paints), glue, and gasoline. Inhalants produce significant behavioral and psychological changes that may be variable or even seemingly opposite, depending both on the individual and the substance. Among these behavioral changes are aggressiveness, apathy, and poor judgment. Inhalants also produce neurological signs and symptoms, including dizziness, incoordination, slurred speech, unsteady gait, tremor, weakness, and stupor or coma. Hallucinations often result from inhalant use, and injury may occur because of impaired judgment. Death may occasionally occur from lung or heart complications. Long-term use of inhalants can lead to permanent neurological damage including brain atrophy and dysfunction. Inhalants are most often used by adolescents, frequently as part of group activities. Inhalant use is widespread and potentially dangerous, but only a relatively small proportion of users become dependent. Inhalants are frequently used in settings in which other drugs are not readily available. The ready availability of organic solvents makes controlling legal access to these drugs very difficult.

Cannabis (Marijuana)

Cannabis, also called hemp or "pot" or "weed," is a plant whose leaves, stems, and resin contain a variety of psychoactive substances that may be smoked or eaten. The effects of cannabis use include euphoria and impairments in memory, judgment, sensory perceptions, and motor skills. Hallucinations may occur, but symptoms of anxiety and dysphoria are more common psychiatric consequences. Cannabis is not regarded as a hallucinogen. While physiological dependence on cannabis probably does not occur, psychological dependence is not uncommon and may have a significant negative effect on personal and social functioning.

MULTIPLE DRUGS, MULTIPLE DIAGNOSES

Out of the dozens of substances that humans commonly abuse, this chapter has focused on the four most commonly used and widely abused: nicotine, alcohol, cocaine, and opiates. In line with the consumer society of the late 20th century, in which few people limit their consumption to one product, it is not at all unusual for any combination of these and other substances to be abused simultaneously. One important study that addressed multiple drug use was the Treatment Outcome Prospective Study (TOPS), which reported its findings in 1989 (Hubbard et al.). TOPS enrolled 10,000 participants in methadone programs and ambulatory and inpatient treatment centers. Thirty percent were women and 25% were under 21 years of age; the majority were male and over 21 years old. A large proportion of all enrolled participants were members of U.S. ethnic minorities. Thirty-one percent had been referred to their programs by the courts. In an analysis of multidrug use, methadone clinic enrollees differed somewhat from those in other treatment programs. Not surprisingly, the participants in methadone clinics were primarily heroin users; but even in methadone programs, 20% of individuals were heavy users of multiple drugs, and 50% used alcohol, cocaine, or marijuana in addition to heroin. Participants in non-methadone programs were even more likely to be multiple-drug users.

While multidrug abuse is a real and growing problem, it is also important to realize that many drug-dependent clients have other psychiatric problems in addition to drug dependence. The Epidemiologic Catchment Area Study found that more than 50% of substance-abusing individuals also had other psychiatric diagnoses. This study and others have reported a strong link between anxiety disorders, depression, mania, schizophrenia, and substance use (Beeder & Millman, 1992). Personality disorders are very common, with borderline and antisocial personalities strongly represented, the latter especially in opiate abusers (Nace, Davis, & Gaspari, 1991). Not surprisingly, it may be difficult for even experienced psychiatric diagnosticians to decide whether depression or anxiety is caused by drug dependence or was a problem before the dependence began. Some clients use substances to self-medicate their symptoms of depression or to suppress hallucinations. In such an individual, effective treatment of the primary underlying psychiatric diagnosis may occasionally eliminate the major motivation to use drugs. In the majority of dually diagnosed individuals, the combination of abuse and other psychiatric disorders merely complicates both diagnosis and treatment. Potentially successful programs, such as 12-step programs or methadone treatment, may be resisted by paranoid or antisocial clients. Dually diagnosed persons take immense amount of staff time in programs that are increasingly underfunded and understaffed. An equally important concern is that substance abuse may be significantly underrecognized in clients with other psychiatric disorders. The failure to recognize a comorbid substance abuse diagnosis may greatly interfere with treatment effectiveness for the presenting psychiatric problem (Beeder & Millman, 1992).

SUBSTANCE ABUSE AS A SOCIAL PROBLEM

Substance abuse is a serious and perplexing social problem that is by no means solely (or perhaps even primarily) psychiatric in its nature. The issues surrounding substance abuse raise important questions about law, individual rights and freedom, and the social role of productive work versus the pursuit of pleasure. Substance abuse challenges society to address issues of homelessness, poverty, alienation, and the spread of infectious diseases, including hepatitis B, AIDS, and tuberculosis including its multidrug-resistant forms. There is no easy answer to the nearly universal and timeless problem of substance abuse. Strict controls have yet to work, perhaps because, as some have argued, they have not yet been strict enough or perhaps because, as others claim, criminal elements have achieved too great an influence over politicians and police. Some have argued for moving beyond limited methadone maintenance to a legalization of virtually all abused substances as long as access is restricted to adult use only. These arguments were first made over 150 years ago by the English political philosopher John Stuart Mill, and they continue to prove attractive to liberal and conservative Americans alike. There is much logic on the side of legalization, including the reality that prohibitions have had at best a small influence on the volume of drug use. However, neither political nor public opinion support legalization, and it seems highly unlikely that the United States will adopt drug legalization as public policy in the near future.

Siegel (1989) has proposed an equally radical but quite different solution to addressing the seemingly irrepressible human need for intoxication. In his view, legal-

ization is flawed, at least in part because drugs are not safe, their use would likely increase under legalization, and the process of legalization puts "the government seal of approval on such appealing yet imperfect substances" (p. 299). Instead of legalizing current substances, Siegel proposes that society devote some of its scientific skill to developing safer and better ones. Even assuming that the "perfect drug" could be found—a drug highly appealing and safe for short- and long-term use—it is unclear that society is likely to endorse its legal use. Still, at this time there are no "good" drugs: Each has its health risks, its tolerance, its withdrawal symptoms, and its devoted users. This reality is unlikely to change as far into the 21st century as it is now possible to see.

IMPACT OF DRUG USE/ABUSE ON FAMILIES

The impact of substance abuse goes beyond the individual abuser. Each person is a member of a family unit, a social group, and society, such that the result of addiction and chemical dependency extend to those in the person's immediate and sometimes not-so-immediate environment.

Family Dysfunction

Father

He weaves past into the house, where he slumps into his overstuffed chair and falls asleep. . . . All evening, until our bedtimes, we tiptoe past him, as past a snoring dragon. Then we curl in our fearful sheets, listening. Eventually he wakes with a grunt, Mother slings accusations at him, he snarls back, she yells, he growls, their voices clashing. Before long, she retreats to their bedroom, sobbing —not from the blows of fists, for he never strikes her, but from the force of words. . . .Whatever my brother and sister and mother may be thinking on their own rumpled pillows, I lie there hating him, loving him, fearing him, knowing I have failed him. I tell myself he drinks to ease an ache that gnaws at his belly, an ache I must have caused by disappointing him somehow, a murderous ache I should be able to relieve by doing all my chores, earning A's in school, winning baseball games, fixing the broken washer and the burst pipes, bringing in money to fill his empty wallet. . . .

When the drink made him weepy, Father would pack a bag and kiss each of us children on the head, and announce from the front door that he was moving out. "Where to?" we demanded, fearful each time that he would leave for good as Mr. Sampson had roared away for good in his diesel truck. "Someplace where I won't get hounded every minute," Father would answer, his jaw quivering. . . . We bawled and bawled, wondering if he would ever come back. He always did come back, a day or a week later, but each time there was a sliver less of him.

(Sanders, 1989, p. 73)

The effects of alcoholism on families has been well documented. Family disruption related to alcoholism is a serious, complex, and pervasive social problem. Alcoholism is linked to violence, disrupted family roles, impaired family communication, and some physical and psychological illnesses such as depression, GI disturbances, and asthma/emphysema (Lindeman, Hawks, & Bartek, 1994). Similarly, consequences of alcoholism all too often result in chaotic, disorganized, and dysfunctional family units. Children reared in homes where one parent is an alco-

holic exhibit stress and express a lack of ability to get along with others as well as a lack of feelings of attachment toward their parents. Adolescents from alcoholic families are reported to exhibit low levels of warmth, awareness, understanding, trust, respect, and kindness toward others when compared to adolescents from families without alcohol abuse (Scavnicky-Mylant, 1990). Characteristics inherent in the diagnosis of *altered family processes: alcoholism* are presented in the accompanying display. Major defining characteristics of this nursing diagnosis are also presented. Review of these family characteristics indicates that the family milieu is such that the needs of family members cannot be met without dealing first with the alcohol abuse and the family characteristics that support the abuse. While less research exists on family dysfunction when drugs other than alcohol are

---

CONCEPTS INHERENT IN THE DEFINITION OF THE NURSING DIAGNOSIS ALTERED FAMILY PROCESSES: ALCOHOLISM

◆ Affects psychosocial function of family

◆ Dysfunction

◆ Denial of problem

◆ Chronicity

◆ Pervades all family functions

◆ Conflict

◆ Disorganization of family unit

◆ Ineffective problem-solving style

◆ Family experiences series of crises

◆ Difficulty in escaping dysfunctional system

◆ Insidious process

◆ Affects spiritual functioning of family

◆ Creates lifetime self-perpetuating pattern

◆ Lack of protective, stable family unit

◆ Ineffective support systems

◆ Affects physiological functioning of family members

From "The Alcoholic Family: A Nursing Diagnosis Validation Study," by Lindeman, M., Hawks, J. H., and Bartek, J. K., 1994, *Nursing Diagnosis, 5,* pp. 65–73. Used with permission.

EXAMPLES OF THE DEFINING CHARACTERISTICS OF THE NURSING DIAGNOSIS ALTERED FAMILY PROCESSES: ALCOHOLISM

◆ Deterioration in family relationships

◆ Disturbed family dynamics

◆ Marital problems

◆ Ineffective spousal communication

◆ Inconsistent parenting

◆ Family denial

◆ Intimacy dysfunction

◆ Closed communication system

◆ Loss of control of drinking

◆ Rationalization

◆ Broken promises

◆ Inability to meet emotional needs of members

◆ Manipulation

◆ Inappropriate expression of anger

◆ Dependency

◆ Enabling behaviors

◆ Decreased self-esteem

◆ Frustration

◆ Powerlessness

◆ Tension

◆ Insecurity

From "The Alcoholic Family: A Nursing Diagnosis Validation Study," by Lindeman, M., Hawks, J. H., and Bartek, J. K., 1994, *Nursing Diagnosis, 5,* pp. 65–73. Used with permission.

involved, the dysfunctional family unit is the same in any situation where the need to obtain drugs/chemicals takes precedence over the need to nurture and support the development of each family member.

Codependence

Codependence is a term used to describe the cluster of behaviors exhibited by family members/significant others (most often a spouse) of one who is chemically addicted that serve to enable the alcoholic or addict to continue using the substance. Codependent behaviors serve to satisfy the needs of the family member to feel loved, important, and needed. The codependent behaviors of a spouse of an alcoholic typically are those enabling behaviors that permit the alcoholic to avoid the logical consequences of drinking. For example, if a husband is unable to go to work due to a hangover and his wife calls his office while he sleeps to tell his co-workers that he has the flu and cannot come to work today, the wife has enabled the alcoholic to be irresponsible. Further, examination of the dynamics of her motivations will almost always demonstrate that she has a need to do good things for others and defines her own self-worth only in terms of caring for and caring about others *at the exclusion of her own needs for self-development and fulfillment*. Codependence should not be confused with altruistic, prosocial behaviors that are performed on the basis of a genuine desire to serve the greater good by acts of kindness and compassion. The difference is that the codependent person performs the acts to meet her own needs and loses her sense of self by defining her self-worth in relation to what others think. The codependent person lacks ability to form intimate relationships with others, as she develops only one part of her personality to the exclusion of others.

Family members who assist an alcoholic or drug addict in maintaining addictive behaviors only aide their loved one in the general downward spiral of chemical dependence. These family members must be taught how to let the addict suffer the logical consequences of addictive behaviors and to remove themselves personally from the disease, the behaviors, and the shame that the addict experiences. Family members need help to realize that there is hope for recovery only if and when the addict himself is willing to stop the addiction. Enabling behaviors serve only to keep the addict from having to confront his behaviors and further keep the enabler from coming to terms with her own unmet needs for acknowledgment, love, intimacy, and personal growth.

A nurse working with any family where alcohol or drugs are used must become familiar with the dynamics of codependence and the means to assist family members even when the addicted individual refuses help. National self-help groups such as Alanon and Alateen (which help family members, friends, and teens who have an alcoholic

relative or friend), Cocaine Anonymous, Narcotics Anonymous, and Co-dependents Anonymous are some of the many groups to which referrals can be made.

NURSING THEORY AND PSYCHOLOGICAL THEORY

Nurses may use any nursing theory in understanding the addicted client and in planning interventions. In some cases, a psychological theory may also be used to guide practice. Theory helps the nurse put the complex problems faced by clients and families in perspective. In addition, theory helps the nurse understand the addiction and accompanying behaviors as well as helps to frame interventions in light of that understanding. An example follows:

> If the nurse seeks to understand the drinking behavior of an alcoholic, she can frame the behavior in terms of behavioral theory: heavy-drinking behaviors related to a positive reinforcement history for drinking behaviors. Here, the nurse will look at the societal reinforcements for drinking—drinking heavily at parties, being taken out for drinks after work, and so on—as factors that contributed to alcoholism. Interventions would be aimed at changing environmental factors that reinforced drinking. In contrast, the same nurse can frame the heavy-drinking behaviors in terms of psychoanalytic theory and view the heavy-drinking behaviors as related to unmet needs for oral gratification. Here, the heavy-drinking behaviors are seen as symptoms of an underlying problem, and interventions would be aimed at meeting the developmental needs from the psychoanalytic perspective.

Interpersonal nursing theory guides the nurse to see the addict as an individual, a human being who has succumbed to the effects of a chemical and lost much of his humanity in the process—as William Burroughs asked when describing his addicted life, "who or what was left to visit?" It is difficult to establish a relationship with one who is chemically dependent; however, the individual's recovery is almost certainly dependent upon his ability to bond with others and to find a life worth living outside the drug world. Interpersonal theory suggests that the nurse approach the client as a caring human being, placing the full responsibility for the client's recovery in his own hands. The nurse can then provide caring, support, and, above all, honesty in all matters relating to recovery. One theme that seems to recur in work with addicted persons is that they do not see themselves as worthy of other persons' caring and attention. Years of abuse lead the person to lose self-esteem; many describe themselves as merely a shell. It is the goal of nursing interventions, then, to assist the client to regain himself, to find the humanness that was once there and literally build a new life.

N U R S I N G   P R O C E S S

A nurse in any setting in virtually every field of nursing will encounter chemical dependency in the course of routine work. Clearly, one recognizes that a nurse working in a chemical dependency unit will encounter addictions. However, few stop to recognize that every nurse in an emergency department, on a medical floor, in home care, or in the schools will be faced with alcohol or drug dependency.

To be adequately prepared to meet the needs of the client and family, the nurse must first make herself ready and willing to view chemical dependency as a disease and know that the client who wishes to recover has options that only he can take. The nurse can play a major role in directing the client to recovery programs and directing the family members to deal with their own dysfunction whether or not the client chooses to deal with his addiction.

◢ ASSESSMENT

Assessment begins with a client history. The nurse should always inquire about use of alcohol and other substances. The nurse should begin with questions such as "Do you drink alcohol?" If the answer is "yes," follow-up questions such as "How much do you drink each week?" "Do you drink every day?" "Have you ever had trouble at work related to your drinking?" and "Have you missed work or school over the last month because of drinking?" should be asked to obtain a clearer picture of the degree to which alcohol plays a role in the client's life. Further questions such as "Do you take medications regularly?" "Do you use street drugs?" and "Have you used street drugs in the past?" help the nurse to obtain information regarding other addictive drugs. Lastly, questions about smoking and caffeine use are also indicated.

If the client has been using addictive substances regularly or if the client is admitted to a chemical dependency treatment unit, the nurse must assess closely for specific symptoms of withdrawal, described earlier in this chapter.

◢ NURSING DIAGNOSIS

There are several nursing diagnoses that are common in situations of addictions. These relate to both client and family. A list is presented in the accompanying display.

◢ OUTCOME IDENTIFICATION

The expected outcome of treatment for any chemical dependence is that the client chooses recovery and estab-

---

COMMONLY USED NURSING DIAGNOSES FOR CLIENTS ADDICTED TO CHEMICAL SUBSTANCES

PSYCHOSOCIAL DIAGNOSES

◆ *Ineffective individual coping*

◆ *Altered family processes*

◆ *Altered self-esteem*

◆ *Social isolation*

◆ *Powerlessness*

◆ *Hopelessness*

◆ *Spiritual distress*

PHYSIOLOGICAL DIAGNOSES

◆ *Altered nutrition, less than body requirements*

◆ *Risk for infection*

---

lishes a lifestyle that does not require use of addictive substances. There are, however, several outcomes of care viewing the recovery as a life-long process with several steps leading to complete recovery. A first expected outcome is the safe withdrawal from the addictive substance. A second outcome is that the client will choose recovery and begin to plan changes in his life based on finding needed supports to avoid using the substance. A third expected outcome is that the client will remain free of the substance, first for one day, then for every other day of his life.

Caring for families, the nurse may identify an expected outcome that the family members will not take on the addict's illness; rather, the family will provide support for recovery and seek healthy family functioning whether the addict chooses recovery or not.

◢ PLANNING/INTERVENTIONS

Interventions will be based on the setting in which the nurse finds herself and the availability of drug treatment programs. In many situations, the nurse will function in a collaborative role rather than as the primary care provider.

Nursing interventions include establishing a relationship with the client that is based on trust, grounded in reality, and characterized by firm kindness. Remembering that denial is the most commonly used defense mechanism by one who is addicted, the nurse must approach the client in a manner to challenge such denial.

Nursing interventions, then, must encourage a successful treatment plan: helping the client to make significant changes in lifestyle, friends, job, and so on are needed. Referrals to groups such as AA along with encouragement to enter into a long-term program (such as a 12-step program) are important nursing activities.

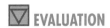 **EVALUATION**

Evaluation is based on expected outcomes. Many persons addicted to alcohol and/or drugs choose recovery, but many do so only after several tries. The nurse must always be ready to help a client toward recovery at the level that the client wants.

CASE STUDY/CARE PLAN

In the excerpts presented in the discussion of alcoholism and its effects on families, Sanders and his father represent a family that could be encountered by a nurse. In his younger years, the father is presented as a man consumed by alcoholism: a husband/father who slips into the garage or barn to drink, who sleeps in a drunken stupor on the living room couch, who fights with his wife, who packs his bags to leave the family home, who then returns to his dysfunctional home. This father, however, stayed dry for 15 years, following the death of his own brother from alcohol abuse. The father's retirement signaled a return to his previous home (Mississippi) and a return to drinking. We are told, "He gave up his identity along with his job." Sanders visits his father only to discover, quite unexpectedly, that his father has resumed drinking and that his mother has been too distraught (or codependent) to tell her son that the father's illness has reemerged.

Based on the son's interpretation, the nurse would want to validate that the drinking behavior resumed because of a loss of direction and/or self-esteem.

Further, the nurse would assess the personal significance to the father of his move back to Mississippi: What are the factors (social, environmental, familial) in

Mississippi that contribute to drinking behaviors of this man? His personal history is important. Further, the wife's behavior is important to assess. Her son writes she is "distraught." Assessment of her level of stress, her support, and verbal/physical abuse needs to be performed.

Imagine nurses are giving care to the Kerwin family, a family with an alcoholic father. The father, a retired mechanic, has moved the family to a smaller town. His increased drinking has disrupted family functioning. This family is going through similar experiences as those described by Sanders. The son has called a community health nurse to assist the family.

ASSESSMENT

The Kerwin family is undergoing confusion. The father of the family is an alcoholic, and his drinking has disrupted family functioning. The father drinks in secrecy, but he is overtly impaired. The mother and wife alternates between anger, tears, and frustration. The father is drinking heavily, apparently as a result of his retirement from work.

NURSING DIAGNOSIS Father: *ineffective individual coping*: related to situational crisis (loss of social role and loss of support system), as evidenced by inability to meet role expectations (of father and retiree)

Outcomes	Planning/Interventions	Evaluation
◆ Client will willingly participate in a treatment program within the next 3 weeks. ◆ Client will choose recovery. ◆ Client will identify: (1) one negative effect of excessive alcohol consumption and (2) two positive personal strengths.	◆ Approach the client nonjudgmentally and establish a professional relationship. ◆ Discuss alcoholism as a disease that is treatable. ◆ Encourage the client to self-admit to a treatment program. ◆ Offer referral to the program. ◆ Provide firm grounding in reality when the client uses denial by pointing out his behaviors and their effects.	The client began to think about his drinking as an illness; he admitted that the drinking was out of his control. He stated he could choose whether or not to take a drink, but if he did take but one drink, he could not choose when to stop drinking.

Continued

Outcomes	Planning/Interventions	Evaluation
◆ Client will identify one behavior other than drinking to deal with life stressors.	◆ Encourage client to talk about himself and his life. ◆ Point out personal strengths and positive traits, such as the fact that client stopped drinking for 15 years, he has his physical health at this time, and he has a good understanding of his disease. ◆ Introduce client to AA, encourage him to talk with his AA sponsor; help him to see that AA is a support group where individuals help each other to stop drinking.	Within 2 weeks, client entered a program and began attending AA.

NURSING DIAGNOSIS Mother: *fear,* related to living in unknown/unpredictable situations due to spouse's drinking behavior

Outcomes	Planning/Interventions	Evaluation
◆ Within 1 week, client will verbalize her fears. ◆ Within 2 weeks, client will identify codependent behaviors and begin to take steps to meet her own needs for safety and security.	◆ Provide positive encouragement for client to talk with nurse: remain nonjudgmental, establish trust, and use interpersonal communication to affirm positive regard. ◆ Provide information on the functioning of alcoholic families; assess client's desire to participate in a support program; and encourage her to accept Alanon groups by explaining that many others in her situation have found support there. ◆ Reaffirm client's personal integrity by letting her make her own choices. Give the control of decisions and treatment to her. Let her know you are there to assist.	Client almost immediately opened up to the nurse. She disclosed personal information regarding herself and her family. She is unhappy and is willing to consider a change but is afraid. She accepted information about Alanon. She asked the nurse to introduce her to one person from Alanon.

NURSING DIAGNOSIS Family: *altered family processes*: alcoholism, related to abuse of alcohol, as evidenced by deterioration in family relationships, ineffective spousal communication, denial of problems, and enabling behaviors

Outcomes	Planning/Interventions	Evaluation
◆ The family members will acknowledge to each other that they have an alcoholic member and that this fact has affected their functioning for years.	◆ Visit with each family member individually and ask the family members if they would like to meet with the nurse as a group. ◆ Provide information on the behaviors common to alcoholic families: enabling behaviors, use of denial, inability to communicate with one another, and fear of family violence.	Within 3 weeks time, the nurse had established a nurse-client relationship with each family member. The family members listened to and received written information on the behaviors of alcoholic families but were not willing to talk with the nurse or any other counselor as a group.

Continued

CRITICAL THINKING BAND

ASSESSMENT

What other factors (e.g., input from the father's former coworkers) would help give a complete assessment picture of the father's apparent substance abuse?

NURSING DIAGNOSIS

How can a nurse be truly holistic with this family?

Outcomes

There were several clients in this situation. How often do we consider spouses, partners, children, and friends in treatment plans? How often should we?

Planning/Interventions

How do nurses deal with "solutionless" problems?

Evaluation

How do you help a family or individual begin a lifelong process of recovery? Is the nurse's work ever done?

〰 KEY CONCEPTS

♦ Substance abuse has been a part of human society since early human history.

♦ Most abused substances can be classified as stimulants, hallucinogens, or CNS depressants.

♦ Drug use refers to the taking of the drug; abuse refers to a maladaptive pattern of continued use despite real or potential harm.

♦ Tolerance is an acquired resistance to a drug's effects; withdrawal is a condition that occurs when stopping a drug results in a drug-specific set of symptoms that would be relieved by taking additional doses of the drug.

♦ Nicotine is the most commonly abused substance in the United States, with clear addictive properties.

♦ Alcohol abuse is typically diagnosed when alcohol use leads to work problems, hazardous practices, legal difficulties, or continuing use in the face of physical or social problems.

♦ Ninety percent of alcoholics have significant medical problems in addition to their alcohol dependence; thus, nurses come into contact with alcoholics in virtually every nursing specialty.

♦ Screening questionnaires like the CAGE provide a means of identifying those who require referral.

♦ Treatment for alcohol dependence begins with a drug detoxification and is followed by counseling, group support, and medication.

♦ Alcoholics Anonymous (AA), based on 12 steps, provides individuals with group support and a method of learning to live without drinking.

♦ Cocaine, which affects the brain's reward centers, produces a high that includes a feeling of improved self-image and increased euphoria. In the form of crack, cocaine has exceedingly high addictive potential.

♦ Tolerance to cocaine is common, with persons reporting that their initial experiences of pleasure and euphoria are almost never replicated with continuing use.

♦ Opiates, which have important medical uses in relieving pain and apprehension, are widely abused because of their euphoric properties.

♦ The opiate addict has a need for increasingly higher doses and experiences distressing symptoms that occur anytime between 6 and 24 hours after the previous dose.

♦ Opiate addiction is a complex physical, psychological, and social phenomenon; treatment involves detoxification and helping the person to find human and spiritual content in a life that has been devoid of everything but the opiate subculture.

♦ Multidrug use is a growing problem in the United States.

♦ Many individuals who abuse substances have other psychiatric diagnoses as well.

♦ Codependence is a term used to describe the behaviors of family members who enable the addicted person to maintain the addiction while serving to satisfy the family members' needs to feel loved, important, and needed.

♦ Drug abuse affects families and is linked to violence, disrupted family roles, and impaired family communications.

◆ Both nursing theory and psychological theory guide the nurse in understanding the client and family and in planning interventions.

REVIEW QUESTIONS AND ACTIVITIES

1. Describe the nature of substance abuse in your home town, in your local high school, and on your college campus.

2. List the commonly abused substances in your region.

3. Identify factors that contribute to use and continued abuse of drugs in your community.

4. Identify community efforts to prevent as well as to treat drug abuse.

5. Identity the effects, withdrawal, and patterns of abuse for nicotine, alcohol, cocaine, and opiates.

6. Explain the major treatment approaches for drug dependence.

7. Examine the effects of alcohol or drug abuse on families and children in your community. What is being done to support families/children? What could the nurse do as a client advocate?

8. Use nursing theory to develop a care plan/treatment approach for a client you have seen with drug dependency.

EXPLORING THE WEB

◆ Visit this text's "Online Companion™" on the Internet at **http://www.DelmarNursing.com** for further information on substance use and abuse.

◆ What organizations or professional journals could you search for information on addictions?

◆ Check the sites of some of the major nursing organizations, such as North American Nursing Diagnosis Association and National League for Nursing. Do they include pages that might offer you information on substance abuse and addiction?

◆ What resources are available through the Internet for families and/or health care professionals needing advice or counseling for substance abuse? Are phone numbers and addresses given?

◆ Is there a listing on the Internet of books, videos, or other media on addictions and substance abuse? Are these resources available in your local library or through purchase over the Web?

◆ What resources are listed for caregivers and health care professionals? Can you find specific information on codependency?

REFERENCES

Alterman, A. I., O'Brien, C. P., McLellan, A. T., August, D. S., Snider, E. C., Droba, M., Cornish, J. W., Hall, C. P., Raphaelson, A. H., Schrade, F. X. (1994). Effectiveness and costs of inpatient versus day hospital cocaine rehabilitation. *Journal of Nervous and Mental Disease, 182,* 157–163.

American Psychiatric Association. (1994). *Diagnostic and Statistical Manual of Mental Disorders* Fourth Edition Washington, DC American Psychiatric Association, 1994.

Bauer, L. O. (1992). Psychobiology of craving. In J. Lowinson, P. Ruiz, R. Millman, & J. Langrod (Eds.), *Substance abuse: A comprehensive textbook* (2nd ed., pp. 51–55). Baltimore: Williams & Wilkins.

Beeder, A. B., & Millman, R. B. (1992). Treatment of patients with psychopathology and substance abuse. In J. Lowinson, P. Ruiz, R. Millman, & J. Langrod (Eds.), *Substance abuse: A comprehensive textbook* (2nd ed., pp. 675–689). Baltimore: Williams & Wilkins.

Boscarino, J. (1980). Factors related to stable and unstable affiliation with Alcoholics Anonymous. *International Journal of Addiction, 15,* 839–848.

Bower, B. (1994). Assaults may amplify female alcoholism. *Science News, 146,* 5.

Bower, B. (1995). Brain data fuel alcoholism gene clash. *Science News, 148,* 20.

Brain, P. F., & Coward, G. A. (1989). A review of the history, actions, and legitimate uses of cocaine. *Journal of Substance Abuse, 1,* 431–451.

Chang, G., & Kosten, T. (1992). Emergency management of acute drug intoxication. In J. Lowinson, P. Ruiz, R. Millman, & J. Langrod (Eds.), *Substance abuse: A comprehensive textbook* (2nd ed., pp. 437–445). Baltimore: Williams & Wilkins.

Charness, M. E. (1992). Molecular mechanisms of ethanol intoxication, tolerance, and physical dependence. In J. H. Mendelson & N. K. Mello (Eds.), *Medical diagnosis and treatment of alcoholism* (pp. 155–199). New York: McGraw-Hill.

Duckert, F. (1987). Recruitment into treatment and effects of treatment for female problem drinkers. *Addictive Behaviors, 12,* 137–150.

Edwards, J. A., Wesnes, K., Warburton, D. M., & Gale, A. (1985). Evidence of more rapid stimulus evaluation following cigarette smoking. *Addictive Behaviors, 10,* 113–126.

Emrick, C. D. (1987). Alcoholics Anonymous affiliation process and effectiveness as treatment. *Alcohol, Clinical and Experimental Research, 11,* 416–423.

Ewing, J. A. (1984). Detecting alcoholism: The CAGE questionnaire. *Journal of the American Medical Association, 252,* 1905–1907.

Frezza, M., Di Padova, C., Pozzato, G., Terpin, M., Bargona, E., Lieber, C. S. (1990). High blood alcohol levels in women: The role of decreased gastric alcohol dehydrogenase activity and first-pass metabolism. *New England Journal of Medicine, 322,* 95–99.

Fuller, R. K., Branchley, L., & Brightwell, D. R. (1986). Disulfiram treatment of alcoholism: A Veteran's Administration cooperative study. *Journal of the American Medical Association, 256,* 1449–1455.

Gardner, E. L. (1992). Brain reward mechanisms. In J. Lowinson, P. Ruiz, R. Millman, & J. Langrod (Eds.), *Substance abuse: A comprehensive textbook* (2nd ed., p. 76). Baltimore: Williams & Wilkins.

Gold, M. S. (1992). Cocaine (and crack): Clinical aspects. In J. Lowinson, P. Ruiz, R. Millman, & J. Langrod (Eds.), *Substance abuse: A comprehensive textbook* (2nd ed., pp. 205–206). Baltimore: Williams & Wilkins.

Goldstein, D. B., Chin, J. H., & Lyon, R. C. (1982). Ethanol disordering of spin-labeled mouse brain membranes—correlation with genetically-determined ethanol sensitivity of mice. *Proceedings of the National Academy of Science USA, 79,* 4231–4233.

Goodwin, D. W. (1992). Alcohol: Clinical aspects. In J. Lowinson, P. Ruiz, R. Millman, & J. Langrod (Eds.), *Substance abuse: A comprehensive textbook* (2nd ed.). Baltimore: Williams & Wilkins.

Grinspoon, L., & Bakalar, J. B. (1992). Marihuana. In J. Lowinson, P. Ruiz, R. Millman, & J. Langrod (Eds.), *Substance abuse: A comprehensive textbook* (2nd ed., pp. 236–246). Baltimore: Williams & Wilkins.

Grunberg, N. E. (1990). The inverse relationship between tobacco use and body weight. In L. T. Koslowski, H. M. Annis, & H. D. Cappell (Eds.), *Research advances in alcohol and drug problems* (Vol. 10, pp. 273–315). New York: Plenum.

Heath, R. G. (1964). Pleasure response of human beings to direct stimulation of the brain. In R. G. Heath (Ed.), *The role of pleasure in behavior* (pp. 219–243). New York: Hoeber.

Hitzig, P. (1993). Combined dopamine and serotonin agonists: A synergistic approach to alcoholism and other addictive behaviors. *Maryland Medical Journal, 42,* 156–157.

Hubbard, R. I., Marsden, M. E., Rachal, J. V., Harwood, H. J., Cavannaugh, E. R., & Ginzburg, H. M. (1989). *Drug abuse treatment: A national study of effectiveness.* Chapel Hill, NC: University of North Carolina Press.

Hughes, P. H., Coletti, S. D., Neri, R. L., Urmann, C. F., Stahl, S., Aialian, D. M., & Anthony, J. C. (1995). Retaining cocaine abusing women in a therapeutic community: The effect of a child live-in program. *American Journal of Public Health, 85,* 1149–1152.

Jaffe, J. H. (1990). Drug addiction and drug abuse. In A. G. Gilman, T. W. Rall, A. S. Nies, & P. Taylor (Eds.), *Goodman and Gilman's the pharmacological basis of therapeutics* (8th ed., pp. 311–331). New York: Pergamon.

Jaffe, J. H. (1992). Opiates: Clinical aspects. In J. Lowinson, P. Ruiz, R. Millman, & J. Langrod (Eds.), *Substance abuse: A comprehensive textbook* (2nd ed., p. 188). Baltimore: Williams & Wilkins.

Jarvik, M. E., & Schneider, N. G. (1992). Nicotine. In J. Lowinson, P. Ruiz, R. Millman, & J. Langrod (Eds.), *Substance abuse: A comprehensive textbook* (2nd ed., pp. 334–356). Baltimore: Williams & Wilkins.

Jellinek, E. M. (1960). *The disease concept of alcoholism.* New Brunswick, NJ: Jillhouse.

Jesinski, D. R., Johnson, R. E., & Henningfield, J. E. (1984). Abuse liability assessment in human subjects. *Trends in Pharmacological Science, 5,* 96–200.

Johnston, L. M. (1985). Tobacco smoking and nicotine. *Lancet, 2,* 742.

Joseph, H., & Appel, P. (1985). Alcoholism and methadone treatment: Consequences for the patient and the program. *American Journal of Drug and Alcohol Abuse, 11,* 37–53.

Kornetsky, C. (1985). Brain-stimulation reward: A model for the neuronal bases for drug-induced euphoria. *National Institute on Drug Abuse Research Monograph Series, 62,* 30–50.

Korsten, M. A., & Lieber, C. S. (1992). The gastrointestinal effects of alcohol. In J. H. Mendelson & N. K. Mello (Eds.), *Medical diagnosis and treatment of alcoholism* (pp. 289–339). New York: McGraw-Hill.

Kranzler, H. R., Burleson, J. A., Del Boca, F. K., Babor, T. F., Korner, P., Brown, J., & Bohn, M. J. (1994). Buspirone treatment of anxious alcoholics. A placebo-controlled trial. *Archives of General Psychiatry, 51,* 720–731.

Kranzler, H. R., Burleson, J. A., Korner, P., Del Boca, F. K., Bohn, M. J., Brown, J., & Liebowitz, N. (1995). Placebo-controlled trial of fluoxetine as an adjunct to relapse prevention in alcoholics. *American Journal of Psychiatry, 152,* 391–397.

Lender, M. E., & Martin, J. K. (1987). *Drinking in America: A history.* New York: Free Press.

Lex, B. W. (1992). Alcohol problems in special populations. In J. H. Mendelson & N. K. Mello (Eds.), *Medical diagnosis and treatment of alcoholism* (pp. 71–154). New York: McGraw-Hill.

Lindeman, M., Hawks, J. H., & Bartek, J. K. (1994). The alcoholic family: A nursing diagnosis validation study. *Nursing Diagnosis, 5,* 65–73.

Lowinson, J. H., Marion, I. J., Joseph, H., & Dole, V. P. (1992). Methadone maintenance. In J. Lowinson, P. Ruiz, R. Millman, & J. Langrod (Eds.), *Substance abuse: A comprehensive textbook* (2nd ed., pp. 550–561). Baltimore: Williams & Wilkins.

Medical Letter. (1995). Naltrexone for alcohol dependence. *Medical Letter on Drugs and Therapeutics, 37,* 64–66.

Musto, D. F. (1992). Historical perspectives on alcohol and drug abuse. In J. Lowinson, P. Ruiz, R. Millman, & J. Langrod (Eds.), *Substance abuse: A comprehensive textbook* (2nd ed.). Baltimore: Williams & Wilkins.

Nace, E. P., Davis, C. W., & Gaspari, J. P. (1991). Axis II comorbidity in substance abusers. *American Journal of Psychiatry, 148*, 118–120.

O'Malley, S. S., Jaffe, A. J., Chang, G., Schottenfeld, R. S., Meyer, R. E., & Rounsaville, B. (1992). Naltrexone and coping skills therapy for alcohol dependence: A controlled study. *Archives of General Psychiatry, 49*, 881–887.

Pfaffmann, C. (1960). The pleasures of sensation. *Psychological Review, 67*, 253–268.

Prochaska, J. O., Velicer, W. F., di Clemente, C. C., & Fava, J. (1988). Measuring processes of change: Applications to the cessation of smoking. *Journal of Consulting and Clinical Psychology, 56*, 520–528.

Raloff, J. (1994). Cigarettes: Are they doubly addictive? *Science News, 145*, 294.

Rinaldi, R. C., Steindler, E. M., Wilford, B. B., & Goodwin, D. (1988). Clarification and standardization of substance abuse terminology. *Journal of the American Medical Association, 259*, 555–567.

Robins, L. N. (1979). Addict careers. In R. I. Dupont, A. Goldstein, & J. O'Donnell (Eds.), *Handbook on drug abuse* (pp. 325–336). Washington, DC: U.S. Government Printing Office.

Rosencrans, J. A., & Chance, W. T. (1977). Cholinergic and non-cholinergic aspects of the discriminative stimulus properties of nicotine. In H. Lai (Ed.), *Discriminative stimulus properties of drugs* (pp. 155–186). New York: Plenum.

Scavnicky-Mylant, M. (1990). The process of coping among young adult children of alcoholics. *Journal of Studies on Alcohol, 43*, 119–128.

Schuckit, M. A. (1992). Treatment of alcoholism in office and outpatient settings. In J. H. Mendelson & N. K. Mello (Eds.), *Medical diagnosis and treatment of alcoholism* (pp. 363–392). New York: McGraw-Hill.

Schuckit, M. A., & Irwin, M. (1988). Diagnosis of alcoholism. *Medical Clinics of North America, 72*, 1133–1153.

Schwartz, J. L. (1987). *Review and evaluation of smoking cessation methods: The United States and Canada, 1978–85.* U.S.

Department of Health and Human Services. Public Health Services. National Institute of Health. Washington DC: U.S. Government Printing Office.

Shiffman, S., Read, L., Maltese, J., Rapkin, D., & Jarvik, M. E. (1985). Preventing relapse in exsmokers. In G. A. Marlatt & J. R. Gordon (Eds.), *Relapse prevention: Maintenance strategies in the treatment of addictive behaviors.* New York: Guilford.

Siegel, R. K. (1989). *Intoxication.* New York: EP Dutton.

Vaillant, G. E. (1982). Natural history of male alcoholism. *Archives of General Psychiatry, 39*, 127–133.

Vanicelli, M., & Nash, L. (1984). Effect of sex bias on women's studies on alcoholism. *Alcoholism, Clinical and Experimental Research, 8*, 334–336.

Victor, M. (1992). The effects of alcohol on the nervous system. In J. H. Mendelson & N. K. Mello (Eds.), *Medical diagnosis and treatment of alcoholism* (pp. 201–262). New York: McGraw-Hill.

Vining, E., Kosten, T. R., & Kleber, H. G. (1988). Clinical utility of rapid clonidine-naltrexone detoxification for opioid abusers. *British Journal of Addiction, 83*, 567–575.

Weiss, R. D., Mirin, S. M., Michael, J. I., & Sollogrub, A. C. (1986). Psychopathology in chronic cocaine abusers. *American Journal of Drug and Alcohol Abuse, 12*, 17–29.

Woods, G. (1993). Drug abuse in society. Santa Barbara, CA: ABC-CLIO.

Zimring, F. E., & Hawkins, G. (1992). *The search for rational drug control.* Cambridge: Cambridge University Press.

≋ LITERARY REFERENCES

Burroughs, W. (1960). Deposition: Testimony concerning a sickness. *Evergreen Review, 4*, 18.

Clark, R. W. (1980). *Freud: The man and the cause.* New York: Random House.

Freud, S. (1975/1960). *Letters of Sigmund Freud.* (J. Stern, Trans.). New York: Basic Books.

Sanders, S. R. (November 1989). Under the influence. *Harper's Magazine*, pp. 68–75.

Svevo, I. (1958). *Confessions of Zeno.* New York: Vintage.

Twain, M. (1987). *Adventures of Huckleberry Finn.* Berkeley, CA: University of California Press.

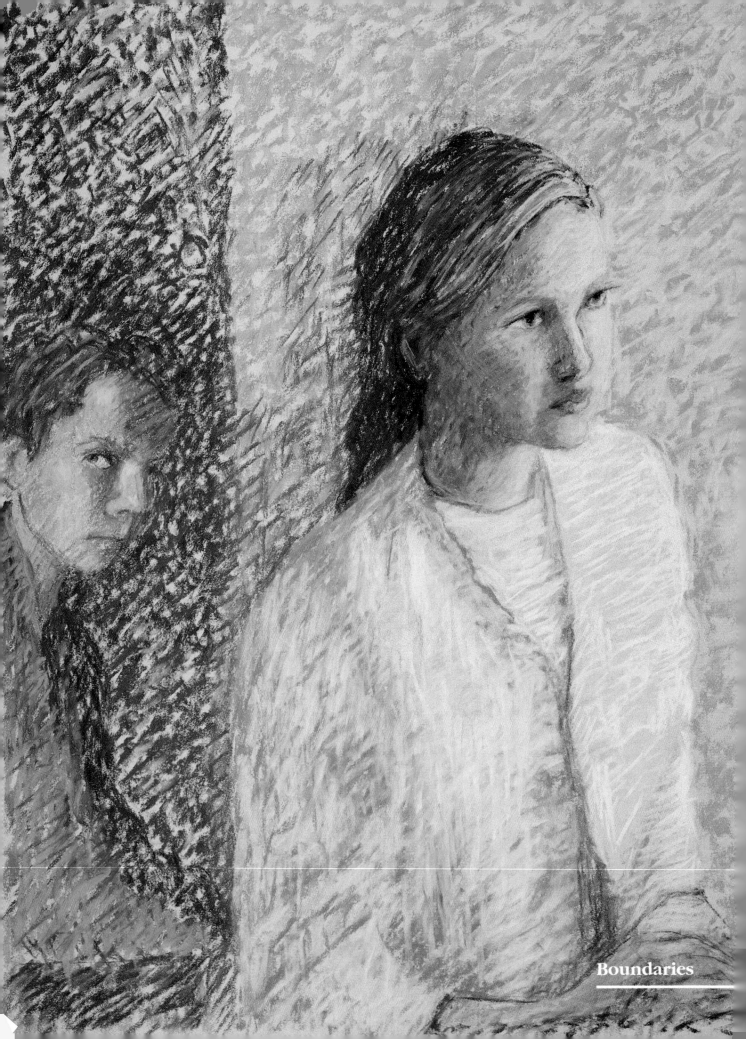

Boundaries

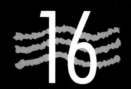
THE CLIENT WITH A PERSONALITY DISORDER

Noreen Cavan Frisch

Lawrence E. Frisch

Personality and You

Consider the following:
- ◆ What qualities do you present to others?
- ◆ How would your best friend describe you?
- ◆ How would your teachers/boss describe you?

Can you identify any experiences that you believe shaped your personality?

Is your personality like that of one of your parents? Your siblings?

Recognize that each person has a number of characteristics that make up who he is and how he presents himself to the world. In this chapter, we will explore personality characteristics that are dysfunctional and learn how to identify normal variations from disorders.

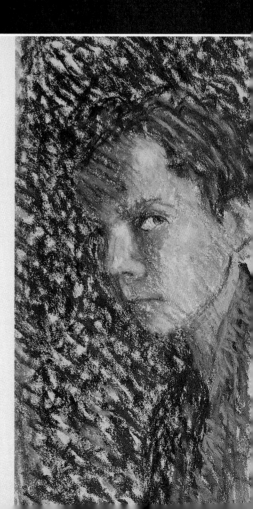

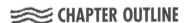 **CHAPTER OUTLINE**

DRAMATIC AND EMOTIONAL PERSONALITY CLUSTER

Borderline Personality Disorder
Etiology

Narcissistic Personality Disorder
Etiology

Histrionic Personality Disorder
Etiology

Antisocial Personality Disorder
Etiology

ODD AND ECCENTRIC PERSONALITY CLUSTER

Schizoid Personality Disorder
Etiology

Schizotypal Personality Disorder
Etiology

Paranoid Personality Disorder
Etiology

ANXIETY- AND FEAR-BASED PERSONALITY CLUSTER

Obsessive-Compulsive Personality Disorder
Etiology

Avoidant Personality Disorder
Etiology

Dependent Personality Disorder
Etiology

Passive-Aggressive or Negativistic Personality Disorder
Etiology

NURSING PERSPECTIVES

NURSING THEORY

▽ **NURSING PROCESS**

▽ **CASE STUDY/CARE PLAN**

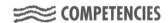 **COMPETENCIES**

Upon completion of this chapter, the reader should be able to:

1. Define personality, personality trait, and personality disorder.
2. Differentiate between a person with eccentric personality traits and a person with a personality disorder.
3. Identify characteristics of specific personality disorders.
4. Describe how early childhood influences can affect personality development.
5. Use nursing theory to understand a client with a personality disorder and to plan appropriate nursing interventions.

≋ KEY TERMS

Antisocial Personality Disorder Behavior pattern characterized by violence, impulsiveness, dishonesty, carelessness, and irresponsibility.

Avoidant Personality Disorder Behavior pattern characterized by social inhibition, feelings of inadequacy, and shyness.

Borderline Personality Disorder Behavior pattern characterized by unstable interpersonal relationships and self-image, efforts to avoid being abandoned, and impulsive actions.

Dependent Personality Disorder Behavior pattern characterized by clinging and submissiveness.

Histrionic Personality Disorder Behavior pattern characterized by excesses of emotional expression and a desire to be the center of attention.

Narcissistic Personality Disorder Behavior pattern characterized in part by lack of empathy for others and a grandiose sense of self-importance.

Obsessive-Compulsive Personality Disorder Behavior pattern characterized by preoccupation with order, cleanliness, control, and perfectionism.

Paranoid Personality Disorder Behavior pattern characterized by persistent yet unfounded fear of exploitation or harm by others.

Passive-Aggressive Personality Disorder Behavior pattern characterized by pervasive negativity along with passive resistance to social/occupational demands; procrastination; and stubbornness.

Personality Habitual patterns and qualities of behavior expressed by physical and mental activities and attitudes; the distinctive individual qualities of a person.

Personality Disorder Pervasive and inflexible pattern of behavior demonstrating unhealthy characteristics that limit the individual's ability to function in society.

Personality Traits Qualities of behavior that make a person unique.

Schizoid Personality Disorder Behavior pattern characterized by lack of emotion and close friendships and detachment from persons and events in the immediate environment.

Schizotypal Personality Disorder Behavior pattern characterized by inability to form close relationships and a pattern of cognitive and perceptual distortions and eccentricities.

A dictionary definition of **personality** reads the "habitual patterns and qualities of behavior of any individual as expressed by physical and mental activities and attitudes; distinctive individual qualities of a person" (Webster, 1982, p. 1062). Every person has his own personality, and by this we mean that each individual has characteristic **personality traits** or qualities that make him unique. Living in a society as diverse as the modern United States, one can observe a wide variation in personality traits. Some persons are shy and retiring, others loud and boisterous; some persons are full of humor, others rather morose; some are spontaneous in action, others thoughtful and considered. All of these traits could be used to describe a person's personality, and each individual has a number of characteristics contributing to his personality as a whole. Personality traits tend to be stable patterns over time and influence how a person looks, behaves, and reacts to life's events.

Clusters of personality traits are sometimes used to describe a person's personality style. An individual might be described as flexible, resourceful, and compassionate if he has a style that exhibits these rather healthy characteristics. In contrast, some individuals have developed personality styles that demonstrate unhealthy characteristics —styles that limit the ability to function in society. Such an individual is said to have a personality disorder.

A **personality disorder** is defined by the fourth edition of the *Diagnostic and Statistical Manual* (DSM-IV) as "an enduring pattern of inner experience and behavior that deviates markedly from the expectations of the individual's culture, is pervasive and inflexible, has an onset in adolescence or early adulthood, is stable over time, and leads to distress or impairment" (American Psychiatric Association, 1994, p. 629). As detailed in Chapter 4 of this text, personality disorders are identified on Axis II of DSM. In general, personality disorders seem to derive from interactions among an individual's temperament, family up-bringing, and life experiences. In turn, they strongly color an affected individual's reaction to stress, illness, and other psychiatric disorders. The multiaxial approach has been adopted by DSM to emphasize that Axis I disorders (primary psychiatric diagnoses such as Depression, Mania, Schizophrenia, Panic Disorder) are constant across all personality types, but their impact on the individual and their management are strongly influenced by underlying personality factors.

There are several personality disorders identified in DSM that present rather commonly to the nurse in both psychiatric and general nursing practice. These personality disorders are categorized into three clusters, each with somewhat similar characteristics. The clusters are based on behaviors observed and are (1) dramatic and emotional, (2) odd and eccentric, and (3) anxiety and fear based. Table 16-1 offers a summary of personality disorders grouped by cluster. The important factor for the nurse to understand is that a personality disorder is identified only

Table 16-1 Personality Disorders by Descriptive Category

DESCRIPTION	PERSONALITY DISORDER
Dramatic and emotional	Borderline Personality Disorder Narcissistic Personality Disorder Histrionic Personality Disorder Antisocial Personality Disorder
Odd and eccentric	Schizoid Personality Disorder Schizotypal Personality Disorder Paranoid Personality Disorder
Anxiety and fear based	Obsessive-Compulsive Personality Disorder Avoidant Personality Disorder Dependent Personality Disorder Passive-Aggressive or Negativistic Personality Disorder*

Passive-Aggressive Personality Disorder was removed from the list of personality disorders in DSM-IV and is included in DSM-IV as a category requiring further study.

if the cluster of personality traits observed clearly leads to distress or impairment. Many, even most, persons have some elements of a disordered personality in their own makeups. While these personality elements may cause occasional personal or social difficulties, unless they constitute "inflexible and pervasive" patterns *and* lead to "clinically significant distress or impairment," they do not constitute a personality disorder.

This chapter identifies and describes 11 personality disorders in detail. The clinical descriptions of personality disorders are often dry and remote, and nurses may approach the understanding of personality disorders as purely an exercise in memorizing lengthy names and unusual characteristics and behaviors. These conditions are too interesting, vivid, and important to be studied in this abstract way, however. In an effort to bring the reader some "flavor" of these disorders, this presentation provides the name of the personality disorder followed by a literary excerpt that presents behaviors consistent with the personalty disorder described. A textbook description of the disorder then follows.

DRAMATIC AND EMOTIONAL PERSONALITY CLUSTER

The common theme of these personality disorders is the inability to establish and maintain close interpersonal relationships. The individual with one of these personality disorders exhibits labile mood swings, for example, going from laughter to tears in seconds. Behavior often appears calculated or cunning to accomplish a goal, such as maintaining the attention of others or gaining power or domination over others.

Borderline Personality Disorder

Annie

She was laughing. At first he thought she might be crying, but she was laughing. . . .

She laughed and kicked her legs and gave off an air, an odor, of intense fleshy heat. I won't survive this one, she giggled. . . .

At Christmas, somehow, they lost contact with each other. Days passed. Twelve days. Fifteen. His widowed mother came to visit them in the big red-brick colonial in Lathrup Park, and his wife's sister and her husband and two young children, and his oldest boy, a freshman at Swarthmore, brought his Japanese roommate home with him; life grew dense, robustly complicated. He telephoned her at the apartment but no one answered. . . .

A girl in a raw unfinished painting. Like the crude canvases on exhibit at the gallery, that day he had drifted by: something vulgar and exciting about the mere droop of a shoulder, the indifference of a strand of hair blown into her eyes. And the dirt-edged fingernails. And the shoes with the run-over heels. She was raw, unfinished, lazy, slangy, vulgar, crude, mouthing in her cheerful insouciant voice certain words and phrases [he] would never have said aloud in the presence of a member of the opposite sex; but at the same time it excited him to know that she was highly intelligent, and really well-educated, with a master's degree in art history and a studied, if rather flippant, familiarity with the monstrousness of contemporary art. He could not determine whether she was as impoverished as she appeared or whether it was a pose, an act. . . .

It excited him to imagine her haphazard, promiscuous life; he knew she was entirely without guilt or shame or self-consciousness, as if, born of a different generation, she were of a different species as well. . . .

In early March he saw her again, but only for lunch. She insisted he return to the gallery to see their current show—ugly, frantic, oversized hunks of sheet metal and aluminum, seemingly thrown at will onto the floor. . . .

He led her to his car. They were both smiling. Where are we going? she asked. . . .

He watched her face as he drove along Wash-

burn Lane, which was graveled and tranquil and hilly. Is this—? Do you live—? she asked. He brought her to the big red-brick colonial he had bought nearly fifteen years ago; it seemed to him that the house had never looked more handsome, and the surrounding trees and blossoming shrubs had never looked more beautiful. . . .

But—Where is—Aren't you afraid—?

There's no one home, he said.

He led her through the foyer, into the living room with its thick wine-colored rug, its gleaming furniture, its many windows. He led her through the formal dining room and into the walnut-paneled recreation room where his wife had hung lithographs and had arranged innumerable plants, some of them hanging from the ceiling in clay pots, spidery-leafed, lovely. He saw the girl's eyes dart from place to place. . . .

She asked him why he had brought her here and he said he didn't know. . . .

Then she kicked about, and laughed, and chattered. He was sleepy, pleasantly sleepy. He did not mind her chatter, her high spirits. While she spoke of one thing or another . . . he watched through half-closed eyes the play of shadows on the ceiling. . . .

His snoring disturbed him. For an instant he woke, then sank again into a warm grayish ether . . . then his snoring woke him again and he sat up.

Annie?

Her things were still lying on the floor. The red blouse lay draped across a chintz-covered easy chair whose bright red and orange flowers, glazed, dramatic, seemed to be throbbing with energy. Annie? Are you in the bathroom?

The bathroom door was ajar, the light was not on. He got up. He saw that it was after two. A mild sensation of panic rose in his chest, for no reason. He was safe. They were safe here. No one would be home for hours. . . . The house was silent. It was empty.

He thought: What if she steals something?

But that was ridiculous and cruel. Annie would never do anything like that.

No one was in this bathroom, which was his wife's. He went to a closet and got a robe and put it on, and went out into the hallway, calling Annie?—Honey?—and knew, before he turned the

knob to his own bathroom, that she was in there and that she would not respond. Annie? What's wrong?

The light switch to the bathroom operated a fan; the fan was on; he pressed his ear against the door and listened. Had she taken a shower? He didn't think so. Had not heard any noises. Annie, he said, rattling the knob, are you in there, is anything wrong? He waited. He heard the fan whirring. Annie? His voice was edged with impatience. Annie, will you unlock the door? Is anything wrong?

She said something—the words were sharp and unintelligible.

Annie? What? What did you say? . . .

Again her high, sharp voice. It sounded like an animal's shriek. But the words were unintelligible. . . .

He heard the lock being turned, suddenly.

He opened the door.

She must have taken the razor blade out of his razor, which she had found in the medicine cabinet. Must have leaned over the sink and made one quick, deft, hard slash with it—cutting the fingers of her right hand also. The razor blade slipped from her then and fell into the sink. There was blood on the powder-blue porcelain of the sink and the toilet, and on the fluffy black rug, and on the mirror, and on the blue-and-white tiled walls. When he opened the door and saw her, she screamed, made a move as if to strike him with her bleeding arm, and for an instant he could not think: could not think: what had happened, what was happening, what had this girl done to him? Her face was wet and distorted. Ugly. She was sobbing, whimpering. There was blood, bright blood, smeared on her breasts and belly and thighs: he had never seen anything so repulsive in his life. . . .

He was paralyzed. Yet, in the next instant, a part of him came to life. He grabbed a towel and wrapped it around her arm, struggling with her. Stop! Stand still! For God's sake! . . .

Why did you do it? Why? Why? You're crazy! You're sick! This is a—this is a terrible, terrible— a terrible thing, a crazy thing—

Her teeth were chattering. She had begun to shiver convulsively . . . I hate you—I don't want to live—

She pushed past him, she staggered into the bedroom. The towel came loose. He ran after her and grabbed her and held the towel against the wound again, wrapping it tight, so tight she flinched. His brain reeled. He saw blood, splotches of blood, starlike splashes on the carpet, on the yellow satin bedspread that had been pulled onto the floor. . . .

After some time the bleeding was under control. He got another towel, from his wife's bathroom, and wrapped it around her arm again. It stained, but not so quickly. The bleeding was under control; She was not going to die.

He had forced her to sit down. He crouched over her, breathing hard, holding her in place. What if she sprang up, what if she ran away?— through the house? He held her still. She was spiritless, weak. Her eyes were closed. In a softer voice he said, as if speaking to a child: Poor Annie, poor sweet girl, why did you do it, why, why did you want to hurt yourself, why did you do something so ugly? . . . It was an ugly, ugly thing to do.*

(Oates, 1981, pp. 509–518)

This excerpt from *The Tryst* is profoundly shocking. The reader certainly agrees with John that Annie's cutting herself is as ugly as it is totally unexpected. Why, indeed, did Annie want to hurt herself? One very plausible explanation is that Annie has the psychological condition known as **Borderline Personality Disorder** (BPD). The essential features of BPD are patterns of unstable interpersonal relationships and self-image, efforts to avoid being abandoned, and impulsive actions. Annie's impulsive swings of emotion from childish laughter to abject despondency are highly characteristic of BPD. Recurrent self-mutilating behavior, especially cutting, is another important BPD characteristic. It seems likely that Annie chose to cut herself out of fear of rejection: Finding herself suddenly in the physical setting of a traditional middle-class marriage—expensive suburban house, custom-decorated bedroom, manicured lawns, grown children, and an aging lover—she surely recognized a relationship with little future.

Borderline individuals develop a life-long pattern of "unstable and intense interpersonal relationships" accompanied by "frantic efforts to avoid real or imagined abandonment." They frequently have "marked reactivity of moods (e.g., intense episodic dysphoria, irritability, or anxiety usually lasting a few hours and only rarely more

---

*"The Tryst" Copyright © 1981 by Joyce Carol Oates, Inc., from SENTIMENTAL EDUCATION by Joyce Carol Oates. Used by permission of Dutton Signet, a division of Penguin Books USA, Inc.

ESSENTIAL FEATURES OF BORDERLINE PERSONALITY DISORDER

◆ Frantic efforts to avoid real or imagined abandonment

◆ Pattern of unstable interpersonal relationships

◆ Unstable self-image or sense of self

◆ Impulsivity in at least two areas that are potentially self-damaging (spending, sex, substance abuse, reckless driving, binge eating)

◆ Recurrent suicidal behaviors, gestures, or threats or self-mutilating behavior

◆ Chronic feelings of emptiness

◆ Inappropriate anger or difficulty controlling anger

◆ Transient, stress-related paranoid ideation

Reprinted with permission from the *Diagnostic and Statistical Manual of Mental Disorders*, Fourth Edition. Copyright 1994 American Psychiatric Association.

than a few days" (American Psychiatric Association, 1994, p. 654). Like Annie, many borderline individuals enter (often repeatedly) into imprudent sexual liaisons, and they also commonly display other impulsive behavior: substance use, reckless spending, unsafe driving, binge eating. Borderline persons are frequently angry, most often with those closest to them or trying to help them. Depression, a sense of emptiness, and an "unstable self-image or sense of self" are other frequent accompaniments of BPD. Annie's appearance and behavior—"raw, unfinished, lazy, slangy, vulgar, crude"—might suggest an "unstable self-image" or might merely reflect what could be considered her Bohemian "artsy" lifestyle. Unlike Annie, who apparently has finished her master's degree, persons with BPD may often have a history of giving up or quitting projects prior to achieving success (e.g., quitting school right before graduation).

Etiology

It is generally assumed that BPD is an acquired condition deriving from the experience of growing up in a chaotic and often violent family. First-degree relatives (parents, siblings, children) of individuals with BPD are about five times more likely to have this diagnosis than are less closely related individuals. This tendency for the disorder to cluster in families could be due to either environmental or genetic factors, but most experts currently stress the importance of environmental determinants. Such determinants include chaos in the family, which may manifest as fighting, infidelity, suicide or suicide attempts, and problems with the law, including imprisonment. It is perhaps not surprising that individuals with BPD are much more likely to suffer from mood disorders (depression), substance abuse disorders, or other associated personality disorders, particularly Antisocial Personality Disorder, than are individuals without BPD. One author describes the family history of the borderline personality as a "disaster a day" and likens the resultant family life to the plot of a television soap opera (Benjamin, 1993). Issues of abandonment are common, and most adults with BPD have some history of feeling abandoned, fearful, and unprotected as children. A childhood history of physical and/or sexual abuse is also common.

The concept "borderline" derives from observations made during psychoanalysis: Under the stress of psychoanalytic treatment, these individuals often develop characteristics of psychosis, such as losing touch with reality, hallucinations, and/or delusions. This potential for developing dissociative symptoms under stress remains one of the DSM-IV defining criteria. To early psychiatrists, these individuals seemed to be "borderline" between persons with "neurosis" (a term now rarely used) and psychosis. It is estimated that about 2% of the general population will meet criteria for a diagnosis of BPD; the majority of persons diagnosed are women (American Psychiatric Association, 1994).

As clients, borderline individuals are often very difficult, demanding, and emotional. They are frequently annoyed *with* and angry *at* their nurses and physicians, and in response, they may provoke angry and rejecting responses from their caretakers. Because individuals with BPD have difficulty maintaining healthy relationships with anyone, including health care providers, they often receive fragmented (and expensive) care in multiple facilities. One authority states:

> The medical setting provides fertile soil for borderline people to experience regressive emotional states. They are unclear as to the source of the physical and emotional discomfort of illness, tending to blame their pain on others; and they may react to painful interventions as specifically motivated hostile acts. Borderline patients are intolerant of groups in general and become confused in the hospital where their care is divided among a variety of doctors, nurses, consultants, and other medical personnel. They respond by simplifying this collection of persons into allies and enemies and proceed with desperate attempts to enlist the former to save them from the latter.
>
> (Nardo, 1986, pp. 59–60)

The major physical risk for individuals with BPD is suicide. While attempts are much more common than completed suicides, there is a real risk of suicide success, either intentional or unintentional. Because of extreme emotional lability and the frequent association with substance abuse, suicide may be very difficult to predict or prevent in BPD, as was seen in Annie's case. Although the overall pattern of behavior in BPD is quite stable over time, the intensity of borderline behavior often decreases with age. Borderline individuals tend to become relatively more functional and to have less risk of attempted and completed suicide as they reach their 30s, 40s, and beyond (American Psychiatric Association, 1994).

Narcissistic Personality Disorder

Mr. Neville

"There," he said, as they stepped out into a lakeside restaurant surrounded by potted hydrangeas. "That wasn't too bad, was it?"

"I am actually quite glad to be surrounded by all these waiters and bottles and millionaires," Edith confessed. "At least I assume they are millionaires?"

"That is what they would like you to assume, certainly. And if money talks, as it is supposed to, then they are certainly making the right amount of noise."

He settled her at a table in the shade of a striped awning, picked up the menu which an attentive waiter had immediately placed before him, and said, "I should have the duck if I were you. . . ."

His own duck dispatched by means of a few expertly calculated incisions, he leaned back to light a cigar. . . . Tilted back in his chair Mr. Neville watched her face. "Let me see," he said mildly. "Let me see if I can imagine what your life is like. You live in London. You have a comfortable income. You go to drink parties and dinner parties and publishers' parties. You do not really enjoy any of this. . . . You come home alone. You are fussy about your house. You have had lovers but not half as many as your friends have had; they, of course, credit you with none at all and worry about you rather ostentatiously. You are aware of this. And yet you have a secret life, Edith. . . ."

Mr. Neville deposited the ash of his cigar carefully in the ashtray.

"Of course, you will say that this is none of my business. . . . Whatever arrangements we may come to must leave these considerations scrupulously unexamined."

"Arrangements?" echoed Edith.

Mr. Neville sat forward and put his hands on the table. He seemed, suddenly, somewhat younger and less controlled than usual. It had been easy to think of him as a wealthy man in his fifties, fastidious, careful, leisured, attractive in a bloodless sort of way, the kind of man who gave great thought to his way of life, a man . . . who would undoubtedly have a fine library but whom it was somehow difficult to imagine in any other room of a house.

"I think you should marry me, Edith," he said.

She stared at him, her eyes widening in disbelief.

"I have a lot of business overseas," he went on, . . . "And I like to entertain. I am away a certain amount of the time. But I dislike having to come back to a house only occupied by the couple who live in it when I am not there. You would fit perfectly into that setting. . . ."

"You make it sound like a job specification," she said. *"And I have not applied for the job."**

(Brookner, 1984, pp. 160–164)

In the novel *Hotel du Lac*, Edith is a successful writer of popular romantic fiction who finds herself confined in a dreary Swiss lake-side hotel for several early winter weeks. In the excerpt quoted here, a fellow Englishman and hotel guest, Mr. Neville, has just invited her to take a lake cruise, and the two of them have stopped for dinner. Edith has just met Mr. Neville, but she is astonished by his remarkably accurate knowledge of her personal life, which he seems to have deduced from careful observation. Impressed with his observational skills, at one point in the novel she asks him if he is a psychiatrist. He is, instead, a wealthy divorced businessman living alone in a large English country house. Before they have spent no more than a few hours together, Mr. Neville astounds Edith by proposing marriage, but solely as a mutually beneficial business-like arrangement.

In many ways, Mr. Neville seems to Edith to be a character out of one of her romantic novels: He is sophisticated, rich, handsome "in a bloodless sort of way," impeccably dressed, self-assured, and seemingly kind. He is, above all, very sure of his own attractiveness, and he proposes marriage with virtually no emotion, only appearing "suddenly, somewhat . . . less controlled than usual." Mr. Neville is quite insistent that neither his nor Edith's "secret life" should be affected by their marriage or even be discussed between them: "We must leave

these considerations scrupulously unexamined." As he explains to her during another conversation, he expects that both would continue to have extramarital affairs. Explicit lack of empathy is central to Mr. Neville's personal philosophy, for as he explains to Edith, "Without a huge emotional investment [in others], one can do whatever one pleases. . . . One can be as pleasant or as ruthless as one wants . . . if one is prepared to . . . simply please oneself" (Brookner, 1984, pp. 94–95). Although Mr. Neville sometimes appeared kindly but in an arrogantly self-assured way, "Edith . . . knew . . . there was a flaw in his ability to feel" (p. 97):

"You know," she said . . . "I find that smile of yours just the faintest bit unamiable."

His smile broadened. "When you get to know me better," he remarked, "you will realize just how unamiable it really is."

(Brookner, 1984, p. 102)

The essential features of **Narcissistic Personality Disorder** are self-centeredness and inflated self-esteem, both beginning by early adulthood. Individuals with Narcissistic Personality Disorder typically overestimate their abilities, feel superior to others, and demand admiration. They invariably expect special treatment and, like Mr. Neville, have a lack of empathy toward others (American Psychiatric Association, 1994). Unlike the fictional Mr. Neville, these individuals are often highly sensitive to the criticism of others and, like Mr. Neville, frequently have difficulty in establishing close relationships.

---

*From HOTEL DU LAC by Anita Brookner. Copyright © 1984 by Anita Brookner. Reprinted by permission of Pantheon Books, a division of Random House, Inc.

ESSENTIAL FEATURES OF NARCISSISTIC PERSONALITY DISORDER

◆ Has a grandiose sense of self-importance

◆ Is preoccupied with fantasies of unlimited success, power, brilliance, beauty, or ideal love

◆ Believes he or she is unique and special and should only associate with others who are special or high-status people

◆ Requires admiration of others

◆ Has a sense of entitlement

◆ Is interpersonally exploitive

◆ Lacks empathy

◆ Shows arrogance

Reprinted with permission from the *Diagnostic and Statistical Manual of Mental Disorders*, Fourth Edition. Copyright 1994 American Psychiatric Association.

Mr. Neville indeed lacks empathy and is unwilling to recognize or identify with the feelings and needs of others. This characteristic of lacking empathy is one of the defining criteria for Narcissistic Personality Disorder. While DSM-IV requires that only five of nine criteria be present, Mr. Neville seems to meet at least six in addition to lack of empathy: (1) He has a grandiose sense of self-importance; (2) he believes he is special and unique and should associate with other special or high-status people; (3) he requires excessive admiration; (4) he has a sense of entitlement, that is, unreasonable expectations of especially favorable treatment or automatic compliance with his expectations; (5) he is interpersonally exploitative; (6) and he shows arrogant, haughty behaviors or attitudes. He does not seem to be particularly envious of others (another DSM-IV criterion). And he does not seem preoccupied with fantasies of unlimited success, power, brilliance, beauty, or ideal love, though perhaps an unromantic marriage to Edith might, for him, represent "ideal love" (American Psychiatric Association, 1994, p. 661).

Etiology

The developmental history of persons with Narcissistic Personality Disorder typically shows a pattern of selfless love and adoration from a significant adult, such that the child escapes reality-based experiences. At the same time, the child experiences an ever-present threat of criticism for not being perfect. Benjamin (1993) states that the "rich and famous are particularly vulnerable to developing Narcissistic Personality Disorder in adulthood" (p. 146) because of the attention, devotion, and nurturance given celebrities by the American public.

To others, narcissistic individuals appear arrogant, conceited, insensitive, and ruthless. Unlike individuals with BPD, who are relatively susceptible to psychotic episodes, narcissistic persons have developed a stable personality structure, but the rigidity of that personality hides extreme vulnerability to any experience that threatens their sense of self-perfection. Narcissistic individuals often use fantasy and daydreams to cope with such stressful experience; the content of these daydreams and fantasies frequently incorporates themes of self-admiration, power, revenge, and personal entitlement (Raskin & Novacek, 1991). Under stress, narcissistic individuals may demonstrate varying degrees of anxiety or depression. Physical illness is often a severe challenge for narcissistic individuals who typically have as much trouble with medical and nursing practitioners as they do with their own illness. Narcissistic persons are often highly critical and competitive, and caregivers can readily come into conflict with them if the providers allow their own feelings of authority or importance to come to the surface. Along with illness, aging is a major stress for those with Narcissistic Personality Disorder. These individuals are often

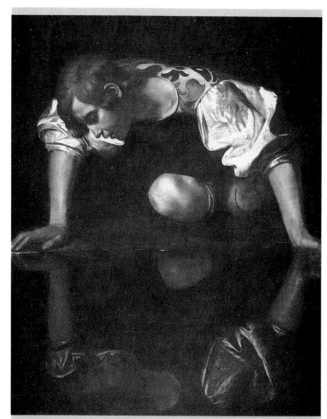

Narcissus by Caravaggio Galleria Nazionale d'Arte Antica (Pal. Barberini-Corsini), Rome, Italy. Courtesy Scala/Art Resource, NY.

Narcissus is the youth who believes he is so beautiful that he spends his days admiring his own image. In this painting, Narcissus is depicted as a handsome young man of the era. Today, we would be more likely to see narcissistic behavior at the health club, where both young and old strive for physical perfection, and some become so engrossed in their own beauty and attractiveness that they find little time for developing interpersonal relationships.

extraordinarily reluctant to accept or accommodate to the declining capabilities brought on by aging. To deal with a client who has a Narcissistic Personality Disorder, the nurse must understand the personality dynamics behind the person's anger and criticism. The nurse should take an unemotional but supportive approach.

In comparison to other personality disorders, Narcissistic Personality Disorder is relatively rare. The prevalence of Narcissistic Personality Disorder in the general population is estimated to be less than 1%, with a majority of those diagnosed being male (American Psychiatric Association, 1994). However, since many individuals with this disorder have significant difficulties adjusting to life stresses, Narcissistic Personality Disorder will be seen with more frequency in mental health practice than expected given the 1% figure.

Histrionic Personality Disorder

Who Is She?

"And who is she? What does she do?"

"She's an English girl, an actress: sings at the Lady Windermere—hot stuff, believe me!"

"That doesn't sound much like an English girl, I must say."

"Eventually she's got a bit of French in her. Her mother was French."

A few minutes later, Sally herself arrived.

"Am I terribly late, Fritz darling?"

"Only half of an hour, I suppose," Fritz drawled, beaming with proprietary pleasure. "May I introduce Mr. Isherwood—Miss Bowles? Mr. Isherwood is commonly known as Chris."

"I'm not," I said. "Fritz is about the only person who's ever called me Chris in my life."

Sally laughed. She was dressed in black silk, with a small cape over her shoulders and a little cap like a page-boy's stuck jauntily on one side of her head:

"Do you mind if I use your telephone, sweet?"

"Sure. Go right ahead." Fritz caught my eye. "Come into the other room, Chris. I want to show you something." He was evidently longing to hear my first impressions of Sally, his new acquisition.

"For heaven's sake, don't leave me alone with this man!" she exclaimed. "Or he'll seduce me down the telephone. He's most terribly passionate."

As she dialed the number, I noticed that her finger-nails were painted emerald green, a colour unfortunately chosen, for it called attention to her hands, which were much stained by cigarette-smoking and as dirty as a little girl's. She was dark enough to be Fritz's sister. Her face was long and thin, powdered dead white. She had very large brown eyes which should have been darker, to match her hair and the pencil she used for her eyebrows.

"Hiloo," she cooed, pursing her brilliant cherry lips as though she was going to kiss the mouth-piece: "Ist dass Du, mein Liebling?" Her mouth opened in a fatuously sweet smile. Fritz and I sat watching her, like a performance at the theatre. "Was wollen wir machen, Morgen Abend? Oh, Wie wunderbar . . . Nein, nein, ich werde bleiben Heute Abend zu Hause. Ja, ja, ich werde wirklich bleiben zu Hause. . . . Auf Wiedersehen, mein Liebling. . . ."

She hung up the receiver and turned to us triumphantly.

"That's the man I slept with last night," she announced. "He makes love marvelously. He's an absolute genius at business and he's terribly rich—" She came and sat down on the sofa beside Fritz, sinking back into the cushions with a sigh: "Give me some coffee, will you, darling? I'm simply dying of thirst."*

(Isherwood, 1989, pp. 22–23)

Sally's personality is characterized by dramatic extremes of expression; being around her seems to Fritz and Christopher "like [watching] a performance at the theater." This sense of performance strongly suggests that Sally has **Histrionic Personality Disorder**. Both Sally's behavior and appearance are quite typical of this disorder: dramatic dress, striking makeup, theatrical entrance, seductive boasting about sexual promiscuity. Individuals with Histrionic Personality Disorder constantly seek attention through excesses of emotional expression. They crave being the center of attention and, like Sally, often gain attention by talking or behaving seductively and dressing in ways that call attention to themselves. Speech in

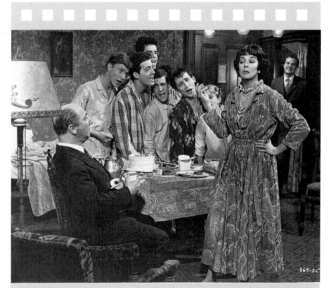

Gypsy. Source: Warner Brothers/Courtesy Kobal.

A histrionic personality, Mama Rose, finds herself to be the center of attention.

ESSENTIAL FEATURES OF HISTRIONIC PERSONALITY DISORDER

◆ Is uncomfortable in situations where he or she is not the center of attention

◆ Displays inappropriate sexually seductive or provocative behavior

◆ Has rapid shifts of emotion

◆ Uses physical appearance to draw attention to self

◆ Shows dramatization or exaggerated expression of emotion

◆ Is suggestible

◆ Considers relationships to be more intimate than they really are

Reprinted with permission from the *Diagnostic and Statistical Manual of Mental Disorders*, Fourth Edition. Copyright 1994 American Psychiatric Association.

Histrionic Personality Disorder is dramatic, exaggerated, but shallow: For Sally, everyone is "darling" or "sweet," or (since this episode was set in pre–World War II Berlin) "liebling." Sally is not just thirsty, but "simply dying of thirst." Individuals with this disorder are often highly suggestible: Later in the story, Christopher says to Sally, "What I really like about you is that you're so awfully easy to take in. People who never get taken in are so dreary" (Isherwood, 1989, p. 69). Histrionic persons may frequently cause embarrassment to others by dramatic public displays of affection directed toward individuals they know only distantly.

There is clearly some similarity between Histrionic Personality Disorder and BPD: Both are characterized by rapid emotional swings, seductive behavior, and inability to form close interpersonal relationships. The distinguishing borderline characteristic is marked shifts in feelings about others, usually based on some perception of rejection. Histrionic individuals also shift emotions rapidly (e.g., moving almost instantaneously from loud laughter to tears), but their primary aim is to keep themselves the focus of attention. It is not uncommon for persons to have characteristics of both Borderline and Histrionic Personality Disorders, and certain DSM-IV Axis I disorders (particularly Somatization Disorder, Conversion Disorder, and Major Depressive Disorder) are relatively common among histrionic individuals (Benjamin, 1993).

Etiology

The adult with Histrionic Personality Disorder has probably been brought up with the sense that his or her value is based on good looks and ability to entertain others.

Histrionic personality is sometimes an asset in a theatrical career, but for most individuals, Histrionic Personality Disorder seriously interferes with life goals and intimate relationships. For both the German, Fritz, and the Englishman, Christopher, Sally's behavior was intriguingly exotic: "She's got a bit of French in her," Fritz offers in trying to explain Sally's histrionic performances. Cultures certainly differ in the degree of flamboyance and emotional expressiveness considered normal. These cultural differences always need to be considered before making any personality disorder diagnosis, but it is likely that Sally's extremes of expression would fall outside the norms in any modern culture. All personality disorder diagnoses require that the condition lead to "significant distress or impairment in social, occupational, or other important areas of functioning" (American Psychiatric Association, 1994, p. 633). Isherwood's (1989) account of Sally Bowles paints her as generally successful and happy, though at one point she observes: "Sometimes I feel I'm no damn use at anything. . . . Why, I can't even keep a man faithful to me for the inside of a month" (p. 41). Despite Isherwood's sympathetic portrayal, it seems inevitable that Sally's histrionic personality will eventually cause her significant distress or functional impairment.

Data from the general population estimate the prevalence of Histrionic Personality Disorder to be 2% to 3%, with some studies reporting equal prevalence among males and females and other studies of clinical populations reporting a higher prevalence among women (American Psychiatric Association, 1994). Histrionic personality in men differs somewhat from that in women. The male histrionic typically focuses on "macho" behavior and talk, often involving physical or athletic prowess. In men, Histrionic Personality Disorder may seem to overlap with Narcissistic Personality Disorder. The histrionic male seeks continually to be the center of attention, while the narcissistic male primarily seeks power and domination over others.

⊚ *REFLECTIVE THINKING*

Histrionic Personality Disorder

In health care settings, a person with Histrionic Personality Disorder will become frustrated easily when he is not able to maintain attention on himself. You must both understand the client's need for attention and provide realistic care, such as setting limits regarding your availability and taking time to let the client know what is possible and not possible. How could you ensure that your nursing care remains objective and appropriate when caring for a client with a histrionic personality who seems to be in need of constant attention?

Antisocial Personality Disorder

Confessions of a "Con Man"

I am only able to live in conditions that leave my spirit and imagination completely free; and so it is that the memory of my years in prison is actually less hateful to me than the recollection of the slavery and fear to which my sensitive boyish soul was subjected through the ostensibly honourable discipline in the small square white schoolhouse down there in the town. And . . . it is not surprising that I soon hit on the idea of escaping from school more often than on Sundays and holidays.

In carrying out this idea I was helped a good deal by a playful diversion I had long indulged in —the imitation of my father's handwriting. A father is the natural and nearest model for the growing boy who is striving to adapt himself to the adult world. Similarity of physique and the mystery of their relationship incline the boy to admire in his parent's conduct all that he himself is still incapable of and to strive to imitate it—or rather it is, perhaps, his very admiration that unconsciously leads him to develop along the lines heredity has laid down. Even when I was still making great hens' tracks on my lined slate, I already dreamed of guiding a steel pen with my father's swiftness and sureness; and many were the pages I covered later with efforts to copy his hand from memory, my fingers grasping the pen in the same delicate fashion as his. His writing was not, in fact, hard to imitate, for my poor father wrote a childish, copybook and, quite undeveloped hand, its only peculiarity being that the letters were very tiny and separated by long hairlines to an extent I have never seen anywhere else. This mannerism I quickly mastered to perfection. As for the signature "E. Krull," in contrast to the angular Gothic letters of the text it had a Latin cast. It was surrounded by a perfect cloud of flourishes, which at first sight looked difficult to copy, but were in reality so simple in conception that with them I succeeded best of all. The lower half of the E made a wide sweep to the right, in whose ample lap, so to speak, the short syllable of the last name was neatly cradled. . . . The whole signature was higher than it was long, it was naive and baroque; thus it lent itself so well to my purpose that in the end its inventor would have certified my product as his own.

But what was more obvious, once I had acquired this skill for my own entertainment, than to put it to work in the interests of my intellectual freedom? "On the 7th instant," I wrote, "my son Felix was afflicted by severe stomach cramps which compelled him to stay away from school, to the regret of yours— E. Krull." And again: "An infected gumboil, together with a sprained right arm, compelled Felix to keep his room from the 10th to the 14th of this month. Therefore, much to our regret, he was unable to attend school. Respectfully yours—E. Krull." When this succeeded, nothing prevented me from spending the school hours of one day or even of several wandering freely outside the town or lying stretched out in a green field, in the whispering shade of the leaves, dreaming the dreams of youth.*

(Mann, 1970, pp. 31–33)

Used as an adjective, the word *confidence* in this excerpt means to swindle or cheat. Today, the slang term "con man" is more frequently used. It certainly is natural, as Felix states, for a young boy to seek to imitate his father; however, this is hardly an excuse for forgery. As he grows up, Felix constantly manipulates, lies, steals, seduces—all without remorse, even when (as he casually indicates in the excerpt) he ends up in prison as a result. Unlike many persons with **Antisocial Personality Disorder**, Felix seems never to have been violent. Felix manipulates his way out of military draft to avoid the inconvenience of service; others with Antisocial Personality Disorder thrive on the opportunities for violent behavior that military service provides. Much fiction and many films focus on the violence associated with this disorder. *Pulp Fiction, Reservoir Dogs*, and *The Godfather* are three films that depict remorseless violence. Chapter 32 in this text lists a number of other films, some requiring quite a strong stomach to watch. Felix Krull reminds us that violence, while common, is not necessary for a diagnosis of Antisocial Personality Disorder to be made: Persistent disregard for the rights and well-being of others can manifest itself through charm and manipulation as well as through violence.

Along with a pattern of "pervasive . . . disregard for and violation of the rights of others," at least three of the characteristics in the accompanying display must be present to diagnose Antisocial Personality Disorder.

In addition, the person's antisocial behavior must have begun before age 15 and at that time have met the criteria for Adolescent Conduct Disorder (Chapter 22).

---

*From CONFESSIONS OF FELIX KRULL, CONFIDENCE MAN by Thomas Mann, Denver Lindley, trans. Copyright © 1955 by Alfred A. Knopf Inc. Reprinted by permission of the publisher.

ESSENTIAL FEATURES OF ANTISOCIAL PERSONALITY DISORDER

◆ A pervasive pattern of disregard for and violation of the rights of others

◆ Repeated acts that are grounds for arrest

◆ Repeated lying, use of aliases, or conning others

◆ Impulsivity or failure to plan ahead

◆ Repeated physical fights or assaults

◆ Reckless disregard for safety of self or others

◆ Failure to sustain consistent work behavior or honor financial obligations

◆ Lack of remorse [at] having hurt, mistreated, or stolen from another

Reprinted with permission from the *Diagnostic and Statistical Manual of Mental Disorders*, Fourth Edition. Copyright 1994 American Psychiatric Association.

Etiology

Family history of adults with Antisocial Personality Disorder shows a pattern of violence, neglect, and, frequently, alcoholism. The child may have been a victim of physical abuse or have watched violent parents in their interactions with each other. Adolescent Conduct Disorder—a prerequisite to the adult diagnosis—includes such behaviors as bullying, cruelty to people and animals, stealing or otherwise damaging property, truancy, and running away from home. It has been suggested that adults with Antisocial Personality Disorder often have had inordinate control over their families when they were children and adolescents, often because of parental negligence or absence (Benjamin, 1993). In this way, patterns of coercion may begin at a very early age. Environment clearly plays an important role in the development of Adolescent Conduct Disorder and Antisocial Personality Disorder. Adoption studies indicate that both genetic and environmental factors contribute to risk for this disorder, which clearly has a tendency to occur repeatedly in families (American Psychiatric Association, 1994).

Fox Butterfield has written about a single remarkably violent family in which the disorder can be traced back as far as 1820. Summing up the current evidence for how antisocial behavior is transmitted from generation to generation, he comments:

Everything criminologists have learned in recent research is that most adolescents who become delinquents, and the overwhelming majority of adults who commit violent crimes, started very young.

They were the impulsive, aggressive, irritable children who would not obey their parents, bullied their neighbors and acted out when they got to school. Because they were accustomed to getting their way by physical force, they see no reason to change. They actually like the way they act, and this makes it increasingly difficult to reverse their antisocial proclivities. . . . Many factors go into producing personality: temperament, the genetic component you are born with; the neighborhood in which you grow up; and perhaps most important, the style of your parents.

(Butterfield, 1994, p. 327)

Antisocial Personality Disorder is one of the conditions specifically studied in the Epidemiologic Catchment Area (ECA) Study of psychiatric disorders in the community (see Chapter 7). One of the major findings of the ECA study was that less than half of persons with Antisocial Personality Disorder have significant criminal records. The most common symptoms are "job troubles (94%), violence (85%), multiple moving traffic offenses (72%), and severe marital difficulties (desertion, multiple separations or divorces, multiple infidelities, found in 67%)" (Robins, Tipp, & Przybeck, 1991, p. 260). The ECA study also clearly showed that this disorder tends to improve with age: The average duration of symptoms was 19 years, but almost no individuals displayed significant antisocial behavior after their mid-30s (Robins et al., 1991). Men have a significantly higher prevalence of Antisocial Personality Disorder than do women, but the ECA study data suggest that the prevalence may be rising among women. The overall prevalence of the disorder may also be increasing (Robins et al., 1991, p. 271). The prevalence is currently estimated to be about 3% in males and 1% in females (American Psychiatric Association, 1994).

Since substance abuse is very much a part of this disorder, nurses working in settings in which substance-abusing clients are treated, including emergency rooms, are particularly likely to encounter persons with Antisocial Personality Disorder. The client will view the nurse like anyone else, as a means of achieving his own goals. The client will look for alliances to obtain outcomes, such as admission to the hospital, a prescription for drugs, and relief from symptoms of illness. Violence and conning are very much a part of the lives of these individuals, and if the client does not get his way, nurses may on occasion be at physical risk from clients with this disorder. The nurse must recognize when she is dealing with a client with Antisocial Personality Disorder. Setting limits may require more than the nurse stating that something is so; the nurse may need to work with a team, including hospital security, when telling a client with antisocial personality that she cannot provide what he wants. (See also Chapter 30 for discussion on dealing with a violent client.)

★ NURSING TIP

Clients with Dramatic and Emotional Personality Disorders

The nurse caring for a client with any of the disorders from this cluster often becomes frustrated and angry because the client demands an excessive amount of time and attention. It often seems that, compared to other clients on a unit, the client with any of the personality disorders in this cluster has a minor problem and the nurse wants to give care to the other (seemingly more deserving) clients. Nurses should remember that clients with personality disorders have diagnosable problems; they cannot change who they are. These clients cannot graciously wait until the nurse attends to others; it is not part of their make-up to do so. The nurse will need to set limits, state clearly what she can and cannot do, and keep to her schedule. When the client complains about or criticizes the nurse, the nurse must understand that this, too, is part of the personality dynamics. Nurses must work as a team in caring for such individuals; each must avoid talking with other caregivers in a manner that criticizes the client for being who he is.

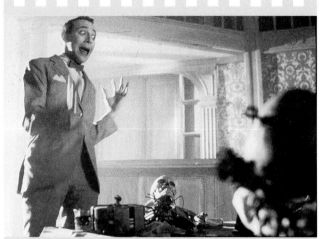

Pee Wee's Big Adventure. Source: Warner Brothers/Courtesy Kobal.

Personality disorders are often difficult to assess and diagnose. While it may be hard to place Pee Wee Herman in a DSM-IV category, one can readily recognize Pee Wee as an odd personality type.

ODD AND ECCENTRIC PERSONALITY CLUSTER

Individuals in this cluster have the characteristic of seeming unusual. They are often described by others as "different" or "somewhat odd." They tend to remain isolated from others, unconcerned about how others perceive them, and develop living patterns that appear disconnected and independent. Those with Paranoid Personality Disorder have a suspiciousness of others as well as an inability to trust.

Schizoid Personality Disorder

Paul

It was Paul's afternoon to appear before the faculty of the Pittsburgh High School to account for his various misdemeanors. He had been suspended a week ago, and his father had called at the Principal's office and confessed his perplexity about his son. Paul entered the faculty-room suave and smiling. His clothes were a trifle outgrown, and the tan velvet on the collar of his open overcoat was frayed and worn, but for all that there was something of the dandy about him, and he wore an opal pin in his neatly knotted black four-in-hand, and a red carnation in his buttonhole. This latter adornment the faculty somehow felt was not properly significant of the contrite spirit befitting a boy under the ban of suspension. . . .

When questioned by the Principal as to why he was there, Paul stated, politely enough, that he wanted to come back to school. This was a lie, but Paul was accustomed to lying; found it indeed, indispensable for overcoming friction. His teachers were asked to state their respective charges against him, which they did with such a rancor and aggrievedness as evinced that this was not a usual case. Disorder and impertinence were among the offenses named, yet each of his instructors felt that it was scarcely possible to put into words the real cause of the trouble, which lay in a sort of hysterically defiant manner of the boy's, in the contempt which they all knew he felt for them, and which he seemingly made not the least effort to conceal. Once, when he had been making a synopsis of a paragraph at the blackboard, his English teacher had stepped to his side and attempted to guide his hand. Paul had started back with a shudder and thrust his hands violently behind him. . . . In one way and another he had made all his teachers, men and women alike, conscious of the same feeling of physical aversion. In one class he habitually sat with his hand shading his eyes; in another he always looked out of the window during the recitation; in another he made a running commentary on the lecture, with humorous intent.

His teachers felt this afternoon that his whole attitude was symbolized by his shrug and his flippantly red carnation flower, and they fell upon him without mercy, his English teacher leading the pack. He stood through it smiling, his pale lips parted over his white teeth. (His lips were continually twitching, and he had a habit of raising his eyebrows that was contemptuous and irritating to the last degree.) Older boys than Paul had broken down and shed tears under that ordeal, but his set smile did not once desert him . . . Paul was always smiling, always glancing about him seeming to feel that people might be watching him and trying to detect something. This conscious expression, since it was so far as possible from boyish mirthfulness, was usually attributed to insolence or "smartness." . . .

His teachers were in despair, and his drawing master voiced the feeling of them all when he declared there was something about the boy which none of them understood. He added: "I don't really believe that smile of his comes altogether from insolence; there's something sort of haunted about it. The boy is not strong, for one thing. There is something wrong about the fellow."

(Cather, 1948, pp. 183–185)

Persons with **Schizoid Personality Disorder** are characterized by marked detachment from persons and events around them. They show little emotion, develop few close friendships, and most commonly spend time by themselves. In Willa Cather's description of "Paul's Case," Paul's teachers were struck, and somewhat offended, at how little impact their criticism seemed to make on him. This lack of concern about either criticism or praise is one of the major characteristics of the schizoid personality. Schizoid individuals "usually display a 'bland' exterior without visible emotional reactivity and rarely reciprocate gestures or facial expressions such as smiles or nods. . . . They often display a constricted affect and appear cold and aloof" (American Psychiatric Association, 1994, p. 638). Paul exhibits a clear presence of aloofness and shows he does not care about the opinions of others, even his teachers. He responds neither to social cues of how to behave in class nor to social cues of how to behave in his current disciplinary hearing.

Paul's teachers are remarkably angry at him, but they have begun to recognize that his behavior does not

---

ESSENTIAL FEATURES OF SCHIZOID PERSONALITY DISORDER

◆ Demonstrates pervasive pattern of detachment from social relationships

◆ Exhibits restricted range of emotions

◆ Must have four or more of the following:

  – Neither desires nor enjoys close relationships, including being part of a family

  – Chooses solitary activities

  – Has little (if any) interest in sexual experiences

  – Takes pleasure in few (if any) activities

  – Lacks close friends

  – Appears indifferent to praise or criticism

  – Shows emotional coldness

Reprinted with permission from the *Diagnostic and Statistical Manual of Mental Disorders*, Fourth Edition. Copyright 1994 American Psychiatric Association.

---

merely derive from insolence or disrespect, such as one might see with Antisocial Personality Disorder, a much more common disorder. Paul's art teacher would seem to have gotten it nearly right: "I don't really believe that smile of his comes altogether from insolence; . . . There is something wrong about the fellow."

Persons with Schizoid Personality Disorder might often inspire the comment, "there is something wrong about [him or her]." They do not seem to obtain satisfaction from being members of a family or social group. They are described as loners and therefore choose occupations and activities that call for a solitary lifestyle. Persons with Schizoid Personality Disorder seem oblivious to the subtleties of social interaction. They do not respond appropriately to social cues, coming across as inept or self-absorbed. Children and adolescents with Schizoid Personality Disorder stand out from their peers as loners and underachievers in school.

Etiology

Benjamin (1993) suggests that the child with Schizoid Personality Disorder would likely have grown up in a home that was orderly and formal, without much warmth, play, or spontaneous social interaction. The person with Schizoid Personality Disorder remains unattached to self or to others and probably learned behaviors from a parent who was withdrawn. The person with Schizoid Personality Disorder learns to "expect nothing and give nothing" (Benjamin, 1993, p. 345).

In comparison to disorders in the dramatic and emotional cluster, Schizoid Personality Disorder is quite uncommon. As the name implies, persons with this disorder may sometimes closely resemble individuals with early Schizophrenia. Most persons who develop Schizophrenia gradually take on "negative" symptoms resembling, but ultimately more severe than, those of schizoid personality. As illustrated in Chapter 11, the contrast between preschizophrenic and postschizophrenic personality can be remarkable. In contrast, the personality of schizoid individuals remains constant from early adolescence or childhood. Thus, Schizophrenia and Schizoid Personality Disorder can often be differentiated by their age of onset and the presence or absence of a premorbid normal state. Still, it is frequently not initially possible to distinguish early Schizophrenia from a Schizoid Personality Disorder, and only time allows the distinction to be made: Schizophrenia is almost invariably relentlessly progressive, in contrast to the stable personality disorder. In reality, however, the two conditions are not completely separate; some individuals who develop Schizophrenia seem to have had a long-standing schizoid personality. The relatively frequent occurrence of Schizoid Personality Disorder in relatives of individuals with Schizophrenia further suggests a significant etiologic association between the two. Like many other personality disorders, Schizoid Personality Disorder is diagnosed more frequently in males than females.

Nursing care for a client with Schizoid Personality Disorder is always marked by the inability to establish a nurse-client relationship. The client may describe a sense of being isolated, yet be unable to share emotions or experiences with others. The best nursing approach is to offer time and support to the client unconditionally; the client will be unable to respond in the way others do. Again, the nurse must be aware of the fact that the client is unable to change his basic personality. He may learn to change some behavioral characteristics, and care should be directed to changing behavior that is causing the most disruption to the client's life, without attempting to change the client's personality.

Schizotypal Personality Disorder

Egaeus

My baptismal name is Egaeus; that of my family I will not mention. Yet there are no towers in the land more time-honored than my gloomy, gray, hereditary halls. Our line has been called a race of visionaries; and in many striking particulars—in the character of the family mansion—in the . . . gallery of antique paintings . . . and, lastly, in the very peculiar nature of the library's contents, there is more than sufficient evidence to warrant that belief.

The recollections of my earliest years are connected with that chamber, and with its volumes—of which latter I will say no more. Here died my mother. Herein I was born. But it is mere idleness to say that I had not lived before—that the soul has no previous existence. You deny it?—let us not argue the matter. Convinced myself, I seek not to convince. There is, however, a remembrance of aerial forms—of spiritual and meaning which will not be excluded; a memory like a shadow, vague, variable, indefinite, unsteady; and like a shadow, too, in the impossibility of my getting rid of it while the sunlight of my reason shall exist. . . .

It is singular that as years rolled away, and the noon of manhood found me still in the mansion of my fathers . . . the realities of the world affected me as visions . . . while the wild ideas of the land of dreams became . . . my every-day existence. . . .

To muse for long unwearied hours with my attention riveted to some frivolous device on the margin, or in the typography of a book; to become absorbed for the better part of a summer's day, in a quaint shadow falling upon the tapestry, or upon the door; to lose myself for an entire night in watching the steady flame of a lamp; . . . to repeat monotonously some common word, until the sound, by dint of frequent repetition, ceased to convey any idea whatever of the mind; . . . such were a few of the most common and least pernicious vagaries induced by a condition of the mental faculties . . . certainly bidding defiance to anything like analysis or explanation. . . . In the strange anomaly of my existence, feelings with me, had never been of the heart, and my passions always were of the mind.

(Poe, 1983, pp. 208–213)

Edgar Allan Poe's character Egaeus illustrates many of the features of **Schizotypal Personality Disorder**. Egaeus lacks the ability to form close relationships. His passions are only "of the mind"; he becomes engaged to his cousin Berenice when "*in an evil moment*, I spoke to her of marriage." His thoughts and language are distinctly odd; his speech is vague, difficult to follow, and overelaborate, probably even for Poe's time. He describes himself and his family as "visionaries," very likely meaning that they held unusual or superstitious beliefs, perhaps of magic or sorcery or communicating with the dead. Not only does Egaeus believe strongly in reincarnation, he speaks of hearing and seeing "aerial forms" (ghosts) too vivid to ignore "while the sunlight of my reason shall exist." He may not be obviously paranoid or suspicious, but he seems so confident that his beliefs in reincarnation will be challenged that he directly accuses the reader of not working hard enough to believe him: "It is mere idleness to say that I had not lived before. . . . You deny it? [reincarnation and spiritualism]—let us not argue the matter. Convinced myself, I seek not to convince." Egaeus is certainly far from friendly.

In addition to social and interpersonal deficits in close relationships, the DSM-IV diagnosis of Schizotypal Personality Disorder requires a pattern of cognitive and perceptual distortions and eccentricities. These characteristics need to be traceable, as they are in Egaeus, to early adulthood and include at least five of nine diagnostic features. Such features include ideas of reference, odd or magical thinking, unusual perceptual experiences, odd speech, suspiciousness or paranoia, inappropriate affect, odd or eccentric behavior, lack of close friends, and excessive social anxiety. The individual with Schizotypal Personality Disorder shares with the person with Schizoid Personality Disorder a distinctly odd personality and a lack of close personal relationships. The schizotypal individual tends to have stranger and more overt thought processes along with magical thinking, paranoia, odd speech, and distorted (but not psychotic) beliefs. The schizoid individual withdraws into a cold, silent self, whereas the schizotypal individual enters a world that strikes us as bizarre and disordered.

ESSENTIAL FEATURES OF SCHIZOTYPAL PERSONALITY DISORDER

- Demonstrates pervasive pattern of acute discomfort with social and interpersonal relationships
- Exhibits cognitive or perceptual distortions and eccentricities of behavior
- Must exhibit five of the following:
  - Ideas of reference
  - Odd beliefs or magical thinking
  - Unusual perceptual experiences
  - Odd thinking and speech
  - Suspiciousness or paranoid ideation
  - Behavior or appearance that is odd, eccentric, or peculiar
  - Lack of close friends
  - Excessive social anxiety

Reprinted with permission from the *Diagnostic and Statistical Manual of Mental Disorders*, Fourth Edition. Copyright 1994 American Psychiatric Association.

Etiology

The cause of Schizotypal Personality Disorder is not known. There is, as in Egaeus's case, some tendency for the personality type to be found in more than one family member, but whether this represents a genetic clustering or the results of common upbringing is unknown. Schizophrenia (see Chapter 11) is also seen more commonly among the relatives of schizotypal individuals. However, most persons with Schizotypal Personality Disorder maintain their personalities throughout adult life without developing Schizophrenia. Schizotypal disorder is slightly more common in men than in women. Studies suggest that up to 3% of the population may suffer from Schizotypal Personality Disorder, making it perhaps the most common of the "odd" personalities.

The nursing approach for a client with schizotypal personality is similar to the approach for a client with schizoid personality. The nurse should provide unconditional acceptance to the client for the person he is and not attempt to change the underlying personality. Characteristics and behaviors that cause the client difficulty can be addressed, and the client can be helped to focus on these specific behaviors. For example, if the client has difficulty communicating with others at work, a socialization group focusing on social communication skills might be helpful. If the client uses strange language that makes it difficult for others to understand him, the nurse may provide realistic feedback as to why others do not understand the client. The nurse's focus is on the behavior, not the personality.

Paranoid Personality Disorder

Ivan

His coat collar turned up, Ivan Gromov was splashing his way through the mud of alleys and back lanes one autumn morning to collect a fine from some tradesman or other. He was in a black mood as he always was in the mornings. In a certain alley he came across two convicts wearing foot-irons and escorted by four guards with rifles. Gromov had met convicts often enough before—they had always made him feel sympathetic and uncomfortable—but now this latest encounter had a peculiarly weird effect on him. Somehow it suddenly dawned on him that he himself might be clapped in irons and similarly hauled off to prison through the mud. He was passing the post office on his way home after paying this call when he met a police inspector of his acquaintance who gave him good day and walked a few steps down the street with

SIMILAR WORDS, DIFFERENT MEANINGS

1. What is the difference between the DSM diagnoses, *Schizophrenia* and two personality disorders with very similar names: *Schizoid* and *Schizotypal*?

   – *Schizophrenia* is a serious mental disorder that most commonly develops fairly suddenly in individuals who were previously quite normal. It tends to progress with time and to become dominated by "negative" symptoms that produce social withdrawal and significant impairment in cognitive and personal functioning.

   – *Schizoid Personality Disorder* is a long-standing stable disorder characterized by aloofness and reluctance to enter into social relationships. Persons with Schizoid Personality Disorder are loners who lack the ability for emotional involvement with others. While school failure is common, overall cognitive skills are generally unimpaired; occupational functioning may be surprisingly normal if an affected individual finds a job that allows him to function independently of others.

   – Persons with *Schizotypal Personality Disorder* share many of the features of Schizoid Personality Disorder. While also aloof and detached, schizotypal persons seem stranger than do those with schizoid personalities. Schizotypal individuals often have bizarre or mystical beliefs, odd speech and thinking patterns, and unusual behavior or dress. They often have some features that suggest Schizophrenia: Ideas of reference (beliefs that natural or historical phenomena have direct personal meaning) often occur, as do paranoia and suspiciousness. When present, both the ideas of reference and the paranoia are less intense than found in persons with Schizo-

phrenia. When observed over time, symptoms of Schizotypal Personality Disorder are highly stable, in contrast to the steady worsening of individuals with Schizophrenia.

2. How are these disorders similar?

   – All three conditions—Schizophrenia, Schizoid Personality Disorder, and Schizotypal Personality Disorder—share marked detachment, oddness of behavior, and social dysfunction. Schizotypal Personality Disorder has even more similarities with Schizophrenia, which may include paranoia and ideas of reference.

3. How are these disorders different?

   – Schizophrenia differs from the two personality disorders by being a dynamic, evolving illness. Most persons with Schizophrenia have normal personalities before they become ill; during the first months or years of their illness, they commonly experience serious loss of social and cognitive abilities. While persons with the two personality disorders may also be very socially handicapped, their conditions can often be traced to earliest childhood and are highly stable.

4. Can these three disorders coexist?

   – Yes. The odd ideas, beliefs, speech, and behavior of individuals with Schizotypal Personality Disorder may at times make it difficult to distinguish them from persons with Schizophrenia. Also, some individuals with either Schizoid or (especially) Schizotypal Personality Disorder may go on to develop Schizophrenia. Most schizotypal individuals could also meet criteria for Schizoid Personality Disorder, but in addition, they have the marked eccentricities of thought or behavior (or both) that characterize Schizotypal Personality Disorder.

---

him. This somehow struck Gromov as suspicious. . . . Was it so difficult to commit a crime accidentally and against one's will? Can false accusations —can judicial miscarriages, for that matter—really be ruled out? And hasn't immemorial folk wisdom taught that going to jail is like being poor; there isn't much you can do to escape from either? . . .

He began seeking seclusion and avoiding people. . . . He was afraid of trickery: of having a

bribe slipped surreptitiously into his pocket and then being caught, of making a chance error tantamount to forgery with official papers, or of losing someone else's money. . . .

In the early morning before sunrise some stove-makers called on his landlady. They had come to rebuild the kitchen stove, as Gromov was well aware, but his fears told him that they were policemen in stove-makers' clothing. Stealing out of the flat, he dashed panic-stricken down the street without hat or coat. Barking dogs chased him, a man shouted somewhere behind him, the wind whistled in his ears, and Gromov thought that all the violence on earth had coiled itself together behind his back and was pursuing him.

(Chekhov, 1971, pp. 125–127)

The Russian writer Chekhov, trained as a physician, was a keen observer of personality and personality types. In this excerpt from a short story, Ivan is convincingly portrayed as a man overcome by paranoia. Ivan begins to suspect that he might have done, or be accused of having done, something wrong. His fears of wrongful accusation increase steadily until his paranoia becomes so overwhelming that he finds himself committed to "Ward 6"— a primitive psychiatric hospital. Fearing imprisonment, Ivan ends up under psychiatric confinement.

Individuals with **Paranoid Personality Disorder** share Ivan's fears of others and their motives. From an early age, they tend to suspect that they are being exploited, or doubt the trustworthiness of friends. Essential characteristics of Paranoid Personality Disorder are listed in the accompanying display.

Chekhov implies that Ivan's symptoms are of fairly recent origin: "[Ivan] Gromov had met convicts often enough before—they had always made him feel sympathetic and uncomfortable—but now this latest encounter had a peculiarly weird effect on him. Somehow it suddenly dawned on him that he himself might be clapped in irons and similarly hauled off to prison through the mud." Today, the sudden development of paranoid ideas would strongly suggest chronic substance use, most commonly cocaine. Other medical conditions involving the central nervous system, particularly in the elderly, may also evoke paranoia. Chekhov provides little certainty about Ivan's actual diagnosis: He might have had a primary psychiatric disorder, or he might have been suffering from neurosyphilis, a common cause of paranoid delusions in the 19th century and still occasionally seen today. Individuals with Paranoid Personality Disorder have many of Ivan's traits but most commonly in a milder and more persistent form. Like Ivan, individuals with Paranoid Personality Disorder not infrequently develop brief psychoses under stress. Consider the example below:

A 60 year-old woman was brought to the psychiatric emergency room with a clinical picture suggesting paranoid schizophrenia. There was no previous history prior to several days before the visit when she became intensely delusional and agitated, fearing for her life. In the exploration of her persecutory thoughts, she reported that her persecutors had begun their assault by throwing her to the ground, taking her breath, and "wrenching" her chest. An

---

ESSENTIAL FEATURES OF PARANOID PERSONALITY DISORDER

◆ Suspect, without sufficient basis, that others are exploiting, harming, or deceiving them

◆ Be preoccupied with unjustified doubts about the loyalty or trustworthiness of friends or associates

◆ Be reluctant to confide in others because of unwarranted fears that the information will be used maliciously against them

◆ Read hidden or demeaning or threatening meanings into benign remarks or events

◆ Persistently bear grudges

◆ Perceive attacks on their character or reputation that are not apparent to others

◆ Have recurrent suspicions, without justification, regarding fidelity of spouse or sexual partner

Reprinted with permission from the *Diagnostic and Statistical Manual of Mental Disorders*, Fourth Edition. Copyright 1994 American Psychiatric Association.

---

electrocardiogram revealed a recent anterior wall myocardial infarction. When her medical illness was explained and she was transferred to the cardiac care unit, her agitation and delusions disappeared, revealing her chronic but stable paranoid personality [disorder].

(Nardo, 1986, p. 62)

In this fascinating case, a woman with a long-standing but unrecognized Paranoid Personality Disorder became psychotic under the stress of physical illness. Entering into her world, her caretakers were able to recognize the source of her decompensation: an acute myocardial infarction that had indeed thrown her to the ground and "wrenched" her chest several days before. Her delusional and psychotic response to this illness delayed treatment, but thoughtful and empathic interviewing allowed appropriate care to be given and full recovery to be made. In a setting lacking such able psychiatric assessment, this woman's delusions and evident psychosis would almost certainly have resulted in inappropriate care. Such, very possibly, was the fictional Ivan's fate in "Ward 6."

Etiology

Psychoanalysts believe that the childhood history of an adult with Paranoid Personality Disorder not infrequently includes a controlling parent who was abusive, cruel, and/or sadistic. From these experiences, the child learns to be fearful and mistrusting. In a very harsh

SIMILAR WORDS, DIFFERENT MEANINGS

1. What is the difference between the DSM diagnoses, *Paranoid Schizophrenia* and *Paranoid Personality Disorder*

   – *Paranoid Schizophrenia* is a term that applies to individuals with Schizophrenia whose delusions have paranoid content. These persons typically believe that others are intent on causing them harm, and because the paranoia is part of a psychotic disorder, it is expressed in bizarre thoughts and hallucinations. Persons afflicted with the paranoid type of Schizophrenia often experience their paranoid fears as voices threatening persecution or harm. Unlike other forms of Schizophrenia, the paranoid form generally leaves cognitive skills and emotional expression intact: These persons can become strongly aroused by their fear and as a result are often dangerous to others. As with other forms of Schizophrenia, the paranoid variety generally develops in an individual whose preillness functioning was relatively normal.

   – Individuals with *Paranoid Personality Disorder* display a long-standing aloofness and unwillingness to trust others. They are suspicious, hypersensitive, and often hostile. This hostility frequently manifests itself as intense jealousy, particularly in marital relationships. While individuals with this disorder may occasionally act out their paranoia either through individual violence or as members of a potentially violent "cult," persons with Paranoid Personality Disorder are generally more likely to express their disorder verbally. While stress may bring on brief periods of psychosis, paranoid beliefs tend to be more unpleasant than irrational or bizarre; hallucinations and unpredictable behavior are generally absent.

2. How are these disorders similar?

   – Paranoia—the expression of distrust and suspiciousness—is common to both Paranoid Schizophrenia and Paranoid Personality Disorder. Individuals with either disorder can be very difficult to work with, either as a professional or as a family member.

3. How are these disorders different?

   – Paranoid Schizophrenia generally develops in an individual who was relatively normal before the onset of her illness. Paranoid Personality Disorder is a pervasive form of behavior that can often be traced to adolescence or even childhood and remains largely stable through a lifetime.

4. Can an individual have both Paranoid Schizophrenia and Paranoid Personality Disorder?

   – Yes. Some people who develop Paranoid Schizophrenia have had a history of Paranoid Personality Disorder.

✴ NURSING TIP

Clients with Odd and Eccentric Personality Disorders

The nurse must approach clients with these personality disorders with the realization that the client will not respond to the nurse's efforts to build a relationship with the client. These clients are socially isolated, their behaviors lead others to avoid them, and they may have difficulties at work or school. They may seek mental health care because they are in distress for another reason, as, for example, the woman who experienced acute heart disease and became psychotic; or they may suffer from an Axis I disorder, depression being one of the most common. Clients with odd and eccentric personality disorders are frequently referred for mental health evaluation when they come up against a rigid system (e.g., schools, as in Paul's case in the excerpt under Schizoid Personality at the beginning of this section) where others notice the unusual aspects of the person's behavior and believe something is seriously wrong. The nurse should focus on the behaviors that are most disturbing or causing the most difficulty for the client and assess for other coexisting psychiatric and medical disorders.

upbringing the child also learns not to ask for help, not to cry, and to remain independent (Benjamin, 1993). Paranoid Personality Disorder occurs in up to 2.5% of the general population and much more frequently in both outpatient and inpatient psychiatric settings (American Psychiatric Association, 1994).

To care for a client with Paranoid Personality Disorder is challenging for the nurse. The nurse must understand that the client is suspicious, that he has longstanding patterns of interaction that will make him unable to respond to the nurse's offer of communication. The nurse should provide care and information to the client in a non-emotional and matter-of-fact manner. If the client is in for care because his behavior patterns are making life too difficult, the nurse should focus on the behaviors. For example, the client frequently does not know how he comes across to others. The nurse can provide clear and honest feedback. As with clients who have paranoid delusions (see Chapter 11), the nurse should not try to talk the client out of unfounded fears. Such discussions will only lead to the client becoming defensive.

ANXIETY- AND FEAR-BASED PERSONALITY CLUSTER

Persons with this cluster of personality disorders appear anxious or express fears that inhibit setting or attaining goals. This fear is not the suspiciousness of Paranoid Personality Disorder; rather, it is the fear that inhibits setting or attaining goals, or the fear of criticism or rejection.

Obsessive-Compulsive Personality Disorder

Akaky Akakyevitch

It would be hard to find a man who lived in his work as did Akaky Akakyevitch. To say that he was zealous in his work is not enough; no, he loved his work. In it, in that copying, he found a varied and agreeable world of his own. There was a look of enjoyment on his face; certain letters were favorites with him, and when he came to them he was delighted; he chuckled to himself and winked and moved his lips, so that it seemed as though every letter his pen was forming could be read in his face. If rewards had been given according to the measure of zeal in the service, he might to his amazement have even found himself a civil councillor; but all he gained in the service, as the wits, his fellow-clerks expressed it, was a buckle in his

button-hole and a pain in his back. It cannot be said, however, that no notice had ever been taken of him. One director, being a good-natured man and anxious to reward him for his long service, sent him something a little more important than his ordinary copying; he was instructed from a finished document to make some sort of report for another office; the work consisted only of altering the headings and in places changing the first person into the third. This cost him such an effort that it threw him into a regular perspiration: he mopped his brow and said at last. "No, better let me copy something."

From that time forth they left him to go on copying forever. It seemed as though nothing in the world existed for him outside his copying. . . . On reaching home, he would sit down at once to the table, hurriedly sup his soup and eat a piece of beef with an onion; he did not notice the taste at all, but ate it all up together with the flies and anything else that Providence chanced to send him. When he felt that his stomach was beginning to be full, he would rise up from the table, get out a bottle of ink and set to copying the papers he had brought home with him. When he had none to do, he would make a copy expressly for his own pleasure, particularly if the document were remarkable not for the beauty of its style but for the fact of its being addressed to some new or important personage. . . .

Akaky Akakyevitch had for some time been feeling that his back and shoulders were particularly nipped by the cold. . . . He wondered at last whether there were any defects in his overcoat. After examining it thoroughly in the privacy of his home, he discovered that in two or three places, to wit on the back and the shoulders, it had become a regular sieve; the cloth was so worn that you could see through it. . . . Its collar had been growing smaller year by year as it served to patch the other parts. . . .

Then Akaky Akakyevitch saw that there was no escape from a new overcoat and he was utterly depressed. How indeed, for what, with what money could he get it? . . . Akaky Akakyevitch had the habit every time he spent a ruble of putting aside two kopecks in a little locked-up box with a slit in the lid for slipping the money in. At the end of every half-year he would inspect the pile of coppers *there and change them for small silver. He had done this for a long time, and in the course of many years the sum had mounted up to forty rubles. . . . Another two or three months of partial fasting and Akaky Akakyevitch had actually saved up nearly eighty rubles.**

(Gogol, 1957, pp. 237–250)

This story, by the famous 19th-century Russian author Nicolai Gogol, is a reminder of how tedious it was to carry out business activities before the invention of type-writers, photocopiers, and word processing. Akaky is clearly preoccupied with his work, the proper performance of which demands compulsive attention. But, as his supervisors and fellow clerks observe, Akaky's compulsiveness goes beyond the requirements of his job. He has excluded leisure and friendships from his life, and he invariably takes his work home with him. Unlike a modern "workaholic," he is not trying to impress his supervisors or to distinguish himself by the quantity or quality of his work. As Gogol portrays him, Akaky is driven by physical and psychological need to copy documents. The content is irrelevant to him; he has interest only in the physical form of the numbers and letters he writes, and perhaps in the identity of the persons to whom the documents are addressed. His compulsive-ness extends to his personal finances. He carefully taxes himself 2% of all that he spends, but he has no long-term plans for how to use the money he saves. Individuals with **Obsessive-Compulsive Personality Disorder** tend, like Akaky, to hoard their money, and, also like him, they frequently find it difficult to discard old and worn-out possessions.

Such preoccupation with order, cleanliness, control, and perfectionism are characteristic of persons with Obsessive-Compulsive Personality Disorder. Persons with Obsessive-Compulsive Personality Disorder attempt to maintain control by attention to trivia, rules, detail, and procedures to the point where the reason for the activity is lost in the attention to form. Like Akaky, persons with Obsessive-Compulsive Personality Disorder are loyal to their work and may avoid leisure or pleasurable pursuits. Persons with this disorder often seem highly inflexible. As a result, they may initially have difficulty accepting the experience of physical illness. Hospitalization, medical visits, and other necessities of illness (and of aging) potentially threaten long-established routines and may be experienced as highly disruptive. With careful counseling, however, persons with Obsessive-Compulsive Personality

---

ESSENTIAL FEATURES OF OBSESSIVE-COMPULSIVE PERSONALITY DISORDER
◆ Is preoccupied with details, lists, rules, organization, or schedules
◆ Aspires to perfectionism that interferes with task completion
◆ Is excessively devoted to work and productivity
◆ Is overconscientious, scrupulous, and inflexible about matters of morality, ethics, or values
◆ Is unable to discard worn-out and worthless objects
◆ Is reluctant to delegate tasks
◆ Adopts a miserly spending style
◆ Is rigid and stubborn

Reprinted with permission from the *Diagnostic and Statistical Manual of Mental Disorders*, Fourth Edition. Copyright 1994 American Psychiatric Association.

Disorder can make extraordinarily compliant clients, especially when disorders like diabetes require careful self-management.

It is important to recognize that, despite a very similar name, Obsessive-Compulsive Personality Disorder is distinct from Obsessive-Compulsive Disorder. In DSM-IV, Obsessive-Compulsive Disorder is an Axis I anxiety diagnosis, whereas Obsessive-Compulsive Personality Disorder is an Axis II description of personality traits.

Etiology

Developmental history of an adult with Obsessive-Compulsive Personality Disorder often reveals a family in which it was expected that the child be perfect and adhere closely to rules. Adults report little warmth in their childhood homes and describe frequent punishment for failure to be perfect. Under such circumstances, praise is rarely received, and the child is strongly motivated to strive for carefully correct performance merely to avoid criticism (Benjamin, 1993). As noted previously, under some circumstances such as adjustment to the requirements of physical illness, the presence of obsessive-compulsive traits may be an asset. Despite the value of careful attention to detail, the constant striving for perfection that is characteristic of a personality disorder causes significant impairment in functioning. While many persons have some obsessive-compulsive traits, the prevalence of frank Obsessive-Compulsive Personality Disorder in adults is only about 1%; the diagnosis is

---

*"The Overcoat," from THE OVERCOAT & OTHER TALES OF GOOD AND EVIL by Nicolai Gogol. Copyright © 1957 by David Magarshack. Used by permission of Doubleday, a division of Bantam Doubleday Dell Publishing Group, Inc.

SIMILAR WORDS, DIFFERENT MEANINGS

1. What is the difference between the DSM diagnoses, *Obsessive-Compulsive Disorder* and *Obsessive-Compulsive Personality Disorder*?

– *Obsessive-Compulsive Disorder* (OCD) is one of the anxiety disorders. Although OCD may develop at any time in life, it tends to begin relatively acutely and may often improve either spontaneously or with therapy. The symptoms of OCD occur under quite specific stimuli (e.g., with fears of self-contamination), and the affected individual tries to relieve these symptoms by certain repeated actions (such as hand-washing). The person who suffers from OCD generally recognizes that his fears are out of proportion to any real threat but without therapy is often powerless to control those fears.

– *Obsessive-Compulsive Personality Disorder* (OCPD) is an Axis II disorder in DSM-IV. This means that it has developmental origins that can generally be traced back to young adulthood or even to childhood. Persons with OCPD tend to be rigid, perfectionistic, and distinctly uncomfortable if others fail to follow the patterns of activity or behavior that they demand. Individuals with OCPD often do not work well with others because they have great difficulty sharing or delegating. Individuals with OCPD typically lack interpersonal flexibility or the ability to negotiate.

2. How are these disorders similar?

– Obsessive-Compulsive Disorder and OCPD may share patterns of rigidity; individuals with either disorder may hoard personal effects, clothing, or other items.

3. How are these disorders different?

– In general, OCD and OCPD are quite distinct. The individual with OCD is usually psychologically normal except in situations that evoke their obsessions or compulsions. Consequently, many affected persons manage to successfully hide their symptoms from friends and family. A person with OCD symptoms that involve fear of contamination may be very uncomfortable if, for example, food is placed back on the table after having fallen on the floor. She may not care in the least if the candles are knocked off the table or the chairs are arranged in any arbitrary order. In contrast, an individual with OCPD may be exceedingly uncomfortable if papers, books, or furniture are moved in any way. She may insist on a rigid order of activities: For example, soup must never be eaten before salad; the television must never be turned on before the windows are opened and the laundry folded. The rigidity of OCPD is generally extreme, unrelated to the specific anxieties or fears that characterize OCD, and applies to virtually all aspects of life and behavior.

4. Can a person have both OCD and OCPD?

– Yes. Howard Hughes, described in the chapter on Obsessive-Compulsive Disorder, almost certainly also had characteristics of OCPD.

---

made twice as often for males as for females (American Psychiatric Association, 1994).

Clients with Obsessive-Compulsive Personality Disorder expect attention to detail. The nurse should recognize that order and rules are important to the client. The client is often prepared to do what is right for his health, but he expects clear and unconfused directions. When obsessive-compulsive behaviors cause personal difficulties, for example at work, school, or in hospital settings wherein the client is not in control, the nurse may assist the client to adapt by allowing the client to arrange aspects of the environment. The nurse also has a role in helping family members, teachers, and significant others in understanding why order is so important to the client.

Avoidant Personality Disorder

Laura

Laura is seated in the delicate ivory chair at the small claw-foot table. She wears a dress of soft violet material for a kimono—her hair is tied back from her forehead with a ribbon. She is washing and polishing her collection of glass. Amanda [her mother] appears on the fire escape steps. At the sound of her ascent, Laura catches her breath, thrusts the bowl of ornaments away, and seats herself stiffly before the diagram of the typewriter keyboard as though it held her spellbound. . . .

LAURA: Hello, Mother, I was—[She makes a nervous gesture toward the chart on the wall. Amanda leans against the shut door and stares at Laura with a martyred look.]

AMANDA: Deception? Deception? [She slowly removes her hat and gloves, continuing the sweet suffering stare. She lets the hat and gloves fall on the floor—a bit of acting.]

LAURA: [shakily]: How was the D.A.R. meeting?

[Amanda slowly opens her purse and removes a dainty white handkerchief which she shakes out delicately and delicately touches to her lips and nostrils.]

Didn't you go to the D.A.R. meeting, Mother?

AMANDA: [faintly, almost inaudibly];—No.— No. [then more forcibly:] I did not have the strength —to go to the D.A.R. In fact, I did not have the courage! I wanted to find a hole in the ground and hide myself in it forever! [She crosses slowly to the wall and removes the diagram of the typewriter keyboard. She holds it in front of her for a second, staring at it sweetly and sorrowfully—then bites her lips and tears it in two pieces.]

LAURA: [faintly] Why did you do that, Mother?

[Amanda repeats the same procedure with the chart of the Gregg Alphabet.]

Why are you—

AMANDA: Why? Why? How old are you, Laura?

LAURA: Mother, you know my age.

AMANDA: I thought that you were an adult; it seems that I was mistaken. [She crosses slowly to the sofa and sinks down and stares at Laura.]

LAURA: Please don't stare at me, Mother.

[Amanda closes her eyes and lowers her head. There is a ten second pause.]

AMANDA: What are we going to do, what is going to become of us, what is the future?

[There is another pause.]

LAURA: Has something happened, Mother?

[Amanda draws a long breath, takes out the handkerchief again, goes through the dabbing process.]

AMANDA: I'll be all right in a minute, I'm just bewildered—[she hesitates.]—by life. . . .

LAURA: Mother, I wish that you would tell me what's happened!

AMANDA: I went to the typing instructor and introduced myself as your mother. She didn't know who you were. "Wingfield," she said, "We don't

have any such student enrolled at the school!"

I assured her she did, that you had been going to classes since early in January.

"I wonder," she said, "If you could be talking about that terribly shy little girl who dropped out of school after only a few days' attendance?"

"No," I said, "Laura, my daughter, has been going to school every day for the past six weeks!"

"Excuse me," she said. She took the attendance book out and there was your name, unmistakably printed, and all the dates you were absent until they decided that you had dropped out of school.

"I still said, No, there must have been some mistake! There must have been some mix-up in the records!"

And she said, "No—I remember her perfectly now. Her hands shook so that she couldn't hit the right keys! The first time we gave a speed test, she broke down completely—was sick at the stomach and almost had to be carried into the wash room! After that morning she never showed up any more. We phoned the house but never got any answer." . . .

Laura, where have you been going when you've gone out pretending that you were going to business college?

LAURA: I've just been going out walking.*

(Williams, 1971, pp. 151–153)

The major features of **Avoidant Personality Disorder** are social inhibition and feelings of inadequacy. Persons with this disorder avoid interpersonal situations at work or school that could lead to criticism or rejection. Affected individuals are shy, inhibited, and sometimes described as "invisible." They may turn down offers of advancement to avoid the risk of criticism or defeat. The affected individual perceives herself to be unappealing or inferior to others and is typically unwilling to take normal risks involved with employment or interpersonal relationships. This description fits Laura exceedingly well: She is shy, fearful, and, as becomes evident later in the play, unable to form relationships outside of the childlike imaginary world in which she lives. As her brother Tom observes:

Laura is different from other girls. . . . She's terribly shy and lives in a world of her own and those things make her seem a little peculiar to people outside the house. . . . She lives in a world of her own—

---

*By Tennessee Williams, from THE GLASS MENAGERIE. Copyright © 1945 by Tennessee Williams and Edwin D. Williams. Reprinted by permission of New Directions Publishing Corp.

a world of little glass ornaments. . . . She plays old phonograph records and—that's about all.

(Williams, 1971, p. 153)

Etiology

A person with Avoidant Personality Disorder often has a childhood history of being in a family where the opinions of others were held in high importance and the opinion of the child not highly regarded or noticed. As a result, the child is socialized to believe that public exposure can result in humiliation. The individual has a desire to be sociable but also a fear that being close to others may bring rejection and/or humiliation. The family is the sole source of support for the person with Avoidant Personality Disorder, even if the family is critical and rejecting. The person with Avoidant Personality Disorder fears that those outside the family will reject him even more than does his own family (Benjamin, 1993).

Individuals with Avoidant Personality Disorder often perceive criticism when it is not intended by others. As with Laura, shyness is a major feature that often begins in early childhood and may increase significantly in adolescence. In contrast, normal childhood shyness decreases through adolescence and young adulthood. Shyness is a far more common trait than full-blown Avoidant Personality Disorder, a condition with a prevalence in the general population of something under 1%. Unlike many other personality disorders, this diagnosis is equally common among males as among females.

A client with Avoidant Personality Disorder will come across as shy and unwilling to try new things. The client's only source of support will be, as in Laura's case, her immediate family or very close friends. The nurse must engage the client's significant others in efforts to provide care. It is sometimes helpful to assist family members to understand the avoidant behaviors and help them to encourage the client to try out new things, as in Laura's case, going to school. The client may be receptive to establishing a relationship with the nurse, but the client will not give up her family supports or seek independence.

Dependent Personality Disorder

Eveline

She was about to explore another life with Frank. Frank was very kind, manly, open-hearted. She was to go away with him by the night-boat to be his wife and to live with him in Buenos Ayres where he had a home waiting for her. . . . Of course, her father had found out the affair and had forbidden her to have anything to say to him. . . . After that she had to meet her lover secretly.

The evening deepened in the avenue. The white of two letters in her lap grew indistinct. One was to [her brother]; the other was to her father. . . . As she mused the pitiful vision of her mother's life laid its spell on the very quick of her being—that life of commonplace sacrifices closing in final craziness. . . .

She stood up in a sudden impulse of terror. Escape! She must escape! Frank would save her. . . .

She stood among the swaying crowd in the station at the North Wall. He held her hand and she knew that he was speaking to her, saying something about the passage over and over again. . . . She answered nothing. She felt her cheek pale and cold and, out of a maze of distress, she prayed to God to direct her, to show her what was her duty. The boat blew a long mournful whistle into the mist. If she went, to-morrow she would be on the sea with Frank, steaming towards Buenos Ayres. . . . A bell clanged upon her heart. She felt him seize her hand:—Come!

No! No! No! It was impossible. Her hands clutched the iron in frenzy. Amid the seas she sent a cry of anguish!

—Eveline! Evy!

He rushed beyond the barrier and called to her to follow. He was shouted at to go on but he still called to her. She set her white face to him, passive, like a helpless animal. Her eyes gave him no sign of love or farewell or recognition.*

(Joyce, 1967, pp. 38–41)

> ## ESSENTIAL FEATURES OF
> ## AVOIDANT PERSONALITY DISORDER
>
> ◆ Is unwilling to get involved with people unless certain of being liked
>
> ◆ Shows restraint in intimate relationships for fear of being shamed or ridiculed
>
> ◆ Is inhibited in interpersonal relationships because of feelings of inadequacy
>
> ◆ Views self as socially inept and inferior to others
>
> ◆ Is unusually reluctant to take personal risks
>
> Reprinted with permission from the *Diagnostic and Statistical Manual of Mental Disorders*, Fourth Edition. Copyright 1994 American Psychiatric Association.

*"Eveline," from DUBLINERS by James Joyce. Copyright 1916 by B. W. Heubsch. Definitive text Copyright © 1967 by the Estate of James Joyce. Used by permission of Viking Penguin, a division of Penguin Books, USA Inc.

ESSENTIAL FEATURES OF DEPENDENT PERSONALITY DISORDER

◆ Has difficulty making everyday decisions
◆ Needs others to assume responsibility for major areas of his or her life
◆ Has difficulty expressing disagreement
◆ Has difficulty initiating projects
◆ Goes to excessive lengths to obtain nurturance from others
◆ Feels uncomfortable or helpless when alone
◆ Urgently seeks relationships as a source of care or support
◆ Is unrealistically preoccupied with fears of being left to take care of self

Reprinted with permission from the *Diagnostic and Statistical Manual of Mental Disorders*, Fourth Edition. Copyright 1994 American Psychiatric Association.

In this excerpt from Joyce's famous story in *The Dubliners*, Eveline is unable to decide or to act. She is in love with Frank, who has promised her a new life in Argentina, far from dreary, oppressive Ireland, but she cannot decide to go with him. She knows that women have been betrayed by men who promise marriage and then desert them far from their homes and family. Her own home offers little future other than the uncertain possibility of a dreary marriage to an unromantic, perhaps physically abusive husband. In the novel, Eveline stays with her father in Dublin, not because she chooses that life but because she cannot choose. She lets her father dictate her life, and despite almost escaping, in the end she cannot make the separation from her past. The story leaves her both uncomfortable and helpless but unable to respond with either "farewell or recognition."

A person with **Dependent Personality Disorder** has a need to be taken care of by others. The individual is clinging and submissive and fears separation from the known. Such persons have trouble making decisions and have difficulty expressing disagreements with others. They feel unable to function alone and are not independent. They are willing to do what others want, particularly if such actions lead to others caring for them. As with other personality disorders, these characteristics must be present in sufficient degree that they significantly interfere with personal or social functioning.

Etiology

One theory of Dependent Personality Disorder is that, in early childhood, parents did not stop nurturing the child when it was developmentally appropriate to do so. Instead of letting the toddler do things on his own, the caregivers offer too much protectiveness. The child becomes incompetent and begins to believe that he cannot do anything. There is overwhelming parental control and the only option for the developing child is submission. In clinical settings, the diagnosis is made more often for females than for males. Dependent Personality Disorder is one of the most frequently reported personality disorders encountered in mental health clinics (American Psychiatric Association, 1994). Individuals with highly dependent personalities frequently use illness to gain support and attention. There is potentially a strong tendency for individuals with Dependent Personality Disorder to develop Axis I somatoform disorders, especially when somatization brings them attention and support.

Nurses who encounter persons with Dependent Personality Disorder often become frustrated because the client does not demonstrate age-appropriate independence. Nurses must recognize that the client may, indeed, live a life of having others take charge. The client may come into nursing care only when he is physically ill or needs nurses to provide care because no one else in his world will do so at a given point in time. The nurse must set limits regarding what the nurse will do for the client and what the client is expected to do for himself.

Passive-Aggressive or Negativistic Personality Disorder

I Am a Spiteful Man

I am a spiteful man . . . I have been living like that for a long time now—twenty years. I am forty now. I used to be in the civil service, but no longer am. I was a spiteful official. I was rude and took pleasure in being so. . . .

When petitioners would come to my desk for information I used to grind my teeth at them, and feel intense enjoyment when I succeeded in distressing someone. I was almost always successful. For the most part they were all timid people—of course, they were petitioners. But among the fops there was one officer in particular I could not endure. He simply would not be humble, and clanged his sword in a disgusting way. I carried on a war with him for eighteen months over that sword. At last I got the better of him. He left off clanking it. . . .

I was lying when I said just now that I was a spiteful official. I was lying out of spite. I was simply indulging myself with the petitioners and with the officer, but I could never really become spiteful. . . . Not only could I not become spiteful, I could

*not become anything: neither spiteful nor kind,
neither a rascal nor an honest man, neither a hero
nor an insect. . . . I am forty years old now, and
forty years, after all is a whole lifetime; . . . Who
does live beyond forty? Answer that, sincerely and
honestly. I will tell you who do: fools and worthless
people do. . . . I have a right to say so, for I shall go
on living to sixty myself. I'll live till seventy! till
eighty!**

(Dostoevsky, 1960, pp. 3–5)

In "Notes from Underground," Dostoevsky has created a character who is remarkable for his perversity and negative outlook on life. Few if any literary characters prior to "Notes" have been portrayed to be as unlikable and pathetic as is the narrator of this excerpt. One of the reasons it is so hard to respond positively to "the Underground Man" is the passive-aggressive way in which his self-hatred expresses itself. Passive-aggressive behavior creates anger in the persons to whom it is directed, and even the reader ultimately reacts with annoyance and anger. The DSM-IV description of **Passive-Aggressive Personality Disorder** reflects Dostoevsky's character with remarkable accuracy: "These individuals . . . may be sullen, irritable, impatient, argumentative, cynical, skeptical, and contrary . . . [They may] feel cheated, unappreciated, and misunderstood and chronically complain to others" (American Psychiatric Association, 1994, p. 733). In DSM-IV, Passive-Aggressive Personality Disorder was removed from the list of personality disorders and placed on the list of disorders requiring further research and investigation. While a diagnosis of Passive-Aggressive Personality Disorder cannot be made (the correct diagnosis at this time is Personality Disorder, Not Otherwise Specified), the authors have included Passive-Aggressive Personality Disorder in this chapter because passive-aggressive behavior is seen relatively frequently in health care settings. The official diagnosis requires study to ensure consistency in definition and diagnosis, but the concept of the passive-aggressive individual is useful for the nurse to understand.

The individual with Passive-Aggressive Personality Disorder typically displays a combination of pervasive negativity with passive resistance to social and/or occupational demands. Such resistance to demands is often characterized by procrastination, stubbornness, and intentional inefficiency, particularly in response to demands made by authority figures. Passive-Aggressive Personality Disorder is sometimes also called negativistic personality disorder.

---

*From NOTES FROM UNDERGROUND AND THE GRAND INQUISITOR by Fyodor Dostoevsky, translated by Ralph E. Matlaw, Translation copyright © 1960, 1988 by E. P. Dutton. Used by permission of Dutton Signet, a division of Penguin Books, USA Inc.

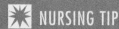 **NURSING TIP**

Clients with Anxiety- and Fear-Based Personality Disorders

Nurses must approach clients with this cluster of personality disorders from a perspective of caring and understanding. The client's anxieties, obsessions, and fears of failure are very real. The nurse may be able to help the client cope with his environment by giving the client control wherever possible and encouraging the client to manage his environment in his own way. Persons with an avoidant personality will need great patience and encouragement to take on even small responsibilities.

Etiology

The developmental history of persons with Passive-Aggressive Personality Disorder may include the abrupt loss of infantile and child nurturance followed by the imposition of unfair or excessive developmental demands. This developmental scenario may most frequently occur when a first-born child is displaced by the birth of a younger sibling. His resultant anger at being frustrated by his life events may be expressed passively. The child ultimately learns indirect ways of dealing with parents/authorities by taking a long time to complete tasks or doing them with obvious flaws (Benjamin, 1993).

To provide care to one with a passive-aggressive personality, the nurse must first evaluate her own feelings in reaction to the passive-aggressiveness. Typically, nurses find themselves angry at the client, and the client seems uncaring, devious, and even cruel. The nurse must have the ability to step back and recognize the passive-aggressive behavior and understand that the client's behavior is likely motivated by a negative view of self and the world. The individual with Passive-Aggressive Personality Disorder is unhappy with himself and with others in his life and will demonstrate his unhappiness through chronic complaints.

Individuals with Passive-Aggressive Personality Disorder almost always provoke anger in others, including their nurses.

NURSING PERSPECTIVES

As emphasized in several of the individual discussions preceding, nurses will likely encounter persons with personality disorders in virtually every area of practice. More often than not, the personality disorder is not the reason for the client's coming to medical or nursing attention; rather, the client presents for care of some other concurrent condition. The client with a personality disorder may present in a clinic with vague complaints or may present at a counseling center with depression. One author suggests that "early indicators that a personality disorder may be present include difficulty establishing a nurse-client relationship, disagreements among team members, a reluctance by the nurse to provide client care, or difficulty accomplishing treatment objectives" (Godfrey, 1991, p. 590). The goals of nursing care are first to recognize that the client has a personality disorder and second to provide care to minimize the negative impact of the client's behaviors.

NURSING THEORY

The Modeling and Role-Modeling Theory (Erickson, Tomlin, & Swain, 1983), with its emphasis on psychosocial development, will assist the nurse to explore the client's early experiences and to understand how such experiences impact on personality development and behavior patterns. For example, the character Eveline in the excerpt that illustrates dependent personality would be a case where knowledge of early years and adolescent development could form the basis for treatment choices. Presumably, Eveline (a young adult) has never been given choices over matters that affect her life. As a child, Eveline had no control over her lack of choices, but as an adult, Eveline could take some control over her own life. However, Eveline would have to be in enough discomfort (mental or physical) that she would be motivated to try something new, and she would have to trust someone enough to believe that that person would provide support to her during her process of changing. Counseling based on modeling her world would direct the nurse to see the events from Eveline's perspective and would ensure that the nurse interacting with Eveline understood that Eveline's condition is based on fear of independence and lack of self-esteem.

Martha Rogers's theory of unitary human beings has been used to assist psychiatric nurses to understand and intervene with clients with Borderline Personality Disorder (Thompson, 1990). The borderline client's behaviors, which include "rapid, radical shifts in mood, perception and behavior" (Thompson, 1990, p. 7), were interpreted from within the framework of human and environmental energy fields. The client with a borderline personality was viewed as having an energy field whose wave patterns change at an unusually rapid rate, which in turn affects the environmental energy field. This may explain why nursing staff often find the borderline client difficult to care for. It was proposed, however, that the nurse could maintain a sense of her own patterning and approach the client with a sense of calm. The interaction of the two energy fields could help produce calm in the client. Further, psychiatric nurses could attend to the environmental energy field, providing a borderline client with a space/room that the client could decorate and use as his own "personal space." Such an intervention would provide the client with both the security of having his own space and the safety of having an environment he can control. Use of Rogers's theory guides the nurse to a different understanding of clients with personality disorders and has great relevance in selection of interventions.

NURSING PROCESS

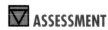 ASSESSMENT

Assessment of a client's behaviors through observation and history taking may suggest the presence of a personality disorder. A diagnosis of a personality disorder may be tentatively made by the nurse and confirmed through psychiatric evaluation. In some instances, psychological tests further add to data and to diagnostic certainty (Wiggins & Pincus, 1994). Personality disorders, by definition, develop in young adulthood or earlier in life. Personal history is therefore quite important to obtain, and often the client history can be augmented with information gathered through interview of family members, teachers, or others significant to the individual's life.

▽ NURSING DIAGNOSIS

Whether or not a personality disorder is formally diagnosed, the nursing process typically results in the formulation of one or more nursing diagnoses. Table 16-2

Table 16-2 Selected Personality Disorders with Expected Nursing Diagnoses

DISORDER	COMMON NURSING DIAGNOSES
Borderline Personality Disorder	*Violence, risk for: self-directed or directed at others* *Ineffective coping: individual* *Self-esteem, chronic low* *Impaired social interactions* *Hopelessness*
Narcissistic Personality Disorder	*Impaired social interactions* *Ineffective coping: individual* *Ineffective denial*
Histrionic Personality Disorder	*Impaired social interactions* *Ineffective coping: individual*
Antisocial Personality Disorder	*Violence, risk for: directed at others* *Ineffective denial* *Impaired social interactions*
Schizoid Personality Disorder	*Impaired social interactions* *Loneliness, risk for* *Ineffective coping: individual*
Paranoid Personality Disorder	*Fear* *Anxiety*
Obsessive-Compulsive Personality Disorder	*Anxiety* *Fear* *Self-esteem, chronic low*
Avoidant Personality Disorder	*Fear* *Loneliness, risk for* *Ineffective coping: individual*
Dependent Personality Disorder	*Self-esteem, chronic low* *Fear*
Passive-Aggressive or Negativistic Personality Disorder	*Ineffective coping: individual* *Self-esteem, chronic low* *Anxiety*

lists common nursing diagnoses for clients with the DSM diagnoses of various personality disorders.

▽ OUTCOME IDENTIFICATION

The goal of nursing care is to minimize the negative and self-defeating behaviors clients present. A positive outcome of care is that the client will experience a reduction in extreme behaviors and will increase effective coping strategies. The nurse must accept the client as he is and understand that the client will be unable to change his basic personality.

▽ PLANNING/INTERVENTIONS

Some basic principles apply to all clients with personality disorders. The nurse must make clear what the nurse can and cannot do and approach the client in a professional, supportive, and nonjudgmental manner. Nurses must work with each other and the health care team to avoid being caught up in the client's manipulative behaviors, which could pit one staff member against another. The best nursing approach is one characterized by clear communication and expectations, setting limits when needed, and providing both structure and support. The nurse should recognize that clients with personality disorders are among the most "difficult" clients seen in clinical

⑤ RESEARCH HIGHLIGHT

Nurses' Attitudes Toward Clients with Personality Disorders

1. Researchers observed nurses' responses to clients in group settings. In all, 20 groups involving 164 clients and 17 nurses were observed. Findings indicate that nurses respond to clients diagnosed with Borderline Personality Disorder in a less empathic manner than they respond to other clients (Fraser & Gallop, 1993).
2. A total of 117 clients were assessed by nurses and psychiatric residents for the degree of management difficulty the clients posed for the professionals. The nurses and residents both agreed that self-harm behaviors, violence toward others, and behaviors to sabotage treatment made the client "difficult to treat." In addition, the nurses felt that inability to form a therapeutic alliance with the nurse was an important factor in making the client "difficult" (Gallop, Lancee, & Shugar, 1993).

practice (see the Research Highlight on the previous page). The nurse will need a high degree of patience to provide comprehensive and accepted care in the presence of significant traits of personality disorders.

In some cases, the nurse may recommend and/or initiate treatment for one of these Axis II disorders. Psychotherapy is felt to be the treatment of choice for persons with schizoid, borderline, histrionic, narcissistic, dependent, passive-aggressive, and avoidant personality disorders (Andrews, 1993; Higgitt & Fonagy, 1992). However, research evidence for the effectiveness of psychotherapy in these conditions is based largely on case reports and is not strong. Other reports indicate that cognitive-behavioral therapy is successful in treating borderline (Linehan, 1987) and avoidant (Alden, 1989) personality disorders. (For a discussion of psychotherapy and cognitive-behavioral therapy, see Chapter 28 on individual therapy.) Table 16-3 lists suggested nursing interventions for working with clients with personality disorders.

▽ EVALUATION

As in all nursing care, evaluation is based on identified outcomes. The nurse should evaluate care realistically and recognize that if the client has been exposed to significant stress, care will be required over a time period of several weeks.

Table 16-3 Suggested Nursing Interventions for Clients with Personality Disorders

INTERVENTION	RATIONALE
Contract with client for specific behaviors; adhere to the terms of the contract.	Giving the client structure; making expectations known.
Assist client to explore and identify emotions.	Promoting the expression of feelings.
Withdraw attention from acting-out behavior (provided that safety of client and others is maintained).	Decreasing attention paid to negative behaviors.
Establish limits on your availability as a nurse. Set mutually agreed-upon goals and keep to them.	Keeping realistic standards.
Point out when client's attempts to manipulate are counterproductive.	Educating client on the effects of own behavior.
Focus on the fact that client's behaviors are a problem, not the client himself.	Promoting the view that the client is respected as a person.
Discuss coping strategies.	Assisting the client to explore alternate methods of dealing with stressors or problems.

CASE STUDY/CARE PLAN

For the case study, we will consider a character similar to "Annie" from the excerpt depicting Borderline Personality Disorder. June is a 24-year-old woman being seen after a suicide attempt. After the episode of her suicidal attempt/gesture, June is brought to a facility for physical treatment and psychiatric evaluation.

ASSESSMENT

June is a highly intelligent young woman. Her interests are eclectic and changeable: contemporary art and music, old classic cars, married men. She is care less about her personal appearance but is able to attract a wide variety of gentlemen who are enticed by her reckless spirit and her energy. Her most recent social meeting is with Bill, a married stockbroker. Bill is horrified to find that June has attempted suicide. He finds her in his office, bleeding profusely from self-inflicted razor blade wounds to the wrists. June is making shrieking sounds, is shivering, and does not respond to Bill. Bill dials 911 to get June help. Her wrists are carefully stitched in the emergency room, and she is admitted to the psychiatric unit of the general hospital. She is minimally communicative.

NURSING DIAGNOSIS *Risk for violence: self-directed*, as evidenced by recent self-destructive behavior

Outcomes	Planning/Interventions	Evaluation
◆ June will remain safely hospitalized for the next 3 days.	◆ Discuss with June the need to remain safe during her hospitalization.	June remained safe in hospital and did not further harm herself.

Continued

Outcomes	Planning/Interventions	Evaluation
◆ June will not mutilate herself further and will leave her current wounds alone during the next 5 days.	◆ Assist June in orienting herself to her room; explain the need for hospital care in relation to her need for safety. ◆ Supervise June closely. ◆ Clarify with June appropriate and expected behaviors specific to self-mutilation. ◆ Discuss healing with June. ◆ Gently set limits with June that she should leave her wounds alone and not further harm herself.	June did not disturb her wounds for 3 days.

NURSING DIAGNOSIS   *Impaired social interaction*, related to altered thought processes, as evidenced by inability to form supportive personal relationships with others

Outcomes	Planning/Interventions	Evaluation
◆ June will begin to communicate with her primary nurse within 24 hours.	◆ Offer self as truly interested in June. ◆ Express unconditional acceptance in interactions with June. ◆ Discuss potential breakdowns in communication that June may find frustrating; explore how the nurse can foster communication.	June was very slow to trust anyone. She refused to communicate for 3 days. She gradually opened up on day 4 to the nurse who sat quietly with June 30 minutes twice a day. The nurse praised June for her communication efforts.

NURSING DIAGNOSIS   *Ineffective individual coping*, related to past behaviors of inflicting harm to self in stress-producing situations

Outcomes	Planning/Interventions	Evaluation
◆ Within 5 days, June will identify one cue that led her to her most recent self-mutilating behavior; June will identify two alternative behaviors other than directing violence toward self.	◆ Discuss with June the factors/situations and feelings that led up to her harming self. ◆ Encourage June to express her feelings and anxieties. ◆ Discuss behaviors to use when feeling out of control—phone call to primary nurse; identify a support system. ◆ Identify with June resources she can immediately access including psych and crisis "hotlines."	The nurse continued to explore with June what precipitated the injury and what cues were present. June could not identify a specific cue but did state she felt great anxiety at the time. June could not identify two alternative behaviors but did agree that she could and would call the nurse or the psych hotline at the hospital if she felt "desperate."

CRITICAL THINKING BAND

ASSESSMENT

What additional assessment information would be pertinent in planning care for June?

NURSING DIAGNOSIS

In determining appropriate diagnoses, how does the nurse balance actual with potential problems? In the absence of client input, can a nurse determine the diagnosis of *spiritual distress*?

Outcomes

Beyond safety, how do outcomes get prioritized? Do you agree with the priority order of outcomes as listed for June?

Planning/Interventions

In addition to being self-destructive, June also had a variety of unattractive characteristics. How can a nurse be truly therapeutic when faced with such characteristics? What should the nurse do when a client acts in an embarrassing and inappropriate manner? How can a nurse best communicate with a noncommunicative client? Is nonverbal communication really noncommunicative?

Evaluation

What is June's long-term outcome likely to be?

≋ KEY CONCEPTS

♦ The term *personality* includes patterns of individual behavior expressed by physical and mental activities and attitudes.

♦ Personality style describes a cluster of personality traits exhibited by an individual.

♦ A personality disorder is described when a person has a personality style that deviates from the individual's culture and leads to distress or impairment.

♦ Personality disorders are divided into three clusters: odd and eccentric, dramatic and emotional, and anxiety and fear based.

♦ Nurses must recognize personality disorders in their clients and know that difficulty in establishing a nurse-client relationship, disagreement among team members regarding the client, personal reluctance to care for the client, or difficulty in reaching treatment goals may be warning signs that a personality disorder may be present.

♦ Psychotherapy and cognitive-behavioral therapy are thought to be the treatments of choice for personality disorders.

♦ Nursing theory directs the nurse to evaluate childhood development and its influence on personality development; further nursing theory directs the nurse to evaluate the client's current environment and its effect on behaviors.

≋ REVIEW QUESTIONS AND ACTIVITIES

1. Describe how the behaviors of unstable interpersonal relationships and self-image, efforts to avoid being abandoned, and impulsive acting out might be displayed by a woman with Borderline Personality Disorder who is brought to a hospital emergency room for treatment and evaluation of fainting and weakness.

2. Mr. R., a middle-aged man with a diagnosis of gastric ulcer, is in hospital care for evaluation of his ulcer. The nurse notes he has an air of self-importance, demands the nurse's time and attention, and expects particularly favorable treatment. Given that he has a narcissistic personality, what should the nurse expect related to Mr. R.'s being told he must accommodate his lifestyle and eating to his physical condition?

3. What would be a good approach for you as a nurse to use in establishing a therapeutic relationship with a client who has Histrionic Personality Disorder?

4. Identify at least one person you know who has characteristics of Antisocial Personality Disorder. Which characteristics? Explain.

5. Differentiate between Obsessive-Compulsive Personality Disorder and Obsessive-Compulsive Disorder.

6. Examine the DSM-IV structure. Explain how Axis II disorders affect treatment and outcome for clients with both Axis I and Axis II disease.

EXPLORING THE WEB

◆ Visit this text's "Online Companion™" on the Internet at **http://www.DelmarNursing.com** for further information on personality disorders.

◆ Search the Web for specific disorders such as Borderline Personality Disorder (BPD), Obsessive-Compulsive Personality Disorder (OCPD), or Antisocial Personality Disorder.

◆ What other key terms might you search for related information (e.g., schizophrenia, paranoia)?

◆ What sites could you recommend to families who live with members suffering from personality disorders and who are looking for self-help, chat rooms, or other electronic information sources?

◆ Is there a listing on the Internet of books, videos, or other media on personality disorders?

REFERENCES

Alden, L. (1989). Short-term structured treatment for avoidant personality disorder. *Journal of Consulting and Clinical Psychology, 57*, 756–764.

American Psychiatric Association. *Diagnostic and Statistical Manual of Mental Disorders*, Fourth Edition. Washington, DC. American Psychiatric Association, 1994.

Andrews, G. (1993). The benefits of psychotherapy. In N. Sartorius, G. Girolamo, G. Andrews, G. A. German, & L. Eisenberg (Eds.), *Treatment of mental disorders: A review of effectiveness* (pp. 235–247). Washington, DC: American Psychiatric Press.

Benjamin, L. S. (1993). *Interpersonal diagnosis and treatment of personality disorders*. New York: Guilford.

Butterfield, F. (1994). All God's children: The Bosket family and the American tradition of violence (p. 327). New York: Knopf.

Erickson, H., Tomlin, E., & Swain, M. A. (1983). *The modeling and role-modeling theory: A paradigm for nursing*. Lexington, SC: Pine.

Fraser, K., & Gallop, R. (1993). Nurses' confirming/disconfirming responses to patients diagnosed with borderline personality disorder. *Archives of Psychiatric Nursing, 7*, 336–341.

Gallop, R., Lancee, W., & Shugar, G. (1993). Residents' and nurses' perceptions of difficult to treat short-stay patients. *Hospital and Community Psychiatry, 44*, 352–357.

Godfrey, M. (1991). Clients with personality disorders. In G. McFarland & M. D. Thomas (Eds.), *Psychiatric mental health nursing, application of the nursing process* (pp. 589–594). Philadelphia: Lippincott.

Guralnik, D. B. (Ed.). (1982). *Webster's new world dictionary of the American language*. New York: Simon & Schuster.

Higgitt, A., & Fonagy, P. (1992). Psychotherapy in borderline and narcissistic personality disorder. *British Journal of Psychiatry, 161*, 23–43.

Linehan, M. M. (1987). Dialectical behavioral therapy: A cognitive behavioral approach to parasuicide. *Journal of Personality Disorders, 1*, 228–333.

Nardo, J. M. (1986). The personality in the medical setting: A psychodynamic understanding. In H. K. Brodie & J. L. Houpt (Eds.), *Consultation-liaison psychiatry and behavioral medicine*. New York: Basic Books.

Raskin, R., & Novacek, J. (1991). Narcissism and the use of fantasy. *Journal of Clinical Psychiatry, 47*, 490–499.

Robins, L. N., Tipp, J., & Przybeck, T. (1991). Antisocial personality. In L. N. Robins & D. A. Regier (Eds.), *Psychiatric disorders in America*. New York: Free Press.

Thompson, J. E. (1990). Finding the borderline's border: Can Martha Rogers help? *Perspective in Psychiatric Care, 26*, 7–10.

Wiggins, J. S., & Pincus, A. L. (1994). Personality structure and the structure of personality disorders. In P. Costa, Jr. & T. A. Widiger (Eds.), *Personality disorders and the five factor model of personality* (pp. 73–94). Washington, DC: American Psychological Association.

LITERARY REFERENCES

Brookner, A. (1984). *Hotel du Lac*. New York: Bantam Books.

Cather, W. (1948). Paul's case. In *Youth and the bright medusa* (pp. 183–185). New York: Random House.

Chekhov, A. (1971). Ward 6. In *The Oxford Chekhov* (Vol. VI, pp. 125–127). (Richard Hingley, Trans.). London: Oxford University Press.

Dostoevsky, F. (1960). Notes from underground. In *Notes from underground and the Grand Inquisitor* (pp. 3–5) (R. E. Matlaw, Trans.). New York: Dutton Signet.

Gogol, N. (1957). The overcoat. In *The overcoat and other tales of good and evil* (pp. 237–250). New York: Bantam Doubleday Dell.

Isherwood, C. (1989). Sally Bowles. In *Berlin Stories* (pp. 22–23). New York: New Directions Publishing.

Joyce, J. (1967). Eveline. In *The Dubliners* (pp. 38–41). New York: Penguin Books.

Mann, T. (1970). *Confessions of Felix Krull, confidence man* (D. Lindley, Trans.). New York: Knopf.

Oates, J. C. (1981). The tryst. In *Sentimental education* (pp. 509–518). New York: Dutton Signet.

Poe, E. A. (1945/1983). Berenice. In P. V. D. Stern (Ed.), *Viking portable library* (pp. 208–213). New York: Viking.

Williams, T. (1971). The glass menagerie. In *The theater of Tennessee Williams* (pp. 151–153). New York: New Directions.

SUGGESTED READINGS

Bornstein, R. F. (1993). *The dependent personality*. New York: Guilford Press.

Clarkin, J. F., Marziali, E., & Munroe-Blum, H. (1992). *Borderline personality disorder: Clinical and empirical perspectives*. New York: Guilford Press.

Guntrip, D. (1968). *Schizoid phenomena, object relations, and the self*. New York: International Universities Press.

Kantor, M. (1993). *Distancing: A guide to avoidance and avoidant personality disorders*. Westport, CT: Praeger.

Krohn, A. (1978). *Hysteria, the elusive neurosis*. New York: International Universities Press.

Lykken, D. T. (1995). *The antisocial personalities*. Hillsdale, NJ: Lawrence Erlbaum Associates.

Shapiro, D. (1981). *Autonomy and rigid character*. New York: Basic Books.

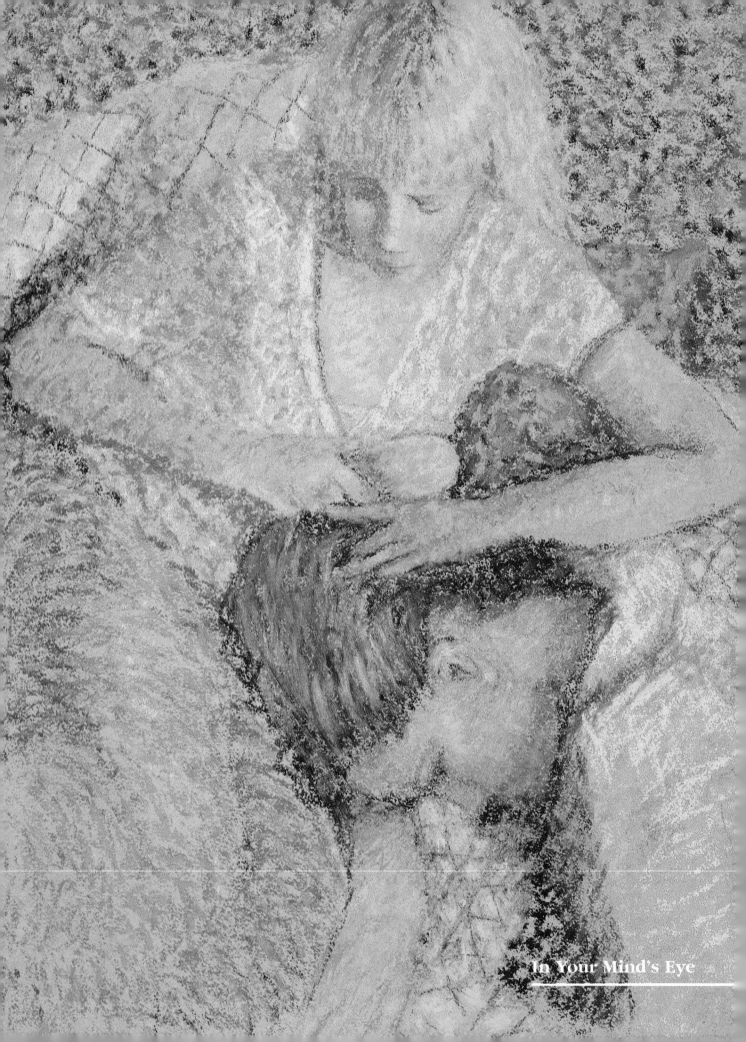

In Your Mind's Eye

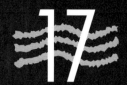

Chapter

17

THE CLIENT EXPERIENCING A PSYCHOSOMATIC ILLNESS

Noreen Cavan Frisch

Lawrence E. Frisch

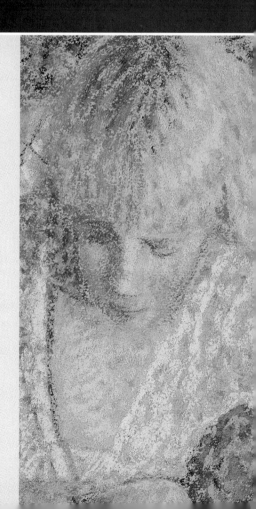

It's All in His Head

During an evening change-of-shift report, the day-shift nurse on a general medical-surgical unit makes the following observations:

> In room 123 is Mr. S., a 37-year-old man admitted 2 days ago with severe back pain. He has been on bedrest and is being worked up for diagnosis. He complains of severe pain and inability to move that are not relieved by pain medication and muscle relaxants. He has also been complaining of intermittent paresthesias of the lower extremities. His neurological examinations and MRI are normal. The day-shift nurse says, "There is nothing wrong with him, we should discharge him. It's all in his head."

◆ What is *your* reaction to this report?
◆ What are your feelings about this client?
◆ Do you have any explanations for what is going on with Mr. S.?
◆ How do you think a nurse should react to this report and to Mr. S.?

In this chapter, you will learn of the psychological underpinnings of physical symptoms and specific psychiatric disorders that present as physical symptoms.

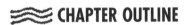 **CHAPTER OUTLINE**

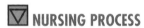
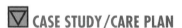
COMPETENCIES

Upon completion of this chapter, the reader should be able to:

1. Define somatoform disorders and distinguish among Somatization Disorder, Hypochondriasis, and Conversion Disorder.

2. Define Factitious Disorder (Munchausen's Syndrome) and Munchausen's Syndrome by Proxy.

3. Describe the presenting characteristics of an individual with Somatization Disorder who comes to an acute-care clinic for diagnosis and treatment.

4. Distinguish between Hypochondriasis and Anxiety Disorder.

5. Cite the major theoretical explanations for Hypochondriasis (psychoanalytic, behavioral, and biological).

6. Describe principles for the effective treatment of Hypochondriasis.

7. Provide an explanation for treatment of Conversion Disorder through direct explanation of the underlying conflict.

8. Differentiate between Factitious Disorder and malingering.

9. Utilize the nursing process and nursing theory to plan care for clients experiencing psychosomatic illness.

10. Use techniques of introspection and self-reflection to examine your own feelings with regard to clients whose physical complaints are results of psychiatric illness.

≋ KEY TERMS

Conversion Disorder   Condition in which an individual exhibits physical symptoms that cannot be explained by any medical or neurological conditions.

Factitious Disorder   Condition marked by physical or psychological symptoms that are intentionally and knowingly produced by an individual in order to gain attention; also known as Munchausen's Syndrome.

Hypochondriasis   Condition marked by preoccupation with fear of having a serious disease, based on misinterpretation of bodily symptoms or functions.

Malingering   Fabrication of symptoms with the intent of achieving some objective goal.

Munchausen's Syndrome   Another term for Factitious Disorder.

Munchausen's Syndrome by Proxy   Form of child abuse marked by a caregiver falsely giving reports of a child's illness that result in unnecessary medical investigations or treatments.

Somatization Disorder   Somatoform disorder in which there are multiple physical complaints without an apparent physiological cause.

Somatoform Disorder   Psychiatric condition manifested in physical rather than psychological symptoms.

This chapter considers a group of psychiatric disorders that have in common an emphasis on *physical* rather than *psychological* symptoms. Persons with these disorders typically present to one or more primary care providers and are usually managed without ever being seen by mental health practitioners. Clients with **somatoform disorders**, as this group of disorders is called, present with a variety of symptoms: symptoms not infrequently puzzling to their caretakers, highly disruptive to the lives of their sufferers, and often very difficult to distinguish from those of serious or life-threatening illness. Collectively, clients with the somatoform disorders are among the most difficult seen in general clinical practice. They are often dissatisfied with their care providers, and they are frequently certain that they have some serious condition that remains undiagnosed and untreated. Clients with somatoform disorders often move from provider to provider seeking new diagnoses and treatments. These clients truly believe they are seriously ill, and they make every effort to convince family members, nurses, and doctors of their need for care. Their efforts may result in hospitalizations, diagnostic procedures, and heroic treatments; rarely do they result in cure.

The somatoform disorders are a group of conditions in which symptoms suggest the presence of a general medical condition, but careful evaluation fails to find any evidence of a physical disorder sufficient to explain the complaints. Most experts feel that psychological factors account for the symptoms of somatoform disorders. This chapter will consider three such disorders: Somatization Disorder, Hypochondriasis, and Conversion Disorder.

While disorders of another group, factitious disorders, are not classified as somatoform in the *Diagnostic and Statistical Manual,* fourth edition (DSM-IV; American Psychiatric Association, 1994), they will also be discussed in this chapter because they share certain similarities with the somatoform disorders. Persons with somatoform

☯ *REFLECTIVE THINKING*

Feigning Illness

Some individuals purposefully try to deceive their health care providers and injure themselves to produce physical symptoms.

- ◆ Why do you think someone would want to be ill?

- ◆ Can you provide a reason why someone would take a drug or toxin to produce symptoms?

Try to understand the behaviors from the client's perspective. Talk to others in your class about such behaviors. Remember that in order to give care, a nurse must be willing to understand the client's subjective experiences.

disorders truly believe themselves to be physically sick; they do not attempt to deceive their caretakers. In contrast, persons with factitious disorders typically fabricate their complaints and may even create physical findings, sometimes injuring themselves by secretly self-administering drugs or toxins. In contrast to individuals with somatoform disorders, who honestly believe themselves to be physically ill, persons with factitious disorders purposefully try to deceive their caretakers into diagnosing and treating one or more medical conditions.

HISTORY OF SOMATOFORM DISORDERS

The terminology in this chapter derives from DSM-IV, but medical practitioners have recognized somatoform disorders for hundreds, if not thousands, of years. The term *hysteria* was commonly applied to these conditions, particularly when they occurred in women. The ancient Greeks and Romans commonly used the diagnosis of hysteria, probably in turn having borrowed the concept from the more ancient Egyptians. The term itself is Greek, deriving from the word *hystera*, meaning "uterus." In these ancient cultures, hysteria was thought to occur when, under certain conditions, the uterus migrated from its usual place and attached itself to other bodily organs (Veith, 1965).

While for many centuries hysteria remained incompletely defined, its presumed origin in the uterus seems to have remained unchallenged until the late 17th century when Thomas Willis (best known for his description of the brain's blood supply—still today called the Circle of Willis) suggested that many cases of hysteria had their origin in the brain. Willis's equally famous contemporary Thomas Sydenham emphasized the importance of hysteria: "Of all the chronic diseases hysteria . . . is the commonest" (Veith, 1965, p. 137). He developed a highly sophisticated "modern" view of this illness—that some persons experienced symptoms of "hysterical origin," that is, their pain and other symptoms had origins in the mind, not the body.

Over the next 200 years, ideas that the condition of hysteria was caused by the brain became accepted among many influential European and American physicians. The spectrum of hysterical symptoms was more accurately defined, and advances in medicine and neurology helped to more accurately distinguish organic from hysterical symptoms. The study of hysteria reached its clinical apex in Paris under the tutelage of Jean-Martin Charcot. Between 1862 and 1882 Charcot worked at the Salpêtriére Hospital, a huge asylum for neurologically and psychiatrically ill women. Faced with large numbers of ill persons, some with organic and others with hysterical symptoms, Charcot was able to define clinical characteristics of hysteria and increasingly to separate them from their organic "look-alikes." As a professor at the University

---

DIAGNOSTIC CRITERIA FOR SOMATIZATION DISORDER

1. A history of many physical complaints beginning before age 30 years that occur over a period of several years and result in treatment being sought or significant impairment in social, occupational, or other important areas of functioning.

2. A series of symptoms to include:
   - *Four pain symptoms*: A history of pain related to at least four different sites or functions (e.g., head, abdomen, back, joints, extremities, chest, rectum; during menstruation, during sexual intercourse, or during urination).
   - *Two gastrointestinal symptoms*: A history of at least two gastrointestinal symptoms other than pain (e.g., nausea, bloating, vomiting other than during pregnancy, diarrhea, or intolerance of several different foods).
   - *One sexual symptom*: Examples are sexual indifference, erectile or ejaculatory dysfunction, irregular menses, excessive menstrual bleeding, and vomiting throughout pregnancy.
   - *One pseudoneurological symptom*: A history of at least one symptom or deficit suggesting a neurological condition not limited to pain (conversion symptoms such as impaired coordination or balance, paralysis or localized weakness, difficulty swallowing or lump in throat, aphonia, urinary retention, hallucinations, loss of touch or pain sensation, double vision, blindness, deafness, or seizures; dissociative symptoms such as amnesia; or loss of consciousness other than fainting).

3. The symptoms cannot be explained fully by physical conditions, including drugs of abuse or medications.

4. The symptoms are not intentionally produced or feigned.

Reprinted with permission from the *Diagnostic and Statistical Manual of Mental Disorders*, Fourth Edition. Copyright 1994 American Psychiatric Association.

---

of Paris, Charcot's personal fame attracted attention to the study of neurological disorders in general and of hysteria in particular (Veith, 1965).

But as medical practice became more sophisticated, it proved difficult to have no uniformly accepted theory of *how* mental processes could so strongly affect the physical body. The most influential of these theories was developed by the Viennese neurologist Sigmund Freud. Freud's brief study with Charcot was influential in directing his interest and attention to the causes of hysteria. On his return to Vienna, Freud began to search for psychological causes of hysteria in repressed memories of childhood events. He and his colleagues sought these repressed memories in dreams and through hypnosis. When such memories were explained to hysterical patients, their symptoms often seemed to improve or disappear. This clinical improvement was taken as evidence of the correctness of Freud's theories regarding the importance of unconscious, often sexually related memories in causing hysteria. While these "psychoanalytic" theories are no longer the only modern views of hysteria, through Freud's work, it has become widely accepted that early childhood events may have lasting effects on mental and physical health.

SOMATIZATION DISORDER

Current psychiatric thinking has separated the diagnosis of Somatization Disorder from the general concept of hysteria. **Somatization Disorder** is a somatoform disorder in which there are multiple physical complaints without an apparent physiological cause. While most of the manifestations of hysteria are included in the diagnosis of Somatization Disorder, specific symptoms and behaviors are required for this diagnosis to be made. DSM-IV requires that four basic criteria be met in order to diagnose Somatization Disorder; these are listed in the accompanying display.

The complex diagnostic criteria reflect the great variety of symptoms that persons with Somatization Disorder manifest. While the Countess in the following description does not describe enough symptoms to qualify for the diagnosis of Somatization Disorder by these criteria, the author, a physician who studied with Charcot in the 1880s, colorfully captures much of the flavor of this disorder:

What Is the Matter with Me?

One of my last cases of appendicitis was, I think, the Countess who came to consult me, on the recommendation of Charcot, as she said. He used to send me patients now and then and I was of course most anxious to do my very best for her. . . . At first she did not know if she had appendicitis, nor did [I], but soon she was sure that she had it, and I that she had not. When I told her so with unwise abruptness she became very agitated. Professor Charcot had told her I was sure to

find out what was the matter with her and that I would help her, and instead of that . . . she burst into tears. . . .

"What is the matter with me?" she sobbed, stretching out her two empty hands towards me with a gesture of despair. . . .

She ceased to cry instantly. Wiping the last tears from her big eyes she said bravely:

"I can stand anything. I have already stood so much, don't be afraid, I am not going to cry any more. What is the matter with me?"

"Colitis."

Her eyes grew even larger than before, though I would have thought that to be impossible.

"Colitis! That is exactly what I always thought! I am sure you are right! Tell me what is colitis?" I took good care to avoid that question, for I did not know it myself, nor did anybody else in those days. But I told her it lasted long and was difficult to cure, and I was right there. The Countess smiled amiably at me. And her husband who said it was nothing but nerves!*

(Munthe, 1975, pp. 43–46)

The Countess is under 30 years old and has at least one gastrointestinal symptom (colitis) as well as pain. These symptoms are part of the spectrum of Somatization Disorder, and one suspects that further questioning of this woman could generate additional symptoms. In another example of Somatization Disorder, Alice James (the Countess's American contemporary) spent virtually her whole life as an invalid, the victim of pain, unexplained paralysis, menstrual disorder, and seemingly endless "doctor shopping." Alice's illness is vividly revealed in letters to family members, including her brother, the famous Harvard psychologist William James. A selection of these letters appears following:

To Have a Tornado Going on Within One

December 23, 1884

Dear William

. . . My doctor came last week and examined me for an hour with a conscientiousness that my diaphragm has not hitherto been used to. When he came to the end he was as inscrutable as they

---

*From *The Story of San Michele*, by A. Munthe, 1975, London: John Murray (Publishers, Ltd). Reprinted with permission.

always are and the little he told me I was too tired to understand. He is coming next week when as there won't be as much percussing and stethoscoping to be done I can get more out of him. I shall not tell you till then what he told me. I think he takes the gout as a foregone conclusion simply and is deciding what other complications there are. Meanwhile he has left me a pill of which he thinks all the world and I am to have my spine sponged with salt-water. I was much disappointed by his lack of remedial suggestions. . . .

Always affectly
Alice

January 31, 1885

My dear Aunt Kate.

. . . My doctor turned out as usual a fiasco an unprincipled one too. I could get nothing out of him and he slipped thro' my cramped and clinging grasp as skillfully as if his physical conformation had been that of an eel instead of a Dutch cheese —The gout he looks upon as a small part of my trouble, "it being complicated with an excessive nervous sensibility," but I could get no suggestions of any sort as to climate, baths, or diet from him. The truth was he was entirely puzzled about me and had not the manliness to say so. I got from him however a very thorough examination. He said I had no organic trouble, that my organs were simply disturbed in their functions. My legs are produced by a functional disturbance of the lower half of the spine. "Is this produced by gout?" "Oh! dear me yes I have seen people with their legs powerless for years from this cause!" He assured me that it did not lead to paralysis, a grim spectre which has been staring me in the face for a long time. My legs have been entirely useless for anything more than hobbling about the room for three months and a half and most of the time excessively painful. I asked the doctor whether it was not unusual for a person to be so ill and have no organic trouble and he said, "yes, very unusual indeed." . . .

Yrs. as always
A.

November 21st, 23rd and 24th, 1885

My dearest Aunt,

Whether I am much better or not, I don't know, I am gradually getting stronger and am able to do a great deal more, but as always happens as my physical strength increases my nervous distress and susceptibility grows with it, so that from an inside view it is somewhat of an exchange of evils. To have a tornado going on within one, whilst one is chained to a sofa, is no joke, I can assure you. . . .

Always very affectly yr
A.

January 3rd, 4th, 1886

Dear William,

. . . Until lately every joint in my body was constantly pierced with rheumatic pains flying from my head to my feet, from my stomach to my hands, how I should have lived without salicene I don't know. The same betterment has taken place since I came to London that was so wonderfully marked when I was here four yrs. ago. . . .

Always
Yr. loving sister
A.

September 10th, 1886

My dear William

. . . I thought it wrong, being so ill as I was last autumn, not to see a physician and find out whether my legs were getting to be a habit or not, so I called in Townsend who gave just the same diagnosis as Drs. Torrey and Garrod, a gouty diathesis complicated by an abnormally sensitive nervous organisation, the legs neurosis brought about by anxiety and strain. He assured me that they could not, the legs, be hurried that time would do it, assisted by his medicines, but I found that they were very strong tonics and that it was going to be only the old Neftel system, drugs instead of battery so I gave him up. I was very glad that I went to him however, as he gave me much good advice and relieved my mind about the genuiness of my legs. He said what I have been told often before

*that I should be much better at any rate, when
I reached middle life, this seems highly probable as
I have had sixteen periods the last year. . . .*

> *Yr loving sister
> Alice—*

June 16, 1887

Dear William and Alice,

    *. . . I have been running down very much the
last six weeks, and had a bad little illness last
week; but Katharine is come to the rescue. . . .
Before K. arrived I fell so low as to send for an
M.D. who had been variously and highly recommended. After examining my heart, which he
seemed to consider an unnecessarily vivacious
organ, he looked at me and asked, "Does the protuberance of your eyeballs increase rapidly?" I am
only sorry, not to be able to gratify William, by
saying that my reply was "Yes"; but truth forbids.
He also remarked, "You won't die, but you will
live, suffering to the end." . . .*

> *Your's as ever
> Alice.*

November 15, 1887

Dear Aunt Kate.

    *. . . I have constant "attacks" of all descrip-
tions, more frequent than ever, but not so bad at
the time and I get up from them quicker and feel
stronger in the intervals. They are extremely incon-
venient and I much prefer the rarer kind. My new
doctor . . . gave a very remarkable diagnosis of my
case and nature after seeing me once for 20 minutes during which time I lay with my eyes shut in
explosions of laughter owing to the comicality of
his manner. I shall give him a good trial. . . .*

> *Always your loving niece
> A*

(Yeazell, 1981, pp. 100–109)

While it is risky to attempt diagnosis more than 100 years
after the fact, it seems unlikely that "gout" would today be
considered a reasonable diagnosis for Alice. It also seems
very improbable that multiple distinguished American and
English physicians of this very sophisticated age would

have overlooked an organic cause for her difficulty walking. While, for example, a disease such as rheumatoid
arthritis might have explained many of Alice's extremity
pains, photographs still available today show no evidence
of deformity and make such illnesses unlikely. One doctor even asked about "protuberance of your eyeballs,"
very likely entertaining a diagnosis of hyperthyroidism as
a cause of her leg weakness and "abnormally sensitive
nervous organisation." DSM-IV stresses the need to
exclude complex medical problems such as hyperthyroidism, which may masquerade as Somatization
Disorder (American Psychiatric Association, 1994). Today,
it is highly likely that Alice's lengthy illness, with its
"'attacks' of all descriptions . . . every joint in my body . . .
constantly pierced with rheumatic pains flying from my
head to my feet, from my stomach to my hands . . . sixteen periods in one year" and unexplained paralysis,
would be diagnosed as Somatization Disorder.

    Clients with Somatization Disorder frequently
describe their illness dramatically, sometimes with inappropriate laughter (as Alice describes in her
November 15, 1887, letter). Both the Countess and Alice
emphasize multiple contacts with physicians, and Alice
details a seemingly endless parade of diagnostic and therapeutic efforts. In modern times, these women likely
would have received an extensive battery of diagnostic
testing, including x-rays, hospitalizations, and even
surgery. Alice tried numerous pills, electrical treatments,
and physical therapies. Today, she would have had far
more treatments from which to choose, but her chances
of receiving benefits from modern treatments are probably no higher now than a century ago.

Epidemiology and Cause

    Somatization Disorder occurs far more frequently
among women than men. The Epidemiologic Catchment
Area Study found a gender ratio of 10 to 1, but overall
found Somatization Disorder to be rare, occurring in only
0.13% of individuals (Robins & Regier, 1991). Other studies have found Somatization Disorder in up to 2% of
women (American Psychiatric Association, 1994).

    The exact cause of Somatization Disorder is not
known, but it clearly tends to occur in families. In women,
the disorder not only is familial but also occurs frequently
in families in which Antisocial Personality Disorder can be
diagnosed in both female and male relatives (Guze,
Cloninger, Martin, et al., 1985). Such clustering in families
does not establish whether Somatization Disorder is
caused by genetics, environment, or some combination of
both. Studies have often been used to try to separate the
genetic and environmental causes of complex psychological disorders. These studies often involve twins who were
separated early in life and reared in different families. Such
twin studies on Somatization Disorder have concluded

that both heredity and environment contribute to the development of the disorder (Bohman, Cloninger, von Knorring, et al., 1984).

Neuropsychological testing has shown patterns of cerebral dysfunction that seem to be typical of Somatization Disorder. In comparison to normal controls, individuals with Somatization Disorder have subtle but unique abnormalities on tests of non-dominant-hemisphere function (Flor-Henry, Fromm-Auch, Tapper, et al., 1981). While such findings are of interest, they do not allow much understanding of the causation of Somatization Disorder. Some authors have suggested that individuals with this disorder learn at an early age to express emotional distress through somatization. Such complaints may bring them support and comfort that they may not otherwise receive (Quill, 1985).

Treatment

As implied earlier, effective treatment for Somatization Disorder is difficult. There are a series of challenges to be overcome in managing individuals with Somatization Disorder. First is establishing the diagnosis. Screening instruments can be useful in suggesting the diagnosis of Somatization Disorder. However, even when the diagnosis is made with reasonable certainty, clinicians must always be alert to the continuing possibility of undiagnosed physical illness. Somatization Disorder frequently remains a tentative diagnosis subject to modification if new symptoms or signs emerge. A diagnosis of Somatization Disorder does not protect individuals from other independent conditions. After years of suffering without any medical explanation, Alice James was found to have breast cancer, from which she eventually died; her last years were spent in severe pain, but she was seemingly happy that she had finally developed a medically diagnosable illness.

Keeping an appropriate level of vigilance in the face of seemingly endless subjective complaints is yet another challenge in caring for these clients. Most authorities recommend that persons with Somatization Disorder be encouraged to make regular scheduled clinical visits at which their problems and symptoms are reviewed. Such regular visits offer support without requiring clients to have new or more severe symptoms in order to receive medical or nursing attention.

Finally, caretaker fatigue is a major challenge in managing the needs of these clients. Clients with Somatization Disorder can be exceedingly demanding, manipulative, and occasionally seductive. It is probable that care for this problem is best given by a team of professionals, perhaps including one or more nurses, physicians, and mental health workers. Effective communication between client and provider and among varied providers is a major challenge in providing quality care.

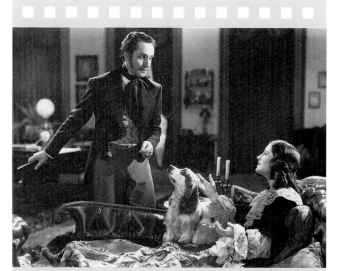

The Barretts of Wimpole Street. Source: MGM/Courtesy Kobal.

Elizabeth Barrett spent much of her youth in bed with undiagnosed somatic symptoms until she fell in love with Robert Browning. She improved greatly after their marriage, and both went on to become major 19th-century English poets.

Psychotherapy

While there have been many claims for specific treatment methods, none has been shown to be uniquely effective (Kellner, 1989b). Three therapeutic goals seem to be of value for any approach to treatment (Martin & Yutzy, 1994):

1. Establishing a firm therapeutic alliance with the client
2. Educating the client regarding the manifestations of Somatization Disorder
3. Providing consistent reassurance to the client

One of the major problems with psychotherapy for this disorder is that many clients do not believe they are psychologically ill. Their symptoms feel physical, and they are often highly reluctant to accept either psychiatric diagnosis or treatment. Both individual and group therapy have been tried, but there is little other than anecdotal data to suggest benefit from either approach. At least one study suggests that primary health care providers can effectively care for clients with Somatization Disorder, utilizing where necessary the consultative services of a psychiatrist (Smith, Monson, & Ray, 1986). This study randomly divided clients into a "usual care" group and a group followed by primary care providers with explicit therapeutic goals set by a psychiatric consultant. The consultant psychiatrist specifically suggested that clients be seen regularly by appointment (so as not to require the presence of symptoms in order to be given medical care), be examined carefully on each visit, and not be subjected to extensive investigations or to hospitalization unless medically essential. While outcomes were largely measured in terms of cost of care, clients treated with such a medically oriented approach seemed to do well and incurred significantly fewer medical expenses.

HYPOCHONDRIASIS

Hypochondriasis is, like hysteria, a condition that has been diagnosed for hundreds, if not thousands, of years. As with hysteria, the medical meaning of Hypochondriasis has changed significantly over the centuries. Only since the early 1820s has this diagnosis come to resemble the current definition (Veith, 1965). Presently, Hypochondriasis is regarded as "the preoccupation with the fear of having, or the idea that one has, a serious disease based on the person's misinterpretation of bodily symptoms or bodily functions" (American Psychiatric Association, 1994, p. 445). Persons with Anxiety Disorder also have fears, including sometimes fears that they may become ill or die; however, Hypochondriasis differs from Anxiety Disorder in that persons with Hypochondriasis have anxieties limited to fear of illness, *and* their fear arises from actual bodily symptoms rather than from more general concerns about contamination. The DSM-IV criteria for Hypochondriasis are presented in the accompanying display.

It is also important that comprehensive medical evaluation reveal no medical condition to account for the symptoms. While Hypochondriasis may still exist in persons who have definable general medical conditions, concerns about health in persons with such conditions are most often *not* Hypochondriasis but, rather, represent either appropriate worries about sickness or a form of affective disorder. As noted in the accompanying display, the belief in or about illness must not be delusional. This means that individuals with Hypochondriasis typically recognize that their worries are out of proportion to the probability that they truly have the feared illness or condition. Delusional individuals cannot be dissuaded from the conviction that they are ill, no matter how improbable the illness given their symptoms and signs.

Persons with Hypochondriasis differ somewhat in the content of their fears and worries. Some focus their concerns on a single disease (cancer or heart disease) and seek confirmation of their fears in minimal symptoms or alterations of normal bodily function. Others focus on a variety of symptoms—a cough, a skipped heart beat, skin blemishes or moles, fatigue. In either case, clinical reassurance (from examination or often from multiple non-invasive and invasive tests) is temporary at best. The worries about health recur and tend to become a major focus of the individual's life and daily routine. It often becomes difficult for persons with Hypochondriasis to function normally in their social and occupational roles, and this disorder can lead to invalidism. While DSM-IV criteria usually allow a clear distinction between Hypochondriasis and Somatization Disorder, both of the cases of Somatization Disorder discussed earlier in this chapter might be equally well taken as examples of Hypochondriasis: the Countess with her focus on "appendicitis" and "colitis" and Alice James with her multiple somatic complaints leading to a life as an invalid. Hypochondriasis and invalidism seemed to have occurred with some frequency in the latter years of the 19th century, seemingly often among the very famous. For example, Charles Darwin had numerous anxieties about his health, which lasted from his youth into very old age:

Darwin

I was also troubled with palpitations and pain about the heart, and like many a young ignorant man, especially one with a smattering of medical knowledge, was convinced that I had heart disease. I did not consult any doctor, as I fully expected to hear the verdict that I was not fit for the voyage, and I was resolved to go at all hazards.

(Colp, 1977, p. 9)

Here is an excerpt from one of several recent biographies focusing on the famous biologist's enigmatic lifelong "illnesses":

Charles Darwin suffered chronic ill-health from the age of thirty until he was sixty. During the last decade of his life, however, he was much better, and he lived to be seventy-three. In the

---

DIAGNOSTIC CRITERIA FOR HYPOCHONDRIASIS

♦ Preoccupation with fears of having, or the idea that one has, a serious disease based on the person's misinterpretation of bodily symptoms.

♦ The preoccupation persists despite appropriate medical evaluation and reassurance.

♦ The belief in the first criterion is not of delusional intensity.

♦ The preoccupation causes clinically significant distress or impairment in social, occupational, or other important areas of functioning.

♦ The duration of the disturbance is at least 6 months.

♦ The preoccupation is not better accounted for by another psychological disorder.

Reprinted with permission from the *Diagnostic and Statistical Manual of Mental Disorders*, Fourth Edition. Copyright 1994 American Psychiatric Association.

Darwin archives there are plentiful papers giving detailed information about his condition, often monthly and for some periods even day by day.

The symptoms on which attention has tended to be concentrated and with which in later years Darwin himself was constantly preoccupied are the gastric ones, which afflicted him especially at night. They included flatulence, gastric pain and a symptom variously referred to as sickness and vomiting.

By far the most complete description of the symptoms is given in a long account Darwin wrote on 20 May 1865. Representative extracts from the first half, with his numerous insertions placed here in brackets, run as follows: "For 25 years extreme spasmodic daily and nightly flatulence; occasional vomiting, on two occasions prolonged during months. Vomiting preceded by shivering (hysterical crying) dying sensations (or half-faint) . . . ringing in ears, treading on air and vision (focus and black dots) . . . (nervousness when E. leaves me)— What I vomit intensely acid, slimy (sometimes bitter) consider teeth. Doctors (puzzled) say suppressed gout—No organic mischief. . . ."

During the course of his life Darwin consulted most of the leading physicians and surgeons of his day, but none of them ever found anything organically wrong. Although a number of physical illnesses that could not have been diagnosed last century have since been proposed—for example chronic cholecystitis, hiatus hernia, arsenic poisoning . . . nearly every medically qualified man who has written on the subject is inclined to the view, with a variable degree of conviction, that Darwin's symptoms were mainly, if not entirely, psychogenic.*

(Bowlby, 1991, pp. 6–8)

Epidemiology and Cause

Very little is known about the epidemiology of Hypochondriasis. The Epidemiologic Catchment Area Study did not ask about this condition, but the prevalence of Hypochondriasis in general medical practice is said to range from 4% to 9% (American Psychiatric Association, 1994). It is likely that Hypochondriasis is similarly much more prevalent than is Somatization Disorder.

Almost all current theories suggest that Hypochon-

*From CHARLES DARWIN: A New Life by John Bowlby. Copyright © 1990 by R. P. L. Bowlby, R. J. M. Bowlby, and A. Gatling. Reprinted by permission of W. W. Norton & Company, Inc.

driasis is a condition resulting from psychological causes. Psychoanalysts have a number of causative theories that include the concept that repressed anger and hostility are displaced into physical symptoms so that they can be safely, if indirectly, communicated to others (Brown & Vaillant, 1981). Freud's emphasis was on the displacement of sexual drive into "narcissistic libido," a more complex theory that also suggested that Hypochondriasis reflects the repression and redirection of feelings toward others (Nemiah, 1985). Other psychological theories suggest that the hypochondriacal individual has low self-esteem and finds it easier to believe there is something wrong with his body than with his fundamental personality makeup (McCranie, 1979).

More recent theories suggest that hypochondriacal behavior is learned through the repetition of rewards—either the attention of parents and caretakers or rewards from internal stimuli resulting from anxiety: "Hypochondriasis can then be characterized by a vicious cycle of anxiety and somatic sensations leading to more anxiety, and with more frequent repetitions of this cycle, an overlearned pattern of behavior occurs in a rapid and predictable sequence" (Iezzi & Adams, 1993, p. 177). Both from such personal experience and from watching others who gain attention via their physical symptoms, an individual may come to develop Hypochondriasis.

A currently influential alternative view of Hypochondriasis is that these individuals learn to be excessively sensitive to normal bodily sensations, and this sensitivity may be further enhanced by fear resulting from the incorrect perception of the significance of such sensations (Barsky & Klerman, 1983). Some psychologists believe that such hypersensitivity may have a neurophysiological basis in reduced central nervous system (CNS) inhibition of sensations that originate in somatic or visceral neural pathways (Ludwig, 1972).

Treatment

As with Somatization Disorder, no firm data suggest that any one psychotherapeutic approach to Hypochondriasis is superior. Some data, however, indicate that persons who enter therapy early in the course of Hypochondriasis have a better prognosis and outcome than do those who continue to receive only somatic evaluations and treatments (Kellner, 1983). The principles of effective treatment have been summarized by Kellner (1989a) and are presented in the accompanying display.

Success in treatment requires that the individual abandon any belief that she has a dangerous undiagnosed condition. This is often the greatest therapeutic challenge, usually accomplished only after establishment of client trust in the health care providers, reassurance regarding physical health, and the individual's understanding of how her own perception of her body leads to overemphasis on symptoms and illness.

PRINCIPLES OF EFFECTIVE TREATMENT FOR HYPOCHONDRIASIS

◆ A physical examination and medical reassurance should precede the onset of treatment and be repeated as needed during the treatment process, especially when new symptoms develop.

◆ Any concurrent psychiatric disorders (particularly anxiety and depression) should be treated as indicated.

◆ The individual should be thoroughly educated about the nature and significance of hypochondriasis. It is important to emphasize the individual's basic good health. Symptoms should be acknowledged as real not imaginary; prolonged; troublesome; but not serious or dangerous.

◆ The individual needs to come to understand how his or her perception of bodily sensations leads to overemphasis on illness and symptoms. Psychotherapy may focus on learning to ignore such symptoms through retraining.

From *Treatment of Psychiatric Disorders: A Task Force Report of the American Psychiatric Association* (Vol. 3), by R. Kellner, 1989, Washington, DC: American Psychiatric Association. Reprinted with permission.

DIAGNOSTIC CRITERIA FOR CONVERSION DISORDER

◆ One or more symptoms or deficits affecting voluntary motor or sensory function that suggest a neurological or other general medical condition.

◆ Psychological factors are judged to be associated with the symptom or deficit because the initiation or exacerbation of the symptom or deficit is preceded by conflicts or other stressors.

◆ The symptom or deficit is not intentionally produced or feigned.

◆ The symptom or deficit cannot, after appropriate investigation, be fully explained by a general medical condition, the direct effects of a substance, or a culturally sanctioned behavior or experience.

◆ The symptom or deficit causes clinically significant distress or impairment or warrants medical evaluation.

◆ The symptom or deficit is not limited to pain or sexual dysfunction, does not occur exclusively during the course of Somatization Disorder, and is not better accounted for by another mental disorder.

Reprinted with permission from the *Diagnostic and Statistical Manual of Mental Disorders*, Fourth Edition. Copyright 1994 American Psychiatric Association.

CONVERSION DISORDER

The DSM-IV concept of **Conversion Disorder** includes most of the dramatic manifestations of the old diagnosis of *hysteria*. Conversion Disorder is a condition in which patients exhibit symptoms that cannot be explained by any medical or neurological condition. These symptoms often include seizures (convulsions) but may include "impaired coordination or balance, paralysis or localized weakness, aphonia, difficulty swallowing or a sensation of a lump in the throat, and urinary retention. Sensory symptoms of deficits include loss of touch or pain sensation, double vision, blindness, deafness, and hallucinations" (American Psychiatric Association, 1994, p. 452). The specific diagnostic criteria are presented in the accompanying display.

While there are many possible conversion symptoms, the most common are loss of vision, loss of hearing, limb paralysis, and glove and stocking anesthesia, i.e., numbness of hands and feet. Two specific features are central to the concept of Conversion Disorder:

1. no medical condition explains the observed symptoms, and

2. symptoms occur as the result of psychological factors

The concept of conversion derives from psychoanalytic ideas that an individual with these symptoms is caught between conflicting desires or needs, some or all of which may be unrecognized or unconscious. The emergence of physical symptoms is thought to keep the unconscious conflict from surfacing into consciousness, where the resultant anxiety might be too strong for the individual to manage. The following excerpt from a play illustrates these concepts. In this play written soon after World War II, the American soldier Coney has become paralyzed after a South Seas battle with Japanese forces in which his fellow soldier, Finch, is killed. Coney could have helped Finch get medical help, but chose instead to run to safety, taking with him maps that could not be allowed to fall into enemy hands. The doctor soon recognizes that Coney's paralysis resulted from repressed memories of his flight and Finch's death. Coney is dimly aware of the psychological conflicts that led to his paralysis, but can describe them only vaguely as a "bad feeling." By helping Coney remember the details of Finch's death, the doctor is eventually able to bring the "bad feeling" out into the open and to cure Coney of his Conversion Disorder:

Why Can't You Walk, Coney?

CONEY [turning] I should have stayed with him.

DOCTOR If you'd stayed with him the maps would be lost. The maps were your job and the job comes first. . . .

CONEY He's dead. . . .

DOCTOR Finch knew he had to get those maps. He told you to take them and go, didn't he? Didn't he, Coney? . . .

CONEY I shouldn't've left him. . . .

DOCTOR Coney, do you remember how you got off that island? . . .

CONEY I remember being taken off the plane.

DOCTOR You weren't shot, were you?

CONEY No.

DOCTOR Then why can't you walk, Coney?

CONEY I don't know. I don't know. . . .

DOCTOR Do you remember waking up in the hospital? Do you remember waking up with that bad feeling?

CONEY Yes.

[Slight pause. The Doctor walks next to the bed.]

DOCTOR Coney, when did you first get that bad feeling?

CONEY It was—I don't know.

DOCTOR Coney—[He sits down] did you first get it right after Finch was shot?

CONEY No.

DOCTOR What did you think of when Finch was shot?

CONEY I don't know.

DOCTOR You said you remember everything that happened. And you do. You remember that too. You remember how you felt when Finch was shot, don't you, Coney? Don't you?

CONEY [sitting bolt upright] Yes. [A long pause. His hands twist his robe and then lay still. With dead, flat tones] When we were looking for the map case, he said—he started to say: You lousy yellow Jew bastard. He only said you lousy yellow jerk, but he started to say you lousy yellow Jew bastard. So I knew. I knew.

DOCTOR You knew what?

CONEY I knew he'd lied when—when he said he didn't care. When he said people were people to him. I knew he lied. I knew he hated me because I was a Jew so—I was glad when he was shot.

[The Doctor straightens up.]

DOCTOR Did you leave him there because you were glad?

CONEY Oh, no!

DOCTOR You got over it.

CONEY I was—I was sorry I felt glad. I was ashamed.

DOCTOR Did you leave him because you were ashamed?

CONEY No.

DOCTOR Because you were afraid?

CONEY No.

DOCTOR No. You left him because that was what you had to do. Because you were a good soldier. [Pause] You left him and you ran through the jungle, didn't you? . . .

CONEY Yes.

DOCTOR So your legs were all right.

CONEY Yes. . . .

DOCTOR And you remember now, you remember that nothing happened to your legs at all, did it?

CONEY No, sir.

DOCTOR But you had to be carried here.

CONEY Yes, sir.

DOCTOR Why?

CONEY Because I can't walk.

DOCTOR Why can't you walk?

CONEY I don't know.

DOCTOR I do. It's because you didn't want to, isn't it Coney? Because you knew if you couldn't walk, then you couldn't leave Finch. That's it, isn't it?*

(Laurents, 1946, pp. 56–63)

Epidemiology and Cause

The epidemiology of Conversion Disorder is incompletely understood, partly because of the difficulties of defining the condition and hence establishing accurate diagnosis. Few patients can afford the intensive evaluation and treatment of psychoanalysis, and hence it is likely that milder forms of conversion go unrecognized and untreated. One study found that 25% of hospitalized women (many of whom were in the hospital only for nor-

---

*From HOME OF THE BRAVE, by Arthur Laurents. Copyright © 1946 by Arthur Laurents. Reprinted by permission of Random House, Inc.

mal childbirth) had previously suffered from one or more conversion symptoms (Cloninger, 1985). Another report indicated that conversion symptoms are not at all unusual among hospitalized patients (Folks, Ford, & Regan, 1984). More recent community studies have provided much lower but highly variable estimates of the prevalence of Conversion Disorder, ranging from 11 to 300 per 100,000 persons (Martin & Yutzy, 1994). Some of this variability seems to be explained by social class and status. While Freud thought Conversion Disorder to be rare among the poor, current research indicates that clients with Conversion Disorder are much more likely to be poor, uneducated, and often from rural backgrounds (Iezzi & Adams, 1993). There is much debate about whether or not Conversion Disorder is found more frequently in women, but at least some current evidence suggests a relatively equal sex distribution (Iezzi & Adams, 1993).

The classical psychoanalytic theories of Conversion Disorder stress trauma due to childhood sexual experiences, real or imagined. Repression of the feelings associated with such sexual trauma leads to the bizarre symptoms often seen in conversion. Psychoanalytic theory assumes that through repression, childhood memories become unconscious but still need to be expressed in some overt way. Since bringing these memories into consciousness would cause great anxiety and fear, they manifest themselves as conversion symptoms. More recent psychoanalysts have suggested that strong nonsexual feelings of aggression or dependency (such as Coney's conflict and anger in the excerpt quoted previously) can also result in conversion symptoms.

Not all psychologists accept psychoanalytic explanations for Conversion Disorder. Some psychologists have viewed conversion symptoms as primarily manipulative, as a means to get attention or care (Kimball & Blindt, 1982). Others see these symptoms as learned responses to behavior that is reinforced by others (Nemiah, 1985).

Some neuropsychologists have focused on one of the characteristic features of Conversion Disorder: a surprising indifference that many clients show toward their symptoms. This indifference is often termed *la belle indifference* and is particularly striking when encountered. For example, persons who find themselves unable to move or see seem remarkably unconcerned about the disability. Such indifference, while highly characteristic of Conversion Disorder, can also be seen in medically ill clients whose symptoms give rise to strong denial. Some studies have suggested that in individuals with Conversion Disorder, such indifference is not solely psychological in origin but results from CNS inhibition of sensory inputs. In this theory, clients with Conversion Disorder have localized brain dysfunction that affects sensory perception and reduces their likelihood of recognizing the seriousness of their symptoms (Iezzi & Adams, 1993). Multiple studies suggesting that conversion symptoms are far more likely to occur on the left side of the body than is explainable by chance

may add weight to such a neurophysiological theory of Conversion Disorder (Bishop, Mobley, & Far, 1978).

Treatment

The recognition that an individual's physical symptoms and signs are due to conversion often makes caretakers angry. Nurses need to identify this anger and approach the client without confrontation. For most individuals, symptoms resolve without any treatment (Folks et al., 1984). If symptoms do persist for long periods of time, chronicity and poor outcome may develop. While there is no clear role for hypnosis or for interview under partial sedation (narcoanalysis with amobarbital), these techniques are still occasionally used. Acute conversion often responds, as did Coney's in the excerpt above, to direct explanation of the underlying psychological conflicts. More chronic conversion symptoms are more difficult to treat with such explanation and may require prolonged therapy. "Faith healing" and exorcism have been traditional approaches to conversion symptoms, and these emotionally charged catharses are often effective in relieving symptoms.

FACTITIOUS DISORDER

As noted earlier in this chapter, **Factitious Disorder** involves physical or psychological symptoms that are intentionally produced in order to gain attention from potential caregivers. The *intention* to fabricate symptoms distinguishes factitious disorders from the somatoform disorders. **Malingering** also involves the fabrication of symptoms, but here the purpose is to achieve some objective goal such as financial compensation or avoiding work. Individuals with Factitious Disorder may present with a complex mixture of real and feigned symptoms, for example, fabricated seizures in a person with prior epilepsy and an abnormal electroencephalogram. This complex interweaving of truth and falsehood is often accompanied by dramatic embellishment of details and by outright lies. While DSM-IV uses the term Factitious Disorder, many clinicians prefer to call this disorder **Munchausen's Syndrome**, a name suggested in 1951 when Asher first clearly described persons with this dramatic condition:

The patient showing the syndrome is admitted to hospital with apparent acute illness supported by a plausible and dramatic history. Usually his story is largely made up of falsehoods; he is found to have attended, and deceived, an astounding number of other hospitals . . . It is almost impossible to be certain of the diagnosis at first, and it requires a bold casualty officer to refuse admission. . . . It must be recognized that these patients are often quite ill, although their illness is shrouded by duplicity and *distortion. . . . Often a real organic lesion from the past has left some genuine physical signs which the patient uses. . . . Most cases resemble organic emergencies. Well-known varieties are: 1. The acute abdominal type . . . 2. The haemorrhagic type, who specialise in bleeding from lungs or stomach . . . 3. The neurological type, presenting with paroxysmal headache, loss of consciousness or peculiar fits. The most remarkable feature of the syndrome is the apparent senselessness of it. Unlike the malingerer, who may gain a definite end, these patients often seem to gain nothing except the discomfiture of unnecessary investigations or operations. Their initial tolerance to the more brutish hospital measures is remarkable, yet they commonly discharge themselves after a few days with operation wounds scarcely healed, or intravenous drips still running.**

(Asher, 1951, p. 340)

Munchausen's Syndrome is named after an 18th-century personage, Baron Munchausen, whose devious exploits, fabrications, and trickeries—real and imagined—were widely popularized in Europe and have remained of sufficient interest to serve as the subject of director Terry Gilliam's 1989 film, *The Adventures of Baron Munchausen.* Factitious Disorder seems to be relatively rare, but most nurses eventually encounter one or more patients with this condition.

While Munchausen's Syndrome is probably more common, there has been increasing interest in another Factitious Disorder known as **Munchausen's Syndrome by Proxy**. This is a form of child abuse in which a parent, usually the mother, falsely reports a story of childhood illness that may result in unnecessary medical investigations or treatments. As in Munchausen's Syndrome, the reports of illness may contain elaborate falsifications, and clinical personnel may fail to recognize the deception for many months or years. Frequently, harm may come to a child from either unnecessary interventions or the parent's efforts to induce the appearance of symptoms through various toxins, drugs, or physical manipulations.

⊙◎ *REFLECTIVE THINKING*

Munchausen's Syndrome by Proxy

Consider the discussion of Munchausen's Syndrome by Proxy. How would you react to a parent who has intentionally induced symptoms in his child, so the child appears ill?

⚠ **NURSING ALERT!**

Munchausen's Syndrome by Proxy

Munchausen's Syndrome by Proxy is, like any other form of child abuse, reportable to Children's Protective Services.

Epidemiology and Cause

The actual prevalence of Factitious Disorder is not known, due to both the fact that the diagnosis may not be made and the fact that the chronic forms of the disorder may be overreported when a client who is diagnosed by one provider moves on to obtain care somewhere else and is reported again. The disorder, however, is more common among men than among women (American Psychiatric Association, 1994).

The factors leading to Factitious Disorder are unclear, but possible predisposing factors listed in DSM-IV include the presence of other mental disorders and/or general medical conditions during childhood or adolescence that led to extensive treatments and hospitalizations; a grudge against the medical profession; employment in medically related work; the presence of a severe personality disorder; and an important relationship with a physician in the past.

Treatment

The nature of the disorder makes it almost impossible to treat, and treatment is almost always unsatisfactory. Clients, particularly those who develop a chronic form of the disorder, develop lifelong patterns of hospitalization, willingness to submit to invasive diagnostic and surgical procedures, and an unending list of symptoms. When the factitious nature of the symptoms is discovered, the clients will most often discharge themselves against medical advice and move to other clinics and other locations to receive care where they are not known.

NURSING CARE AND SOMATOFORM DISORDERS

One of the great challenges in nursing is to care for and care about a difficult client—a client who does not respond in the manner expected or one who does not have the same values and goals that nurses generally hold. While all nursing theories and stated philosophies of nursing include care of each individual as a unique and whole person, nurses frequently find themselves to be judgmental, particularly when it comes to caring for a client with a somatoform disorder. The client with such a disorder tests the patience of nurses and the ethic that nursing must provide unconditional *care*. It is important to explore nurses' experiences with such clients and to understand the nurses' feelings and attitudes. Further, it is

⊙⊙ *REFLECTIVE THINKING*

Somatoform Disorder

Take a moment to stop and reflect on the information you have read in the chapter so far and ask yourself the following questions:

◆ What emotions have you experienced? List them for yourself and reflect on the source of each.

◆ Do the descriptions of somataform disorders make you angry? If yes, what is the source of your anger?

◆ Do you find the clients described are believable?

◆ Can you begin to understand the world experience of someone who is suffering from any one of these disorders?

◆ How much do you value health, rather than illness, in yourself? In others?

◆ How much do you value independence in yourself? In others?

Consider your answers and recognize that there are no right or wrong answers to these questions. Know that if you know yourself and understand your reactions to clients with these disorders, you will be in a much better position to provide professional and therapeutic care.

equally important to revisit basic nursing philosophies that underlie modern theories of care.

Nurses and other health care providers have limited resources (time, energy, emotions, and finances) with which to provide care to clients. Studies have indicated that there are persons who "overutilize" health care services. For example, data such as the finding that 13% of adults in an HMO made 31% of the office visits and accounted for 35% of hospital admissions and 30% of the surgeries (McFarland et al., 1985) lead many to conclude that such clients are indeed taking and/or demanding more than their "fair share." Health care providers, particularly primary care providers, find themselves frustrated with such clients. These clients seem to demand something of them that they are unable and/or unwilling to give. Nursing authors comment, "If you often feel frustrated by somatizing patients, you're hardly alone" (Ford, Katon, & Lipkin, 1993, p. 31). Each nurse must explore the personal meaning of this frustration, recognizing that clients with somatoform disorders are psychiatrically ill and greatly in need of care. For many, the frustration comes from not knowing what to do and from being uncomfortable with the psychiatric nature of the physical problem. The following discussion of nursing theory and approaches may help to empower nurses to provide quality, professional care.

NURSING THEORY

Nursing as caring is an important concept when dealing with clients with somatoform disorders. Caring means that the nurse will try to understand the client as she is, accept her personality, her complaints, and her need for care. Often, clients with somatization have low self-esteem, repressed hostility, and guilt derived from a dysfunctional family background (Roberts, 1994). A nurse must see through the presenting symptoms in order to begin caring for the person behind the presenting illness.

Caring means that the nurse will bring a presence, an acceptance, and a sense of compassion and concern. Watson's Theory of Human Care draws attention to the need for care, not cure. However, another important component of Watson's theory is that "caring can be effectively demonstrated and practiced only interpersonally" (Talento, 1995). Clients with somatoform disorders will not enter into relationships readily or readily express emotions. The challenge, then, is to give care and to present a healing presence without making demands on the client that he be someone or something he is unable to be.

In addition to the concept of nursing as caring, some of the ideas basic to the Modeling and Role-Modeling Theory (Erickson, Tomlin, & Swain, 1983) are also helpful. Modeling the client's world means understanding the world from the client's perspective. A nurse must attempt to know the client's subjective experience of her illness, her disability, her needs for care and services. More than likely, much of the nurse's frustration with the somatizing client is the nurse's inability to comprehend how and why the client reacts to her life situations in the manner she does. The best advice coming from the Modeling and Role-Modeling Theory is to *listen* to the client and begin to build a nurse-client relationship based on trust. Nurses need to understand that by building such a relationship they are, indeed, providing nursing care. Further, from the perspective of this theory, when a client is in impoverishment, that is, in a state where she is unable to mobilize any of her own resources to deal with life's stressors (see Chapter 3), the nurse is guided to provide direct physical care. It becomes clear that a client presenting with Somatization Disorder is quite often in impoverishment. At that time, direct nursing care would be offered by a nurse using this theory.

The Special Case of Factitious Disorder

Many of the nursing approaches and nursing theories discussed previously for somatoform disorders also apply to clients with Factitious Disorder. However, there seems an even greater reluctance on the part of nurses to truly *care* for clients who feign illnesses. A recent report from a group of critical care nurses, presented in the Research Highlight on the following page, describes the nurses' reactions to a client with significant psychiatric disease. The nurses were angry (in their words, "furious")

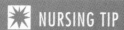 **NURSING TIP**

Caring for Someone with a Somatoform Disorder

Following are ways to provide a healing presence without demanding the client be someone he is not:

- Know yourself
- Read the descriptions of the somatoform disorders
- Reread them
- Tell yourself and your colleagues that these clients are psychiatrically ill
- Try to empathize with the client by feeling and understanding the client's pain
- Consider the client's day-to-day life
- Compare the client's life to your own
- Tell yourself to remember you became a nurse to care about people and to provide compassion

REFLECTIVE THINKING

Factitious Disorder

How can nurses manage their personal feelings in order to provide sensitive nursing care to clients presenting with Factitious Disorder?

- How would you react to the client?
- Does your institution have counseling or support services that nurses might use if faced with a situation such as that described in the Research Highlight?

and in a state of "shock and disbelief" that they had been fooled by this client. These nurses recommended that all who provided care to a client with Factitious Disorder participate in discussion sessions to explore their own feelings and reactions and share their perceptions of the situation. Clearly, there is an important aspect of caring for the caregiver here, in that nurses need support from one another in dealing with such a difficult and hard-to-comprehend client. These nurses tended to blame themselves for having been taken in by a client who was lying; they felt betrayed. It would perhaps be helpful if these nurses remembered that clients with factitious disorders are excellent actors. These clients do "take people in"; the acting and lying are part of the illness. Questions these critical care nurses could ask themselves are:

- Does this client need a nurse?
- Do I believe that this client is ill?

RESEARCH HIGHLIGHT

Nurses' Reactions to a Client with Factitious Disorder

STUDY PROBLEM/PURPOSE

In 1994, a group of critical care nurses found themselves providing care to a client who was eventually diagnosed as having Factitious Disorder. These nurses described their own experiences and feelings regarding their involvement with this client.

METHODS

The client was a 35-year old woman who presented to the hospital emergency room with progressive hematuria. The client gave a detailed history of an injury to the lower back following an assault. She also provided a medical history of having had multiple surgeries and procedures. The client's hematuria could not be controlled, and ultimately the client was scheduled for and gave consent for a second nephrectomy. A nurse then discovered that the client had vials of urokinase and streptokinase in a tote bag, along with syringes. Her bleeding and need for surgery was a result of her self-medication.

FINDINGS

The nurses' reactions first included feelings of anger and betrayal. Some of the staff became furious with the client; others became angry with themselves. Many felt shock and disbelief. Some nurses had feelings so strong that even after support groups and educational sessions on Factitious Disorder, they preferred not to be assigned to the client.

IMPLICATIONS

These nurses warn that nurses who have not been able to effectively deal with their own feelings about Factitious Disorder may be "adversely affected in their nursing careers." The recommendations that come from this report are that nurses must be knowledgeable and prepared to care for individuals with behaviors they cannot understand. Nurses must find ways to assist each other in dealing with such clients who are psychiatrically ill.

From "Addiction to Surgery," by M. Miller and S. Cabeza-Stradi, 1994, *Critical Care Nurse, 14,* pp. 44–47.

- Can a mental disorder ever take precedence over physical problems?
- How do I feel when the client does not want to get well?

There is a very important need for nurses outside of psychiatry to have compassion for and understanding of a client whose disorder is not physical in nature.

NURSING PROCESS

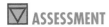 **ASSESSMENT**

Nursing care must begin with an assessment of the client, both his physical condition and the psychosocial aspects of his functioning. While the nurse will be working in a collaborative role with physicians and other professionals in any case as complicated as a somatoform or factitious disorder, specific nursing assessment includes questioning about the family history and family interaction patterns, sociocultural history and its influence on values and beliefs, current life stressors and past methods of coping, and the significance of the current illness/symptoms to the client. Assessment questions are presented in the display on the next page.

NURSING DIAGNOSIS

In addition to the nursing diagnoses related to the specific physical condition/symptoms displayed by the client, the psychosocial nursing diagnoses that need to be considered include the following:

♦ *body image disturbance*

♦ *self-esteem disturbance*

♦ *ineffective individual coping*

♦ *hopelessness*

♦ *powerlessness*

♦ *spiritual distress*

♦ *social isolation*

Nursing diagnoses specifically for the family may also include *altered family processes* and *caregiver role strain*. Each of these diagnoses, when validated, could lead to specific interventions based on the client's readiness to acknowledge feelings and accept a path toward greater health. For example, the client that relates she feels socially isolated and wishes to engage in more frequent interactions with others can be assisted to identify means to accomplish this within the parameters of her lifestyle and symptoms. The client who relates she has a poor image of her own body may be encouraged to see the positive qualities and strengths she does have. Consideration of the nursing diagnoses listed helps the

nurse consider the range of problems his client may face and then helps in determining what appropriate nursing actions to take.

OUTCOME IDENTIFICATION

Outcome for clients with somatoform or factitious disorders will not realistically be perfect physical and psychological health. Short-term treatment goals make more sense, for example, stating as an outcome that a client who has Somatization Disorder "will maintain independent functioning in between weekly visits to the clinic" may be a realistic goal. The nurse should discuss outcomes with the client and set out mutually agreed-upon goals. Goals should focus on care, not cure.

PLANNING/INTERVENTIONS

In all cases, the nurse should begin by establishing a caring and trusting nurse-client relationship, understanding full well that many of these clients will not reciprocate. In many cases, listening to the client and attempting to understand the client's experience is the best nursing intervention one has to offer. In cases where specific diagnoses (such as social isolation) and goals are identified, nursing interventions will be to work with the client to solve the identified problem (for example, wanting increased interaction with others).

Financial resources almost inevitably become a source of concern for clients who cannot work and must pay bills for numerous health care problems. Nurses must be aware of community services and will need to make referrals to social workers and others who can assist the client to obtain health care and services to meet other basic needs.

EVALUATION

Evaluate care for somatizing clients based on short-term, identifiable goals. Ask the client what he thinks can be expected and continue to offer compassionate care, recognizing that these are chronic diseases that require management over time.

ASSESSMENT QUESTIONS FOR SOMATIZING CLIENTS

FAMILY HISTORY

Please tell me about your family:

◆ Who do you consider to be your family?

◆ Do you live with family members? Friends? By yourself?

◆ Do other members of your family have medical illnesses?

◆ Does anyone in your family have the same symptoms as you?

◆ Where do members of your family go to receive care?

◆ Who have you told that you are ill?

◆ How often do you interact with family members/significant others?

◆ Has the interaction changed since you have become ill?

SOCIOCULTURAL HISTORY

◆ How do you interpret your illness/symptoms?

◆ Have you known others who have similar problems?

◆ How is your illness/symptom interpreted within your family? By your friends?

◆ How does your illness/symptom affect how others treat you?

◆ Do members of your family share the same values? Or are they different in their thinking?

CURRENT STRESSORS

◆ What are the current stresses in your life?

◆ What would you do if you needed medical attention in the middle of the night?

◆ What would you say is your method of dealing with stress?

◆ Do you have health insurance?

◆ Are you able to obtain the care you think you need?

◆ What do you expect from care in this hospital (clinic)?

SIGNIFICANCE OF THE SOMATIZATION

◆ How do you interpret your symptoms?

◆ What is the significance of this hospitalization for you?

◆ Have you experienced these or similar symptoms in the past?

CASE STUDY/CARE PLAN

Similar to the descriptions of health/illness in the letters of Alice James, we will consider Betty as a modern-day woman who is coming to a clinic for a work-up for the following symptoms: functional disturbance of lower extremities, including weakness, intermittent partial paralysis and numbness of lower extremities, and pain with movement; multiple vague discomforts, including head and foot pain; stomach pain; and episodes of nausea and vomiting, "heart trouble," and palpitations.

ASSESSMENT

Betty has had multiple medical work-ups and evaluations. She has seen several subspecialists, and there is no known physiological cause for all of her symp-

toms; however, she does carry a diagnosis of gout. Betty readily talks about her symptoms and seems pleased that her nurse wants to hear of her situation. However, Betty does not wish to talk about any feelings or her family background. Betty has been suffering with various physical complaints for 20 years and believes her symptoms have worsened with time. Betty expresses a sense that she will never get better but does not express feelings of despair or sadness when describing this. Betty denies stress in her life, although she does admit to having few friends and no support system. Further, there are few activities Betty enjoys. She rarely leaves her house and receives no visitors. When the nurse asked Betty, "If you were sick in the middle of the night and needed help, do you have a friend you could call who would come to help you?" Betty responded, "No, there is no one to call."

NURSING DIAGNOSIS *Social isolation*, related to inability to engage in satisfying personal relationships, as evidenced by absence of supportive significant others

Outcomes	Planning/Interventions	Evaluation
◆ Betty will reciprocate in establishing a nurse-client relationship. ◆ Betty will interact with one individual who is not a member of the health care team during the week in between regular visits to the clinic.	◆ Establish a positive nurse-client relationship by offering time to meet with Betty each week, expressing positive regard, and listening to her experiences. ◆ Help Betty to identify someone she could consider a friend—a neighbor, a relative—someone with whom she could interact. Explore the ways Betty could reach out to this person—by telephone, letter writing. ◆ Given Betty's physical health, explore with her the option of interacting with persons over the World Wide Web through e-mail, discussion groups, and chat rooms.	Betty seemed quite willing to talk with the nurse, although her interactions seemed guarded and she did not disclose more about herself and family. When Betty arrived at the clinic, she did ask to see the nurse. Betty was unwilling or unable to identify a person with whom she could interact other than the nurse and health care workers at the clinic; however, she did become interested in computer-based communications. She had a computer and began to interact via a discussion group related to literature. Betty related that she enjoyed this activity.

NURSING DIAGNOSIS *Powerlessness*, related to lifestyle of helplessness, as evidenced by passivity

Outcomes	Planning/Interventions	Evaluation
◆ Betty will feel in control of some aspects of her life within 2 months. ◆ With your help, Betty will identify two of her day-to-day activities over which she has choices.	◆ Provide caring interactions and support. ◆ Engage Betty in conversation and reflection regarding what she does and how she can make some decisions.	Betty stated she has choices over what she reads and what she eats. She has only begun to see that even given her physical symptoms, she does have some choices. The condition of powerlessness still exists; continued interventions are needed.

CRITICAL THINKING BAND

ASSESSMENT

What other factors in Betty's environment should be considered when planning her care? Should the nurse pursue questions about Betty's family?

NURSING DIAGNOSIS

Are there other diagnoses that would apply to Betty?

Continued

Outcomes	**Planning/Interventions**	**Evaluation**
Do you believe a nurse can enter into a relationship with Betty? What are the obstacles? Do you think Betty is trustworthy?	What can you really do to empower another person? Do you think helping someone make choices in day-to-day life has anything to do with powerlessness?	Does it seem like a good idea to bring social interaction to someone via the Internet? What else could be done?

KEY CONCEPTS

◆ Somatoform disorders are a group of conditions in which symptoms suggest the presence of a general medical condition but evaluations fail to find evidence of physical problems to explain the complaint.

◆ Somatoform disorders are highly disruptive to the lives of their sufferers, puzzling to health care providers, and difficult to distinguish from major physical illnesses.

◆ Somatization Disorder exists when there is a history of physical complaints beginning before age 30, with a series of specific symptoms that cannot be explained and are not intentionally produced.

◆ Somatization Disorder is usually treated in general medical clinics, not mental health clinics; regularly scheduled appointments are recommended.

◆ Conversion Disorder has two specific features: no medical condition explains the symptoms and the symptoms occur as a result of psychological factors.

◆ *La belle indifference* is a characteristic of at least some clients with Conversion Disorder, describing the fact that they show surprising indifference toward their symptoms.

◆ Acute Conversion Disorder may respond to direct explanation of the psychological conflicts leading to the symptoms.

◆ Factitious Disorder (or Munchausen's Syndrome) involves a physical symptom intentionally produced to gain attention from a caretaker.

◆ Munchausen's Syndrome by Proxy is a form of child abuse whereby an individual (usually a parent) intentionally produces symptoms of illness in a child under his or her care.

◆ Nurses must examine their own feelings in relation to being asked to provide care to clients with somatoform and factitious disorders.

◆ The goal of nurse-client interactions dealing with clients who have somatoform and factitious disorders should be *care* and not *cure*.

REVIEW QUESTIONS AND ACTIVITIES

1. Describe the differences between Somatization Disorder, Conversion Disorder, Hypochondriasis, and Factitious Disorder.

2. Explain the principles of treatment for managing clients with Somatization Disorder in a general medical clinic.

3. Do you believe a nurse practitioner is in the best position to care for somatizing clients?

4. What would you tell the critical care nurses quoted in this chapter regarding care of a client with Factitious Disorder?

5. Which nursing theories do you believe are most beneficial when working with a client with Somatoform Disorder?

EXPLORING THE WEB

◆ Visit this text's "Online Companion™" on the Internet at **http://www.DelmarNursing.com** for further information on psychosomatic illness.

◆ What sites could you recommend to families who are looking for self-help, chat rooms, or other electronic information sources?

◆ Is there a listing of books, videos, or other media on somatoform disorders?

◆ What other key terms might you search (e.g., Hypochondriasis, Conversion Disorder, Factitious Disorder, Munchausen's Syndrome)?

REFERENCES

American Psychiatric Association *Diagnostic and Statistical Manual of Mental Disorders*, Fourth Edition. Washington, DC. American Psychiatric Association, 1994.

Barsky, A. J., & Klerman, G. L. (1983). Overview: Hypochondriasis, bodily complaints and somatic styles. *American Journal of Psychiatry, 140*, 273–283.

Bishop, E. R., Jr., Mobley, M. C., & Far, W. F., Jr. (1978). Lateralization of conversion symptoms. *Comprehensive Psychiatry, 19*, 393–396.

Bohman, M., Cloninger, C. R., von Knorring, A. L., & Siquardsson, S. (1984). An adoption study of somatoform disorders, III: Cross-fostering analysis and genetic relationship to alcoholism and criminality. *Archives of General Psychiatry, 41*, 872–878.

Brown, H. N., & Vaillant, G. E. (1981). Hypochondriasis. *Archives of Internal Medicine, 141*, 723–726.

Cloninger, C. R. (1985). Somatoform and dissociate disorders. In G. Winokur & P. J. Clayton (Eds.), *The medical basis of psychiatry* (pp. 123–151). Philadelphia: WB Saunders.

Erickson, H., Tomlin, E., & Swain, M. (1983). *Modeling and role-modeling: A theory and paradigm for nursing*. Lexington, KY: Pine Press.

Flor-Henry, P., Fromm-Auch, D., Tapper, M., Schopflocher, D. (1981). A neuropsychological study of the stable syndrome of hysteria. *Biological Psychiatry, 16*, 601–626.

Folks, D. G., Ford, C. V., & Regan, W. M. (1984). Conversion symptoms in a general hospital. *Psychosomatics, 25*, 285–295.

Ford, C., Katon, W., & Lipkin, M., Jr. (1993). Managing somatization and hypochondriasis. *Patient Care, 27*, 31–34, 37, 40.

Guze, S. B., Cloninger, C. R., Martin, R. L., & Clayton, P. J. (1985). A follow-up and family study of Briquet's syndrome. *British Journal of Psychiatry, 149*, 17–23.

Iezzi, A., & Adams, H. E. (1993). Somatoform and factitious disorders. In P. B. Surker & H. E. Adams (Eds.), *Comprehensive handbook of psychopathology* (2nd ed., p. 170). New York: Plenum.

Kellner, R. (1989a). Hypochondriasis and body dysmorphic disorders. In *Treatments of psychiatric disorders: A Task Force Report of the American Psychiatric Association* (Vol. 3). Washington, DC: American Psychiatric Association.

Kellner, R. (1989b). Somatization disorder. In *Treatments of psychiatric disorders: A Task Force Report of the American Psychiatric Association* (Vol. 3, pp. 2155–2171). Washington, DC: American Psychiatric Association.

Kellner, R. (1983). The prognosis of treated hypochondriasis: A clinical study. *Acta Psychiatrica Scandinavica, 67*, 69–79.

Kimball, C. P., & Blindt, K. (1982). Some thoughts on conversion. *Psychosomatics, 23*, 547–549.

Ludwig, A. M. (1972). Hysteria: A neurobiological theory. *Archives of General Psychiatry, 17*, 771–777.

Martin, R. M., & Yutzy, S. H. (1994). Somatoform disorders. In R. E. Hales, S. C. Yudofsky, & J. A. Talbott (Eds.), *The American Psychiatric Press textbook of psychiatry* (2nd ed.). Washington, DC: American Psychiatric Association.

McCranie, E. J. (1979). Hypochondriacal neurosis. *Psychomatics, 20*, 11–15.

McFarland, B., et al. (1985). Utilization patterns among long term enrollees in a prepaid group practice health maintenance organization. *Medicare Care, 23*, 762–767.

Miller, M., & Cabeza-Stradi, S. (1994). Addiction to surgery: A nursing dilemma. *Critical Care Nurse, 14*, 44–47.

Nemiah, J. C. (1985). Somatoform disorders. In H. I. Kaplan & B. J. Saddock (Eds.), *Comprehensive textbook of psychiatry* (4th ed., pp. 924–942). Baltimore: Williams & Wilkins.

Quill, T. E. (1985). Somatization disorder. One of medicine's blind spots. *Journal of the American Medical Association, 254*, 3075–3079.

Roberts, S. (1994). Somatization in primary care: The common presentation of psychosocial problems through physical complaints. *Nurse Practitioner, 19*, 47–55.

Robins, L. N., & Regier, D. A. (1991). *Psychiatric disorders in America*. New York: Free Press.

Smith, G. R., Monson, R. A., & Ray, D. C. (1986). Psychiatric consultation in somatization disorder. *New England Journal of Medicine, 314*, 1407–1413.

Talento, B. (1995). Jean Watson. In J. George (Ed.), *Nursing theories, the base for professional practice* (4th ed., pp. 317–333). Norwalk, CT: Appleton & Lange.

Veith, I. (1965). *Hysteria: The history of a disease*. Chicago: University of Chicago Press.

LITERARY REFERENCES

Asher, R. (1951). Munchausen syndrome. *The Lancet, 1*, pp. 339–341.

Bowlby, J. (1991). *Charles Darwin: A new life*. New York: W. W. Norton.

Colp, R. (1977). *To be an invalid*. Chicago: University of Chicago Press.

Laurents, A. (1946). *Home of the brave*. New York: Random House.

Munthe, A. (1975). *The story of San Michele*. London: John Murray Publishers.

Yeazell, R. B. (Ed.). (1981). *The death and letters of Alice James*. Berkley, CA: University of California Press.

SUGGESTED READINGS

Asaad, C. (1996). *Psychosomatic disorders: Theoretical and clinical aspects*. New York: Brunner Mazel Publishers.

Levin, A., & Sheridan, M. S. (1995). *Munchausen syndrome by proxy: Issues in diagnosis and treatment*. New York: Lexington Books.

Shorter, E. (1994). *From the mind to the body: The cultural origins of psychosomatic symptoms*. New York: Free Press.

Trowbridge, B. (1996). *The hidden meaning of illness: Disease as symbol and metaphor*. Virginia Beach, VA: A.R.E. Press.

Vrettos, A. (1995). *Somatic fictions: Imagining illness in Victorian cultures*. Stanford, CA: Stanford University Press.

Wolman, B. (1988). *Psychosomatic disorders*. New York: Plenum Medical Book Co.

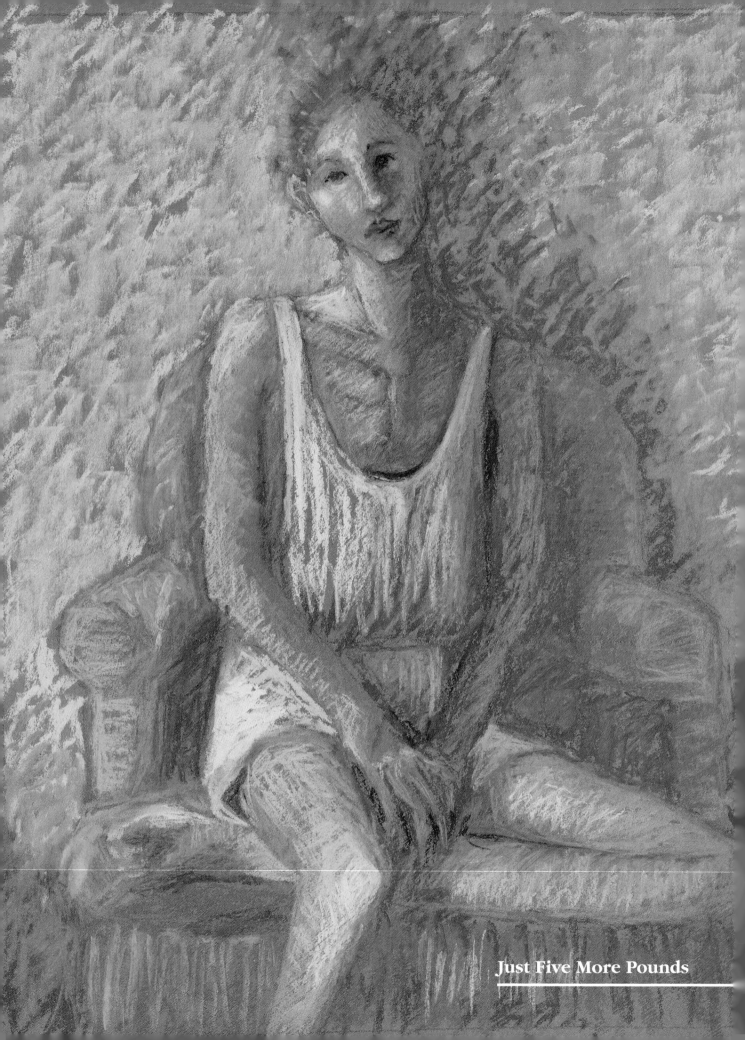

Just Five More Pounds

Chapter

18

THE CLIENT WITH DISORDERS OF SELF-REGULATION
Sleep Disorders, Eating Disorders, Sexual Disorders

Noreen Cavan Frisch

Lawrence E. Frisch

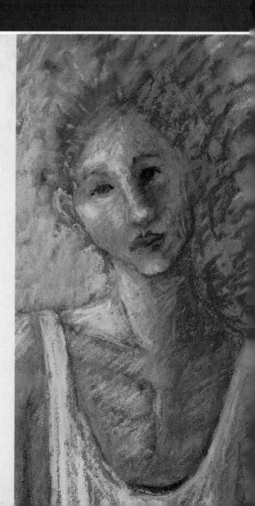

Finding Balance

Many people these days talk about finding balance in the hectic world of modern life. The idea of balance assumes that people are able to regulate their activities in a way that produces or promotes health. Consider your own life in terms of a balance between needs for sleep, exercise, and rest.

♦ Do you meet your physiological needs in these areas? If not, what is stopping you from finding your own balance in this regard?

Consider your own need for food and nutrition. Nutrients are essential for physical health; social aspects of food and eating contribute to mental health.

♦ Do you meet your physical and social needs in relation to your food and eating habits?

♦ Are there aspects of your food habits you would like to change? If yes, what do you need to do to make the change?

Lastly, consider your own sexual identity and needs for intimacy.

♦ Have you found a balance in your relationships that results in personal health?

As you reflect on your own life and lifestyle, examine how much or how little you believe you can control your own behaviors in areas of sleep, eating, and sexuality. In this chapter, we will examine common disorders, many quite debilitating, that can be grouped as disorders of regulation. Being honest about your own ability and success in these areas will assist you to learn about these disorders and provide empathy to clients.

CHAPTER OUTLINE

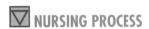
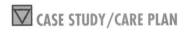
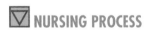
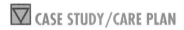
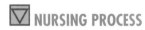
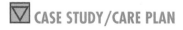
COMPETENCIES

Upon completion of this chapter, the reader should be able to:

1. Describe normal sleep cycles and changes in sleep cycles expected in aging.
2. Assess clients for the presence of Insomnia.
3. Provide a sleep hygiene regimen for clients with disturbed sleep.
4. Define Primary Hypersomnia.
5. Identify parasomnias and provide appropriate nursing interventions and support.
6. Assess clients for the presence of Bulimia Nervosa and Anorexia Nervosa.
7. Plan nursing care for clients with eating disorders, including nutritional rehabilitation, psychotherapy, maintenance, and follow-up care.
8. Assess clients for *altered sexuality, sexual dysfunction*, and sexual disorders.
9. Utilize nursing theory and the nursing process in planning and providing care for clients with disorders of regulation.

KEY TERMS

Anorexia Nervosa Psychological eating disorder characterized by profound disturbance in body image, failure to maintain minimum weight, and obsession with weight despite underweight status.

Bulimia Nervosa Psychological eating disorder characterized by fasting, binging, purging (by either self-induced vomiting or misuse of laxatives, diuretics, or enemas), and lack of extreme weight loss.

Cataplexy Sudden loss of muscle power at times of sudden emotion.

Dyssomnia Condition where there is an abnormality in the amount, quality, or timing of sleep.

Exhibitionism Exposing one's genitals to a stranger.

Fetishism Sexual arousal occurring from contact with a nonliving object, often an article of clothing.

Frotteurism Recurrent sexual touching of a nonconsenting individual, usually a stranger and usually in a crowded public place.

Gender Dysphoria Condition existing when an individual has a strong desire to live as the opposite sex.

Gender Identity Internal sense that one is female or male.

Gender Identity Disorder Condition in which an individual feels him- or herself to be a member of the opposite sex and desires gender change.

Gender Role Learned expressions of femaleness and maleness.

Hypoactive Sexual Desire Disorder Significant distress or disturbance in interpersonal relationships when the sexual desire is truly less than would be normal for an individual.

Insomnia Sleep disorder characterized by difficulty in initiating or maintaining sleep.

Narcolepsy Sleep disorder characterized by frequent irresistible urges for sleep, hallucinatory dreamlike states, and episodes of cataplexy.

Nightmare Exceedingly vivid dream from which the sleeper wakens in fear, often sweating and with heart racing, and is able to recall the dream.

Normal Sexual Behavior Any sexual act that is consensual, lacks force, is mutually satisfying to both partners, and is conducted in private [for adults].

Paraphilia Disorder of sexual interest, arousal, and orgasm.

Parasomnia Condition where the person suffers from profoundly disturbed sleep, most commonly nightmares, sleep terrors, or sleepwalking.

Pedophilia Sexual interests directed primarily or exclusively toward children.

Primary Hypersomnia Severe daytime sleepiness despite normal nighttime sleep patterns that interferes with daily activities; a condition that cannot be explained by any other sleep, medical, or pharmacological cause.

Primary Insomnia Condition in which an individual can fall asleep easily and remain asleep for several hours but does not feel rested upon waking.

Sexual Dysfunction Condition existing when a person experiences a change with any aspect of sexuality that is viewed as unsatisfying, unrewarding, or inadequate.

Sexual Masochism Disorder characterized by sexual excitement resulting from fantasies or behaviors about being the recipient of physical abuse or humiliation.

Sexual Sadism Disorder characterized by sexual excitement resulting from persistent fantasies or behaviors involving infliction of suffering on others.

Sleep Hygiene Specific activities that assist many persons to achieve restful sleep.

Sleep Latency Time it takes to fall asleep.

Sleep Paralysis Sensation of being unable to move, speak, or breathe during sleep.

Sleep Terrors Parasomnia in which there is *no recall* of the sleep-related event.

Sleepwalking Pattern of sleep behavior usually including getting out of bed, walking around in the bedroom or on occasion outside of the bedroom, and then returning to bed.

Transvestic Fetishism Cross dressing or fantasies about cross dressing.

Voyeurism Observing or fantasizing about observing others disrobing, naked, or involved in sexual activity.

Sleep, eating, and sexual function are basic human drives that are closely related to good physical and mental health. Both psychological disorders and physical illnesses often manifest as disturbances in any or all of these functions. But, even in the absence of more general psychiatric or physiological diagnoses, independent disorders of sleep, eating, and sexual function can occur. These disorders may present in psychiatric nursing practice or in the course of giving care to clients in other settings. The purpose of this chapter is to provide an introduction to some of the most common of such disorders of regulation.

SLEEP DISORDERS

So Inestimable a Jewel

Do but consider what an excellent thing sleep is: it is so inestimable a jewel that, if a tyrant would give his crown for an hour's slumber, it cannot be bought; of so beautiful a shape is it, that though a man lie with an Empress, his heart cannot beat quiet till he leaves her embracements to be at rest with the other: yea, so greatly indebted are

◎◎ *REFLECTIVE THINKING*

Sleepiness

Have you ever experienced a situation where:

♦ You were driving home from a trip late at night feeling tired and unable to stay awake. You opened the car window to let cold air in, turned the radio up, yawned, and continued to drive?

♦ You could not stay awake in a class lecture, and even though you tried to listen to the topic or discussion, you found your head nodding and your eyes closing?

♦ You went to bed early the night before an important event knowing that a good night's sleep would help you during the event, only to find you could not get to sleep until the early hours of the morning?

If you have experienced any of the above (and almost all of us have), you have an understanding of the feelings of sleep deprivation, sleepiness at times when you need to be awake, and arousal at times when you need to be asleep. Consider these isolated incidents from your own life as compounded or exaggerated when you think of the day-to-day lives of persons with sleep disorders.

*we to this kinsman of death, that we owe . . . half
our life to him: and there is good cause why we
should do so: for sleep is the golden chain that ties
health and our bodies together. Who complains of
want? of wounds? of cares? of great men's oppres-
sions? of captivity? whilst he sleepeth? Beggars in
their beds take as much pleasure as kings: can we
therefore surfeit of this delicate ambrosia?*

(Dekker, 1982, p. 138)

While sleep is not always the exquisite release from daily cares that Thomas Dekker describes, he is certainly correct in describing high-quality sleep as "an excellent thing." As common as sleep is in everyone's life, it is remarkable how much is still unknown about its nature and functions. The physiological function of sleep remains a mystery, and there is remarkably little evidence that even prolonged sleep deprivation is physically harmful, at least in young and healthy individuals. Nonetheless, most people feel highly unwell when they are deprived of sleep.

In recent years, many hospitals and medical centers have developed sleep study programs to evaluate persons who complain of sleep-related disorders. Sleep has become a scientific and medical study of its own, and many nurses now work exclusively with individuals whose only problem is disturbed sleep. The discussion in this section on sleep disorders is divided into two parts: the first addressing **dyssomnias**, those conditions where there is an abnormality in the amount, quality, or timing of sleep, and the second addressing **parasomnias**, those conditions where the client exhibits abnormal behavioral or physiological events in association with sleep. First, however, normal sleep cycles are reviewed.

Normal Sleep Cycles

There are five sleep stages identified by changes in brain wave patterns that are measured by electro-encephalographic (EEG) recordings. Stages 1 through 4 are characterized by increasingly slow brain wave patterns and coincide with deepened sleep. Stage 5 is rapid-eye-movement (REM) sleep and is characterized by vivid dreams and a comparably faster brain wave pattern that resembles awake states. Persons typically pass through each of the five stages in cycles of 1 to 2 hours. There is marked individual variation in the time spent in each sleep cycle; however, most persons will experience all of the sleep stages in the course of a night's sleep. Older adults experience sleep pattern changes with aging and will awaken several times during the night. Sleep is needed for body restoration and repair, and the subjective sense of being well rested is central to a person's perception of well-being. Temporary disruption of sleep patterns requires nursing support and attention; true sleep disorders require both accurate nursing assessment and care as well as referral and specialist evaluation and treatment.

Dyssomnias

The conditions discussed following represent the most common abnormalities of amount, quality, and timing of sleep; they are insomnias and daytime sleepiness.

Insomnia is a sleep disorder characterized by difficulty in initiating or maintaining sleep. Insomnia is considered a psychological problem if it lasts sufficiently long (1 month or more) and leads to impairment in functioning. The term **Primary Insomnia** is given to the condition in which there are no known external causes of the inability to sleep; for example, there are psychological disorders (Post-Traumatic Stress Disorder), physical disorders (those resulting in pain or discomfort), or medications and/or substances (caffeine) that affect sleep. Primary Insomnia refers only to those situations where there is no other condition responsible for the sleep difficulties. The following passage describes the experience:

Insomnia

*It's three or four in the morning.
There's a bird squawking and beating
its wings in the chimney, louder*

*than the jealous noise of dreams:
a boy turning into a dog.
The changing profile of a man on the wall.*

*These have nothing to do
with my life here in bed, next to
this other dreamer: he lifts his head,*

*looks me in the eye, rows away.
He hears the bird but prefers to think
it's hallucination. I kick the sheets away,*

*spend the night eliminating
possibilities. I don't want to walk
around with this bird's bad dream.*

*Anyway, it's another day.
There's dew on the stack of logs.
There's the sound of wings*

*trying to fly. A strong smell of ash
lifts through the house.
A lime-colored sun wheels through the sky.**

(Mishkin, 1982, pp. 251–252)

---

*Reprinted with permission of Quarterly Review of Literature. Poetry Book Series, Vol. 26.

In her poem entitled "Insomnia," Julia Mishkin describes a sleepless night during which the softest of noises— the sound of a bird fluttering in the fireplace chimney —is enough to keep her awake and actively engaged in the process of "eliminating possibilities." Her sleeping partner apparently wakes up enough to listen, concludes the sounds are imaginary, and "rows away" back to sleep, leaving the poet alone in bed with her night thoughts. She might choose to get up, get a flashlight, and check the chimney, but she does not "want to walk around," she tells us, "with this bird's bad dream." In contrast, the famous 19th-century novelist Charles Dickens spent his sleepless nights far from his own chimney, walking around dark and dangerous London until he too found himself seemingly in the middle of someone else's nightmare:

Night Walks

Some years ago, a temporary inability to sleep, referable to a distressing impression, caused me to walk about the streets all night, for a series of several nights. The disorder might have taken a long time to conquer, if it had been faintly experimented on in bed; but, it was soon defeated by the brisk treatment of getting up directly after lying down, and going out, and coming home tired at sunrise.

. . . My principal object being to get through the night, the pursuit of it brought me into sympathetic relations with people who have no other object every night of the year.

The month was March, and the weather damp, cloudy, and cold. The sun not rising before half-past five, the night perspective looked sufficiently long at half-past twelve: which was about my time for confronting it.

The restlessness of a great city, and the way in which it tumbles and tosses before it can get to sleep, formed one of the first entertainments offered to the contemplation of us houseless people. It lasted about two hours. . . .

When a church clock strikes, on houseless ears in the dead of night, it may at first be mistaken for company and hailed as such. . . .

Once—it was after leaving the Abbey and turning my face north—I came to the great steps of St. Martin's church as the clock was striking Three. Suddenly, a thing that in a moment more I should have trodden upon without seeing, rose up at my

feet with a cry of loneliness and houselessness, struck out of it by the bell, the like of which I never heard. We then stood face to face looking at one another, frightened by one another. The creature was like a beetle-browed hair-lipped youth of twenty.

(Dickens, 1982, pp. 3–12)

Both Mishkin and Dickens describe common experiences of sleeplessness: a desire to sleep, preoccupation with thoughts upon retiring, an interest in getting up and walking about (repressed by the poet and indulged in by the novelist), and a sense of the waking night world as threatening and ultimately nightmare-like.

On occasion, almost everyone experiences difficulties getting to sleep or staying asleep. Even a few days of insomnia, as Dickens describes, while acutely unpleasant, are far from abnormal. Insomnia is considered a psychological problem if it lasts sufficiently long to impair functioning. While impairment may result from complaints of daytime sleepiness, individuals with insomnia rarely have objectively detectable daytime sleepiness (American Psychiatric Association, 1994). In many individuals, insomnia does lead to anxiety, arousal, and preoccupation with the process of falling to sleep. As Dickens observed about his brief bout with insomnia, "the disorder might have taken a long time to conquer, if it had been faintly experimented on in bed." An astute psychologist, Dickens recognized that worrying about sleeplessness while in bed can prolong an episode of insomnia. Some individuals fall asleep easily and remain asleep through the night but do not feel in the morning as if they have had a restful or restorative night of sleep.

Primary Insomnia is usually diagnosed on the basis of an individual's subjective complaint, but quality and quantity of sleep are difficult to judge objectively outside the sleep laboratory. Many people overestimate the amount of sleep they need and underestimate the amount they actually get during a restless night. Requirements for sleep vary widely. Most adults need the traditional 7 to 9 hours of sleep a night, but some adults are "short sleepers" and function well on only 3 or 4 hours. Persons who function well despite little sleep are not diagnosed with Primary Insomnia.

Primary Insomnia is diagnosed only when no other psychological, medical, or substance-related condition is responsible for sleep difficulties. Substance use is often a cause of sleep disturbance. Alcohol and caffeine are both commonly associated with sleep disorders, and use of stimulant drugs such as diet pills, amphetamines, and cocaine may be falsely denied. While prescription sleep medications (most commonly benzodiazepines) may have a role in short-term treatment of insomnia, their side effects may include insomnia, especially when long-term usage leads to habituation and withdrawal symptoms. Mood disorders, both depression and mania, may affect the need for and quality of sleep, and these must be carefully excluded in evaluating and treating sleep complaints.

Primary Insomnia in the Elderly: Special Considerations

The National Institutes of Health (NIH) convened an expert panel on sleep disturbance in older people (1990). This panel reached a number of conclusions. First, sleep problems are common but probably not inevitable among older individuals. As the panelists observed:

A large proportion of older people are at risk for disturbances of sleep that may be caused by many factors such as retirement and changes in social patterns, death of spouse and close friends, increased use of medications, concurrent diseases and changes in circadian rhythms. While changes in sleep patterns have been viewed as part of the normal aging process, new information indicates that many of these disturbances may be related to pathological processes that are associated with aging.

(NIH, 1990, p. 2)

Estimates are that disturbances of sleep, including but not limited to Primary Insomnia, afflict more than half of the people age 65 years and older who live at home and about two-thirds of those who live in long-term-care facilities. In addition to affecting the quality of life, troubled sleep has been associated with excess mortality among the elderly, though a causal relationship has not been proven. Multiple drug treatment of the elderly is extremely common, and sedative-hypnotics are among the most frequently prescribed medications for these individuals. There is currently little evidence that medications are useful in improving the sleep of the older individual, and they may be particularly harmful by increasing the risk of falls and by interacting with other prescription and nonprescription medications. Over-the-counter sleep preparations such as diphenhydramine may be troublesome in the elderly person since they have anticholinergic effects that may influence vision and excretory function. The effectiveness of such over-the-counter substances for inducing sleep in older persons remains unproven.

Insomnia is often treated with techniques of **sleep hygiene**—specific activities that assist many persons to achieve restful sleep. While there is no standard sleep hygiene regimen, the recommendations presented in the accompanying display are often employed and are felt to

---

TECHNIQUES OF SLEEP HYGIENE

◆ Restrict bed and bedroom to sleep and sexual activities. Do not read, watch television, or do other activities in bed. If sleepless, do not lie in bed for hours staring at the walls or clock. If you do not fall asleep after 15 or 20 minutes, it is best to get up and do something quiet until you become drowsy.

◆ Try to get up at the same time each day, regardless of when you went to bed. This will help establish a sleep-wake rhythm.

◆ Exercise each day, preferably in late afternoon or early evening.

◆ Make sure the bedroom is quiet, dark, and comfortable in temperature (around 65°F).

◆ A light snack may help, possibly with warm milk; a heavy meal will not. If gastroesophageal reflux (an occasional physical cause of insomnia) has been diagnosed, never eat within 3 hours of sleeping.

◆ Avoid daytime napping.

◆ Caffeine in the evening disturbs sleep, even if you do not think so! Alcohol causes fragmented sleep, especially if consumed immediately before sleep but also earlier in the day.

◆ If your alarm clock's ticking keeps you awake at night, get a quieter one. Position the clock so that you cannot see it.

◆ It is sometimes possible to break the cycle of insomnia by deliberately staying awake for an entire night.

✳ NURSING TIP

Melatonin

While not proven to be useful in treating insomnia, melatonin has been shown useful when jet travel, shift work (common in hospital employment), or other temporary factors disrupt the normal daynight sleepiness cycle.

---

be clinically useful. With the use of sleep hygiene techniques, most people should be able to overcome Primary Insomnia after a short period. The use of medications, including the over-the-counter drug melatonin, is of unproven benefit.

RESEARCH HIGHLIGHT

Sleep Concerns Among Older Adults

STUDY PROBLEM/PURPOSE

To evaluate sleep patterns and sleep problems of healthy, older adults.

METHODS

A sample of 84 participants who were 60 to 90 years of age, over half of whom were identified as having concerns about their sleep.

FINDINGS

Qualitative evaluations indicated that factors such as physical discomfort, external environments, emotional worries, and changes in sleep patterns were the primary issues. Gender differences emerged, in that men expressed being more concerned than women over external stimuli that affected sleep. These stimuli included noises (often attributed to spouse), uncomfortable room temperature, and poor air quality. The nature of emotional discomforts that kept these participants awake were different among men and women in the sample. Men expressed concerns regarding vivid dreams and nightmares whereas women attributed trouble falling asleep to worry over family, health, and finances.

IMPLICATIONS

Nurses must be sensitive to the possibility that sleep patterns and difficulties may vary along gender lines.

From "Use of Across-Method Triangulation in Study of Sleep Concerns of Healthy Older Adults," by M. Floyd, 1993, *Advances in Nursing Science, 16,* pp. 70–80.

Daytime Sleepiness

Three conditions where a person experiences excessive sleepiness during the day, often unrelated to the amount and quality of sleep at night are discussed following. These are Primary Hypersomnia, Narcolepsy, and Breathing-Related Sleep Disorder. To begin the discussion, consider the following:

He's Gone to Sleep Again

"Damn that boy, he's gone to sleep again."

So the stout gentleman put on his spectacles, and Mr. Pickwick pulled out his glass, and everybody stood up in the carriage, and looked over somebody else's shoulder at the evolutions of the military.

"Joe, Joe!" said the stout gentleman, when the citadel was taken, and the besiegers and besieged sat down to dinner. "Damn that boy, he's gone to sleep again. Be good enough to pinch him, Sir—in the leg, if you please; nothing else wakes him—thank you. Undo the hamper, Joe."

The fat boy, who had been effectually roused by the compression of a portion of his leg, between the finger and thumb of Mr. Winkle, rolled off the box again, and proceeded to unpack the hamper, with more expedition that could have been expected from his previous inactivity. . . .

"Now, Joe, knives and forks." The knives and forks were handed in, and the ladies and gentlemen inside, and Mr. Winkle on the box, were each furnished with those useful implements.

"Now, Joe, the fowls. Damn that boy; he's gone to sleep again. Joe!, Joe! . . .

"Very extraordinary boy, that," said Mr. Pickwick, "does he always sleep in this way?"

"Sleep!" said the old gentleman, "he's always asleep. Goes on errands fast asleep, and snores as he waits at table." . . .

As the Pickwickians turned round to take a last glimpse of it, the setting sun . . . fell upon the form of the fat boy. His head was sunk upon his bosom; and he slumbered again.

(Dickens, 1969, pp. 64–69)

Remaining awake when fatigued is among the hardest of human activities:

Captain Harold Doud, attached to the Japanese Army from 1934 to 1935, tells of his conversation with a Captain Teshima. During peacetime maneuvers the troops "twice went three days and two nights without sleep except what could be snatched during ten-minute halts and brief lulls in the situation. Sometimes the men slept while walking. Our junior lieutenant caused much amusement by marching squarely into a lumber pile on the side of the road while sound asleep." When camp was finally struck, still no one got a chance to sleep; they were all assigned to outpost and patrol duty. "'But why not let some of them sleep?" I asked. "Oh no!" he said. "That is not necessary. They already know how to sleep. They need training in how to stay awake.'"

(Benedict, 1974, p. 181)

Joe, the "fat boy" in Charles Dickens's *The Pickwick Papers*, has profound daytime sleepiness, marked obesity, and loud snoring. He falls asleep in a moment and sleeps through every possible daytime disturbance, including military drills and the firing of cannons. Joe has been thought to have a Breathing-Related Sleep Disorder, "Pickwickian syndrome," a condition of alveolar hypoventilation secondary to massive obesity. Individuals with Pickwickian syndrome breathe very shallowly and are sleepy because of CO_2 narcosis: They breathe so little they are unable to blow off CO_2, which in the resulting high concentrations acts very much like a general anesthetic and produces sleepiness. This life-threatening medical syndrome was named after Dickens's vivid description in *The Pickwick Papers*. Whether or not he is truly Pickwickian, Joe snores loudly and may have obstructive sleep apnea, another cause of daytime sleepiness. Obstructive sleep apnea is a Breathing-Related Sleep Disorder caused by upper airway obstruction during sleep. In the novel, Joe receives from Charles Dickens a colorful 19th-century description of his sleep disorder; from a modern perspective he also needs a careful medical evaluation and probably a sleep laboratory study to determine the cause of his recurrent sleep attacks.

Even after such a comprehensive evaluation, some individuals have no obvious explanation for daytime sleepiness. Their nighttime sleep is normal, so they are not suffering from insomnia. They do not have obstructive sleep apnea, are not Pickwickian, and have no psychological disorder such as depression that can account for their symptoms. They do not have a substance-related disorder such as occurs in users of depressant drugs or those on withdrawal from stimulants. They do not suffer from another sleep disorder, yet the condition exists and results in impairment of daily activities; these individuals have **Primary Hypersomnia**—daytime sleepiness for which there is no external or physiological explanation.

In Primary Hypersomnia, formal sleep studies are essentially normal except that **sleep latency** (the time it takes to fall asleep) is decreased, consistent with increased daytime sleepiness. No REM sleep occurs during daytime sleep episodes. Primary Hypersomnia is relatively rare but does occur in about 10% of persons referred to sleep centers for evaluation (American Psychiatric Association, 1994). One of the most critical issues in management is to ensure that persons with excessive daytime sleepiness not engage in activities, particularly driving, since a sleep attack could put them or others at risk. Many states have laws requiring health care professionals to report individuals with potential for loss of consciousness during driving.

Treatment for daytime sleepiness is not well established; however, stimulant drugs may be useful. Careful medical and sleep evaluation can assist in excluding potentially treatable physiological conditions such as obstructive sleep apnea.

Narcolepsy is another primary sleep disorder in which individuals frequently have three different and quite striking sleep-related symptoms. First, like Joe, they have the frequent recurrence of irresistible need for brief episodes of sleep. They awaken from these feeling remarkably refreshed and rarely report daytime sleepiness except immediately prior to one of these episodes. Second, narcoleptic persons often have vivid dreamlike states as they are falling asleep or waking up. These states typically include hallucinatory experiences in which elements of the real world around them are mixed with dream images. **Sleep paralysis**—the sensation of being unable to move, speak, or breathe—may accompany these states and may provoke great fear. Third, individuals with Narcolepsy may have episodes of **cataplexy**, which is defined as the sudden loss of muscle power at times of sudden emotion, often laughter or fear. These persons may drop things or even fall to the ground, but unlike a simple faint, they never lose consciousness during a cataleptic episode.

Narcolepsy is rare, occurring in only about one per thousand individuals. Since there is strong evidence for a hereditary predisposition, Narcolepsy is relatively common among close relatives of affected individuals. The disorder is diagnosed on the basis of a history that includes sleep attacks, usually with cataplexy or hallucinations and/or sleep paralysis. Formal sleep studies confirm the diagnosis by measuring how long it takes the individual to fall asleep. The consequences of Narcolepsy can be severe. Individuals with this disorder should generally not drive or operate dangerous machinery, as they are at risk for falling asleep and injuring themselves or others. There is a significant association with other psychological disorders, including Major Depressive Disorder. Treatment involves daytime use of stimulant drugs, typically amphetamines. These are controlled substances, have some risk of abuse, and need to be monitored carefully.

Parasomnias

Individuals with parasomnias suffer from profoundly disturbed sleep, most commonly nightmares, sleep terrors, or sleepwalking. Of the three conditions, nightmares would seem to be the most common, occasionally affecting up to half of all persons.

Nightmares are exceedingly vivid dreams from which the individual wakens in fear, often with signs of autonomic nervous system hyperactivity: sweating, and tachycardia. The content of nightmares is often inherently frightening: a physical attack or pursuit by another person, animal, or frightening "monster." One of the important characteristics of nightmares is that, on awakening, the individual has good recall of the nightmare content. This recall is often accompanied by persistent anxiety that may inhibit return to sleep. Persons with recurrent nightmares that interfere with sleep and social functioning may have Nightmare Disorder, a DSM-IV diagnosis.

Sleep terrors are a related parasomnia in which there is *no recall* of the sleep-related event. Individuals experiencing sleep terrors rouse suddenly from sleep with a cry or scream. They typically sit up in bed in apparent terror: sweaty, pupils dilated, tachypneic, and tachycardic. Usually, the affected individual cannot be awakened during a terror but gradually calms and returns to sleep. If awakened at the time, he has only fragmentary recall of the episode without prominent dream imagery, and on arising in the morning, has virtually no memory of what may have happened. Some individuals with sleep terrors will have prominent physical activity including motions of physical fighting. In such cases, the distinction between sleep terrors and sleepwalking may become blurred. Sleep terrors are fairly commonly seen in children and typically resolve by adolescence. Adult-onset sleep terrors may also occur.

A Scream in the Night

The car door opened. "Wssht" said Miss Finan, scuttling out again. "I've just remembered. Not last night, but two weeks ago. And once before that. A scream, you said?"

Mrs. Hazlitt stood up. Almost unable to speak, for the tears that suddenly wrenched her throat, she described it.

"That's it, just what I told my niece on the phone next morning. Like nothing human, and yet it was. I'd taken my Seconal too early, so there I was wide awake again, lying there just thinking, when it came. 'Auntie,' she tried to tell me, 'it was just one of the sireens. Or hoodlums maybe.'" Miss Finan reached up very slowly and settled her hat. . . . "But I've laid awake on this street too many years, I said, not to know what I hear. . . . Like somebody in a fit, it was. We'd a sexton at church taken that way, with epilepsy once. And it stopped short like that, just as if somebody'd clapped a hand over its mouth, poor devil."*

(Calisher, 1982, p. 40)

Mrs. Hazlitt and her elderly neighbor are discussing a strange and curiously recurrent night noise that Mrs. Hazlitt fears might be the scream of a neighbor in danger.

Miss Finan is struck by how short the sound was and speculates that it might have come from some neighbor experiencing an epileptic seizure. It seems likely that these women heard a neighbor suffering from sleep terrors, a condition in which the sleeper awakens screaming.

Whereas nightmares are difficult to confuse with other disorders, night terrors have a more extensive differential diagnosis. Central nervous system injury, infection, or tumor can occasionally produce night terror–like episodes. Epileptic seizures not infrequently occur during sleep and, as the elderly Miss Finan suggests, can be difficult to distinguish from night terrors. Often only EEG studies at home or in the sleep laboratory can make this distinction. Medications, particularly in the elderly, can produce symptoms of either nightmares or night terrors that disappear or are greatly attenuated with drug withdrawal.

Sleepwalking involves a pattern of behavior usually including getting out of bed, walking around in the bedroom or on occasion outside of the bedroom, and then returning to bed. During these episodes, the individual is not fully conscious but on occasion may perform remarkably coherent activities such as eating or talking. Some persons may be able to carry on rudimentary conversations during a sleepwalking episode. Sometimes sleepwalking behaviors are bizarre and stereotyped, occasionally including behavior like urinating in unusual places. Episodes of this sort require careful evaluation, often with ambulatory EEG monitoring, to distinguish them from temporal lobe epilepsy. Like persons with sleep terrors, sleepwalkers are difficult to arouse during an episode and if awakened are often confused and without any specific recall of the events that led to their behaviors. In the morning, they have little or no recall of what has happened to them. Sometimes, the affected individual may awaken spontaneously in the middle of a sleepwalking episode, occasionally completely out of her house and in a strange environment. Frequently, a sleepwalker awakens in the morning to find herself sleeping in an entirely different bed or room than where she fell asleep the previous night. Sleepwalking occurs in up to 7% of individuals and, like sleep terrors, is much more common in children than in adults (American Psychiatric Association, 1994).

Treatment is rarely indicated for sleep terrors. Nightmares often necessitate reassurance, especially in children. Occasionally nightmares reflect significant anxieties or unrecognized traumatic experiences. Sympathetic interviewing and counseling may be effective in evaluating and treating nightmares. Sleepwalking potentially poses some danger to the sleepwalker, and good management often requires special efforts to ensure protection from injury during an episode. Such protection is particularly important if the sleepwalker ventures out of the house or is at risk of falling down stairs.

---

*Reprinted by permission of Donadio & Ashworth, Inc. Copyright 1982 Hortense Calisher.

NURSING PROCESS

All standardized nursing history tools include questions related to a client's sleep and rest patterns. *Sleep pattern disturbance* was accepted as a nursing diagnosis in the 1970s, indicating the nursing role in maintenance of sleep in support of the general health and well-being of clients. The nurse has a clear role in assessment. Care of one who is diagnosed with a sleep disorder will be collaborative, and the nurse will participate in an interdisciplinary team providing treatment.

▽ ASSESSMENT

The nurse must always assess the client's sleeping patterns in completing any nursing history. Suggestions for obtaining information are presented in the accompanying display.

▽ NURSING DIAGNOSIS

The nurse must first determine if the client has a sleep pattern disturbance that can be addressed by nursing care or if the client requires referral to a sleep specialist. If the client experiences *sleep pattern disturbance* (the condition where he is unable to obtain restorative sleep) or is experiencing nightmares or sleep terrors, the nurse may make the nursing diagnoses and begin intervention. However, if the nurse suspects that the client has a Breathing-Related Sleep Disorder, Narcolepsy, or episodes of sleepwalking, the nurse should make a referral to a sleep specialist.

▽ OUTCOME IDENTIFICATION

If the nurse is initiating treatment for a *sleep pattern disturbance*, such as Primary Insomnia, the expected outcome will be that within 2 weeks the client will experience restorative sleep and will describe falling asleep easily and waking up feeling rested. If the nurse is initiating treatment for a condition such as nightmares, the expected outcome is that the client will understand the disorder and establish means of coping with it within his family.

▽ PLANNING/INTERVENTIONS

For Primary Insomnia, the best intervention is a standard sleep hygiene protocol, such as the one presented in a previous display. The nurse should educate the client and family about the condition and explain that a sleep hygiene protocol is a series of techniques that have been

ASSESSMENT OF SLEEP PATTERNS

It is not enough to ask, "Did you sleep well last night?" A nurse must inquire if the client has/had difficulty falling asleep, experiences early awakening without the ability to return to sleep, and feels well rested in the morning. Further, the nurse should ask if the client feels fatigued and sleepy during the day. Questions for the nurse to ask are:

◆ How long does it take you to fall asleep at night?

◆ Do you awaken during the night? If yes, how many times in a typical night?

◆ If you do awaken at night, can you get back to sleep?

◆ Do you feel well rested in the morning?

◆ Do you have enough energy to perform your tasks during the day?

◆ Do you find yourself nodding off or sleeping during classes or meetings or while watching TV or movies?

Evaluate with the client whether there have been any environmental changes associated with the bedroom or household that could be influencing changes in sleep cycle. Questions for the nurse to ask are:

◆ Have you changed where you sleep?

◆ Have there been any changes in your household that could affect your sleeping?

◆ Have there been any changes in your environment (neighbors, traffic) that could affect your sleeping?

Determine whether there have been any emotional stressors that could be contributing to an inability to sleep. A question for the nurse to ask is:

◆ Do you find yourself awake at night worrying about a problem or an upcoming activity?

useful to many. The nurse should then help the client to individualize the protocol to fit his own environment and personality. Further, the nurse may suggest complementary modalities, such as guided relaxation, music therapy, or massage, that have been helpful for many who are unable to get to sleep (see Chapter 31 for complementary modalities).

For a client experiencing nightmares or sleep terrors, the nurse has two important interventions. First, support and reassurance for the anxiety that these conditions provoke are needed. The nurse should develop a supportive relationship with both the client and family and help the family to maintain a sense of calm regarding the disorder. Second, the nurse should provide education on the disorder to the client and family so that they have a better understanding of the condition. If the nurse suspects the nightmares or sleep terrors are a result of other trauma,

anxieties, or delusions, the nurse must refer the client for further assessment and evaluation.

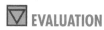 **EVALUATION**

Evaluation of nursing care will be done on the basis of achieving expected outcomes. The nurse should remember that the subjective experience of sleep, sleepiness, and rest is of utmost importance; that is, the outcomes may not be directly observed. The nurse must validate with the client that there has or has not been improvement.

CASE STUDY/CARE PLAN

Fred is a 65-year-old, retired man who lives with his wife in a comfortable home they have owned for over 40 years. He is an active member of his community, being involved in civic clubs and church activities. Fred is in good health, as is his wife. They have a stable retirement income. They have two grown children and three grandchildren who live in another city. Fred makes an appointment to talk with the nurse at the Senior Citizens' Center because he is unable to sleep at night and explains that the problem has been worsening over the last 2 weeks.

ASSESSMENT

Taking a detailed nursing history, the nurse learns that Fred has several concerns over his sleep patterns:

Specifically, Fred explains that he just does not "sleep well anymore." He says, "I wake up several times during the night, sometimes I have dreams that I am with several other people—but I can't quite make out or remember what the dreams are about. Noise in the neighborhood bothers me—when I hear a bus go down the street I can't go back to sleep." Fred stays in bed about 7 hours but believes he gets very little sleep; he gets up in the morning feeling tired and tries to nap in the afternoon to keep himself going.

Upon further questioning, the nurse learns that Fred often eats a snack before retiring; takes a daily walk, usually in the morning; sleeps with his wife in their bedroom, where they have a TV on which they often watch a late show before going to sleep. He retires at about 11:00 P.M.

NURSING DIAGNOSIS *Sleep pattern disturbance*, related to subjective reports of not sleeping well, waking up during the night, awakening during the night without ability to go back to sleep, and feeling tired in the morning and throughout the day

Outcomes	Planning/Interventions	Evaluation
By 2 weeks time, Fred will experience restful sleep and feel rested upon awakening.	◆ Establish a sleep hygiene protocol with Fred that includes: – Taking some form of physical exercise, such as Fred's daily walk, in the early evening. – Eating an evening meal around 7:00 P.M. and then having only a drink of warm milk before bedtime. – Keeping his bed reserved for sleep, therefore watching TV in the living room and retiring to bed when feeling sleepy.	With establishment of the change in patterns, Fred reported he was able to sleep better at night. Within 2 weeks, Fred felt he had received restful sleep for the first time in months.

Continued

Outcomes	Planning/Interventions	Evaluation
	– Running a fan in the bedroom to provide good circulation of air and to provide a background "white" noise that could help eliminate disturbances of street noise.	Fred also reported feeling reassured that it was "normal" for him to be awakening frequently during the night. Fred did not know that most people develop different sleeping patterns in their 60s than they had in their 40s.
	– Refraining from afternoon naps, at least until nighttime sleep is reestablished.	
	◆ Educate Fred on what is known regarding sleep patterns in persons of his age group.	

CRITICAL THINKING BAND

ASSESSMENT

Would you also question Fred's wife about his sleeping patterns? What questions should you ask about the physical environment of Fred's bedroom?

NURSING DIAGNOSIS

Are there other diagnoses the nurse should look for in Fred? How do we know the nurse is not missing something important in Fred's emotional life?

Outcomes	Planning/Interventions	Evaluation
Is it too much to expect that the nurse and Fred together can change this pattern?	How should the nurse provide this sleep hygiene protocol to Fred? Should she write it out? Put it on a graph? Put it on a timetable? How would the nurse decide? Should Fred's wife be involved? In what way?	If the interventions used did not work, what else could the nurse do or suggest?

EATING DISORDERS

Two eating disorders are described in this chapter: Bulimia Nervosa and Anorexia Nervosa. Before reading about this ever-prevalent problem, read and consider the Reflective Thinking on body image and self worth.

Bulimia Nervosa

Food Frenzy

As I opened the refrigerator door, my stomach growled with anticipation. . . . Suddenly, I realized I'd gone too far. In two minutes I had destroyed an all-day effort to avoid eating. Well, no need to get depressed. I might as well eat my fill of everything now. I'll just have to get rid of it later. I knew how. I'd done it dozens of times before.

Mindlessly, I began shoveling handfuls of food into my mouth. I devoured huge amounts of leftovers from Christmas dinner, breakfast, and even from days before. . . .

(O'Neill, 1982, pp. xii–xiv)

✇ REFLECTIVE THINKING

Body Image and Self Worth

How a person perceives her body is influenced by what it looks like to her and what it looks like to others. Our society teaches us through media and social pressures that body image is important. Feeling attractive is an important part of self-worth, and for many, feeling attractive means matching a certain ideal appearance.

Most of us will never be able to look like this ideal, but the message we get is that we risk social failure if we do not try hard enough. When we believe this message, we may feel incompetent and depressed and have low self-esteem because we cannot meet impossible standards of appearance.

Women and men need to develop personal skills that will help them feel good about themselves without placing undue emphasis on physical appearance. No one should rely on dieting, exercising, and dressing to determine their self-worth.

⭐ NURSING TIP

Body Image

Here are some hints that can help in developing a positive body image:

◆ Learn to like yourself as you are.

◆ Set realistic goals.

◆ Learn about good nutrition and exercise.

◆ If you are a woman, expect that you may experience normal monthly changes in weight and shape.

◆ Listen to your body. Eat when you are hungry, and only then.

◆ When life proves stressful, learn to ask for support from friends and family.

Remember the Three As:

Attention: Listen to and respond to internal cues; know when your body is hungry and when it is tired.

Appreciation: Honor and appreciate the pleasures your body can provide.

Acceptance: Accept yourself for what you are. Do not long for the unattainable; having a wish "magically" come true does not lead to happiness but leads to more unattainable wishes.

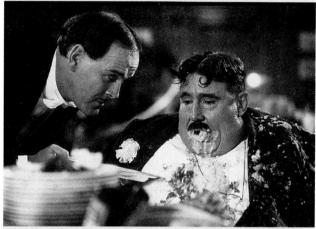

The Meaning of Life. Source: Universal/Courtesy Kobal.

Binging and purging, common in many eating disorders, are generally hidden behaviors, rarely observed by the nurse.

In this episode, the author describes the experience of what DSM-IV now terms **Bulimia Nervosa**. Fasting, binging, and purging, three major aspects of Bulimia Nervosa, are illustrated. There is the ever-present risk of discovery by parents or other family members. DSM-IV states that the prevalence of Bulimia Nervosa among adolescent and young adult females is approximately 1% to 3%, with a much lower prevalence among males (American Psychiatric Association, 1994). Several cross-sectional studies have offered somewhat lower prevalence estimates (Hoek, 1991; Warheit, Langer, Zimmerman, & Biafora, 1993).

Bulimia Nervosa is characterized by a preoccupation with weight and bodily appearance and by recurrent episodes of binge eating dominated, as in the excerpt previous, by lack of control. The young woman, Cherry Boone goes to the refrigerator intending only to sample the Christmas dinner. She finds herself unable to stop eating and relies on purging to achieve weight control. The diagnosis of the disorder requires both binge eating and the presence of behaviors intended to restrict weight gain, most commonly self-induced vomiting, fasting, and excessive exercise. Laxative abuse and misuse of other drugs and medications may also occur. Bulimia Nervosa may occur alone or may be associated with other psychologi-

cal diagnoses including Anorexia Nervosa, Major Depressive Disorder, Substance Abuse, Obsessive-Compulsive Disorder, and Borderline Personality Disorder. While DSM-IV requires that the full spectrum of binging and purging behaviors be present at least twice weekly for 3 months to make the diagnosis, many individuals report milder or less frequent manifestations of the eating disorder. Not surprisingly, these manifestations may be much more common than fully developed Bulimia Nervosa (Langer, Warheit, & Zimmerman, 1991).

The consequences of Bulimia Nervosa depend on its severity, duration, and associated psychological disorders. Recurrent vomiting leads to erosion of dental enamel and tooth decay and may occasionally result in stone formation in the salivary glands. Salivary gland enlargement is common and, along with enamel erosion, may be a helpful diagnostic clue when physical examination is performed for some unrelated reason. Frequent vomiting and weight loss may lead to electrolyte disturbances that can result in dangerous or fatal heart arrhythmias (Roseborough & Felix, 1994).

Depression often complicates bulimia and may lead to suicide attempts or to completed suicide. Bulimic individuals commonly use psychoactive substances that affect appetite and weight. Tobacco is probably the most common of such abused substances, but bulimia is also strikingly common among cocaine abusers (Walfish, Stenmark, Sarco, Shealy, & Krone, 1992). Nurses and other health professionals must be vigilant to detect bulimia in a variety of clinical settings and to recognize complications of bulimia as causes of otherwise-unexplained serious illness (Myer & O'Brien, 1993). While bulimic individuals may be very evasive in their actual

> ### ✳ NURSING TIP
>
> ### Screening Questions for Persons with Bulimia
>
> **1.** Are you satisfied with your eating patterns?
> **2.** Do you ever eat in secret?
>
> Note that 100% of persons with Bulimia Nervosa will answer no to question 1 and/or yes to question 2.

binging and purging activities, direct clinical questioning seems to be remarkably effective in screening for bulimia. Freund and coworkers have suggested that two specific questions are particularly useful (Freund, Graham, Lesky, & Moskowitz, 1993). In these authors' study, a "no" response to the question "Are you satisfied with your eating patterns?" or a "yes" response to "Do you ever eat in secret?" had a sensitivity of 1.00 and a specificity of 0.90 for bulimia. In other words, 100% of bulimic individuals were either unsatisfied with their eating patterns or reported eating in secret (or both). Only 10% of non-bulimic persons answered similarly. Because Bulimia Nervosa is rare in most clinical settings, positive answers to such screening questions are most commonly "false positives," detecting individuals who, on further questioning, do not have bulimia. Nonetheless, a significant proportion of positive answers will come from individuals who *do* have bulimia. Consequently, the authors strongly endorse the incorporation of these two screening questions into routine clinical interviews, especially for women, whose risk of bulimia is substantially higher than for men.

Treatment

Both psychological and pharmacological treatments for Bulimia Nervosa have been used and studied. Numerous studies have shown that antidepressant medications, particularly selective serotonin reuptake inhibitors, are useful in the management of bulimia (Crow & Mitchell, 1994). Various forms of psychotherapy have been used for bulimia, and in one study, structured cognitive-behavioral therapy was found to be more effective than antidepressants alone (Pyle et al., 1990). Multiple studies, including a number of good experimental quality, have shown cognitive-behavioral therapy to have good short-term benefit in reducing the frequency and severity of bulimic symptoms (Wilson, 1995).

Anorexia Nervosa

There is a strong association between Bulimia Nervosa and Anorexia Nervosa, an association illustrated by another quote from *Starving for Attention*:

I'll Tell You If I Need a Doctor!

"There is nothing wrong with me! I'm just thin! I don't feel sick and I don't need to see the doctor! . . . "It's my body!" I argued. "I know how I feel, and I'm not sick! I'm not hurting anyone else by being thin, so why should it bother you? I'll tell you if I need a doctor."

(O'Neill, 1982, p. 55)

In the first excerpt from *Starving for Attention*, Cherry Boone describes the binging and purging of Bulimia Nervosa. In this second excerpt, she argues with her parents, who have discovered how emaciated she is. They begin a medical evaluation that results in the additional diagnosis of Anorexia Nervosa. **Anorexia Nervosa**, frequently termed *anorexia*, is a serious medical-psychological condition characterized by a profound disturbance in body image. Persons with Anorexia Nervosa view themselves as undesirably fat even when they, like Cherry, become clinically emaciated. These individuals do not lose their appetite for food (the strict meaning of the word *anorexia*), but, like Cherry, actively starve themselves in an effort to keep from gaining weight. Some anorexic individuals control their weight through dieting and exercising alone; others combine this restriction with episodes of binge eating and purging.

Anorexia results in profound bodily changes. The most apparent change is weight loss, which may reach levels of profound emaciation before being detected by friends, family members, or even health care providers. The diagnosis of Anorexia Nervosa requires that weight be 15% below that expected for age and height, but many anorexic individuals experience much greater weight loss. In women, malnutrition typically results in menstrual dysfunction; most women stop menstruating altogether. The skin becomes dry and frequently is covered with fine downy hair called lanugo. Because of fat loss and metabolic changes, anorexic individuals frequently complain of feeling cold. Recurrent syncope is not uncommon, and cardiac dysrhythmias may occur from electrolyte imbalance. Bradycardia is almost always present, partly due to the commonly associated rigorous exercise regimens adopted by many anorexics but probably also as a direct response to starvation (Kollai, Bonyhay, Jokkel, & Szonyi, 1994). Osteoporosis is common and may result in bone fractures (Salisbury & Mitchell, 1991).

In addition to 15% weight loss and cessation of menstrual cycle (in women), requirements for diagnosis include documentation of an intense fear of gaining weight *and* either a disturbed experience of body weight or shape *or* denial of the seriousness of the individual's current low weight (American Psychiatric Association, 1994). Cherry's "There is nothing wrong with me! I'm just thin! I don't feel sick and I don't need to see the doctor!" is a highly typical response of anorexic individuals when challenged with the reality of their physical emaciation.

Differential Diagnosis

Weight loss alone does not permit a diagnosis of Anorexia Nervosa. Weight loss can occur from a wide variety of medical and psychiatric conditions, including intestinal malabsorption, brain tumors (Chipkevitch, 1994), cancer, chronic bacterial infections, human immunodeficiency virus– (HIV-) associated conditions, and autoimmune disorders. Depressed, schizophrenic, and obsessive-compulsive individuals may sometimes experience significant weight loss as a manifestation of their psychological conditions. On occasion, distinguishing these psychological conditions from Anorexia Nervosa may be difficult. Usually, medical and psychiatric consultation can rapidly establish a diagnosis of Anorexia Nervosa by ruling out other potential causes of weight loss.

The Perceived Need for Weight Control

The precise cause of Anorexia Nervosa remains unknown. Psychoanalysts have stressed that weight control in Anorexia Nervosa derives from a desire to suppress adult sexual development and responsibility (Wilson, Hogan, & Mintz, 1985). Such desire for suppression in turn is thought to derive from early childhood sexual experiences, perhaps including seeing the mother's abdomen enlarge during pregnancy.

The psychoanalytic view is only one of a number of competing psychological explanations for Anorexia Nervosa. It has long been taught by some psychologists that Anorexia Nervosa is a developmental disorder deriving from disordered family structure and functioning. Family systems theorists have suggested that the condition arises in a family structure characterized by marital discord, strong emphasis on control, and overprotectiveness. More socially-oriented theorists have stressed how pressures to achieve success, competence, and societally defined attractiveness can lead, especially in women, to compulsive efforts to control weight. This is especially true given strong social identification of thinness with attractiveness (Palmer, 1990).

Other theorists stress that anorexic individuals manifest very strong perfectionist tendencies and that failing to achieve complete control in other aspects of their lives leads them to attempt to gain full control of their eating and weight. Cherry had a particularly strong need for control and perfection. In other chapters of her book, she describes experiences of growing up in a Hollywood environment that strongly emphasized personal appearance. She and her sisters performed on television with their father, Pat Boone, a nationally famous popular singer and celebrity. While anecdotes do support the concept that a perfectionistic upbringing in high-achieving families may lead to eating disorders, more formal studies of families of anorexic individuals fail to show any distinct pattern of family interaction (Rastam & Gillberg, 1991).

In contrast to psychodynamic explanations, other psychologists have offered cognitive and behavioral models. Some of these emphasize the important role that film, photography, and, especially, advertising images of thinness play in leading to anorexia (Bruch, 1978). Bruch has further suggested that anorexic individuals have a combination of poor self-esteem, distorted self-image, and an inability to process *interoceptive stimuli* such as the sensations of being hungry and full (Bruch, 1973). Such discussions of self-image and misperceived stimuli raise the possibility that a definable neurological or endocrine abnormality underlies some cases of anorexia (Braun & Chouinard, 1992). This possibility of organic causation has been considered for many years with varying degrees of enthusiasm. For example, between 1920 and 1945, physicians commonly regarded anorexia as an endocrine disorder and experimented with numerous (unsuccessful) hormonal treatments (Vanderycken & Van Deth, 1994). More recent evaluations of individuals with anorexia reveal significant abnormalities in all major neuroendocrine pathways and in a variety of major neurotransmitter systems (Study Group on Anorexia Nervosa, 1995). Whether any or all of these abnormalities are a *cause* of anorexia or merely *result from* the disorder remains unknown. Aberrations in luteinizing hormone (LH), follicle-stimulating hormone (FSH), and gonadotrophin-releasing hormone (GnRH) (all hormones involved in regulating sexual function) are common in anorexia, and, like the loss of periods in affected women, may occur *before* significant weight loss takes place (Pope & Hudson, 1989). Reported neurotransmitter abnormalities suggest that there may be a link between Anorexia Nervosa and Major Depressive Disorder, but it remains unclear whether these findings are primary abnormalities or are the result of starvation.

Genetic studies have often been used to help distinguish organic (hereditary) from environmental causes of psychological disorders. Such studies, while difficult to perform without bias, do suggest that some individuals may be genetically predisposed to develop anorexia (Strober, 1991). Twin studies, for example, show that when one sibling has anorexia, there are higher rates of anorexia in identical (monozygotic) than in fraternal (dizygotic) sibling twins. Such studies suggest a definite genetic contribution to the development of anorexia (Treasure & Holland, 1990).

Joughin and colleagues have emphasized that anorexia may sometimes present in individuals over the age of 30 years (Joughin, Crisp, Gowers, & Bhat, 1991). Anorexia in this older age group may be much harder to diagnose, partly because it is often an unsuspected diagnosis, and may have a significantly worse prognosis than when it occurs in adolescence and young adulthood.

History of Anorexia as a Disorder

Anorexia is not a "new" disorder. Modern understanding of anorexia began in 1868 when William Gull addressed the British Medical Association on the subject of mesenteric tuberculosis (Gull, 1868). In an era in which systemic tuberculosis frequently caused profound weight loss, he cautioned his fellow doctors against assuming that all anorexic patients suffered from tuberculosis. In his lecture he briefly described "young women emaciated to the last degree through hysteric apepsia," a reference frequently taken to be the first scientific recognition of anorexia. Five years later, a French psychiatrist and contemporary of Charcot, Ernest Lasègue, wrote a paper describing eight individuals age 18 to 32 years who today would be recognized as having Anorexia Nervosa. He even used the word "anorexia" in his description, though influenced by the terminology of his era, he called the condition "hysterical anorexia." But while Gull and Lasègue were the first to provide clinical descriptions of anorexia, the famous Romantic poet George Byron (1788 to 1824) almost certainly suffered from anorexia more than 60 years before his countryman Gull described the disorder:

> Born with a club foot and being a "fat bashful boy," Bryon suffered on account of his outward appearance. His notorious sexual escapades during his adolescence, however, seem to indicate that women found him attractive. . . . He was obviously upset about his fatness and decided to drastically reduce weight. About this endeavour he made a bet with an acquaintance, which he won by a fanatic regime of strict dieting and violent exercise. Within a few months . . . acquaintances found, according to his own saying, "great difficulty in acknowledging me to be the same person." The weight reduction did not satisfy. Like a "leguminous-eating ascetic," as he called himself, he persevered anxiously to remain so. . . . For the rest of his life he remained obsessed by fear of fatness and preoccupied with food. . . . Initially his diet consisted of biscuits and soda water, later of purely vegetarian meals or potatoes mashed in vinegar. To appease his hunger he chewed tobacco or smoked cigars, but occasionally gave himself up to an abundant meal (then "I gorge like an Arab or a Boa snake," he wrote). For this reason Byron took refuge in vomiting and purgative pills or consumed quantities of vinegar. . . . At the end of his life . . . he was described as "unnaturally thin."
>
> (Vanderycken & Van Deth, 1994, pp. 227–228)

At times, Byron's food preoccupations seem to have made their way into his poetry. For example, his satirical poem "Don Juan" describes an episode of cannibalism among shipwrecked sailors who "perish'd, suffering madly,/ For having us'd their appetites so sadly" (from Lord Byron, "Don Juan," Canto 2, LXXX). In Byron's poem, as in his life, eating led to suffering, even "suffering madly."

Treatment

Numerous medications have been studied for treatment of anorexia: hormones, antidepressants, antipsychotics, and gastrointestinal motility enhancers. None has shown any consistent benefit (Crow & Mitchell, 1994). Where depression coexists, antidepressants are likely to be of significant benefit, but these may have only limited effect on the

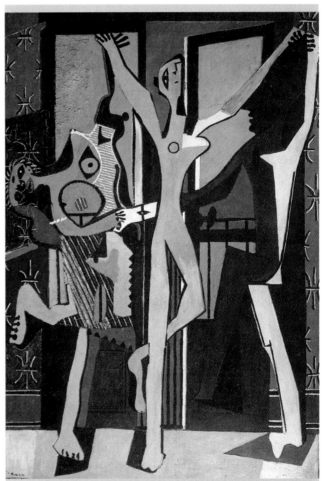

Three Dancers by Picasso. Source: © 1988 Estate of Pablo Picasso/ Artists Rights Society (ARS), New York

Only the still-large left breast suggests that this remarkably thin, hairless, central dancer does not have anorexia. Picasso's interests are primarily in the forms and colors of his canvas, but surely it was the anorexic appearance of this woman that caught his artistic fancy.

anorexic process itself. One group of researchers found strong evidence for the co-occurrence of Anorexia Nervosa and Obsessive-Compulsive Disorder (Thiel, Broocks, Ohlmeier, Jacoby, & Schussler, 1995). These authors also found that obsessive-compulsive symptoms were more likely in clients whose anorexia was most severe. Since Obsessive-Compulsive Disorder is typically drug responsive (Chapter 10), certain clients may benefit significantly from carefully chosen pharmacotherapy. For most individuals, however, psychotherapy is the mainstay of treatment. Profoundly emaciated individuals are almost invariably hos-pitalized and managed with a combination of behavioral therapy and, where necessary, forced feeding (Agras, 1987). Cognitive therapy, clearly effective in bulimia, is thought to be helpful in Anorexia, especially in combination with behavioral approaches (Powers & Powers, 1984). When the individual is severely emaciated, efforts to restore positive nutritional balance take precedence over psychological issues. The nurse's role is often to ensure that the individual receives and retains appropriate nourishment. Most of these individuals will receive care from a team, including experts in psychiatry or psychology, nursing, and nutrition.

NURSING PROCESS

The majority of affected individuals may be treated as outpatients, and the nurse often has an important role in this setting. Frequently, as in the inpatient setting, a team of professionals work together to supervise the affected individual's recovery. Therapeutic goals will differ from program to program but will certainly include the necessity of ensuring adequate caloric intake and documenting weight gain. Individuals with eating disorders are typically made exceedingly anxious by eating and will often try to deceive their caretakers by hiding food or falsifying their weight. The nurse will have to balance her important "policing" role with the likewise-important task of gaining the individual's trust and confidence (Chitty, 1991). Further important tasks in the management of these clients include addressing needs for exercise (usually at a level much less than the individual had previously engaged in), building self-esteem, and helping the individual to achieve a more normal sense of body image.

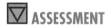 **ASSESSMENT**

The nurse will begin with an assessment and then identify nursing diagnoses that present for the individual client. The nurse will need to know the weight history, eating and purging experiences, and the degree of distress and/or anxiety the client is experiencing (Love & Seaton, 1991). Further, the nurse should identify the motivation for treatment, understanding that most individuals with eating disorders are highly ambivalent toward treatment. Love and Seaton advise that motivation can be considered as inversely proportional to the level of ambivalence the client experiences. Listing the advantages and disadvantages of treatment can serve to explore background and readiness for change.

NURSING DIAGNOSIS

Common nursing diagnoses associated with eating disorders are presented in the accompanying display. The nurse can focus care on these human responses to the eating disorder and begin to plan interventions aimed at the client's priority of need.

OUTCOME IDENTIFICATION

The nurse must identify realistic outcomes of care, recognizing that eating disorders are complex, chronic diseases. It is best to focus on short-term outcomes, such as the client will take in 1,200 calories per day for the next week; the client will gain weight to return to a regular menstrual cycle; or the client will identify one positive aspect of her body unrelated to weight.

PLANNING/INTERVENTIONS

Nursing care can be viewed as taking place during four stages of treatment: nutritional rehabilitation,

---

**COMMON NURSING DIAGNOSES
FOR PERSONS
WITH EATING DISORDERS**

Altered nutrition: less than body requirements
Impaired body image
Low self-esteem
Social isolation
Impaired health maintenance

North American Nursing Diagnosis Association (1996).
*NANDA Nursing Diagnoses: Definitions & Classification
1997–1998.* Philadelphia: NANDA.

psychotherapy, maintenance, and follow-up care (Cahill, 1994). The first, nutritional rehabilitation, begins with diagnosis and sometimes with hospital admission. The priority here is to establish nutrition adequate to stop starvation. During this phase, the nurse may need to take on the role of guardian and promote the client's physical well-being by monitoring food intake and weight gain (Irwin, 1993). Once an appropriate eating pattern is established, the client will enter a stage of treatment focusing on psychotherapy. Interventions that raise self-esteem and increase assertiveness are helpful, as are recreational therapies that provide a balance of exercise with rest and nutrition. Group and individual therapy would be initiated during this phase. Maintenance involves the client in learning to monitor and take control of her own eating patterns (Cahill, 1994). The client must develop internal strategies to meet her needs for nutrition and her desire to feel good about herself. The nurse should remember that personal stress and anxiety seem to increase the client's need to eat less and/or purge or vomit. Stress reduction techniques, then, may prove appropriate in helping the client find balances in her life. Further, it has been noted that persons with eating disorders frequently have little or no experiences with events or services that put one in touch with one's own body, for example with massage therapy, having a professional manicure, or having one's hair shampooed at a salon (Irwin, 1993). These activities may help the client to focus on her body in a positive way and can be encouraged. Above all, nurses interacting with clients with eating disorders can offer presence, role modeling of healthy eating/exercise behaviors, and emotional and psychological support. Further, nurses provide flexibility, empathy, and rational limit setting for one who is out of control but has a strong need to be in control (Love & Seaton, 1991).

▽ EVALUATION

Evaluation of the individual nursing care plans is done on the basis of stated outcomes. In evaluating treat-ment, however, the nurse must recognize the numerous challenges that still exist in dealing with this complex disorder.

☮ NURSING ALERT!

Challenges of Eating Disorders

Both Bulimia and Anorexia Nervosa are potentially fatal disorders. Death in anorexia occurs at a rate much higher than in the population as a whole; approximately 5.6% of anorexics die each decade, a strikingly high figure given the relatively young age at which this disorder typically begins (Sullivan, 1995). Weight more than 60% below ideal and marked muscle weakness may be important risk factors for acute mortality in anorexia (Okabe, 1993). Eckert, Halmi, Marchi, Grove, and Crosby (1994) reported a 10-year follow-up study of 76 severely affected female anorexic individuals. Five of these persons had died, and only 18 (24%) were fully recovered, 41% remained bulimic, and 42% had a relapse with further weight loss within the first year after discharge from the hospital. A similar study from Germany used explicit criteria for good outcome: weight above 85% of ideal and normal menstrual function. Of 81 clients, 69% were found to have a good outcome at a mean follow-up time of 11.7 years; 22 of the original 103 clients either were lost to follow-up (19) or had died (3). Ten percent were bulimic, and 18% had persistent anorexia (Remschmidt, Wienand, & Wewetzer, 1990). It is clearly difficult to evaluate the effectiveness of treatment in a disorder whose recovery rate varies from 24% to 69%, but the significant ongoing mortality in anorexia emphasizes the importance of both defining effective treatment and ensuring careful follow-up.

CASE STUDY/CARE PLAN

Marcia is a 22-year-old university student who comes to the student health center for evaluation of upper respiratory symptoms. She has been coughing and has had "cold symptoms" for 3 days. She is uncomfortable and unable to sleep well at night because coughing keeps her awake. She expresses worry that she will not do well on her upcoming tests because she is not able to adequately prepare for them.

ASSESSMENT

Taking her history, the nurse, David, documents that Marcia is 5 feet 7 inches tall and weighs 95 pounds. Inquiring about recent weight gain or loss, the nurse learns that Marcia has just gained 5 pounds, and Marcia expresses some concern over that fact. The nurse begins to ask questions regarding nutrition and food intake, to which Marcia responds, "I've come here for my cold, I don't want to talk with you about my eating!"

Continued

NURSING DIAGNOSES

- *Ineffective breathing pattern*, related to cough, cold symptoms
- *Fear*, related to uncertainty over ability to perform on upcoming exams
- *Altered nutrition: less than body requirements*, related to inadequate food intake as evidenced by body weight under ideal (diagnosis needing validation)

Outcomes	Planning/Interventions	Evaluation
• Cough and cold symptoms will subside.	• Treat for cold and cough symptoms by increasing fluids, increasing ability to sleep.	Marcia's physical health problem improved and she returned to the clinic for follow-up.
• Marcia will feel in control of her physical symptoms and attend to her studies.	• Provide reassurance to Marcia that she will feel better soon and will be able to return to her normal pattern by providing information on what to expect from the physical illness.	The nurse was unable to validate whether an eating disorder existed.
• Marcia will return to the clinic in a few days for further interaction with the nurse.	• Plan to discuss Marcia's eating habits when Marcia returns to the clinic.	

CRITICAL THINKING BAND

ASSESSMENT

What other factors (family, friends, daily habits, sleep patterns) would you assess to get a more complete picture of Marcia's health?

NURSING DIAGNOSIS

Why did the nurse focus only on the cold and cough? Do you think there is enough information to make a diagnosis of an eating disorder?

Outcomes

Are these the outcomes you would have written? How do we really plan care for a chronic condition? Is it appropriate to merely suggest that the client return? Is the nurse trying to establish trust or do you think something else is going on?

Planning/Interventions

How would you go about obtaining enough information to validate a diagnosis of altered nutrition?

Evaluation

What do you think would have happened if the nurse focused on Marcia's weight during this first encounter? How long do you think it will take to be able to diagnose and address Marcia's weight and eating patterns?

SEXUAL DISORDERS

Sexuality is part of any person's personality. It is an important dimension of a person, and influences how that person views herself and presents herself to others. It is quite impossible to define "normal" sexual behaviors and attitudes, as these are highly dependent on personal/family values, culture, and societal views. Sexual identity includes **gender identity** (internal sense that one is male or female) and **gender role** (learned expressions of male-

ness or femaleness). One author suggests that **normal sexual behavior** [for adults] is any sexual act that is consensual, lacks force, is mutually satisfying to both partners, and is conducted in private (Goldstein, 1976).

Sexual dysfunction occurs when a person experiences problems with any aspect of sexuality. According to the North American Nursing Diagnosis Association (NANDA, 1996), sexual dysfunction is "the state in which an individual experiences a change in sexual function that is viewed as unsatisfying, unrewarding, or inadequate"

(p. 41). Some persons with sexual dysfunction will readily seek counseling; however, many will be reluctant to discuss sexual concerns with anyone. Nurses and health care providers must be willing to take a sexual history in their general assessments of individuals to determine if their clients are experiencing sexual dysfunction or some identified sexual disorder.

Taking a Sexual History

The nurse must remember that sexuality is among the most personal and private areas of human life, and few individuals will volunteer information about sexual functioning or sexual thoughts unless explicitly asked. Many nurses and doctors are uncomfortable asking questions related to sexuality, and as a result, these questions frequently remain unaddressed during clinical encounters. Nurses should evaluate their own feelings regarding discussing sexuality and attempt to identify personal factors that may help or inhibit one's ability to provide care.

Many persons seek medical care with somatic complaints as an excuse to discuss issues of sexual functioning but are too embarrassed to raise their sexual concerns unless asked specifically about them. As a result, taking a sexual history is a highly important task in a clinical nursing evaluation. The sexual history may be quite brief or it may include a wide variety of questions; the length of the interview should be tailored to the client's interest, need, and presenting concerns.

Three important topics of the sexual history are sexual functioning; sexual thoughts, fantasies, and behaviors; and sexual preferences. While many, if not most, individuals are sexually involved and sexually competent, have sexual thoughts and behaviors, and are comfortable with their sexual choices and gender assignment, a careful sexual history will occasionally discover problems in one or more of these areas of sexual being. Further, once the nurse asks questions that open the topic of sexuality as appropriate for discussion, clients may be able to express needs for education/information or the desire for sex counseling and/or support.

Specific Sexual Disorders

Sexual disorders fall into two basic categories: (1) disorders of sexual functioning and (2) **paraphilias**, or disorders of sexual thought, fantasy, and behavior. The disorders of functioning include difficulties with sexual interest, arousal, and orgasm. Paraphilias include Exhibitionism, Fetishism, Pedophilia, Sadism, and Masochism. These terms are defined more explicitly later in this section. DSM-IV also includes a third category, termed Gender Identity Disorder, which is considered briefly in this chapter.

Disorders of Sexual Functioning

The human sexual response typically occurs in four sequential stages: sexual interest or desire, sexual excitement, orgasm, and resolution. Sexual dysfunction may manifest itself as a disorder of interest or desire, a physical disorder of erection in men or vaginismus in women, a dysfunction in orgasmic response, or in men premature ejaculation and in women a painful response to intercourse. These dysfunctions correspond fairly closely to the stages of sexual response. Sexual dysfunctions may be entirely somatic—that is, have no discernible physical cause—or may clearly be the result of a physical disorder. Whatever their causation, as with most psychological conditions, a diagnosis of dysfunction or disorder is made only when the observed problem causes significant discomfort to the involved individual or couple. Many individuals report sexual "difficulties" that they integrate quite comfortably into their lives. In taking a sexual history, the nurse must be alert to the human responses of both accommodation and denial. Many individuals come to accept or accommodate aspects of their lives—including what might otherwise be termed sexual dysfunction—that would prove difficult for others to accept. For some, however, such accommodation really represents a form of denial: The problem actually is causing problems in personal life or relationships, but acknowledging this reality would prove too painful. Accommodation is usually a healthy response, whereas denial is generally dysfunctional. The nurse should not overlook the presence of denial, but she should be very careful to avoid challenging or threatening this psychological defense mechanism without a clear psychotherapeutic plan.

Disorders of desire. There is a wide variation in normal human sexual interest, and this variation is in turn influenced by a huge variety of extrapersonal factors, including age, health, leisure, and availability of potential partners. On occasion, disorders of sexual desire reflect other sexual disorders: If intercourse is painful, nonorgasmic, or consistently embarrassing (as with premature ejaculation), there will be decreased motivation to seek sexual opportunities. The San Francisco newspaper columnist Arthur Hoppe not infrequently found variations in human sexual interest to be apt subjects for his satirical humor:

Dr. Pettibone

Dr. Homer T. Pettibone is executive director of the United Anti-Sex Drive, a social-consciousness-raising organization. "Once again . . . we are appealing to sectarians of all faiths . . . to see sex for what it is. It is a monumental waste of time."

Dr. Pettibone said the most recent studies showed that Americans, who are not even French, devoted 3.2 hours per day—or 20 percent of their waking time—to thinking about, talking about, reading about, viewing depictions of, preparing for, attempting to avoid or indulging in (on fleeting occasions) sex.

"Any individual who renounces sex thereby immediately increases his or her overall efficiency 20 percent," he pointed out. "And that's seven days a week. Here at last is the secret to power, fame and fortune in one easy step."

Members of Dr. Pettibone's organization are only too eager to testify to the benefits of celibacy: "I was a poor, friendless $100-a-week stock clerk until I gave up sex," says Bert L. of Flint, Mich. "With the time I saved I was able to complete a correspondence course in accounting. I am now a bookkeeper for a large pet firm. Last year alone, I was able to embezzle $43,578 and two parakeets."*

(Hoppe, 1979, p. 35)

While Dr. Pettibone, Bert L., and the easy adoption of celibacy are probably equally products of Hoppe's imagination, his essay emphasizes the important interplay of sexual thoughts, sexual fantasies, and sexual desire. Outside of religious orders, relatively few people choose, like Bert L. of Flint, Mich., to purposefully renounce sex drive, and for some individuals with a disorder of sexual desire, an endocrinological dysfunction may contribute to symptoms. For example, elevations of the hormone prolactin—sometimes due to a small pituitary tumor—may greatly reduce libido or sexual interest. In both men and women, testosterone levels seem to be directly linked to sexual drive, and any process that leads to a reduction in testosterone, such as prolactin excess or "normal" aging, may decrease sexual interest. There is currently an increasing interest in androgen supplementation [most commonly testosterone and dihydroepiandrosterone sulfate (DHEAS)] to counteract the effects of aging on sexual function.

However, most persons with what DSM-IV terms **Hypoactive Sexual Desire Disorder** are not elderly and have no demonstrable hormonal abnormalities. The disorder is diagnosed when the affected individual reports significant distress or disturbance in interpersonal relationships and when the evaluating clinician assesses subjectively that sexual desire is truly less than would be normal for that individual. Because there is such a wide range of normal sexual interest, interpersonal difficulties often result when two sexual partners have significantly different levels of interest that are well within the normal

range. For instance, one partner may have an "excessive" interest or need for sexual expression. While the other partner's sexual desire may be completely normal, interpersonal difficulties arise from unwillingness (or inability) to meet unusually frequent sexual demands. The evaluating clinician must also be careful to ask about physical conditions, affective disorders, and, especially, substance use; each of these may have a significant effect on sexual desire.

Premature ejaculation. Premature Ejaculation is defined as male orgasm and ejaculation taking place with minimal physical stimulation and before it is expected or desired. Premature Ejaculation, one of the most common sexual dysfunctions, may cause significant psychological distress for both sexual partners. Because there are no standards for the duration of any of the four stages of sexual functioning, Premature Ejaculation has to be defined subjectively. Almost all men experience significant variability in the length of time between arousal and ejaculation; in general, that time is shortest in youth, with a new partner, under situations of poor privacy, and after relatively long sexual abstinence. It is not unusual for any of a variety of circumstances to lead to relatively brief and self-limited episodes of premature ejaculation. A disorder of Premature Ejaculation should be defined only when the complaint is persistent, psychologically troublesome, and not due to a chemical substance (some medications and opioid withdrawal can occasionally be causes).

For many men, the reassurance of a normal examination is sufficient to relieve an episode of premature ejaculation. As with other sexual disorders, there is often an element of ongoing anxiety about performance that can respond to brief counseling. Often, this counseling can involve the sexual partner, who may not have a complete understanding of the frequently self-limited nature of this disorder. The use of condoms may somewhat decrease physical sensation and moderately prolong the time between penetration and ejaculation. In many circumstances, especially when symptoms have been prolonged and particularly troublesome, specialized evaluation and treatment are indicated. Often reflecting the work of the sexual therapists Masters and Johnson, sexual counselors have developed fairly standardized protocols for the management of common disorders of sexual functioning, including premature ejaculation. Confronted with a client whose symptoms do not readily respond to reassurance, the nurse should urge consultation with an experienced sex therapist.

Paraphilias

Sexuality is such a private part of human life that most persons know very little about unusual sexual behavior. Some paraphilias and their definitions are found in the display on the following page; selected paraphilias are discussed in the following box.

---

*From A. Hoppe, April 17, 1979, © *San Francisco Chronicle*, p. 35. Reprinted with permission.

PARAPHILIAS

- **Exhibitionism:** Exposing one's genitals to a stranger. This exposure may actually occur or it may be only a sexually exciting fantasy.

- **Fetishism:** Sexual arousal occurring from contact with a nonliving object, often an article of clothing. Individuals with fetishism often cannot achieve sexual excitement without the presence of such objects.

- **Frotteurism:** Recurrent sexual touching of a nonconsenting individual, usually a stranger and usually in a crowded public place.

- **Pedophilia:** Sexual interests directed primarily or exclusively toward children. As with other paraphilias, there may only be recurrent fantasies or urges but no abnormal behavior.

- **Sexual Masochism:** Sexual excitement resulting from being the recipient of physical suffering. Masochistic individuals may overtly seek out forms of physical abuse (commonly by asking to be beaten, bound, or otherwise physically humiliated) or they may only fantasize about such experiences.

- **Sexual Sadism:** Sexual excitement resulting from fantasizing about or participating in the infliction of suffering on others. In its extreme forms, Sexual Sadism may result in severe injury or even death.

- **Voyeurism:** Observing or fantasizing about observing others disrobing, naked, or involved in sexual activity.

- **Transvestic Fetishism:** Cross dressing or fantasies about cross dressing; usually a male dressing in women's clothes. Transvestic Fetishism varies from the wearing of a single inconspicuous item of clothing to complete cross dressing.

- **Other paraphilias:** Urophilia (fascination with urine and urination), necrophilia (real or fantasized sexual interests in the dead), zoophilia (sexual involvement with animals), and telephonic scatologia (sexual excitement from obscene telephone calls).

Exhibitionism. Many women have, at some time in their lives, been confronted by Exhibitionism, or a male exposing himself. When asked to describe the sexual excitement deriving from their behavior, some exhibitionists describe a desire to shock their victims, whereas others

fantasize that their displays will result in sexual interest. Exhibitionism rarely results in any response other than fear or disgust, and most exhibitionists do not pursue their sexual overtures more aggressively. Rape, for example, almost never results from an exhibitionistic encounter. Unless arrested, few exhibitionists come to professional attention, and outside a forensic setting, few nurses will come into clinical contact with this paraphilia.

Transvestic Fetishism. In recent years, cross dressing has been sympathetically portrayed in popular films. *The Crying Game* (1992) featured a homosexual transvestite who astonishes both the movie's hero and audience by revealing his male identity. While some homosexuals do dress as women, individuals with Transvestic Fetishism are more commonly heterosexual males. The movie *Ed Wood* (1994) offers a convincing view of Transvestic Fetishism. In this film, Ed Wood (a real-life 1950s novelist and director of low-budget films) is sympathetically portrayed as an otherwise normal heterosexual who is possessed by the desire to wear women's clothing. Rudolph Grey's biography of Ed Wood includes lengthy interviews with Wood's wife, Kathy, and with numerous Hollywood actors and friends:

Nightmare of Ecstasy

KATHY WOOD: When he was a kid growing up in Poughkeepsie, he was always interested in the movies, especially the westerns. . . . Eddie told me that his mother did dress him as a girl when he was two, three or four, So maybe she's responsible. . . . He didn't embarrass me too much with it . . . it was kind of a put-on half the time. . . . And nobody took offense at it. Nobody at all.

JOE ROBERTSON: We were both in the Marine Corps, he was in the invasion of Tarawa. 4000 Marines went in. . . . 400 came out. He was one of the 400. He was wearing pink panties and a pink bra underneath his battle fatigues. And he said to me, "Thank God Joe I got out, because I wanted to be killed. I didn't want to be wounded because I could never explain my pink panties and pink bra." . . .

DOLORES FULLER: Ed knew Danny Kaye, who was also a transvestite. . . . And he'd [Wood] say he could write much better if he could wear my angora sweater. He would work for hours, sitting there, saying that it felt good. . . .

HARRY THOMAS: . . . Ed said, "Harry, come over and pick up the script." So he gave me the address, I went over there and knocked on the *door. This beautifully dressed person comes to the door. Polished nails, hair all grown down. I said, "Oh, I beg your pardon, is your brother home?" "You mean Eddie?" "Yes, Eddie, is he home?" She says, "Oh, come in and have a cup of tea, he'll be here in a little while." I sat there, and she poured me a cup of tea, she was prancing around and changing garments, the ermine coat, all this, and I said, "I'm getting a little perturbed. I have a lot of appointments, do you think he'll be very much longer?" She says, "Oh, no, he'll be here soon." Suddenly, she comes out of a sliding door, and says, "I am Ed Wood."**

(Gray, 1992, pp. 16–42)

Other films with significant cross-dressing scenes include *Paris is Burning* (1991), a documentary about New York City transvestite dances; *Philadelphia* (1993); and *Just One of the Girls* (1993). The last of these describes a high school student who cross dresses to avoid a run-in with the neighborhood tough. In his female guise he meets, and eventually wins the heart of, the school's prettiest girl. *Just One of the Girls* effectively conveys one of the major characteristics of Transvestic Fetishism: the common onset of this disorder in adolescence. Cross dressing often begins in private, and, as in *Ed Wood* and *Just One of the Girls*, the individual does not "come out" publically until late adolescence or young adulthood. For some cross dressers, the involved articles of clothing are erotic fetishes —sources of sexual excitement. However, as both *Ed Wood* and *Nightmare of Ecstasy* convincingly show, the wearing of female clothing is frequently experienced as more a source of emotional comfort.

While, like Ed Wood, most persons with Transvestic Fetishism are fully comfortable as social and sexual males, occasional cross-dressing individuals do develop a strong desire to live as a female. DSM-IV categorizes these persons—some of whom may eventually seek sex changing surgery—as **gender dysphoric**. Whether or not they are comfortable with their genetic gender assignment, transvestic fetishists may find illness and hospitalization particularly distressing. Like Marine Corporal Ed Wood at age 18, cross dressers may fear discovery if they are injured or become ill: "I didn't want to be wounded because I could never explain my pink panties and pink bra." Worse, they may fear the hospital as a place where cross dressing, an important source of comfort, can be neither acknowledged nor practiced. A thorough history can help the nurse recognize a client's special needs for comforting objects or clothing.

**From *Nightmares of Ecstasy: The Life and Art of Edward D. Wood, Jr.*, by R. Gray, 1994, Portland, OR: Feral House Press. Reprinted with permission.*

Sexual Sadism and Sexual Masochism. Sexual Sadism is defined as persistent fantasies or behaviors involving the infliction of suffering on others. Sexual Masochism is a reciprocal disorder in which fantasies and/or behaviors involve being the recipient of physical abuse or humiliation. The word *sadism* derives from the family name of Donatien-Alphonse-François de Sade, whose sexual exploits and writings led to his lengthy imprisonment in 18th-century France and, ever since, to his great notoriety as a writer and exemplar of evil. Sade's multiple imprisonments were for debt, attempted poisoning, and sodomy (until the present century, a serious crime throughout Europe). He had also been accused but not convicted of beating, cutting, and otherwise abusing prostitutes. Released from the Bastille during the French Revolution, he narrowly escaped a death sentence, was finally rejailed in 1801, and was committed to a mental institution 2 years later. Apparently quite sane but regarded as a serious moral menace, he remained comfortably housed in this asylum until his death in 1814 —"helping to stage plays which the hospital's director regarded as a form of therapy" (de Sade/D. Coward trans., 1992, p. xv). There is little in the historical record to prove that Sade's actual behavior was particularly vicious, and he claimed as much in a letter to his wife (whose family had aggressively sought his imprisonment):

Yes, I am a libertine, I admit it freely. I have dreamed of doing everything that it is possible to dream of in that line. But I most certainly have not done all the things I dreamt of and never shall.

(de Sade/D. Coward. trans., 1992, p. xvii)

Whatever his actual behavior, Sade's writings were, and remain, profoundly shocking in their imaginings of sexual violence. The *Misfortunes of Virtue* was written while he was imprisoned in the Bastille and is far less "sadistic" than much of his later work. Part of the plot involves a young servant woman, Sophie, who is falsely accused of murdering the woman for whom she works. The victim's son, the real murderer, surprises Sophie in the woods, ties her to a tree, and assisted by friends proceeds to punish her for his mother's murder. Sade's writing combines murder, bondage, flagellation, and a fascination with the victim's suffering. These are the elements of sadism, and even if Sade had "most certainly . . . not done all the things [he] dreamt of," others at that time and since have both fantasized and enacted scenes of sexual sadism.

Sadism and masochism are often combined in the same individual. One of the most striking sadomasochists of recent times was Percy Grainger, a famous pianist and composer who died in 1961:

Grainger was one of the eccentrics of music —a gangling figure with an aquiline face and a formidable mop of hair; a vegetarian; a health

faddist; a man who likely as not would hike from
concert to concert with a knapsack on his back,
and a whale of a pianist. . . . Grainger was one
of the most gifted pianists of the century . . . who
forged his own style and expressed it with amazing
skill, personality and vigor.

(Schonberg, 1992, pp. 12–13)

Unlike Sade, whose sadism probably expressed itself primarily with prostitutes and in his imagination, Grainger seems to have confined his sadomasochistic behavior to ongoing relationships, including his 33-year marriage. In his will, Grainger directed "that the flesh be removed from my bones and the flesh destroyed" (Bird, 1976, p. 248). This dying request (never granted) symbolized much of his behavior in life:

> *Grainger liked to flagellate himself or to be*
> *beaten by another. . . . These acts were obsessively*
> *documented in his letters to his lover, the pianist*
> *Karen Holten (with whom he seems also to have*
> *enjoyed normal sexual relations) . . . in reality he*
> *practised such monstrosities on himself, branding*
> *his own nipple with a hot key and forcing needles*
> *through his breasts.*
>
> *(B. Morton in T. P. Lewis, pp. 33–34)*

Grainger's sadomasochism appears to have been confined to relationships with consenting partners. There seems no evidence that either he or his several partners were ever seriously injured or that he imposed his sexual preferences on others without due warning. Long before their marriage, for example, his wife-to-be received a lengthy letter detailing his sexual appetites and fascinations: "Despite many statements to the contrary, [she] did walk into wedlock fully aware of Grainger's lust for bizarre, even brutal sex acts" (Gillies & Pear, 1994, pp. 94–100).

It is likely that some individuals express Sexual Sadism or Sexual Masochism only in fantasy. For others, pornography may be a vehicle for such sexual drives. Yet others may find themselves subject to sadistic or masochistic urges that they strive to repress; some of these individuals may seek therapy and in this manner come to clinical attention. Others may become the perpetrators of sexual crimes on nonconsenting victims. While the majority of sexual sadists are probably harmless—like Sade, expressing themselves more in fantasy than in reality—there is no doubt that some sadistic individuals represent very dangerous risks to society. Psychiatrists and psychiatric nurses may play a role in evaluating the societal risk posed by sadistic individuals who have committed sex crimes. This task is exceedingly

difficult and risks wrongly imprisoning a person who *may* pose little risk of perpetrating serious harm. There is limited evidence that Sexual Sadism can be modified by treatment, and for some individuals, lengthy incarceration may be society's best protection against dangerous behavior. When such behavior results in harm to others, and when there is little motivation for change, incarceration may offer the only hope of preventing catastrophe.

The average nurse is relatively unlikely to be involved in ongoing treatment of these individuals, many of whom will be treated in specialist or forensic psychiatric units. It is important to recognize that paraphilic behavior often seems bizarre, repulsive, "perverted," and physically and morally offensive. It is not wrong for the nurse to be shocked or offended by the behavior of some individuals. Sadism, particularly when directed against nonconsenting victims, is revolting, as is child sexual abuse, sometimes an accompaniment of Pedophilia. Occasionally, paraphilias seem quite harmless and even of some social value as stimuli to artistic creativity. For example, while the idea of Pedophilia is deeply disturbing to most adults, it is well to remember that one of this era's most popular books, *Alice in Wonderland*, was written by Charles Dodgson (pen name, Lewis Carroll), a shy bachelor whose passion was to befriend young girls and photograph them nude (Cohen, 1979).

We do not yet know what causes some individuals to act criminally, aggressively, or *evilly*, but as an editorialist for the *Lancet* observed, perhaps in the not distant future "evil . . . may even prove reversible" (Anonymous, 1996, p. 1). In pursuit of such a potentially optimistic vision, one of humankind's goals must be to identify and, where possible, to correct the genetic, social, and psychological antecedents of evil behavior. Our survival as a society requires no less.

As with many other psychological disorders manifesting primarily as unusual behavior, the cause of paraphilias remains unknown. Psychoanalytic theory traces Fetishism and cross dressing to severe castration anxiety during the oedipal phase of early childhood, with the chosen object replacing the missing penis. Other explanations for paraphilias also focus on early childhood experiences and evoke pleasurable reactions to early cross dressing or sexual encounters with other children as sources of subsequent transvestism or Pedophilia (Becker & Kavoussi, 1994). Ed Wood's wife suggested a similar etiology for his cross dressing: "his mother did dress him as a girl when he was two, three or four, So maybe she's responsible." These conditions are very deeply a part of the individual's self image, probably indeed implying an origin in early childhood. While insight-oriented psychotherapy has occasionally proven effective with paraphilias, programs that combine behaviorally oriented counseling with appropriate pharmacological interventions may be the most effective (Marshall, Jones, Ward, Johnston, & Barbaree, 1991).

Other Disorders

DSM-IV recognizes **Gender Identity Disorder**, a condition in which an individual feels him- or herself to be a member of the opposite sex and desires gender change, as a psychiatric disorder. Homosexuality is not defined as a disorder because it has become clear that a psychiatric disorder, by definition, requires that the individual experi-ence some degree of personal, vocational, or social dys-function. However, there are some individuals who have difficulty in accepting their sexual orientation, whether it be heterosexual or homosexual; these persons do qualify for a sexual disorder diagnosis, but only on the basis of their distress. Sexual and Gender Identity Disorders imply marked, persistent distress about sexual orientation.

N U R S I N G   P R O C E S S

No matter where the nurse works in clinical practice, she will encounter individuals in various states of sexual dysfunction or disorder. It is the nurse's role to support clients in their quest for physical and emotional health, and this most certainly includes sexual health. All aspects of human sexuality can be affected by illness or injury, and illness or injury may cause a change in perception of self or in participation in sexual activity (Lubkin, 1990).

Should any of the diagnoses of sexual disorders discussed in this chapter be uncovered, the nurse will function in a collaborative role and will refer the client to a sex therapist or other specialist. In other cases, however, assessment will indicate that the client has neither a dysfunction nor a disorder but, rather, wishes to discuss a sexual concern. The nurse will be able to provide an empathic under-standing of the issues raised and relay needed information.

▽ ASSESSMENT

The nursing role is to identify in conjunction with the client whether a dysfunction or disorder exists and to refer to the most appropriate resource for the client's care.

▽ NURSING DIAGNOSIS

The nursing diagnosis of *altered sexuality patterns* has been defined as the state in which an "individual expresses concern regarding his/her sexuality" (NANDA,

---

DEFINITIONS AND PROPOSED DEFINING CHARACTERISTICS OF THE NURSING DIAGNOSIS ALTERED SEXUALITY PATTERNS

DEFINITION

The state in which an individual expresses concern regarding his or her sexuality

DEFINING CHARACTERISTICS

1. Men

- Inability to have or sustain an erection

- Problems with ejaculation

- Decreased desire for sexual activities

- Lack of sensation

- Confusion about sexual preference

- Concerns about changes in relationships

- Concerns about changes in roles

- Concerns about how one appears to others

- Feelings of being different

2. Women

- Decreased desire for sexual activities

- Inability to have an orgasm

- Concerns about changes in relationships

- Concerns about how one appears to others

- Fear of pain with intercourse

- Confusion about sexual preference

- Concerns about changes in rules

- Fear of becoming pregnant

- Fear of reproductive infection

- Decreased vaginal lubrication

- Lack of sensation

- Lack of privacy

- Fear of vaginal infection

- Pain with movement

- Fatigue

- Feelings of being different

From "Validating Gender-Specific Defining Characteristics of Altered Sexuality," by P. LeMone and J. Weber, 1995, *Nursing Diagnosis,* 6, pp. 64–69.

1996, p. 47). It has been difficult for nurses to differenti-ate this diagnosis from the general diagnosis of *sexual dysfunction.* One researcher has suggested that one diag-nosis, *altered sexuality patterns,* be used by nurses to encompass both a change in sexual patterns and the con-cerns related to that change (LeMone, 1993). Further, LeMone has conducted a gender-specific validation study of the meaning of the new, proposed nursing diagnosis of *altered sexuality patterns.* The display on the previous page presents both the definitions and defining charac-teristics of these diagnoses. These defining characteristics represent the consensus definitions of *altered sexuality patterns* and provide a basis for nurses to plan general nursing care.

 OUTCOME IDENTIFICATION

The nurse planning independent nursing care for the client with *altered sexuality patterns* will identify outcomes with the client. For example, if a client wishes to discuss

a sexual concern, the outcome will be that the client was given opportunity to discuss and reflect on his sexuality.

 PLANNING/INTERVENTIONS

Nursing theories that provide for unconditional accep-tance and support may prove most helpful in guiding nursing care, as issues of a sexual nature will rarely be dis-cussed in situations other than those of complete trust. The most commonly used nursing intervention for the diagno-sis of *altered sexuality patterns* is active listening.

 EVALUATION

Individuals who present with a psychiatric diagnosis of sexual disorder will require referral to a psychiatrist, psychologist, or sex therapist. Therefore, in addition to knowledge of sexual health and dysfunction, it is essen-tial that the nurse have knowledge of the identified sex-ual disorders. Follow-up with other health care team members will help ensure continuity of care.

CASE STUDY/CARE PLAN

Ken is an 18-year-old man. He comes to see a nurse for an employment physical. In the process of taking a general nursing history, the nurse asks ques-tions related to sexual health. Specifically, she asks Ken if he is sexually active and if he has any concerns over matters of sexual health. Ken responds that, indeed, he does have some concerns. He describes having ambivalence over his sexual preferences; he has had a personal history of both heterosexual and homosexual encounters. He is not sure which is more comfortable for him. He feels pressured to decide what

his preferences are. He discloses that he has always been somewhat "preoccupied" with academic and work successes, so that he has had somewhat limited social interactions. He does not feel that he has a strong sexual drive and states he has never had any-one with whom he could discuss these issues. His fam-ily includes parents (married and living together), two brothers who are both heterosexual, and one young sister who is 11 years old. Ken believes that no one in his family would either understand or support his exploring his sexual concerns.

NURSING DIAGNOSIS *Altered sexuality patterns,* related to conflicts with sexual orientation, as evidenced by reported concerns over sexual behaviors and activities

Outcomes	Planning/Interventions	Evaluation
Client will explore his own sexuality and will reflect on issues to gain insight regarding his uncomfortable feelings.	◆ Let the client know that the nurse is willing to talk about these matters as a professional. Make sure he knows that all discussions are/will be confiden-tial and that the nurse can assist him in exploring his concerns and his feelings.	Ken returned to talk with the nurse for three appointments. He talked freely only after the first meeting. He disclosed that he had felt pressure from peers and his par-ents to declare his sexual preference and that he believed that sexuality was not as important to him as it seemed to be to
	◆ Make an appointment for Ken to talk with the nurse the following week.	
	◆ Provide a safe environment where Ken can describe his very personal, sexual concerns in the presence of a caring professional.	

Continued

Outcomes	**Planning/Interventions**	**Evaluation**
	◆ Encourage Ken to discuss his sexuality as well as his relationships with others in both a social and a sexual sense.	others. He stated he did not need to deal with these issues with the nurse again, although he was grateful for the opportunity to explore them. He stated he felt much less anxious about his sexuality at this time.
	◆ Help Ken understand where the "pressure to decide" on his personal sexual preferences is coming from.	

CRITICAL THINKING BAND

ASSESSMENT

Do you feel that Ken's current sexual status needs further exploration? Does it seem worthwhile to assess other aspects of his life as well?

NURSING DIAGNOSIS

Is this the correct diagnosis? Could you make another diagnosis based on the information you have been given?

Outcomes	**Planning/Interventions**	**Evaluation**
Is it appropriate to have as an outcome that the client will explore something rather than that the client will do something? Why or why not?	Should the nurse be thinking of something else?	Is this client ready to terminate sessions with the nurse? Have the nurse and client achieved a good outcome?

≋ KEY CONCEPTS

◆ Sleep occurs in five stages, with marked individual variation in time spent in each sleep cycle. Stage 5 sleep is rapid-eye-movement (REM) sleep, during which dreams occur.

◆ Insomnia is a psychiatric problem when it lasts 1 month or longer and leads to impairment of functioning.

◆ Older persons experience changing of their sleep patterns and are at risk for insomnia.

◆ Sleep hygiene techniques are useful in treating insomnia.

◆ Persons with Primary Hypersomnia should not engage in activities where a sleep attack could pose a threat to self or others (such as driving).

◆ Parasomnias include nightmares, sleep terrors, and sleepwalking.

◆ Eating disorders of bulimia and anorexia are often complicated by a concurrent diagnosis of depression, low self-esteem, and the client's strong denial of the problem.

◆ Care of clients with eating disorders includes nutritional rehabilitation, psychotherapy, maintenance, and follow-up.

◆ Sexuality is part of each person's personality and influences how each person views self and presents self to others.

◆ Sexual dysfunction is a state in which a person experiences a change in sexual function that he or she views as unsatisfying, unrewarding, or inadequate.

◆ A client's sexual history includes sexual functioning; sexual thoughts, fantasies, and behaviors; and sexual preferences.

◆ There are two categories of sexual disorders: disorders of sexual functioning and paraphilias.

◆ The nursing role in sexual disorders/paraphilias is most often one of assessment and referral.

〰 REVIEW QUESTIONS AND ACTIVITIES

1. How would you assess the adequacy of sleep/rest and activity for a person in a nursing home?

2. Present a sleep hygiene regimen for your 60-year-old home health client whom you are following for hypertension.

3. What are the day-to-day risks for a person suffering from Hypersomnia?

4. How would you tell the mother of 4-year-old Joey to support him during the time he is experiencing night terrors?

5. What can you do as a nurse regarding primary prevention of Bulimia Nervosa and Anorexia Nervosa?

6. What nursing diagnosis/interventions are likely present/appropriate for clients with eating disorders?

7. How does a nurse balance her roles to "monitor food intake" and to build trust with an anorexic client?

8. Define *altered sexuality patterns*, sexual dysfunction, and sexual disorder.

9. Examine your own feelings, attitudes, and beliefs about sexual expression and appropriate sexuality. What will you do when you encounter a client with views quite different from your own?

⚛ EXPLORING THE WEB

◆ Visit this text's "Online Companion™" on the Internet at **http://www.DelmarNursing.com** for further information on disorders of self-regulation.

◆ Search specific key terms such as bulimia nervosa, anorexia nervosa, narcolepsy, insomnia, paraphilia, sadism, and fetishism; what information can you find?

◆ What sites could you recommend to families who are looking for self-help, chat rooms, or other electronic information sources?

◆ Is there a listing on the Internet of books, videos, or other media on disorders of self-regulation? Are these resources available in your local library or through purchase over the Web?

〰 REFERENCES

Agras, S. (1987). *Eating disorders*. New York: Pergamon.

American Psychiatric Association. (1994). *Diagnostic and statistical manual* (4th ed.). Washington, DC: Author.

Anonymous. (1996). Pandora and the problem of evil. *The Lancet, 347*, 1.

Becker, J.V., & Kavoussi, R. J. (1994). Sexual and gender identity disorders. In R. E. Hales, S. C. Yudofsky, & J. A. Talbott (Eds.), *The American Psychiatric Press textbook of psychiatry* (2nd ed., pp. 666–667). Washington DC: American Psychiatric Association.

Braun, C. M., & Chouinard, M. J. (1992). Is anorexia nervosa a neuropsychological disease? *Neuropsychological Review, 3*, 171–212.

Bruch, H. (1973). *Eating disorders*. New York: Basic Books.

Bruch, H. (1978). *The golden cage: The enigma of anorexia nervosa*. Cambridge, MA: Harvard University Press.

Cahill, C. (1994). Implementing an inpatient eating disorders program. *Perspectives in Psychiatric Care, 30*, 26–29.

Chipkevitch, E. (1994). Brain tumors and anorexia nervosa syndrome. *Brain and Development, 16*, 175–179, 180–182.

Chitty, K. K. (1991). The primary prevention role of nurse in eating disorders. *Nursing Clinics of North America, 26*, 789–800.

Crow, S. J., & Mitchell, J. E. (1994). Rational therapy of eating disorders. *Drugs, 48*, 372–379.

Eckert, E. D., Halmi, K. A., Marchi, P., Grove, W., & Crosby, R. (1994). Ten-year follow-up of anorexia nervosa: Clinical course and outcome. *Psychological Medicine, 25*, 143–156.

Freund, K. M., Graham, S. M., Lesky, L. G., & Moskowitz, M. A. (1993). Detection of bulimia in a primary care setting. *Journal of General Internal Medicine, 8*, 236–242.

Goldstein, B. (1976). *Human sexuality*. New York: McGraw Hill.

Gull, W. W. (1868). The address in medicine delivered before the annual meeting of the British Medical Association, at Oxford. *Lancet, 2* , 171–176.

Hoek, H. W. (1991). The incidence and prevalence of anorexia nervosa and bulimia nervosa in primary care. *Psychological Medicine, 21*, 455–460.

Irwin, E. G. (1993). A focused overview of anorexia and bulimia. *Archives of Psychiatric Nursing, 7*, 347–352.

Joughin, N. A., Crisp, A. H., Gowers, S. G., & Bhat, A. V. (1991). The clinical features of late onset anorexia nervosa. *Postgraduate Medical Journal, 67*, 973–977.

Kollai, M., Bonyhay, I., Jokkel, G., & Szonyi, L. (1994). Cardiac vagal hyperactivity in adolescent anorexia nervosa. *European Heart Journal, 15*, 1113–1118.

Langer, L. M., Warheit, G. J., & Zimmerman, R. S. (1991). Epidemiological study of problem eating behaviors and related attitudes in the general population. *Addictive Behaviors, 16*, 67–73.

LeMone, P. (1993). Validation of the defining characteristics of *altered sexuality patterns. Nursing Diagnosis, 4*, 56–62.

LeMone, P., & Weber, J. (1995). Validating gender-specific defining characteristics of *altered sexuality. Nursing Diagnosis, 6*, 64–69.

Love, C. C., & Seaton, H. (1991). Eating disorders: Highlights of nursing assessment and therapeutics. *Nursing Clinics of North America, 26*, 677–697.

Lubkin, I. (1990). *Chronic illness: Impact and interventions*. Boston: Jones and Bartlett.

Marshall, W. L., Jones, R., Ward, T., Johnston, P., & Barbaree, R. E. (1991). Treatment outcome with sex offenders. *Clinical Psychology Review, 11*, 465–485.

Myer, S. A., & O'Brien, A. (1993). Multisystem complications of bulimia: A critical care case. *Dimensions of Critical Care Nursing, 12*, 194–203.

National Institutes of Health (NIH). (1990). *The treatment of sleep disorders of older people*. NIH Consensus Statement, March 26–28, 8(3), 1–22. Bethesda, MD: Author.

North American Nursing Diagnosis Association (NANDA). (1996). *Nursing diagnosis: Definitions and classification 1997–1998.* Philadelphia: Author.

Okabe, K. (1993). Assessment of emaciation in relation to threat to life in anorexia nervosa. *Internal Medicine, 32,* 837–842.

Palmer, T. A. (1990). Anorexia nervosa, bulimia nervosa: Causal theories and treatment. *Nurse Practitioner, 15,* 12, 14–16, 18, 21.

Pope, H. G., & Hudson, J. I. (1989). Eating disorders. In H. I. Kaplan & B. J. Sadock (Eds.), *Comprehensive textbook of psychiatry* (20th ed., pp. 1854–1864). Baltimore, MD: Williams & Wilkins.

Powers, P. S., & Powers, H. P. (1984). Inpatient treatment of anorexia nervosa. *Psychosomatics, 25,* 512–527.

Pyle, R. L., Mitchell, J. E., & Eckert, E. D., Hatsukami, D., Pomeroy, C., & Zimmerman, R. (1990). Maintenance treatment and 6-month outcome for bulimic patients who respond to initial treatment. *American Journal of Psychiatry, 147,* 871–887.

Rastam, M., & Gillberg, C. (1991). The family background in anorexia nervosa: A population-based study. *Journal of the American Academy of Child and Adolescent Psychiatry, 30,* 238–239.

Remschmidt, H., Wienand, F., & Wewetzer, C. (1990). The long-term course of anorexia nervosa. In H. Remschmidt & M. Schmidt (Eds.), *Anorexia nervosa* (pp. 127–136). Toronto: Hogrefe & Huber.

Roseborough, G. S., & Felix, W. A. (1994). Disseminated intravascular coagulation complicating gastric perforation in a bulimic woman. *Canadian Journal of Surgery, 37,* 55–58.

Salisbury, J. J., & Mitchell, J. E. (1991). Bone mineral density and anorexia nervosa in women. *American Journal of Psychiatry, 148,* 768–777.

Strober M. (1991). Family-genetic studies of eating disorders. *Journal of Clinical Psychiatry, 52*(Suppl.), 9–12.

Study Group on Anorexia Nervosa. (1995). Anorexia nervosa: Directions for future research. *Journal of Eating Disorders, 17,* 235–241.

Sullivan, P. F. (1995). Mortality in anorexia nervosa. *American Journal of Psychiatry, 152,* 1073–1074.

Thiel, A., Broocks, A., Ohlmeier, M., Jacoby, G. I., & Schussler, G. (1995). Obsessive-compulsive disorder among patients with anorexia nervosa and bulimia nervosa. *American Journal of Psychiatry, 152,* 72–75.

Treasure, J., & Holland, A. (1990). Genetic vulnerability to eating disorders: Evidence from twin and family studies. In H. Remschmidt & M. H. Schmidt (Eds.), *Anorexia nervosa* (pp. 59–68). Toronto: Hogrefe & Huber.

Vanderycken, W., & Van Deth, R. (1994). *From fasting saints to anorexic girls.* New York: New York University Press.

Walfish, S., Stenmark, D. E., Sarco, D., Shealy, J. S., & Krone, A. M. (1992). Incidence of bulimia in substance misusing women in residential treatment. *International Journal of the Addictions, 27,* 425–433.

Warheit, G. J., Langer, L. M., Zimmerman, R. S., & Biafora, F. A. (1993). Prevalence of bulimic behaviors and bulimia among a sample of the general population. *American Journal of Epidemiology, 137,* 569–576.

Wilson, C. P., Hogan, C. C., & Mintz, I. L. (1985). *Fear of being fat: The treatment of anorexia nervosa and bulimia.* New York: Jason Aronson.

Wilson, G. T. (1995). Psychological treatment of binge eating and bulimia nervosa. *Journal of Mental Health, 4,* 451–457.

≋ LITERARY REFERENCES

Benedict, R. (1974). *The chrysanthemum and the sword.* New York: New American Library.

Bird, J. (1976). *Percy Grainger.* London: Paul Elek.

Calisher, H. (1982). The scream on Fifty-seventh Street. In J. C. Oates (Ed.), *Night walks: A bedside companion* (p. 40). Princeton: Ontario Review Press.

Cohen, M. N. (1979). *Lewis Carroll, photography of children.* Philadelphia: Rosenbach Foundation and Clarkson W. Potter, Inc. Publishers.

Dekker, T. (1982). On sleep. In J. C. Oates (Ed.), *Night walks: A bedside companion* (p. 138). Princeton: Ontario Review Press.

Dickens, C. (1982). Night walks. In J. C. Oates (Ed.), *Night walks: A bedside companion* (pp. 3–12). Princeton: Ontario Review Press.

Dickens, C. (1969). *The posthumous papers of the Pickwick Club.* New York: Oxford University Press.

Gillies, M., & Pear, D. (1994). *The all-round man: Selected papers of Percy Grainger, 1914–1961.* London: Clarendon Press.

Gray, R. (1994). *Nightmares of ecstasy: The life and art of Edward D. Wood, Jr.* Portland, OR: Feral House.

Hoppe, A. (1979). *The San Francisco Chronicle,* April 17, p. 35.

Mishkin, J. (1982). Insomnia. In J. C. Oates (Ed.), *Night walks: A bedside companion* (pp. 251–252). Princeton: Ontario Review Press.

Morton, B. (1992). To half fight nature: Percy Grainger. In T. P. Lewis (Ed.), *A source guide to the music of Percy Grainger* (pp. 32–37). White Plains, NY: ProAM Music Resources.

O'Neill, S. B. (1982). *Starving for attention.* New York: Continuum.

Sade, Marquis de. (1992). *The misfortune of virtue, and other early tales* (D. Coward, Trans./Ed.). Oxford: Oxford University Press.

Schonberg, H. C. (1992). Percy Grainger. In T. P. Lewis (Ed.), *A source guide to the music of Percy Grainger* (pp. 12–13). White Plains, NY: ProAM Music Resources.

Vanderycken, W., & Van Deth, R. (1994). *From fasting saints to anorexic girls.* New York: New York University Press.

≋ SUGGESTED READINGS

Antrobus, J. S. (Ed.). (1992). *The neuropsychology of sleep and dreaming.* Hillsdale, NJ: Erlbaum.

Hesse-Biber, S. J. (1996). *Am I thin enough yet?: The cult of thinness and the commercialization of identity.* New York: Oxford University Press.

Monk, T. H. (Ed.). (1991). *Sleep, sleepiness, and performance.* Chichester, England: Wiley.

Poorman, S. G. (1988). *Human sexuality and the nursing process.* New York: Appleton and Lange.

Stumkard, A. J., & Baum, A. (Eds.). (1989). *Eating, sleeping, and sex.* Hillsdale, NJ: Erlbaum.

Thompson, S. B. N. (1993). *Eating disorders: A guide for health professionals.* London: Chapman and Hall.

Wincz, J. P., & Carey, M. P. (1991). *Sexual dysfunction.* New York: Guilford.

Unit

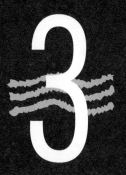

SPECIAL POPULATIONS

What are the psychological challenges facing physically ill persons? Why should we be concerned about the mental health needs of persons in jail? Do children and adolescents have unique mental health concerns? How can the nurse recognize elderly people suffering from Alzheimer's disease? Violence continues to be a daily experience of many individuals, especially women and youth. What are the mental health implications of our culture of violence?

These questions reflect the content of the six chapters on *Special Populations.*

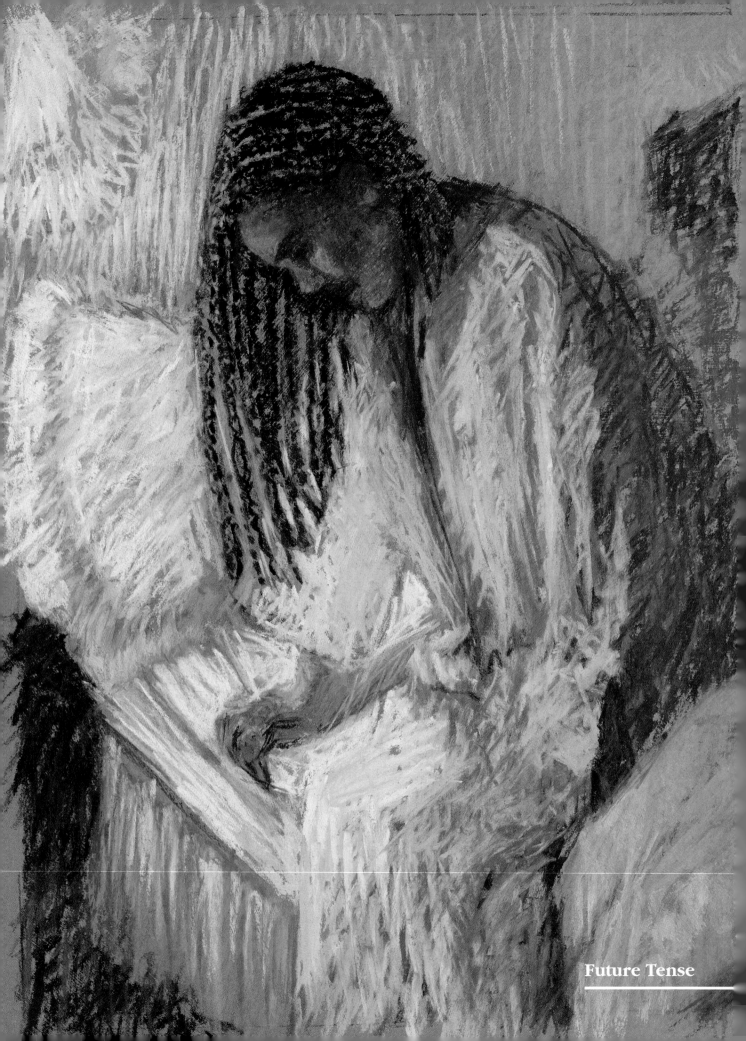

Future Tense

Chapter

19

THE PHYSICALLY ILL CLIENT EXPERIENCING EMOTIONAL DISTRESS

Noreen Cavan Frisch

Lawrence E. Frisch

Physical Illness and Emotional Health

Think about a time when you were physically ill, particularly a time when your illness was serious or lasted a long time. How did your physical illness affect your emotions and mood?

Did you experience any of the following?
◆ Fear
◆ Shame
◆ Guilt
◆ Depression
◆ Anger
◆ Loneliness

Most nurses today recognize the connection between body and mind. When there is a physical illness, one can expect effects on emotions or mood, and these effects may have an impact on prognosis for recovery from the physical illness.

In this chapter, we will explore the sometimes dramatic emotional outcomes of physical illnesses, to provide you with heightened awareness of your clients' needs for psychological support.

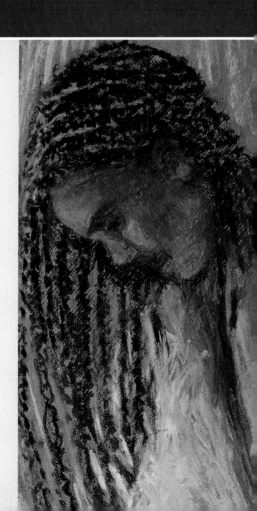

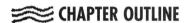 **CHAPTER OUTLINE**

IMPACT OF EMOTIONS ON HEALTH

DSM-IV AND PHYSICAL ILLNESS

PSYCHOLOGICAL RESPONSES TO PHYSICAL ILLNESS

Cancer

Cardiovascular Disease

Chronic Pain

Movement and Neurological Disorders

FAMILY RESPONSES TO SIGNIFICANT ILLNESS

NURSING ROLES

Liaison Psychiatric Nursing

Psychiatric Home Care

NURSING THEORY

PSYCHIATRIC NURSING AND MIND-BODY MEDICINE

Psychoneuroimmunology

FUTURE DIRECTIONS

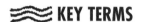 **COMPETENCIES**

Upon completion of this chapter, the reader should be able to:

1. Identify those situations where a physical illness produces emotional stress to the point where a client may present with psychological symptoms.

2. Describe the common reactions clients have to cancer, heart disease, chronic pain, and neurological disorders that may require mental health and psychological adjustments.

3. Describe the role of the psychiatric liaison nurse.

4. Describe the role of the community mental health nurse in home care settings.

5. Describe the emerging field of body-mind medicine and its effects on holistic nursing care.

6. Utilize nursing theory to complete holistic nursing assessments and provide interventions in situations where the client is facing both physical and psychiatric symptoms.

KEY TERMS

Liaison Psychiatry/Liaison Psychiatric Nursing Practice concerned with the study, diagnosis, treatment, and prevention of psychiatric illness in the physically ill and of psychological factors affecting physical conditions.

Mind Modulation Processes by which thoughts, feelings, attitudes, and emotions are converted by the brain into neurohormonal messenger molecules.

There are important aspects of psychiatric mental health nursing practice involving clients with primarily somatic (or physical) illness. Somatic illness, particularly when chronic or life threatening, may often be a source of great stress. Individuals must call on all of their adaptive strengths to cope with the challenges of illness, and occasionally these strengths are insufficient to prevent the emergence of psychiatric symptoms. Anxiety, depression, or even psychosis may develop in individuals facing serious physical health problems. In such cases, it is usually clear that the physical illness preceded psychiatric symptoms. A major goal of this chapter is to increase nurses' sensitivity to psychological complications of physical illness so that timely—and sometimes life-saving—psychiatric care can be sought and provided.

IMPACT OF EMOTIONS ON HEALTH

The following excerpt is presented as a clear example of a case where emotional response to physical illness profoundly impacted the client's prognosis. The client is delusionally obsessed with death following a heart attack. Prior to his hospitalization for cardiac disease, this individual had no history of mental illness. His physician suspected depression when the client appeared to "give up" on rehabilitation. A consulting psychiatrist recognized the seriousness of the client's symptoms but was unable to offer help because of the family's resistance to intervention. This case is a striking example of a significant psychiatric disorder deriving from a physical illness:

The Killing Fear of Death

Julian Davies is a sixty-three-year-old architect who has suffered his second heart attack. . . . I was asked to see Julian Davies by his cardiologist, Samuel Medwar, because Dr. Medwar felt his patient had given up and was not participating in the program of rehabilitation, in spite of being in a stable physiological condition without serious aftereffects. I saw Mr. Davies three weeks after his heart attack.

A short, obese, bald man, reclining in his pajamas and silk bathrobe in a huge leather chair in his suburban home, Mr. Davies greeted me with a nod of the head and a downcast gaze. His wife hovered around him, straightening the blanket on his lap, refilling his water glass, offering him advice not to overexert himself, and regarding me with obvious suspicion.

I first asked Mr. Davies about his physical condition, and he assured me that he felt no pain or other serious symptoms. I then told him that he

seemed to me somewhat depressed. He shrugged. I asked if he felt hopeless. He nodded. I asked if he had given up. He said, "Maybe." I asked why. Mr. Davies looked directly at me for the first time since I had entered the room. He told me that he knew he would die from his heart condition, and therefore he believed there was no good reason to follow the rehabilitation program. Mr. Davies reached out and grabbed my arm. His eyes were dilated, and his face was covered with perspiration. He seemed terrified. . . .

Mr. Davies's mother had died in childbirth when he was eleven. He recalled his mother's death as a horrendous blow to the family, a crushing loss that had left him deeply wounded. His father had died a lingering death after a heart attack twenty years ago, weakening over the course of months, developing arrhythmia followed by heart failure, and finally dying from a pulmonary embolus. Mr. Davies confided to me that he felt helpless to prevent his condition from following the downhill course his father had taken. At night he awoke in terror that he would stop breathing or die in his sleep. He was obsessed with the fear.

Mr. Davies could not talk to his wife about his alarming thoughts. He accepted her deep concern and mothering as an additional sign that his condition was critical, or as he told me, "terminal." He could not accept the reassurance of his cardiologist, which he interpreted as professional dissembling. Before I left Mr. Davies, I asked him specifically if he were convinced he would die. He told me, again with horror in his gaze, that he was convinced. . . .

After returning to my office, I called Dr. Medwar to express my concern that Mr. Davies had in fact given up and had a delusional conviction that he would die . . . I recommended a brief psychiatric hospitalization, which I argued should be arranged as soon as possible. Dr. Medwar visited Mr. Davies but was unable to convince him either to enter a psychiatric hospital or to see me again. I called his home, but his wife refused to let me speak to him.

Two weeks later, Dr. Medwar called to tell me Mr. Davies had died suddenly, without a clear-cut cause, a day after he had examined him and found his condition unchanged. . . . That same day Dr. Medwar had tried to talk Mrs. Davies into letting me or another psychiatrist visit the house . . . Mrs. Davies had refused the request. Dr. Medwar was unable to change Mrs. Davies's mind, even though he reviewed the medical evidence with her and concluded that Mr. Davies was not in life-threatening ["physical"] danger but rather had developed an obsession.

(Kleinman, 1988, pp. 149–150)

Depression is not uncommon after serious or life-threatening illness. The consulting psychiatrist recognized that this client's symptoms (such as expression of hopelessness, awakening at night in terror, and experiencing fear and anxiety) were not only those of depression. The psychiatrist recognized that Mr. Davies was profoundly convinced he would die from his illness. This kind of delusion can be so powerful that it leads, as here, to the client's death without any recognizable physical cause. Had Mr. and Mrs. Davies agreed to psychiatric hospitalization, it is possible that Mr. Davies could have overcome his delusional beliefs and survived his illness.

DSM-IV AND PHYSICAL ILLNESS

As described in Chapter 4, the *Diagnostic and Statistical Manual,* fourth edition (DSM-IV) uses the description Axis III to indicate that a physical condition is importantly related to the described psychological disorder. In the case of depression, DSM-IV distinguishes two forms of depression occurring in the face of physical illness (American Psychiatric Association, 1994). The first is Mood Disorder Due to a General Medical Condition. These disorders are typically diagnosed when brain dysfunction directly influences the client's feelings, for example, poststroke, when it is thought that depression can be produced by a direct neurological effect as well as through the individual's recognition of loss of functioning. In the preceding excerpt, Mr. Davies does not have a Mood Disorder Due to a General Medical Condition, for as DSM-IV states, "when sadness, guilt, insomnia, or weight loss are present in a person with a recent myocardial infarction, each symptom would count toward a Major Depressive Episode because these are not clearly and fully accounted for by the physiological effects of a myocardial infarction" (American Psychiatric Association, 1994, p. 323). Individuals like Mr. Davies would be assigned an Axis III diagnosis along with the appropriate primary Axis I psychiatric diagnosis. For example, Mr. Davies could be assigned Major Depressive

---

*EXCERPTS AS SUBMITTED from THE ILLNESS NARRATIVES by ARTHUR KLEINMAN. Copyright © 1988 by BasicBooks, Inc. Reprinted by permission of BasicBooks, a division of HarperCollins Publishers, Inc.

Disorder as an Axis I diagnosis and Diseases of the Circulatory System (Myocardial Infarction) as an Axis III diagnosis. While this notation may seem cumbersome, it calls attention to the fact that the management of psychiatric disorders complicating general medical illness is an important therapeutic role (American Psychiatric Association, 1994):

Major Depressive Disorder may be associated with chronic general medical conditions. Up to 20%–25% of individuals with certain general medical conditions (e.g. diabetes, myocardial infarction, carcinomas, stroke) will develop Major Depressive Disorder during the course of their general medical condition. The management of the general medical condition is more complex and the prognosis is less favorable if Major Depressive Disorder is present (p. 341).

PSYCHOLOGICAL RESPONSES TO PHYSICAL ILLNESS

As illustrated in the case of Mr. Davies, clients may have strong psychological responses to their physical illnesses. While "minor" illnesses can occasionally trigger such responses, such responses are far more common when individuals are confronted with threats to life or ongoing well-being. This section will consider four common serious conditions: cancer, heart disease, chronic pain, and neurological disorders. While the threats that each of these conditions present are similar—loss of autonomy, loss of livelihood, risk of death, and interference with social relationships—each is threatening in a different way and may lead to differing responses. Of course, every individual's illness and response are unique and must be approached individually and without preconception. The case examples provided through excerpts are given to help the nurse understand some of the many ways in which individuals may react to the stress of physical illness.

Cancer

A diagnosis of cancer can have a profound impact on a person's emotions and future life. Some clients describe receiving the diagnosis of cancer as a life-changing event, similar to the crisis events described in Chapter 9. From the day of diagnosis forward, these people become cancer survivors, and their diagnoses mark turning points in their lives. The reader may remember from Chapter 9 (focusing on crisis) the excerpt describing Stewart Alsop's experiences after being diagnosed with leukemia. Alsop had met Winston Churchill on two occasions and regarded him as a personal hero. Churchill led his country, England, through World War II partly through his great public speeches, which gave people courage despite the serious threat of defeat by Nazi Germany and the Axis Powers. In facing his own risk of death, Alsop tried to adopt Churchill's courageous attitude:

We Will Fight Amongst the Platelets

I wrote my letter as a takeoff on Winston's [Churchill] famous speech of defiance. "We will fight amongst the platelets," I wrote, "We will fight in the bone marrow. We will fight in the peripheral blood. We will never surrender."

Having written this, I began, for the first time in about fifty years, to cry. I was utterly astonished, and also dismayed. I was brought up to believe that for a man to weep in public is the ultimate indignity, a proof of unmanliness. Only my elderly roommate was in the room, and he hadn't noticed. I ducked into our tiny shared bathroom, and closed the door, and sat down on the toilet, and turned on the bath water, so that nobody could hear me, and cried my heart out. Then I dried my eyes on the toilet paper and felt a good deal better.*

(Alsop, 1973, p. 68)

Early in his fight against cancer Alsop tried to battle his own fears and depression by calling on his war memories, his youthful need for courage in the face of death, and his admiration for Churchill's coolness under severe threat. The nurse can recognize Alsop's behavior as his method of coping with significant stress. War memories, of the battles and the courage needed during these times, are a means many persons have to help them deal with fears, and Alsop predictably uses his past coping style to deal with his present situation. When these actions cannot make his situation better and alleviate his anxiety and fears, Alsop reverts to a heretofore unused coping method—he cries. Even though he acknowledges that he believes crying is unmanly, he does report that crying makes him feel better. The nurse must be aware of the fact that many clients in Alsop's situation feel overwhelmed by feelings of fear, depression, and powerlessness and find that their past coping patterns do not help.

The nurse has clues that privacy is more important to Alsop than interaction at the time he goes to the bathroom and cries in private. A caring nurse might approach him later in the evening when he is alone, and perhaps more stable emotionally, to spend time with him. Alsop is not in a position to meet demands that he behave in any particular way or that he talk. The nurse can offer self and express interest in his experience and feelings.

The following excerpt describes how another young

⊚⊚ *REFLECTIVE THINKING*

Supporting the Client without Hope

Consider Alsop's statements about his fight against cancer. He writes his letter of defiance and then begins to cry. His crying is an expression of hopelessness—unable to be manly and fearing inability to conquer his disease, he cries.

◆ What do you think a caring nurse could do to assist and support this client?

◆ Is privacy more important to Alsop than support of another human being?

◆ Considering his need for privacy when crying, what would you do if you were the nurse?

client with cancer expressed his frustrations with the discomfort and perceived insensitivity he experienced during a long hospitalization for chemotherapy. He had brought a Halloween mask with him into the hospital and used it in a practical joke.

My Breakfast Nurse

Immediately after [the chemotherapy nurse] left, I ran toward the bathroom. I started vomiting as I entered. Two hours later I limped back to bed. On Wednesday morning I finally did what I had often thought of doing during the last six months. During several chemo sessions . . . my breakfast nurse had appeared visibly nervous whenever I was around.

I awoke with the sun. Soon the breakfast carts began clanking down the hallway. Still tasting the remains of nausea, I nevertheless grinned as I stumbled towards the closet. I pulled out my Ape-Face.

Back in bed, I slipped the rubberband attachment over my head and then pulled the blue blanket over my head . . . I could feel her getting closer and closer. Finally the magic moment as she pulled my blanket away.

"Oh, shit. Oh, my God. Oh, no," she yelled and ran from the room. I smiled and lay back in bed. I had scored another victory against passivity and dependence.*

(Howe, 1982, pp. 147–148)

---

*From *Stay of Execution*, by S. Alsop, 1973, HarperCollins. Reprinted with permission.

---

*From *Do Not Go Gentle*, by H. Howe, 1982, New York: Norton.

෴ *REFLECTIVE THINKING*

Exploring Your Reaction to Very Ill Clients

A young man expresses his own victory against passivity and dependence by playing a practical joke on the breakfast nurse. However, he believes that the nurse is uncomfortable around him. He does not feel good about himself, so he is particularly sensitive to the fact that the nurse is not comfortable in his presence.

◆ Are there clients with whom you are uncomfortable?

◆ Are there settings where you believe you cannot give care to clients?

◆ Can you give a specific example where you thought your feelings left you unable to care for a particular client?

◆ Are you able to discuss your feelings about clients with other nurses?

Psychiatric nursing is as much a practice of understanding as it is of providing care.

◆ How would you decide what methods of coping to suggest to a client?

◆ What if a client insists that none of these methods work for her?

Consider which of the coping methods listed above you might use if you were diagnosed with cancer.

෴ *REFLECTIVE THINKING*

How Clients Report Coping with Cancer

Clients describe several methods of coping with the diagnosis and treatment of cancer:

◆ Writing (a letter, journal, poem)
◆ Crying
◆ Laughing
◆ Using humor (practical jokes) for relief
◆ Taking control of treatment
◆ Regaining power
◆ Obtaining information
◆ Talking with others
◆ Receiving support from significant others

This highly sensitive young man somehow felt that his "breakfast nurse" perceived that chemotherapy had turned him into something ugly or frightening. He felt her to be "visibly nervous whenever I was around," and as a result, he decided to transform himself, if only for a few moments, into the monster that he thought she perceived him to be. Her response might have been laughter and a hug as she realized what he was trying to tell her with his "practical joke." Instead, she proved that he had correctly read her anxieties and insecurity.

While all nurses may try to give compassionate care to all clients, most nurses can identify situations where they cannot give care to a particular client or to a client with a particular illness. It is important to know yourself and understand those situations where you must seek help from other nurses to ensure that all clients receive the care they need.

Alsop and the young man in the other excerpt each found a means to surmount the threat of cancer and the fear and indignity that accompany its treatment. Only some persons achieve such success; for others, the diagnosis of cancer leads to significant depression. In the following excerpt, the novelist and poet May Sarton

describes the weeks following her mastectomy. While she emphasizes that depression preceded her cancer diagnosis, that depression certainly was made worse by illness. It seems unlikely that the doctors and nurses who worked with her knew how depressed she was; very likely, her supportive network of friends and her strong love of nature allowed her to overcome depression and facilitate her own healing:

Tuesday, June 26th

The operation was on the eighteenth and I came home yesterday welcomed by dear Martha and Marita who have been holding the fort here.

The York hospital, small, intimate, and kind, was an ideal place for me to be, especially as I was on their new plan, Joint Practice, where nurses are given unusual powers and work closely with the surgeon. The operation was not bad at all, a modified radical mastectomy . . . modified meaning that they found no malignancy in the lymph glands. It looks as though I am in the clear.

I had a room of my own until the last night, and it was soon full of flowers, glorious flowers, among them a bunch of many sprays of delphinium, several blues, and white peonies. Another was a basket with six African violets of shades of pink and lavender. The first day Heidi brought a little bunch from her garden, and later on Martha and Marita brought me samples from my garden, one day two clematis, one deep purple and one white, another day, Siberian iris. The flowers were a constant joy. I opened my eyes to find them there, silent presences, and I slept a lot, grateful for the loss of consciousness.

The flowers helped, the visible sign of the love of many, many friends, and the great elm tree I looked at from the window helped too, its long branches waving gently in the wind. One evening an oriole came to rest there and sing. The changing skies and the admirable steadfast tree did me a lot of good. I needed it, for I had imagined that the loss of a breast would create catharsis, that I would emerge like a phoenix from the fire, reborn, with all things made new, especially the pain in my heart. I had imagined that real pain, physical pain, and physical loss would take the place of mental anguish and the loss of love. Not so. It is all to be begun again, the long excruciating journey through pain and rejection, through anger and not understanding, toward some regained sense of my self. . . .

What I am fighting now is depression, but it is not, I think, wholly and perhaps at all, the result of the shock of a major operation on the body. . . . It is that I feel devalued and abandoned at the center of my being. I sometimes feel that everyone else manages to grow up and harden in the right way to survive, whereas I have remained a terribly vulnerable infant. When poetry is alive in me I can handle it, use it, feel worthy of being part of the universe. When I can't as now, when the source is all silted up by pain, I think I should have been done away with at birth. . . .

One of the insights that has come to me through the operation is that physical disability rouses the will, so much so that extra power seems to be given in overcoming it, power beyond what is needed. . . . Whereas depression, mental anguish, destroy the will or numb it. So they are much harder to handle. I sometimes wonder whether I shall ever fully recover the sense of myself and of my powers as a writer and as a person after last year. . . .

What the mastectomy does to each individual woman is, at least temporarily, to attack her womanhood at its most vulnerable, to devalue her in her own eyes as a woman. And each woman has to meet this and make herself whole again in her own way . . . I would like to believe when I die that I have given myself away like a tree that sows

seeds every spring and never counts the loss, because it is not loss, it is adding to future life. It is the tree's way of being. Strongly rooted perhaps, but spilling out its treasure on the wind. *

(Sarton, 1980, pp. 118–140)

Sarton clearly exhibits depression; she expresses feeling depressed, devalued, abandoned, and being vulnerable. Further, she states, "I should have been done away with at birth," expressing that the cancer, its treatment, and the surgery have destroyed her will. It seems, though, that her depression never gave way to complete despair; she found joy in her flowers and recognized them as expressions of love and connectedness. In contrast to Sarton, some clients with cancer may be both depressed and suicidal. The following extraordinary account describes how a young man's deepest depression occurred not on diagnosis of cancer but when his chemotherapy had concluded and he was ready to leave the hospital. His nursing assistant and, ultimately, his family were able to provide support that allowed him to recover his physical and mental health. It seems unlikely that during a lengthy hospital stay anyone had recognized the seriousness and depth of his depression.

Excerpt from VITAL SIGNS by Fitzhugh Mullan, M.D.

Friends in the hospital congratulated me on my impending departure. I had made it through therapy and, after two months, was going home, where things would be better. I didn't feel that way about it at all. I had arrived at the hospital seemingly healthy, mentally intact, and ready to do battle. Now I was leaving the hospital in a wheelchair, emaciated, unable to swallow, troubled by breathing, and acutely depressed. I didn't miss my trips to the chemotherapy unit, but my last morning of radiation therapy, the day before I was to leave the hospital, I suffered an incredible spasm of anxiety. Crying did no good. Vomiting, spitting, and belching were in no way cathartic. There seemed to be no avenue of escape from the constant fear and nausea that I felt.

I began studying the screens on the two windows in my private ninth-floor room. Would I have the strength to remove them? Was there anything that I could lift that was heavy enough to punch through them? I didn't care so much where

---

*From RECOVERING, A JOURNAL by May Sarton. Copyright © 1980 by May Sarton. Reprinted by permission of W. W. Norton & Company, Inc.

I landed or who discovered that I was missing as I did what the mechanism would be to get the windows cleared. I still had enough sense of what was going on inside my head to call the nursing station and ask for help. It was seven in the morning, Judy would be busy with Meghan, so I called Dad and asked him to come to the hospital as soon as he could. He was there by eight o'clock. In the meantime, a corpsman named Al who had been a steady friend sat beside my bed and held my hand. I hugged Dad when he arrived.

I had no idea of what was happening that day except that my life, or what was left of it, was coming to a head. In spite of my abhorrence of the hospital I feared leaving it. The burning radiation and the noxious chemicals were what I had come to believe in—in spite of their poisonous effects. Deep within me I could not accept being cut adrift to fend for myself. I had become a slave of my therapies. Even though I understood the need to terminate them, I think I would have doggedly climbed onto the radiation table daily until the rays had burned a hole clean through me. Leaving Tower Nine through the window became more appealing than abandoning the poisons. I wanted to live at any cost, so badly, in fact, that I was prepared to die.*

(Mullan, 1983, pp. 57–58)

ASSESSMENT QUESTIONS FOR CLIENTS UNDERGOING TREATMENT FOR CANCER

- ◆ Who are the significant people in your life?
- ◆ Do you have friends or family in town who are available to help you? Do you have someone you can call at any time?
- ◆ Do you belong to any groups?
- ◆ Can you ask others for help when you need it?
- ◆ What choices are available to you to enhance your healing?
- ◆ What information would you like to have about your cancer, its treatment, and recovery?
- ◆ How do your cancer and its treatment interfere with your life goals?
- ◆ How do your cancer and its treatment interfere with your family functioning?
- ◆ How hopeful are you about recovering?
- ◆ What is the most important or powerful thing in your life?
- ◆ How has your cancer influenced your faith or beliefs?

Perhaps nurses are more aware of the relationship between depression and cancer now than they were when Mullan was a patient. Nurses are alert to signs of hopelessness and depression and have come to value the role of support groups for both client and family. However, as noted in Chapter 12 (focusing on depression), the suicide rate among cancer sufferers remains high. These excerpts illustrate that cancer provokes significant responses in individual clients. It is never adequate to treat the tumor alone; the client must be evaluated to uncover his response to the condition so that appropriate supportive interventions can be offered. The accompanying display provides examples of assessment questions for determining client responses. These questions are offered as examples that will help the nurse not only to initiate discussion and obtain information but also to stimulate nurse-client discussion about issues of the client's support system, his knowledge of the disease, his beliefs, and his spiritual health. The questions thus constitute both assessment and intervention, as the nurse will be able to provide support by asking these questions and through the resulting conversations to explore the client's subjective experience of the cancer.

Cardiovascular Disease

Clients are frequently depressed after a heart attack as they face the fear that resuming their preattack personal, vocational, and sexual activities may represent a physical risk of pain, breathing difficulty, or even sudden death. For many, preinfarction life patterns of eating, smoking, stress, and drinking may need to be changed if subsequent cardiac events are to be avoided. Such dramatic changes in lifestyle may provoke anxiety or depression. Some myocardial infarctions are truly life threatening in their severity. The following excerpt from a book by Martha Weinman Lear describes her husband's heart attack and hospitalization:

---

*Excerpt from "The Seige" from VITAL SIGNS: A YOUNG DOCTOR'S STRUGGLE WITH CANCER by Fitzhugh Mullan, M.D. Copyright © 1983 by Fitzhugh Mullan, M.D. Reprinted by permission of Farrar, Straus & Giroux, Inc.

Dr. Lear*

He awoke at 7 A.M. with pain in his chest. The sort of pain that might cause panic if one were not a doctor, as he was, and did not know, as he knew, that it was heartburn.

He went into the kitchen to get some Coke, whose secret syrups often relieve heartburn. The refrigerator door seemed heavy, and he noted that he was having trouble unscrewing the bottle cap. Finally he wrenched it off, cursing the defective cap. He poured some liquid, took a sip. The pain did not go away. Another sip; still no relief.

Now he grew more attentive. He stood motionless, observing symptoms. His breath was coming hard. He felt faint. He was sweating, though the August morning was still cool. He put fingers to his pulse. It was rapid and weak. A powerful burning sensation was beginning to spread through his chest, radiating upward into his throat. Into his arm? No. But the pain was growing worse. Now it was crushing—"crushing," just as it is always described. And worse even than the pain was the sensation of losing all power, a terrifying seepage of strength. He could feel the entire degenerative process accelerating. He was growing fainter, faster. The pulse was growing weaker, faster. He was sweating much more profusely now—a heavy, clammy sweat. He felt that the life juices were draining from his body. He felt that he was about to die. . . .

I'll be damned, he thought. I can't believe it. . . .

He made his way back to the bedroom, clutching walls for support. He eased himself onto the bed, picked up the telephone receiver and, with fingers that felt like foreign objects, dialed the Manhattan emergency number.

A woman's voice, twangy: "This is 911. Can I help you?"

He spoke slowly, struggling to enunciate each word clearly:

"My name is Dr. Harold Lear. I live at - - - - - . I am having a heart attack. My doctor's name is - - - - - . I am too weak to look up his number. Please call him and tell him to come right away."

"Sir, I'm sorry. This is 911. I can't call your doctor. . . . This is strictly an emergency service . . . I can't call your doctor. We don't do that."

Now he felt not panic, but a certain professional urgency. A familiar statistic plucked at his brain like an advertising slogan: 50 percent of all coronary victims die in the first ten minutes. "Thank you," he said to 911, and hung up.

Slowly he tugged on a robe, staggered back into the foyer and pressed for the elevator. . . . Suddenly he knew that if he did not lie down he would fall. He lowered himself to the floor. When the elevator door opened, he rolled out into the lobby and said to the startled doorman, "Get a wheelchair. Get me to the emergency room. I am having a heart attack."

"An ambulance, Doctor? Shouldn't we get an ambulance?"

"No. No time. A wheelchair." Then he lost clarity.

He was next aware of being in a wheelchair that was careening down the street. His head was way back, resting against a softness that seemed to be a belly. He did not know whose it was, but he was so pleased to have that belly for support.

The hospital—his hospital, where he was on staff—was nearby, a few blocks from his home. He felt the wheelchair take a corner with a wild side-to-side lurch and go rattling on toward the emergency room. Though his mind was floating and he could not keep his eyes open, that curiously disengaged observer within him reached automatically for the pulse. He could no longer detect any beat. He was very cold, very clammy, and he knew that he was in shock.

I am dying now, he thought. I am dying in a creaky wheelchair that is rattling down the avenue, half a block from the emergency room. Isn't this silly? And then: Well, if I am dying, why isn't my life flashing in front of me? Nothing is flashing. Where is my life?

The apartment-house doorman, who was steering the wheelchair, and a janitor, who was running alongside, recalled later that he was smiling. They wondered why. . . .

---

*From *Heartsounds* by Martha Weinman Lear; published by Simon & Schuster, New York, 1980. Reprinted by permission of the author.

Then, dimly, he felt himself being lifted onto a stretcher, sensed noise and light and a sudden commotion about him. . . . He understood that at this moment he was no more than a body with pathology. They were not treating a person; they were treating an acute coronary case in severe shock. They were racing, very quickly, against time. He himself had run this race so often, working in just this detached silent way on nameless, faceless bodies with pathologies. He did not resent the impersonality. He simply noted it. But one of the medical team, a young woman who was taking his blood pressure, seemed concerned about him. She patted him on the shoulder. She said, "How do you feel?" It was the only departure from this cool efficiency, and he felt achingly grateful for it. . . .

(Later—he thought it was the same day, but it may have been the next—she came up to the coronary-care unit, and took his hand and said, "How are you doing, Dr. Lear?" and smiled at him. He never knew her name, and he never forgot her.) . . .

Now administrative forces descended upon him. They asked about next-of-kin.

His wife was out of the country, he said.

Where?

He wasn't sure.

Children?

His son was traveling too. He could not remember his daughter's married name.

Siblings? None. Parents? None. Finally he gave them the name of a friend. . . .

He remembered thinking, just before he passed into a long, deep sleep, How can I get hold of Martha? I've got to get hold of Martha, because if I die without telling her, she will never forgive me.

He knew this was the logic of a deranged mind. A nurse wondered, as his street escorts had wondered earlier, why he was smiling.

(Lear, 1980, pp. 11–15)

In this passage, Dr. Lear suffers a severe heart attack and manages, despite an apparently unresponsive emergency system, to get himself transported to the nearby hospital in time to survive. Although in shock and nearly unconscious, he manages to stay in control of at least his means of transportation until he eventually finds his way to the hospital's emergency and intensive care units. Once under expert care, he seems willing to adopt a more passive role. Whether his chances of survival would have been less (as the narrative implies) had he asked 911 to send an ambulance, this certainly would have been a more conventional way to enter the hospital than the one he chose. Despite his surgeon's "take charge" attitude and behavior, this narrative emphasizes that Dr. Lear found great comfort in two episodes of human touch, mere physical contact with the "belly" of the doorman pushing his wheelchair and the kindness of one woman of the emergency department team.

Telling the story later, Dr. Lear's wife emphasizes his puzzling smile and offers some explanations for his behaviors. It would have been easy to misinterpret Dr. Lear's smile as a sign of complete self-control and detachment. In reality, his smile meant just the opposite: a sense of life—his life—being far more out of control than he was accustomed to. The smile expressed an ironic lack of trust in fate and the people on whom his life depended. Rather than an expression of self-confidence, Dr. Lear's smile was the nearest he could allow himself to a statement of fear and uncertainty. The nurse who saw his smile and wondered at it could perhaps best have responded by telling this brave, frightened, and lonely man something like, "You've fought hard for your life; give us your trust and let's get the healing of your heart started."

For some individuals who experience a heart attack, a smile observed by the nurse can most often be a sign of denial. Denial is a common response to life-threatening illness; indeed, Dr. Lear was in denial when he went to the refrigerator to treat his coronary ischemia with a soft drink. In describing a nursing study of adjustment following a heart attack, Johnson (1991) reported that "rather than face what had happened and the uncertainty of the future many of the informants continued to distance themselves by refusing to believe that the heart attack happened or by denying the diagnosis":

*Afterwards, it didn't seem like I had a heart attack. It didn't seem real. I thought, "Somebody else had it." It was funny.**

(Johnson, 1991, p. 25)

One of the important milestones in recovering from a heart attack, as with other severe physical illness, seems to be coming to terms with the question "why did it happen to *me*?" Johnson reports numerous similar comments from recovering cardiac clients:

---

*Johnson, J., Learning to Live Again: The process of adjustment following a heart attack." In J. M. Morse & J. L. Johnson (Eds.), *The Illness Experience*, pp. 25–85. Copyright © 1991 by Sage Publications. Reprinted by permission of Sage Publications, Inc.

I kept thinking about it for about the first month after I got home . . . just going over in my mind "Why did this have to happen?" And then I'd sit and ponder over it. . . .

I felt mad because I did all the right things. I thought, "I walk up and down eight flights. I swim every day. I walk whenever I can." I'd been doing all the right things. I'd also been watching my diet like mad . . . I've always been interested in nutrition.

(Johnson, 1991, p. 31)

For some, this questioning turns to self-blame and guilt:

It's the old story I guess . . . I've worked, I've put in long hours, lots of worry, frustration, lots of stress. I've worked for this heart attack, and I got it. I mean it's mine. I've worked for this, and I guess you could say I got what I deserved. . . .

I don't know how a person can opt out of not taking responsibility. And more so for a heart attack than cancer. I wouldn't feel the same way if I had cancer. I would say, "Hey, why me?" Or if I had been hit by a car, I could say, "Why me?" But I can't honestly say "Why me?" with a heart attack. I guess one could almost say I had it coming.

(Johnson, 1991, p. 32)

There is a widespread belief that heart disease can be avoided via risk factor control; as a result, people who suffer heart attacks frequently do feel guilty, as if they "had it coming" or "got what they deserved." Through the questioning process of taking a nursing history, caretakers may contribute to this guilt instead of helping to dissipate it: "Some of the informants found the scrutiny of the health professionals distressing":

There is a lot of finger pointing. You go along with them. And you start to think, "Something I did must have been wrong." "Cause you're told this immediately. They tell you, 'Well, let's see what you did that was wrong. Why did you get a heart attack?'"

(Johnson, 1991, p. 33)

Guilt is, of course, a major symptom of depression, and nurses need to be careful to avoid adding to guilty feelings.

The nurse must understand that offering the client a chance to express the range of his feelings is extremely important and perhaps is the most valuable intervention the nurse has to offer. Often, fear is the hardest emotion

✳ NURSING TIP

Dealing with Client Guilt

1. Accept the client where he is; practice the art of unconditional acceptance.

2. Establish trust; demonstrate that you as the nurse are trustworthy by keeping appointments, doing everything you have promised to do, and letting the client know you have made time to be with him to meet his needs.

3. Ask yourself the following:
   - Do you really believe the client is at fault if he has had a heart attack?
   - How does your answer to the preceding question affect your ability to give care?

to express. This may be truest for individuals like Dr. Lear, who have such a strong need to seem (and be) in control. Fear may arise at any time in the course of a heart attack, and the resulting adrenergic stimulation may put clients at increased risk for arrhythmia. While the coronary care unit experience can be particularly fear provoking, leaving the hospital may be as traumatic for some heart attack sufferers as it was for Fitzhugh Mullan after his chemotherapy hospitalization:

I Was Afraid to Leave

I was afraid to leave. I thought, you know, "What if I have another heart attack?" At the hospital I'd be attended to right away . . . I mean, they bring you your pills at a certain time, and you're looked after pretty good. And then you think, "Gee, when you go home, you're on your own. Am I going to make it? Am I going to manage?" Yes, it was a worry. Oh, the first week I think I was so scared at home. I was scared of having another heart attack and not getting to the hospital in time.

(Johnson, 1991, p. 43)

In recent years, length of hospital stay for persons with myocardial infarction has been dropping significantly. It is unclear how shortening hospital stays will affect the fear and anxiety associated with leaving the hospital: Perhaps if clients have shorter hospital stays, they will be less likely to identify the hospital with safety. Nonetheless, returning home is often a time for anxiety and depression. This may be particularly true if there is nowhere to go outside the home:

Sitting at Home

I find the worst part about it is sitting at home being idle. It is very frustrating. I guess I was a workaholic to a point. And to sit and not do anything, well. Like, when I was discharged I said, "Well, now I can go home. I can do some exercises." I was overweight. I knew that without having been told. I could do some exercises to strengthen, and as soon as I talked to my doctor, he says, "You don't do anything." I says, "Well, can't I?" He says, "You can go and you can walk, but you're not to leave the house." For the first week, I was housebound, I couldn't go anywhere . . . I found it very frustrating to get up and not to have a purpose in life except to maybe exist until the next day.

(Johnson, 1991, p. 44)

This sense of restriction, of being without "a purpose in life except to maybe exist," is also a part of depression. Depression becomes a greater risk when postinfarction heart failure or angina restricts physical activity:

One Day

One day I started getting the angina. I mentioned it to them at the clinic. I had done, you know, the beds and tidied the bathrooms, and then in the afternoon, I went down, and I ironed, and they said, "Well, you know, you should iron maybe two pieces at a time to begin with." And here I stood there for half an hour. But I was so mad at myself. I kept on saying, "I'm sure I can do half an hour's ironing."

(Johnson, 1991, pp. 48–49)

When a client is in recovery from a serious illness or physical crisis, such as the woman in the preceding example, the physiological limitations of recovery affect the client's autonomy. In the example, the client could no longer perform her household tasks without triggering her angina. She expressed anger and frustration at being unable to perform "half an hour's ironing" without feeling exhausted.

The nurse must explain that recovery often takes more time than both the client and nurse would like. It is important for the nurse to help the client pace activities. In this case, the nurse could state, "You have learned that the activity you tried doing was too much. How can you pace yourself to remain active without being at risk for angina? Let's look at a typical day together." When entering this conversation, the nurse must acknowledge the client's frustration and the risk of giving up. Sharing that many clients feel the same way is helpful. The nurse should remember to accept the client where she is and work together to maintain hope and establish a rehabilitation plan.

Some clients may simply be unable to cope. For one of the 14 participants in Johnson's study, depression proved overwhelming:

She Gave Up

She experienced numerous setbacks in the adjustment process and she was constantly setting goals and failing to meet them. Eventually she was no longer able to face perpetual disappointment. She stopped setting goals, refused to monitor her progress, and abandoned attempts. . . . Although . . . by no means the most ill of the informants, she believed that she would not improve . . . and at the time of the last interview she said she had given up.

(Johnson, 1991, p. 85)

Johnson does not tell more about this informant's outcome and in particular whether a diagnosis of depression was formally made and treated.

The nurse's role in caring for clients with cardiovascular disease may be to ensure that the client is evaluated and treated holistically. Clearly, the life-threatening nature of the disease requires immediate and vigilant attention to the physiological state. However, recovery requires careful attention to the human response to both the illness and its treatment: caring for the emotions of depression, anxiety, guilt, and loneliness (as expressed by clients in the preceding excerpts) and assisting the client to make necessary changes in lifestyle that are conducive to continuing recovery and health. The nurse, in her role as a caring professional, can offer the client the chance to express emotions, examine the meaning of the illness and treatments, and provide support through establishment of a positive nurse-client relationship.

Chronic Pain

Those who experience significant pain have to make adjustments to daily living unlike any other group of clients. Often, the illness is not life-threatening, but it is ever present and impacts on virtually every one of the individual's social roles. The following is a description of a case being reviewed by a group of professionals in a chronic pain clinic. A psychiatrist is describing the case conference:

A Case Conference

Helen Winthrop Bell is a twenty-nine-year-old minister's wife from a rural area in Georgia. She has had chronic pain in her arms for six years. She has undergone eight surgical procedures, has been treated with more than two dozen medications—two of them prescribed narcotics to which she briefly became addicted—and has been in the care of four different primary care physicians. She has already "failed" two local pain clinics. Mrs. Bell is at the end of her first week in the inpatient pain unit. The discussion of her case at the pain conference lasts thirty-six minutes. First, the anesthesiology resident reviews the past medical history and the results of X-rays, nerve and muscle tests, blood studies, and various physical examinations. Then one of the behavioral psychologists reads the results of the psychological test battery: depression, anxiety, bodily preoccupation, hysterical personality traits, and very substantial anger. Everyone shakes his head knowingly, and a few jokes are told to indicate what an extremely hostile and difficult patient Mrs. Bell is. It is noted that the pain seems to be an effective way for her to get angry at her husband. The social worker reports that Mrs. Bell is extremely difficult to interview. She denies all problems, even though there are reports in the medical records that she doesn't like her life as a minister's wife and has been on the verge of considering divorce. . . . The senior psychologist adds that the couple's sex life reportedly has come to a halt and that the patient's pain has been observed by the ward staff to worsen at the times her husband visits. He interprets this as evidence that the patient is "using" her pain to manipulate her marital relationship. The nurses jump in at this point with further impressions of the relationship between the Bells: evidence, it turns out, that is greatly contradictory. They have been observed arguing, but also holding hands and praying together. . . .

The chief anesthesiologist admits that nothing has seemed to work, including the nerve blocks and analgesics. . . . The junior behavioral psychologist points out . . . that the patient uses her anger to undermine the treatment program. [A] nurse breaks in, saying: "We all know what chronic pain patients are like: they are all angry and self-destructive. What's so special about Mrs. Bell?" The head nurse says she is special because she is so hostile and negative. Maybe we should discharge her before she causes a major problem on the unit, she suggests. "Do you psychiatrists have anything you want to add?" asks the chief anesthesiologist. "We only have a few minutes, because we have three other cases to get to," he cautions.

That's where I came in when I participated in this pain conference one spring afternoon in 1979. I could have told the group that Mrs. Bell satisfied the diagnostic criteria for major depressive disorder, a treatable psychiatric disorder. But she had met these criteria for three years and had been treated on numerous occasions with appropriate doses of antidepressant medication without significant effect on her depression or pain. I could have told them that I had also interviewed her husband and had found him to be even more profoundly depressed than his wife . . . I could have told the group about my interview with Mrs. Bell, which was fairly typical of her interactions with the staff. Mrs. Bell did not want to speak to me. She told me that she did not have a psychiatric problem nor any other problem except for her pain . . . I asked her how she had learned to deal with the anger "created by the pain," the rage that was so visible to me. Mrs. Bell shouted at me to leave the room, accusing me of provoking her and yelling that she was most definitely not angry. . . .

I could also have reported a chat I had with Helen Bell's older sister, Agatha, who told me that Helen had been angry all her life; before the pain it was her relationship with their parents and with her that elicited Helen's anger. She also told me that anger was often expressed indirectly through chronic bodily complaints: first, headaches or backaches; later, her arm and shoulder pain. Agatha Winthrop told me that in their family no problems of a personal or family kind could be openly talked out.

I decided, given the very limited time, there was nothing further to be gained reviewing these problems. I told my colleagues, rather, that in my view we were part of the problem. I pointed out that the pain center itself had now been taken up in the angry, self-defeating relationships that characterized Mrs. Bell's life. We were now in the same situation as her many doctors, her husband, her sister, and other family members. . . .

I couldn't get any further. The chief anesthesiologist thanked me for my interventions, reminded me that time had run out, and asked if I didn't really want to see her receive the latest psychopharmacologic agent. He gently chided me for my utopian suggestion. Mrs. Bell was here on the ward and "something has to be done with her now."*

(Kleinman, 1988, pp. 175–180)

Pain is one of the fundamental responses to physiological dysfunction. All persons experience pain with injury, illness, surgery, childbirth, and sometimes for no discernible reason. For most persons, pain is a transient experience, sometimes requiring powerful medication for its alleviation. The pain of chronic disorders, such as arthritis or cancer, can frequently be controlled by appropriate interventions. One of the major achievements of health care in the last half of the 20th century has been the development of new forms of analgesia allowing most clients with severe somatic and visceral pain, even terminal cancer sufferers, to experience much pain relief. Nonetheless, there are individuals, like Mrs. Bell, whose agonizing pain seems to completely resist medical and psychological efforts at relief. In recent years, multidisciplinary "pain clinics" have been formed

to bring the broadest scope of expertise to the problems of these individuals. Many of these clinics and their associated inpatient facilities function better as professional groups than does the one that Kleinman describes. While Kleinman is clearly annoyed at the chief anesthesiologist's domineering behavior, some readers may interpret Kleinman's description of nurses' "jumping in" and "breaking in" as a devaluing of nursing participation and as further evidence of this particular group's serious therapeutic dysfunction. But, of course, this dysfunction was precisely Kleinman's point: Mrs. Bell's pain is so tied up with her personal and social relationships that she draws everyone around her into her world of pain. An inpatient "pain unit" as torn by role and personal conflicts as this one is likely incapable of handling a client as tortured and complex as Mrs. Bell.

DSM-IV includes a diagnosis of Pain Disorder in the category of Somatoform Disorder (see Chapter 17 for a discussion of the other somatoform disorders). This diagnosis recognizes that many patients, like Mrs. Bell, have no distinct physical condition that satisfactorily explains their pain. These individuals are given the DSM diagnosis Pain Disorder Associated with Psychological Factors, or, where physical diagnoses clearly contribute to the pain, Pain Disorder Associated with Both Psychological Factors and a General Medical Condition. The DSM-IV diagnostic criteria for Pain Disorder are listed in the accompanying display.

---

෬ REFLECTIVE THINKING

Can the Treatment Team Be Part of the Problem?

Consider the case conference described in the preceding excerpt. The psychiatrist suggests that the treatment team is part of the client's continued difficulty, that the pain center staff had been taken up in the angry, self-defeating relationships that haunted the client's life.

Can you describe the difference between a treatment team that works to meet the client's needs and a treatment team that demands that the client receive treatment offered and get well?

Identify at least two examples of comments reportedly made by professionals at the case conference that were judgmental and uncaring. Restate each one in a manner that exemplifies human caring. What do you think the difference would be for the treatment team? For the client?

DIAGNOSTIC CRITERIA FOR PAIN DISORDER

◆ Pain in one or more anatomic sites is the predominant focus of the clinical presentation and is of sufficient severity to warrant clinical attention.

◆ The pain causes clinically significant distress or impairment in social, occupational, or other important areas of functioning.

◆ Psychological factors are judged to have an important role in the onset, severity, exacerbation, or maintenance of the pain.

◆ The symptom or deficit is not intentionally produced or feigned (as in Factitious Disorder or Malingering).

◆ The pain is not better accounted for by a mood, anxiety, or psychotic disorder. This disorder is not diagnosed if criteria for Somatization Disorder are met.

Reprinted with permission from the *Diagnostic and Statistical Manual of Mental Disorders*, Fourth Edition. Copyright 1994 American Psychiatric Association.

As implied in Kleinman's description of Mrs. Bell's evaluation, treatment of individuals with Pain Disorder is difficult and complex. There is always a temptation to use yet another surgical procedure or "the latest psycho-pharmacologic agent." Well-functioning multidisciplinary assessment and treatment teams are indispensable tools in the management of these seriously troubled clients and their families. These teams evaluate the meaning of the pain for the individuals. Interventions are planned that may not eliminate the pain but, rather, help the client to control the pain while having a life, as opposed to living in a situation where the pain controls every aspect of the individual's living. A nurse's role in management of chronic pain is, first and foremost, to provide a caring and compassionate response to the client's situation. Second, the nurse must work with others in a functional treatment team to help the client find interventions that allow the client to manage his life. Complementary treatments such as those described in Chapter 30 offer nonpharmaco-logical interventions, such as hypnosis, guided relaxation, therapeutic touch, and acupuncture, that are helpful to some persons with chronic pain.

Movement and Neurological Disorders

Movement and sensation are so much a part of every-day experience that impairment of these functions is felt as a particularly profound loss. Visual and hearing impairments pose a severe threat to full social and vocational participation. The following excerpt describes the experiences of progressive visual loss from the perspective of a man entering a rehabilitation program for the newly visually impaired.

Ordinary Daylight

I had become incapable of dealing with my approaching blindness, and I signed up for a four-month residency with others also going blind. We all wanted to learn, with varying degrees of desperation, how to survive. . . . As difficult as the word rehabilitation *was to handle, the word* blind *was worse. It was fraught with archetypal night-mares: beggars with tin cups, the useless, helpless, hopeless dregs of humanity. It was a word I still couldn't say, not to my friends or my family. . . .*

I had been going downhill fast. Print looked as if it had been soaked in a bathtub. On my bad days, it looked eaten by acid. Sometimes, I could see headlines, but even they swam in and out of blind spots. Everything else appeared as in a dazzling snowstorm—gauzy and colorless. Already the blind areas, the scotomas, were widening consider-

*ably, like puddles in a heavy rain. I was frightened by the blanks, the no sights, which registered only by the notable absence of things I knew were there. Still, there was much I could see and do . . . and because I was adept at hiding my impairment, I appeared ridiculously normal, especially at St. Paul's.**

(Potock, 1980, p. 55)

Potock vividly describes the experience of gradual visual loss: With some residual vision, he does not feel truly part of the blind world, but yet he finds himself unable to function usefully in the seeing world. The words he uses—*desperation, nightmares, hopeless, frightened*—reflect depression and are understandable responses to profound loss. Depression might be even more acute for Potock than others because prior to becoming blind he was an artist, a painter: He both lived and made his living through his eyes. Potock has come to St. Paul's Rehabilitation Center to begin to reconfigure his life for a future without sight. While at St. Paul's, he discovers that he is not alone in his loss, and he begins to take on a new identity as a blind adult.

Many neurological conditions, of which stroke is likely the most common, result in loss of motor function. This loss may be sudden (as in stroke) or gradual, such as occurs with multiple sclerosis. Postencephalitic parkin-sonism is one of the rare causes of motor loss, but it can result in profound functional impairment that is none-theless compatible with long survival. The following description of Rolando P., provided by Oliver Sacks, gives a sense of the tremendous grief and loss that can accompany a life impaired by neurological dysfunction. For Rolando, human support—initially his mother's and then a therapist's—was the thread that kept him from despair:

Rolando

Rolando P. was born in New York in 1917, the youngest son of a newly immigrated and very musical Italian family. He showed unusual vivac-ity and precocity as a child, acquiring speech and motor skills at an exceptionally early age. He was an active, inquisitive, affectionate and talkative child, until at thirty months of age his life was sud-denly cut across by a virulent attack of encephalitis lethargica, *which presented itself as an intense drowsiness lasting eighteen weeks, initially accom-panied by high fever and influenzal symptoms.*

---

*From ORDINARY DAYLIGHT. Copyright © 1980 by Andrew Potock.

As he awoke from the sleeping-sickness, it became evident that a profound change had occurred, for he now showed a completely masked and expressionless face, and had great difficulty in moving or talking. . . . He was generally taken to be mentally defective, except by his very observant and understanding mother, who would say: "My Rolando is no fool—he is as sharp and bright as he ever used to be. He has just come to a stop inside." . . .

"Rolando is not stupid," said a report in 1924. "He absorbs everything, but nothing can come out." This impression of him as purely absorptive, as a sort of unfathomable, black and hungry hole was to be echoed over the next forty years by all who observed him closely. . . .

The next third of a century, in a back ward of the hospital, was completely eventless in the most literal sense of the word. . . .

I examined Mr P. and talked to him several times between 1965 and 1969. He was a powerfully built man at this time, who appeared far younger than his fifty-odd years; he would easily have passed for half his actual age. He would always be tied in his wheelchair, to prevent an otherwise irresistible tendency to fall forwards. . . .

His voice was so soft as to be inaudible: sudden effort and excitement, however, rendered exclamatory speech possible for a few seconds. Thus, when I asked him whether his salivation disturbed him much, he exclaimed loudly: "You bet it does! It's one hell of a problem!" immediately afterwards relapsing into virtual aphonia [inability to speak]. . . .

His best moods and functioning are brought out by his family, when they take him home for occasional weekends or holidays. In particular Mr P. likes the hi-fi and swimming pool at his brother's country home. Very remarkable, Mr P. can swim the length of the pool, and shows a great diminution of his Parkinsonism in the water; he apparently swims with an ease and fluency which he can never achieve when he moves on dry land. . . . But Mr P.'s favourite occupation is to sit on the porch, watching the wild life which teems in the garden, or gazing at the wide prospects of upstate New York. Mr P. is always intensely depressed when he returns from the country, and the senti-

ments he expresses are always the same: "What a goddamn relief to get out of this place! . . . I've been shut up in places since the day I was born . . . I've been shut up in this illness since the day I was born. . . . That's a hell of a life for someone to have. . . . Why the hell couldn't I have died as a kid? . . ."

Despite progressive age and arthritis [Rolando's mother] would visit Rolando every Sunday without fail. . . . By the summer of 1972, however, Mrs. P. had become so disabled by arthritis that she was no longer able to come to the hospital. The cessation of her visits was followed by a severe emotional crisis in her son—two months of grief, pining, depression and rage, and during this period he lost twenty pounds. Mercifully, however, his loss was mitigated by a physiotherapist we had on the staff, a woman who combined the skills of her craft with an exceptionally warm and loving nature. . . . Under this benign and healing influence, Rolando's wound began to heal over—he became calmer and better-humoured, gained weight and slept well.

Unfortunately, at the start of February, his beloved physiotherapist was dismissed from her job (along with almost a third of the hospital staff) as a result of economies dictated by the recent Federal Budget. . . . Towards the end of February his state changed again, and he moved into a settled and almost inaccessible corpse-like apathy; he became profoundly Parkinsonian once again, but beneath the physiological Parkinsonian mask one could see a worse mask, of hopelessness and despair; he lost his appetite and ceased to eat; he ceased to express any hopes or regrets; he lay awake at nights, with wide-open, dull eyes. It was evident that he was dying, and had lost the will to live. . . .

A single episode (in early March) sticks in my mind: the medical staff, extremely alert for "organic disease" (but seemingly blind to despairs of the soul), arranged for Rolando to have a battery of "tests," and I was on the ward, that morning, when the diagnostic trolley came up, laden with syringes and tubes for blood, and accompanied by a brisk, white-coated technician. At first, passively, apathetically, Rolando let his arm be taken for blood, but then he suddenly burst out in an unforgettable, white-hot passion of

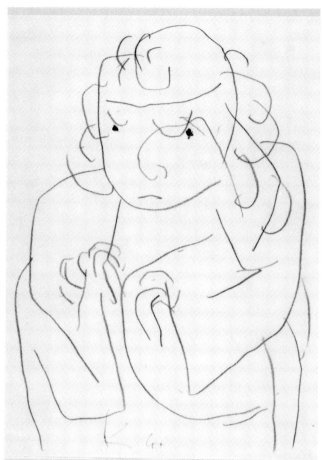

Detaillierte Passion: ein Gestalter.
Source: Courtesy of Kunstmuseum Bern, Paul-Klee-Stiftung.
© 1988 Artists Rights Society (ARS), New York/VG Bild-Kunst, Bonn.

This cartoon-like figure looks with a mixture of anger and disbelief at deformed hands and fingers. This drawing was made only a few months before Klee's death from scleroderma, a collagen vascular disorder associated with severe arthritis and loss of mobility. Prior to being struck by this disorder in 1935, Klee's paintings and drawings were full of exuberant and inventive line and color. Here is one of the most beloved of modern artists contemplating his own disability—and imminent death.

outrage. He pushed the trolley and the technician violently away, and yelled: . . . "Don't you have eyes and ears in your head? Can't you see I'm dying of grief? For Chrissake let me die in peace!" These were the last words which Rolando ever spoke. He died in his sleep, or his stupor, just four days later.*

(Sacks, 1983, pp. 105–118)

*From *Awakenings*, by O. Sacks, 1983, New York: Dutton. Reprinted with permission.

While Rolando's tragic story involves a rare disorder, his grief, desperation, and loss of will to live are not uncommon among persons devastated by neurological disease. Oliver Sacks, the neurologist who described Rolando's life and death, wrote tellingly of despairs of the soul. As Sacks implies, Rolando's death was due to more than just depression: Cut off from the few persons who truly mattered to him, Rolando entered into spiritual impoverishment. Without extraordinary nursing intervention to restore his will to live, Rolando's death was inevitable. A nurse has an important role in both understanding the sense of despair that clients may be feeling and ensuring that other members of treatment teams take human despair into account. Nurses should not hesitate to examine a client's personal interpretation of *hopelessness, powerlessness,* and *distress of the human spirit.* The first intervention in regard to these conditions is to acknowledge their importance and relevance to health for every person and to take the time to learn of the client's personal, subjective experiences of living life restricted by physical impairments. When the client is unable to express his experience and feelings verbally, the nurse must learn to understand human expressions through nonverbal, individual means. Nursing theory, as discussed later in this chapter, can serve as a guide for nurses in providing expressions of caring that are important for clients with neurological disorders.

FAMILY RESPONSES TO SIGNIFICANT ILLNESS

It is important to recognize that the stresses of chronic disease involve not just those who experience illness but also family members whose lives are affected through their roles as the caretakers for ill family members. Spouses and parents are most often greatly affected by illness in a close family member, and these persons may feel particularly vulnerable when attention is given to the involved individual but not to their own needs or to the adjustments required of the family accommodating the needs of one very ill person. In the next excerpt, a woman describes the profound impact the illness of her son had on the family:

The Williams Family

Mavis Williams is a forty-nine-year old architect and mother of three. She is a single head of household; eight years ago she and her husband of fifteen years divorced. Her oldest child, Andrew, age twenty-three, suffers from inherited muscular dystrophy. Now in a wheelchair, he is progressively losing control of his speech, arms, and upper body. The disorder first appeared when he was nine years old, but it seriously accelerated when he was twelve. It is incurable. His neurologist's prognosis is a slow decline of motor activity over three to five years, with subsequent mental deterioration and death. I met Mrs. Williams not through clinical consultation but in the course of a field research project. I had administered several questionnaires to her to ascertain her reaction to her son's illness and to obtain her evaluation of its effect on their family.

"Dr. Kleinman, I hope you don't mind me saying this to you, but I found the questions ridiculous. I filled in all the little boxes, but I think the questions are superficial. You really want to know what impact my son's illness has had? All right then, you need to get at the way it has torn us apart, divided me from my husband, affected each and every one of us and our plans and dreams. When the questionnaire says, "Has the effect on your relationships with your spouse or your children been minimal, moderate, serious," or whatever it says—you know the question I mean— what does that have to do with a family turned into a cauldron? With explosions of rage, with a daily grief that sucks your eyes dry, with turning away hurt and empty? It is the totality of its effects, its all-encompassingness that you should study. And especially its deep currents of desperation and failure. There is a little voice in me which, if I knew you better, would scream at you: Doctor, it has murdered this family!

There is no stability; we can't work it through. Andrew's illness doesn't end. It tortures him, it does the same to us. John, my husband, blamed me. It seems to come from my side of the family. John collapsed, literally collapsed. He couldn't handle it or do anything for any of us, even himself. He ran away and drank. He was no help, no help at all. But I can't really blame him. Who can expect to meet a test like this? It is the daily struggle to stay on top of it. I blame me for being absolutely, totally incapable of separating any part of me from Andrew's suffering. I have no free space, no private and protected place to get away and call my own. It has taken all of me. What is a mother to do? Between this horror and working to support the family I have, I really have, no—no— time! Zero time for me.

Look at Barbara and Kim [her other children]. What have their lives been like? Guilt because they are normal. Anger, intense anger because Andrew has required so much of my time and energy. I have had, I'll admit, precious little left over for them. But they can't express any of this. How can you, when the person responsible is dying slowly, day by day, in front of your eyes? So they can't express it to him; they take it out on me! Like John does, like Andrew does, like I want to also—since there is no one else strong enough to take it.

OK, tell me. How do you convert this into a +3 or −3 answer, to a decimal? How do you compare it with other people's reactions? I insist it is illegitimate to make comparisons. We are not things. This is not an "interpersonal problem," a "family stress"—this is a calamity! I do not exaggerate. Before Andrew's disaster we were like everyone else: some days good, some bad. Then we had problems. But looking back, that was a kind of paradise I can hardly believe was real. Now we are burning up. I sometimes think we are all dying, not just Andy. Even my parents and brothers and sisters have been more than "affected," Dr. Kleinman. You look around you—you look! This, what you see, this tomb, our family's tomb.

(Kleinman, 1988, pp. 183–184)

Nurses are familiar with the nursing diagnoses of *altered family processes* and *ineffective family coping. Altered family processes* is the diagnosis used when a family that is functioning well encounters an event or situation requiring an adjustment. Significant illness of any family member requires adjustment of those who are to provide care. If the illness is chronic, no matter how well the family attempts to adjust and cope, the problem may be so overwhelming that the family's coping is ineffective.

In recent years, the diagnosis of *caregiver role strain* has been added to the North American Nursing Diagnosis Association (NANDA) taxonomy to identify the difficult roles family members experience when providing care over time. The difficulty in identifying the diagnosis of *caregiver role strain* is that the nurse may not be in a position to provide or arrange for respite care. The nurse may be able to identify the problem, but without well-developed community resources, there may be little the nurse can provide to an individual other than understanding and validation of the difficult situation and problem solving to help the caregiver look for alternatives of action. On the community level, however, the nurse can advocate for appropriate support services for families caring for chronically ill

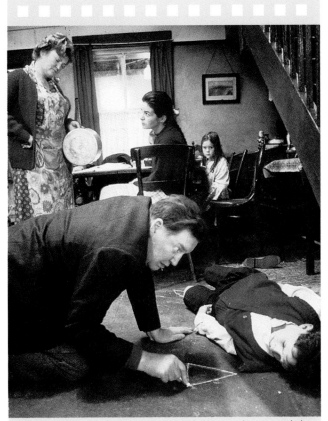

My Left Foot. Source: Granada/Miramax/Courtesy Kobal.

Physical illness, here cerebral palsy, poses immense challenges for a family. *My Left Foot* is an adaptation of a true story about a severely handicapped young man who develops into a serious artist because of his family's love and perseverance.

individuals, such as support groups, respite care, and volunteer programs to help meet needs of family members.

NURSING ROLES

There are two nursing roles in regard to assisting clients with physical illness who have strong emotional reactions. The first is liaison psychiatric nursing, a field that developed in the 1960s in which psychiatric professionals serve as consultants to health care providers in the general medical settings. The second, emerging role is that of the psychiatric nurse specialist in home care. Each is discussed following.

Liaison Psychiatric Nursing

Over the past several decades, the disciplines of **liaison psychiatry/liaison psychiatric nursing** have

arisen to provide nonpsychiatric health care providers, particularly those working in general hospital settings, with consultation about clients whose problems involve both physical and psychological symptoms. One expert has defined liaison psychiatry as being concerned with the study, diagnosis, treatment, and prevention of psychiatric illness in the physically ill and of psychological factors affecting physical conditions (Pasnau, 1982). Consultation-liaison nursing seems to have begun at Duke University in the 1960s when psychiatric nurses made their skills and expertise available to assist nurses working on other hospital units (Johnson, 1963). In a classic book describing this nursing specialty, Lewis and Levy (1982) described the major goals of psychiatric liaison nursing, which are presented in the accompanying display.

These roles remain important today as nurses in general hospital and clinic settings continue to encounter clients with emotional and psychiatric symptoms and reactions that impede recovery from physical disease. It is particularly interesting to note the emphasis in Lewis and Levy's writings on the need for nurses to educate and support one another and to encourage each other to accept those situations where immediate recovery will not be possible. These goals are articulated today by nursing organizations and nursing support groups that declare "nurses have a responsibility to nurture each other" (AHNA, 1995). One role of the psychiatric liaison nurse is to help other nurses work as a team and to support healthy work relationships and goals.

GOALS OF PSYCHIATRIC LIAISON NURSING

◆ To demonstrate and to teach mental health concepts and their application to clinical nursing practice

◆ To effect appropriate psychiatric and nursing intervention

◆ To support nurses in continuing to provide quality nursing care

◆ To promote and to develop the professional and personal self-esteem of the nurse

◆ To encourage among the members of the nursing staff tolerance of situations in which immediate and/or effective intervention or resolution is unattainable

From *Psychiatric Liaison Nursing*, by A. Lewis and J. Levy, 1982, Reston, VA: Reston. Reprinted with permission.

Psychiatric Home Care

While all still appropriate, the psychiatric liaison nursing roles evolved in the general hospital setting at a time during which relatively lengthy hospitalizations for general medical conditions were not uncommon. In today's economic climate, diagnostic evaluations often take place outside hospitals, and clients move rapidly in and out of the inpatient setting in which liaison nursing initially developed. There is little doubt that the psychiatric nurse has an important contribution to make to an increasingly ambulatory model of patient care. New roles are developing in the field of community psychiatric care and for psychiatric nursing in home health care (see also Chapter 29).

The psychiatric clinical nurse specialist in home care takes responsibility to monitor and follow clients who are chronically mentally ill as well as those clients and families who are dealing with psychosocial crises (Mellon, 1994). Particularly during times when early hospital discharge leaves clients and families feeling vulnerable, the nurse with psychiatric experience has much to offer in areas of prevention and wellness care. In some settings, psychiatric nurses have defined specialized populations with whom they work; for example, some provide mental health services to the elderly in their homes (Harper, 1989; Thobaben & Kozlak, 1990), others develop programs to support persons with acquired immuno-deficiency syndrome (AIDS) (Frey, Oman, Robins, & Smith, 1991), while others accept referrals from accident and emergency units (Storer, Whitworth, Salkovskis, & Atha, 1987).

NURSING THEORY

All nursing theories call upon nurses to view the client holistically. Adaptation theories, such as those of Callista Roy or Helen Erickson and colleagues, address directly the need for the client to react to stress in some way that returns the self to a state of homeostasis. This thinking fits well with the notion that any client adapts to physical disease and that his adaptation includes changes on both an emotional and a physical level. Understanding the connections between mind and body will assist a nurse in making holistic assessments and providing interventions that meet the client's need for peace and harmony. The Modeling and Role-Modeling theory specifically calls upon nurses to assess the client's physical state and to further assess the client's needs, worries, and wants to facilitate the nurse's evaluation of the client's emotional reactions to physical illness and events surrounding treatment. The numerous case examples in this chapter emphasize the great need to evaluate the client's emotional, physical, and attitudinal states in working with clients for whom somatic illness is the primary factor in seeking care. Table 19-1 summarizes the nursing process for clients with emotional responses to physical illness using the Modeling and Role-Modeling Theory.

Further, the nursing theories that emphasize human caring are also relevant to the nurse providing care to clients with physical illness. The case examples in this chapter emphasize client feelings of abandonment, loneliness, rejection, and depression. These feelings are rather common human responses to life's situations that the clients believe no one else can really understand. The presence of a caring nurse—the therapeutic presence of another human being who provides connection—is an intervention all too often lacking in current health care settings. The nurse using theories of human caring can validate that caring in and of itself is an important and worthy activity. The case example of Rolando exemplifies the need for human care and may help the reader to remember how crucial care can be for health and, ultimately, for survival.

✺ RESEARCH HIGHLIGHT

Community Psychiatric Nursing Follow-up Care and Effect on Utilization of Services

STUDY PROBLEM/PURPOSE

In a general hospital accident and emergency department, 99 patients were referred to a community psychiatric nurse (CPN) for follow-up care.

METHODS

Subjects were divided into two groups: those who had received psychiatric care previously and those who had not. The CPN followed all subjects for 6 months.

FINDINGS

Data on utilization of care indicated that for the group with a psychiatric history, the CPN follow-up care resulted in a substantial reduction in use of other services; in the group without psychiatric history, the CPN services showed a decrease in use of services at follow-up.

IMPLICATIONS

The authors conclude that CPN services are cost-effective and impact on the client's recovery to health.

From "Community and Psychiatric Nursing Intervention in an Accident and Emergency Department: A Clinical Pilot Study" by D. Storer, R. Whitworth, P. Salkovskis, and C. Atha, 1987, *Journal of Advanced Nursing, 12*, pp. 215–222.

Table 19-1 Summary of Nursing Process for Clients with Physical Illness, with Emotional Responses Using Modeling and Role-Modeling Theory

NURSING PROCESS STEP	NURSING ACTION BASED ON MODELING AND ROLE-MODELING THEORY
Assessment	What is the meaning of the illness to the client? What are the client's needs, worries, and wants? What does the client want the nurse to do? Is the client able to cope with the illness and treatment? What support does the client need?
Diagnosis	Nursing diagnoses written based on preceding assessment. *Examples: Ineffective individual coping,* related to feeling overwhelmed by the demands of treatment; *fear* of disease and treatment regime; *hopelessness,* related to lack of sense of future/belief that recovery is not possible.
Outcomes	The client will be able to cope effectively with illness; the client will receive treatment and move toward recovery or the ability to live with illness as part of his life.
Interventions (begin with the five aims)	**1.** Build trust. **2.** Promote positive orientation. **3.** Promote perceived control. **4.** Promote strengths. **5.** Set mutual goals that are health related.
Evaluation	Mutual evaluation of client's condition.

PSYCHIATRIC NURSING AND MIND-BODY MEDICINE

In a chapter focusing on mental health nursing involving clients with somatic illness, it is important to acknowledge the emerging research on mind-body medicine—the connection between thought, emotion, and physical functioning. Nurses have long intuited that the mind and body function as one such that factors influencing the mind have profound effects on physiological processes. However, only in the late 1980s did a new field of scientific inquiry emerge to study and evaluate how the mind can affect physiology.

Rossi used the term **mind modulation** to refer to those processes by which thoughts, feelings, attitudes, and emotions are converted by the brain into neurohormonal messenger molecules (Rossi, 1986). Thus, Rossi provides explanations for how the mind modulates biochemical functions through several of the body's systems. For example, the mind affects the autonomic nervous system in the following ways: Images and thoughts are generated in the frontal cortex; these images and thoughts are transmitted through areas of the limbic-hypothalamic system to the neurotransmitters that regulate the autonomic nervous system branches; the neurotransmitters (norepinephrine and acetylcholine) initiate the biochemical changes within different tissues down to the cellular level, resulting in either sympathetic or parasympathetic responses. Further, neurotransmitters act as messenger molecules, crossing nerve cell junctional gaps and fitting onto receptors in the cell walls, changing the receptor molecular structure (Dossey, 1995). These explanations help nurses to understand why interventions such as imagery, relaxation, music therapy, and hypnosis produce effects in that the interventions permit calming influences of the client's parasympathetic system to take over in situations that would otherwise be stress inducing (Dossey, 1995).

Data from others' work continue to suggest profound mind-body connections. Dossey reports that state of mind is statistically associated with morbidity and mortality. The "Black Monday" syndrome is a powerful example. In the United States, more persons die of heart attacks on Mondays than any other day of the week (Rabkin, Mathewon, & Tate, 1980); and more persons have heart attacks between the hours of 8:00 AM and 9:00 AM than at any other time (Kolata, 1986). These observations led others to study and conclude that one factor—job satisfaction—is the single most important risk factor in predicting (or perhaps preventing) heart attack (Dossey, 1991). While at least one investigation has not concluded that job satisfaction has such a predictive risk (Hlatky et al., 1995), other research continues to suggest that the client's faith in the treatment, perception of support, and sense of hope can, indeed, affect clinical outcome (Dossey, 1991).

Psychoneuroimmunology

Psychoneuroimmunology (PNI) is a branch of scientific study that "seeks to understand the mind-body connection" (Schwartz, 1994, p. 4). Psychoneuroimmunology is based on a theoretical model of the relationships between psychological factors and immune function via the hypothalamic pituitary axis of the sympathetic nervous system. Based on Selye's General Adaptation (or Stress) Syndrome, the model suggests that psychosocial stressors influence health via the hypothalamic pituitary axis by affecting the secretions of glucocorticoids, which can suppress immune function (Schwartz, 1994). While the field of study is new and there are significant methodological problems with the design and conduct of related work (Lloyd, 1996), PNI has led many to rethink traditional ideas that the mind and body are separate. Indeed, as early as 1986, Pert, of the National Institutes of Health, wrote: "The more we know about neuropeptides, the harder it is to think in the traditional terms of a mind and a body. It makes more sense to speak of a single integrated entity, a '*body*mind' (Pert, 1986, p. 9).

Nurses must take into account the meaning of a body-mind connection in all aspects of nursing care. There are many ways to do so, but the authors suggest that nurses begin with the following:

1. Examine how attitudes—such as feelings of hope or despair, love or fear, perceptions of an event as a crisis or a challenge, feelings of personal control or powerlessness—can influence an individual client's recovery.

2. Treat every client in a holistic manner, that is, ensure that the nursing assessment not only is of the client's physical state and mental status but also includes an understanding of the client's attitudes, fears, challenges, and supports.

3. When the client has physical disease that affects emotions, take time to understand the emotions. Accept the client as he is, never judging that one reaction is appropriate or is better than another.

FUTURE DIRECTIONS

Every nurse who is caring for a client in a holistic manner recognizes that the body and the mind are, indeed, one and that any illness in the physical body affects the client's psychoemotional state and that the psychoemotional state in turn affects the recovery and healing of a physical problem

Today more than ever, professional nurses are playing a key role in the understanding and care of clients experiencing emotional distress in relation to physical conditions. A nursing intervention in psychiatric nursing can sometimes be as elementary as a hug and a smile or as complex as performing one of the complementary modalities described in Chapter 30, such as guided imagery. The growing field of PNI is changing the way health professionals look at and treat clients. As the body of evidence that physical health can be influenced and seriously affected by mental and emotional health grows, nurses will need to be more sensitive to the psychological complications of physical illness in order to arrange for and, if appropriate, provide timely psychiatric care. Nurses in psychiatric liaison services will be called upon to assess clients in the general medical setting and to assist other nurses in establishing the appropriate approach to care. Over the next few years, the number of

psychiatric nurses working in home care is expected to grow. These nurses will play a critical role in bringing the awareness of the body-mind relationship to others working to support client care.

KEY CONCEPTS

◆ Persons must call upon their adaptive strengths when facing chronic or life-threatening illnesses. Occasionally, these strengths are insufficient to prevent the emergence of psychiatric symptoms.

◆ It has been clearly documented that clients with certain physical illnesses face serious emotional adjustments. These conditions are cancer, heart disease, chronic pain, and neurological disorders.

◆ Liaison psychiatric nursing has emerged as a means for psychiatric professionals to provide consultation in general medical settings regarding clients whose problems involve both physical and psychological symptoms.

◆ Community psychiatric nursing is a developing role within home care to provide mental health services to clients with primarily physical conditions.

◆ Nursing theory serves to guide nurses in providing holistic care that addresses the connections between body, mind, and emotions.

◆ Body-mind medicine is an emerging area of scientific study of the connections and relationships between thoughts, emotions, and physical conditions.

REVIEW QUESTIONS AND ACTIVITIES

1. Describe the reaction of a client you have known who was facing a life-threatening illness. What nursing supports did this client require? What kind of services would you provide?

2. What are the means you have as a nurse to meet the emotional needs of clients in the general medical setting?

3. Consider the case presented in this chapter of Mrs. Bell, attending a clinic for patients with chronic pain. What could you do as a nurse to address the dysfunctional work of the team attending to her pain?

4. Describe the clues apparent in assessing that a client who presents with psychological symptoms has a physical disorder.

5. What nursing theories assist you in your assessment of the client with psychological and physical symptoms?

6. How is the field of body-mind medicine reflected in your work as a holistic nurse?

EXPLORING THE WEB

◆ Visit this text's "Online Companion™" on the Internet at **http://www.DelmarNursing.com** for further information on physical conditions and emotional distress.

◆ What sites could you recommend to families and individuals coping with illness and emotional distress who are looking for self-help, chat rooms, or other electronic information sources?

◆ What other key terms might you search to find information about emotional distress related to illness (e.g., faith, hope, chronic illness, grieving)?

REFERENCES

American Holistic Nurses Association (AHNA). (1995). *Code of ethics for holistic nurses*. Raleigh, NC: Author.

American Psychiatric Association *Diagnostic and Statistical Manual of Mental Disorders*, Fourth Edition, Washington, DC. American Psychiatric Association, 1994.

Dossey, B. (1995). The psychophysiology of bodymind healing. In B. Dossey, L. Keegan, C. Guzzetta, & L. Kolkmeier (Eds.), *Holistic nursing: A handbook for practice* (pp. 77–95). Rockville, MD: Aspen.

Dossey, L. (1991). *Meaning and medicine*. New York: Bantam Books.

Frey, D., Oman, K., Robins, J., & Smith, E. J. (1991). Psychiatric home care with AIDS patients. *Journal of Home Health Care Practice, 3*, 34–45.

Harper, M. S. (1989). Providing mental health services in the homes of the elderly. *Caring, 8*, 4–6, 8–9, 52–53.

Hlatky, M. A., Lam, L. C., Lee, K. L., Clapp-Channing, N. E., Williams, R. B., Pryor, R. B., Califf, A. M., & Mark, D. B. (1995). Job strain and the prevalence and outcome of coronary artery disease. *Circulation, 92*, 327–333.

Johnson, B. S. (1963). Psychiatric nurse consultant in a general hospital. *Nursing Outlook, 11*, 728–729.

Johnson, J. (1991). Learning to live again: The process of adjustment following a heart attack. In J. M. Morse & J. L. Johnson (Eds.), (pp. 25–85) *The illness experience*. Newbury Park, CA: Sage.

Kolata, G. (1986, July). Heart attacks at 9:00 A.M. *Science*, 417–418.

Lewis, A., & Levy, J. (1982). *Psychiatric liaison nursing*. Reston, VA: Reston.

Lloyd, R. (1996). New directions in psychoneuroimmunology: A critique. *Advances, 12*, 5–12.

Mellon, S. K. (1994). Mental health clinical nurse specialists in home care for the 90s. *Issues in Mental Health Nursing, 15*, 220–237.

Pasnau, R. O. (1982). Consultation-liaison psychiatry at the crossroads: In search of a definition for the 1980's. *Hospital Community Psychiatry, 33*, 989–995.

Pert, C. (1986). The wisdom of the receptors: Neuropeptides, the emotions, and bodymind. *Advances, 3*, 8–16.

Rabkin, S. W., Mathewson, A. L., & Tate, R. B. (1980). Chronobiology of cardiac sudden death in men. *Journal of the American Medical Association, 244*, 1357–1358.

Rossi, E. (1986). *The psychobiology of mind-body healing*. New York: Norton.

Schwartz, C. E. (1994). New directions in psychoneuro-immunology, introduction: Old methodological challenges and new mind-body link in psychoneuroimmunology. *Advances, 10*, 4–7.

Storer, D., Whitworth, R., Salkovskis, P., & Atha, C. (1987). Community and psychiatric nursing intervention in an accident and emergency department: A clinical pilot study. *Journal of Advanced Nursing, 12*, 215–222.

Thobaben, M., & Kozlak, J. (1990). Home health care's unique role in serving the elderly mentally ill. *Home Healthcare Nurse, 8*, 37–39.

LITERARY REFERENCES

Alsop, S. (1973). *Stay of execution*. New York: HarperCollins.

Howe, H. (1982). *Do not go gentle*. New York: Norton.

Johnson, J. (1991). Learning to live again: The process of adjustment following a heart attack. In J. M. Morse & J. L. Johnson (Eds.), (pp. 25–85). *The illness experience*. Newbury Park, CA: Sage.

Kleinman, A. (1988). *The illness narratives: Suffering, healing, and the human condition*. New York: BasicBooks.

Lear, M. W. (1980). *Heartsounds*. New York: Simon & Schuster.

Mullan, F. (1983). *Vital signs: A young doctor's struggle with cancer*. New York: Farrar, Strauss, and Giroux.

Potock, A. (1980). *Ordinary daylight*. New York: Holt, Rinehart & Winston.

Sacks, O. (1983). *Awakenings*. New York: Dutton (Obelisk paperback).

Sarton, M. (1980). *Recovering, a journal*. New York: Norton.

SUGGESTED READINGS

Ferrell, B. R. (1996). *Suffering*. Boston: Jones and Bartlett.

Kleinman, A. (1988). *The illness narratives: Suffering, healing, and the human condition*. New York: BasicBooks.

Lubkin, I. M. (1986). *Chronic illness: Impact and interventions*. Boston: Jones and Bartlett.

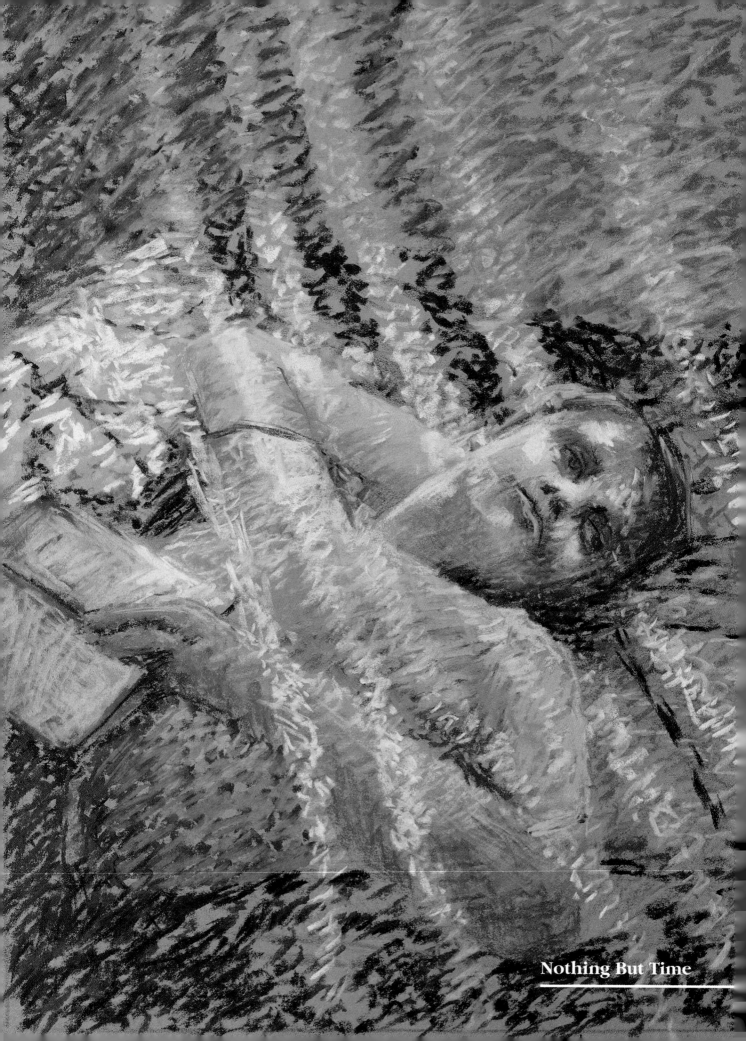

Nothing But Time

Chapter
20

FORGOTTEN POPULATIONS
The Homeless and the Incarcerated

Noreen Cavan Frisch

Lawrence E. Frisch

Walking Down the Street

Walk down the street in any major U. S. city and notice the persons sitting in doorways, sleeping in subway stations, and asking for food. Consider what you know, what you feel, and what you believe about your encounters with these persons.

What you know
- ◆ Where do these homeless persons come from?
- ◆ How did they become "down and out"?
- ◆ What are their day-to-day lives like?

What you feel
- ◆ Do you feel any of the following: anger, fear, repulsion, sadness, and/or annoyance?

Walking down the same city street, notice the construction of a new prison (a very common sight now in the United States). Reflect on the following:
- ◆ Why did the United States become the world leader in incarceration?
- ◆ Who are the persons in jails?
- ◆ Are you prepared to provide nursing services to the incarcerated?
- ◆ What need do you think the incarcerated have for care, safety, and rehabilitation?

What you believe
- ◆ Examine your own beliefs about individual and societal responsibilities regarding the homeless and the prison population. Before reading on, reflect on your beliefs and feelings regarding both the homeless and the incarcerated. In order to provide nursing care, one must be able and willing to see the world from the perspective of one's own clients. Information in this chapter may help you to be aware of a new perspective.

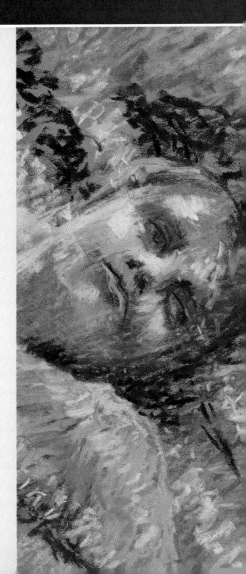

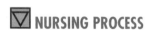 **CHAPTER OUTLINE**

THE HOMELESS

Mental Illness

Physical Illness

Health Care Needs

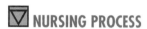 **NURSING PROCESS**

THE INCARCERATED

The Prison Population

Mental Health Needs

Mental Health Services
 Risk of Suicide
 Substance Abuse/Addiction

▽ **NURSING PROCESS**

ADVOCACY FOR FORGOTTEN POPULATIONS

Prevention

≋ **COMPETENCIES**

Upon completion of this chapter, the reader should be able to:

1. Describe the economic and social factors leading to the number of homeless persons currently in the United States.
2. Assess the basic needs of the homeless population.
3. Describe nursing services and interventions helpful in meeting the needs of the homeless from an individual and a community nursing perspective.
4. Describe the changing and growing population of prisoners in the United States.
5. Identify the major mental health needs and risks of the prison population.
6. Describe the nursing services and interventions helpful in meeting the needs of the incarcerated.

≋ **KEY TERMS**

Deinstitutionalization Movement of clients and mental health services from state mental hospitals into community settings.

Homelessness Condition of being without shelter or a permanent place to live.

Incarcerated Condition of being in a jail or other correctional institution.

NIMBY Syndrome Literally, "not in my backyard." Condition of persons or groups who state support for services for the homeless or for underprivileged groups but who refuse to allow such services in their own neighborhoods.

⊚⊚ *REFLECTIVE THINKING*

Cost of Housing/Cost of Drugs

In many cities it has become cheaper to buy cocaine than to purchase a room for the night.

◆ Has this knowledge affected planning for services in your community?

◆ Consider discussing this issue with those providing social services to the homeless in your community.

⊚⊚ *REFLECTIVE THINKING*

Services for the Homeless

As you review statistics on the homeless, inquire about the services that are available in your own community:

◆ Are there mental health services for the homeless? Where?

◆ Is there someone to do screening and mental health evaluations for the homeless?

their more affluent peers, must choose how to allocate their scarce funds among competing priorities. While food, clothing, and housing are major needs for everyone, many of the poorest spend a significant proportion (or even all) of their available income on intoxicants. For many of the homeless, the cost of alcohol or cocaine is less than the cost of a night in a hotel room. It may not be surprising, then, that individuals choose to spend their money on substances rather than the more costly housing (Jencks, 1994b). Though cocaine has by no means directly caused America's current homeless problem, its availability as a relatively inexpensive and highly mood-enhancing stimulant has had a huge impact on the lives of many of the poor. There is recent evidence as well that in some urban areas crack is becoming less the "drug of choice" for the homeless and is being replaced by alcohol and heroin (Massing, 1996). If such a drug "transition" is indeed occurring, it remains uncertain how it will affect the problems and living conditions of the homeless. Drug and alcohol dependency—both have been prominent features of American poverty life for generations—continue to be part of the cause of today's burden of homelessness.

Mental Illness

While not all of the homeless are mentally ill, mental illness is common and widespread in the homeless population. Not surprisingly, substance-related disorders and depression are among the most common diagnoses that affect the homeless. Urine screening of New York City homeless showed positive tests for cocaine in 66% and for all tested substances combined in 80% (Cuomo, 1993). Further, another study reported a 26.6% prevalence of Major Depressive Disorder, more than five times higher than that found in the general population (Kales, Barone, Bixler, Miljkovic, & Kales, 1995). The few reported studies of smaller, more rural areas have also suggested high rates of substance-related disorders. Relatively few studies have focused on homeless women, but those that have been reported suggest that psychi-

atric disorders are not uncommon among this group. Random interviews with women in St. Louis shelters found substance abuse diagnoses in a third. Post-traumatic Stress Disorder was equally common. In contrast, Bipolar Disorder and Schizophrenia were decidedly uncommon (Smith, North, & Spitznagel, 1993). The women in these St. Louis shelters were relatively young and frequently had young children living with them. While Schizophrenia was not common among the women in the St. Louis study, individuals with Schizophrenia may frequently find themselves homeless. An epidemiologic study of schizophrenic women found that these women were more likely to be homeless if they had inadequate family support, had associated substance abuse problems, or had an additional diagnosis of Antisocial Personality Disorder (Caton et al., 1995).

Homelessness is a problem outside the United States as well, but comparable studies from other countries have shown somewhat differing findings. For example, a British study researched an estimated 80% to 90% of the homeless in one moderate-sized community. Only 34% of this population admitted to substance abuse problems (compared to 66% to 80% of individuals in U.S. studies), but many had previously been residents of psychiatric hospitals, prisons, or both (Shanks, George, Westlake, & al-Kalai, 1994). Although homelessness is not exclusively an American problem, it is possible that the association with substance abuse is higher in this country than in some others.

Physical Illness

Many of the homeless have significant chronic medical conditions, including alcoholic liver disease, tuberculosis, and acquired immunodeficiency syndrome (AIDS) (Jencks, 1994b). These conditions require ongoing medical care, but that care often requires development of therapeutic relationships with health care providers. Many homeless individuals have great difficulty maintaining any sort of ongoing relationship, and as a result, both their physical and mental health may suffer seriously:

The homeless have almost as much trouble maintaining relationships with loved ones as with employers. More than half the Chicago homeless told Rossi that they had no good friends, and 36 percent reported no friends at all. A third also said they had no contact with their relatives, even though they almost all had kin in the Chicago area.

(Jencks, 1994a, p. 22)

The combination of ill health and social isolation can be particularly debilitating. Marked psychological distress, sometimes manifested by suicidal ideation, is not unusual among the homeless and is made much worse by social isolation (Schutt, Meschede, & Rierdan, 1994).

Health Care Needs

While 65% of one homeless population in England had a source of primary health care (Shanks et al., 1994), American homeless are more likely to use public hospital emergency rooms for health care. This reliance on emergency rooms prevents any continuity of care and limits opportunities for preventive intervention. There have

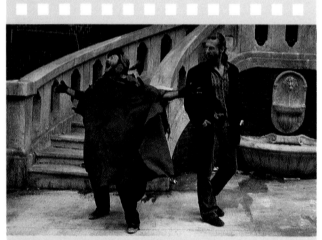

The Fisher King. Source: Columbia Tri-Star Films/Courtesy Kobal.

Pervasive social stereotypes, such as "all homeless people are lazy" or "street people are psychotic," can cloud people's ability to be sensitive to someone who is homeless and in need of psychiatric care. Often, we judge a homeless person's character without knowing who she is or where she comes from. In *The Fisher King*, Robin Williams plays a kindhearted homeless man with bipolar (manic-depressive) psychosis. He yells at invisible people on the street and believes that a headless horseman is after him. This man was once a professor and scholar, but the murder of his wife in a restaurant shooting spree stripped him of his ability to cope with life as he knew it.

been some efforts to develop programs to meet the special physical health care needs of homeless populations as well as programs specifically focused on mental health needs. One such program emphasizing mental health services reported in a 1-year follow-up evaluation that program completers (48% of the total) were able to find secure housing and remain off the streets (Murray, Baier, North, Lato, & Eskew, 1995). Another program worked primarily with inner city chemically dependent homeless clients (Bennett & Scholler-Jaquish, 1994). While outcome measures were less clearly defined for this program, the authors observed that innovative and caring efforts can at least connect the homeless to sources of primary health care, allowing some to overcome substance dependency and homelessness. Carling has reported on the efforts of the Center for Community Change Through Housing and Support in Vermont, a state with a strong reputation for innovate community-based management of mental illness (Carling, 1993). The center described efforts to develop housing for mentally ill individuals through various community actions, efforts often frustrated by the **NIMBY** (not in my backyard) **syndrome**. Jencks observes, "most Americans want the homeless off the streets, but no one wants them next door" (Jencks, 1994b, p. 117).

Comprehensively addressing the mental health needs of the homeless is an enormous challenge. Over many decades, Americans have tended to view the poor as either "worthy" or "unworthy" of public support. Children and their mothers have generally been regarded as worthy, while their fathers, the elderly, criminals, the insane, and substance abusers have frequently been regarded as unworthy—those who are regarded as chiefly having themselves to blame for misfortune. While through the 1970s and 1980s Americans remained relatively generous in providing programs for the worthy poor, more recent attitudes supporting reduced governmental roles in civic life have made it unlikely that current programs for either

⊚⊚ *REFLECTIVE THINKING*

NIMBY

While most compassionate Americans want services for homeless individuals, many persons do not want such services provided in their own neighborhoods.

♦ Provide at least three reasons why a person might reject a plan to provide services next to his own home.

♦ How do you assess the validity of the reasons you provided in response to the preceding item?

♦ What do you believe is the best direction for your community to take in developing services for the homeless?

the worthy or the unworthy will be maintained, much less expanded. It is unlikely that any society can eliminate poverty, much less mental illness, substance abuse, and homelessness. However, it seems unlikely that American society can continue to ignore the plight of the homeless. Jencks comments,

> our dilemma, both as individuals and as a society, is to reconcile the claims of compassion and prudence. When I ponder that problem I often think of a homeless woman whom Elliot Liebow quotes at the end of *Tell Them Who I Am*: "I'm 53 years old," Shirley says. "I failed at two marriages and I failed at

every job I ever had. Is that any reason I have to live on the street?"*

(Jencks, 1994b, p. 122)

Most nurses, the authors of this textbook hope, would say to Shirley, "No, that is no reason you should have to live on the street." Surely, a just and civil society can provide more for its poor—even its unworthy poor—than ours has provided in recent years.

---

*From *The Homeless* by Christopher Jencks, 1994, Cambridge, MA: Harvard University Press.

NURSING PROCESS

Nursing interventions for the homeless may be directed toward either the individual person or the community as a whole. Individual assessments and care plans are made as with any client; however, the client's condition of homelessness and poverty poses obvious challenges when choosing acceptable and realistic interventions and providing follow-up care. The homeless tend to see their needs in concrete terms—jobs, food, shelter (Mulkern & Bradley, 1986)—and this perspective must be taken into account. Many nurses view the nursing role with the homeless as one of advocacy for the homeless population, and here the nurse works with the community as a client in efforts to establish appropriate services and support for the population. The following sections on the nursing process include the community perspective (see also Chapter 29).

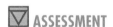 ASSESSMENT

It is important for nurses to evaluate both individual clients and the homeless population as a group in their own communities. The homeless are not a homogeneous group. Estimates of the prevalence of alcoholism and/or chemical dependency among the homeless are 50% to 70% (Fischer & Breakey, 1992). Other studies indicate that the severely and persistently mentally ill are highly represented among the homeless, with over half the individuals in one study carrying diagnoses of Schizophrenia or Bipolar Disorder (Murray et al., 1995). Each homeless person should be evaluated at a point of care (shelters, soup kitchens, or any other setting where the nurse may encounter clients receiving social services). Nursing assessment usually begins with evaluation of physical health related to basic needs for food or clothing and evaluation of communicable disease, chronic conditions, and skin problems. Psychiatric assessment should include

questions regarding any previous hospitalizations, diagnoses, or recommended treatments. Further, the nurse may ask questions to determine if there have been psychiatric symptoms, such as: "Have you ever heard voices that others cannot hear?" "Have you ever had visions and seen things others could not see?" "Do you believe you have special powers others do not have?" "Have you ever felt that your mind is out of your control?" If a nurse works in a community facility for the homeless, over time, that nurse will be able to document the population the facility is serving.

NURSING DIAGNOSIS

There are several nursing diagnoses that apply to the mental health and social needs of the homeless. *Ineffective individual coping: alcoholism or chemical dependency* is a diagnosis that will be made for any person whose homeless life is being complicated by drugs. Those with psychoses or diagnosable psychiatric disease could be given a DSM-IV (American Psychiatric Association, 1994) diagnosis as well as nursing diagnoses of *altered thought processes* or *impaired sensory perceptions: hallucinations*. For many homeless persons, the nursing diagnoses of *social isolation*, *hopelessness*, and *powerlessness* can be made as well.

OUTCOME IDENTIFICATION

Outcomes of nursing care will be individualized and depend on the diagnosis made. A priority for each person may be that the individual receive services dealing with his or her primary problem, for example, as a result of nursing assessment and intervention, client A will receive services for alcoholism and client B will receive services for untreated Schizophrenia. Given that the homeless as a group do not have access to services, an outcome of nursing assessment and diagnosis may be that nurses work with other community workers and mental health workers to develop services for this population.

▽ PLANNING/INTERVENTIONS

Several successful interventions have been reported by nurses in their work and advocacy with the homeless. Nurses dealing with the severely and persistently mentally

---

🌀 RESEARCH HIGHLIGHT

Transitional Residential Program

STUDY PROBLEM/PURPOSE

Stabilization of psychiatric disease among homeless individuals.

METHODS

A transitional residential program was designed for homeless persons who were diagnosed as severely and persistently mentally ill (SPMI). Over a 5-year period, 228 persons had been admitted to the program. Psychiatric diagnoses of these persons included Schizophrenia, Bipolar Disorder, Substance Abuse Disorder, and dual diagnoses. About half of the clients carried a diagnosis of Schizophrenia and half carried the diagnosis of Bipolar Disorder.

The residential center provided an individual treatment plan for each client, within the context of supervised housing and a 24-hour-a-day staff. Programs included supervision of daily activities, support in securing housing and/or pensions, and referrals for psychiatric care.

FINDINGS

Measurable outcomes of the program were that the client complete the program, find secure housing, and receive a disability pension or employment. Forty-eight percent of the clients completed the program and were discharged with successful outcomes, with an average length of stay of 90 days.

IMPLICATIONS

The program appears successful in assisting about half of the clients to achieve successful treatment goals. The researchers noted a lack of association between psychiatric diagnosis and outcome. The emphasis that seems most important is not clinical psychiatric solutions, but, rather, community-level interventions, empowerment, and alliances with services for the homeless. Psychiatric stabilization, however, must occur within a setting that is safe and secure, such as the setting of a residential program.

From "Components of an Effective Transitional Residential Program for Homeless Mentally Ill Clients," R. Murray, M. Baier, C. North, M. Lato, and C. Eskew, 1994, *Archives of Psychiatric Nursing, 9*, pp. 152–157.

🌀 RESEARCH HIGHLIGHT

The Winner's Group

STUDY PROBLEM/PURPOSE

Nurses working in a facility operating through a church in an urban, inner city area report on outcomes of a self-help group for homeless chemically dependent persons.

METHODS

The facility is described as a holistic ministry, providing a soup kitchen, a neighborhood pantry, a children's program, and social worker assistance, as well as health care offered through a nurse-managed clinic. Nurses assessed that homeless individuals who sought care for chemical dependency had difficulty finding and obtaining services. The nurses, along with other counselors, set up a self-help group as an intervention to help clients identify their chemical dependency, to instill hope, and to introduce knowledge that chemical dependency is a treatable disease.

The group met weekly for 12 weeks, having two facilitators and open sessions for those who wished to participate. Attendance averaged four persons per session. All members present participated in group discussions.

FINDINGS

The nurses reported that, as meetings progressed, group members opened up and shared their personal stories with one another. Some group members believed that their homelessness was a result of their chemical dependency.

Outcomes for each group member varied, but one member was accepted at a group home, two members were admitted to long-term treatment through the Veterans Administration, and two others attended Alcoholics Anonymous meetings. Group members asserted a desire to make lifestyle changes.

IMPLICATIONS

Nurses concluded that the self-help group was successful and recommended that nurses offer services for the homeless in places that permit immediate access and support.

From "The Winner's Group: A Self-Help Group for Homeless Chemically Dependent Persons," by J. B. Bennett and A. Scholler-Jaquish, 1994, *Journal of Psychosocial Nursing and Mental Health Services, 33*, pp. 14–19.

ill who are homeless reported that transitional residential programs are needed to stabilize the client's mental illness and to teach living skills (Hawthorne, Fals-Stewart, & Lohr, 1994; Murray et al., 1995). Within the context of offering a transitional residential program with 24-hour-a-day staff and client stays of over 90 days, the nurses found that interventions that encouraged clients to identify their own needs and goals and approaches that maximized client autonomy were most helpful (Murray et al., 1995).

Other nurses dealing with chemically dependent homeless individuals reported that a weekly self-help support group facilitated by the nurse was useful in assisting clients to acknowledge the effects of their drinking/drug abuse and that this group served as a stimulus for some clients to enter chemical dependency treatment (Bennett & Scholler-Jaquish, 1994).

Other homeless clients benefit from knowledge of how to negotiate the system, since some persons are eligible for services and assistance but have been unable to apply for aide. Providing knowledge of how to apply for services, job retraining, and transitional living programs is important.

Lastly, nursing care that treats the client with respect and dignity and offers authentic person-to-person interactions is an intervention that addresses the diagnoses of *social isolation* and *self esteem disturbance.* The nurse must always remember that the homeless are shunned by most of society and that a relationship with a caring nurse may be the first step for some in caring about self.

Clearly, other nursing interventions for the homeless are the range of activities within any community to advocate for services such as shelters, food, and health care. Nurses throughout the country are participating in community activities that aim to assist those in greatest need.

EVALUATION

Nursing evaluation is always done based on stated outcomes. Individuals may begin to receive needed care and treatment because of nursing assessment and referral. Community services can be improved and have been due to the efforts of many caring individuals. The two preceding Research Highlights illustrate successful nursing interventions with this population.

THE INCARCERATED

Another significant forgotten population in the United States is the **incarcerated**, or what some see as the most unworthy of the unworthy poor. While jail life is far from pleasant for most, Jencks (1994b) astutely observes that a 1980 survey "found that those who had spent time in both [homeless] shelters and jails rated the jails superior to the shelters on cleanliness, safety, privacy, and food quality" (p. 45). The irony of these findings is that, like homeless shelters, jails are rarely clean, safe, or private. As Columbia University's David Rothman emphasizes, they are also far from cheap:

> It was once commonplace to observe that a year in jail was as expensive as a year at Harvard, but by now jail costs in many cities are much higher. Maintaining one inmate for one year in New York City costs $58,000, at least twice the tuition and living expenses at a private university.
>
> (Rothman, 1994, p. 34)

A complete accounting for the reasons behind such very high costs is beyond the scope of this discussion. Clearly, the need for close supervision of inmates plays a role, as does the legal requirement to provide health care. As Rothman (1994) observes, New York City spends over $50 million a year on court-ordered treatment for inmates with AIDS, some of whom must be housed in special isolation cells, each of which cost $450,000 to construct.

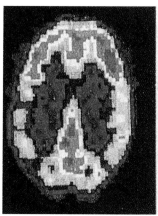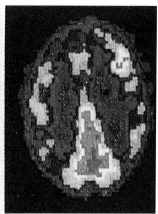

Persons who commit murder make up only a small percentage of inmates, but most murderers spend many years in prison. Neurophysiologists have studied murderers using PET scanning. These PET scan images show less activity in the frontal cortex (top ⅓ of the image) when a murderer (right) is compared with a control subject (left). Decreased frontal lobe activity may reflect impaired regulation of aggressive impulses. *Courtesy of Drs. Adrian Raine and Monte S. Buchsbaum. From "Seeking the Criminal Element" by W. Wayt Gibbs. 1995, Scientific American, March, p. 103.*

The Prison Population

In recent years, the United States has invested enormously in providing incarceration for a remarkably high percentage of its population. Between 1980 and 1990, the number of adults on probation or parole more than doubled. The U.S. federal and state prison population has almost tripled in the same period and now likely numbers a million or more (Rothman, 1994). This significant growth in the prison population has affected black Americans far more than whites; for example, 57% of young black men in Baltimore are in prison, on probation, on parole, or under a warrant for arrest. Some believe that the extraordinary growth of the prison and postprison population is a factor in the decreasing urban incidence of violent crime, but this growth has above all had a huge impact on the nation's prisons themselves. Overcrowding, poor services, and outdated facilities have given rise to numerous court orders for improvements, new services, and new construction. The eventual result will likely be a better equipped, better staffed prison system. Court-imposed requirements to deliver health and mental health services will provide opportunities and challenges to health care professionals, including nurses. Whether or not history will regard as wise social policy America's decision to become the world's leader in imprisonment, it is a decision that will affect nursing and nurses in the 1990s and beyond.

Mental Health Needs

While there have been some studies of mental health needs among prison residents, there is little definitive data on psychiatric diagnoses and needs in prisoners (Steadman, Holohan, & Dvoskin, 1991). It should come as no surprise, however, that the prevalence of substance abuse diagnoses is high in American prisons; one of the major causes for recent increases in the jail population has been an increased emphasis on mandatory sentences for possession and selling of illegal substances, particularly crack cocaine. Other diagnoses seen among prisoners include psychoses, personality disorders, and organic disorders (Gunn, Maden, & Swinton, 1991). Depression, sometimes with significant suicide potential, is commonly found. One study suggested that up to 15% of prisoners had not only a diagnosable psychiatric condition but also severe or significant functional impairment (Steadman et al., 1991). Individuals accused of committing crimes but unable to stand trial because of legal insanity may be treated in high-security forensic units within the mental health system. Other psychotic individuals may be judged competent to stand trial and after conviction may be sent to prisons. The psychiatric needs of both of these groups may be extensive. Another group of prisoners with potentially unique mental health needs is the developmentally disabled, some of whom are in prison and others of whom may, like some psychotic defendants, be judged incompetent to stand trial. Many of these individuals are dually diagnosed with both developmental and psychiatric disorders.

While jails may be required by law or court ruling to provide mental health care to psychotic inmates, such severely ill persons are relatively rare in prison populations (as they are in the population at large). Only 5% to 8% of California inmates were judged psychotic in one survey, and others have described prevalences not much different from those of the community at large (Lamb & Grant, 1982; Jerrell & Komisaruk, 1991). Indeed, mental health services ranked thirteenth on a list of prison deficiencies that have given rise to court orders for change. Far more common are overcrowding, fire hazard, inadequate medical care, and poor food (Kerle, 1991). Still, two of the major mental health challenges in prison care are providing care to those who are psychotic and preventing in-prison suicide.

Mental Health Services

Prior to deinstitutionalization, prisons could often readily transfer inmates to nearby mental institutions for evaluation and treatment. Rules governing committal apply to prisoners as well as to the population at large: There must be a strong presumption of potential harm to self or others. Today, in most settings, such transfers are not feasible, and as a result, prisons must provide their own procedures for internal psychiatric evaluation and treatment. Large state and federal prisons can (and do) employ psychiatric staff, including psychiatric nurses, psychologists, and psychiatrists. City and county jails may have much more difficulty dealing with psychotic inmates because these individuals, while mentally ill, may not be judged to be any danger to themselves and, being in jail, may pose little risk to others. Resources for in-prison mental health services are very limited in some facilities. When psychiatric care can be provided, prisoners do not lose their civil rights protections so that in the absence of risk to themselves or others, they cannot be medicated without their express consent.

Risk of Suicide

Suicide is among the most important mental health concerns in the prison population. City and county jails have higher risk of attempted and completed inmate suicide because they have much higher turnover than do federal or state penitentiaries. Many inmates are brought to local jails immediately after arrest, often under the influence of various substances and with relatively

NURSING ALERT!

Suicide Risk among Prison Inmates

Indicators that suicide risk is high include:

- ◆ History of alcoholism and/or drug abuse, intoxication
- ◆ Young age with diagnoses of Conduct Disorder, depression, and substance abuse
- ◆ Being under the influence of drugs or alcohol
- ◆ Being held for the short term in a high-turnover holding facility

unknown psychiatric histories. Such "pass-through" inmates often come at night, when staffing needs for close supervision may be stretched and personnel for psychiatric assessment may be unavailable. Adolescents held in adult jails may be particularly susceptible to suicide. While not inconsequential in larger, more stable prison populations, studies suggest that suicide risk is greatest in facilities with rapid inmate turnover (Winfree & Wooldredge, 1991). The subject of suicide in prison was discussed earlier in this text (Chapter 14).

Suicide is a major source of legal liability for prison administrators and health care workers. Nurses working in prisons must maintain a high index of suspicion for suicide risk. Close supervision, especially of recently arrived inmates, those with histories of psychiatric disorders, or those who appear psychotic or inebriated, can usually prevent suicide attempts.

Substance Abuse/Addiction

Since substance-related disorders are a major cause of arrest, many incarcerated individuals are at significant risk of undergoing withdrawal while in jail. Alcohol and opioids (separately or together) are the most likely substances to produce withdrawal. The management of withdrawal syndromes is discussed elsewhere in this text (Chapter 15). In many prison settings, withdrawal may be managed by transfer to an acute-care medical setting, but the nurse needs to be able to recognize signs of impending withdrawal so that the inmate's condition can be monitored and the need for transfer assessed in a timely manner.

NURSING PROCESS

Nurses working within the penal system will provide direct care to clients, the major nursing role being provision of primary care and direct screening services. Client needs, both physical and mental, should be assessed, and appropriate nursing interventions initiated. The American Nurses Association (ANA, 1995) has published Standards of Nursing Practice for nurses working in correctional facilities. These standards declare that "ensuring inmates' human rights is of major importance. . . . Justice, a cardinal concept guiding the nursing profession, mandates that all persons receive nursing services that are equitable in terms of accessibility, availability, and quality" (p. 5). Nurses will apply the nursing process to complete assessments and make diagnoses and will follow up care based on outcome identification. The following guidelines have been taken from the ANA Standards of Practice.

◈ ASSESSMENT

Priority data collected are determined by the client's immediate needs. Nurses will assess physical conditions and emotional state. Data collection involves the client, significant others, health care providers, and other criminal justice system personnel.

◈ NURSING DIAGNOSIS

The nurse makes diagnoses based on assessment data collected. These diagnoses are documented so that a plan of care may be developed. Emotional and social diagnoses that are relatively common in the prison population include *ineffective individual coping, hopelessness, risk for suicide, risk for violence, self esteem disturbance,* and *social isolation.*

◈ OUTCOME IDENTIFICATION

Outcomes are based on unique factors of the individual as well as the setting. For example, length of stay, overall safety, and lack of information about prior health needs will affect the nurse's ability to provide care. Nonetheless, the nurse will identify outcomes that are realistic within the setting and include a time estimate for attainment.

PLANNING/INTERVENTIONS

Appropriate nursing interventions and actions for clients within the prison system will be quite similar to those for clients outside the prison system. For example, the client who is addicted to alcohol will need medical services during the withdrawal period and follow-up care that will support sobriety. Attendance at Alcoholics Anonymous meetings is possible in many prison settings, as is individual counseling from an addictions worker. For the client who is depressed, particularly the client at risk for suicide, the nurse should request mental health services and initiate careful monitoring with the correctional facility staff to prevent suicide.

EVALUATION

Evaluation of nursing services is based on initial outcomes. The nurse should gather data and monitor outcomes systematically. Revisions in diagnoses and in care plans are made during evaluation.

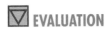

ADVOCACY FOR FORGOTTEN POPULATIONS

With either population, the homeless or the incarcerated, nurses will find themselves in the role of client advocate. The nurse will often be the first person to discover that the basic needs of the client are not being met within the system designed to provide care. Advocacy may take on several roles, and these may include working within the system to provide additional services, working to shift funds from one service to another, and overt political action demanding that community and social services be developed.

Prevention

One approach to nursing services for both the homeless and the incarcerated is to consider these "forgotten" populations within the context of society as a whole. Many believe that the considerable increase in the numbers among both groups is a direct result of social ills—poverty, powerlessness, and the individual's inability to take a place in society. Nurses have suggested that any nursing diagnosis could be considered at the level of the individual, family, and/or community such that diagnoses such as *powerlessness* or *ineffective coping* could be attributed to a community at large (Warren, 1991) and a nursing role in serving communities could be described and validated. If this idea of community diagnoses is developed, nurses can consider interventions aimed at improving the community's ability to meet the needs of its members. For example, nurses have suggested a new nursing diagnosis of "impaired ability to participate in workforce" as a potential diagnosis (Coler, 1996), relating to the problems faced by unemployed and underemployed youth, who frequently choose a lifestyle of drugs and crime when they perceive they have no option of being productive, employed members of a community. Nursing in the community may take on roles that overlap with the community developer or social worker.

KEY CONCEPTS

- At least four factors have contributed to the increased numbers of homeless persons in the United States: deinstitutionalization, loss of jobs for unskilled workers, loss of low-cost housing, and crack cocaine.
- Mental illness, most specifically chemical addiction, major depression, Bipolar Disorder, and Schizophrenia, is found in higher prevalence among the homeless than among the population at large.
- Physical illness among the homeless includes liver disease, tuberculosis, and AIDS.
- Health care for the homeless is often sporadic and provided only through emergency rooms.
- Health care is mandated for prisoners in most settings but is not mandated for the homeless.
- Mental illness seen in the prison population includes chemical dependency, psychoses, personality disorders, and organic disorders.
- Suicide potential is high among prisoners, particularly in "pass-through," or holding, jails.
- Nurses working with these "forgotten" populations take on roles of assessment, referral, direct service, advocacy, and prevention.

REVIEW QUESTIONS AND ACTIVITIES

1. Learn about the homeless population in your own community.
   a. Where do the homeless persons come from?
   b. Where and how do these people receive health care?
   c. Are there shelters? Who uses them?
   d. Are there nurses working with the homeless in your community?

2. Examine what is known about the prison population in your state.

    a. What is the number of prisoners?

    b. How are health care and mental health care being provided?

3. What role do you believe professional nursing has in addressing major societal problems?

⚛ EXPLORING THE WEB

◆ Visit this text's "Online Companion™" on the Internet at **http://www.DelmarNursing.com** for further information on the relationship of homelessness and incarceration to mental health.

◆ Search using the key terms "mental health and homelessness" and then "homeless mental." How different are the results of each search?

◆ Do you notice sites about the homeless in other countries? Which countries? Are the issues different from those in the United States?

◆ What types of mental health issues concerning the incarcerated have you found when searching the Web? What key terms do you use to search?

◆ What organizations or journals could you search for information on mental health concerns of the homeless and incarcerated?

〰 REFERENCES

American Nurses Association. (1995). *Scope and standards of nursing practice in correctional facilities.* Washington, DC: Author.

American Psychiatric Association *Diagnostic and Statistical Manual of Mental Disorders*, Fourth Edition. Washington, DC. American Psychiatric Association, 1994.

Bennett, J. B., & Scholler-Jaquish, A. (1994). The winner's group: A self-help group for homeless chemically dependent persons. *Journal of Psychosocial Nursing and Mental Health Services, 33,* 14–19.

Carling, P. J. (1993). Housing and supports for persons with mental illness: Emerging approaches to research and practice. *Hospital and Community Psychiatry, 44,* 439–449.

Caton, C. L., Shrout, P. E., Dominguez, B., Eagle, P. F., Opler, L. A., & Cournos, F. (1995). Risk factors for homelessness among women with schizophrenia. *American Journal of Public Health, 84,* 1153–1156.

Coler, M. (1996). Community diagnoses. Presentation at the 12th conference on nursing diagnoses. Pittsburgh, PA.

Cuomo, A. (Ed.) (1993). *The way home: A new direction in social policy.* New York: New York City Commission on the Homeless.

Fischer, P. J., & Breakey, W. R. (1992). The epidemiology of alcohol, drug and mental disorders among homeless persons. *American Psychologist, 46,* 1115–1128.

Gunn, J., Maden, A., & Swinton, M. (1991). Treatment needs of prisoners with psychiatric disorders. *British Medical Journal, 303,* 338–341.

Hawthorne, W., Fals-Stewart, W., & Lohr, I. (1994). A treatment outcome study of community-based residential care. *Hospital and Community Psychiatry, 45,* 152–155.

Jencks, C. (1994a, April 21). The homeless. *New York Review of Books, 41,* 20–27.

Jencks, C. (1994b). *The homeless.* Cambridge, MA: Harvard University Press.

Jerrell, J. M., & Komisaruk, R. (1991). Public policy issues in the delivery of mental health services in a jail setting. In J. A. Thompson & G. L. Mays (Eds.), *American jails: Public policy issues* (pp. 100–115). Chicago: Nelson-Hall.

Kales, J. P., Barone, M. A., Bixler, E. O., Miljkovic, M. M., & Kales, J. D. (1995). Mental illness and substance abuse among sheltered homeless persons in lower-density population areas. *Psychiatric Services, 46,* 592–595.

Kerle, K. E. (1991). Introduction. In J. A. Thompson & G. L. Mays (Eds.), *American jails: Public policy issues* (p. x). Chicago: Nelson-Hall.

Lamb, H. R., & Grant, R. W. (1982). The mentally ill in an urban county jail. *Archives of General Psychiatry, 39,* 17–22.

Massing, M. (1996, February 1). Crime and drugs: The new myths. *New York Review of Books, 43,* 16–22.

Mulkern, V., & Bradley, V. (1986). Service utilization and service preference of homeless persons. *Psychosocial Rehabilitation Journal, 10,* 23–31.

Murray, R., Baier, M., North, C., Lato, M., & Eskew, C. (1995). Components of an effective transitional residential program for homeless mentally ill clients. *Archives of Psychiatric Nursing, 9,* 152–157.

Robins, L. N., & Regier, D. A. (Eds.). (1991). *Psychiatric Disorders in America.* New York: Free Press.

Rothman, D. J. (1994, February 17). The crime of punishment. *New York Review of Books, 41,* 34–38.

Schutt, R. K., Meschede, T., & Rierdan, J. (1994). Distress, suicidal thoughts, and social support among homeless adults. *Journal of Health and Social Behavior, 35,* 134–142.

Shanks, N. J., George, S. L., Westlake, L., & al-Kalai, D. (1994). Who are the homeless? *Public Health, 108,* 11–19.

Smith, E. M., North, C. S., & Spitznagel, E. L. (1993). Alcohol, drugs, and psychiatric comorbidity among homeless women: An epidemiologic study. *Journal of Clinical Psychiatry, 54,* 82–87.

Steadman, H. J., Holohan, E. J., Jr., & Dvoskin, J. (1991). Estimating mental health needs and service utilization among prison inmates. *Bulletin of the American Academy of Psychiatry Law, 19,* 297–307.

Warren, J. (1991). Implications of introducing axes into a classification system. In R. M. Carroll-Johnson (Ed.), *Classification of nursing diagnoses: Proceedings of the ninth conference* (pp. 38–44). Philadelphia: Lippincott.

Winfree, L. T., Jr., & Wooldredge, J. D. (1991). Exploring suicides and deaths by natural causes in America's large jails. In J. A. Thompson & G. L. Mays (Eds.), *American jails: Public policy issues.* Chicago: Nelson-Hall.

〰 SUGGESTED READINGS

Thompson, J. A., & Mays, G. L. (1991). *American jails: Public policy issues.* Chicago: Nelson-Hall.

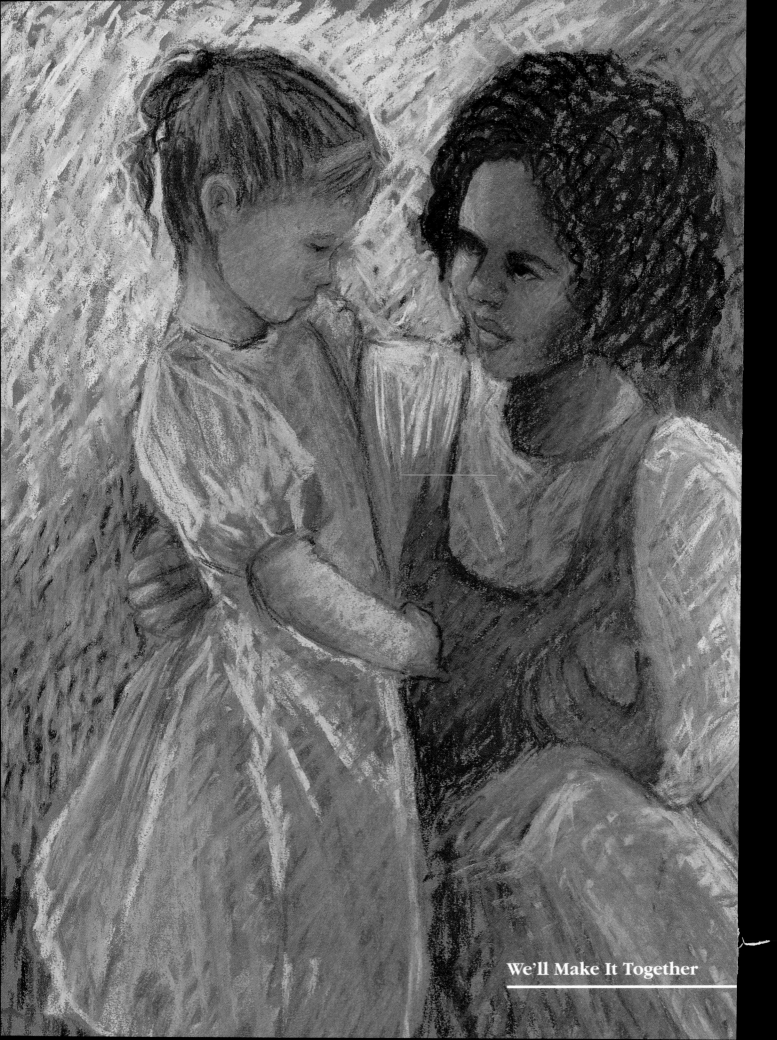

We'll Make It Together

THE CHILD

Nicki Potts

Working with Children Who Have Emotional Disorders

Working with children who have mental health or emotional disorders is challenging and requires you to be self-aware. Use the following questions to examine your personal feelings:

- How do I feel toward caregivers who seem to neglect or abuse or who are overcoercive or overpermissive with their children?
- What are my feelings about children who lie, steal, act aggressively toward others or animals, withdraw from others, or set fires?
- Have I ever been in the presence of a depressed child? How did I feel?
- How do I feel when caring for a hyperactive child?
- How do I feel about physical abuse of children? Verbal abuse? Sexual abuse?
- Have I ever been in the presence of an autistic child? How did I feel during the encounter? After the encounter?

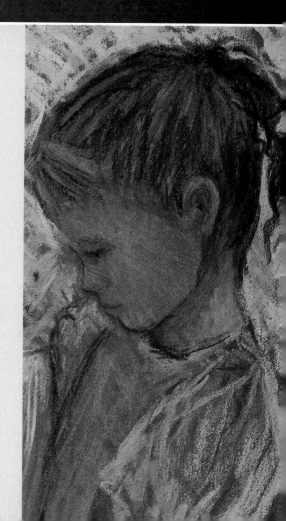

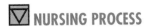

CHAPTER OUTLINE

CHILDHOOD DISORDERS

Autistic Disorder

Attention-Deficit Hyperactivity Disorder (ADHD)

Conduct Disorder

Depression

Anxiety Disorders
    Separation Anxiety Disorder
    Post-Traumatic Stress Disorder (PTSD)

▽ NURSING PROCESS

▽ CASE STUDY/CARE PLAN

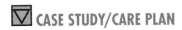

COMPETENCIES

Upon completion of this chapter, the reader should be able to:

1. Discuss the prevalence of and risk factors for emotional disorders in children.

2. Explain how to assess the emotional, social, and educational needs and problems of children and their families.

3. Describe the common psychiatric disorders of childhood.

4. Apply the nursing process to children with psychiatric disorders through assessment, diagnosis, outcome identification, planning individualized care, and evaluating care based on outcomes.

5. Describe various treatment modalities relevant to the care of children with these disorders.

KEY TERMS

Anhedonia Persistently depressed mood and loss of interest or pleasure in almost all activities.

Echolalia An involuntary, parrotlike repetition of words spoken by others.

Morbid Ideation Thinking of matters of a gruesome or unwholesome nature.

Play Therapy Therapeutic technique using games and toys to help children express their feelings, explore relationships, and attempt new solutions to problems.

Routinely we hear social comment from every quarter about the troubling picture of childhood today. The problems experienced by children are the products of multiple and complex causes. For example, over the past two decades, fundamental changes in our economy have reduced traditional job opportunities and earnings for low-skilled workers. Paralleling the decline of employment and income for many workers has been the rise in the number of single-parent households, accounting for 20% of all families, and half of these live below the poverty line. Nearly 4 million children are living in "severely distressed neighborhoods," areas with high levels of four or more of the following factors: poverty, unemployment, single-parent households, high school dropouts, and welfare recipients. Children who grow up in such communities are more likely to experience negative physical and emotional health outcomes (Palfrey, 1995). The numbers of children with mental health issues, transitory or severe, will probably continue to expand; yet, the resources for intervention become less adequate with each day. In fact, recent studies estimate that some type of diagnosable mental disorder affects between 17% and 22% of the 6 million children under the age of 18 years (U.S. Department of Health and Human Services, 1990). Yet, less than one-fifth, or 2 million, who need mental health treatment actually receive it.

The nurse may well be the single most important resource coming in routine contact with these children in need, through the schools, the clinics, the physicians' offices, and the hospitals. We must vow to become more productive and more active in identification of these children in need—the earlier the better. Indeed, our society would benefit if nurses would take it upon themselves to intervene more aggressively in the mental health of children.

CHILDHOOD DISORDERS

The emotional disorders described in this chapter are those that usually arise and are first evident during infancy or childhood.

Autistic Disorder

The essential features of Autistic Disorder are a qualitative impairment in verbal and nonverbal communication, in reciprocal social interactions, and in imaginative activity before the age of 3 years. Typically, there is no period of normal development during the first 3 years. Autistic disorders are very rare (2 to 5 cases per 10,000) and are four to five times more common in boys than in girls. Among the most notable symptoms are nondeveloped or poorly developed verbal and nonverbal skills, abnormalities in speech patterns, impaired ability to sustain a conversation, lack of empathy, and an inability to

RESEARCH HIGHLIGHT

Worries of School-Age Children

STUDY PROBLEM/PURPOSE

To determine how worrisome some situations are for school-aged children and if their caregivers can identify how worrisome the situations would be for their children.

METHODS

A convenience sample of 48 children (7 to 11 years old), 40 mothers, and 8 fathers completed a 27-item questionnaire titled "What Worries You (Your Child) the Most." The child was asked to rate the events on a Likert scale using a facial drawing with a broadly smiling affect (1 = no worry at all) to a tearing affect (5 = most worry possible) and then to rank order the items. The questionnaire for caregivers contained the same items as the child questionnaire.

FINDINGS

For the most part, caregivers knew what would worry their children the most. Having a caregiver die and not being able to see were worries that both children and caregivers recognized. However, caregivers underestimated the importance of pets and adequate family income to the child. There were significant differences in child and caregiver perceptions of three items ranked among the most worrisome: being asked to take drugs, being in a war, and hearing caregivers quarrel.

IMPLICATIONS

Findings indicate that considerable discrepancies can exist between what the caregiver and the child perceive as worrisome. Nurses can help caregivers and children become more aligned in their perceptions and actions to counteract childrens' worries.

From "Worries of School-Age Children," by J. A. Neff and J. Dale, 1996, *Journal of the Society of Pediatric Nurses, 1*(1), 27–32.

make friends. Impaired social interactions include a lack of awareness of the existence or feelings of others and being oblivious to another's distress. There may be marked impairment in the use of nonverbal behaviors such as eye contact to regulate social interaction and communication. Autistic children demonstrate an absence of attachment behaviors that are characteristic of normal children. They do not stay close to their caregivers and may not even show any acknowledgment of their caregivers' return after an absence. They do not seem to use their caregivers for comfort and fail to seek bodily contact to gain comfort or security (Rutter, 1983).

The impairment in communication affects both verbal and nonverbal skills. There may be a delay in or total lack of development of spoken language, as well as a disturbance in the comprehension of language. If speech is present, **echolalia**, or repeating exactly what is heard, nonsense rhyming, and other idiosyncratic language forms, may predominate. The child displays abnormal nonverbal communication, such as stiffening when held, not smiling, and a fixed stare. Imaginative play is often absent or markedly impaired. Autistic children are often preoccupied with one narrow interest, such as train schedules or baseball statistics. They insist on sameness and become very disturbed over changes in their surroundings and alterations in their routines. For example, if their toys are accidentally moved out of place, they are unable to adjust to the change and may scream or have a temper tantrum. There is often an insistence on following the same routine or ritual. Stereotypical body movements include rocking or swaying and clapping or flicking of the fingers. There may be a fascination with movement, such as with an electric fan, the opening and closing of doors, or the spinning wheels of a toy. The child is often attached to some inanimate object, for example, a rubber band or a piece of string. Mental retardation is associated with autistic disorder in 75% of the cases; however, the deficits in language and socialization make it difficult to obtain an accurate estimate of intellectual potential.

The cause(s) of autism is speculative. Genetic causes have been implicated; however, what exactly is inherited is not clear. Abnormal neurochemical findings have been associated with autism. Theories of etiology have also focused on a variety of other possibilities: brain injury, deficits in the reticular activating system, and structural cerebellar changes. Contrary to theories in vogue in the past, autism is not induced by caregivers.

Different treatment approaches have been advocated for autistic children, but success has been limited. Gains in speech acquisition and modification of destructive behavior and aggression have been reported with behavior therapy. Neuroleptics or antipsychotics have been somewhat effective in reducing self-injurious behavior, outwardly directed aggression, stereotypical behavior, and social withdrawal.

The prognosis for autistic children is guarded. A better prognosis is associated with higher intelligence and the ability to acquire speech. Only a small percentage of children are able to go on as adults to lead marginal, self-sufficient lives. Two researchers (Massie & Rosenthal, 1984) have advocated that early diagnosis and intervention seem to be related to long-term improvement. They have proposed that if treatment is initiated early, a significant number of children will improve. They state that 42 months is the upper age limit for intervening effectively in an autistic disorder. Based on viewing home movies of infants later diagnosed as autistic, Massie and Rosenthal assert that signs of autism can be identified as early as 6 months of age. Their criteria include the infant's somber mood, avoidance of caregiver gaze, resistance to being held, stereotypical behavior such as rocking or swaying, and emotional distancing from caregivers.

Most of us are familiar with *Rain Man*, a film depicting autism. Rare is the first-person exposition of the experience. Donna Williams's story of her early life as an autistic child provides revealing insight in her book *Nobody Nowhere* (Williams, 1992). Her journey is remarkable because so few have made the transition from autism to near normalcy. Following is her description of a dream depicting the nature of her world as she remembers it when she was 3 years old:

Nobody Nowhere

I would face the light shining through the window and rub my eyes furiously. There they were. The bright fluffy colors moving through the white. I discovered the air was full of spots. People would walk by, obstructing my magical view of nothingness. I'd move past them. They'd gabble. My attention would be firmly set on my desire to lose myself in the spots, and I'd ignore the gabble. I learned eventually to lose myself in anything I desired—the patterns on the wallpaper or carpet. Even people became no problem. Their words became a mumbling jumble. I could look through them until I wasn't there, and then, later, I learned to lose myself in them. Other people's expectations for me to respond to them was a problem. This would have required my understanding what was said, but I was too happy losing myself to want to be dragged back by something as two-dimensional as understanding. For the first three and a half years of my life ... my language consisted of repeating what others said, complete with intonation and inflection of those I came to think of as "the world." The world seemed to be impatient, annoying, callous and unrelenting. I learned to respond to it as such, crying, squealing, ignoring it, and running away. The more I became aware of the world around me, the more I became afraid. Other people were my enemies, and reaching out to me was their weapon.

I never hugged either of my caregivers; neither was I hugged. I didn't like anyone coming too close to me, let alone touching me. I felt that all touching was pain, and I was frightened. For many years

I played with, touched, and chewed on my own hair. Touching other children's hair was the only friendly physical contact I would make.*
(Williams, 1992, pp. 3–5, 8–9)

At the end of the book Williams presents suggestions for helping an autistic child. Some of these ideas may seem new and may benefit child psychiatric nurses. She states that the best way to give things to such a child is to place them near with no expectation of response or a thanks. To expect a thank you or a response is to alienate the child. Physical touch should be initiated by the child, or at least the child should be given a choice about being touched. Allow the child privacy and space. She explains that only the unthreatening nature of privacy and open space inspires the courage to explore the physical surroundings; otherwise, it is easier for the child to remain in the mental world. The child needs to know he is being listened to when he speaks and that the listener understands the seriousness of what he is trying to communicate and the courage it takes to try to speak. The listener should convey understanding of what the child is trying to communicate by symbolic gesture or replaying his actions. This would have given Williams the hope and courage to keep trying to communicate. Further, Williams states that love, kindness, and affection were her greatest fears. When these were offered to her, she became frustrated by trying to live up to their efforts, and her sense of inadequacy and hopelessness was compounded. And, finally, for those who have strived to help people like herself, she admonishes that their efforts are not useless. Williams's experiences and her telling of them open a window into the mind of the autistic child.

The following excerpts are about a deeply disturbed 5-year-old boy named Dibs who exhibits autisticlike behaviors. Virginia Axline, Dibs's psychiatrist, is telling the story of Dibs's search for the self through the process of psychotherapy. It turned out that Dibs did not have an autistic disorder but was, in fact, an exceptionally gifted child who was rejected and emotionally deprived by both his mother and father.

Dibs in Search of Self

"Come on, Dibs. It's time to go now. It's time for lunch," the teacher said patiently. Dibs did not move. His resistance was unwavering. Like a small fury Dibs was at her, his small fists striking out at her, scratching, trying to bite, screaming. "No go home! No go home! No go home!" It was the same

---

*From *Nobody Nowhere* by D. Williams, 1992, New York: Avon Books. Reprinted with permission.

cry every day. Dibs had been in this private school for almost two years. The teachers had tried their best to establish a relationship with him ... Dibs seemed determined to keep all people at bay. When he started school, he did not talk and he never ventured off his chair. He sat there mute and unmoving all morning. When anyone approached him, he would huddle up in a ball on the floor and not move. He never looked directly into anyone's eyes. He never answered when anyone spoke to him.

(Axline, 1964, pp. 13–14)

When Dibs's mother met with Dr. Axline, she talked about how difficult Dibs was as an infant and her disappointment in him:

"He is a really difficult child to understand. I have tried. Really, I have tried. But I have failed. From the beginning, when he was an infant, I could not understand him. I still don't understand him. He was such a heartache—such a disappointment from the moment of his birth. When he was born he was so different. So big and ugly. Such a big, shapeless chunk of a thing! Not responsive at all. In fact, he rejected me from the moment he was born. He would stiffen and cry every time I picked him up!"

(Axline, 1964, pp. 85–86)

Although we may not encounter autism often, we will observe autisticlike behaviors in many children, and our actions may be guided by the same set of principles proposed by Donna Williams.

Attention-Deficit Hyperactivity Disorder (ADHD)

This disorder is much more frequent in boys than girls and may occur in 3% to 5% of school-age children. The essential feature of this disorder is a persistent pattern of inattention and/or hyperactivity-impulsivity that is developmentally inappropriate. Some hyperactive-impulsive or inattentive symptoms that caused impairment must have been present before the age of 7. The DSM-IV criteria for ADHD include:

◆ Six or more symptoms of inattention that have persisted for at least 6 months to a degree that is maladaptive and inconsistent with developmental level OR

◆ Six or more symptoms of hyperactivity-impulsivity that have persisted at least 6 months to a degree that is maladaptive and inconsistent with developmental level

Impairment from the symptoms must occur in two or more settings, for example, at school and at home. Additionally, there must be evidence of interference with developmentally appropriate social, academic, or occupational functioning.

The child with ADHD has difficulty sustaining attention, is fidgety, is easily distracted, has difficulty awaiting his turn, impulsively blurts out answers to questions, shifts from one uncompleted activity to another, talks excessively, intrudes on others, often appears to be not listening, has difficulty organizing tasks and activities, loses items regularly, and often engages in physically dangerous activities without considering the consequences. He often avoids or is reluctant to perform tasks that require sustained mental effort or close concentration, such as paperwork or homework. He is easily distracted by extraneous stimuli that are ignored by others, such as traffic noises and background conversation.

SYMPTOMS OF ATTENTION DEFICIT HYPERACTIVITY DISORDER

INATTENTION

◆ Fails to give attention to details/careless mistakes in school/work

◆ Cannot sustain attention

◆ Does not seem to listen when spoken to directly

◆ Does not follow through on instruction

◆ Has difficulty organizing a task

◆ Avoids tasks that require sustained mental effort

◆ Loses things

◆ Is easily distracted

◆ Is forgetful

HYPERACTIVITY

◆ Fidgets with hands/feet

◆ Leaves seat in classroom or in situations where being seated is expected

◆ Runs or climbs excessively

◆ Has difficulty in quiet play

◆ Talks excessively

IMPULSIVITY

◆ Blurts out answers before questions are completed

◆ Has difficulty awaiting turn

◆ Interrupts or intrudes

Performance at school is usually impaired, and the group situation of the typical classroom tends to exaggerate the attentional difficulties. The child with hyperactivity appears to be "bouncing off the walls," "on the go," or as if "driven by a motor." Gross motor activity such as excessive running and climbing is seen in younger children with ADHD. Older children and adolescents appear restless and fidgety, frequently getting up while doing homework or eating and making excessive noise during quiet activities. They have difficulty engaging quietly in leisure activities such as reading a book or watching a movie.

Some children with ADHD are also described as "colicky," temperamentally difficult, and overactive from a very early age, with sleep and feeding problems. The identification of many children with this problem commonly occurs when they enter kindergarten or elementary school. They are often reported as being uncontrollable, refusing to sit still, being boisterous and inattentive, and refusing to follow directions. They often provoke anger in others and rarely learn from their mistakes. Recent studies seem to link untreated ADHD to lowered self-esteem, lowered social success, and potentially to violence and criminal behavior.

Successful treatment of ADHD involves a multimodal approach. Medication in conjunction with academic and behavioral management offers the most effective long-term results. A program that gives structure to the child's environment helps in academic and social learning. Such a program includes teaching caregivers how to structure the child's environment and help the child manage his own behavior. Several controversial therapies have been proposed in the past, but there is no evidence to support their effectiveness. These therapies include elimination of certain food items, such as chocolate, sugar, and food additives and colorings, and the administration of megavitamin and mineral supplements.

Conduct Disorder

Conduct disorder is the most common reason for referral for pediatric psychiatric evaluation, and the number of cases is increasing (American Psychiatric Association, 1994). Recent estimates of the prevalence of the disorder suggest 6% to 16% of boys and 2% to 9% of girls are involved. The essential feature of this disorder is a persistent pattern of behavior in which the basic rights of others or the major age-appropriate societal norms or rules are violated. The conduct or behavior is more serious than the ordinary noncompliant and antisocial behavior common in the course of normal growth and development. Antisocial behaviors exist on a continuum of overt acts (fighting) to covert acts (embezzling) and, in isolation, do not suggest a psychiatric disorder. The Conduct Disorder diagnosis should be applied only when the antisocial behaviors are symptomatic of an underlying dysfunction within the individual and not simply a reaction to one's social context, such as impoverished, high-crime situations.

The behaviors seen in this disorder fall into four main groups: (1) aggressive conduct that causes or threatens physical harm to other people or animals, (2) nonaggressive conduct that causes property loss or damage, (3) deceitfulness or theft, and (4) serious violations of rules. To meet the DSM-IV (American Psychiatric Association, 1994) diagnostic criteria for Conduct Disorder, a child must demonstrate at least three of the following behaviors during the past 12 months, with at least one in the past 6 months:

- Bullying, threatening, or intimidating others
- Initiating frequent physical fights
- Using a weapon that can cause physical harm, such as a bat, brick, knife, or gun
- Being physically cruel to people or animals
- Stealing while confronting the victim
- Forcing someone into sexual activity
- Deliberately destroying other's property
- Breaking into someone else's house, building, or car
- Lying to obtain goods or to avoid obligations
- Staying out at night despite caregiver prohibitions
- Running away from home overnight
- Being truant from school

The behavior patterns manifest themselves in virtually all areas of the child's life, at home, at school, in the community, and with peers. Children with a conduct disorder have little concern or empathy for other people and lack feelings of guilt or remorse. Projection is a common defense mechanism. They typically blame others for their difficulties and feel unfairly treated. Low self-esteem is manifested by a "tough guy" image. Characteristics include poor frustration tolerance, irritability, and frequent temper outbursts. Symptoms of anxiety and depression are common. Suicidal ideation, suicide attempts, and completed suicides occur at a higher than expected rate in the child with a conduct disorder. The use of tobacco, alcohol, and illegal substances as well as participation in sexual activity occurs earlier than the peer group's expected age. Academic achievement is often below the level expected on the basis of age and intelligence.

Two subtypes of Conduct Disorder are distinguished based on the age at onset. The childhood-onset type is defined by the presence of at least one of the diagnostic behaviors prior to the age of 10. These children are usually male, display physical aggression, have disturbed peer relationships, and are more likely to develop adult antisocial personality disorder. The adolescent-onset type is defined by the absence of any diagnostic behaviors before the age of 10 years. These individuals are less likely to be aggressive, more likely to have normal peer

---

✳ NURSING TIP

Helping Children Who Exhibit Unacceptable Behavior

- ◆ Praise accomplishments through touch, verbal affection, or small rewards such as stickers or stars on an activity calendar.
- ◆ Model desirable traits, such as sharing and honesty.
- ◆ Acknowledge positive or desirable behaviors.
- ◆ Correct unacceptable or undesirable behaviors immediately and calmly.
- ◆ Communicate that the behavior, not the child, is unacceptable.
- ◆ Have the child help determine acceptable behavior parameters.
- ◆ Explain expectations in clear terms.
- ◆ Ensure that the child understands expectations by asking the child to repeat instructions.
- ◆ Be certain that expectations are within the child's developmental parameters.
- ◆ Clearly outline consequences for unacceptable behaviors, and follow through on their implementation.

Table 21-1   Age-Specific Symptoms of Depression

AGE	SYMPTOMS
Preschoolers: 2½–5 years	Less exuberance in play
	Lower assertiveness than peers
	Frequent complaints of stomachaches
	Increased clinginess and whiny behavior around primary caregiver
	Greater fearfulness than peers about separating from caregiver
	Fear of abandonment
School-age children: 5–10 years	Complaints of not having friends
	Picked on by peers
	Deeply sad facial expressions and unwillingness to talk about sad feelings
	Frequent complaints of headaches
	Frequent tantrums with caregivers
	Unusual combativeness and argumentativeness
	Frequent fights with peers
	Inappropriate behavior in school, i.e., class clown, bad guy
Preteens: 10–13 years	Excessive self-recrimination and expressions of low self-esteem
	Persistent sadness, inhibition
	Isolation from peers
	Isolation from family
	Inability to sleep
	Excessive sleep
	Eating disorders

---

relationships, and less likely to develop adult antisocial personality disorder.

Many different approaches have been used in the treatment of children with conduct disorders. Individual therapy has not been shown to be especially effective in resolving the behavioral problems; however, this therapy is useful in establishing a trusting relationship necessary for a positive outcome. Training in problem-solving skills helps some children in modifying maladaptive styles of relating and behaving. The use of medication to treat symptoms of aggression in conduct disorders is controversial. Although lithium and haloperidol (Haldol) have been effective in decreasing aggression, it is not clear if these drugs are effective in conduct-disordered children (Stewart, Myers, & Burket, 1990). The most effective treatment results have been obtained with caregiver management training in which caregivers are taught to promote prosocial behaviors and to place limits on unwanted behaviors (Webster-Stratton, 1991).

Depression

Views on childhood depression have changed dramatically in recent years. Prior to the 1970s it was thought that children could not become depressed. In fact, the *Diagnostic and Statistical Manual-II* (American Psychiatric Association, 1968) did not include childhood

depression. Many argued that depression involves feelings of hopelessness and helplessness about the future and that children do not have the ability to hypothetically think about the future; therefore, they do not experience depression. However, researchers have now shown that prepubertal children do suffer mood disorders not unlike those affecting adults (Kazdin, 1990). The American Academy of Child and Adolescent Psychiatry estimates the number of children with depression to be about 5%. Although many symptoms of depression are the same for adults and children, there are some differences having to do with a child's stage of development. Table 21-1 presents these age-specific symptoms of depression.

Persistently depressed mood and loss of interest or pleasure in almost all activities (**anhedonia**) are key criteria for diagnosing a major depressive episode. In children, an irritable or cranky mood may develop rather than a depressed mood. Children with moderate or severe depression look distinctly unhappy. The distinction between a depressed child and an unhappy child can be made by determining the duration of the sad mood. A depressed child has sad or irritable feelings that persist for most of the day nearly every day for at least 2 consecutive weeks. Information about duration should be sought from several sources, for example, caregivers, teachers, and the child. It is often difficult for caregivers to be objective about their child's depression. Depressed children are unable to describe what they do for fun. Seemingly pleasurable activities or events are perceived without anticipation.

In order to be diagnosed with Major Depression per DSM-IV, the child must also experience at least four of the following symptoms: (1) changes in eating habits indicated by weight loss or gain; (2) sleep difficulties; (3) psychomotor retardation; (4) lowered self-esteem, feelings of worthlessness or guilt; (5) difficulty thinking, concentrating, or making decisions; and (6) recurrent thoughts of death, suicide ideation, or wishes to be dead. Children are poor reporters of appetite reduction and often do not report this symptom. Loss of weight or failure to make expected weight gains are usually mentioned by caregivers. A large number of depressed children have difficulty sleeping. They report difficulty falling asleep and, more rarely, wake up in the middle of the night or in early morning and cannot return to sleep. Generally, the child is more aware of sleep disturbance than the caregivers realize. When asked, "Do you have trouble sleeping?" children can describe their problems with accuracy. Depressed children are often hypoactive, particularly in moderate or severe depression. They may sit with a slumped posture and stare at the floor. Retardation of speech is also common. They answer questions in one- or two-word sentences delivered in a monotone. Complaints of fatigue, which are rarely heard from normal children, are expressed by depressed children. They report taking voluntary naps or feeling too tired to engage in activities they usually enjoy.

Lowered self-esteem is an area that is difficult to explore given that children develop only an abstract idea of self-concept around the ages of 6 to 9 years. Children will describe themselves in negative terms such as "stupid" or "not popular" or admit that friends call them derogatory nicknames. Difficulty concentrating often leads to poor school performance. A noticeable drop in grades is a red flag that depression may be the problem. Social withdrawal is another prominent symptom of depression. In asking about friendships, the nurse needs to determine what the child was like before the depression began and to keep in mind what is developmentally appropriate. **Morbid ideation**, or thoughts of a gruesome or unwholesome nature, may center around a real event such as the death of a pet or grandparent. The difference between a normal grief reaction and morbid ideation is qualitative and quantitative. The theme of death recurs repeatedly.

Depressed children may show morbid ideation without a precipitating event.

Associated symptoms of depression include irritability, weeping or feeling like crying, and somatic complaints. Irritable children respond with angry outbursts over minor events. Crying is seen often in the child 6 to 8 years of age, yet children of all ages often report episodes in which they feel like crying. The most common somatic complaints are stomachaches, headaches, and leg pains that have no organic cause (Poznanski, 1982).

Many depressed children contemplate suicide; however, few prepubertal children actually kill themselves. Yet, the incidence of suicide in children has been rising since the 1950s. Suicide is now the third leading cause of death in young people under 20 years of age in the United States, preceded only by unintentional injuries and homicide (National Safety Council, 1993). Among preadolescents, jumping from heights is the most common method of death, followed by self-poisoning, hanging, stabbing, and running into traffic. Episodes of self-poisoning that occur after the age of 6 years are less likely to be accidental and should be treated as if the behavior had suicidal potential (Kazdin, 1990).

Nurses in a variety of practice settings may discover children at risk for depression or who are depressed. Those in schools are in a unique position to identify depression. Problems in school performance may be the only unmistakable cue that something is wrong. Teachers and caregivers may be unaware that aggression, inattention, and overactivity may signal depression.

🌀 NURSING ALERT!

Assessing Children for Suicidal Behavior

When assessing suicidal behavior of a child:

◆ Carefully explore the child's life during the 48 to 72 hours prior to the threat or attempt.

◆ Identify precipitating events.

◆ Determine the degree of premeditation or impulsivity.

◆ Assess intent by evaluating the possibility of rescue as foreseen by the child.

◆ Judge intent according to:

  – The margin of error allowed by the child in terms of method used or proposed

  – The closeness or remoteness of available help

  – Whether the child called for help after the attempt

  – Whether the child calculated correctly if the family would return in time to discover the attempt

Anxiety Disorders

Separation Anxiety Disorder

The essential feature of this disorder is excessive anxiety concerning separation from home or from those to whom the child is attached. The problem is not uncommon, occurring among 4% of all children (American Psychiatric Association, 1994). In most cases, the child has difficulty separating from the mother. Children with Separation Anxiety Disorder express fear about harm coming to a major attachment figure or of being separated from this individual and never being reunited. They may be uncomfortable when traveling alone from familiar areas and may avoid going places by themselves. They may be reluctant or refuse to go to school or camp or to visit or sleep at friends' homes. Younger children may be unable to stay in a room by themselves and may "shadow" or follow the caregiver, from whom they are afraid to be separated. Bedtime can be difficult because these children may insist that someone stay with them until they fall asleep. Worrying is common and relates to the possibility of harm coming to themselves or their caregivers. They may even have nightmares to this effect. Physical complaints are common when separation occurs or is anticipated. Specific phobias are not uncommon, for example, fear of the dark, monsters, kidnappers, and burglars. The onset of the anxiety symptoms commonly occurs following a major stressor such as the death of a relative or pet, a change in schools, or a move to a new city.

Post-Traumatic Stress Disorder (PTSD)

This anxiety disorder has received considerable attention during the past decade as investigators have explored the effects of trauma on children and as our culture has continued to exhibit so much violence. Affecting at least 1% of all children in the United States (American Psychiatric Association, 1994), the prevalence seems likely to increase. Post-Traumatic Stress Disorder results from exposure to extreme traumatic stress perceived by the child as dangerous. Life-threatening situations, sexually traumatic events such as abuse, and witnessing the traumatic death of a close friend or family member place a child at risk for PTSD. The child's response to the event involves intense fear, helplessness, horror, or disorganized or agitated behavior. This disorder is characterized by recurrent and intrusive recollections and dreams of the event, as well as psychological and physiological distress in situations resembling or symbolizing the original trauma. In younger children, distressing dreams of the event may change into generalized nightmares of monsters, of rescuing others, or of threats to self or others. Children usually do not have the sense that they are reliving the past, but rather they re-experience the trauma through play. Symptoms of this disorder include diminished responsiveness to the external world (psychic numbing), reduced interest in activities, reduced ability to feel emotions, the sense of a foreshortened future, and increased arousal as seen in sleep problems, hypervigilance, and exaggerated startle response. It may be difficult for children to report reduced interest in previously enjoyed activities and constriction of affect; therefore, caregivers, teachers, and other observers should be asked about these symptoms. A sense of a foreshortened future may be manifested by the belief that life will be too short to include becoming an adult. Children may also experience various physical symptoms such as stomachaches and headaches.

NURSING PROCESS

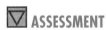 ASSESSMENT

There are many levels of mental health assessment, the earliest of which is screening for risk. Screening involves understanding the forces or factors that put children at risk for poor outcomes.

When a child is referred for psychological services, both the child and family are assessed. Assessment of the family should occur before assessment of the child. This focus on the family rather than the child initially gives the message that everyone is involved in the problem and its solutions and decreases some of the pressure placed on the child. The assessment process varies depending on the age and developmental level of the child, the nurse's skills, and the clinical setting. Assessment data should be gathered from multiple sources, including interviews with the child and with members of the nuclear and extended families, observations of the child in interactions with others, caregivers reports of the child's behavior, data gathered from questionnaires or behavior checklists, and interviews with teachers.

The nurse gathers in-depth information about the nature and extent of the child's problem in order to generate nursing diagnoses and a plan of care. Three means for collecting data are (1) the nurse's therapeutic use of self, (2) gathering information from the child and family,

NURSING ALERT!

Risk Factors for Childhood Emotional Disorders

- ◆ Poverty
- ◆ Minority status
- ◆ Homelessness
- ◆ Severe caregiver conflicts or divorce
- ◆ Caregiver psychopathology or substance abuse
- ◆ Physical or sexual abuse
- ◆ Chronic illness or disability of caregivers

and (3) use of specific techniques or tools (Bumbalo & Siemon, 1983). The nurse's use of self may be the most important communication method, because establishment of trust and rapport are necessary for obtaining complete and valid data. A child and family are more likely to be open and honest if trust and mutual respect have been established with the nurse and the nurse is viewed as one who will understand and can help resolve the child's and family's concerns.

The child and family are also an important source of information. They can provide an invaluable history of the problem as well as information about school performance, relationships with peers, and family relationships. It is sometimes more productive to interview the older child without the caregivers present, because the child might be angry with them for being referred to treatment or may not be willing to disclose certain information in front of caregivers. Because the child is part of a family system, observations of the child should also be made in the family context. This can be accomplished by seeing the child with the caregivers and having an interview with the extended family, including the siblings, grandparents, other care-takers, and so on. Although there are no truly unique skills necessary to assess a child, the usual methods of observation and history taking need to be adapted for the child's age and developmental level. Assessment of the young child requires a nurse who is comfortable with play techniques and is able to use concrete language skills. The school-age child is better able to verbalize than the younger child; however, he may still feel more comfortable engaged in an activity such as a board game or clay modeling as he talks. This aged child often reveals his personality, conflicts, and feelings through play, drawings, and stories.

The third method for collecting data involves specific techniques and tools. The child's drawings, games, puppet and doll play, standardized tests, and various rating scales, questionnaires, and checklists provide additional data. Standardized measures should be used to augment other data collection methods, not to stand alone as a source of information (Bumbalo & Siemon, 1983).

Throughout the assessment interview, the nurse gathers information in the following areas:

- ◆ Presenting problem: onset, severity, duration, impact
- ◆ Health history: birth history, allergies, illnesses, past medical problems, surgeries, current health problems, previous and current medications
- ◆ School and social history: school performance; relationships with peers, teachers, and family; living arrangements; play activities
- ◆ Developmental history and status of child and family
- ◆ Psychiatric history: history of psychiatric disorders, substance abuse problems, organic mental disorders in the child and family members
- ◆ Physical assessment and exam
- ◆ Mental status exam: appearance, motor behavior and coordination, thought process and content, speech and language, emotional status, manner of relating to examiner

Ideally, the assessment of the child and family culminates in the formation of both nursing and medical diagnoses. The validity of the nursing diagnoses depends on the accuracy of the information obtained in the assessment. Once the assessment data have been gathered, the next step is to determine if the behavior and symptoms are maladaptive. When assessing a child's behavior, it is important to remember that it should be measured against the usual developmental responses characteristic of a certain age and a child's unique temperament and personality. For example, a temper tantrum may express the normal negativism of a toddler; on the other hand, temper tantrums on slight provocation in a 6-year-old child may indicate psychological disturbance.

Several characteristics of behaviors are used to define serious emotional disorders. First is that the disordered behaviors extend beyond age appropriateness for either the type or frequency of the behavior. Many behaviors that appear dysfunctional are normal behaviors for certain periods of development. Second, the disordered behaviors are of such intensity that they become detrimental to the child's functioning. Most acting-out behaviors do not seriously impair the child's functioning, even though the child may experience consequences of his behavior. However, behaviors that are self or other destructive create a situation in which the child's or another's safety becomes a reason for seeking treatment. The third characteristic is that the behaviors often deviate from social or cultural norms. Hearing voices, vandalism, cruelty to

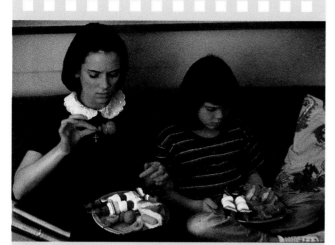

Mermaids. Source: Orion Pictures/Courtesy Kobal.

Among the most poignant of human truths is that children cannot choose the families or the life circumstances into which they are born. In the film *Mermaids*, Charlotte and Kate live with a personality-disordered mother whose fear of close relationships results in numerous precipitous moves from one town to the next. *Mermaids* paints a realistic, if at times overly optimistic and humorous, picture of children's lives in a profoundly dysfunctional family.

animals, firesetting, and similar behaviors are deviant in that they defy socially or culturally acceptable norms. These three criteria are not exhaustive; yet, they provide an initial guideline to distinguish behaviors indicative of normal development from those reflecting more serious disorders.

▽ NURSING DIAGNOSIS

Following are several common diagnoses that deal with issues and problems facing children.

Anxiety

Children who are anxious may appear very active. Gentle touch and redirection is often helpful to reduce anxiety and restore self-control. When this does not work, the child may have to be placed in a less stimulating environment. Children may experience anxiety because of fear of separating from their caregivers. Explore the child's fear of separating from the caregiver as well as the caregiver's possible fears of separation from the child. Caregivers may be so frustrated with the child's clinging and demanding behaviors that they need assistance in problem solving.

Impaired Social Interaction

The behavior of some children is intrusive and immature. Conveying acceptance of the child separate from the behavior increases feelings of self-worth. The child must know which behaviors are and are not acceptable and the consequences of unacceptable behavior. Children can learn appropriate social skills in their relationships with nurses, in group therapy, and by role playing. For the child with an anxiety disorder, social interactions can be impaired because of excessive self-consciousness and inability to interact with unfamiliar people.

Ineffective Individual Coping

Ineffective coping involves the inability to utilize an adaptive problem-solving approach when confronted by anticipated and unanticipated life events. Children must develop effective coping strategies appropriate to each phase of development. For example, a young child may withdraw from unsatisfactory play situations. The child's ability to use effective coping strategies grows in direct relation to developmental progress. When the child has not learned effective coping skills, dysfunctional behaviors may develop.

Risk for Violence

Children need to learn ways of handling conflict without becoming aggressive toward self or others. However, most children in inpatient psychiatric units have a limited notion of feelings, usually only identifying anger, and an equally limited way to express themselves. Risk for violence is highest when children are not able to express feelings through other than physical means or react in a manner inconsistent with their developmental age and the severity of the situation.

Self-Esteem Disturbance

Decreased self-esteem underlies many dysfunctional behaviors. How a child feels about himself is largely determined by how he is regarded by others. A child develops positive self-esteem through positive relationships with others, beginning in infancy with attachment to caregivers and broadening throughout childhood. When a child is confronted with consistent negative or rejecting communication, his perception of self-worth is diminished. The child can eventually adopt behaviors indicative of low self-esteem: excessive need for reassurance from caregivers, poor eye contact, self-derogatory verbalizations, lack of initiative, somatic complaints such as stomach- and headaches, withdrawal from friends or family, depression, and aggressive or attention-getting behavior.

▽ OUTCOME IDENTIFICATION

The nurse can help the caregivers and child to establish realistic and achievable goals that take into account the child's developmental level and family situation. Areas of concentration can include having the child focus on learning effective coping strategies for developmental age, learning appropriate means for expressing self and getting needs met, and beginning to identify own strengths as opposed to concentrating on weaknesses. For children experiencing anxiety, short-term outcomes can include steps such as the child staying with the sitter for 2 hours with minimal distress. For children needing help with social interactions, caregivers should be taught to gradually encourage small contributions from the child in social settings until the child is able to participate more fully. Focusing on and praising small, intermediate successes will increase the child's self-confidence while decreasing self-consciousness.

In in-patient units, outcomes need to be targeted to tasks that the child can achieve within the boundaries of the setting. To help reduce anxiety, for instance, an attachment object such as a favorite doll or blanket can be offered to reduce fears about separation. To realize improved social interaction, the child can attend groups with the nurse and other children, where the nurse can facilitate and support the child's efforts to interact with others.

Identifying adaptive coping skills that the child can use in the face of anxiety is another important outcome. This can be achieved through practice via role play, which facilitates the use of adaptive behaviors in the face of stressful situations. Caregivers can to be taught to give positive reinforcement for appropriate, desired behaviors.

▽ PLANNING/INTERVENTIONS

When working with children with emotional problems, the nurse may react as if the child were part of her family of origin or her current family. In this situation, the nurse needs help to identify personal experiences that limit her perception of the child. In working with the family, the nurse should avoid taking a critical position but should attempt to establish a collaborative relationship in problem solving and intervention. The nurse's capacity for empathy is limited by reacting to the child and family from her own beliefs, values, and stereotypes. When working with families from different cultural backgrounds, the nurse must guard against imposing her own cultural assumptions about child-rearing. When helping caregivers to alter their child-rearing behaviors, it is important to remember that these behaviors are usually based on the child-rearing practices that the caregivers experienced as children. Because their beliefs about child rearing tend to be based on long-standing experiences, simply teaching new approaches is not adequate. They

need to talk about their reactions to these new ideas. Nurses may need help to deal with their feelings toward caregivers who seem to neglect or abuse or who are over-coercive or overpermissive with their children. However, in most cases, we need to remember that caregivers are doing the best job they can with their children. Additionally, they often describe feelings of guilt, anxiety, denial, and embarrassment when confronted with the decision to obtain psychiatric services for their child. Thus, support and understanding are essential to establishing a trusting relationship with the family.

Once the assessment has been completed and nursing diagnoses formulated, a plan of care is developed. Intervention is optimally aimed at two levels, the family and the child. The family members, especially the caregivers, need assistance in changing their responses to the child. The child needs to learn more adaptive coping skills. A variety of treatment modalities exist that are effective in caring for a child with an emotional problem.

A continuum of options exists for managing behavior that is escalating or getting out of control. The least restrictive is teaching and encouraging acceptable ways for children to express themselves and to get their needs met. Then, procedures such as time-outs (quiet time spent alone in a nonstimulating environment) can be used if needed. As a last resort, holding and seclusion may be used. When behavior has been out of control, the child should be encouraged to review the situation in order to gain insight into what happened, why it happened, and how to avoid this loss of control in the future (Antoinette, Tyengar, & Puig-Antich, 1990).

One of the most important nursing interventions to improve self-esteem is to help the child identify and promote his strengths rather than weaknesses. Caregivers need to identify methods they can use to help their child gain a more positive self-esteem, such as listening to their child, having realistic expectations, offering praise for accomplishments, and the like. The nurse can encourage the child to engage in activities in which he is likely to succeed and to focus on aspects of his life for which positive feelings exist.

Play Therapy

Most younger children find it difficult to express themselves verbally. Their limited vocabularies restrict the ability to identify feelings and concerns. **Play therapy** is one of the most useful techniques for expressing feelings, exploring relationships, and attempting new solutions to problems. Play provides an opportunity for developing a therapeutic relationship between the nurse and child. Therapeutic play provides the opportunity for hidden and threatening content to be presented. Play can serve additional functions. The child can learn basic skills and social skills, explore the environment, release excess energy, and imitate and acquire adult roles. Toys that are imaginative and age appropriate should be offered to the child, such as blocks, a play house, dolls that represent family members, trucks, cars, and soldiers. The child is urged to play without any directions from the nurse. The nurse should not guide the play or make interpretations that link the play to the child's life experiences.

Individual Therapy

A child enters therapy with a different perspective than does an adult. Many adults enter therapy willingly because they realize they have problems for which they need help. Children tend not to see themselves as having problems; therefore, the need for therapy may not be recognized. Often the child believes that he has been forced into treatment against his will by his caregivers. The nurse is seen as having allied herself with the caregivers, so the child may distrust her also. In order to develop a trusting relationship with the child, the nurse needs to avoid taking sides. Communicating a sense of acceptance of the child separate from his unacceptable behavior is essential.

Another characteristic of children in therapy is that they often perceive the nurse as an all-powerful, all-knowing adult to whom they look for direction. Thus, the nurse becomes a powerful role model whose verbal and nonverbal behaviors must be consistent to gain the child's respect. Additionally, a child's cognitive level and language abilities necessitate the need to act out feelings and situations. The nurse must use methods that provide the vehicle for the safe acting out of feelings, such as role playing, games, and journals.

Family Therapy

Family therapy is an especially important treatment for children with psychiatric disorders. Child disorders cannot be fully understood without exploring the family context. Family therapy is based on the premise that the behavior of one person cannot be changed without bringing about change in the entire family. Studies have shown that treating the family system produces more rapid and enduring changes. For additional information on family therapy, refer to Chapter 27.

Psychopharmacology

Psychopharmacology is one aspect of a treatment program for children. The use of psychotropic medications in this population often arouses controversy about efficacy, side effects, and long-term impact on growth and development. Several issues are important to consider when discussing pediatric psychopharmacology. One issue is the risk-to-benefit ratio: The benefit to the child must outweigh the risks. The possibility of toxicity, the

---

☏☏ *REFLECTIVE THINKING*

Are We Overmedicating Children?

Sometimes medication is requested by a caregiver or teacher in order to make a child more manageable or to enhance cognitive development. Do you think this is an appropriate request? Why or why not? In your opinion, what situations would merit medicating a child in order to achieve behavior control?

---

possibility of paradoxical reactions, and the possibility of adverse effects on the child's cognitive and social development must be considered when assessing the risks. Ideally, medication should either not impair learning or should improve a child's ability to benefit from learning experiences.

The fact that a child is growing and developing makes any period of less than optimal functioning of greater importance than in an adult. For an adult to be "zonked" for a few weeks due to medications is not good but usually does not have grave implications. For a child, however, to be excessively sedated or socially unresponsive for a period of weeks or even months may have severe implications for the child's development. Another issue is that children, whose metabolic and neurological systems are still developing, react differently to medications than do adults. Dosages of medications for children should be based on research with children, rather than extrapolated from standard doses for adults. Unfortunately, such data are often not available. Finally, legal issues must be considered in the use of psychotropic medications. It is important to have the informed consent and informed cooperation of both the child and caregivers in any medication trial. Caregivers often have extremely strong feelings about the use of psychoactive medications in their children; therefore, it is essential that they be well informed about the risks and benefits and about their right to accept or reject the recommendation for medication, and that they truly give informed consent. The child and caregivers should also have an opportunity to discuss their feelings about medications. It must be remembered that medication is not the sole treatment indicated. The complexity of emotional problems demands an integrated approach involving various therapies: psychodynamic (individual, family, or group), behavioral, milieu, medication, and resources in the family and school.

Antipsychotics (Neuroleptics)

Antipsychotic drugs, or neuroleptics, have proven clinically effective in treating thought disorders, hallucinations, delusions, overwhelming anxiety, and severe agitation. They are primarily indicated for children with schizophrenic disorders, psychotic reactions secondary to major affective disorders, and autism presenting with stereotypic and withdrawal symptoms and self-abuse. Side effects from the antipsychotic drugs are numerous. Extrapyramidal symptoms, a Parkinson-like syndrome involving drooling, involuntary hand movements, and an inability to remain still develop in at least one-fourth of children treated with neuroleptics. This syndrome is rarely seen in preschool children but is more common in school-age children and adolescents. Therefore, caregivers should be taught to continually monitor for these adverse side effects by assessing for muscle rigidity, inability to remain still, vague subjective complaints such as a need to move, and any abnormal involuntary movements. These side effects should be reported to the physician for possible reduction in the medication dosage and/or the addition of an anti-Parkinson or anticholinergic agent such as Cogentin or Artane. Anticholinergic side effects include dry mouth, blurred vision, constipation, and urinary retention, so caregivers need to assess bladder and bowel elimination, especially in younger children (Gadow, 1992).

The most problematic side effect of the antipsychotics is the development of tardive dyskinesia, which occurs in approximately 20% to 30% of children treated long term. Early signs are characterized by tongue movement or increased blinking. Later signs involve tongue protrusion and unusual mouth movements such as sucking, smacking lips, or chewing jaw movements. The treatment for tardive dyskinesia involves decreasing or discontinuing the medication if possible. However, the most effective treatment is prevention, specifically, regular assessment for beginning side effects, regular reevaluation of drug dosage, drug-free holidays when appropriate, and maintenance on the lowest effective dosage.

Antidepressant Drugs

Tricyclic antidepressants (TCAs) were developed in the 1950s to treat depression and gained acceptance for use with children in the 1960s. These drugs frequently affect the cardiovascular system, and children are more susceptible than adults to the cardiotoxic effects of increased blood pressure and tachycardia. The sudden deaths of several children treated with desipramine (Norpramin) from 1987 to 1990 have raised concerns about the safety of this drug and similar ones. Although the deaths in some cases appear to have been related to preexisting heart conditions, the resulting controversy has led some health care providers to stop using desipramine as a first line of treatment. Tricyclic antidepressants are still prescribed, but only after a child has had a complete cardiac examination and continues with follow-up electrocardiograms. The serotonin reuptake inhibitors (SRIs)

and the selective SRIs (SSRIs), such as fluoxetine (Prozac) and sertraline (Zoloft), which are used with adults, are being tested with children in the United States and abroad, and early results are encouraging.

Nurses have an important role in educating caregivers about the potential risk of cardiac toxicity and standstill associated with TCAs. Teaching should include keeping the medication out of reach of younger children to prevent accidental overdosage and ensuring that the severely depressed child or adolescent does not have access to the medication to prevent suicide.

Mood Stabilizers

Lithium carbonate and carbamazepine (Tegretol) are effective in treating mania in bipolar disorder. Lithium blood levels should be determined while the child is taking the medication because the therapeutic dose is, in many instances, near toxic level. Tegretol has also been used to treat self-injurious behavior in organically impaired children.

Stimulants

Stimulant medications are used to treat the signs and symptoms of attention-deficit disorder and ADHD. These medications act on the central nervous system and stimulate the reticular activating system. Methylphenidate (Ritalin), dextroamphetamine (Dexedrine), and magnesium pemoline (Cylert) are most commonly prescribed and have

---

⚠ NURSING ALERT!

Medication Safety and Children

◆ Encourage caregivers to always keep medications locked away and out of reach of children.

◆ Closely monitor all medication courses for side effects including uncontrollable tics and body movements, change in affect, change in activity or sleeping patterns, blurred vision, change in elimination patterns, and the like. Notify physician immediately of any untoward side effects.

◆ Encourage caregivers to keep careful record of medication administration and immediately report side effects or changes in the child's behavior.

◆ Warn caregivers of signs of toxicity/overdose, and ensure that they have the phone number for poison control.

been shown to increase children's ability to be attentive, to improve classroom behavior, and to increase social acceptance. Long-term stimulant side effects may include growth suppression and weight loss. Some think the decreased growth rate is a short-term problem; however, others have reported a drop in height of 2% in children who receive an average of 40 mg in 24 hours for 2 to 4 years. The growth of children receiving stimulants should be monitored. Appetite suppression can lead to significant weight loss in some children, and providers often recommend drug-free holidays to allow children to gain weight. In other words, on weekends, holidays, and during summer vacation, the child would not take the medication, thus encouraging weight gain (Vatz & Weinberg, 1993).

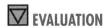 **EVALUATION**

Evaluation of the effectiveness of the interventions and care plan should include not only the child's progress toward achieving targeted outcomes but the family unit's progress toward a more healthy, supportive, and interactive relationship with the child. Progress in many instances may be slow, requiring weeks or months or even years to realize, so it is important for the nurse to help the family view their successes in increments and to maintain realistic expectations of the outcomes they will see. It is also critical for the family and child to view together their successes and failures, so they can mutually agree on what tactics are most effective and those that should be changed.

CASE STUDY/CARE PLAN

Jean, 10 years old, was admitted to a child and adolescent inpatient psychiatric unit. Her admission was part of a court evaluation for stealing cigarettes from a convenience store, her second infraction with the law in a year. Jean's caregivers divorced when she was 3 years old, after many years of conflict and fighting. Jean now lives with her mother and 6-year-old brother because her father, with whom she lived for the past 7 years, was sentenced to prison for robbery. She no longer attends public school, having been expelled for threatening her teacher with a knife and smoking and drinking alcohol on school premises. Jean's mother reports that at home Jean frequently fights with her brother, has threatened him, and has stayed out all night for several nights at a time.

ASSESSMENT

Jean has had a continued pattern of antisocial behaviors, including violation of rules, theft, bullying, and aggression with a weapon toward others, and she lacks feelings of guilt or remorse. She has used tobacco and alcohol earlier than her peer group's expected age. Low self-esteem is manifested by a "tough girl" demeanor. Her level of academic achievement is low in relation to her age and IQ. She exhibits the following characteristics: poor impulse control, poor frustration tolerance, irritability, and frequent temper outbursts.

NURSING DIAGNOSIS *Risk for violence: self-directed or directed at others*, related to negative caregiver role models and dysfunctional family dynamics, as evidenced by poor impulse control

Outcomes	Planning/Interventions	Evaluation
◆ Jean will not harm herself, others, or other's property.	◆ Communicate expected behavior to Jean; state limits firmly; offer substitute behaviors.	Many conduct-disordered clients are adept at becoming socialized to the milieu and may show rapid "improvement." Because of shortened hospital stays, it may be necessary to evaluate short-term goals as opposed to intermediate or long-term goals.
	◆ Explain the consequences of unacceptable behaviors.	
	◆ Set limits that are not negotiable to ensure safety.	
	◆ State the reasons for limits.	
◆ Jean will learn to express anger appropriately.	◆ Give positive reinforcement for appropriate behaviors and observation of limits.	

Continued

Outcomes	Planning/Interventions	Evaluation
	◆ Ignore misbehavior every time it occurs.	Evaluation is made of the behavioral changes in the client. This is accomplished by determining if the goals of treatment have been achieved.
	◆ Redirect violent behavior with physical outlets.	
	◆ Use time-outs for unacceptable behaviors.	
		Evaluate the following areas for improvement: prevention of harm to self, others, or other's property; ability to express anger in an appropriate manner; development of more adaptive coping strategies to deal with anger and feelings of aggression.

NURSING DIAGNOSIS *Self-esteem disturbance*, related to lack of positive feedback and unsatisfactory caregiver/child relationship, as evidenced by "tough girl" demeanor, denial of problems, and projection of responsibility

Outcomes	Planning/Interventions	Evaluation
◆ Jean will demonstrate increased feelings of self-worth by verbalizing positive statements about self and exhibiting more appropriate, acceptable behaviors.	◆ Plan activities that allow for success.	Evaluate the following for improvement: ability to verbalize positive statements about self; ability to interact with others without engaging in manipulation; less blaming of others.
	◆ Praise appropriate behaviors in front of others.	
	◆ Identify Jean's perceptions of any strengths or special qualities she values.	
	◆ Assist her in developing more effective social skills.	

NURSING DIAGNOSIS *Ineffective individual coping*, related to maturational crises, as evidenced by use of manipulative behaviors to express emotions and to get needs met

Outcomes	Planning/Interventions	Evaluation
◆ Jean will verbalize those behaviors that are self-defeating.	◆ When observing manipulative behaviors, confront Jean with these behaviors.	Evaluate progress by looking to Jean's new ability to accept responsibility for own behavior and her ability to accept feedback without becoming manipulative.
◆ She will connect her manipulative behaviors to particular feelings or family situations.	◆ Explore the self-defeating nature of these behaviors.	
	◆ Explore what she accomplishes when using these behaviors, i.e., the need to control her environment.	
◆ She will ask directly for needs to be met.	◆ Explore ways to promote a more positive sense of control at home, at school, and with peers.	

CRITICAL THINKING BAND

ASSESSMENT

Do you think that interviewing Jean's teachers or peers might provide additional insight into her troubled behaviors? What environmental factors could you evaluate that might also affect her demeanor?

NURSING DIAGNOSIS

What other nursing diagnoses are applicable to this case?

Outcomes

Do you agree with the nurse's goals for Jean? What other goals would you select?

Planning/Interventions

If the nursing actions directed toward managing Jean's aggressive and manipulative behaviors have been ineffective, what other interventions might be appropriate?

Evaluation

What behavioral changes do you think are realistic over a 2-week period? One month? Six months? Should you include changes in caregiver attitudes when evaluating Jean's progress? How would you do this?

KEY CONCEPTS

- ◆ Children are encountering an increasingly hostile culture resulting in a growing number of children experiencing mental health problems.

- ◆ Mental health resources are currently treating only one of five children requiring treatment, and resources are diminishing at federal, state, and local levels.

- ◆ Disorders identified by the DSM-IV as first becoming evident in infancy or childhood include Autistic Disorder, Attention-Deficit Hyperactivity Disorder, Conduct Disorder, Depression, Separation Anxiety Disorder, and Post-Traumatic Stress Disorder.

- ◆ Nursing assessment of emotional disorders of children includes a basic assessment of both the child and the family.

- ◆ Nursing diagnoses form the basis for interventions. Common diagnoses with children with emotional problems include *anxiety, impaired social interaction, ineffective individual coping, risk for violence,* and *self-esteem disturbance.*

- ◆ Treatment modalities for children include play therapy, individual therapy, family therapy, and psychopharmacology.

REVIEW QUESTIONS AND ACTIVITIES

1. What are the characteristic responses to the environment in children with Autistic Disorder?

2. Describe nursing interventions for children with Autistic Disorder.

3. Discuss the characteristic behaviors of a child with Attention-Deficit Hyperactivity Disorder.

4. What are the common behaviors seen in conduct disorders?

5. What is the most effective treatment of conduct disorders?

6. Describe the clinical manifestations of depression in children.

7. Describe the manifestations of Separation Anxiety Disorder.

8. What are the causes and characteristics of Post-Traumatic Stress Disorder?

9. Discuss the characteristics of behaviors used to define serious emotional disorders.

10. Describe the various treatment modalities used for children with emotional disorders.

11. What psychotrophic medications are most commonly used with children?

⚛ EXPLORING THE WEB

◆ Visit this text's "Online Companion™" on the Internet at **http://www.DelmarNursing.com** for further information on childhood psychiatric disorders such as Attention-Deficit Disorder.

◆ What resources are listed for caregivers and health care professionals?

◆ Search under specific disorders such as Post-Traumatic Stress Disorder, Depression, or Conduct Disorder. What information is available? Is it specific to children?

◆ What children's organizations can you locate that have specific discussion groups addressing the psychiatric needs of children?

≋ REFERENCES

American Psychiatric Association. (1968). *Diagnostic and statistical manual of mental disorders* (2nd ed.). Washington, DC: Author.

American Psychiatric Association. (1994). *Diagnostic and statistical manual of mental disorders* (4th ed.). Washington, DC: Author.

Antoinette, T., Tyengar, S., & Puig-Antich, J. (1990). Is locked seclusion necessary for children under 14? *American Journal of Psychiatry, 147,* 1283–1289.

Bumbalo, J. A., & Siemon, M. K. (1983). Nursing assessment and diagnosis: Mental health problems of children. *Topics in Clinical Nursing, 5*(1), 41–54.

Gadow, K. D. (1992). Pediatric psychopharmacology: A review of recent research. *Journal of Child Psychology and Psychiatry, 33,* 153.

Kazdin, A. E. (1990). Childhood depression. *Journal of Child Psychology and Psychiatry, 31,* 121–160.

Massie, H., & Rosenthal, J. (1984). *Childhood psychosis in the first four years of life.* New York: McGraw-Hill.

National Safety Council. (1993). *Accident facts.* Itasca, IL: Author.

Neff, J. A., & Dale, J. (1996). Worries of school-age children. *Journal of the Society of Pediatric Nurses, 1*(1), 27–32.

Palfrey, J. S. (1995). *Community child health.* Westpoint, CT: Praeger.

Poznaski, E. (1982). The clinical phenomenology of childhood depression. *American Journal of Orthopsychiatry, 52,* 308–313.

Rutter, M. (1983). Cognitive deficits in the pathogenesis of autism. *Journal of Child Psychology and Psychiatry, 24,* 513–531.

Stewart, J. T., Myers, W. C., & Burket, R. C. (1990). A review of pharmacotherapy of aggression in children and adolescents. *Journal of the American Academy of Child and Adolescent Psychiatry, 29,* 269.

U.S. Department of Health and Human Services. (1990). *National plan for research on child and adolescent mental disorders.* Rockville, MD: National Institute of Mental Health.

Vatz, R. E., & Weinberg, L. S. (1993). Treatment of attention-deficit hyperactivity disorder. *JAMA, 269*(18), 2368.

Webster-Stratton, C. (1991). Annotation: Strategies for helping families with conduct disordered children. *Journal of Child Psychology and Psychiatry, 32,* 1047.

〰 LITERARY REFERENCES

Axline, V. M. (1964). *Dibs in search of self.* New York: Houghton Mifflin.

Williams, D. (1992). *Nobody nowhere.* New York: Avon Books.

〰 SUGGESTED READINGS

Dolgan, J. (1990). Depression in children. *Pediatric Annals, 19*(1), 45–50.

Gottlieb, S. E., & Friedman, S. B. (1991). Conduct disorders in children and adolescents. *Pediatric Review, 12*(7), 218–223.

Lewis-Abney, K. (1993). Correlates of family functioning when a child has attention deficit disorder. *Issues in Comprehensive Pediatric Nursing, 16*(3), 175–190.

O'Connell, K. (1996). Attention deficit hyperactivity disorder. *Pediatric Nursing, 22*(1), 30–33.

Ryan, N. (1992). The pharmacologic treatment of child and adolescent depression. *Psychiatric Clinics of North America, 15*(1), 29–37.

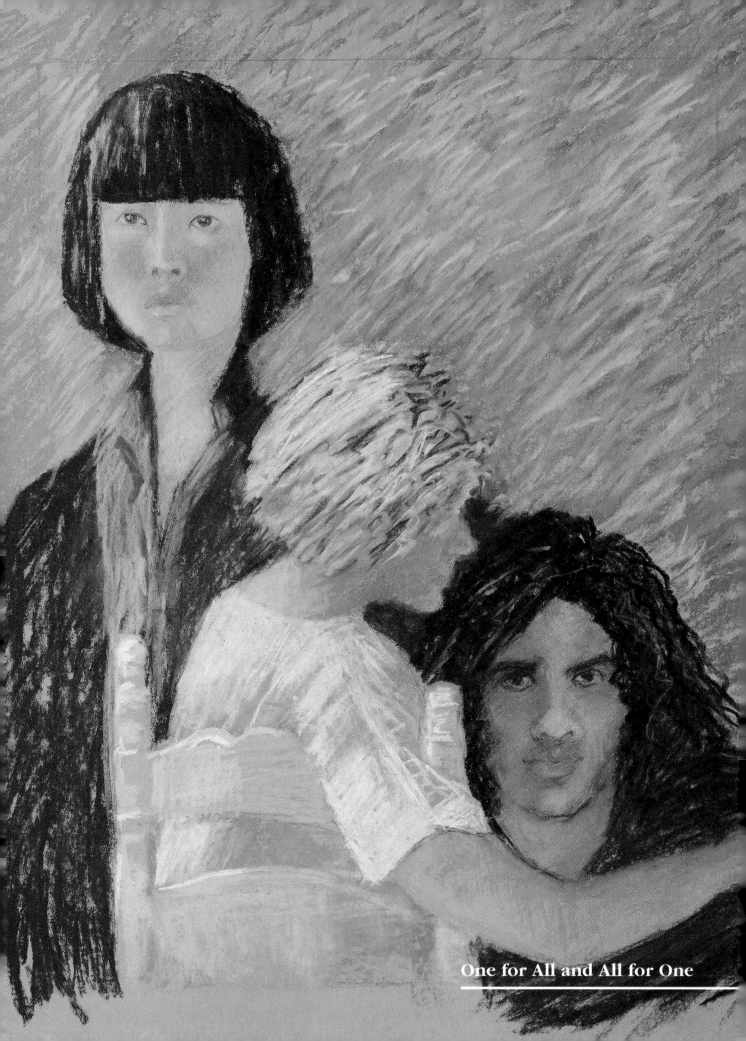

One for All and All for One

Chapter

22

THE ADOLESCENT

Lynn Rew

Transitions in Adolescence

Remember your own transition from childhood to adulthood:
- ◆ What were the significant changes you experienced?
- ◆ What emotions did you experience with these changes?
- ◆ How did significant others respond to these changes?
- ◆ How did this transition affect your sense of personal identity?
- ◆ How did this transition affect your sense of competence and responsibility as an adult?

Keep these experiences in mind as you read this chapter.

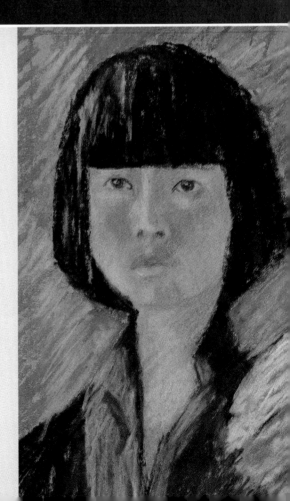

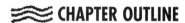 **CHAPTER OUTLINE**

ADOLESCENCE DEFINED

Physical Transitions

Cognitive Transitions

Emotional Transitions

Social Transitions

THEORIES OF ADOLESCENT DEVELOPMENT

Identity Formation

Social Competence

MENTAL HEALTH IN ADOLESCENCE

Mental Health Care Needs

    Needs Related to Physical Transitions

    Needs Related to Cognitive Transitions

    Needs Related to Emotional Transitions

    Needs Related to Social Transitions

NURSING THEORIES

Humanistic Nursing

Health as Expanding Consciousness

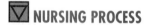 **NURSING PROCESS**

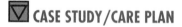 **CASE STUDY/CARE PLAN**

COMPETENCIES

Upon completion of this chapter, the reader should be able to:

1. Differentiate among various definitions of adolescent mental health.

2. Identify the physical, cognitive, emotional, and social transitions of adolescence.

3. Examine concepts and theories about identity formation and social competence.

4. Reflect on your own sense of personal identity and social competence.

5. Identify major mental health needs and concerns of adolescents.

6. Apply the nursing process to the care of adolescent clients.

7. Integrate nursing theories into planning care for the adolescent in need of mental health services.

〰 KEY TERMS

Foreclosure One of four identity statuses; refers to the adolescent's lack of thoroughly exploring alternatives before making a commitment to an adult identity.

Gender Identity An individual's subjective feeling associated with being male or female.

Gender Role Public recognition of one's gender assignment as male or female and the individual's expression of appropriate social behaviors related to that assignment.

Identity Achievement One of the four identity statuses in which an adolescent makes a commitment to an adult identity after a period of exploring alternatives.

Identity Diffusion One of the four identity statuses in which an adolescent avoids making a full commitment to an adult identity and does not reach his or her potential; often associated with restricted emotional expression or detachment from others.

Identity Formation An adolescent's process of finding a place within the larger society, beyond the boundaries of the family.

Moratorium One of the four identity statuses in which an individual delays making a decision about adult identity while exploring various alternatives during adolescence.

Presence Activity of being physically present with another person that begins with the nurse's genuine commitment to caring and nurturing the potential of the client.

Self-awareness Perception of oneself in relation to others and to society's expectations.

Self-efficacy Ability to organize and manage individual responses to the demands of the environment.

Social Competence Degree to which significant others rate an individual as successful at performing expected social tasks.

Status Style used by an adolescent in resolving issues of adult identity.

Suicidal Ideation An individual's process of thinking about reasons for and ways of killing oneself.

Adolescence, the period of transition from childhood to adulthood, is a decade filled with profound and often confusing changes. Dramatic physical and psychological development is typically accompanied by cognitive, emotional, and social changes; decreasing levels of adult supervision; increasing experimentation with adult behaviors and responsibilities; and changes in the social milieu of school and work. All of these can upset an individual's sense of identity and social competence. The purposes of this chapter are threefold: (1) to identify various ways to define mental health during the developmental phase of adolescence, (2) to examine the many ways in which the transitions experienced by adolescents create a need for mental health care, and (3) to demonstrate the application of nursing theories to the care of adolescents with mental health concerns.

ADOLESCENCE DEFINED

In the current American culture, adolescents are viewed as neither children nor adults. The decade of adolescence, conceptualized as the ages of 11 to 20 years, is composed of three arbitrary subphases: early adolescence (ages 11 to 14), middle adolescence (ages 15 to 17), and late adolescence (ages 18 to 20) (Crockett & Petersen, 1993). Early adolescence is evident with the onset of puberty, which involves many biological changes such as height and weight spurts, development of internal and external genitalia, and hair growth. Middle adolescence is characterized by increasing focus on peers and the pressures of conforming to a normative group on the basis of how one dresses, speaks, and acts. Late adolescence is marked by the final shift from preoccupation with appearances and conformity to commitment to roles and responsibilities within the adult society. The transitions from childhood to adolescence can create internal and interpersonal conflict as the adolescent struggles for a concrete personal identity, skills of social competence, and a commitment to play a particular role as an adult within the community.

The central developmental task of adolescence, according to Erikson (1950, 1968), is **identity formation**. The issue of identity concerns finding a place for oneself in the larger society beyond one's family. Adolescents are challenged with finding out who they are and what part they will play in society as responsible adults.

Identity formation begins with an understanding of the self, which starts in early childhood. Early life experiences shape one's development of a personality complete with attitudes and beliefs, talents, capacities, and limitations. Experiences alone and with other people help the child form an awareness of one's separateness as well as relatedness within a social order. As Erikson (1950) conceptualizes it, early childhood allows the individual to tackle the tasks of developing trust, autonomy, initiative, and industry by overcoming mistrust in infancy, shame and doubt as a toddler, and guilt and inferiority during school age. The child who successfully masters these psychosocial tasks and incorporates these qualities into a personality structure is well equipped to face the complexities of adolescent identity formation.

The adolescent whose childhood has been characterized by positive interactions with a loving and supportive family and community and who has developed a strong sense of self-worth and self-esteem experiences this period of transition with some confusion and self-doubt. Emotions go up and down like the proverbial roller coaster. New challenges and problems are stressors that must be met with new coping and problem-solving skills. On the other hand, the adolescent whose childhood has been marred by neglect; emotional, physical, and/or sexual abuse; or some other type of trauma faces even greater confusion and self-doubt during this time of profound change. Scars from a wounded childhood can make the adolescent vulnerable to identity problems and **suicidal ideation**, or thoughts about killing oneself. Others may have to face this time of transition with a diagnosable mental illness carried over from childhood or one that finally erupts full blown with adolescence.

Many adolescents feel confusion and conflict as they resolve the developmental task of identity formation. Emotions swing from wanting to remain within the safety and security of childhood to wanting to experiment with new freedoms associated with being an adult. Behaviors and beliefs that were initially formed and approved by the nuclear family are now exposed to the approval of peers in the larger community. The period of adolescence is necessarily lengthy in our society so that the individual has ample time to explore and incorporate the sense of mastery of psychosocial tasks, including identity formation, into a repertoire of attitudes, beliefs, values, behaviors, and skills that will serve society in a responsible manner. In other societies in which less emphasis is placed on individual identity, the transitional phase of adolescence is less lengthy and less associated with conflict and confusion. At the conclusion of the adolescent phase of development, the individual essentially makes a commitment or statement to society about what he stands for and about his role in the society.

Physical Transitions

The onset of puberty signals the beginning of physical maturation that transforms the child into a sexually mature adult. The physical changes of puberty are set in motion by the production of hormones that direct the development of secondary sexual characteristics and physical functions that permit reproduction. These physi-

cal and biochemical alterations occur within the social context of family and community and within a personal framework of personality and previous experiences.

The physical changes in early adolescence are accompanied by an increasing interest in sexual attractiveness. Those individuals who mature early may experience situations in which older adolescents find them sexually attractive. Yet, the young adolescent is cognitively and socially unprepared for the risks associated with early sexual activity and is at special risk for unwanted pregnancy and sexually transmitted diseases. Middle (ages 15 to 17) and late (ages 18 to 20) adolescents, on the other hand, are cognitively more mature and better able to make decisions about the consequences of their behaviors in social settings with little adult supervision.

Cognitive Transitions

The cognitive, or intellectual, changes that occur in adolescence point to the need for mental health prevention and intervention strategies. In particular, adolescents are often characterized by impulsivity and high risk taking in an attempt to feel good, to be accepted by a peer group, and to experiment with adult behaviors. Decisions about being sexually active, driving motor vehicles without seatbelts or helmets, and using alcohol and other drugs are often made with little thought to the consequences of such behaviors (Vernon, 1991). These high-risk behaviors are potentially destructive not only to the individual but to his or her family and society. For example, females who become pregnant in early or middle adolescence are at high risk for dropping out of school. This has enormous economic implications for them and their children, as a large percentage remain on welfare as adults.

School-based prevention programs, such as sex education that focus on consequences of behaviors rather than on moral dictums, have been successful. The nurse can assist in acknowledging that adolescents have a need to be accepted by a peer group and to feel good but at the same time must have visions for the future so that decisions that may affect the rest of their lives are not left to sudden whims of desire and passion.

Emotional Transitions

The emotional changes that accompany puberty are often characterized by feelings of anxiety and depression. Anxiety about physical changes are related to eating disorders, sleeping problems, and the inability to pay attention in school with subsequent poor performance. Anxiety is also aroused as the adolescent strives to become part of a normative peer group and may face conflicts with expected behaviors that are different from those approved of by caregivers. Increases in anxiety may

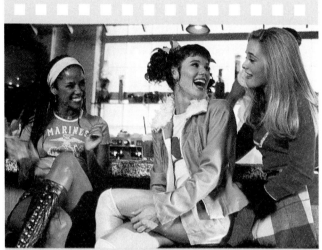

Clueless. Source: Paramount/Courtesy Kobal.

Adolescence is a time for self-exploration and the establishment of a group identity. These young women portrayed in the film *Clueless* share an identity based on little more than clothing and popular culture.

lead the adolescent to engage in other high-risk behavior such as alcohol and drug abuse, gang involvement, or sexual promiscuity.

The lengthy period of adolescence and identity formation is one of exploration, in which the adolescent "tries on" various ways of being alone and with groups. Some individuals adopt identities without exploration, simply hanging on to childhood beliefs and coping strategies, while others remain adrift, making no effort to explore or resolve the issue of identity formation (Josselson, 1994). The complex process of identity formation is addressed in myriad ways in the mental health needs and concerns of adolescents.

Social Transitions

The social milieu of the adolescent includes the family, peer, school, and working environments. This social world contains the opportunities and barriers for the individual to explore various roles and responsibilities associated with being a responsible member of the community (Perry, Kelder, & Komro, 1993). As the child moves into adolescence, he may experience changes within the family structure and function as caregivers and siblings also mature. Stereotypically, adolescents begin to spend more time away from their caregivers and other supervisory adults. They seek out peers who are also engaging in more activities with less adult supervision. Thus they begin to experiment with more adultlike behaviors including working part-time jobs, making their

own decisions about spending money and leisure time, driving motorized vehicles, using alcohol, tobacco, and other drugs, and initiating sexual activities. Engaging in these behaviors may have a variety of consequences for the adolescent, including poor performance at school and work as well as an increase in other risky and violent behavior. According to Jessor (1991), most of these risky behaviors are purposeful and goal oriented. They help adolescents to cope with anxiety and frustration and to gain peer respect and acceptance and are significant in establishing a break with the status of being a child.

Behaviors during early adolescence (ages 11 to 14) are often erratic and impulsive as these youngsters shift their primary role models from caregivers to peers. They tend to resist authority in an effort to gain more independence and autonomy (Pletsch, Johnson, Tosi, Thurston, & Riesch, 1991).

Adolescents and their caregivers experience increasing conflicts around issues such as appropriate attire, school work, curfews, and use of leisure time. Caregiving style has been shown to be related to high-risk behaviors among adolescents. Authoritative caregivers provide clear boundaries and expectations for their children. As a result, the children of such caregivers, in general, engage in less substance abuse, display greater psychosocial maturity, and perform better in school than children whose caregivers are indifferent or uninvolved (Crockett & Petersen, 1993). As depicted in the following excerpt, misunderstanding between caregivers and children can be even more trying when the adolescent has a bona fide need for mental health intervention:

Lisa, Bright and Dark

"Listen to me!" Lisa shouted.

Everyone did.

"I think I'm going crazy," Lisa said again.
"I think I'm going out of my mind. Could we get some help or something?"

"Like what?" her mother asked. "You've mentioned this before, but you never say what you want to do about it."

M. N. [Mary Nell] was startled. This was the first time she'd ever heard Lisa say anything about this.

"Besides," Mrs. Shilling went on, "I think it's very rude of you to discuss this sort of thing when we have guests."

"Oh," M. N. smiled sheepishly, "don't mind me. Really."

"Since you don't pay any attention to me when we're alone," Lisa protested, "I thought you might with other people around."

"All right, all right," Mrs. Shilling sighed.

"What is it you think you need?"

"Well," said Lisa, calmer, quiet but not hopeful, "maybe a psychiatrist or someone. I mean," she added quickly, "it wouldn't have to be an expensive one. Just someone who would understand and know what to do."

"You've seen too many movies," Mr. Shilling said.

"Who else has a psychiatrist, Lisa, in your class?" her mother wanted to know.

"How should I know?" Lisa said, clenching her teeth, trying to smile politely.

(Neufeld, 1970, p. 10)

Lisa and her caregivers illustrate some of the common communication patterns that develop between adolescents and their caregivers. Lisa shouts and deliberately brings up an emotionally laden topic in front of her friend to get her caregivers' attention. This pattern of communication does not necessarily indicate the need for mental health intervention, but in this case, it is a drastic attempt by Lisa to let her caregivers know that she really feels something is wrong with her mental health.

Lisa's mother feels embarrassed about her daughter's outburst in front of one of her friends and does not pass up the opportunity to discipline Lisa in front of Mary Nell by telling her how rude she thinks this type of communication is. Lisa, on the other hand, is trying to be honest and forthright with her caregivers by telling them directly that she thinks she needs to visit a psychiatrist. She adds that the doctor does not need to "be an expensive one," possibly reflecting other previous conflicts with her caregivers over the cost of other requests (not an uncommon area of conflict between caregivers and youth).

Lisa's caregivers continue to either deny that Lisa has a mental health problem or fail to sense her pain and frustration in their last responses. Lisa's father dismisses her request by commenting that she has simply seen too many movies (suggesting that watching movies about people who visit psychiatrists puts "ideas" into her young head). Lisa's mother dismisses her request by asking who else in her class has seen a psychiatrist (suggesting that her outburst and request for help are simply mimicry of some teenaged idol). The story of Lisa's mental illness (Schizophrenia) exemplifies the importance of communication between caregivers and teens as well as the suffering that results when that communication is perceived as a source of caregiver-child conflict.

Transitions from elementary to middle to high school create new opportunities and social stresses for the adolescent. With each transition comes a new set of rules and expectations, creating the need for great adaptability within the individual. Often, adolescents find themselves not only in a new physical environment but also with peers and upperclassmen who were unknown to them in the previous school. Those whose families move from one location to another also experience increased stress in adjusting to new locations and peers. Loneliness may become an everyday experience for the adolescent who feels misunderstood or rejected from the normative group in the new school (Brage, Meredith, & Woodward, 1993).

THEORIES OF ADOLESCENT DEVELOPMENT

Several theoretical approaches can help to clarify the unique phase of life known as adolescence. Two approaches that are of particular relevance to the mental health of adolescents are theories of identity formation and social competence. The concepts central to these theories blend well with nursing approaches to the adolescent client.

Identity Formation

Identity formation is a central concept in the developmental theory of Erikson (1950, 1968). Erikson's theory is related to but different from classical, or Freudian, psychoanalytic theory. Rather than having a focus on psychopathology rooted in one's libido, this psychosocial theory focuses on adaptation and interaction between the individual and the environment or society (Marcia, 1994). According to Erikson, adolescence is the phase in life in which previous childhood tasks of development are revisited and integrated. The first developmental stage of learning to trust oneself and others must be integrated as the adolescent questions what people and which ideas should be trusted and how trustworthy the adolescent himself is. Ultimately, this is a question of identity whose roots extend far back into infancy.

The second developmental stage of autonomy also centers around identity, an identity that is to be revisited in adolescence. The maturing individual, much like the toddler, must face issues of independence and making decisions based on free will. A sense of pride in one's choices and shameless approval of one's peers are important in settling the issue of identity in the second decade of life. Similarly, as the school-age child displays initiative and industry in learning the skills that enable problem solving and coping with the stresses of living, so too does the adolescent resolve again to express initiative and industry in determining an identity and role to which to be committed within the larger society (Erikson, 1968).

Marcia (1994) extended the psychosocial development theory of Erikson by conducting extensive research on the stage of adolescence, in which the crisis of identity versus identity confusion is generally resolved. Marcia believed that identity is a process by which adolescents decide how to take a place in the world as responsible adults who are committed to a particular way of being.

The process is characterized by exploration of alternatives. While much of identity formation takes place in adolescence, significant life changes—such as the birth of a child, marriage, or death of a loved one—call for identity reformulation throughout the life span.

Marcia identified four categories of styles used by adolescents to resolve the issue of identity. These four styles, termed **statuses**, are outlined in Table 22-1. The first status is called **foreclosure**. These individuals have not thoroughly explored the possibilities of identity before making a commitment about adult status. They are closely tied to their families because to question caregiver values would be too threatening and would make them feel guilty. Their families are generally warm, but this is contingent upon the child's decision to follow the family's rules and adhere to their values and beliefs. The second status is characterized by exploring alternatives in search of an adult-sized identity and suffering the crisis and consequences of this exploration This status is called **moratorium** and represents an expected period of delay in making a final decision about identity. The third status is **identity achievement** and involves making a commitment to a specific identity after a period of exploration. Finally, the fourth status, **identity diffusion**, refers to avoiding making commitments and may indicate a need for mental health services. Some of these individuals are socially skilled but are not reaching their intellectual or physical potentials. They may have some or all of the characteristics of individuals with Schizoid Personality Disorder, which is a pattern of restricted emotional expression and detachment from other people (American Psychiatric Association, 1994). Still others may suffer from

Table 22-1	**Four Statuses of Adolescent Identity**	
STATUS	**CHARACTERISTICS**	**EXAMPLES**
Foreclosure	Identity decision made before options explored	Mary Ellen decides to live at home and work in the family dry-cleaning business rather than apply to a college. Her parents show strong approval of this decision even though Mary Ellen has previously expressed an interest in studying music at a nearby university.
Moratorium	Identity decision delayed until options explored	Jeffrey is feeling ambivalent about what to do after high school. His father encourages him to think about medical school and, thus, follow in his father's footsteps. His mother encourages him to do whatever he wants to do. Jeffrey considers going to a community college for a year or two until "I can find myself."
Identity diffusion	Identity decision avoided	Lindsey is a charming 16-year-old. He easily finds an after-school job at a fast-food restaurant but maintains a poor work record and soon leaves to pursue employment at a bakery. His interpersonal relationships lack commitment as he flits from one new girlfriend to another in a few weeks time. His teachers and parents often lament that Lindsey is just not "living up to his potential."
Identity achievement	Identity decision made after options explored	Jill has explored many alternatives when considering what to do after graduating from high school. She recognizes that she has many different interests, including sports, music, and writing. She has been active in a variety of extracurricular activities in high school and won a letter in the Senior Debate Team. This experience taught her to examine issues critically, solve problems creatively, and display self-confidence.

Adapted from *Interventions for Adolescent Identity Development*, edited by S. L. Archer, 1994, Thousand Oaks: Sage Publications.

a more severe type of psychiatric disorder such as Borderline Personality (Marcia, 1994). Individuals with Borderline Personality are impulsive in ways that are potentially self-damaging (e.g., diagnostic criteria include impulsivity in at least two of the following: spending money, reckless driving, sex, substance abuse, and binge eating), display frantic activity to avoid feelings of abandonment, experience unstable interpersonal relationships with others, and suffer from identity disturbance, recurrent suicidal or self-mutilating behaviors, unstable affect, chronic feelings of emptiness, inappropriate anger, and transient paranoid ideas (American Psychiatric Association, 1994).

The majority of adolescents behave as if their status were that of moratorium. That is, adolescence is a time for experimenting with how one might want to be as an adult. These adolescents show wide variety in their experimentation and are sensitive to the responses of others. As a group, they do not necessarily require help for mental health problems related to identity. Such individuals may exhibit experimental behaviors such as wearing dramatic make-up, changing hairstyles (e.g., the 14-year-old boy who shaves his head on a dare from his friends is merely experimenting with autonomy and self-expression), and donning particular fashion styles (e.g., jeans with ragged knees). The behavior represents an honest search for what "fits" and is not indicative of outright rebellion or confusion. After a variable period of moratorium, most adolescents determine who they are, what they like, and what they want to do in the future. Thus, they arrive at the status of identity achievement after a period of exploration. Again, these youngsters seldom need specific mental health interventions directly related to achieving this status, although caregivers may need some direction on appropriate responses to behaviors.

Youth who attain a status of foreclosure or identity diffusion, on the other hand, may well be in need of specific mental health interventions. For example, the child who has been seriously abused or expected to take on adultlike responsibilities throughout childhood may arrive in adolescence holding the belief that he or she is to put self-interests aside and continue to attend to the needs of others. Such an individual may foreclose on an identity or occupation when he really has neither the aptitude nor healthy motivation to pursue such a path. Mental health interventions such as group counseling may be helpful for such a teen to sort out what is part of his or her identity and what is emotional trauma or baggage left over from a wounded childhood. The school nurse may identify such individuals through their consistent serious attitude about the needs of others, often at the expense of their own needs and wishes.

Similarly, the individual who experiences identity diffusion may need specific psychiatric intervention to deal with a serious personality disorder such as one of those identified previously. Again, the school nurse or clinic nurse giving routine physicals should be alert to signs of a more serious underlying condition. For example, an adolescent with disturbed diffusion may exhibit signs of social isolation or feeling empty inside.

Social Competence

Social learning theory is based on the premise that human behavior is motivated and regulated to some degree within the context of social structure. People learn to act in ways that they perceive as rewarding from either their own personal experiences or observing the experiences of others within the social setting. An individual's behaviors are both internally and externally motivated, evaluated, and regulated. Self-efficacy is a central concept in the social learning theory developed by Bandura (1977). Competence in responding to demands from the environment is not attained once and for all nor is it simply a matter of following a prescribed set of rules or instructions. **Self-efficacy**, or competence in managing one's personal response to the environment, involves making judgments about how one organizes and engages in activities when dealing with situations that may be ambiguous and stressful (Bandura & Schunk, 1981). **Self-awareness**, or a perception of one's competence, influences the types of choices or judgments the individual makes in facing demands from the larger society.

Positive mental health in adolescence has been associated with the construct of **social competence**, or "the degree to which significant others rate an individual as successful in solving and completing relevant social tasks" (Compas, 1993, p. 164). Specific skills or competencies that are mastered for positive mental health include understanding how to decode social cues and interpreting these in meaningful ways. Other skills consist of initiating behavioral responses to these cues from a set of alternatives and monitoring the effects of displaying the chosen responses. These skills are complex and related to previous experiences in social interactions and problem solving. These skills also vary with the social context in which the adolescent is acting. For example, decoding, interpreting, and responding to social cues within the adolescent's home may be very different from doing so in school or at a party.

MENTAL HEALTH IN ADOLESCENCE

From a broad psychosocial point of view, mental health can be defined as the absence of psychosocial and behavioral dysfunction and the presence of optimal psychosocial functioning or well-being. Mental health in adolescence is defined differently by mental health professionals, caregivers, society at large, and adolescents themselves. The perspective of mental health professionals, including nurses, is usually based on a theoretical framework such as a theory of personality development, motivation for human behavior, or psychopathology. Caregivers and society at large, in contrast, tend to conceive of adolescent mental health in terms of stable and predictable behaviors and conformity with the rules of social conduct. For example, caregivers and teachers expect youngsters to display increasing self-responsibility in going to school and doing their homework. Adolescents themselves view mental health more subjectively, in terms of their individual well-being and feelings of contentment and happiness (Compas, 1993). For example, an adolescent who spends his time in the company of several friends, is included in social activities, and perceives little intrusion from caregivers and teachers on what he thinks and how he acts may consider himself to be happy and content. On the other hand, when an adolescent does not have peers as a frame of reference for what he is feeling or experiencing, he may feel quite unhappy and even "crazy." The following example of positive mental health comes from an eighth-grader who wants more information about what is "normal." *Deenie*, written by Judy Blume, provides many such examples through the main character of the same name:

Deenie

We're starting a new program in gym. Once a month we're going to have a discussion group with Mrs. Rappoport. It sounds very interesting because Mrs. Rappoport asked us each to write down a question and drop it into a box on her desk. The question could be about anything, she said, especially anything we need to know about sex. She told us not to put our names on the paper. She doesn't want to know who's asking what. It's a good thing too, because I'd never have asked my question if I had to sign my name. I wrote:

Do normal people touch their bodies before they go to sleep and is it all right to do that?

On Tuesday, when we walked into gym, Mrs. Rappoport told us to sit in a circle so we could talk easily. The first questions she discussed were all about menstruation. But I already knew most everything from my booklet. After that she said, "Okay, now I think we can move on to another subject. Here's an interesting question." She read it to us. "Do normal people touch their bodies

RESEARCH HIGHLIGHT

Stress Management Techniques for Adolescent Males

STUDY PROBLEM/PURPOSE

To examine effectiveness of two interventions to teach male adolescents how to cope with stress. Sample included 25 males aged 15 to 16 years who attended a college preparatory school for boys in a midwestern city. All but one (Asian) were Caucasian.

METHODS

Randomly assigned to one of two intervention groups (cognitive intervention or anxiety management training) or to a control group. All were given pre- and posttests to measure anxiety, anger, self-esteem, depression, and anxious self-statements.

FINDINGS

Analysis of pretests indicated no differences in baseline data among the three groups. Analysis of posttests showed there were no significant differences between the two intervention groups. However, there were significant differences between the control group and intervention groups in regard to anxiety, anger, and depression. There were no significant differences among the three groups in self-esteem or anxious self-statements.

IMPLICATIONS

Both cognitive stress reduction training and anxiety management training interventions are effective strategies for adolescent males needing stress management skills. Follow-up measures were done 11 weeks following the study, and males receiving either of the interventions maintained their skills.

From "Comparison of cognitive-behavioral stress management techniques with adolescent boys" by A. A. Hains, 1992, *Journal of Counseling and Development, 70,* 600–605.

before they go to sleep and is it all right to do that?"

I almost died! I glanced around, then smiled a little, because some of the other girls did, and hoped the expression on my face looked like I was trying to figure out who had asked such a thing.*

(Blume, 1973, pp. 82–83)

*Reprinted with permission of Simon & Schuster Books for Young Readers, an imprint of Simon & Schuster Children's Publishing Division, from *Deenie* by Judy Blume. Copyright © 1973 Judy Blume.

Positive mental health consists of two fundamental dimensions. The first of these dimensions is to develop skills that enable the individual to handle stress, manage emotions, and solve problems effectively. The second dimension is to develop skills that enable the individual to be involved in activities that are purposeful and meaningful. These skills are based on obtaining accurate information. As illustrated in the excerpt above, Deenie exhibits a healthy curiosity about her body. She also expresses a social sensitivity to the normative behavior of her peers by smiling and looking around. She has both the courage to ask an important question and the desire to be accepted by her friends. Once developed, such skills enhance feelings of self-esteem and social competence. They are developed within the context of family and other sociocultural factors such as community (e.g., school), ethnicity, and race. Thus, positive mental health, which consists of these two dimensions, can be evaluated from several perspectives: coping skills; level of involvement in meaningful activities; perspectives of different groups such as caregivers, health professionals, and the adolescents themselves; developmental factors; and sociocultural factors (Compas, 1993).

Because the definitions of mental health differ among health professionals, caregivers, and adolescents themselves, misunderstanding and conflict may arise when describing problems and planning for solutions. Mental health professionals may label an adolescent's behavior in a specific way that reflects a theoretical understanding of the complexity of motivation, emotion, and behavior. Such a label may have adverse effects on the adolescent and his family. For example, to label an adolescent as "suicidal" may unleash a host of fears and expectations that are difficult to overcome. The same individual may be viewed by caregivers and teachers as "a loner, lazy, or an underachiever." In terms of the adolescent's personal and subjective view, he may simply feel lonely, sad, confused, and helpless.

Mental Health Care Needs

Adolescents face considerable changes and pressures that are among the most complex of the life cycle (Ferguson, 1993). These changes and pressures converge in ways that challenge the stability and mental health of many, but not all, adolescents. Adolescents who may benefit from mental health care services include those with diagnosable mental illnesses such as Conduct Disorder, mood disorders (including major depression), Schizophrenia, Obsessive-Compulsive Disorder, and Adjustment Disorder, as well as those adolescents who engage in high-risk behaviors that make them vulnerable to mental health problems, such as substance use and abuse, irresponsible use of motor vehicles, and early initiation of sexual activity.

The most recent Institute of Medicine report (1989) indicates that 12% of youth under age 18 (7.5 million children in the United States) have diagnosable mental illness and 70% to 80% of those in need are underserved or not receiving services. Studies conducted on adolescents' use of mental health services in the 1970s and 1980s indicate that less than 2% of the adolescent population received services while estimates of need ranged from 5% to 22% of the adolescent population (Burns, 1991). In a school-based survey of 17,193 adolescents, nearly 25% identified themselves as having a serious problem such as emotional distress or suicidal ideation, and those who decided they needed professional help had a history of abuse, physical health problems, and suicidal ideation (Saunders, Resnick, Hoberman, & Blum, 1994).

Current estimates are that between 11 and 14 million (17% to 22%) American children under the age of 18 have behavioral, emotional, or developmental problems (Institute of Medicine, 1989). Many disorders that originate and are diagnosed first in childhood (e.g., autism, Conduct Disorder, and Attention-Deficit/Hyperactivity Disorder) continue into adolescence and adulthood (Kazdin, 1993). Conduct Disorder, for example, is one of the most frequently diagnosed psychiatric conditions in children and adolescents. Prevalence rates are 6% to 16% for males and 2% to 9% for females under age 18 (American Psychiatric Association, 1994). Conduct Disorder is characterized in childhood by aggression toward one's peers. In the adolescent-onset type (absence of diagnosis before age 10), aggression is less common, but the individual may engage in delinquent behaviors such as lying, stealing, and truancy from school, usually with little expression of guilt or remorse. Conduct Disorder is often associated with other risk-taking behaviors such as those noted previously.

Other disorders, such as Anorexia Nervosa and Bulimia Nervosa, may be diagnosed first in adolescence. The average age of onset of Anorexia Nervosa is 17, often associated with stressful life events such as leaving home to attend college (American Psychiatric Association, 1994). This disorder is characterized by an intense fear of gaining weight, refusal to maintain acceptable minimum body weight, disturbed body image, and amenorrhea. Bulimia Nervosa, on the other hand, is characterized by recurrence of concern about body shape and weight, binge eating, misuse of laxatives and diuretics, and, often, purging through self-induced vomiting. Each of these conditions is diagnosable in 1% to 3% of the population and occurs more frequently (90%) in females than in males (American Psychiatric Association, 1994).

Depressive disorders are relatively common among adolescents. Depression is often difficult to diagnose, particularly in adolescence, because the symptoms are frequently on a continuum with normal behavior

(Hoberman, 1995). However, it occurs in at least 10% of adolescents and is diagnosed more frequently in girls than in boys. Moodiness in the form of pervasive and persistent sadness is seen in less than 50% of cases, while the majority with the diagnosis have symptoms of anhedonia (that is, they lack enjoyment in or pleasure from the usual activities of daily living), anger, or irritability (Hoberman, 1995). The majority go untreated in spite of other symptoms, including sleep disturbance, weight change, and thoughts of death or suicide.

Suicide is the second leading cause of death among adolescents between the ages of 15 and 24 (Centers for Disease Control, 1995). Suicidal ideation, which includes thinking about the reasons for and ways of killing oneself, and suicide attempts are related to a variety of life events in childhood and adolescence. In general, adolescents who attempt or complete suicide have experienced more turmoil in their families, sexual abuse during adolescence, frequent changes in residence, and having to repeat a grade in school (de Wilde, Kienhorst, Diekstra, & Wolters, 1992). There are significant gender differences in rates of adolescent suicide. While more females admit to having suicidal ideation and make more attempts at suicide, more males actually succeed in completing suicide. These differences have been found to be related to greater feelings of loneliness and experiences of substance abuse in males than in females (Rich, Kirkpatrick-Smith, Bonner, & Jans, 1992). Researchers also found that males express greater fear of social disapproval for having suicidal thoughts while females express more fear of injury.

Expression of suicidal ideation should always be taken seriously. Unfortunately, it is not always easy to identify signs of suicidal ideation. Troubled adolescents who are contemplating suicide rarely ask directly for help. Males, in particular, may ask for help only indirectly by acting out or by withdrawing from usual activities (Dumont, 1991). Preventing suicide in adolescents depends to some extent on identifying those individuals at highest risk. These include those who (1) have other psychiatric problems (particularly substance abuse or depression), (2) have a history of suicide within the family, (3) are experiencing high levels of stress (particularly related to achievement or sexuality), and (4) are experiencing parental rejection, family conflict, or family disruption (Steinberg, 1996).

The following excerpt is from a true story of an adult, named Truddi, who is speaking with her psychotherapist, Stanley, about the turmoil and transitions of her adolescence. Her anguish demonstrates her struggle to form a unique identity as an adult. Her memories of her experiences during adolescence reflect the harsh realities of physical and emotional abuse and the conflict she experiences in seeking her own autonomy yet feeling the need to keep her family intact.

When Rabbit Howls

"Why don't I remember more right this minute?" she screamed suddenly. "When I told my mother I was leaving that house because of the stepfather, what did I tell her? The incidents were so vague, I could never be certain they'd really happened. But until I turned fifteen, 'tell her' rang in my head. I don't know what finally precipitated my telling her—or even our conversation. She didn't look shocked at all, just determined that I mustn't leave her. There I was, looking forward to a new life when she'd spent hers in as much filth as I had, paying him for the roof over my head, for the food that kept me healthy. She'd paid him with herself."

"My mother didn't rant or rave that day, she just said that I was to stay. Things would get better, she'd make him stop. It's impossible for me to believe that she knew what was going on."

As the woman talked, Stanley saw the conflict: a mother's harsh qualities weighed against the good—an inclination to accentuate the good and blame one's self for the harsh.

Her mother, she said, pinched pennies all year because of a tight-fisted man who wouldn't give to his own children or wife, let alone his stepdaughter. The pennies at Christmas bought a wealth of gifts for the children; creatively, beautifully wrapped, even stacked artistically under the perfect tree.

There was more. It amounted to an inability on his client's part to see her own side or to speak in her own defense. Her mother had been perfect, she had not.

Stanley had listened. Now he laid down the clipboards. "You were not responsible for your mother's happiness or unhappiness. Your mother was an adult and her emotions were hers to deal with. You talk about how she scrimped and saved and denied her own needs to feed you, to give you nice holidays. But with your earnings from various jobs, you supported your mother, half brother, and half sisters, a long time before your stepfather eventually left."

"I couldn't really earn a lot after school and lots of times I hurt her. I wasn't an easy child. I screamed and smashed things. I was a malcontent, whom nothing satisfied, one of those people who is happy with nothing and no one."

"Or so your mother told you. You worked," he reminded her, *"as a waitress every afternoon until midnight and every single weekend, during your junior and senior years. And your mother hurt you, didn't she? She beat the hell out of you. And she gave you to your stepfather; she handed you over to him."**

(Chase, 1987, pp. 27–28)

This true story of Truddi Chase in *When Rabbit Howls* provides a rare glimpse into the complexity and resiliency of the human psyche as it struggles with identity formation. From the ages of 2 through 16, Truddi faces unimaginable physical, sexual, and emotional abuse from her stepfather as well as physical and emotional abuse from her own mother. The preceding excerpt depicts one of the internal conflicts Truddi faces as an adolescent. She wants to disclose the truth about her stepfather's molestation of her and, consequently, to be protected from him by her mother, yet she defends her mother and expresses more concern over her mother's victimization than she does over her own. As an adolescent, Truddi cannot yet sort out her responsibility for herself. Her identity as a separate and worthy individual is not part of her self-awareness. The boundaries between herself and her mother are blurred. As an adolescent, Truddi is poorly prepared to face adulthood. Her experiences from childhood include very little development of trust, autonomy, and initiative.

Needs Related to Physical Transitions

As sexual maturation continues, issues related to gender identity, gender role, and sexual preference increase. Gender Identity Disorder is characterized by two major indicators: (1) a persistent and strong identification of self as the other sex and (2) persistent discomfort with being one's assigned sex (American Psychiatric Association, 1994). **Gender identity** refers to the individual's subjective or private experience of gender, while **gender role** is the public recognition of one's gender assignment as biological male or female and the expression of appropriate social behaviors related to that assignment. Several congenital anomalies (e.g., Klinefelter's syndrome in the male and congenital virilizing adrenal hyperplasia in the female) may result in gender "crosscoding" such that there is a discrepancy between the anatomical sex evident at birth and certain behavioral characteristics of being male or female are exhibited by the individual over time (Money, 1994). Those individu-

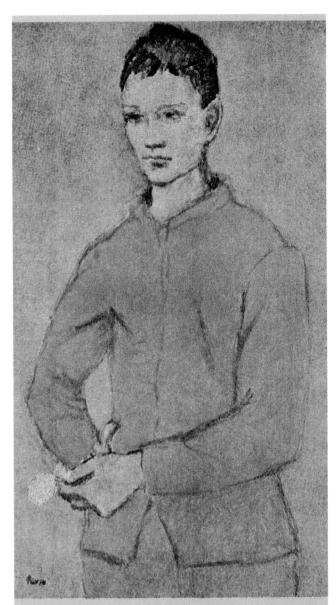

Blue Boy by Picasso. Source: © 1988 Estate of Pablo Picasso/Artists Rights Society (ARS) New York

Picasso's *Blue Boy* depicts a somber young man posed awkwardly as if to represent the state of adolescence. The young man is pensive and thoughtful, at the door of adulthood, yet holding back. While we often think of adolescence in terms of violence or frivolous and uninhibited behavior, *Blue Boy* presents a differing perspective.

als who are uncertain about sexual preferences must overcome social stereotypes and hostile environments when struggling with issues such as homosexuality and bisexuality. Estimates are that 10% of adolescents are either unsure of their sexual orientation or believe they are not heterosexual (Treadway & Yoakam, 1992). Confusion and frustration in coming to terms with gender

---

*From *When Rabbit Howls* by Truddi Chase. Copyright © 1987 by Truddi Chase. Introduction and Epilogue Copyright © 1987 by Robert A Phillips, Jr. Used by permission of Dutton Signet, a division of Penguin Books USA Inc.

identity, gender role, and sexual orientation may lead to feelings of depression and suicidal ideation that require professional intervention.

Other mental health problems are related to the physical transitions of adolescence. Skin problems such as acne may lead to diminished self-esteem and social isolation and loneliness. Eating disorders become more prevalent, particularly among females. Adolescents (both males and females) who participate in sports that require weight limits may develop eating disorders in an effort to meet weight requirements. Adolescents, particularly males, who participate in specific sports associated with strong, muscular physiques may also suffer from mental health problems related to use of anabolic steroids (Crockett & Petersen, 1993).

Other physical problems that may result from accidental injury or illness are of great concern to the adolescent because they are often perceived as a threat to body image and identity. For example, the adolescent who sustains a spinal cord injury resulting from a recreational sport, such as skiing or climbing, faces enormous mental health concerns related to loss of function and the perception that he no longer has a future or would be a desirable companion for peers. Issues of sexuality and reproduction require much sensitivity on the part of health care professionals who counsel these youngsters during rehabilitation.

Needs Related to Cognitive Transitions

Cognitive limitations that the adolescent may have experienced in childhood may continue to be problematic during the many transitions of adolescence. The individual with Attention-Deficit/Hyperactivity Disorder (ADHD) will continue to need mental health assistance during this phase of life. Such limitations will become an essential dimension for the adolescent to integrate into an adult identity, and the young person should be encouraged to ask for assistance with learning disabilities during each new transition.

Academic achievement may continue to be impaired in the adolescent with ADHD and is often a source of conflict with caregivers and teachers. The risk for school drop-out is high, and subsequent ability to find meaningful work decreases. The tendency toward impulsivity and inappropriate social behavior interferes with the adolescent's development of self-efficacy related to skills needed for satisfying social relationships.

Needs Related to Emotional Transitions

The adolescent often experiences transient periods of depression. With the loss of childhood and the associated security of childhood routines and expectations, the adolescent must engage in some normal grieving. However, depression that is marked by increasing withdrawal from

social contact and declining feelings of self-worth may require professional intervention. Such feelings of depression can lead to self-destructive behaviors including suicide. Depression in adolescents may be difficult to spot because these young people often avoid intimacy and are at a stage in life where they spend increasingly smaller amounts of time with family members. Caregivers and teachers should be alert to the possibility of depression as a response to perceived trauma, regardless of its source, in the adolescent. Perceived inadequacy in social relationships, such as dating, or in social competency, such as making the football team or cheerleading squad, can trigger an intense emotional response that, to an adult, may not seem proportional to the stimulus. However, in the life of an adolescent, such disappointments are of paramount importance. The accompanying Nursing Alert identifies some of the life events that place an adolescent at risk for suicide. The adolescent's response to such life events depends on the internal and external resources available. Internal resources include coping skills, intellectual ability, and perceived locus of control. External resources include social support such as satisfying relationships with friends and family members (Rice & Meyer, 1994).

Depression may also result from more traumatic events, such as the loss of a caregiver or friend. When a change in behavioral patterns that is marked by withdrawal from usual activities, excessive sleeping, poor appetite, and sudden outbursts of anger is noted, depression may be the adolescent's problem and he needs professional assistance. The adolescent whose caregiver commits suicide is also at higher risk for suicide when depressed. Such individuals should be encouraged to seek help (refer to Chapters 12 and 14).

It is important not to ignore the warning signs of depression and/or suicide in the adolescent client. Nurses who work with adolescents must be comfortable in talking with them about the possibility of suicide and in responding

---

⚙ NURSING ALERT!

Risk Factors for Adolescent Suicide

- Loss of significant relationship with friend, family member, or pet
- Suicide of a friend, relative, or public figure
- Homophobic response of family members to an adolescent's sexual preference (e.g., rejection)
- Divorce of parents
- Break-up with a girl- or boyfriend
- Unattainment of a significant goal (e.g., acceptance at a particular college)

⚡ NURSING ALERT!

Warning Signs of Potential Adolescent Suicide

- Drastic changes in behavior (e.g., sudden withdrawal in an otherwise socially active person or sudden gregariousness in an otherwise shy person)
- Stated feelings of sadness, loneliness, hopelessness, or despair
- Increased impulsive risk-taking behaviors (e.g., disregard for safety by not wearing seatbelt)
- Alienating behaviors (e.g., withdrawal or aggression)
- Giving away possessions (especially those with special meanings)
- Preoccupation with death or dying
- Sudden changes in personal appearance and hygiene
- Previous suicide attempt or gesture
- Direct suicidal comments such as "I wish I were dead"

seriously to any indications that the adolescent might give. It is a mistake to reassure the individual that everything will turn out all right. What is important is to ask direct questions in a calm manner, refer the person to a professional skilled in crisis intervention, and continue to provide support even after the crisis is past (Steinberg, 1996).

Needs Related to Social Transitions

All of the above transitions occur within the context of social interactions within the family, school, and community. These interactions are characterized by patterns of communication that can lead to mental health or to mental health problems. During the drastic and rapid transi-

⚡ NURSING ALERT!

Nursing Interventions for the Suicidal Adolescent

- Always take seriously the expression of a wish to die.
- Provide a safe environment.
- Obtain a verbal contract that the individual will not do anything to harm himself without talking to you or another responsible adult.
- Check on the adolescent's feelings of safety and control at frequent intervals.

tions of adolescence, communication within the family, between student and teacher, among friends, and with members of the community at large is essential to the mental health and well-being of all. Nurses should bear in mind that adolescents from minority racial and ethnic groups may also experience mental health concerns related to their immigration and acculturation status.

Statistically, adolescents at highest risk for mental health problems are those from single-caregiver homes and homes in which one or more caregivers have a history of alcoholism or drug use, suicide attempts, or antisocial behaviors (Vernon, 1991). Moreover, the adolescent may have grown up in a violent atmosphere with caregivers who fight or batter one another. As they become older and more independent, many adolescents who are the victims of violent homes or abusive families may take matters into their own hands and run away from home to escape the pain of abuse and violence. These youth may become homeless, fall in with gangs, or resort to prostitution, all of which will introduce additional mental and physical health risks. Although the exact number of homeless youth is unknown, some estimates are that the number may be as many as 2 million (Robertson, 1992). Homeless adolescents include not only those who run away from home to escape abuse and neglect but also those who are thrown out of their homes; many of these are youth with long-standing psychiatric and conduct problems (Rotheram-Borus, Parra, Cantwell, Gwadz, & Murphy, 1996). Homeless youth are at increased risk for further sexual abuse, sexually transmitted diseases including acquired immuno-deficiency syndrome (AIDS), injury, substance abuse, and a lifestyle characterized by poverty. Drug addiction or prostitution may lead these youth to encounters with the law. Nurses working in public health settings or detention institutions such as jails and prisons are instrumental in assessing the need for mental health services.

Poverty places the adolescent at risk for mental health problems. Poverty and crowding in inner cities contribute to what Schorr (1988) refers to as "rotten outcomes." For example, by the time many youngsters growing up in crowded cities reach the eighth grade, they have lost hope for meaningful employment in the future. Many have dropped out of school and have turned to the streets for identity and for seeking a way out of the downward spiral of poverty. As adolescents spend more time away from caregivers and family and more time with peers, opportunities to become involved with groups who exhibit high-risk behaviors for violent activity, such as gangs, increases. Gangs are most likely to develop in areas where there is little adult supervision and where violent activity is accepted as the primary means of control (Earls, Cairns, & Mercy, 1993). Homicide may be a standard for acceptance within the peer group and may also be associated with other risky behaviors such as dealing in illicit drugs.

A growing number of adolescents, particularly African Americans, are living in single-caregiver households. The greatest impact of this trend is economic: 75% of African American families who are not in metropolitan areas live below the poverty line (Millstein, Irwin, & Brindis, 1991). In addition, an increasing number of adolescents have been raised as "latchkey children," returning home after school to no adult supervision.

Adolescents are at risk for specific health-related problems, such as early initiation of sexual intercourse and teen-age pregnancy (Schorr, 1988) and sexual victimization, yet little is understood about the impact this has on adolescent development (Esparza & Esperat, 1996). Adolescents are at particularly high risk for date or acquaintance rape. This is the most common type of sexual assault among adolescents and is defined as sexual intercourse involving threat of force or actual force from a perpetrator known to the victim and without the person's consent (Neinstein, Juliani, Shapiro, & Warf, 1996). Health care providers should screen for this type of victimization when treating adolescents for other health-related concerns (Pope & Brucker, 1991). Nurses working with adolescents in schools or other clinical settings should provide educational information on ways to prevent the occurrence of sexual assault (see the accompanying Nursing Tip).

Because sexuality is a major developmental task for adolescents, their naivete and inexperience may increase their vulnerability to nonconsensual sexual activity and reduce their ability to cope with its consequences. In a study of adolescents' perceptions of nonconsensual sexual activity, Telljohann and colleagues (1995) concluded that many youth remain confused about issues of responsibility concerning sexual harassment, rape, and sexual abuse. These researchers added that adolescents need help in building skills for assertive communication as well as knowledge about developing consensual intimate relationships.

In a study of adolescent assaultive behavior and drug use, Vinogradov, Dishotsky, Doty, and Tinklenberg (1988) found that their sample of 63 adolescent males were usually intoxicated during the rape episode or stated they had used alcohol or marijuana on the same day as the rape. Subjects reported that few rapes were premeditated and most were the result of impulsive behavior and not provoked by the female victims. However, these researchers cautioned that these research subjects/rapists had a tendency to subtly blame the victim, and this could lead to psychological trauma for the victims that should influence treatment by health care providers.

The role of communities in providing support for adolescent development was studied by Blyth and Leffert (1995). These researchers found that youth in the 9th to 12th grades experienced different types of community strengths. Youth who were vulnerable benefited more

---

 NURSING TIP

Addressing Sexual Concerns with Adolescents

- Explore the adolescent's sexual preference (self-identity as homosexual, bisexual, or heterosexual).

- Ask open-ended questions about their worries or concerns (e.g., what concerns do you have about your sexual preferences?).

- Use correct anatomical and socially accepted terms for genitalia and sexual expression (e.g., penis and vagina; gay and lesbian).

- Provide accurate and factual information when possible (use books, pamphlets, fact sheets, hotlines).

- Refer adolescents to community resources when appropriate (Planned Parenthood for contraceptive options, Caregivers & Friends of Lesbian and Gays (PFLAG) for support of sexual orientation, etc.).

- Encourage contact with school resources (counselors and nurses).

NURSING TIP

Guidelines for Avoiding Sexual Assault/Rape

Help adolescents prevent sexual assault or rape by offering the following guidelines:

- Avoid hitchhiking or giving rides to hitchhikers/strangers.

- Avoid taking walks (or shopping) alone; go with a friend.

- Walk confidently; avoid looking uncertain about your destination.

- Keep one arm free to defend yourself against an attacker.

- When getting into your car, check back seat for intruders.

- Keep car locked when driving and lock it at your destination.

- Be sure car has sufficient gas to get you to your destination.

- If being followed in your car, drive to a business or the police station.

- Do not open door of house to strangers.

- Do not go to a secluded location on a first date.

from living in communities where other youth engaged in few problem behaviors than from living in communities where youth engaged in more problem behaviors. Healthier communities included those where families were caring and supportive and provided monitoring and discipline to their youth. Such communities also included schools that were perceived as caring and supportive, where a high percentage of youth were committed and motivated to continue to learn and where a high percentage of caregivers were involved. Other strengths within the healthiest communities were the percentage of youth involved in religious services and structured activities, such as sports or music, and the peer norms related to personal values and responsibility.

NURSING THEORIES

As the following nursing theories will demonstrate, communication and caring are important components of all successful interventions, regardless of setting. These theories emphasize the importance of the relationship between nurse and client.

Humanistic Nursing

The Humanistic Nursing Theory of Paterson and Zderad (1988) began in 1960 when these two nurses engaged in discussions with other nurses about their experiences in caring for clients. They were not impressed with the objective nature of empirical science that viewed human beings objectively and as predictable objects. Rather, they believed that their work as nurses would be facilitated by understanding how people experience their existence. Thus, they were led to literature concerning existential philosophy. Humanistic and existential philosophy assert a broad view of human beings and their potential.

According to Paterson and Zderad (1988), "Nursing is an experience lived between human beings" (p. 3). It is a transactional relationship based on an awareness of both nurse and client of self and of each other. A major assumption of this definition of nursing is that human beings are unique and capable of making choices. This philosophical framework is appropriate for understanding the adolescent's struggles with making choices and forging a unique identity for self in society. This perspective also assumes that one person's presence is of value to another person. Nursing is a caring and nurturing response of one human being toward another with the aim of developing more well-being (Praeger & Hogarth, 1985). Within this context, nursing focuses on the whole person rather than on reducing the person to components such as a mind, behavior, or body parts. Such an approach can be very encouraging to the adolescent and can help to consolidate identity.

The goal of humanistic nursing is attainment not of mere health or well-being as a state but of dynamic "more-being." The objective is for the nurse to assist the client to become *more*, to realize a potential not yet attained in the present moment of their interaction. Health is conceptualized as a process of becoming whatever is possible for the human being. Again, this approach is very appropriate for working with adolescents in various settings. Adolescents often resist a concrete set of rules from adults in authority but need the support of adults who understand their developmental phases and who can offer empathic support that encourages the unique development of the individual.

Nursing phenomena, those things that nurses think are important and to which they must pay close attention, are experienced as nurturing, being nurtured, or the process between these two reference points: "It is a quality of being that is expressed in the doing" (Paterson & Zderad, 1988, p. 13). While other theories of nursing may focus on what the nurse does *to* or *for* the client, humanistic nursing focuses on the intersubjective experience. The most important activity for the nurse to engage in may be the use of self, or **presence** with the client. Presence is the activity of being physically present with another person that begins with the nurse's genuine commitment to caring and nurturing the potential of the client. The nurse must hold the belief that an authentic interaction between nurse and client is a valuable opportunity to develop human potential. Communicating caring is the essence of nursing based on this belief and theory. From an existential viewpoint, every action that a nurse takes in relation to the client is a unique event. It is shaped by the experiences and expectations of the individuals relating to one another within the context of nurturing and being nurtured. The physical needs of the client are of basic concern to the nurse. How the client experiences his body, its functioning, and its relationship with the environment are of fundamental importance to the nursing relationship. The nurse is concerned with the client's unique expression of the body related to its position in time and space.

When the nurse goes beyond being an object within the perceptual field of the client, there is an opportunity for the nurse to express authentic presence. The nurse must maintain the commitment to care and to be open to experience the dialogue with the client. The commitment to care and to nurture is accompanied by "a sense of responsibility or regard for what is seen as the patient's vulnerability" (Paterson & Zderad, 1988, p. 28). The dialogue that unfolds between client and nurse represents what Paterson and Zderad refer to as a "call and response" (p. 29). The client calls for nursing care with an expectation that care will be provided or an unmet need will be satisfied. The nurse responds with the intention of providing the care or satisfying the unmet need.

Paterson and Zderad (1988) outline 12 behaviors that nurses perform in providing comfort to a client. These are directly applicable to the nursing care of the adolescent

---

HUMANISTIC NURSING BEHAVIORS

1. The nurse introduces herself to the client and refers to the client by name. The use of names supports the dignity, worth, and individual identity of the client and is essential for an authentic subject-subject relationship.

2. The nurse provides information about the client's situation as it is sought by the client or when the nurse perceives the client is puzzled about what is happening. This action on the part of the nurse is based on the existential belief that the client has the right to know and make choices about his own life, and such choices are shaped by honest information.

3. The nurse accepts the client's expression of feelings by verbalizing this acceptance when appropriate. This also validates that the client has a right to feelings and can learn appropriate ways to express feelings.

4. The nurse accepts the client's expression of feelings by staying with the client or doing something for the client when a verbal expression of acceptance by the nurse is not appropriate. The message conveyed here is that the feeling the client is experiencing is valid but a better method of expressing the feeling is socially desirable. By remaining with the client, the nurse validates the feeling and may model a more appropriate behavioral expression.

5. The nurse expresses authentic positive feelings for the client when appropriate. The purpose of this action is to refute negative self-concepts that the client may hold.

6. The nurse supports the client's rights to have loving relationships with family members, staff, and other clients.

7. The nurse shows respect for clients as persons who have rights to make choices as their capabilities permit.

8. The nurse helps clients consider current expression of feelings and behaviors in the light of previous life experiences. This behavior enables clients to formulate self-understanding by recognition of patterns that may be helpful or unhelpful to their healing.

9. The nurse encourages clients to express themselves openly so that the nurse can respond in a helpful and therapeutic manner.

10. The nurse verifies the intuitive grasp of how the client experiences events by asking questions and making comments to the client, then observing the client's response.

11. The nurse encourages realistic (not false) hope through discussing the positive outcomes that might occur if the client were to engage in a therapeutic opportunity.

12. The nurse supports the client's self-image with concrete examples.

Adapted from *Humanistic Nursing*, by J. G. Paterson and L. T. Zderad, 1988, New York: National League of Nursing.

---

with a psychiatric mental health problem and are outlined in the accompanying display.

The case example that follows is an application of these 12 behaviors in providing nursing care for Juanita, an Hispanic girl 14 years of age who was hospitalized in an adolescent psychiatric hospital for an eating disorder, Anorexia Nervosa. Juanita's primary nurse exhibited these behaviors upon Juanita's admission to the unit.

CASE EXAMPLE   *Juanita*

Introduction: "Hi, Juanita, may I call you that? My name is Ann and I will be your nurse until 11 o'clock tonight."

Information: "I would like to show you around the unit and tell you about our routines here. We think it is important for you to know about us as we also try to learn what can be helpful to you. I hope you understand that any time you have questions about what is happening here, you can ask me or any of the other nurses."

Accepting feelings: After Ann makes the above statements, Juanita stomps her feet, pulls her hair, and says, "I don't want to know anything about this place and I don't want to be here!" Ann responds, "Juanita, I understand that you are frustrated and angry about being in the hospital. I hope you will continue to tell us how you feel about yourself and your treatment here. We will help you find more ways to express your

Continued

feelings directly so you won't have to feel like pulling your hair and stomping your feet so hard."

Staying with the client: Ann points to two chairs and a sofa in the recreation room and says to Juanita, "I would like to spend a few more minutes with you. Would you care to sit in a chair or on the sofa?"

Authentic positive feelings: Juanita shrugs her shoulders, then flops down on the sofa, looking at the floor and folding her arms across her chest. Ann responds, "Thank you for taking the time to be with me. It really helps me to do my job if I can get to know you a little better. I think you have a beautiful name. Is there a story behind it?"

Support loving relationships: Juanita is silent for a few seconds, then shrugs her shoulders again and says softly, "I was named after my grandmother." Ann says, "You must feel very special to have a family with such traditions. Tell me more about your grandmother."

Respect for choices: Juanita's posture relaxes a little. She begins to confide slowly, "Yeah, I like my grandmother, but she lives in Mexico. I wish I could live with her instead of with my mom and step-dad." Ann responds, "It sounds as if you have given this some thought. What do you think would be best about living with your grandmother?"

Previous life experiences: Juanita says, "She doesn't hassle me. My folks just hassle me all the time. Grandmother just likes me the way I am." Ann replies, "It sounds as if some things have happened with your fam-

ily that make you feel frustrated and angry."

Encourages open expression: Juanita unfolds her arms and pounds her fists firmly into the sofa cushions. "No kidding! Sometimes I just wish I could hit them [parents], they make me so mad. They just nag at me all the time and they won't listen. They will never understand me the way Grandmother does."

Intuitive grasp: Ann replies, "It seems like you feel misunderstood by your parents and unable to find safe ways to please them."

Encourages realistic hope: Ann continues, "I hope we can help you find some new ways to tell your parents how strongly you feel about how they treat you and what you would like for them to change. We have several people on staff here who are pretty good about that. Tell me about some of the ways you have already tried to tell your parents about how they hassle and nag at you."

Encourages self-image: Juanita begins to glance occasionally at Ann and to list ways in which she has fallen short of pleasing her parents. Ann identifies the strengths in this list of complaints and states, "Juanita, what you are telling me is that you are a good student even though you don't make straight A's and that you are also a fine musician even though you didn't make first violin in the orchestra. While you are here I hope we can help you see that these are real positive skills that you have already developed and that you don't have to be so hard on yourself by trying to be perfect."

Health as Expanding Consciousness

The nursing theory of Margaret Newman (1994) offers a similar view of the relationship between client and nurse. This theory may be of special relevance for the adolescent who suffers from a diagnosed mental illness such as depression or Conduct Disorder. Rather than viewing disease as an objective entity, Newman conceptualizes disease within the whole person and focuses on the pattern that the individual expresses within the environment. Human health is an experience of consciousness that follows a rhythmic pattern of order and disorder. Disease is not something to get rid of but something to incorporate into one's understanding of self.

Nursing care given within Newman's framework focuses on helping the client to experience congruence between emotional and physical feelings. As in humanistic nursing, the nurse offers *presence* to the client by being physically and emotionally committed to the client through an authentic relationship. When working with a hospitalized adolescent, the focus of nursing is not on treatment of the disease but on helping the client understand the meaning of his pattern of health and how it fits

into the scheme of the universe. Nursing is an expression of caring for the client, whatever manifestation of health is present.

The adolescent client who is depressed is manifesting a particular pattern or expression of how she fits into the world. Through a caring relationship, the nurse helps the client to expand her consciousness about this unique experience. By listening to the client's words and nonverbal communication, the nurse can help the adolescent to connect the emotional feelings to thoughts about self-identity and self-worth. Through mere presence, staying quietly and securely with the client, the nurse affirms the client's right to feel depressed. Through continued interaction, the nurse also assists the adolescent in connecting physical distress, such as inability to sleep or eat, with the emotions and thoughts that may seem disordered and threatening. Throughout the nurse-client interaction, the focus is on the rights of the client to express himself through appropriate feelings and behaviors without the nurse judging them as sick or crazy or wrong. As the client becomes more consciously aware of the connections between emotions, thoughts, and behaviors, the client begins to experience health in a different, and perhaps better, way.

NURSING PROCESS

▽ ASSESSMENT

Transitions are of central importance to nursing intervention and care and are therefore necessarily a focus in the assessment of adolescents. Nurses interact frequently with clients during periods of transition, not only in the developmental phase of adolescence but also in transitional situations such as acute illness or death, which may occur at any stage of life. In a comprehensive review of nursing literature on the topic of transitions, Schumacher and Meleis (1994) identified three types of indicators of healthy transitions that can be useful to nurses during the assessment process: subjective well-being, role mastery, and well-being of relationships. In addition, these researchers also identified three nursing measures to assist clients with transitions: assessment of readiness, preparation for transition, and role supplementation. Assessment of readiness includes identifying the meaning of the transitional experience to the client. In the adolescent, for example, the transition from junior high to high school may be desirable or dreaded. Similarly, expectations about the transition may vary from those that are realistic to those that are extremely unrealistic. The adolescent whose expectations are unrealistic is poorly prepared for such a transition. Preparation for the transition includes education and skill development. The developmental phase of adolescence is filled with opportunities to learn and master skills for adult living. Role supplementation provides additional experience in mastering skills required for a healthy transition.

Nurses have opportunities to work with adolescents in many settings. For example, the school nurse is in an optimum position to provide education and guidance in promoting positive mental health. The school nurse has the advantage of observing and listening to adolescents in one of their usual social settings and can thus plan and intervene with groups as well as individuals. Nurses may also work with adolescents in health care facilities such as drug treatment and rehabilitation centers, psychiatric hospitals, and general hospitals and clinics. Again, nurses should be well prepared to identify the usual as well as the more serious mental health needs of adolescents.

✴ NURSING TIP

Assessing Mental Health of Adolescents

The following should be assessed when planning nursing care for the adolescent with a history of physical, emotional, or sexual abuse:

◆ Experience of flashbacks. These are fragments of memory that may appear suddenly with no conscious forethought.

◆ Feelings of anger or hostility that are expressed in self-mutilation or threat of injury to others.

◆ Ability to concentrate on tasks at hand.

◆ Experiences of amnesia in past or present. These may indicate lack of coherent identity formation due to severe abuse.

◆ Body memories that interfere with physical examination or development of intimacy with others (e.g., nervous twitches, nausea, pain with no stimuli).

◆ Withdrawal from social situations, especially those involving close interpersonal contact.

◆ Lack of appropriate affect (e.g., numb response to painful stimuli).

◆ Ability to maintain eye contact with another person.

◆ Feelings of safety and control in social situations.

◆ Strategies for coping with anxiety-producing situations and memories.

▽ NURSING DIAGNOSIS

The most common nursing diagnoses seen in adolescents relate to the effects of the developmental changes that the adolescent is experiencing. *Body image disturbance* and *altered role performance* can be common responses from individuals who are struggling to cope with the often overwhelming transitions that occur in the few short years of adolescence. Clients who have suffered abuse may be diagnosed with *self-esteem disturbance* if they harbor lingering feelings of shame or blame themselves for their past experiences; such a teen will need assistance in exploring the past in an effort to effectively move forward in the present and in developing or realizing a self-concept that is acceptable to his current state of mind. Teens who have been victims of abuse or violence may also exhibit related symptoms, such as *sleep pattern disturbances* related to memories of abuse as evidenced by anxiety, restlessness, and flashbacks and *altered thought processes* related to past experiences as evidenced by lack of concentration or fear of being victimized.

Working with Adolescents

A nurse working in an alcohol treatment center may be viewed with more credibility if he wears jeans and a sport shirt rather than a suit and tie and introduces himself to his client(s) as Jim rather than as Mr. Brown. Similarly, a sincere effort to understand and use the jargon of adolescents in conversations with clients can convey acceptance. However, the nurse should proceed cautiously so that he does not come across to the client as mocking the language or mannerisms of youth. Also, if the nurse is clearly not comfortable with narrowing the gap between age and professional status in this way, the adolescent will quickly recognize this, and credibility will be lost.

Adolescents are also particularly vulnerable to experiencing *social isolation* or *impaired social interaction* related to past experiences, comfort level with peers, and self-perception of abilities in social contexts. These individuals will need interventions designed to focus on their positive qualities while developing skills that will help them achieve their desired level of social integration.

▽ OUTCOME IDENTIFICATION

Identifying outcomes for adolescents receiving mental health care is critical for developing an attainable and realistic plan of care. The first step typically involves having the adolescent acknowledge the need for care and agreeing to be a partner in that care. Mutually

---

👓 *REFLECTIVE THINKING*

The Role of the School Nurse

Imagine that you are the school nurse responsible for maintaining the health records and responding to the health care needs of a suburban middle school. This school is located in a fairly affluent neighborhood and has students who are predominantly Caucasian, Asian, Mexican-American, and African American (in decreasing order of prevalence).

◆ Which transitions of adolescence are you most likely to encounter with these students?

◆ What mental health care concerns would you be most likely to encounter on a daily basis in this setting?

◆ What kinds of mental health programs would be appropriate for students in this school?

---

outlining targeted outcomes respects the adolescent's independence while providing needed guidance; it also ensures that the adolescent's expectations of progress and success will be realistic and in line with what is likely to occur.

The nurse must be careful to ensure that outcomes are realizable in terms of the targeted mental health state that the client is capable of achieving and that appropriate time frames are identified. Goals that are realistic and attainable ensure success, while goals that are long term and ambiguous may contribute to greater anxiety and confusion.

▽ PLANNING/INTERVENTIONS

Nursing science remains in a state of infancy concerning which interventions work and which do not for many mental health needs of adolescents. In general, however, interventions that are based on a sincere interest in and respect for the adolescent as an individual and adolescence as a genuine phase of development will be most helpful. When working with young adolescents in particular, the nurse should be as concrete as possible in providing information about treatment plans and in communicating expectations about behavior. To enhance the chances of success, the nurse should find out about the adolescent's interests and favorite activities when planning interventions. Activities that are managed by the adolescent, such as keeping a journal, listening to music, and practicing guided imagery, may be most appropriate for individuals who need to maintain a feeling of control. Adolescents needing assistance in role identity and self-confidence may find reassurance with a nurse and family who help set limits and offer guidance.

Meeting the mental health needs of children and adolescents provides a unique challenge to nursing and other health care professions. As society becomes more complex with rapid changes in technology, the adolescent faces an increasingly difficult crisis in forging an identity that incorporates skills for survival and for finding meaning and purpose in life. Research is needed to identify the genetic and environmental influences on adolescent development and behavior. Strategies must be developed to strengthen the family, school, and community interactions with youth in assisting them with the crisis of identity formation. Multidisciplinary interventions that are culturally appropriate must be investigated to promote optimum physical and mental health for youth in the second decade of life.

Longitudinal studies need to be done to explore how cognitive, emotional, and social transitions are experienced relative to health (National Institute of Nursing Research, 1993). The influence of peers in developing health-promoting lifestyles and in reducing high-risk behaviors also needs to be studied. Nurses in school- and community-based clinics have a tremendous responsibility for identifying the mental health care problems and needs of adolescents and in proposing innovative ways to provide useful services.

▽ EVALUATION

When evaluating the success of the nursing care plan and the effectiveness of the interventions, the nurse should look at the progress the teen has made toward realizing the targeted outcomes that were mutually agreed upon. Successes can be judged in increments and should be shared with the adolescent and family so that all can feel a sense of accomplishment. If certain goals are not met, the nurse, adolescent, and family should jointly review what the expectations were at the outset of care and reassess how realistic the targeted goals were. An evaluation of resources available and family support may also indicate additional areas that could be called upon to increase chances of success in reaching goals.

CASE STUDY/CARE PLAN

The following excerpt provides data on which a case study and nursing care plan can be devised. The fictionalized plan that follows the excerpt is based on how the nurse could respond to an adolescent client whose childhood experiences were similar to those of Truddi.

When Rabbit Howls

"I'm scared to think of the hedgerow nearest the house, of the chicken house or the fields. There was never a day of peace, nothing was safe. I was fifteen when I dared complain to my mother for the first time, to tell her I couldn't spend one more day in that house, that I was leaving. About the only thing I recall when my mother and I confronted my stepfather with those years of hell was that he broke a broom over my back in his rage. He hurled a bowl of fresh made apple sauce at someone. That day, his killing instincts went full-throttle. I knew that if he got his hands on any one of us, he'd choke us until we had no more breath. My mother held him off with the rifle; she explained in deadly quiet tones that he had to leave."

"At some point afterward my half brother, who was twelve, found a small hole carved in the door of the closet separating my bedroom from that of my mother and stepfather. There was a pile of old sawdust on the floor under the hole. I felt shock, and then I felt dirty and immobile."

. . . "I was so ashamed. I just shook, realising that while I hid in my room all those years in what I believed was privacy, my stepfather had stood there on the other side of the wall, peering through the knothole. In short, the bastard had made himself privy to my every movement."

She shrugged and shuddered at the same time. "Right now, what bothers me most is the pink thing in the flicks [flashbacks]. It's there with all that wiry brush around it and it seems to pertain to me, and yet it doesn't. The flicks won't stand still long enough."

"What pink thing?" Stanley asked innocently, and she tried to describe her stepfather's male organ with a look of utter helplessness. Her hands balled into fists and she pounded them on yoga-positioned kneecaps.

"It's like the animals, we lived on a farm, we had animals. I know we did! But I can't remember a single god-damned one, and I know they were there. I hate animals, always have, always will, something about animals and my stepfather and me, but every time I think of them or him lately, I run, I go crazy."

(Chase, 1990, pp. 97–98)

ASSESSMENT

Ms. Ivanhoe is a 15-year-old high school junior. Similar to Truddi in the preceding excerpt, she was sexually abused by her stepfather between the ages of 6 and 14 years. Last year her mother and stepfather were divorced and the abuse came to an end. Since that time, Ms. Ivanhoe has had difficulty sleeping. She awakens nearly every night with nightmares, and sometimes during the day she experiences flashbacks to those nights when her sleep was interrupted by her stepfather's sexual advances. She avoids going out with boys who ask her to accompany them on dates. In the past 6 months, Ms. Ivanhoe has had increasing difficulty paying attention in school and startles easily when other students move around the classroom.

Continued

NURSING DIAGNOSIS *Sleep pattern disturbance*, related to psychological stress, as evidenced by interrupted sleep and nightmares

Outcomes	Planning/Interventions	Evaluation
• The client will acknowledge that her sleep pattern is disturbed. • The client will verbalize her anxiety and fear about sexual abuse. • The client will identify the daytime flashbacks as memories of childhood sexual abuse. • The client will identify at least two relaxation strategies that will enhance her ability to sleep at night. • The client will practice at least two relaxation strategies.	The nurse will assist the client in acknowledging that her nightmares frighten her and remind her of the past by: • Being present with Ms. Ivanhoe when she talks about the nightmares and flashbacks. • Using active and empathetic listening. • Communicating her acceptance of Ms. Ivanhoe regardless of the content of her nightmares. • Teaching Ms. Ivanhoe two relaxation techniques: (1) using music that she enjoys and (2) using a mental image she describes as peaceful to her.	At the end of 4 weeks Ms. Ivanhoe was able to state that she understood the relationship between her nightmares and flashbacks and her memories of sexual abuse as a child. She gradually began to trust the nurse and provided more details of the abuse, which were similar to the images in her nightmares and flashbacks. At first she had difficulty relaxing with music before going to bed, but after 3 weeks she found a recording of flute music that helped her feel calm. Ms. Ivanhoe also practiced using a mental image of herself resting on a warm beach and reported that this helped her to relax and fall asleep.

NURSING DIAGNOSIS *Social isolation*, related to inability to engage in satisfying personal relationships, as evidenced by insecurity and fear of being alone with others

Outcomes	Planning/Interventions	Evaluation
• The client will acknowledge her fear of being alone with boys. • The client will state how her current behavior around boys is related to early experiences of abuse. • The client will identify goals for future relationships with boys.	• The nurse supports the client's right to have loving relationships. • The nurse helps Ms. Ivanhoe consider how her current behavior is related to previous experience. • The nurse encourages realistic hope for developing healthy relationships outside her family. • The nurse demonstrates two ways in which Ms. Ivanhoe can feel safe in the company of boys: (1) by writing self-affirmative statements such as "I am respectable and have a right to say no about anything that makes me uncomfortable" and (2) by role playing a situation in which she will	During the first week of treatment, Ms. Ivanhoe refused to talk about going out with boys, but gradually she began to trust the nurse and to say that she was afraid to be alone with boys but she didn't really know why. During the second week of treatment, the nurse encouraged Ms. Ivanhoe to identify things about boys that scared her. After making a short list, Ms.

Outcomes	Planning/Interventions	Evaluation
◆ The client will demonstrate at least two ways in which she can feel safe around male peers.	say to a boy, "I do not want to be alone with you right now, I feel uncomfortable." ◆ The nurse facilitates Ms. Ivanhoe's self-understanding by describing the pattern of current behavior as it relates to fear of childhood abuse.	Ivanhoe began to say that she thought she was afraid they would harm her the way her stepfather had. During the third and fourth weeks, Ms. Ivanhoe began talking daily with the nurse about her fear of boys and how they might harm her. She also wrote self-affirmations daily and reported that this made her feel stronger and more secure. She role-played affirmations with the female nurse and at the end of 4 weeks asked if she could role-play with a male nurse or doctor.

NURSING DIAGNOSIS   *Altered thought processes*, related to previous experiences of abuse, as evidenced by distractibility

Outcomes	Planning/Interventions	Evaluation
◆ The client will state how difficult it is for her to feel safe in the classroom. ◆ The client will identify how her lack of concentration is related to her fear of being victimized. ◆ The client will demonstrate at least two ways in which she can concentrate on material presented in the classroom. ◆ The client will feel more relaxed in a classroom setting.	◆ The nurse will encourage the client to verbalize her feelings about paying attention in the classroom through the nurse's presence and active listening. ◆ The nurse will assist the client in connecting her feelings to past experiences of abuse and her need to be vigilant. ◆ The nurse will assist the client in increasing her concentration through meditation and relaxation exercises.	During the first week, Ms. Ivanhoe had difficulty paying attention to what the nurse was saying to her. As the nurse continued to remain with her, Ms. Ivanhoe began to tell the nurse that she was confused about what she should be doing at school. In the second week of treatment, the nurse taught Ms. Ivanhoe a progressive relaxation exercise, and while she was relaxed, Ms. Ivanhoe began to relate her thoughts about being a bad person and deserving the abuse. By the end of the fourth week, she was able to practice progressive relaxation on her own and was able to sit for a period of 30 minutes and read without being startled.

Continued

NURSING DIAGNOSIS *Self-esteem disturbance*, related to sexual abuse, as evidenced by feelings of shame/guilt

Outcomes	Planning/Interventions	Evaluation
◆ The client will verbalize her feelings about the sexual abuse. ◆ The client will state with conviction that she was not to blame for the abuse. ◆ The client will identify at least two ways in which she can share her feelings with her mother. ◆ The client will demonstrate at least two behaviors that reflect a positive self-image.	◆ The nurse will encourage the client to express her feelings orally (through the nurse's active listening), in writing (in a daily journal), and by sculpting clay. ◆ The nurse will acknowledge that the client's feelings are appropriate and will not judge her. ◆ The nurse will role-play with the client ways in which she can tell her mother about her feelings about the abuse and about herself. ◆ The nurse will reflect to the client the client's ability to express herself appropriately in writing, speaking, and sculpting.	At the end of the first week of treatment, Ms. Ivanhoe was writing in her journal daily and beginning to state how she felt about herself and her responsibility for allowing her stepfather to abuse her. By the end of the third week, she had made six clay sculptures of her as a small helpless child and increasing in size and strength to portray herself as a mature and capable young woman. Ms. Ivanhoe role-played with the nurse how to talk to her mother, and at the end of four weeks asked the nurse to help her confront her mother with her feelings.

CRITICAL THINKING BAND

ASSESSMENT

What additional information might the nurse need to plan more comprehensive and holistic care for this client? What other health care team members should be brought into the assessment loop?

NURSING DIAGNOSIS

What other nursing diagnoses might be made in this situation?

Outcomes	Planning/Interventions	Evaluation
How realistic are these outcomes? What would the nurse do if the client could not concentrate or trust the nurse enough to participate in setting goals for nursing care? What additional outcomes might be met as the client began to respond to the nurse? How would the outcomes change if the client did not feel that she could trust the nurse?	What specific skills does the nurse need to care for this client? How can previous experiences of the nurse help or hinder her ability to care for this client? What kind of environment will facilitate these nursing interventions?	What kind of outcomes might have been achieved if the nurse had only a few days to work with this client? How might the outcomes have been different if the primary nurse had gone on a 2-week vacation in the middle of Ms. Ivanhoe's treatment? What can the nurse do to reinforce her care plan after the client leaves the treatment facility?

〰 KEY CONCEPTS

◆ Adolescence is a transitional phase of development, with significant changes occurring in physical, emotional, cognitive, and social dimensions.

◆ Identity formation is a major developmental task for the adolescent.

◆ Positive mental health is optimal psychosocial competence or well-being.

◆ Mental health concerns in adolescence include diagnosable problems such as depression and Conduct Disorder as well as distress related to cognitive, emotional, and social transitions.

◆ Adolescents at highest risk for mental health problems are from families in which at least one parent has a history of alcoholism, drug use, suicide attempts, or antisocial and/or violent behavior.

◆ Poverty also places adolescents at risk for mental health problems including school drop-out, gang involvement, and substance abuse.

◆ Sexual development, identity, and orientation are issues central to the mental health of adolescents.

◆ Suicidal ideation and behavior are the most serious outcomes related to adolescent mental health problems and may be related to childhood abuse, neglect, and homelessness.

◆ Nursing interventions for adolescents with mental health problems are based on developing an authentic caring relationship between nurse and client and on increasing the adolescent's conscious awareness of connections between experiences, feelings, and behaviors.

〰 REVIEW QUESTIONS AND ACTIVITIES

1. How might the difference between an adolescent's subjective feeling of mental health and a mental health professional's (e.g., school counselor) definition of mental health lead to conflict between these two individuals?

2. What effect could an adolescent's relocation from Texas to New Jersey during high school have on that person's identity formation?

3. How might a person's experiences with emotional abuse in childhood affect his feelings of self-efficacy or competence as an adolescent?

4. How did your personal experiences with peers' evaluations during adolescence contribute to your role as an adult?

5. What are the effects of loneliness on the adolescent?

6. How can Paterson and Zderad's theory of humanistic nursing help you plan your interactions with adolescent clients?

7. How can Newman's theory of health as expanding consciousness help you to understand mental health in adolescents?

8. List the various nursing interventions that might be helpful to an adolescent who is struggling with identity formation.

⚛ EXPLORING THE WEB

◆ Visit this text's "Online Companion™" on the Internet at **http://www.DelmarNursing.com** for further information on adolescents with psychiatric disorders.

◆ Do the resource organizations listed in this chapter also have Web sites? What types of information do they provide? Do they seem more targeted to the adolescent or to the care provider?

◆ What sites can you find that offer information on suicide prevention? Do they also offer separate tips, chat lines, or resources specific to adolescents?

◆ Can you locate organizations on the Internet that have specific discussion groups addressing the psychiatric needs of adolescents?

〰 REFERENCES

American Psychiatric Association *Diagnostic and Statistical Manual of Mental Disorders*, Fourth Edition, Washington, DC: American Psychiatric Association, 1994.

Bandura, A. (1977). *Social learning theory.* Englewood Cliffs, NJ: Prentice-Hall.

Bandura, A., & Schunk, D. H. (1981). Cultivating competence, self-efficacy, and intrinsic interest through proximal self-motivation. *Journal of Personality and Social Psychology, 41,* 586–598.

Blyth, D. A., & Leffert, N. (1995). Communities as contexts for adolescent development: An empirical analysis. *Journal of Adolescent Research, 10*(1), 64–87.

Brack, C. J., Orr, D. P., & Ingersoll, G. (1988). Pubertal maturation and adolescent self-esteem. *Journal of Adolescent Health Care, 9,* 280–285.

Brage, D., Meredith, W., & Woodward, J. (1993). Correlates of loneliness among midwestern adolescents. *Adolescence, 28,* 685–693.

Burns, B. J. (1991). Mental health service use by adolescents in the 1970s and 1980s. *Journal of the American Academy of Child and Adolescent Psychiatry, 30,* 144–150.

Centers for Disease Control. (1995). Suicide among children, adolescents and young adults—United States, 1980–1992. *MMWR, 44,* 289–291.

Compas, B. E. (1993). Promoting positive mental health during adolescence. In S. G. Millstein, A. C. Petersen, & E. O. Nightingale (Eds.), *Promoting the health of adolescents* (pp. 159–179). New York: Oxford University Press.

Crockett, L. J., & Petersen, A. C. (1993). Adolescent development: Health risks and opportunities for health promotion. In S. G. Millstein, A. C. Petersen, & E. O. Nightingale (Eds.), *Promoting the health of adolescents* (pp. 13–37). New York: Oxford University Press.

De Wilde, E. J., Kienhorst, C. W. M., Diekstra, R. F. W., & Wolters, W. H. G. (1992). The relationship between adolescent suicidal behavior and life events in childhood and adolescence. *American Journal of Psychiatry, 149*(1), 45–51.

Dumont, L. (1991). *Surviving adolescence: Helping your child through the struggle to adulthood.* New York: Villard Books.

Earls, F., Cairns, R. B., & Mercy, J. A. (1993). The control of violence and the promotion of nonviolence in adolescents. In S. G. Millstein, A. C. Petersen, & E. O. Nightingale (Eds.), *Promoting the health of adolescents* (pp. 285–304). New York: Oxford University Press.

Erikson, E. (1950). *Childhood and society.* New York: Norton.

Erikson, E. (1968). *Identity: Youth and crisis.* New York: Norton.

Esparza, D. V., & Esperat, M. C. R. (1996). The effects of childhood sexual abuse on minority adolescent mothers. *JOGNN, 25,* 321–328.

Ferguson, J. (1993). Youth at the threshold of the 21st century: The demographic situation. *Journal of Adolescent Health, 14,* 638–644.

Hains, A. A. (1992). Comparison of cognitive-behavioral stress management techniques with adolescent boys. *Journal of Counseling and Development, 70,* 600–605.

Hoberman, H. M. (1995). *Suicide and depression in children and adolescents: Clinical characteristics, assessment, and intervention approaches.* Lecture in Child and Adolescent Psychiatry, School of Medicine, University of Minnesota, September 23, 1995.

Jessor, R. (1991). Risk behavior in adolescence: A psychosocial framework for understanding and action. *Journal of Adolescent Health Care, 12,* 597–605.

Josselson, R. (1994). The theory of identity development and the question of intervention. In S. L. Archer (Ed.), *Interventions for adolescent identity development* (pp. 12–25). Thousand Oaks, CA: Sage Publications.

Institute of Medicine. (1989). *Research on children and adolescents with mental, behavioral, and developmental disorders.* Washington, DC: National Academy Press.

Kazdin, A. E. (1993). Adolescent mental health: Prevention and treatment programs. *American Psychologist, 48,* 127–141.

Marcia, J. E. (1994). Identity and psychotherapy. In S. L. Archer (Ed.), *Interventions for adolescent identity development* (pp. 29–46). Thousand Oaks, CA: Sage Publications.

Millstein, S. G., Irwin, C. E., & Brindis, C. D. (1991). Sociodemographic trends and projections in the adolescent population. In W. R. Hendee (Ed.), *The health of adolescents* (pp. 1–15). San Francisco: Jossey-Bass.

Money, J. (1994). The concept of gender identity disorder in childhood and adolescence after 39 years. *Journal of Sex & Marital Therapy, 20,* 163–177.

National Institute of Nursing Research. (1993). *Health promotion for older children and adolescents.* Report of the NINR Priority Expert Panel on Health Promotion. Bethesda, MD: U.S. Department of Health and Human Services.

Neinstein, L. S., Juliani, M. A., Shapiro, J., & Warf, C. (1996). Rape and sexual abuse. In L. S. Neinstein (Ed.), *Adolescent health care: A practical guide* (3rd ed., pp. 1143–1172). Baltimore, MD: Williams & Wilkins.

Newman, M. A. (1994). *Health as expanding consciousness* (2nd ed.). New York: National League for Nursing Press.

Parker, B., McFarlane, J., Soeken, K., Torres, S., & Campbell, D. (1993). Physical and emotional abuse in pregnancy: A comparison of adult and teenage women. *Nursing Research, 42,* 173–178.

Paterson, J. G., & Zderad, L. T. (1988). *Humanistic nursing.* New York: National League for Nursing.

Perry, C. L., Kelder, S. H., & Komro, K. A. (1993). The social world of adolescents: Family, peers, schools, and the community. In S. G. Millstein, A. C. Petersen, & E. O. Nightingale (Eds.), *Promoting the health of adolescents* (pp. 73–96). New York: Oxford University Press.

Pletsch, P. K., Johnson, M. K., Tosi, C. B., Thurston, C. A., & Riesch, S. K. (1991). Self-image among early adolescents: Revisited. *Journal of Community Health Nursing, 8,* 215–231.

Pope, C., & Brucker, M. C. (1991). Adolescents as victims: An overview of the special impact of sexual abuse. *NAACOGs Clinical Issues, 2,* 263–270.

Praeger, S. G., & Hogarth, C. R. (1985). Josephine E. Paterson and Loretta T. Zderad. In J. B. George (Ed.), *Nursing theories* (2nd ed., pp. 287–299). Englewood Cliffs, NJ: Prentice-Hall.

Rice, K. G., & Meyer, A. L. (1994). Preventing depression among young adolescents: Preliminary process results of a psychoeducational intervention program. *Journal of Counseling & Development, 73,* 145–152.

Rich, A. R., Kirkpatrick-Smith, J., Bonner, R. L., & Jans, F. (1992). Gender differences in the psychosocial correlates of suicidal ideation among adolescents. *Suicide and Life-Threatening Behavior, 22,* 364–373.

Riggs, S., & Cheng, T. (1988). Adolescents' willingness to use a school-based clinic in view of expressed health concerns. *Journal of Adolescent Health Care, 9,* 208–213.

Robertson, J. M. (1992). Homeless and runaway youths: A review of the literature. In J. M. Robertson & M. Greenblatt (Eds.), *Homelessness: A national perspective* (pp. 287–297). New York: Plenum.

Rotheram-Borus, M. J., Parra, M., Cantwell, C., Gwadz, M., & Murphy, D. A. (1996). In R. J. DiClemente, W. B. Hansen, & L. E. Ponton (Eds.), *Handbook of adolescent health risk behavior* (pp. 369–391). New York: Plenum.

Saunders, S. M., Resnick, M. D., Hoberman, H. M., & Blum, R. W. (1994). Formal help-seeking behavior of adolescents identifying themselves as having mental health problems. *Journal of the American Academy of Child and Adolescent Psychiatry, 33,* 718–728.

Sells, C. W., & Blum, R. W. (1996). Current trends in adolescent health. In R. J. DiClemente, W. B. Hansen, & L. E. Ponton (Eds.), *Handbook of adolescent health risk behavior.* New York: Plenum.

Steinberg, L. (1996). *Adolescence* (4th ed.). New York: McGraw-Hill.

Telljohann, S. K., Price, J. H., Summers, J., Everett, S. A., & Casler, S. (1995). High school students' perceptions of nonconsensual sexual activity. *Journal of School Health, 65,* 107–112.

Treadway, L., & Yoakam, J. (1992). Creating a safer school environment for lesbian and gay students. *Journal of School Health, 62,* 352–357.

Vernon, M. E. L. (1991). Life-style, risk taking, and out-of-control behavior. In W. R. Hendee (Ed.), *The health of adolescents* (pp. 162–185). San Francisco: Jossey-Bass.

Vinogradov, S., Dishotsky, N. I., Doty, A. K., & Tinklenberg, J. R. (1988). Patterns of behavior in adolescent rape. *American Journal of Orthopsychiatry, 58,* 179–187.

〰 LITERARY REFERENCES

Blume, J. (1973). *Deenie.* New York: Dell.

Chase, T. (1990). *When rabbit howls.* New York: Jove Books.

Neufeld, J. (1970). *Lisa, bright and dark.* New York: Penguin Books.

〰 SUGGESTED READINGS

Barker, L. A., & Adelman, H. S. (1994). Mental health and help-seeking among ethnic minority adolescents. *Journal of Adolescence, 17,* 251–263.

Barron, C. R., & Yoest, P. (1994). Emotional distress and coping with a stressful relationship in adolescent boys. *Journal of Pediatric Nursing, 9*(1), 13–20.

Bensinger, J. S., & Natenshon, A. H. (1991). Difficulties in recognizing adolescent health issues. In W. R. Hendee (Ed.), *The health of adolescents* (pp. 381–410). San Francisco: Jossey-Bass.

Brindis, C. D. (1993). What it will take: Placing adolescents on the American national agenda for the 1990s. *Journal of Adolescent Health, 14,* 527–530.

Brooks-Gunn, J. (1992). The impact of puberty and sexual activity upon the health and education of adolescent girls and boys. In S. S. Klein (Ed.), *Sex equity and sexuality in education.* Albany, NY: State University of New York Press.

Brooks-Gunn, J., Attie, I., Burrow, C., Rosso, J. T., & Warren, M. P. (1989). The impact of puberty on body and eating concerns in athletic and nonathletic contexts. *Journal of Early Adolescence, 9,* 269–290.

Hibbard, R. A., Brack, C. J., Rauch, S., & Orr, D. P. (1988). Abuse, feelings, and health behaviors in a student population. *AJDC, 142,* 326–330.

Lester, D. (1993). *The cruelest death: The enigma of adolescent suicide.* Philadelphia: Charles Press.

Martin-Causey, T., & Hinkle, J. S. (1995). Multimodal therapy with an aggressive preadolescent: A demonstration of effectiveness and accountability. *Journal of Counseling & Development, 73,* 305–310.

Millstein, S. G., Petersen, A. C., & Nightingale, E. O. (Eds.). (1993). *Promoting the health of adolescents.* New York: Oxford University Press.

Renshaw, D. C. (1991). Child-on-child sex abuse. *Medical Aspects of Human Sexuality, 25*(6), 60–62.

Resnick, M. D., Harris, L. J., & Blum, R. W. (1993). The impact of caring and connectedness on adolescent health and well-being. *Paediatric Child Health, 29S,* 53–59.

Reuler, J. B. (1991). Outreach health services for street youth. *Journal of Adolescent Health, 12,* 561–566.

Schneider, M. B., Friedman, S. B., & Fisher, M. (1995). Stated and unstated reasons for visiting a high school nurse's office. *Journal of Adolescent Health, 16,* 35–40.

Schorr, L. B. (1988). *Within our reach: Breaking the cycle of disadvantage.* New York: Anchor/Doubleday.

Schumacher, K. L., & Meleis, A. I. (1994). Transitions: A central concept in nursing. *IMAGE: Journal of Nursing Scholarship, 26,* 119–127.

〰 RESOURCES FOR ADOLESCENTS WITH MENTAL HEALTH CONCERNS

National Coalition Against Sexual Assault: 217-753-4117
123 S. 7th, Suite 500
Springfield, IL 62701

AIDS Hotline: 1-800-342 AIDS

Suicide and Runaway Hotline: 1-800-621-4000

Survivors of Suicide (SOS): 414-442-4638
3251 N. 78th Street
Milwaukee, WI 53222

Gay and Lesbian Community Services Center: 213-993-7400
1625 North Schrader Boulevard
Los Angeles, CA 98828-9998

Federation of Parents and Friends of Lesbians and Gays: 202-638-4200, FAX: 202-638-0243
1101 14th Street NW/Suite 1030
Washington, DC 20005

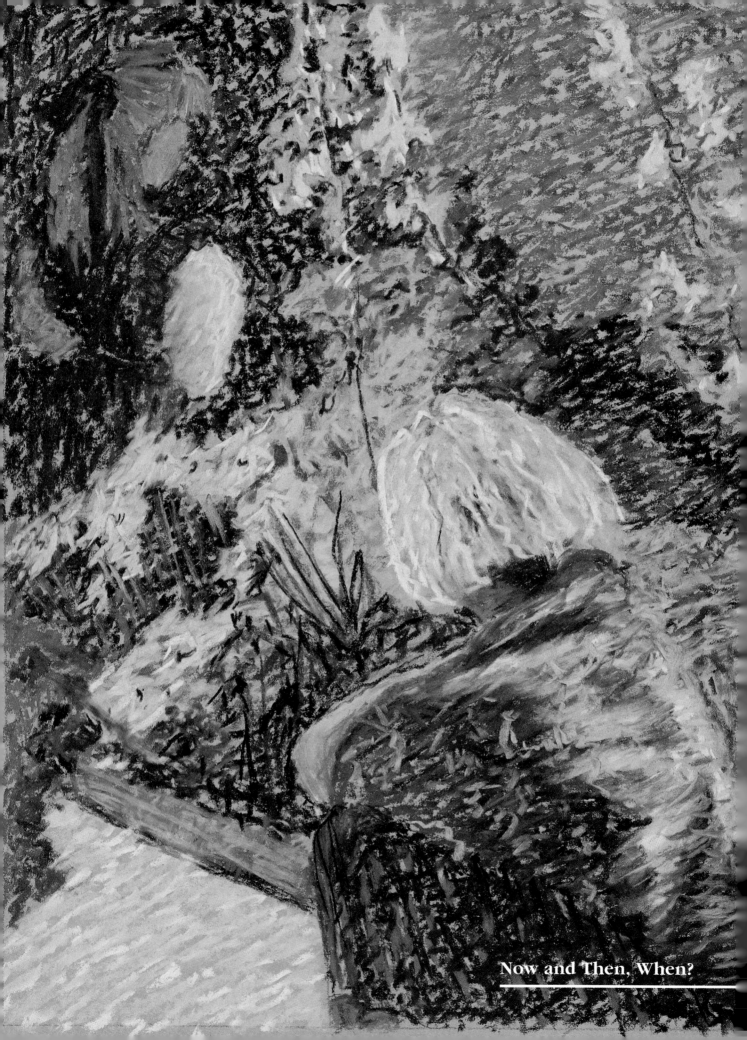

Now and Then, When?

Chapter

23

THE ELDERLY

Brenda P. Johnson

The Person Within

Consider the following situations and how they might change your perception of who *you* are:

◆ How would you feel if you woke up tomorrow and realized that no one was still alive who had known you as a child?

◆ Choose a residence, three favorite possessions, and three characteristics that you would like to have into your old age. Now imagine that these are all suddenly taken away from you; how would you feel?

◆ Suppose you gradually start losing things several times a day at home, at school, or at work. Your friends and family tell you it must just be stress but you feel that something else is wrong. Your doctor tells you that you need to "get more rest." Your mental function continues to deteriorate until you are totally dependent upon someone else for dressing, bathing, and eating. You do not recognize any of your friends or family and are only able to mumble "Take me home . . . I don't live here . . . I need to go home." What would your emotional response be?

Many individuals find themselves in such situations as they age; reflect on these as you read this chapter.

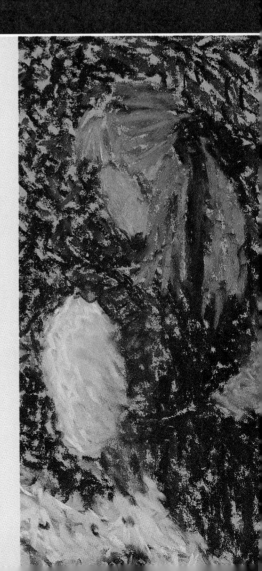

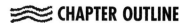 **CHAPTER OUTLINE**

MENTAL HEALTH IN THE AGED

COGNITION IN THE ELDERLY

DELIRIUM

Characteristics

Diagnosis and Pathophysiology

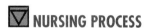 **NURSING PROCESS**

DEPRESSION

Theories of Depression

Characteristics and Diagnoses

Subtypes of Depression
    Major Clinical Depression
    Dysthymic Disorder
    Adjustment Disorder with a Depressed Mood
    Grief and Depression

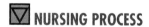 **NURSING PROCESS**

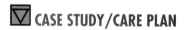 **CASE STUDY/CARE PLAN**

DEMENTIA

Alzheimer's Disease
    Characteristics and Prevalence
    Diagnosis and Pathophysiology

Vascular Dementias
    Characteristics and Prevalence
    Diagnosis and Pathophysiology

Other Dementias
    Symptoms and Sequelae

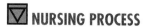 **NURSING PROCESS**

CARING FOR THE CAREGIVERS

Honesty with the Diagnosis

Relationship Tensions

Financial and Legal Affairs

Use of Community Resources

Guilt Over Nursing Home Placement

Humor

The Positive Aspects

FUTURE DIRECTIONS

≋ **COMPETENCIES**

Upon completion of this chapter, the reader should be able to:

1. Recognize the interconnected role that physical health and family support systems play in the mental health of older adults.

2. Identify pathological processes that are responsible for the disorders of cognition and affect most commonly seen in the older adult.

3. Analyze how ageist stereotypes and socioeconomic factors affect the occurrence of mental illness in the elderly.

4. Describe the most common physiological causes (risk factors) of delirium and acute confusional states in the elderly.

5. Envision and illustrate ways in which severe memory loss pose a challenge to self-concept and human dignity.

6. Propose nursing interventions for demented elders and their caregivers that are derived from a caring framework.

7. Identify environmental and physiological risk factors for depression in the elderly.

8. Explain the basis for treatment modalities of depression in older adults.

≈≈ KEY TERMS

Aphasia   Difficulty or inability to recall words.

Catastrophic Reaction   Severe overreaction out of proportion to the stimulus.

Cognition   Process by which a person "knows the world" and interacts with it.

Confabulation   Intentional efforts to cover up memory losses or gaps.

Confusion   Multidimensional phenomenon incorporating changes in both cognition and behavior.

Delirium   Acute change in a person's level of consciousness and cognition that develops over a short period of time.

Dementia   Gradual onset of multiple cognitive changes in memory, abstract thinking, judgment, and perception that often results in a progressive decline in intellectual functioning and decreased capacity to perform daily activities.

Mutuality   Client involvement in the therapeutic relationship.

History has given us countless examples of powerful, creative, and productive elders. Michelangelo was appointed chief architect of St. Peter's Cathedral in Rome at the age of 71 and over the next 18 years, until his death at 89, he personally supervised the creation of the vast main body of the church. Picasso was painting until the day he died, at the age of 91 (Dychtwald, 1989).

The "elderly" are often characterized as anyone over the age of 65. However, life as experienced by an 85-year-old is often as different from the experience of a 65-year-old as is an adolescent's from a child's. The significance of differentiating the "old-old" from the "young-old" is heightened by the growing numbers of the very old. Persons 85 years of age and older (old-old) constitute the fastest growing segment of the United States population. While the proportion of those over 65 has increased by 24% since 1960, the proportion of those aged 85 years and older has risen 174%. And the number of centenarians is steadily growing!

While old age is not synonymous with illness and disability, the number of chronic illnesses grows steadily with age. Although the elderly experience fewer acute illnesses, most older persons have at least one chronic illness, such as arthritis, hypertension, diabetes, or a hearing or visual impairment (Eliopoulos, 1997). Among the old-old, multiple chronic conditions are commonplace. Chronic illness is responsible for some degree of limitation in personal care activities among 49% of older adults (Eliopoulos, 1997). Although less than 5% of the older population is institutionalized at any given time, about one in four adults will spend some time in a nursing home during the last years of their lives (Eliopoulos, 1997, p. 40). When a combination of physical illnesses such as heart disease, stroke, and Alzheimer's disease results in the inability of individuals to care for themselves, self-esteem and personal identity can be greatly affected. This change is made worse by stereotypical attitudes of those who do not look beyond the physical decline to see the person inside the failing body.

The following poem was found in a bedside table of a geriatric ward in a hospital in Ireland. It was written by an anonymous "Crabbit Old Woman" and first appeared in the Christmas issue of *Beacon House News*, the magazine of the Northern Ireland Association for Mental Health.

A Crabbit Old Woman

What do you see nurses, what do you see?
Are you thinking when you are looking at me?
A crabbit old woman, not very wise,
Uncertain of habit, with far-away eyes;
Who dribbles her food and makes no reply
When you say in a loud voice "I do wish you'd try."
Who seems not to notice the things that you do,
And forever is losing a stocking or shoe.
Who, unresisting or not, lets you do as you will
When bathing and feeding the long day to fill.
Is that what you are thinking, is that what you see?
Then open your eyes, nurse, you are not looking at me!

I'll tell you who I am as I sit here so still,
As I wee at your bidding, as I eat at your will.
I'm a child of ten with a father and mother,
Brothers and sisters who love one another.
A young girl of sixteen with wings on her feet,
Dreaming that soon now a lover she'll meet.
A bride soon at twenty, my heart gives a leap,
Remembering the vows that I promised to keep.
At twenty-five now I have young of my own,
Who need me to build a secure, happy home.
A woman of thirty, my young now grow fast,
Bound to each other with ties that should last.
At forty my young ones now grown and will be gone,
But my man stays beside me to see I don't mourn.
At fifty once more babies play round my knee,

*Again we know children, my loved ones and
me.*

Dark days are upon me, my husband is dead.
*My young ones are all busy rearing young of
their own,*
*And I think of the years and the love that I've
known.*

I'm an old woman now, and nature is cruel—
'Is hers just to make old age look like a fool.
The body it crumbles, grace and vigor depart.
There now is a stone where I once had a heart.
But inside this carcass a young girl still dwells,
And now and again my battered heart swells.
I remember the joys, I remember the pain,
And I'm loving and living life over again.
I think of the years all too few; gone too fast . . .
I accept the stark fact that nothing can last.
So open your eyes, nurses, open and see
*Not a crabbit old woman; look closer—see
me!**

Anonymous

MENTAL HEALTH IN THE AGED

The elderly are a very heterogeneous group. The influence of an individual's work and home environments and cultural and economic conditions combine to make each person's life experience grow more different from every other with each passing day. The interplay of physiological and sociocultural conditions in combination with individual and family expectations and support to a great extent determine the mental health of an individual in old age.

Mental health decline is not inevitable with aging. In fact, there are some indications that mental illness occurs less frequently in older adults than in young persons. First-time depression in women after age 65 has been thought to be relatively infrequent unless associated with bereavement (Wykle & Musil, 1993). Older women with severe depression are likely to have also experienced depressive episodes when younger. The strongest predictors of depression that manifests for the first time in old age are poor physical health and inadequate social support. The combination of low educational level and socioeconomic position is associated with the greatest rates of depression, putting elderly women and minorities at greatest risk (Wykle & Musil, 1993).

Losses are a frequent and significant occurrence among aged persons. Death, retirement, and physical frailty change dramatically the pattern of one's life. While depressive symptomatology is common among the elderly, it tends to be more transient and to present with milder symptoms as compared to the depression of younger adults. However, this fact should not overshadow the sad reality that suicide has become one of the leading causes of death among older persons.

One reason that depression may be underdiagnosed and undertreated in the elderly is that older persons are less likely to seek treatment for mental health problems through formal mental health care systems. Many older adults with mental illness use physical symptoms as the basis for seeking medical help. Less stigma is often attached to seeking help for physical problems than for mental ones, especially since there is a widespread, unfounded belief that aging and illness go hand in hand.

Another reason that mental illness in the elderly is misunderstood and underrecognized is that many older adults with mental illness are institutionalized in long-term care facilities. Although only a very small percentage of persons over the age of 65 live in nursing homes (approximately 5%), the need for long-term care increases dramatically in the very old, as does the number of chronic illnesses. Twenty-three percent of the over-age-85 population now require nursing home care (Finkel, 1993). Of those admitted to nursing homes, 43% to 60% have some type of mental disorder (Gatz & Smyer, 1992).

Although lower rates of affective disorders, anxiety disorders, and substance abuse are reported for the elderly, the elderly exhibit higher rates of multiple disorders that result in impairments in cognition and memory. The three most prevalent mental disorders of older adults are dementias, delirium, and depression. Due in part to its high metabolic rate, brain tissue is particularly susceptible to the damaging effects of trauma or biochemical abnormalities. Thus, a large number of both temporary and permanent pathologies may result in a cognitive disorder in the older adult. Depression in the elderly has been called "pseudodementia" since more frequently than in younger adults it results in significant impairments in cognition. Higher rates of physical disability and multiple losses place the elderly at risk for depression. Perhaps this fact is illustrated most clearly in those individuals for whom depression and dementia coexist. Many admissions to nursing homes are due to the difficulties of family caregivers in managing the self-care needs and behavioral problems associated with dementias. Certainly the progressive decline in cognitive function may be at least one precipitating factor for the depression.

It is important to understand that mental illness in the elderly is a complex multifactoral problem. Mental health decline is not an inevitable part of aging and there is some evidence that mental illness occurs less frequently in older adults than in younger persons. When it does

---

*Courtesy of Northern Ireland Association for Mental Health

Caring for the Elderly

Remember the following when caring for elderly clients:

◆ Common disorders may affect cognition, which in turn may affect personhood.

◆ A primary goal of nursing care must be to ensure that the dignity and personhood of the elderly client are preserved to the fullest extent possible.

◆ Needs of caregivers must be addressed as important to preserving the pattern, integrity, and dignity of family life.

arise, the symptoms and manifestations are often different and physical illness is often present. The strength of family and social support also plays a very big part in how mentally healthy older adults remain throughout their advancing years and the emotional, economic, and physical losses that these advancing years bring.

COGNITION IN THE ELDERLY

The latter part of the 20th century is known as the Information Age. Just as a computer relies upon stored memory to function, so does the cognitive aspect of the human brain rely upon memory to make decisions. **Cognition** is generally described as the process by which a person "knows the world" and interacts with it. The human brain is far more complex, however, than even the most sophisticated computer circuitry. The linking of geographical areas of the cerebral cortex with specific human functions such as speech and sight has provided the map for 20th century neurology. However, it has become all too evident that such a map can only be a guide and does little to help us actually understand the highly complex interactions, images, and capabilities of the human mind.

Intellectual capacity does not diminish with advancing age. However, the brain as it ages is more susceptible to injury from a variety of external and internal environmental factors. Factors such as drugs, electrolyte imbalances, and ischemia diminish the supply of oxygen and nutrients or alter the chemical or electrical environment needed to sustain adequate brain function. Common symptoms of temporary cognitive dysfunction include a limited attention span, sensory misperceptions (illusions), hallucinations, distorted thoughts, and disturbances of activity patterns and the sleep-wake cycle. Unfortunately, although these symptoms are the result of temporary

injury to brain tissue, unless this trauma can be reversed, permanent brain injury can result. For the elderly, this is a situation that happens all too frequently when changes in orientation, alterations in attention, or agitation is seen not as symptomatic of a physical illness, but as the untreatable consequence of old age or "senility."

Cognitive disorders are divided into four diagnostic categories according to the specific symptoms observed and the disorder causing the impairment: delirium, dementia, amnestic disorders, and other cognitive disorders (American Psychiatric Association, 1994). In general, **delirium** is an acute change in a person's level of consciousness and cognition that develops over a short period of time. Delirium is not usually due to nervous system abnormalities but, rather, to potentially reversible medical abnormalities such as infection, dehydration, or drug toxicities. **Dementia** is a broad diagnostic category that includes multiple physical disorders characterized by alterations in memory, abstract thinking, judgment, and perception; dementia often results in a progressive decline in intellectual functioning and decreased capacity to perform daily activities. Unlike delirium, dementias are characterized by gradual onset, usually over months or years. The common factor in all of the dementing disorders is a significant degree of memory loss and a progressive decline in intellectual functioning to the extent that daily function is affected. Although forgetfulness is a very common complaint of older adults, memory problems severe enough to cause decreased abilities to function in everyday family and social life are not normal at any age. Among the elderly, depression, or feelings of hopelessness and despair, is identified as it is in younger individuals, as a mood disorder. However, among the elderly it results in impairments in cognition more often than it does in a younger population (Figure 23-1).

To care for an older adult experiencing a change in cognitive abilities, the nurse must understand as much as possible about the basis for these impairments. In order to maximize quality of life, the nurse must differentiate between the reversible cognitive impairments for which medical intervention is warranted and those that cannot be reversed and for which assistance with managing the deficits is indicated. Outcomes will be determined mainly by the extent to which the impairment in cognition may be arrested or reversed. After all attempts have been made to correct physiological abnormalities and treat cognitive impairments resulting from depression, nursing care must be directed toward preserving the dignity and integrity of a person's self-hood and the well-being of the family structure to the fullest extent possible. Although most people over the age of 65 do not have persistent severe cognitive impairments (3% of women, 5.6% of men), it is an important health problem that has significant physical, psychological, and social consequences (Jubeck, 1992).

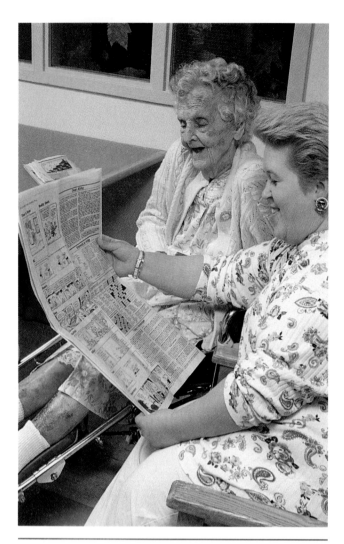

Figure 23-1 **Nurses can assist clients experiencing memory loss by helping orient them to reality (person, time, surroundings, current events, etc.).**

DELIRIUM

Characteristics

Delirium is a potentially reversible state that is characterized as a clouding of consciousness. While memory is usually impaired in both dementia and delirium, a distinguishing feature is that with delirium the level of alertness fluctuates much more so than it does with dementia, and there is usually a significant degree of difficulty in concentrating. Delirious persons may often continuously shift attention from one stimulus to another. Their speech is often difficult to understand because they shift abruptly and inappropriately from one thought to another. It is often difficult to engage such persons in conversation because of their inability to focus or sustain attention on any certain stimulus. Disorientation is more often to time and place rather than to self. Speech may be rambling or incoherent, and the person often experiences distur-

bances in perception, such as illusions or hallucinations. Psychomotor activity often fluctuates from restlessness to lethargy, and emotions from fear and irritability to apathy and anger.

Diagnosis and Pathophysiology

The diagnosis is typically based on observations of the previously described symptoms and identification of medical pathology or drug intoxication or withdrawal. Etiologic general medical conditions include systemic infections, metabolic disorders (e.g., hypoxia, hypercarbia, hypoglycemia), fluid or electrolyte imbalances, hepatic or renal disease, thiamine deficiency, postoperative states, hypertensive encephalopathy, postictal states, and sequelae of head trauma or brain lesions (American Psychiatric Association, 1994, p. 128).

⚡ NURSING ALERT!

Warning Signs of Delirium

- ◆ Rapid fluctuation in level of consciousness (agitated to lethargic)
- ◆ Difficulty in maintaining attention span
- ◆ Illusions or hallucinations
- ◆ Unfocused speech and disorganized thinking
- ◆ Disorientation to place or time
- ◆ Strong emotional reactions
- ◆ Memory problems

PATHOLOGIES THAT MAY CAUSE DELIRIUM

- ◆ Brain tumors
- ◆ Dehydration
- ◆ Drug toxicities or interactions
- ◆ Infections
- ◆ Electrolyte abnormalities
- ◆ Hepatic or renal disease
- ◆ Hypoxia secondary to respiratory or circulatory disorders
- ◆ Hyperthermia or hypothermia
- ◆ Metabolic disorders (especially thyroid and blood glucose abnormalities)
- ◆ Nutritional deficiencies (especially folate, B_{12}, and iron deficiency anemias)

NURSING PROCESS

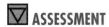ASSESSMENT

Acute confusional states (ACS) is the term often used by nurses to describe the behavioral and cognitive manifestations of delirium. Nurses are often the first to identify sudden changes in behavior or cognition, which are harbingers of medical pathology. Although the term "confused and disoriented" has been a common one used by clinicians in both acute and long-term care, confusion was for some time a largely undefined, undescribed behavioral phenomenon. Wolanin's (1977) groundbreaking work was the first to attempt to define the phenomenon of confusion. A major implication of this study was the finding that sensory deficits (loss of hearing and vision) accounted for much of the changes in behavior and cognition being labeled as confusion.

Subsequent nursing studies have attempted to define and explore ACS from a holistic perspective and to identify risk factors that are amenable to manipulation by nurses. **Confusion** can generally be viewed as a multidimensional phenomenon incorporating changes in both cognition and behavior.

Assessment of risk factors for acute confusion places the nurse in a proactive role of preventing rather than merely identifying delirium. Delirium is a diagnostic term with specific objective criteria that reflect a pathophysiological basis. Acute confusional states may not be the same phenomenon as delirium, although it may incorporate some aspects of that phenomenon. Confusion is more than just cognitive changes. Acute confusional states is a multidimensional phenomenon that incorporates a variety of cognitive and behavioral responses. Older clients are at high risk for developing acute confusion during hospitalization for acute illnesses. The confusion is associated with an increased risk of morbidity and mortality. Confusion is fundamentally a nursing phenomenon; delirium is a medical diagnosis (Vermeersch, 1991).

Tools exist for studying the phenomenon of confusion, the Visual Analogue Scale for Confusion (VAS-C) (Vermeersch, 1990) and the Clinical Assessment of Confusion (CAC-B) (Nagley, 1984). While these tools are adequate for research purposes, they need further refinement for use as a screening tool to detect the onset of confusion or to determine the level of confusion (Vermeersch, 1991). Such tools must sensitively discriminate various levels of cognition, perception, and behaviors. The Mini Mental Status Exam (MMSE) (Folstein, Folstein, & McHugh, 1975) is frequently used as a measure of mental status in the elderly. However, its useful-

🌀 RESEARCH HIGHLIGHT

Study on Confusion

STUDY PROBLEM/PURPOSE

Examine confusion using nurses' and physicians' descriptions of client behavior as noted in records of 30 clients from a large nursing home.

METHODS

Records were searched for descriptions of behaviors of patients labeled as "confused." A grounded theory approach was used for this qualitative study. This meant that as patterns of information emerged during the study, new bits of data were included. For example, observations of clients pointed out the trend of sensory deficits. The investigators rechecked all of the records for evidence of hearing and/or visual loss.

FINDINGS

All of the nouns, adjectives, and verbs describing behaviors were coded into categories. When all data were recorded as one of two categories—cognitive inaccessibility or social inaccessibility—interrater reliability on coding rose from 60% to 90%. Physicians reported behaviors as "confused" that were more indicative of cognitive functions and response to others, such as "poor historian," "incoherent," or "nuisance to staff." Nurses tended to label behaviors as confused that were more indicative of function and activities, such as "client refused medication," "wandering about," "lost," or "agitated."

IMPLICATIONS

A conclusion from this study was that sensory deficits and resulting communication problems accounted for much of what was being labeled as confusion by nurses and physicians.

From "Confusion Study: Use of Grounded Theory As Methodology," in Western Interstate Commission for Higher Education, by M. O. Wolanin, 1977, *Communicating Nursing Research, 8*, pp. 68–75.

ness is limited in that it is a measurement only of changes in cognition and does not assess for other dimensions of delirium or acute confusional states. Any nursing assessment of acute confusion should include baseline as well as ongoing data on cognition, behavior, and functional status (Matthiesen, Silvertsen, Foreman, & Cronin-Stubbs, 1994).

When the term confusion is used to label patient behaviors rather than to describe and investigate the basis for them, the term is being used in error. Implications of research findings suggest a holistic approach to prevention and management of the confused client. This approach emphasizes careful maintenance of physiological homeostasis as well as personal identity with orienting and familiar objects in the environment and the inclusion of significant others in the care of the client.

▽ NURSING DIAGNOSIS

Identification of pathophysiological risk factors for delirium can be described by collaborative nursing diagnoses. Common human responses are those resulting from dehydration, fluid and electrolyte disturbances, drug toxicities, and metabolic disturbances. The inability to attend appropriately to environmental stimuli and to communicate needs and feelings poses a serious threat to dignity and safety. The inability to focus and attend to anything for any length of time results in some degree of inability to care for one's bodily needs (Table 23-1).

▽ OUTCOME IDENTIFICATION

One desired outcome is to diminish the risk of precipitating an acute confusional state by correcting any potential environmental stimulant, such as sensory overstimulation or understimulation for a bedridden client. Another is to correct pathophysiological causes of delirium via collaborative interventions. The prevention or reversal of delirious symptoms is based upon the assessment that the client has maintained or returned to his usual level of alertness and cognitive function.

▽ PLANNING/ INTERVENTIONS

Preventing sensory overstimulation and understimulation is a major factor in preventing or diminishing the severity of acute confusional states in the elderly. Family members may be able to help reduce the severity of confusion seen in acutely ill patients by reading and talking about events and matters going on outside the hospital. Playing familiar music is also a soothing and therapeutic action to take. The research, however, is contradictory in regard to how effective attempts at reorientation are in acute confusional states (Foreman, 1989).

Sleep deprivation is a frequent confounding variable in acute confusional states. In hospitals nurses can control how frequently patients are interrupted during the night. In the great majority of cases this can be accomplished by timing medication administration, vital signs, and other planned aspects of care at the beginning and end of the night shift. Attention to such minor details as turning off suction machines and intentionally lowering the decibel level of the voice can make a significant contribution toward creating an environment conducive to sleep (Tess, 1991).

Hallucinations and memory loss pose a very clear threat to personhood and self-esteem. In order to protect the integrity of an individual's self-concept during acute confusional states, the nurse has a responsibility to explain the physical basis of the delirium to the greatest degree possible to the person experiencing it. Oftentimes simple reassurances that such experiences are not the result of a "psychiatric problem" and that they do not mean that the person is "losing his mind" but rather are the result of the physical illness or drug treatment for which the person is being hospitalized are helpful and comforting.

Impairments in judgment, communication, motor strength, and agility pose grave threats to the independence and dignity of an older adult experiencing an acute

---

Table 23-1 Nursing Diagnoses Often Associated with Acute Confusional States

COLLABORATIVE PATHOPHYSIOLOGICAL RESPONSES	RESPONSES TO BRAIN DYSFUNCTION	THREATS TO DIGNITY AND SAFETY
Electrolyte imbalances	Sensory/perceptual alterations secondary to illusions and hallucinations	Powerlessness
Fluid volume deficit		Personal identity disturbance
Hypothermia/hyperthemia	Communication, impaired verbal	Injury, high risk for
Infection	Thought processes, altered	Self-care deficit
Nutrition: altered, less than body requirements	Sleep pattern disturbance	Incontinence, functional
Tissue perfusion, altered cerebral		Fear
		Anxiety
		Physical mobility, impaired

confusional state. Anticipating the person's need for food and water, elimination, and communication in as private and dignified a manner as possible is a fundamental caring action.

When hospitalized clients become restless during acute confusional states, one concern is that tubes will be dislodged or pulled out. Another is that the client will not have the cognitive capacity to call for assistance before attempting to ambulate (usually to the bathroom) and will be at risk for falling. These concerns about the potential for physical injury as well as the responsibility for carrying out the medical regimen have been the major reasons nurses have given for using restraints on hospitalized clients.

The nurse's privilege to confine or restrict a client's movement by chemical or physical means is legal only within carefully prescribed limitations. The particular setting (nursing home, hospital, or mental health facility) will largely determine the legal parameters. In general, there must be significant threats to an individual's safety, no other alternative for control of the behavior putting the person at risk, and evidence that the least restrictive measures are being used. The use of restraints in nursing homes is controlled by the Nursing Home Reform Law, which is a part of the Omnibus Budget Reconciliation Act (OBRA) of 1987. The influence of OBRA in limiting or preventing the use of restraints is beginning to be reflected in the policies of acute-care hospitals.

Restraint use poses very serious threats to an elderly person's physical well-being. The increased incidence of pneumonia, urinary incontinence, urinary tract infections, and venous thrombosis from immobility is well documented. Older adults have described being physically restrained as a traumatic event outside of the usual range of human experience—feelings of being jailed or of feeling like a caged animal without an escape—and have stated, "I felt like a dog and cried all night" (Strumpf & Evans, 1988). Feelings of being threatened, fear, and helplessness may be exaggerated since the restrained person expects to be safe and protected in the hospital and yet is being restrained over protests and usually cannot understand the rationale for the restraints. Depending

> ### ꩜ *REFLECTIVE THINKING*
>
> #### *The Experience of Being Restrained*
>
> ◆ What questions would you have if you were to awaken in a hospital room, have no memory of how or why you are there, and find yourself tied to the bedframe via a vest restraint?
>
> ◆ What fears would you have if you were sick, tied down to a bed or chair, and completely dependent upon strangers for your every need?

upon the person's interpretation, it is even conceivable that the experience may lead to the development of post-traumatic stress disorder (Sullivan-Marx, 1995). The trauma of the emotional response may be made worse when nurses offer no opportunity for the client to discuss the assault on their personal integrity by ignoring the experience once the person has recovered from the delirious state.

Rather than triggering the response to restrain, behavior associated with delirium and acute confusional states should elicit in-depth assessment, medical consultation, environmental manipulation, and collaborative interventions to reverse physical pathophysiology. The risk of permanent brain damage can only be decreased if there is a timely and competent response to confusion as a symptom of pathology.

▽ EVALUATION

Successful intervention for preventing or reversing delirium or an acute confusional state must be based on the client's everyday level of cognitive and social function. As previously discussed, no instrument has been developed to sensitively discriminate levels of cognitive, behavioral, and social function. Nurses need to include the client's as well as significant others' perceptions of the client's level of function in any evaluation of the effectiveness of treatment for delirium or acute confusional states.

DEPRESSION

The most common mental health problem of old age is depression. Depression is defined as a loss of pleasure in one's usual activities. Old age, on the other hand, is not depressing! Overall, life satisfaction is good among the elderly, even those with one or more functional impairments. The elderly tend to rate their health according to

how much the disorder affects their daily function. In general, they rate their own health higher than health professionals rank it. The elderly often compensate for quite severe impairment to the point that it affects function very little and is not seen, personally, as a major detriment to their overall health and well-being.

The same factors that are associated with life satisfaction in younger years hold true for old age: an adequate income, security, a variety of adequate relationships, good health, and a sense of control over one's life. The prevailing myth that vitality and zest for life naturally wane with advancing years is perhaps the biggest barrier to the appropriate recognition and treatment of depression in the elderly. The widespread belief in this myth of waning vitality in combination with the intermingling of physical illness and multiple losses experienced by the elderly makes the diagnosis and treatment of depression in the elderly particularly challenging.

Theories of Depression

Biological theories attempt to explain the association among neurotransmitters, cortisol levels, physical illness, and depression. There is some evidence that the concentration of the neurotransmitters norepinephrine and serotonin is decreased in old age. However, it is thought that it is not so much the decrease in concentration as it is the decreased sensitivity of the postsynaptic cell receptors to the neurotransmitters that is responsible for the physiological effect on mood. It is by restoring this decreased receptor sensitivity (also referred to as "down regulation") back to normal that the effectiveness of electroconvulsive therapy and many antidepressant drugs is explained. The disregulation of the hypothalamus-pituitary-adrenal feedback loop found more commonly in the elderly is a purported mechanism by which chronic stress is responsible for depression. Chronic stress leads to elevated cortisol levels. Since the normal feedback mechanism that would lower the output of cortisol is thought to diminish in all people as they age, the increasing concentration of cortisol is thought to contribute to depression.

Psychosocial theories also exist to explain the increasing prevalence of depression in old age. Erickson, Erickson, and Kibnick (1987) speculate that depression in the elderly may result from unfulfilled desires or accomplishments. According to this theory, the inability to acquire a sense of integrity in regard to the evaluation of their lives can result in a sense of despair and depression for older adults.

The effect of the sociocultural environment on depression in the elderly is somewhat complex. A supportive social environment has certainly been found to be a buffer for most older adults in protecting them from the multiplicity of environmental stressors and losses that occur with increasing frequency in old age. In fact, some would argue that issues such as poverty, isolation, the loss of role and status, and their effect on the emotional and physical well-being of the aged have been largely ignored. Because science and medicine occupy such a privileged place in society, the "problems" of aging are primarily seen as resulting from physiological decline rather than from a culturally and politically ageist society (Estes & Binney, 1989). However, the health of an aged population is greatly affected by the cultural, political, and physical environments as is health at *any* age!

While financial strain is associated with higher rates of depressive symptomatology in both men and women, social support significantly modifies this effect, particularly in men (Mendes de Leon, Rapp, & Kasl, 1994). However, the elderly may actually be more resistant to social stressors as they anticipate and "rehearse" some of these stressors. For example, it is a well-known fact that most women outlive their husbands. Many women, therefore, have already done some mental preparation as they experience widowhood through other women friends. One aspect of stress that may make the elderly particularly vulnerable is that chronic stress is thought to have more harmful psychological and physiological consequences than do sporadic stressful events. Many of the stressful situations that the elderly experience, such as caregiving for a dependent spouse, financial worries, or fears of crime in their neighborhoods, are chronic, daily stressors.

Characteristics and Diagnoses

The difficulty of correctly identifying depression in the elderly is similar in complexity to the identification and diagnosis of delirium. Depression may be a symptom of certain physical disorders, especially endocrine disorders such as hypothyroidism, pancreatic and adrenal disorders, and cancers of all types. Drugs that may cause depression, such as certain antihypertensives, antianxiety drugs, narcotics, and hormones, are often prescribed for disorders that occur with greater frequency in the elderly. Nutritional deficiencies and the use of alcohol are associated with depressive symptoms as well as delirium.

Depressive symptoms may be emotional, physical, social, and cognitive. They include paranoia, pessimism, sadness, self-degradation, difficulty in concentrating and thinking, and disturbances of appetite and sleep. Sleep difficulties are among the most common and severe symptoms of depression in the elderly along with disturbances in cognition. Once again, the first step in treating the problem becomes one of differentiating the memory loss and change in cognition as a symptom of depression rather than an irreversible dementia or a normal consequence of growing older! Without treatment, there are serious negative consequences for elderly clients, such as cognitive impairments, physical disability, social isolation, substance abuse, and suicide (Capriotti, 1995). Older persons are also far more likely than younger individuals to experience chronic physical or mental illness as a predecessor or comorbid condition with depressive symptomatology (Harper & Grau, 1994).

Subtypes of Depression

Major Clinical Depression

Major clinical depression manifests as a broad range of symptoms in the elderly. These range from psychotic, life-threatening ones to a significant impairment of enjoyment while maintaining the ability to function on a day-to-day basis. The prevalence of major depression among those elderly residing in the community is lower in late life than in midlife. The prevalence rate goes up to 12% to 16% among the medically ill and those residing in long-term care (Blazer, 1990). Bipolar depression with alternating periods of manic and depressive symptoms occurs less commonly in the elderly. When it does occur, the expansive, euphoric mania is found to be expressed more often than in younger adults as angry outbursts or irritability. Antidepressant medication is the mainstay of treating major depression. For those elderly who do not respond favorably to drug treatment or who are experiencing severe, psychotic symptoms, electroconvulsive therapy (ECT) has been found to be particularly effective. Electroconvulsive therapy may, in fact, be safer than medication for some elderly. When memory problems are a significant symptom, however, ECT may be contraindicated since there is some resulting temporary memory loss following each treatment.

Dysthymic Disorder

Chronic, milder forms of depression are called dysthymic disorder and are more common among older persons than is major depression. Symptoms must occur for at least 2 years and be present the majority of the time during those 2 years. Since psychosocial factors are thought to be greatly responsible for this type of depression, counseling often focuses on a restructuring and greater involvement in social activities with an emphasis on the "here and now" rather than on past disappointments or abilities. On the other hand, reminiscence therapy and life review (Butler, 1963) may be considered beneficial in helping the elderly feel more positive about themselves and their lives. Comorbid chronic illness that results in a degree of disability, loss of independence, and, in some cases, chronic pain is frequently a major factor.

Adjustment Disorder with a Depressed Mood

This type of depression is distinguished from the other types in that the symptoms are linked to a specific physical or environmental stressor. Among the elderly, physical illness is the most common stressor. Retirement, financial difficulties, and a change in residence are other frequent precipitants. By definition, the condition is self-limiting. However, because most illness in the elderly is chronic, symptoms may be sporadic, in keeping with the remissions and exacerbations of the physical illness.

Education plays a big role in treating this type of depression. Family members must usually be closely involved in order to recognize the behaviors as depressive symptoms rather than hostility or a worsening of the physical condition. Empathetic family members who can encourage positive thoughts while validating the depressed symptoms can have a very therapeutic effect.

Grief and Depression

Since death and loss are such close companions to the aged, the topic of grief and depression is a complex one. Grief is not considered a mood disorder in the elderly, just as it is not in a younger population. However, more depressive symptomatology is often associated with bereavement in the elderly. In fact, grief may be quite different for the man or woman who has lost a spouse of 50+ years and for whom there was such a complete intertwining of their lives as to make a separation of identities virtually impossible. The same is true for an older adult who loses the last remaining immediate family member or the last remaining person who knew him or her as a child (Figure 23-2).

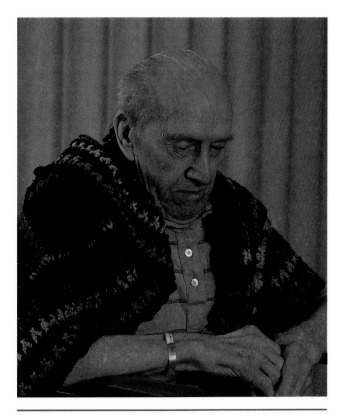

Figure 23-2   Older adults may be particularly saddened by losses of people or situations that have been a part of their lives for many years. Nurses can be supportive of these emotions by showing empathy and taking the time to listen to the client's stories and reminiscences.

Survived by His Wife

Margaret Flanagan
Eyes swollen she lay in their bed—
head covered, legs drawn up,
cold though her forehead was damp—
who had warmed herself on his warm flesh.

Now his absence was a constant companion:
his hairbrushes, his keys,
his clothes still smelling of him
in his closet, covered, like museum

She shuddered, remembering the shoes he wore
Were still beneath the bed
exactly as he left them,
as if covered by a glass case.

All of the things he had handled,
used, inhabited, and finally left
were covered or lying about
like the frames of stolen paintings left behind.

(Flanagan, 1987, p. 103)

NURSING PROCESS

▽ ASSESSMENT

Nurses hold a privileged position because of the unique access they have to the very personal and private parts of people's lives. Knowing the details of an individual's abilities and difficulties with such personal activities as bathing, eating, drinking, and toileting oftentimes provides the bridge by which the symptoms of depression can be assessed. Along with privilege comes the responsibility of acting upon this information with compassion and informed knowledge. There are several key elements that may help unmask the symptoms of depression in the stories of older adults.

The onset and pattern of symptoms may provide clues as to the etiology of the symptoms. These causes could range from the possibility of a dementia rather than a depressive disorder, chronic illness with significant functional impairment and severe pain, or a severe grief response. The nurse must also listen closely to the client's story for possible links of the symptoms to a reversible cause such as a concomitant physical illness or adverse drug reaction. Family history may help determine specific types of depression for which the individual may be at particularly high risk. For example, if someone has a reported history of bipolar depression, the risk of this specific type of depression may be also greater for his or her siblings. Open-ended questions will generally yield the most beneficial information when screening for depression in the elderly. However, when time is limited or whenever warning signs of depression are noted, a screening instrument should be used for further validation.

One such popular instrument designed specifically for screening for depression in the elderly is the short version of the Geriatric Depression Scale (Yesavage & Brink, 1983). When more than five questions are answered as indicated, a high probability of depressive symptoms exists.

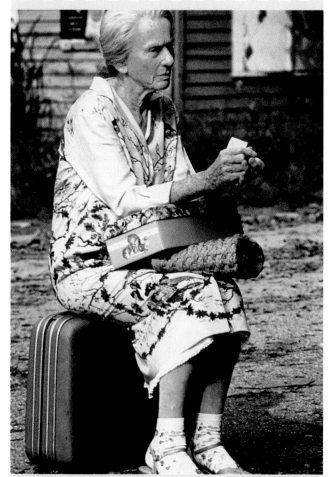

Fried Green Tomotoes. Source: Universal/Courtesy Kobal.

Jessica Tandy plays Ninny Threadgoode in this film. The sometimes harsh realities of aging and loss contrast with Ninny's spirited reminiscences of young womanhood in a small Southern town.

NURSING ALERT!

Warning Signs of Depression in the Older Adult

1. Prolonged grieving
2. Sudden or progressive change in appearance, speech, movement, behaviors, or cognition, as evidenced by:
   - Self-neglect and poor hygiene
   - Weight loss
   - Unwillingness to socialize with family or friends
   - Lack of attention to finances (e.g., paying bills)
   - Complaints of memory loss or difficulty concentrating

GERIATRIC DEPRESSION SCALE

1. Are you basically satisfied with your life? (no)
2. Have you dropped many of your activities and interests? (yes)
3. Do you feel that your life is empty? (yes)
4. Do you often get bored? (yes)
5. Are you in good spirits most of the time? (no)
6. Are you afraid that something bad is going to happen to you? (yes)
7. Do you feel happy most of the time? (no)
8. Do you often feel helpless? (yes)
9. Do you prefer to stay home at night, rather than go out and do new things? (yes)
10. Do you feel that you have more problems with memory than most? (yes)
11. Do you think it is wonderful to be alive now? (no)
12. Do you feel pretty worthless the way you are now? (yes)
13. Do you feel full of energy? (no)
14. Do you feel that your situation is hopeless? (yes)
15. Do you think that most persons are better off than you are? (yes)

Score 1 point for each response that matches the yes or no answer after each question.

From "Development and Validation of a Geriatric Depression Screening Scale: A Preliminary Report," by J. A. Yesavage and T. L. Brink, 1983, *Journal of Psychiatric Research,17*, pp. 37–49, Elsevier Science Ltd., Pergamon Imprint, Oxford, England. Reprinted with permission.

As stated previously, screening instruments do not confirm a diagnosis, but, rather, merely point out the need for a more in-depth assessment or referral. The nurse must also keep in mind that many elderly clients may downplay their emotional feelings due to fear of stigma; careful questioning and observation by the nurse will help uncover true feelings and their impact.

Symptoms of depression in the elderly more commonly manifest as changes in cognition (memory deficits, paranoia, and agitation) and physical symptoms (muscle aches, joint pains, gastrointestinal disturbances, and headache) than they do in younger adults. Weight loss and nutritional deficits are also common symptoms of depression in the elderly.

Nurses must also understand the basis for certain laboratory studies. Physiological indicators of depression may be measured with a Dexamethasone Suppression Test or assay of neurotransmitter metabolites. Reported hallucinations and delusions will usually call for a computed tomography (CT), magnetic resonance imaging (MRI), and an electroencephalogram (EEG) in order to rule out the possibility of organic brain disorders such as brain tumors, hematomas, or hydrocephalus. Laboratory studies such as serum drug levels, complete blood counts, and thyroid function studies are often done to rule out a physical pathological basis for the symptoms. Educating the client about the strong connection between physical illness and depression plays an important role in prevention as well as treatment.

Assessing the risk of suicide should be a high priority. The elderly have the highest rate of suicide of any age group. The primary predictors of suicide seen in both the general population and older adults include being male, Caucasian, depressed, a substance abuser, and unmarried

NURSING ALERT!

Risk Factor Assessment for Suicide

Self-transcendence is thought to be specific to the success of older adults in meeting the multiple changes of later life. Two questions addressing self-transcendence are:

1. Who is most meaningful (important) to you now?
2. What is most meaningful (important) to you now?

The inability to answer these questions warrants further assessment regarding the client's risk of suicide during any type of major transition or crisis.

From "Suicidal Thought and Self-Transcendence in Older Adults," by D. Buchanon, C. Farran, and D. Clark, 1995, *Journal of Psychosocial Nursing and Mental Health Services,* 33(10), pp. 31–34.

or separated (Osgood, 1992). Since cognitive impairments are a common symptom of depression in the elderly, the risk of suicide by drug overdose or gunshot may be greater when judgment and inhibitions are impaired. The older adult's desire for independence and relationships has been well documented in the literature as reflective of a meaningful existence (Nadelson, 1990; Poznanski-Hutchison & Bahr, 1991; Trice, 1990). In studying suicidal thought among a group of older clients hospitalized with a variety of mental illnesses, Buchanon, Farran, and Clark (1995) found that the inability to give meaning to life by moving outside and beyond oneself during times of change, crisis, or suffering was a risk factor for suicide. Adult caregivers of elderly spouses or parents often become socially isolated and are also at risk for depressive symptomatology.

NURSING DIAGNOSIS

The dependency brought on by chronic physical illness or a cognitive impairment can lead to feelings of helplessness and despair, as characterized by the mursing diagnoses *hopelessness*, *self-esteem disturbance*, and *chronic low self-esteem*. These feelings are often compounded by multiple losses brought about by physical frailty or death. A barrage of losses within a short period of time often causes a "spiraling-down" effect that can lead to depressive symptoms. The combination of personality, isolation, and cognitive impairments can also put the elderly person at high risk for self-directed violence, ineffective individual coping, and spiritual distress. Just as with younger individuals, the importance of validating these responses with the depressed older individual and/or family cannot be overemphasized.

OUTCOME IDENTIFICATION

The yardstick by which success is measured in treating depression in the elderly is by nature a highly individual one. A severely depressed individual is not usually capable of setting goals at the onset of treatment. Realistic outcomes for the initial stages of treatment may merely be an increase in food intake or some degree of participation in self-care activities. The final outcome may be to see the depressed older adult return to a level of independence and social interaction that makes life more meaningful for him as well as for his family and loved ones. Consideration must often be given to the effect that irreversible chronic physical or cognitive disorders may have on the individual's capacity for independence and level of activity.

PLANNING/INTERVENTIONS

The need to reinforce that depression is an illness is one that presents itself in a multitude of ways. Caregivers often look to nurses for assistance with the physical complaints and needs of the elder with chronic mental or physical impairments. The nurse must help the caregiver and the depressed elder to recognize the effect that depression can have on physical symptoms such as insomnia, appetite, and memory loss. Living with chronic illness often makes an older person more resigned to the unavailability of effective medical treatment. This attitude, in turn often carries over to an acceptance that things must just be "the way they are" in emotional health as well. Nurses have the responsibility to inform the elderly that not only should they expect the treatment of depression to work but that they have the right to demand adequate treatment!

Drug therapy for depression in the elderly presents a special challenge. While it is often very effective in relieving the depressive symptoms, it is associated with a high incidence of adverse side effects. The key to appropriate drug management is choosing the right drug for the unique combination of depressive symptoms and concomitant physiological disorders. In general, it is the anticholinergic and sedating side effects that must be most closely regulated.

The specific drug must be very carefully chosen. For example, for an elderly man with a history of prostatic enlargement and depressive symptoms of insomnia and agitation, an antidepressant with low potential for anticholinergic side effects and high sedating properties would be the drug of choice. The second-generation antidepressants, serotonin reuptake inhibitors, may offer

⚡ NURSING ALERT!

Medications with Anticholinergic Side Effects

Medications	*Side Effects*
Antihistamines (Benadryl, Phenergan, Seldane, Chlor-Trimeton)	Urinary retention
	Constipation
Tricyclic antidepressants (Elavil, Norpramine, Sinequan, Tofranil, Asendin, Aventil, Pamelor)	Dry mouth and dry eyes
	Orthostatic hypotension
Antipsychotics (Clozapine, Mellaril, Haldol, Navane)	Blurred vision and photophobia
Antiparkinsonians (Artane, Cogentin)	Elevation of intra-ocular pressure
Anticholinergics/ parasympatholytics (Atropine, Bentyl, Robinul, Scopolamine)	Tachycardia

increased safety and an improved side effect profile in the treatment of depression in the elderly.

Safety issues are especially high priorities in cases of irreversible dementias or whenever memory loss is present as a symptom of depression. Nurses must often collaborate with family members in managing behaviors that may threaten the lives of not only the depressed elder but others as well. Driving, leaving the stove on, or smoking in bed may become issues that will require creative strategies for each unique set of circumstances. Regardless of the interventions, focusing on maximizing control and choices plays a central and primary role in the management of depression for older adults. Kivnick (1993) speaks of the importance of the reinforcement and nurturance of the "vital spirit"—those things in life (no matter how seemingly small) that give meaning and pleasure. By helping the depressed person identify those activities and special habits that have given them pleasure through the years and that they can still participate in, the focus is on the positive and not the negative. These pleasures can be any-

thing from drinking coffee out of a favorite mug to reading a newspaper first thing in the morning, cooking a favorite dish, attending religious services, or listening to favorite music while sitting in a warm, sunny spot in a favorite chair. Nightingale (1969) recognized the importance of environmental influences (light, color, movement, and touch) on healing nearly a century ago. Recent studies are reinforcing the validity and importance of these techniques.

EVALUATION

Pharmacotherapy and psychotherapy have been found to be very effective in treating depression in the elderly. The chronic nature of depressive symptomatology, however, may be a complicating factor. Outcomes include a decrease in such depressive symptoms as anxiety and memory loss. Self-perceptions of control and well-being may also be useful indicators of treatment effectiveness.

CASE STUDY/CARE PLAN

The Parkers' son and daughter were very concerned about the health status and living conditions of their parents, 78-year-old Viola Parker and 82-year-old Ernest Parker. Their parents had lived in the same home for the past 35 years. Five years ago Mr. Parker had two myocardial infarctions and Mrs. Parker took over management of the household duties.

The Parkers' children lived in other cities and visited their parents once or twice a year. The Parkers' daughter had noticed that her mother had been sounding very tired and "down" over the telephone for about a month. However, it was not until a long-time neighbor called her to express concern about the trash and papers piling up in the yard that she began to realize what a virtual recluse her mother had become. She immediately called her brother and they made arrangements to visit their parents.

They were shocked at the disheveled appearance of both parents and the cluttered and dirty house (their mother had always been an immaculate housekeeper). After much resistance, they were able to convince both parents to make an appointment with their family doctor. Diagnostics indicated that Mr. Parker was anemic and hypoxic secondary to an exacerbation of his congestive heart failure and malnutrition. He was admitted to the hospital for further diagnostics and treatment. The history and physical for Mrs. Parker revealed no acute physical abnormalities, only a gradual worsening of her osteoarthritis. However, she was admitted to the

geriatric inpatient mental health unit because of noted hallucinations, change in mental status, and an obviously debilitated physical condition.

A multidisciplinary team evaluation found that Mrs. Parker could not perform any activities of daily living (ADL) without assistance. She would eat only a few bites of food at mealtimes and only if someone else put them in her mouth. She had a very flat affect and would answer most questions with "I don't know" or no response at all. She had no interest in visiting her husband three floors away. Based on the multidisciplinary team assessment and thorough medical evaluation, Mrs. Parker was diagnosed with a psychotic major depression that had presented in her case as a pseudodementia. The psychiatrist decided to treat Mrs. Parker with ECT rather than antidepressants due to the severity of her symptoms.

ASSESSMENT

Both Mr. and Mrs. Parker were exhibiting changes in cognition that had been developing over a relatively short period of time (weeks to a month or two). In Mr. Parker the cognitive impairment was manifested as lack of interest in ADL such as bathing, shaving, and dressing, and a lack of judgment and perception that anything was wrong with himself or his wife. Mrs. Parker's

Continued

symptoms manifested as a pseudodementia, with her social withdrawal and complete lack of interest in her own appearance and hygiene as well as in maintaining even basic sanitary conditions in their home. Open-ended questions revealed that Mrs. Parker's long-time friend and confidante had died 8 months before. In the previous few weeks Mrs. Parker has not been sleeping more than 3 hours at a time and often awakened with joint pain. Mrs. Parker had been taking the non-steroidal anti-inflammatory drug (NSAID) prescribed for her arthritic pain only in the middle of the night, when she would awaken in pain because she did not like to take "too much medicine."

(NOTE: Care must be planned individually for Mr. and Mrs. Parker during the acute phase. Discharge plans will obviously be dependent upon the outcome in health and level of independence in self-care for *both* husband and wife and must include consideration of Mr. Parker's condition.) The following care plan is for Mrs. Parker.

NURSING DIAGNOSIS *Altered nutrition: less than body requirements*, related to inability to ingest nutrients, as evidenced by inadequate food intake and need for assistance with feedings

Outcomes	Planning/Interventions	Evaluation
◆ The client will feed herself at least one-half of the meals served her within 1 week.	◆ The nurse will assist her in eating and sit with her during mealtime until she is able to eat without help. If son or daughter is available, they will be encouraged to eat with their mother.	Mrs. Parker responded immediately to ECT therapy by eating two-thirds of her meal.

NURSING DIAGNOSIS *Self-care deficit (bathing/hygiene)*, related to depression and activity intolerance, as evidenced by disheveled appearance

Outcomes	Planning/Interventions	Evaluation
◆ The client will be bathing and dressing herself within 1 week.	◆ The nurse will encourage client to choose time of day for bathing and assist with preparing tub and clothes for her. Nurse will ask daughter to bring in one of her mother's favorite pictures to guide makeup and hair care and nurse will encourage daughter's participation in mother's care.	It took nearly a week and a half for the medication to decrease her joint discomfort, which increased her independence in ADL.

NURSING DIAGNOSIS *Impaired social interaction*

Outcomes	Planning/Interventions	Evaluation
◆ *Short-term goal:* Client will show interest in husband's condition and will engage in brief conversation within 1 week. *Long-term goal:* By discharge client will identify one outside activity (e.g., church choir or Bible study, craft group, volunteering, exercise group) that she would like to attend on a regular basis. Nurse will attempt to engage client in conversations in day room and during mealtimes.	◆ Nurse will take client to visit husband in adjoining hospital unit and client will be assisted as desired to call husband on the phone.	After beginning ECT treatment, client greeted husband with a hug and exclaimed, "I've been so worried about you." She reluctantly (only upon her son's and daughter's insistence and a visit from two women friends) agreed to begin attending a weekly Bible study at her church. Mrs. Parker's daughter decided to start telephoning 3 to 4 times a week in order to encourage her mother's social interaction.

CRITICAL THINKING BAND

ASSESSMENT

What factors of Mr. Parker's care should you consider that will have a direct impact on Mrs. Parker's status and progress? What questions might you ask the Parkers' daughter?

NURSING DIAGNOSIS

Which (if any) of the nursing diagnoses are life threatening? How would you prioritize them?

Outcomes

What outcomes will be evidence of Mrs. Parker's renewed interest in her role as caregiver and household manager?

Planning/Interventions

What is the nurse's role in discharge planning for Mrs. Parker's return to her home and the stress of caregiving?

Evaluation

What avenues exist for follow-up of Mrs. Parker's physical and emotional conditions and her ongoing ability to cope with the chronic stress of caregiving?

DEMENTIA

The essential characteristics of a dementia are the development of multiple cognitive deficits that include an impairment of memory and at least one of the following cognitive disturbances: aphasia, apraxia, agnosia, or a disturbance in executive functioning. This impairment must be significant enough to cause a disturbance in everyday functioning and it must be a decline from a previously higher level of functioning (American Psychiatric Association, 1994, p. 134). Although a variety of disorders are responsible for the development of a dementia, they all share similarities in the way in which symptoms present.

Poor judgment and poor insight are common in dementia. Although affected persons are often aware of their declining abilities, they are generally not able to judge the consequences of the loss of memory and cognition. This presents a great challenge to family members or caregivers faced with figuring out how to curtail activities such as driving or the control of banking and finances for an older individual who is completely unaware of the risks involved (and who is accustomed to independence in such matters for nearly a lifetime!).

Alzheimer's Disease

Characteristics and Prevalence

Approximately 60% of dementia in people over the age of 65 is caused by Alzheimer's disease (Dawes, 1996). Alois Alzheimer has been credited with the first known description of the disease in 1907. Alzheimer's disease (AD) is now often cited as the number 1 mental health problem among our rapidly increasing aging population. Alzheimer's disease is a progressive disorder characterized by stages of increasing impairments and dependency. Although memory impairment is generally characterized as the key diagnostic criteria for AD, the earliest objective signs of the disease may more often be

---

PATHOLOGIES THAT MAY CAUSE DEMENTIA

INFECTIONS

◆ Creutzfeldt-Jakob disease

◆ Human immunodeficiency virus (HIV)

◆ Syphilis

DEGENERATIVE NEUROLOGICAL DISORDERS

◆ Alzheimer's disease

◆ Pick's disease

◆ Huntington's disease

◆ Parkinson's disease

VASCULAR DISORDERS

◆ Ministrokes (cardiovascular accidents)

STRUCTURAL DISORDERS OF BRAIN TISSUE

◆ Normal-pressure hydrocephalus

◆ Subdural hematoma

◆ Head injury

◆ Tumors

of a behavioral type. These may include behaviors such as suspiciousness and paranoia, irritability, aggression or angry outbursts, hoarding, withdrawal, or a report from others of poor performance at work (Oppenheim, 1994). As the disease progresses, gait and motor disturbances may appear along with severe cognitive impairments and behavioral manifestations such as wandering. In the latter stages, the person may become bedridden and nonverbal. The onset of the disease is generally insidious, with the average duration of the illness from onset of symptoms to death being 8 to 10 years (American Psychiatric Association, 1994, p. 142).

Diagnosis and Pathophysiology

The cause of AD is still unknown, although numerous genetic, viral, environmental, and immunologic etiologies are being explored. It has even been suggested that Alzheimer's may be a multitude of disorders. Latest developments in Alzheimer's research have linked disease that occurs early in life (forties to sixties) to a gene on chromosome 21 and late-onset disease to a gene on chromosome 19. Defective genes on chromosomes 1 and 14 have been identified as certain predictors of AD. People with AD are nearly twice as likely as the general population to carry an allele on chromosome 19, which codes for a plasma protein, apolipoprotein E, involved in the transport of cholesterol and other hydrophobic molecules (JAMA, 1995). Evidence is also accumulating that disease risk increases and the age of onset decreases with the number of these alleles found on chromosome 19. Although an association between the ε4 allele and risk of AD has been found, the correlation is not perfect. Thirty-five percent to 50% of persons with AD do not carry an ε4 allele and approximately 24% to 31% of the non-affected adult population carry the defective gene. Genetic testing, therefore, remains a controversial issue, especially in the absence of effective interventions for the prevention and treatment of AD (JAMA, 1995). Much research effort has also been directed toward finding neurotransmitters that might play a specific role in AD. Since the observation of deterioration in the nucleus basalis of Meynert (the primary site of acetylcholine synthesis in the brain), acetylcholine has been the most frequently studied neurotransmitter and seems to hold the most promise for a role in AD treatment (Keltner, 1994, p. 37).

The location of pathological lesions associated with AD in brain tissue complicates the definitive diagnosis of this disorder. Only brain biopsy upon autopsy can identify the accumulation of excessive amounts of amyloid plaques in cortical gray matter and neurons filled with neurofibrillary tangles, hallmarks of AD pathology. Because of the difficulty of obtaining pathological evidence, the diagnosis of AD can be made only when all other etiologies for dementia have been ruled out. The diagnosis, therefore, is typically made via a battery of medical tests that rule out other reversible or irreversible etiologies and a battery of neuropsychological tests that rule out depression as the basis for deficits in memory and cognition.

DIAGNOSTIC CRITERIA FOR DEMENTIA OF THE ALZHEIMER'S TYPE

A. The development of multiple cognitive deficits manifested by both:

1. Memory impairment (impaired ability to learn new information or to recall previously learned information)

2. One (or more) of the following cognitive disturbances:

   a. Aphasia (language disturbance)

   b. Apraxia (impaired ability to carry out motor activities despite intact motor function)

   c. Agnosia (failure to recognize or identify objects despite intact sensory function)

   d. Disturbance in executive functioning (i.e., planning, organizing, sequencing, abstracting)

B. The cognitive deficits in criteria A1 and A2 each cause significant impairment in social or occupational functioning and represent a significant decline from a previous level of functioning.

C. The course is characterized by gradual onset and continuing cognitive decline.

D. The cognitive deficits in criteria A1 and A2 are not due to any of the following:

1. Other central nervous system conditions that cause progressive deficits in memory and cognition (e.g., cerebrovascular disease, Parkinson's disease, Huntington's disease, subdural hematoma, normal-pressure hydrocephalus, brain tumors)

2. Systemic conditions that are known to cause dementia (e.g., hypothyroidism, vitamin B_{12} or folic acid deficiency, niacin deficiency, hypercalcemia, neurosyphilis, HIV infection)

3. Substance-induced conditions

E. The deficits do not occur exclusively during the course of a delirium.

F. The disturbance is not better accounted for by another axis I disorder (e.g., major depressive disorder, schizophrenia).

Reprinted with permission from the *Diagnostic and Statistical Manual of Mental Disorders*, Fourth Edition. Copyright 1994 American Psychiatric Association.

Vascular Dementias

Characteristics and Prevalence

The second most common dementia, often coexisting with AD, is vascular dementia. This type of dementia, often referred to as multi-infarct dementia, accounts for 10% to 20% of all dementias. Hypertension and a history of cardiovascular disease are the greatest risk factors for this disorder. Vascular dementia typically results from the occurrence of multiple small strokes over a period of time. A gradual occlusion and blockage of arteries to the brain usually leads to such a gradual decline in function that each event is not noticed. However, a more severe disruption of cerebral perfusion may result in immediate neurological symptoms, usually including one-sided weakness or focal neurological signs. Although the symptoms are similar to those of AD, the course of vascular dementia tends to be more sporadic. The person may appear to be completely normal for a few hours or days and then suddenly, without warning, become very inappropriately suspicious, belligerent, or forgetful. Signs and symptoms of damage to specific areas of the brain, such as weakness of an extremity or gait abnormalities, often coincide with the behavioral and memory changes. The unpredictability of the person's behavior and impairment in cognition create a "roller coaster" effect on the emotions and coping abilities of the person's loved ones and caregivers.

Diagnosis and Pathophysiology

Multiple medical problems may result in small emboli or strokes. These include atherosclerosis, dysrythmias, and spasms of blood vessels. Contributing risk factors for vascular disease include diabetes mellitus, obesity, smoking, and hypertension. Destruction of brain tissue resulting from the small emboli or strokes may be localized or diffuse. Lesions often appear in both white and gray matter structures, including subcortical regions and nuclei. Evidence of both new and old infarctions may be detected by CT and MRI. The EEG findings may reflect focal lesions in the brain (American Psychiatric Association, 1994, pp. 144, 145). Diagnosis is typically based on a history of cardiovascular disease, reported episodic decline in function, and physical examination of neurological abnormalities.

Other Dementias

A variety of other neurological, metabolic, and infectious disorders are responsible for the remaining types of dementias. Since many of these disorders arise at a younger age, it is not only the elderly that may be affected. These disorders include alcoholic dementia (Korsakoff's syndrome), a condition of unknown etiology called Creutzfeldt-Jakob disease, the human immunodeficiency virus causing acquired immunodeficiency syndrome

---

DIAGNOSTIC CRITERIA FOR VASCULAR DEMENTIA

A. The development of multiple cognitive deficits manifested by both:

1. Memory impairment (impaired ability to learn new information or to recall previously learned information)

2. One (or more) of the following cognitive disturbances:

   a. Aphasia (language disturbance)

   b. Apraxia (impaired ability to carry out motor activities despite intact motor function)

   c. Agnosia (failure to recognize or identify objects despite intact sensory function)

   d. Disturbance in executive functioning (i.e., planning, organizing, sequencing, abstracting)

B. The cognitive deficits in criteria A1 and A2 each cause significant impairment in social or occupational functioning and represent a significant decline from a previous level of functioning.

C. Focal neurological signs and symptoms (e.g., exaggeration of deep tendon reflexes, extensor plantar response, pseudobulbar palsy, gait abnormalities, weakness of an extremity) or laboratory evidence indicative of cerebrovascular disease (e.g., multiple infarctions involving cortex and underlying white matter) that are judged to be etiologically related to the disturbance.

D. The deficits do not occur exclusively during the course of a delirium.

Reprinted with permission from the *Diagnostic and Statistical Manual of Mental Disorders*, Fourth Edition. Copyright 1994 American Psychiatric Association.

(AIDS), a dementia associated with the spirochete causing Lyme's disease, and a dementia associated with the neurological disorders Parkinson's and Huntington's diseases. All of these dementias share similar damage to memory and intellectual function. However, the balance and degree to which behaviors, memory, and judgment or cognition are affected may vary slightly from one disorder to another. For example, there tends to be a blunting of emotion (or at least the ability to display emotion) in Parkinson's disease as contrasted with the often exaggerated and explosive emotions of vascular dementia. Cerebellar and extrapyramidal deficits with myoclonus

⊚⊚ *REFLECTIVE THINKING*

Early Stages of a Dementia

Liz was 68 years old when she first complained of feeling "funny in the head" and a tingling sensation in her arm. Hypertension with possible transient ischemic attacks (TIAs) was diagnosed in the emergency room and she was prescribed antihypertensives and told to follow up with her family doctor. Liz's blood pressure kept fluctuating over the next few weeks and she felt "hazy and tired" as different medications were tried.

Liz and her husband ran a drapery business out of their home. Her husband noticed that Liz was beginning to have difficulty with calculations. A calculator solved this problem for several months, until one day her husband noticed that Liz was completely disregarding any fractions and adding only whole numbers. Liz had always taken pride in her attention to detail, and this kind of oversight was very uncharacteristic of her. Liz's husband, however, attributed this change to her being more tired. She had been having some difficulty sleeping at night and some angry outbursts that her husband also attributed to lack of sleep. One day Bill walked in while Liz was attempting to charge a customer $500 for a $50 job.

Several months later Liz had to be rushed once more to the emergency room, this time because of slurred speech and numbness of her entire left side. She was diagnosed with a CVA.

- ◆ What were the first signs of a cognitive impairment being exhibited by Liz?
- ◆ What possible reversible causes needed to be investigated?
- ◆ How will you answer Bill's question, "Will my wife continue to have mental problems? What can I do to help?"

and other involuntary movements often occur in Creutzfeld-Jakob disease (CJD), along with a rapidly progressive course of dementing symptoms over 4 to 7 months (Wallace, 1993). The time span from onset of symptoms to death of 6 to 12 months is much shorter in CJD than in most other forms of dementia. Twenty-five percent to 30% of all disorders resulting in a dementia are treatable (Lind, 1995). However, the majority of dementias are of an unidentifiable etiology or a chronic, untreatable condition.

Symptoms and Sequelae

How a particular dementia manifests as specific changes in mood, personality, and behavior is probably a combination of the physiology of the condition and the unique personality of the individual. Similarities, however, exist among the variety of manifestations found across all types of dementias.

Memory loss. Even in the absence of disease, some memory loss does seem to occur with advancing age. For example, an older man may forget the name of his best friend's daughter. He is acutely aware of and frustrated by his memory loss and searches his memory until he eventually remembers again. In contrast, however, the demented adult may be completely unaware that he has forgotten—"forgets that he forgets"—or may frequently try to cover up his memory loss. This **confabulation**, or intentional filling in of memory gaps, is not so unlike the tricks we have all used at one time or another when we forget an acquaintance's name upon a chance meeting and attempt to cover it up with conversation that does not require us to speak the person's name. However, in a dementia the extensiveness and frequency with which confabulation is used far exceeds the occasional use made of it during normal, everyday life. Family members are often surprised by the details that their loved one with dementia can remember about weddings, vacations, or events 30 or 40 years before while having no recollection about going to church or the movies 2 days before.

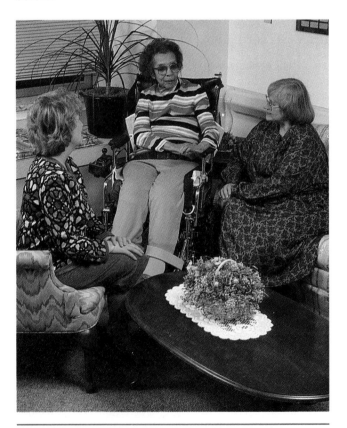

Figure 23-3 Spending time with family and friends helps the older client feel valued and enjoy days that might otherwise be lonely.

In a rare personal account of what it is like to be immersed in the early throes of a dementia, Reverend Robert Davis describes his experience with memory loss in the early stages of this disease:

My Journey into Alzheimer's Disease

I still have the aggravations of daily living. For instance, it is annoying to be unable to remember information such as my license tag. It is embarrassing and irritating to go to a service station and have to make two trips back to the car to check the license plate because I forgot the number between the pump and the cash register. How frightening it is to go into a large, familiar shopping center with crowds and blinking lights and become totally lost! How humiliating it is to be unable to make the right change and ask the cashier to pick the correct coins from my hand!

It is still sometimes terrifying at night. When I let my mind go in order to go to sleep, my mind still slips into blankness and moonlight. However, this is all just surface frustration, brought on by the constant process of losing control at the daily living level. I can either struggle angrily and uselessly against the inevitable, or else I can admit my inadequacy and humbly ask for help. I choose to do the latter and keep a calmer and more peaceful mind. Fortunately, I can still make this choice, but it is possible with the progress of the brain damage that I will lose this ability.*

(Davis, 1989, pp. 56, 57)

As Reverend Davis points out, the ability to choose a response and find a peaceful way to cope with the frustration of memory loss is often lost as the disease progresses. This lack of control in combination with unique personality factors gives life to a broad range of behaviors commonly associated with dementia.

Just as significant as the effect that memory loss may have on behavior but even more difficult to understand is the way in which severe memory loss affects self-identity. Self-concept is the identity each person has acquired of himself over a lifetime. Self-concept is fashioned out of how well persons believe that they have reached their potentials along with the nature and satisfaction of their relationships to both other persons and their environments. This enduring aspect of self is at least partially dependent upon memory. The extent to which varying degrees of memory loss destroy an individual's identity and self-concept is almost solely a matter for conjecture and speculation. If memory and identity are purely subjective states, one can only learn about them through personal accounts made possible by self-reflection. However, the pathologies that result in severe memory loss also hinder the ability for self-reflection and to communicate the personal meaning of such loss. Oliver Sacks (1987) explores the possible ramifications of an extraordinary case of near-complete recent memory loss in a young man in his forties. The medical diagnosis was completely unknown.

The Man Who Mistook His Wife for a Hat

I found an extreme and extraordinary loss of recent memory—so that whatever was said or shown to him was apt to be forgotten in a few seconds' time. Thus I laid out my watch, my tie, and my glasses on the desk, covered them, and asked him to remember these. Then, after a minute's chat, I asked him what I had put under the cover. He remembered none of them—or indeed that I had even asked him to remember.

(Sacks, 1987, p. 27)

I wrote in my notes, "isolated in a single moment of being, with a moat or lacuna of forgetting all round him . . . He is a man without a past (or future), stuck in a constantly changing, meaningless moment" . . . I kept wondering, in this and later notes—unscientifically—about "a lost soul," and how one might establish some continuity, some roots, for he was a man without roots, or rooted only in the remote past.

(Sacks, 1987, p. 29)

Aphasia. The person with dementia commonly has difficulty with the recall of words. This is called **aphasia**. For example, in the midst of a conversation, the individual may not be able to recall the word "car" and will attempt to get the message across by describing the car's purpose, such as "the box that goes everywhere" or "the machine with wheels."

Delayed response time. Simple calculations may be impossible for the person to perform within a reasonable time frame. Being confronted with figuring out the right amount of money at the grocery store, for example, may be terrifying. Not only mental response time but physical response time may often be affected. Driving becomes a

☜☞ *REFLECTIVE THINKING*

Understanding the Aphasic Client

A frustrating and common dilemma that caregivers must often face on a daily basis is interpreting the sometimes garbled sentences of their aphasic loved ones. Would you be able to figure out what the aphasic individual is attempting to say in the following situation?

You are in a crowded mall with an individual who has AD. Suddenly, this person becomes slightly agitated and begins to repeat the phrase "I want . . . box with a top . . . people here . . . I want . . . box with a top . . . people, people, people."

◆ How would you respond?

◆ How would you go about trying to determine what the aphasic person is trying to say?

This may be the person's way of trying to tell you that he wants to go home. Asking simple yes or no questions such as "Are you tired?" and "Do you want to stop at another store?" or finding a quiet spot and saying, "Let's sit here and rest for a minute," may be an appropriate response.

hazardous situation when the person with dementia cannot react quickly enough—not to mention getting lost!

Paranoia. Suspiciousness and paranoia also frequently accompany dementia. When items are "lost" because the person cannot remember where they were last placed, loved ones are often blamed for "stealing" them. This can progress to a rather persistent paranoia that becomes very emotionally draining on family members who are being suspected of wishing to harm their loved one when they are so desperately trying in vain to help. These paranoid ideations may be accompanied by delusions and hallucinations. A daughter describes the sequelae of doorkeys lost by her demented mother:

When I Grow Too Old To Dream

She would take all the keys out of the doors, even the wardrobe keys, and they would be stowed away anywhere. She lost the backdoor key, then attacked the lock with a hammer. She then called to say someone had broken into the house and there was no peace until we were able to get up there to do the necessary repairs. After that we attached the key by a chain to each appropriate door. The wardrobe-door keys were removed altogether. Then there were the bricks piled up at

the back door to be put against it at night. There were pieces of wood and long sticks beside the bed, a whistle (which didn't work) was under her pillow. Again, looking back, I realize she must have felt very insecure which was not like Mom at all.*

(Naughtin, 1992, p. 126)

Catastrophic reactions. Agitation and angry outbursts may build to the point of a **catastrophic reaction**, or severe overreaction out of proportion to the stimulus. As the disease progresses, the individual may have great difficulty completing even the simplest of tasks. For example, it is not uncommon for the person to jump up every few minutes from the dinner table with no apparent purpose but to pace around the room or walk into another. Impulsiveness also takes the form of angry outbursts—oftentimes in response to questions that the person may have difficulty in answering because of memory loss. Thankfully, the outburst is usually short-lived and the anger easily forgotten if the individual can be distracted. However, this is not always the case, and a very volatile situation with verbal and physical outbursts may result in a catastrophic reaction. The emotional outbursts are often precipitated by fatigue and overstimulation. Providing a quiet and more soothing environment or taking the person away from the stimulation may distract the person and prevent or halt the overreaction. A calm tone of voice and soothing touch may also somewhat alleviate the catastrophic response.

Alterations in perception. Some of the most unusual of responses to dementia and the most complex to comprehend are the perceptual problems. These alterations in interpretation of images and sounds take many forms. A husband describes the difficulty his wife, Joyce, had in bathing herself:

The order of washing up and any cleaning became affected by the inability to remember the normal sequence. She was unable to mop the floor unless she cleaned ahead of herself, which meant she walked over the wet floor as she cleaned. The reason for this was simply that she could see what was ahead of her, but not what was behind. Her mind's eye could no longer perceive and recall what was behind. For Joyce, "behind" no longer existed. Her range of vision became the limit of her ability. This then began to affect her ability to shower.

---

*Extracts from *When I Grow Too Old To Dream,* © G. Naughtin and T. Laidler 1992, used with permission of the publishers, HarperCollins *Religious*, Melbourne.

She would go into the shower and wash her hair first. She could put the shampoo into her hands and lift them to her head to apply shampoo, but, not being able to see the soap in her hair, she didn't rinse it out.

She kept the spray of water in front of her running from her breasts and down. She didn't wash her back or up between her legs and she didn't dry the parts she couldn't see.

It seemed as if she were unable to feel that she was wet. She used to come out of the shower and put on her cotton dressing gown. Then it would be very noticeable that she hadn't dried herself because the back of the gown was wet and her hair was still soapy.

*"Come here darling, let's go back into the shower and I'll help you." I would say with a kiss.**

(Naughtin, 1992, p. 110)

Wandering.   A serious safety issue for caregivers arises when the demented person begins to wander. At times, the wandering may merely be from one room to another as the person is looking for something or someone. It may even be an attempt to combat frustration and boredom. Joyce's wandering is described by her husband and caregiver:

Joyce also frequently realised that something was wrong, and her frustration and anger led her to the wandering off into the bush. Our home is surrounded on three sides by forested bushland. There are tracks along which we had walked many hundreds of kilometers together, but always together. The wandering became a daily looking for her, but usually the wrong way, and there was always the danger that she would return while I was searching in the wrong place.

In a strange way, her dementia was a blessing in disguise. After some time, she would forget that she was running away and her mind would simply revert to having a normal walk. She was not lost as the area was very familiar to her. She would return with no idea that anything was wrong. The initial wanderings were of about one to one and a half hours duration, but this slowly decreased in time, because she began to forget her original anger and frustration much more quickly. Eventually she reached a stage where she would go out of the back door, walk up the path, reach the

*edge of the forest, immediately forget what she was doing, and walk back into the house all in about thirty seconds.**

(Naughtin, 1992, pp. 106, 107)

Disinhibition.   Personality is always a major determinant of the way in which physical or emotional problems present and progress in the older adult. Dementia does not change this fact altogether. As pathology worsens, however, there is often a general loss of inhibition that may take a variety of forms. Spontaneous undressing without regard for privacy may occur. Inappropriate sexual overtures to friends or family are not uncommon and can be particularly distressing to caregivers. Episodes of physical or verbal aggressiveness may also occur. A mother describes the effect of her husband's, Les's, disinhibitions and aggressions on both her and her daughter:

Les went through a stage of total rejection of any conversation between my daughter and any males of her age. She was seventeen, at school, making her debut, and she's quite attractive. Kids of that age just talk to one another without it having any particular meaning to it.

I knew he was in one of those moods one day when she was coming home. A boy she knew rode past, came back, and rode with her. It was very hot, so Les only had his underpants on. He got tangled up getting his shorts on, and I had enough time to get out in the street and warn them.

Aggression—physical, verbal and psychological—was a big problem for Les, one I found hard to deal with. We had to hide the gun, because we were a bit worried that he'd either take it to himself or he'd get too aggressive towards others.

It seemed to involve an exaggeration of his basic prejudices. If you look at his life as a child, and the fears and the prejudices he developed then, what you see now are those same prejudices just accentuated, without the social damper that he would normally put on them.

*The problems with my daughter and the general aggressiveness are examples of how his inhibitions began to diminish. Sometimes he becomes totally uninhibited and totally unreasonable. Alzheimer's disease obviously strips away socialization and social understanding.**

(Naughtin, 1992, pp. 160, 166)

---

*Extracts from *When I Grow Too Old To Dream*, © G. Naughtin and T. Laidler 1992, used with permission of the publishers, HarperCollins *Religious*, Melbourne.

NURSING   PROCESS

▽ ASSESSMENT

The older person experiencing significant short-term memory loss and impairments in reasoning, judgment, and overall intellectual ability is nearly always very resistant to acknowledging his or her difficulties and to seeking help. If the individual lives alone, it is often neighbors who first recognize changes in the person's behavior (e.g., leaving garbage to pile up or walking outside only partially dressed). Once family members are involved and start to look more closely into personal and financial matters, a pattern of gradual decline over months and even years in the individual's ability to manage household, financial, and personal affairs usually emerges. The changes noted may be as subtle as gradual withdrawal from social activities (dining out or regular attendance at religious services) or as dramatic as writing checks for household repairs that were never done or a $10,000 check for a $10.95 bill.

The struggle to remain an independent and competent, respectable adult is a very normal and expected response to the mental decline. However, the family's concerns for the person's safety and needs for assistance in personal, household, and financial matters require some type of recognition and identification of the problem. Generally, it is a plea from family that first reaches the ears of a health professional (nurse, physician, or social worker). Oftentimes, the story emerges when the person with a dementia is seeking health care for another physical problem in a clinic or hospital setting.

From a medical perspective, the diagnosis of dementia is one of exclusion. When symptoms of a gradual cognitive decline similar to the pattern previously described occur, a thorough medical workup is indicated. It includes a battery of tests to rule out a reversible cause

for these impairments. Nurses may be the first to recognize risk factors such as nutritional intake or poor management of diabetes as a reversible type of impairment and be responsible for medical consultation.

Common reversible conditions that may be causing the symptoms of dementia include depression or any of the pathophysiological disorders that may cause a delirium.

Completing this first step in assessment usually takes at least 3 to 4 weeks. If a drug toxicity is suspected, it generally takes this long for drugs to be cleared from the older adult, who has diminished renal function and slower excretion rates. If no treatable condition can be identified, an interdisciplinary assessment is required for the diagnosis of dementia.

A complete interdisciplinary assessment is usually performed at a geriatric mental health facility on either an outpatient or inpatient basis. Even though many screening tests for the diagnosis and long-term monitoring of dementia are available, no single instrument is considered to be adequately sensitive to mild degrees of impairment across a broad range of cultures, educational levels, and predementia intelligence levels (Ritchie, 1988). An interdisciplinary assessment has a twofold purpose: validation of an irreversible dementia and identification of level of care required to meet the individual's functional deficits or behavioral manifestations.

Many different screening instruments can be used to measure the various degrees of impairment in at least 12 categories of cognitive function and mental status (McDougall, 1990). Different screening instruments focus on different domains, with few covering all 12.

Precise differentiation of delirium, dementia, or depression is difficult since the presenting symptoms often overlap. Often a combination of screening instruments will be used in an assessment. The difficulty in selecting any one instrument for any one specific purpose is that each instrument measures a different blend of affective function, cognitive function, functional ability, and mental status. Two commonly used tests to differentiate Alzheimer's from other types of dementia are the Brief Cognitive Rating Scale (BCRS) (Reisberg & Ferris, 1988) and the Dementia of the Alzheimer Type Inventory (DAT) (Cummings & Benson, 1986). In a retrospective study of 50 patients, the DAT correctly identified 100% of those individuals with AD and 94% of those individuals without it (Cummings & Benson, 1986). A psychologist is usually responsible for administering the battery of neuropsychological tests used to differentiate types of cognitive impairments and rule out depression as the cause or exacerbating condition.

⚠ NURSING ALERT!

Warning Signs of Dementia

- ◆ Withdrawal from usual social activities
- ◆ Financial misappropriations
- ◆ Neglect of household repairs or maintenance
- ◆ Unusual or bizarre behaviors in dress, personal contacts, business contacts, or correspondence

MEDICAL SCREENING FOR PATHOPHYSIOLOGICAL CAUSES OF COGNITIVE IMPAIRMENT

DIAGNOSTICS

◆ CT/MRI scan of brain to rule out tumor, hematoma, or hydrocephalus

◆ EEG/positron emission tomography scans

◆ Fasting serum glucose to rule out hypoglycemia

◆ Serum calcium, K^+, and Na^+ to identify electrolyte deficits that can cause a change in mental status

◆ Serum B_{12} and folate to identify vitamin deficiencies

◆ Thyroid and renal function studies to identify hyper/hypothyroidism or renal failure

◆ Urinalysis to rule out infection

◆ Complete blood count with differential to rule out anemia and septicemia

◆ Serum drug levels to rule out drug toxicities

MEDICAL INTERVENTIONS

◆ Withdrawal from all nonessential medications to eliminate toxicities or drug interactions (usually takes 2 to 4 weeks for all drugs to be cleared from body tissues)

◆ Administer antibiotics and hydrate (as needed) for infectious disorders

◆ Correct medical disorders and electrolyte imbalances

◆ Surgery for structural abnormalities of brain tissue, such as tumor, hematoma, or hydrocephalus

OUTCOMES

The prognosis will be determined by the cause of the condition. In general, the earlier that treatment is initiated in the course of the abnormality, the better the prognosis. When aggressive interventions are needed to reverse severe alterations in homeostasis, the chances of iatrogenic complications become more likely. Irreversible physiological abnormalities may result in a permanent cognitive impairment.

CATEGORIES OF COGNITIVE FUNCTION

◆ Attention span
◆ Concentration
◆ Intelligence
◆ Judgment
◆ Learning ability
◆ Memory

◆ Orientation
◆ Perception
◆ Problem solving
◆ Psychomotor ability
◆ Reaction time
◆ Social intactness

Conclusions derived from the interdisciplinary assessment can have a variety of meanings for the demented individual and his family. Being labeled with a progressively deteriorating condition for which there is no cure is a difficult experience. A spouse describes her feelings as she first shares her husband's diagnosis of Alzheimer's with others:

Catch a Falling Star

Reactions, once the news is out, are interesting. Our neighbor Veron says, "Hank could not have lost all his expertise unless something was drastically wrong. Alzheimer's explains his present condition."

Others, good friends included, seem to have a father, mother or ancient aunt to whom they compare Hank. Some divulge useful, helpful information.

Mostly, though, it's hard to take. This is not someone from another era we're talking about. This is a contemporary. This is my HUSBAND! I feel we are being put into some antique category. This really hurts.

(Spohr & Bullard, 1995, p. 52)

On the other hand, a definitive diagnosis can also be somewhat of a relief for both the individual experiencing these changes as well as the caregiver unable to make any long-term plans until a diagnosis is made. Joyce's husband said:

When I Grow Too Old To Dream

In my opinion, the best thing that any medical practitioner can do, if he or she suspects possible dementia, is to advise the carer immediately. Do not wait to be sure, for by that time the patient will be on the autopsy table. Tell the carer there is a possibility that the patient could have an irreversible disease of the brain. Further tests and observations may disprove that. I wish I had known earlier about how the deterioration of memory might affect the patient.

Nurses and occupational therapists contribute to an evaluation of the individual's abilities and difficulties in the performance of activities of daily living (ADL). Nurses are usually best able to assess personal self-care activities such as bathing, dressing, eating, toileting, and walking. Occupational therapists usually assess the instrumental activities of daily living (IADL) such as shopping, using a telephone, food preparation, housekeeping, doing laundry, and handling finances.

Taking into consideration the carer's condition or attitude as a reason for not telling them is not really helpful. If it is true that the patient has progressive dementia, the carer is going to find out in any case, the hard way. If the possible diagnosis is later disproved, then the carer will be happy. If not, then the carer will be prepared.

*For me, understanding had to come first. Then, there was acceptance and finally the ability to cope. I feel it would be the same for most people.**

(Naughtin, 1992, p. 113)

▽ NURSING DIAGNOSIS

The level of dependence and specific behaviors that result from the unique blend of personality traits and physical and cognitive impairments will determine the nursing diagnosis profile for the person with chronic dementias. Self-care deficits, altered nutrition, incontinence, fear, and anxiety are common responses.

Chronic dementias not only affect an individual, but also generally change the entire family process. Because of the intense and heavy demands such conditions place on caregivers, the profound effect of caregiving on daily life has been termed "The 36 Hour Day" (Mace, 1983). Common nursing diagnoses for the family and caregiver, therefore, reflect the physical and emotional stresses of caring for every physical need as well as coping with difficult behavioral responses and the safety risk imposed by a person who may wander off at any given moment of the day or night.

Another major factor influencing caregiving needs is the extended period of time for which care will be required. Given the average span of 10 to 15 years for AD, the caregiver must make many decisions regarding future financial, legal, and ethical issues. Emotional adjustments to the role changes brought about by the caregiving relationship and dependent position of the demented loved one will be required. In order to make these adjustments, family members need a great deal of information regarding the usual progression of the disease and types of services available for respite care as well as assistance in the home. *Knowledge deficit* is, therefore, a common nursing diagnosis for families caring for a demented loved one.

▽ OUTCOME IDENTIFICATION

From a strictly biomedical perspective, maintaining the independence and function of the demented older adult is the major therapeutic goal. However, limiting nursing care

---

*Extracts from *When I Grow Too Old To Dream,* © G. Naughtin and T. Laidler 1992, used with permission of the publishers, HarperCollins *Religious,* Melbourne.

NURSING DIAGNOSES FOR THE INDIVIDUAL AND FAMILY EXPERIENCING CHRONIC IMPAIRMENTS IN COGNITION

CLIENT

- ◆ Bathing/hygiene self-care deficit
- ◆ Dressing/grooming self-care deficit
- ◆ Feeding self-care deficit
- ◆ Altered nutrition: less than body requirements
- ◆ Functional incontinence
- ◆ Anxiety
- ◆ Fear
- ◆ Risk for injury
- ◆ Self-esteem disturbance
- ◆ Altered role performance
- ◆ Impaired social interaction
- ◆ Impaired physical mobility
- ◆ Spiritual distress

CAREGIVER/FAMILY

- ◆ Knowledge deficit
- ◆ Fatigue
- ◆ Altered family processes
- ◆ Caregiver role strain
- ◆ Altered role performance
- ◆ Ineffective family coping: compromised
- ◆ Ineffective family coping: disabling

---

to the biomedical model is more akin to the maintenance of a machine than to the care of a human being. In contrast, nursing care from a human caring theory perspective is more strongly focused upon methods and ways of intuiting how dignity and selfhood can be preserved. While this may certainly include attention to independence in daily functions and activities to the fullest extent possible, it is not the only purpose or even the major purpose of nursing care. Many human conditions exist for which there is vulnerability and the threat to autonomy and selfhood. While dementia may be only one such condition, it is a particularly poignant one since there is usually only the rare possibility of a cure and the prognosis generally involves years of gradual decline in the cognitive abilities associated with independence, self-control, and self-identity.

▽ PLANNING/INTERVENTIONS

Watson's (1988) theory of human care nursing can provide a foundation for practice with demented adults that responds to the spiritual and emotional needs as well as the physical ones. As discussed in Chapter 3, Watson views caring as the substance of nursing. The transpersonal exchange of energy between nurse and client is based on the nurse's genuine commitment to dignity, support, warmth, and comfort. This commitment involves both the art and science of nursing.

The art of nursing involves a transcendence or interpretation in order to appreciate the essence of the individual's state of being. The importance to Watson of **mutuality**, or client involvement in the therapeutic relationship, does not rule out the importance of intuition in the art of nursing. This process of "being with" is often referred to as empathy. The intuitive knowing that enables nurses to step inside another's reality even when that person cannot verbalize all his thoughts and feelings has also been called the "art/act" (Chinn & Kramer, 1991). According to Chinn and Kramer, it is this "comprehension of meaning in a singular particular, subjective expression" (p. 10) called the art/act that enables nurses to know what is significant in the moment and to "envision what is possible but not yet real" (p. 10). The art of nursing when combined with the science of nursing allows for judgments to be made about specific caring behaviors that will promote health and dignity for the person with a cognitive impairment in any given situation, experience, or moment.

Viewing Cognitive Impairments from a Caring Framework

The person with memory loss is disconnected from his or her past. In being robbed of the past, the person is stripped of much of his identity, at least identity as others have known it. In order to plan nursing care from the perspective of Watson's (1988) human care theory, the nurse must first understand what it is like for a human being to live in a manner where he is denied of his past and a sense of self-control and identity.

Promoting self-identity in the presence of severe cognitive impairments requires an ongoing collaboration between the nurse and family caregivers. Personal history and experience guides creative problem-solving approaches to managing behaviors, identifying physical needs, and meeting those needs in a way that honors a lifetime of habits and preferences. Several general principles, however, may be useful guides for planning individualized care.

When loss of memory and judgment makes even the most minor of decisions a major obstacle, simplification of the environment and consistency in daily routines may lessen the stress. Identifying lifelong habits in preparing for bedtime, mealtimes, or morning rituals and consistently adhering to them seems to ease the daily frustrations for the person with the impairment as well as for the caregiver. Caregivers have also discovered that simplifying the environment by removing mirrors and any unnecessary clutter or background noises such as television or radio may have a calming influence on the person frustrated by memory loss and alterations in perception. Displaying familiar pictures or objects imbued with mean-

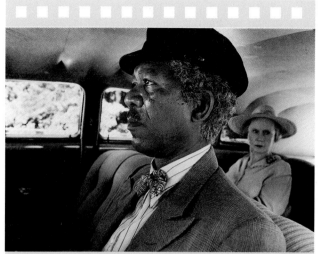

Driving Miss Daisy. Source: Warner Brothers/Courtesy Kobal.

Old age is a time of transition. In *Driving Miss Daisy*, Jessica Tandy's Daisy has to come to an accommodation with her increasing loss of independence and a world that changes greatly in 25 years.

ing may serve as orienting cues. Subtle methods such as these are preferable to more direct attempts at reality orientation, such as correcting or bombarding the person with facts and figures. The latter type of approach relies upon short-term memory, which is the first to go in various forms of dementias. Constant reminders of memory failure result in little or no significant improvement in functional status and may do harm by assaulting the already fragile identity and self-esteem of the older adult with cognitive impairments.

Making the most of remaining abilities is a key element in a healthy and meaningful existence for both the cognitively impaired and their caregivers. The ability to respond and express emotion seems to remain intact after other cognitive abilities have been lost. Emphasizing the affective component of communication (e.g., eye contact, tone of voice, and touch) is generally best received by the demented person. When instructions or specific messages must be conveyed, using language that is simple and direct in structure is usually most effective and least frustrating. Expressing a message in a statement format such as "Let's sit down here" is usually favorable to a question such as "Where would you like to sit when you get tired?" Validation therapy has grown in popularity in recent years as a technique that focuses on the interpersonal aspects of communicating with the individual who is cognitively impaired (Feil, 1989). The primary purpose of this therapy is the validation of feelings rather than reorientation with current facts.

Plenty of exercise is important for overall general health. Many caregivers have found that they can manage to keep a daily walk in the person's routine long after other activities have become unmanageable, so long as the walk is done at the same time of day and over the same route. Maintaining as much social interaction as possible is important for an overall sense of well-being for most individuals. Once again, individuality and life-long preferences must be taken into consideration. Reminiscence therapy is frequently used in long-term care facilities to promote social involvement and self-identity not only among the cognitively impaired but also among the nonimpaired healthy elderly. Familiar items such as articles of clothing, newspaper headlines, old songs, or photographs are used to elicit past memories. A sharing of personal stories associated with these memories is encouraged for the purpose of social interaction and validation of self-worth.

Regardless of communication techniques utilized, as cognition declines there is a significant decline in the ability of persons with cognitive impairments to express their physical needs or discomforts. Subtle changes in behavior, such as agitation or restlessness, are often indications of physical discomfort such as a shoe rubbing a callous, or a full bladder. Knowing the individual and using the process of elimination is often the best way for a caregiver to determine the source of discomfort. At other times, however, agitation may be a more direct response to the daily frustration of living with a cognitive impairment, and distraction may be the most useful way to prevent the behavior from escalating into a catastrophic reaction.

▽ EVALUATION

The progressively declining nature of various dementias makes improvements in function an unlikely goal of nursing care. Therefore, the effectiveness of care must be evaluated from a different perspective. If dignity and comfort are the major goals, listening to the stories of elders and caregivers gives us insight into the fears of those with dementia. A caregiver for persons with dementia noted the following of many of the individuals for whom she had cared: "None of us enjoys being organised and pushed around faster than we can personally manage and not one of us likes to feel that we do not have control over our own lives" (Naughtin, 1992, p. 214). Such stories tell us that fear of loss of dignity and ultimately of control and personality weigh heavily on the person with dementia.

My Journey into Alzheimer's Disease

Just because a person is incontinent or requires feeding does not give some eighteen-year-old twit the right to call them "dearie," or "sweetie." Watching some of the Alzheimer's day care centers featured on television gives me the "willies." I could never bear to be talked to and treated like a child at summer camp. "All right boys and girls, let's all stretch our arms to the music; let's dance the hokey pokey."

I am repulsed by activity directors on cruise ships, much less some twenty-year-old trying to get me to play childish exercises to rock music. I'm sure I would try to get back to my room and if stopped in this attempt I would become churlish and belligerent. If the insensitive director continued to push or become condescending and began to pat my arm, I would probably explode with all the violence pent up in my six-foot-seven frame. If I were then restrained or tied in my chair, my fury would take me right out of my mind.

Why? Is this a result of Alzheimer's disease? No, this is how I would react now in my best state of mind. I cannot stand the beat of rock music or the bouncing around of even senior citizen aerobic exercise classes. Human dignity demands that I have the right of refusal for any activity or entertainment that I do not perceive as entertaining. I deserve the right to withdraw from any situation and to go to a place of quiet and calm that I have appreciated over the years.

(Davis, 1989, p. 102)

Evaluation within a caring framework, therefore, must include the degree to which persons with dementia maintain control and dignity over their lives. The degree to which they remain functional and independent in ADL is one aspect of control and dignity. Since loss of control and resulting frustration may be manifested as a catastrophic reaction, the degree to which such reactions are reduced may be another reflection of how well control and dignity are being maintained. An even more direct evaluative approach may be undertaken in partnership with the demented elder and his primary caregivers. This partnership is formed for the purpose of designing and evaluating care that honors the elder's pattern of habits, lifestyle, and personality traits that have developed over a lifetime and are now threatened by disease. The plan of care will be a continually evolving one as cognitive abilities decline. However, all outcomes will be judged against the degree to which the individual's established pattern is being maintained in the presence of declining cognitive abilities.

CARING FOR THE CAREGIVERS

The "graying of America" is changing the composition of the American family. Most families have members in four generations and some have members in five or six. One of the standards by which modern societies may be judged may be how they respond to the increased numbers of dependent members, both young and old (Burke & Walsh, 1997).

Unlike the familiar rearing of children in which family caregivers are typically young and healthy parents, the caregivers of older persons are often spouses or adult children who may also be struggling with chronic illness. Thirty-five percent of family caregivers for older adults are themselves 65 or older (Wykle, 1994). Women still provide the bulk of caregiving in our society. In fact, a woman today can expect to spend 18 years of her life caring for aging parents (the average amount of time spent caring for children is 17 years!). These women are often referred to as the "sandwich generation" or "the women in the middle," as they try to juggle the needs of adult children, a household, their own personal and career needs, and the physical and emotional needs of a dependent parent or spouse. The mental and physical stresses of caregiving may include isolation and alienation from friends, sleep disturbances, fatigue, and more frequent complaints of stress-related illnesses such as headaches and gastrointestinal disturbances.

Nearly 3 to 4 million older Americans are affected today by permanent cognitive impairments. This figure is expected to rise to nearly 7 million within the next half century. Family members provide as much as 80% of the care required to maintain elders with dementia in their homes (Brady, 1985). The needs of caregivers are a growing responsibility for geropsychiatric nurses both today and in the future.

The changes in roles and relationships established over a lifetime and the practical, legal, financial, and everyday demands of caregiving for a demented loved one exact an emotional and physical toll. Certain themes are expressed repeatedly as caregivers tell their stories of caring for cognitively impaired loved ones (Naughtin, 1992). These themes, presented in what follows, provide much needed insight for nurses providing care to the caregiver.

Honesty with the Diagnosis

A direct approach when informing a person of his diagnosis early in the course of the disease helps both the individual and the family to recognize that they are not going "mad." Caregivers also say that once the diagnosis is made, they benefit from a clear statement regarding the nature of the illness, the likely process of its development, and information about resources that will help them cope both emotionally with role and relationship changes as well as with the practical day-to-day problems.

Relationship Tensions

The insidious onset and delay in diagnosis lead often to much tension between the person with dementia and the primary caregiver when the caregiver holds the demented loved one responsible for personality changes and problem behaviors. Caregivers need reinforcement from professionals and friends and family that these behaviors are not intentional and truly are typical of the disease.

Financial and Legal Affairs

Decisions about legal matters such as wills and powers of attorney are best handled in the early stages of dementia, when the person with dementia can still participate in the decision-making process.

Use of Community Resources

There seems to be a general reluctance to use community support services. Caregivers seem often to feel that this is an admission of failure or see such services as "welfare." Or they may be simply unaware of them. Caregivers do acknowledge the importance of knowing all the variety of options of support available to them. One form of service that is overwhelmingly well received by caregivers is respite or day care. While there often is some initial reluctance to use respite caregivers and persons with dementia struggle with admitting that they are like "all those other people," there is general acceptance once a pattern is established. Caregivers find it vital as pressure mounts.

Psychoeducational programs and support groups are growing in popularity. One advantage of these programs over psychotherapy or personal counseling is that their educational nature takes away the stigma or feelings of failure often attached to the more traditional types of mental health services. There is also usually no cost associated with self-help groups (except for small donations for refreshments or minor associated costs). All groups involve a mutual sharing of emotional support as well as practical tips on everyday problems encountered during caregiving. A recent development is computer "on-line" support groups. An advantage of this type of service is that caregivers may join in the discussion at any time (day or night!) from the convenience of their own homes. Nurses serve as moderators for some of these groups.

Guilt Over Nursing Home Placement

Placing a loved one in permanent residential care is one of the most difficult decisions caregivers must make. The caregiver often experiences much guilt when coaxing the loved one into the ambulance or car that will take the loved one to the facility. Moments of agony often follow as the caregiver must walk away from a loved one pleading not to be left. This is often a scene replayed over and over again in the caregiver's mind. After spending years attending to the loved one's every need, the caregiver often finds the care provided by a nursing home to be very unsatisfactory. This feeling, however, can change over time as the loved one adapts to the new environment and the caregiver begins to recognize the dedication of the staff and the quality of care being given.

Humor

Caregivers often talk about the benefit of being able to see humor in the absurd and of being able to laugh with their loved ones over the uncontrollable.

The Positive Aspects

Caregiving is not only about stress and negative consequences. Caregivers also relate the experience of joyful moments. Of no minor significance is the satisfaction of love, affection, and commitment expressed by the act of caregiving!

FUTURE DIRECTIONS

For the foreseeable future, mental health and aging concerns can be characterized as "high tech/high touch" (Smyer, 1993). New advances in neuroimaging and gene mapping are giving hope for better ways of diagnosing and possibly even treating AD. For at least the near future, however, these new technologies will not take away the need for social support as families care for loved ones with dementia.

The present appproach to the diagnosis of AD can be as accurate as 90% to 95% in moderate to severe cases (Tune, 1993). Discoveries in neuroimaging, however, may prove most useful in improving the ability to diagnose in the early stages and in complex cases where there are several pathologies present (e.g., AD and stroke). The latest research has shown that pathological changes in brain tissue and function in certain areas of the brain are associated with AD (Pearlson et al., 1992; Bondareff, Raval, Woo, Hauser, & Colletti, 1990). The combination of MRI scans for identifying structural changes and PET for measuring decreased cerebral blood flow and decreased glucose metabolism in the temporal/parietal cortex has been found to have 100% diagnostic capabilities (Pearlson et al., 1992). Although there is some evidence that choline-potentiating drugs hold some promise for slowing down the memory loss of AD, in general, effective treat-

ment lags behind discoveries in diagnosis. The emotional consequences, therefore, of earlier and more definitive diagnosis of AD in the absence of effective treatment remain an ethical concern.

Historically, geropsychiatry owes its recognition and growth to the burgeoning interest in AD some 25 years ago. The study of cognitive impairments has received the "lion's share" of attention in this field. The prevalence of and need for research into other mental illnesses experienced by older adults, such as schizophrenia, substance abuse, and anxiety disorders, will be expanding areas of study.

Lastly, much attention to date has been given to mental illness and aging. There is a recognized need for a greater emphasis to be placed on the essence of mental health in old age. Questions are being raised as to how we as a society can nurture, support, and fuel the "vital spirit" of old age. Much more needs to be learned, not only about the factors and forces that allow certain individuals to resist the stresses of aging, but also about those characteristics that contribute to the wisdom and hardiness of old age.

The future holds promise for a more in-depth and broader understanding of both mental health and mental illness in old age. In order to be a part of this future, nurses will need to become active participants in the political and economic issues that will influence the success of this endeavor.

KEY CONCEPTS

- ◆ There is a strong association between physical illness and mental illness in the elderly.

- ◆ Ageist myths and stereotypes are major barriers to the identification and treatment of mental illness in the elderly.

- ◆ Impairments in cognition can be the result of a dementia, delirium, or depression. An incorrect diagnosis can lead to much needless suffering, permanent impairment, and even death.

- ◆ Dementia is generally an irreversible condition characterized by memory loss. Delirium is a harbinger of an acute medical condition and is characterized by a clouding of consciousness. Dementia is slow in onset; delirium is rapid.

- ◆ Intellectual function does not diminish with age. However, the aging brain is more susceptible to injury.

- ◆ Memory deficits pose a serious threat to self-esteem and identity.

- ◆ An interdisciplinary assessment is essential for the diagnosis and management of delirium, depression, and dementia in the older adult.

◆ Severe memory deficits are not the result of normal aging. The first priority is to look for an acute, reversible cause.

◆ Confusion is an important phenomenon for nursing research. Confusion should not be used as a label for the behavioral manifestations of impairments in cognition or memory loss.

◆ Old age is not depressing. However, multiple losses, financial strain, and poor health are risk factors for depression in old age.

◆ Insomnia and physical complaints are frequent symptoms of depression among an aged population.

◆ Pharmacotherapy and psychotherapy have good success rates in treating depression in the elderly.

◆ The risk of suicide is high among the elderly.

◆ Maximizing control and the opportunity for choices should be a major goal of nursing care for the depressed older adult.

REVIEW QUESTIONS AND ACTIVITIES

1. Describe the physiological basis for at least three disorders that result in an irreversible dementia. List one type of dementia that is potentially reversible.

2. Describe three common symptoms of dementia. Explain how the symptoms may affect self-esteem and dignity.

3. Describe the major differences in caring for an older adult with dementia between Watson's caring framework and care from a strictly biomedical perspective.

4. List the components of an interdisciplinary assessment of dementia.

5. What are the distinguishing symptoms that characterize a delirium from a dementia?

6. Describe at least two therapeutic modalities used with cognitively impaired individuals in long-term care.

7. State the common variables associated with acute confusional states.

8. What is confusion? Why can its use as a label for patient behaviors hamper treatment goals?

9. Explain the mechanism of action of antidepressant drugs and anticonvulsant therapy in the treatment of depression in the aged.

10. Identify at least three sociocultural stressors that increase the risk of depression in the elderly.

11. What are some symptoms that characterize depression in the older adult?

12. Describe the adverse effects of antidepressant drugs most commonly experienced by the older adult?

EXPLORING THE WEB

◆ Visit this text's "Online Companion™" on the internet at **http://www.DelmarNursing.com** for further information on mental health and the elderly.

◆ Search the web for specific disorders such as Alzheimer's dementia, delirium, or depression. What information is available? Are there phone numbers and addresses that you can contact for literature?

◆ Is there a listing on the Internet of books, videos, or other media on self-care for caregivers to the elderly? Are these resources available in your local library or through purchase over the web?

◆ Can you locate resources for families needing information on nursing homes or care facilities for elderly clients with mental health needs?

◆ What seniors' organizations can you locate that have specific discussion groups addressing the psychiatric needs of the elderly and their caregivers?

◆ Search government web sites for information on seniors' health care, Medicaid, Medicare, and support groups.

REFERENCES

American College of Medical Genetics/American Society of Human Genetics Working Group on ApoE and Alzheimer Disease. (1995). Statement on use of apolipoprotein E testing for Alzheimer disease. *Journal of the American Medical Association, 20,* 1627–1629.

American Psychiatric Association. (1994). *Diagnostic and Statistical Manual of Mental Disorders* (4th ed.). Washington, DC: Author.

Blazer, D. (1990). *Emotional problems in later life: Intervention strategies for professional caregivers.* New York: Springer.

Bondareff, W., Raval, J., Woo, B., Hauser, D. L., & Colletti, P. M. (1990). Magnetic resonance imaging and the severity of dementia in older adults. *Archives of General Psychiatry, 47*(1), 47–51.

Brady, E. (1985). Parent care as a normative family stress. *The Gerontologist, 25,* 19–29.

Buchanon, D., Farran, C., & Clark, D. (1995). Suicidal thought and self-transcendence in older adults. *Journal of Psychosocial Nursing and Mental Health Services, 33*(10), 31–34.

Burke, M. M., & Walsh, M. B. (1997). *Gerontologic nursing: Wholistic care of the older adult* (2nd ed.). St. Louis: Mosby-Year Book.

Butler, R. N. (1963). The life review: An interpretation of reminiscence in the aged. *Psychiatry, 26,* 65.

Capriotti, T. (1995). Unrecognized depression in the elderly: A nursing assessment challenge. *MedSurg Nursing, 4*(1), 45–54.

Chinn, P. L., & Kramer, M. K. (1991). Nursing's pattern of knowing. In P. L. Chinn & M. K. Kramer (Eds.), *Theory and nursing: A systematic approach* (3rd ed., pp. 1–18). St. Louis, IL: Mosby-Yearbook, Inc.

Cummings, J. L., & Benson, F. (1986). Dementia of the Alzheimer type: An inventory of diagnostic clinical features. *Journal of the American Geriatrics Society, 32*(1), 12–19.

Dawes, B. (1996). Neurological and cognitive function. In A. Leuckenotte (Ed.), *Gerontologic nursing* (pp. 727–766). St. Louis: C.V. Mosby.

Dychtwald, K. (1989). *Age wave.* Los Angeles: Jeremy P. Tarcher, Inc.

Eliopoulos, C. (1997). *Gerontological nursing* (4th ed.). Philadelphia: Lippincott-Raven.

Erickson, E. H., Erickson, J. M., & Kibnick, H. Q. (1987). *Vital involvement in old age.* New York: W.W. Norton.

Estes, C., & Binney, E. (1989). The biomedicalization of aging: Dangers and dilemmas. *The Gerontologist, 29*(5), 587–596.

Feil, N. (1989). *Validation: The Feil method.* Cleveland, OH: Edward Feil Production.

Finkel, S. I. (1993, Winter/Spring). Mental health and aging: A decade of progress. *Generations, 17*(1), 25–30.

Folstein, M., Folstein, S., & McHugh, P. (1975). Mini-mental state: A practical method for grading the cognitive state of patients for the clinician. *Journal of Psychiatric Research, 12*, 189–198.

Foreman, M. (1989). Confusion in the hospitalized elderly: Incidence, onset, and associated factors. *Research in Nursing and Health, 12*, 21–29.

Gatz, M., & Smyer, M. (1992). The mental health system and older adults in the 1990s. *American Psychologist, 47*(6), 741–751.

Harper, M., & Grau, L. (1994). State of the art in geropsychiatric nursing. *Journal of Psychosocial Nursing, 32*(4), 7–12.

Jubeck, M. (1992). Are you sensitive to the cognitive needs of the elderly? *Home Healthcare Nurse, 10*(5), 20–25.

Keltner, N. (1994). Tacrine: A pharmacological approach to Alzheimer's disease. *Journal of Psychosocial Nursing, 32*(3), 37–39.

Kivnick, H. (1993, Winter/Spring). Everyday mental health: A guide to assessing life strengths. *Generations, 17*(1), 13–20.

Lind, A. L. (1995). Delirium, dementia, and other cognitive disorders. In M. O. Hogstel (Ed.), *Geropsychiatric nursing* (2nd ed.). St. Louis: Mosby.

Mace, N. (1983). *The 36 hour day: A family's guide to caring.* Baltimore: John Hopkin's.

Matthiesen, V., Silvertsen, L., Foreman, M. D., & Cronin-Stubbs, D. (1994). Acute confusion: Nursing intervention in older patients. *Orthopaedic Nursing, 13*(2), 21–29.

McDougal, G. (1990). Review of screening instruments for assessing cognitive and mental status in older adults. *Nurse Practitioner, 15*(11), 18–28.

Nadelson, T. (1990). On purpose, successful aging, and the myth of innocence. *Geriatric Psychiatry, 23*(1), 3–12.

Nagley, S. (1984). Prevention of confusion in hospitalized elderly persons. *Dissertation Abstracts International, 45*, 1732. (University Microfilms No. 8420848)

Nightingale, F. (1969). *Notes on nursing.* Unabridged republication of 1st American edition, 1860, by D. Appleton & Company. New York: Dover Publications.

Oppenheim, G. (1994). The earliest signs of Alzheimer's disease. *Journal of Geriatric Psychiatry and Neurology, 7*, 116–120.

Osgood, N. (1992). *Suicide in later life.* New York: Lexington Books.

Pearlson, G. D., Harris, G. J., Powers, R. E., Barton, P. E., Camargo, E. E., Chase, G. A., Noga, J. T., & Tune, L. E. (1992). Quantitative changes in miseal temporal volume, regional cerebral blood flow, and cognition in Alzheimer's disease. *Archives of General Psychiatry, 49*(5), 402–408.

Poznanski-Hutchison, C., & Bahr, R. T., Sr. (1991). Types and meanings of caring behaviors among elderly nursing home residents. *Image: Journal of Nursing Scholarship, 23*, 85–88.

Reisberg, B., & Ferris, S. (1988). Brief cognitive rating scale (BCRS). *Psychopharmacology Bulletin, 24*(4), 629–636.

Ritchie, K. (1988). The screening of cognitive impairment in the elderly: A critical review of current methods. *Journal of Clinical Epidemiology, 41*(7), 635–643.

Strumpf, N. E., & Evans, L. K. (1988). Physical restraint of the hospitalized elderly: Perceptions of patients and nurses. *Nursing Research, 37*, 132–137.

Sullivan-Marx, E. M. (1995). Psychological responses to physical restraint use in older adults. *Journal of Psychosocial Nursing and Mental Health Services, 33*(6), 20–25.

Tess, M. (1991). Acute confusional states in critically ill patients. *Journal of Neuroscience Nursing, 23*(6), 398–402.

Trice, L. B. (1990). Meaningful life experience to the elderly. *Image: The Journal of Nursing Scholarship, 22*, 248–251.

Tune, L. (1993, Winter/Spring). Neuroimaging: Advances and new direction. *Generations, 17*(1), 79–80.

Vermeersch, P. (1990). The clinical assessment of confusion—A. *Applied Nursing Research, 3*(3), 128–133.

Vermeersch, P. (1991). Response to the cognitive and behavioral nature of acute confusional states. *Scholarly Inquiry for Nursing Practice: An International Journal, 5*(1), 17–20.

Wallace, M. (1993). Creutzfeldt-Jakob disease assessment and management. *Journal of Gerontologic Nursing, 19*(11), 15–22.

Watson, J. (1988). Nursing: Human science and human care: A theory of nursing. New York: National League for Nursing.

Wolanin, M. O. (1977). Confusion study: Use of grounded theory as methodology. In Western Interstate Commission for Higher Education. *Communicating Nursing Research, 8*, 68–75.

Wykle, M. L. (1994). The physical and mental health of women caregivers of older adults. *Journal of Psychosocial Nursing, 32*(3), 41–42.

Wykle, M. L., & Musil, C. M. (1993, Winter/Spring). Mental health of older persons: Social and cultural factors. *Generations, 17*(1), 7–12.

Yesavage, J. A., & Brink, T. L. (1983). Development and validation of a geriatric depression screening scale: A preliminary report. *Journal of Psychiatric Research, 17*, 37–49.

≋ LITERARY REFERENCES

Anonymous. *A crabbit old woman.* Northern Ireland Association for Mental Health.

Davis, R. (1989). *My journey into Alzheimer's disease.* Wheaton, IL: Tyndale House Publishers.

Flanagan, M. (1987). Survived by his wife. In *When I am an old woman I shall wear purple* (p. 103). Watsonville, CA: Papier-Mache Press.

Naughtin, B. (1992). *When I grow too old to dream.* North Blackburn, Australia: Collins Dove.

Sacks, O. (1987). *The man who mistook his wife for a hat.* New York: Harper Perennial.

Spohr, B., & Bullard, J. (1995). *Catch a falling star: Living with Alzheimer's.* Seattle, WA: Storm Peak Press.

〰 SUGGESTED READINGS

Brandt, B., & Ugarriza, D. N. (1996). Electroconvulsive therapy and the elderly client. *Journal of Gerontological Nursing, 22*(12), 14–20.

Buckwalter, K. C., Gerdver, L. A., Hall, G. R., Stolley, J. M., Kudart, P., & Rideway, S. (1995). Shining through: The humor and individuality of person's with Alzheimer's disease. *Journal of Gerontological Nursing, 21*(3), 11–16.

Clark, W. G., & Vorst, V. R. (1994). Group therapy with chronically depressed geriatric patients. *Journal of Psychosocial Nursing and Mental Health Services, 32*(5), 9–13.

Goldstein, M. A., & Perkins, C. A. (1993). Mental health and the aging woman. *Clinics in Geriatric Medicine, 9*(1), 191–196.

Gurian, B., & Goisman, R. (1993, Winter/Spring). Anxiety disorders in the elderly. *Generations, 17*(1), 39–42.

Johnson, B. K. (1996). Older adults and sexuality: A multidimensional perspective. *Journal of Gerontological Nursing, 22*(2), 6–15.

LeBarge, E., & Trtanj, F. (1995). A support group for people in the early stages of dementia of the Alzheimer type. *Journal of Applied Gerontology, 14*(3), 289–301.

Mellins, C., Blum, M., Boyd-Davis, S., & Gatz, M. (1993, Winter/Spring). Family network perspective on caregiving. *Generations, 17*(1), 21–24.

Norberg, A. (1996). Caring for demented patients. *Acta Neurol Scand Suppl, 165*, 105–108.

Nursing Clinics of North America. (March 1994). *Issue topic: Alzheimer's Disease, 29*(1).

Reed, P. (1991). Spirituality and mental health in older adults: Extant knowledge for nursing. *Family & Community Health, 14*(2), 14–25.

Roughan, P. A. (1993). Mental health and psychiatric disorders in older women. *Clinics in Geriatric Medicine, 9*(1), 173–190.

Smyer, M. (1993, Winter/Spring). Mental health and aging. Progress and prospects. *Generations, 17*(1), 5.

Steiner, D., & Marcopulos, B. (1991). Depression in the elderly: Characteristics and clinical management. *Nursing Clinics of North America, 26*(3), 585–600.

Taft, L. B., & Barkin, R. L. (1990). Drug abuse? Use and misuse of psychotropic drugs in Alzheimer's care. *Journal of Gerontological Nursing, 16*(8), 4–10.

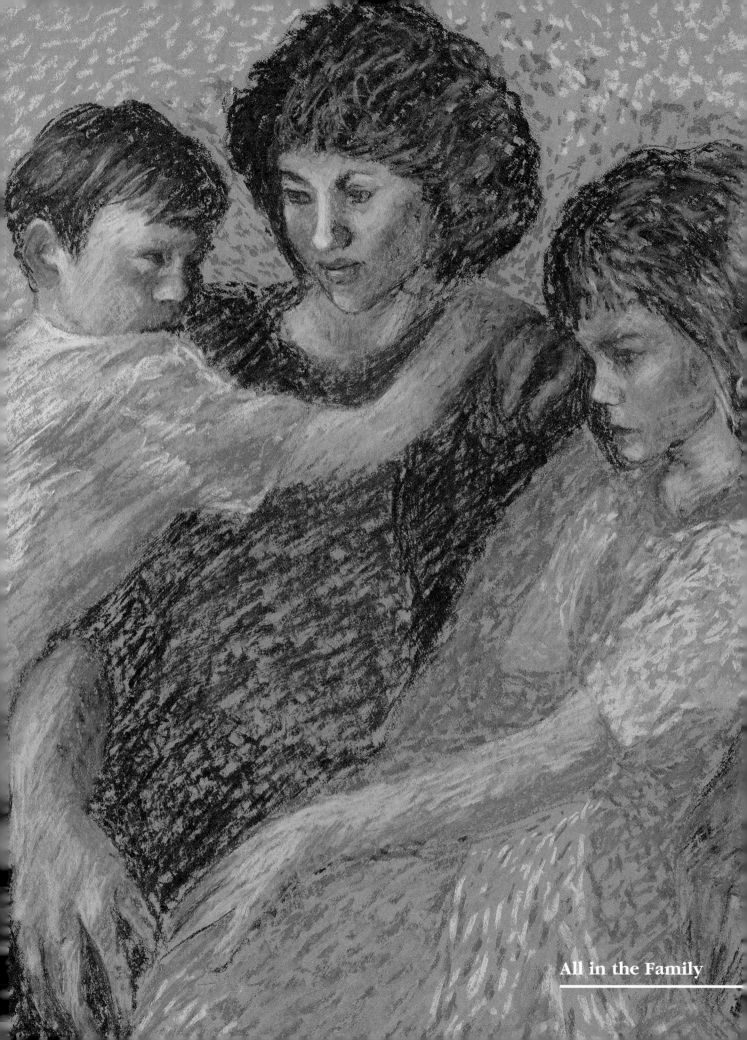

All in the Family

Chapter

24

SURVIVORS OF
VIOLENCE OR ABUSE

Marshelle Thobaben

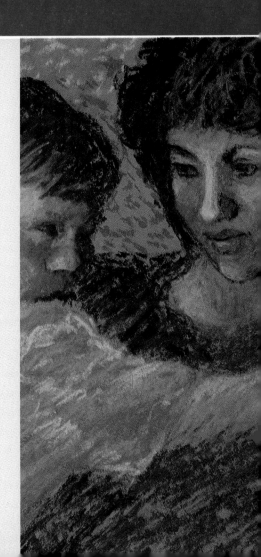

Reflections on Abuse

Consider how you feel about abuse and violence:

♦ What are your beliefs about disciplining a child? Where do they come from?

♦ Do you wonder why women stay in abusive relationships? What are your beliefs based on?

♦ Can you imagine an adult child punishing a frail parent for being incontinent? Have you ever become frustrated while taking care of an older, confused, incontinent client who is at risk for falling?

♦ How would you feel if your client was a gang member who was arrested for killing an innocent person in a drive-by shooting?

♦ Do you think that "date rape" is a crime? Why or why not?

♦ Do you feel you are being intrusive when interviewing clients about the possibility of their involvement in abusive relationships?

♦ Do you believe society has a right to remove children or frail adults from their homes if they are being abused by their family? Under what circumstances would removing them be appropriate?

♦ Do you think the effects of child abuse are different for girls and boys?

♦ Do you think that health care providers who, themselves, have experienced family violence or sexual assault respond differently to abused clients than those who have not?

♦ Have you ever felt that you mistreated a client?

Use the answers to these questions to develop an understanding of your personal attitudes and beliefs about violent and abusive relationships. As you read through this chapter, continue to examine your responses to those discussed.

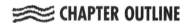 **CHAPTER OUTLINE**

CHILD ABUSE

Child Protective Legislation

Realities of Child Abuse
  Sexual Abuse
  Shaken-Baby Syndrome
  Munchausen Syndrome by Proxy
  Adolescent Abuse
  Community Violence

RAPE

DOMESTIC VIOLENCE

ELDER ABUSE

Legislation

NURSING PERSPECTIVES ON ABUSE AND NEGLECT

Self-Care Deficit Theory

Crisis Intervention Theory

Nursing Responsibilities

▽ **NURSING PROCESS**

▽ **CASE STUDIES/CARE PLANS**

FUTURE DIRECTIONS

COMPETENCIES

Upon completion of this chapter, the reader should be able to:

1. Identify the major theories that explain why interpersonal violence occurs.

2. Identify factors that may contribute to interpersonal violence.

3. Define the general types of family violence: physical, psychological, financial, and sexual abuse and neglect.

4. Identify the typical indicators of abuse and neglect observed in interpersonal relationships and the characteristics of the abusers.

5. Describe the nurse's legal responsibility in regard to child and elder abuse mandatory reporting laws and clients who have been sexually assaulted.

6. Describe the cycle of domestic violence.

7. Utilize crisis intervention techniques in intervening in cases of family violence and sexual assault.

8. Utilize community resources that are available to prevent abuse and to assist the survivors and perpetrators in abusive situations.

9. Apply the nursing process to clients who are abused and neglected by:
  ◆ Performing nursing assessments for abuse and neglect
  ◆ Analyzing data in terms of nursing and crisis theories
  ◆ Formulating individual nursing diagnoses
  ◆ Deriving a plan of care
  ◆ Evaluating care based on resolution of the abuse and neglect

≋ KEY TERMS

Acquaintance (or Date) Rape   Forcible rape or sexual battery that occurs by the victim's acquaintances or dates.

Aggravated Criminal Sexual Assault   Criminal sexual assault in which a weapon is used or displayed; the victim's life or someone else's is endangered or threatened; the perpetrator causes bodily harm to the victim; the assault occurs during the commission of another felony; or force is used to threaten or cause physical harm to the victim.

Child Abuse   Any physical or mental injury, sexual abuse, exploitation, negligent treatment, or maltreatment of a child by a parent or caregiver.

Child Molestation   Sexual involvement with a child, such as oral-genital contact, genital fondling and viewing, or masturbation in front of a child.

Child Pornography   Sexually explicit reproduction of a child's image.

Criminal Sexual Assault   Genital, anal, or oral penetration by a part of the perpetrator's body or by an object using force or without the victim's consent.

Domestic Violence   (often referred to as spousal/partner abuse or battering syndrome) Intentional violent or controlling behavior by a person who is or has been intimate with the victim(s) and may or may not reside in the same household.

Financial Abuse   Theft or conversion of money or anything of value belonging to the elderly by their relatives or caregivers.

Forcible Rape   Forced intercourse or penetration of a body orifice by a penis or other object by a perpetrator.

Gang Rape   Sexual acts that are proximate in time by multiple perpetrators who are either acquaintances of or strangers to the victim.

Incest   Sexual relations between children and blood relatives or surrogate family members.

Mental Injury   Harm to a child's psychological or intellectual functioning; manifested as severe anxiety, depression, withdrawal, or outward aggressive behavior or a combination of these behaviors.

Negligent Treatment   Failure of a parent or caregiver to provide, for reasons other than poverty, adequate food, clothing, shelter, or medical care, which may lead to serious endangerment of the physical health of the child.

Passive Physical Abuse (or Negligence)   Conduct that is careless and a breach of duty that results in injury to the person or is a violation of rights; includes the withholding of medication, medical treatment, food, and personal care necessary for the well-being of the elderly person.

Physical Abuse   Conduct of violence that results in bodily harm or mental stress; includes a spectrum of violence ranging from assault to murder.

Physical Injury   Lacerations, fractured bones, burns, internal injuries, severe bruising, or serious bodily harm.

Psychological Abuse   Simple name calling and verbal assaults in a protracted and systematic effort to dehumanize the victim, sometimes with the goal of driving the victim to insanity or suicide; usually exists in combination with one or more other abuses.

Rape   Act of sexual intercourse in which the person does not give consent; accomplished against a person's will by means of force or fear of immediate and unlawful bodily injury or threatening to retaliate in the future against the victim or other person.

Sexual Abuse (Child)   Employment, use, persuasion, inducement, enticement, or coercion of a child to engage in, or assist another person to engage in, sexually implicit conduct; includes rape, molestation, prostitution, or other forms of sexual exploitation of children or incest with children.

Sexual Abuse (Elder)   Threat of sexual assault or actual sexual battery, rape, incest, sodomy, oral copulation, penetration of genital or anal opening by a foreign object, coerced nudity, and sexually explicit photographing.

Sexual Battery   Activity of a person touching an intimate part (sexual organs, groin, buttocks, breast) of another person, if that touching is against the will of the person touched and is for the purpose of sexual arousal, gratification, or abuse.

Sexual Exploitation   Child pornography, sexually explicit reproduction of a child's image, or child prostitution.

Sexually Explicit Conduct   Actual or simulated sexual intercourse, bestiality, masturbation, lascivious exhibition of the genitals of a person or animal, or sadistic or masochistic abuse.

Spousal Rape   Sexual intercourse against the victim's will by the spouse; accompanied by force, fear of bodily harm, or future retaliation.

Statutory Rape   Sexual activity with a person under the age of consent (in most states, under 16 years of age) and considered to have occurred despite the apparent willingness of the underage person.

Stranger Rape   Aggravated criminal sexual assault, forcible rape, or sexual battery that is committed against a victim by persons not acquainted with the victim.

Violation of Rights   Abuse that occurs when the inalienable rights conferred by the U.S. Constitution and federal statutes are violated by a family member or caregiver; includes such rights as not to have one's property taken without due process, the right to adequate appropriate medical treatment, and the right to freedom of assembly, speech, and religion.

The chapter will focus on interpersonal violence that occurs within families, sexual assaults, and gang violence. For the purposes of this chapter the term *family* goes beyond relationships of blood or marriage to mean interpersonal relationships that have similar dynamics to traditional families. The terms *violence* and *abuse* are often used interchangeably in the professional literature and thus will be used interchangeably in this chapter. The term *victim* is often used to describe the person being abused. This chapter will also use the term *survivor* since it conveys a sense of empowerment for the person in an abusive relationship.

Family violence refers to a range of abusive behaviors among family members. It includes child, sibling, spousal, and elder abuse and neglect. It is often hidden and may continue from one generation to another. Violent and abusive relationships exact a huge toll on the survivors and their family's physical and mental health. They are an indicator that the family is dysfunctional or in a crisis.

There is no single theoretical framework that offers a complete explanation as to why family violence occurs. Studies show that children, domestic partners, and the elderly who are abused and neglected come from all social, economic, and racial groups. There is evidence that family violence is influenced by a complex interaction of personal, psychological, social, and environmental factors. Some experts believe that everyone has the potential of being a family abuser given the right circumstances. The major theoretical frameworks that explain violence are biological, psychoanalytical, social-learning, and sociological.

The biological theoretical frameworks theorize that aggression is an innate characteristic that is either an instinctual drive or neurologically based. Instinctivist biologists believe that aggressive behavior is an instinctual drive and that people, like animals, have a natural fighting instinct that preserves the species. Neurophysiologists hypothesize that violence is caused by brain or hormonal imbalances, specifically the limbic system and neurotransmitters (e.g., epinephrine, norepinephrine, dopamine, acetylcholine, and serotonin) (Campbell &. Humphreys, 1993).

Freud and his followers have theorized that violence lies in the personalities of the abusers. People who are violent have the internal need to discharge hostility and are unable to control the impulsive expression of anger and hostility. Aggressive behavior is a process of displacement that redirects the self-destructive death instinct away from the individual and outward toward others. These theorists posit that ego weakness is caused when an individual's basic needs or drives have been thwarted, usually by the mother during child rearing. Other interpersonal theories suggest that individuals who are violent have personality disorders since people who abuse often are paranoid, sadistic, obsessive-compulsive, excessively jealous, and suspicious (Campbell & Humphreys, 1993).

Social-learning theorists hypothesize that the development of aggressive behavior is part of the socialization process and that it is a learned response. They believe that the stimulation of the neurophysiological mechanisms that enable people to behave violently is under cognitive control and that violence is learned through modeling, observing, direct experience, or practice. The abuser generally has some form of power or control over the victims. Violence is used as a method of persuasion, and the fear of it keeps people in positions of submission. If the use of violence or the threat of it is rewarded by gain in power, it will increase (Campbell & Humphreys, 1993).

A variety of other factors contribute to interpersonal abusive relationships. The sociological theory of family violence proposes that the social environment places stress on the family. Violent families often have multiple problems that deplete their personal resources. When caregivers' physical, financial, and/or emotional resources are strained, there is a higher probability that family conflict will result in violence. Caregivers may also be at higher risk for family violence if they abuse alcohol and other drugs, have chronic physical or mental illnesses, or have inadequate relief from caregiving responsibilities. Dependent family members may be at higher risk for abuse if they are not wanted, have chronic physical, developmental, or mental disabilities, or are terminally ill. Personal crisis, poverty, unemployment, and other stressors can increase the risk of violence (Campbell & Humphreys, 1993).

Clients who experience interpersonal violence or sexual assaults may develop major physical and psychological problems or die.

CHILD ABUSE

Americans have long held the belief that parents are in the best position to provide for the well-being and growth of their children. They have an obligation to raise their children to be responsible citizens. Part of that responsibility involves disciplining children when they misbehave. The moral obligation of parents to use physical force when disciplining their children for misbehavior has roots in the *Holy Bible*:

Proverbs 13:24

He that spareth his rod hateth his son: but he that loveth him chasteneth him betimes.

(*Holy Bible, 1913, p. 695*)

Parents and caregivers who physically discipline children believe that physically punishing children is essential for them to become responsible citizens. Most parents do not intentionally permanently injure their children. Some family violence experts believe that parents who hit their children are modeling that interpersonal violence is acceptable behavior. Spanking children may not be considered physical abuse by legal authorities, but whipping children with belts on their bare skin might legally be considered physical abuse. Psychological abuse, sexual abuse, and severe neglect can be as damaging to children as physical abuse.

Many of us have repeated Mother Goose nursery rhymes, but do we agree with what they say? The following two Mother Goose verses, originally copyrighted in 1916, are still read to and repeated by children. They speak of parents physically disciplining their children.

Little Polly Flinders

Little Polly Flinders
Sat among the cinders
Warming her pretty little toes;
Her mother came and caught her,
Whipped her little daughter
For spoiling her nice new clothes.
(*The Real Mother Goose, 1916, p. 26*)

There Was an Old Woman

There was an old woman who lived
in a shoe.
She had so many children she
didn't know what to do.
She gave them some broth without
any bread.
She whipped them all soundly and
put them to bed.
(*The Real Mother Goose, 1916, p. 117*)

Child Protective Legislation

The United States began legally protecting abused children in 1874. "Little Mary Ellen," as she was known, had been severely neglected and abused by her adoptive parents, the Connollys. Her case was brought to the Supreme Court by Henry Bergh, founder and president of the Society for the Prevention of Cruelty to Animals (SPCA). Mary Ellen gave the following court statement.

My mother and father are both dead. I don't know how old I am. I have no recollection of a time when I did not live with the Connollys. I call Mrs. Connolly mamma. I have never had but one pair of

⤫ *REFLECTIVE THINKING*

The Impact of Nursery Rhymes

What impression do these verses leave children with when they hear them? What words could you substitute when reading them to children? Even though they were written in 1916, they raise some of the questions about disciplining children that society is still debating. Was it appropriate for Polly's mother to whip her because she spoiled her new clothes? The "old woman" neglected and whipped her children because she had too many and did not know what to do. Do you think that she acted as a responsible parent? When is it appropriate for parents to physically punish a child and for what kind of behavior? May they only use their hand, or can they use a belt? Do parents have a right to take their frustrations out on their children as it appeared that the "old woman" did? Would a nurse have to report either "situation" to the child protection agency if she was aware of it?

shoes, but I cannot recollect when that was. I have had no shoes or stockings on this Winter. I have never been allowed to go out of the room where the Connollys were, except in the night time, and then only in the yard. I have never had on a particle of flannel. My bed at night has been only a piece of carpet stretched on the floor underneath a window, and I sleep in my little under-garments with a quilt over me. I am never allowed to play with any children, or to have any company whatever. Mamma (Mrs. Connolly) has a habit of whipping and beating me almost every day. She used to whip me with a twisted whip—a raw hide. The whip always left a black and blue mark on my body. I have now the black and blue marks on my head which were made by mamma, and also a cut on the left side of my forehead which was made by a pair of scissors. (Scissors produced in court.) She struck me with the scissors and cut me; I have no recollection of ever having been kissed by any one—have never been kissed by mamma. I have never been taken on mamma's lap and caressed or petted. I never dared to speak to anybody, because if I did I would get whipped. I have never had, to my recollection, any more clothing than I have at present—a calico dress and a skirt. I have seen stockings and other clothes in our room, but was not allowed to put them on. Whenever mamma went out I was locked up in a bedroom. I do not know for what I was whipped—mamma never said

⚙️ *REFLECTIVE THINKING*

Mary Ellen's Case

How would you feel if Mary Ellen was returned to the Connollys if they agreed to go into therapy and attend parenting classes? What would help Mary Ellen to recover from the abuse? What type of nursing interventions would be appropriate to help her adjust to her new living situation?

anything to me when she whipped me. I do not want to go back to live with mamma, because she beats me so. I have no recollection of ever being on the street in my life.

(U.S. House of Representatives, House Select Committee on Aging, 1981, pp. 225–227)

Mary Ellen was removed from the Connolly home and sent to an asylum, the Sheltering Arms. Mrs. Connolly was found guilty of assault and battery and sentenced to 1 year in the penitentiary at hard labor. Because of the publicity of this case, on December 17, 1874, the New York Society for the Prevention of Cruelty to Children (NYSPEC) was founded to protect children (U.S. House of Representatives, House Select Committee on Aging, 1981, p. 227).

Mary Ellen was severely abused by her adopted family. As extreme as Mary Ellen's situation was, similar and worse situations still exist today.

The following definitions of child abuse and neglect have been adopted from the Victims of Child Abuse Act of 1990.

◆ **Child abuse** is any physical or mental injury, sexual abuse, exploitation, negligent treatment, or maltreatment of a child under the age of 18 (or the age specified by the child protection law of the state in question) by a parent or parent substitute.

◆ **Negligent treatment** is the failure of a parent or parent substitute to provide, for reasons other than poverty, adequate food, clothing, shelter, or medical care to seriously endanger the physical health of the child.

◆ **Physical injury** includes, but is not limited to, lacerations, fractured bones, burns, internal injuries, severe bruising, or serious bodily harm.

◆ **Mental injury** is harm to a child's psychological or intellectual functioning. It may be exhibited by severe anxiety, depression, withdrawal, or outward aggressive behavior or a combination of those behaviors, which may be demonstrated by a change in behavior, emotional response, or cognition.

◆ **Sexual abuse** includes the employment, use, persuasion, inducement, enticement, or coercion of a child to engage in or assist another person to engage in sexually implicit conduct. It is the rape, molestation, prostitution, or other forms of sexual exploitation of children or incest with children.

◆ **Sexually explicit conduct** is actual or simulated sexual intercourse whether with persons of the same sex or of the opposite sex, bestiality, masturbation, lascivious exhibition of the genitals or pubic area of a person or animal, or sadistic or masochistic abuse.

◆ **Child molestation** is sexual involvement such as oral-genital contact, genital fondling and viewing, or masturbation.

◆ **Sexual exploitation** is child pornography, sexually explicit reproduction of a child's image, or child prostitution (U.S. Code Annotated, Title 42, 1990, P.L. 104, pp. 4806–4807).

◆ **Incest** is sexual relations between children and blood relatives or surrogate family members.

If parent-child relationships fail because of child abuse and neglect, as in the case of Mary Ellen, the state has the authority to intervene to protect the children. It took the federal government nearly 100 years after Mary Ellen's tragic situation to pass child protection legislation. In 1974 the federal government passed the Child Abuse Prevention and Treatment Act (P.L. 93-247), which outlined certain requirements each state must meet to be eligible for federal funding. It defined child abuse, determined the appropriate role for public child welfare agen-

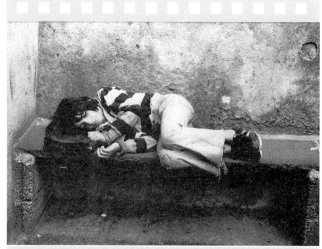

Agent De Poche. Source: United Artists/Courtesy Kobal.

Child neglect is a serious and prevalent problem. The nurse should always be aware of child neglect when working with the young.

cies, and established a set of uniform operating standards for the identification and management of child abuse cases. It also established the National Center on Child Abuse and Neglect (NCCAN).

All states, Washington, D.C., Puerto Rico, and the Virgin Islands have statutes that mandate nurses who know or suspect child abuse to report it. The report is made to an agency designated by the state, usually the county welfare or social service's child protective unit. The laws provide that nurses who report child abuse be protected from civil and criminal liability unless they make a false report. Failure to report is a misdemeanor in many states. Ideally, nurses should tell abusing parents that they are legally required to report the suspected child abuse in an attempt to keep lines of communication open. They should not put themselves at risk for injuries if they think that informing families would lead to personal harm.

The primary purposes of child abuse mandatory reporting laws are to protect children by early identification of abused and neglected children; provide help to abusing families; and identify persons suspected of crimes against children. They also provide data to determine incidences of child abuse and neglect. Public child welfare agencies have the responsibility to protect children from harm and cruelty. Their staff investigates reports of child abuse and neglect. Depending upon the results of their investigations and subsequent court actions, children can be immediately, temporarily, or permanently removed from their parents' custody and placed with relatives or foster care or placed for adoption. The court can

impose certain requirements that parents must comply with to maintain or regain custody of their children, for example, attending parent classes or a drug treatment program.

The federal government established the National Child Abuse and Neglect Data System (NCANDS) to help with the voluntary data collection and analysis of the national incidence of child abuse and neglect. In its 1995 report it documented that 3,140,000 cases of child abuse or neglect were reported to Child Protective Services (CPS) agencies. Of those cases reported, 33% were substantiated, with an estimate of 1,036,000 *confirmed* as victims of child maltreatment. To prove a case, the investigation disposition had to determine that there was sufficient evidence under state law to conclude that child maltreatment had occurred or that the child was at risk of maltreatment. Nationwide, the rate of children reported for child abuse or neglect was 47 per 1000, and 16 children per 1000 were substantiated in 1994. Of the substantiated cases, 21% were physical abuse, 11% sexual abuse, 3% emotional abuse, 49% neglect, and 16% other. Approximately 1271 children were killed, over 3 children each day, as a result of child abuse or neglect. The vast majority of these cases involved children under the age of 5, and almost half were under the age of 1. The report indicated that one of the limitations of the study was that individual states determined their definitions of maltreatment, investigative procedures, and data collection procedures; thus, there was not consistency in the reported statistics among the states (Wiese & Daro, April 1995, p. 18).

Third National Incidence Study of Child Abuse and Neglect (1996) (NIS-3), a government report, provides some important insights into the incidence and distribution of child abuse and neglect. It reported that there was a significant increase in the incidence of child abuse and neglect since its previous study in 1986; the number of seriously injured children had quadrupled; the poorest families had the highest rate of maltreatment; and community professionals were better at recognizing the more subtle cues that indicate potential abusive and neglectful cases. The study did not specifically investigate the causes of abuse and neglect but found that parental illicit drug use was often mentioned in the narrative descriptions of reported cases (Sedlak & Broadhurst, 1996).

Realities of Child Abuse

Child abuse statistics only partially reflect the true incidence of child maltreatment since a vast number remain underreported. Some unsubstantiated reports of child maltreatment may be actual cases of abuse, and many abuse cases are never reported. The decision to report child abuse is often subjective and depends upon the beliefs and observations of the potential reporter. Few family members are willing to admit they have abused or

---

✳ **NURSING TIP**

Child Abuse Reports

The report should carefully document the physical evidence of abuse and neglect without making judgments about the family. Child abuse reports should include the following:

◆ The name of the victim

◆ Current location of the victim

◆ Type of abuse you are reporting

◆ Types of injuries you observed and how severe

◆ Parent or caregiver's account of the injuries

◆ When possible, children's account of their injuries

◆ Why you suspect the child is being abused or neglected

◆ In the client's record, chart your observations and your report to the child protective agency

⑤ RESEARCH HIGHLIGHT

Incidence and Factor Assessment of Abused Children and Adolescents

STUDY PROBLEM/PURPOSE

To explore and describe the documented incidents and factors of physical and sexual abuse of children and adolescents suffering from psychiatric disorders.

METHODS

Retrospective review of the charts of 69 psychiatric clients between the ages of 5 and 16 who had been admitted to and discharged from an inpatient psychiatric children and adolescent unit.

FINDINGS

Results indicated that physical abuse happened most frequently with 0 to 5 years the age of onset, the father the most likely perpetrator, and for a duration of more than 5 years; it was disclosed to either the mother, a school employee, or a health care professional; and removal from the home was the most frequent outcome. The study indicated that the most frequent sexual abuse pattern was age of onset 0 to 5 years with a single perpetrator (likely a male family member), duration of 6 months to less than 5 years, disclosure to both parents, and removal of the child from the home as the most frequent outcome. The study also found that nurses failed to assess and plan treatment based on the comprehensive documenta-

tion of sexual and physical abuse factors. One of the most disquieting findings of this study was the lack of critical information in the charts regarding the abuse. As horrifying to the public as Mary Ellen's abuse and neglect may have been in 1874, today, homicide has become the leading cause of injury-related death in infants younger than 1 year of age. Children under age 5 are often reported as the most likely to experience physical abuse or neglect. Children continue to be sexually abused by parents or parent substitutes. The average age of onset of child sexual abuse is 8 years, with a duration of 5 years. It is estimated that 1 in 4 girls and 1 in 7 boys are sexually abused. The most common form of child sexual abuse is father-(stepfather-) daughter abuse.

IMPLICATIONS

Nurses must be aware of the high incidence of child abuse and neglect and specifically assess physical and emotional signs that may indicate abuse. Sexual and physical abuse findings must be carefully documented and reported to the proper authorities; nursing care must center on preserving the welfare of the child as discovered through the assessment findings. Knowing the trends of abuse and neglect in children as well as the most likely perpetrators and most common situations will aid nurses in more effectively evaluating children and planning care.

From "What Really Happened? Incidence and Factor Assessment of Abused Children and Adolescents," by G. Polk-Walker, 1990, *Journal of Psychosocial Nursing, 28*(11), pp. 17–22.

neglected their child because they are afraid of criminal prosecution, being exposed as unfit parents, or the removal of their children from their home. Abused or neglected children, generally, do not reveal that they have been mistreated, even when they have been badly brutalized. Children who have lived with being abused their whole lives may think it is normal or that they deserve the abuse because they have done something wrong. They may be scared their parents will retaliate against them or desert them. They may feel loyalty to their parents or believe that they will be removed from their parents. They may be too young to report or understand what has happened to them.

For nurses to be able to identify children who are abused and neglected, they need to be familiar with the common symptoms and behaviors that abused or neglected children experience and the common behaviors observed in parents or caregivers who are abusing and neglecting them. Refer to the accompanying displays

for a list of characteristics and behaviors indicative of child abuse or neglect.

Children who are abused and neglected develop physical and psychological problems. Many studies have shown that there is a relationship between children being abused and having problems with family and peer relationships, school performance, emotional development, physical health, sexual behavior, self-esteem, depression and anger, fears, and guilt. If they are not successfully treated for their psychological problems, they may develop *post-trauma response (PTR)* (NANDA) or Post-Traumatic Stress Disorder (PTSD) (DSM-IV). The symptoms of PTR/PTSD in children may last throughout their lives and interfere with their development as responsible adults. Child abuse may also intensify the symptoms of other psychiatric disorders, such as depression, eating disorders, dissociative disorders, attention-deficit hyperactivity disorder, phobias, panic disorder, and separation anxiety disorder (USDVA, National Center for Post-Traumatic Stress Disorder, 1997).

CHARACTERISTICS OF CAREGIVERS WHO ABUSE OR NEGLECT THEIR CHILDREN

◆ Has history of abuse or neglect as a child, reveals concern about having been abandoned and punished by own parents

◆ Uses harsh discipline inappropriate to the child's age

◆ Believes that violence is a way to reduce tension, exhibits violent feelings and behavior, has a low tolerance for frustration, has poor impulse control

◆ Never mentions any good qualities in the child

◆ Fails to respond to the child or responds inappropriately

◆ Is extremely protective or jealous toward the child

◆ Is critical of the child and angry with the child for being injured or sick, shows no concern about the child's injury, treatment, prognosis, or follow-up care, often disappears from the hospital shortly after the child is admitted and tends not to visit the child

◆ Leaves small children alone or abandons them

◆ Significantly misperceives the child, distrusts the child, falsely accuses the child of sexual promiscuity

◆ Has marital difficulties, lives in a chaotic home life

◆ Is insulated from the influence of others, is socially isolated

◆ Has feelings of hopelessness and helplessness

◆ Has personality disorders, misuses alcohol or other drugs

◆ Lacks knowledge of childhood developmental issues

◆ Often neglects own physical health

◆ Attempts to conceal the child's injury, is evasive or contradicts self about the child's injury or illness, protects the identity of person responsible for the child's injuries

◆ Is unable to admit the need for help

◆ Lives in unsanitary or unsafe living conditions

◆ Encourages the child to engage in prostitution or sexual acts in the presence of parent

⚠ NURSING ALERT!

Sibling Abuse

Sibling abuse, or battery of child by a brother, sister, stepbrother, or stepsister, is one of the most common yet underrecognized forms of child abuse. It may be physical, sexual, or psychological. It is frequently minimized by parents as "normal sibling rivalry" and subsequently not recognized or reported (Whipple & Finton, 1995).

Sexual Abuse

Annually, approximately 80,0000 cases of child sexual abuse are reported, but the number of unreported cases is far greater. Child sexual abuse can take place within the family, by a parent, stepparent, sibling, or other relative, or outside the home, by a friend, neighbor, child caregiver, teacher, or random molester. An adult caregiver, who is more powerful, takes advantage of a child for the purpose of sexual gratification. The adult is able to manipulate and intimidate the child. The child, believing she has no choice, usually complies with the adult. It is an abuse of power (AACP, 1995).

It is uncommon for children to admit they are being sexually abused. Some are too young to describe what they have experienced; feel too ashamed or embarrassed; are afraid that no one will believe them; feel loyal or threatened or are bribed by the abuser; feel confused by the attention and feelings accompanying the abuse; blame themselves or believe the abuse is punishment for being bad; or worry about getting into trouble or getting a family member into trouble. As long as the abuser can keep the victim silent, the abuse can continue. Silence protects the abuser and damages the child. Once child protective services has investigated a case, the legal procedures for validating a case can be difficult.

A sexually abused child may not have any obvious signs of physical abuse; the only evidence might be changes in the genital and anal area. Physical evidence of sexual abuse is often harder to observe in boys than in girls because the abuse often involves anal intercourse and injuries to the anus heal quickly. Additionally, boys initially will often not reveal they have been molested, because of the stigma attached to it (Carroll, 1996). The accompanying display includes common symptoms and behaviors observed in sexually abused children. The effects of sexual abuse on children can be devastating. It affects their self-esteem, self concept, and sexual adjustment. They can develop problems such as substance abuse problems, eating disorders, depression, suicidal tendencies, and sexual promiscuity.

Commercial sexual exploitation of children is another form of child sexual abuse. Millions of children are at risk

COMMON CHARACTERISTICS OF CHILD ABUSE AND NEGLECT

CHILD'S SYMPTOMS OF PHYSICAL ABUSE

♦ Bruises and welts in various stages of healing showing the shape of the items used—belt marks, shoe prints—in unusual patterns or clustered

♦ Human bite marks

♦ Burns: on the dorsal surface of the hand (if children burn their hand by accident, they usually burn the palm), by an iron or cigarettes or immersion in scalding liquid (glove or doughnut-shaped burns on the buttocks or genitalia)

♦ Fractures: spiral fractures of upper extremities, skull, jaw, or nasal, X-ray of healed or healing with no history of treatment, or multiple fractures

♦ Malnutrition, failure to thrive

♦ Lacerations and abrasions: injury to the oral mucosa or frontal dental ridge (from having a bottle jabbed into the mouth), or to external genitalia

♦ Shaken-baby (whiplash) syndrome or retinal hemorrhage (from being shaken too hard or cuffed about the head) in infants and toddlers

♦ Repeated injuries, always explained as accidental

♦ Chunks of hair missing from the scalp

CHILD'S SYMPTOMS OF NEGLECT

♦ Malnourished, comes to school hungry; often does not have lunch money

♦ Poor skin care, consistently dirty

♦ Tired, no energy

♦ Clothes dirty or wrong for weather

♦ Lacks needed medical care, glasses, or dental care

♦ Lacks emotional care or attention

♦ Unsupervised for extended periods of time, especially when engaged in dangerous activities

♦ Has been abandoned

CHILD'S BEHAVIOR

♦ Frequently absent, late, or comes to school much too early; hangs around after school is dismissed, causes trouble in school; often has not done homework

♦ Acts unpleasant and demanding, causes trouble or interferes with others, or is unusually shy, avoids other people including children, seems exceptionally fearful of adult authority (or lack of it)

♦ Often does not obey

♦ Behaves wary when in the presence of adults or avoids physical contact with adults or seeks affection from any adult

♦ Appears too anxious to please, seems too ready to let other people say and do things to him or her without protest

♦ Frequently breaks or damages things

♦ Begs or steals food

♦ Uses alcohol or drugs

♦ Engages in vandalism

♦ Engages in sexual misconduct

♦ Resists physical examination/assessment

♦ Wears long sleeves or other concealing clothing to hide injuries

♦ Child or adolescent's story of how an injury occurred is not believable; it does not fit the type or seriousness of the injury

♦ Seems frightened of parents, shows little or no distress at being separated from parents

♦ Reports injury by parents

---

of commercial sexual exploitation or already caught in the megadollar sex industry. Children are scarified to the abuse of power by unscrupulous adults. They are subject to violence and serious health hazards, denied an education, and their childhood and all aspects of their development are undermined. **Child pornography** is the sexually explicit reproduction of a child's image. Advances in technology have made child pornography easier to produce and distribute and more difficult to stop. Computer graphics and global transmission via the Internet means that images can now be transmitted worldwide and downloaded at home. It teaches the child that the body is for sale and can be a first step to prostitution. It involves coercion of and violence toward children. Children from poor communities are the most at risk (World Congress Against Commercial Sexual Exploitation of Children, 1997).

Shaken-Baby Syndrome

Fatal injuries from child abuse result from severe head trauma, trauma to the abdomen and/or thorax,

CHILD'S SYMPTOMS OF SEXUAL ABUSE

VERBAL

◆ Reports to a friend, a teacher, or the authorities that sexual activity with adults has occurred

◆ Physical complaints

◆ Indirect comments or statements about the abuse or statements about being sexually assaulted by parent/parent substitute

PHYSICAL

◆ Itching, bruises, bleeding or pain in the external genitalia, vagina, or anal area, edema of the cervix, vulva, or perineum, or stretched hymen at a very young age

◆ Pain or injury to the mouth

◆ Vaginal or penile discharges: semen or evidence of a sexually transmitted disease

◆ Bladder infections

◆ Pregnancy in an older child

◆ Sexually transmitted diseases (STDs)

BEHAVIORAL

◆ Reluctance or fear of a person or of certain places, such as showers or bathrooms

◆ Torn, stained, or bloody undergarments

◆ Regression to babyish habits, such as thumb sucking or bed wetting

◆ Temper tantrums, aggressive behavior, running away, or engaging in delinquent acts

◆ Acting out sexual or abusive behavior with toys, animals, or people

◆ Preoccupation with sexual organs of self or others with younger children

◆ Sexual promiscuity or prostitution in older children

◆ Change in sleeping patterns, nightmares, or sudden fear of falling asleep

◆ Poor peer relationships, reluctance to participate in sport or other recreational activities

◆ Feelings of guilt, fear, anger, shame, confusion, isolation

◆ Delinquency, truancy, acting out, or runaway behavior

◆ Use of alcohol and other drugs

◆ Phobias, avoidance behavior

◆ Depression, suicidal behavior

◆ Evidence of child pornography

scalding, drowning, suffocation, poisoning, or shaken-baby syndrome (SBS), which is often not recognized by nurses and other health care professionals. The classic features of SBS are retinal hemorrhage and intracranial injury. It occurs when parents or other caregivers violently shake infants by their extremities or shoulders, usually out of frustration and rage over the child's incessant crying. It causes children to have whiplash-induced intracranial and intraocular bleeding but with no external signs of head trauma. Parents or caregivers rarely mention that they forcefully shook their infants, often may withhold the information about how the injury occurred, or may give some other excuse for it. Infants most often present in the emergency room with respiratory difficulty or apnea. It is difficult to diagnose because of the vague symptoms and unreliable history given by parents or other caregivers. It is important for nurses to be alert for SBS because the intracranial hemorrhage and life-threatening cerebral edema need prompt medical treatment. Death or permanent disabilities can result (Jackson & Miller, 1996).

Munchausen Syndrome by Proxy

Munchausen syndrome by proxy (MSP) is another form of child abuse that may go undetected by nurses and other health care professionals. It is a difficult problem to diagnose and treat. Parents invent or directly induce their children's illnesses or symptoms and then seek medical assistance. The parents might report that their children have had seizures or suffer from abdominal pain when the children are well. Children undergo extensive diagnostic procedures or therapeutic regimens needlessly. An indicator of MSP is that the symptoms are not easily detected by the health care professional, only by the history of the parent. Mothers are most often the abusers. Their behavior can be deceptive to nurses because they give the appearance of being caring parents who want to stay with their children and give them care. The reasons for the parents' need to cause their children to become ill is not understood. Once discovered, it is generally necessary to remove the children from the parents in order to protect them. It is estimated that approximately 10% of the children who are victims of MSP die each year (Olds, London, & Ladewig, 1996).

Adolescent Abuse

A number of factors may interfere with nurses' identifying adolescent survivors of abuse. There is a perception by adults, including some health care professionals, that adolescents are less likely to be innocent victims of abuse. They believe that adolescence is a challenging period for parents and the abuse that may occur is deserved. They believe in the stereotype of victims of abuse as small and helpless and the abusers as big and powerful. They believe that adolescents with their greater physical and

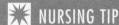

RESEARCH HIGHLIGHT

Physical and Sexual Abuse among Runaway Youths

STUDY PROBLEM/PURPOSE

To determine a correlation between abusive family situations and teens' running away from home.

METHODS

Seventy-eight runaway youths admitted to a shelter were given face-to-face interviews and asked questions related to certain aspects of their current and past situations, including any history of familial abuse. The youths ranged in age from 11 to 17. Approximately 56% were female and 44% were male. The majority were white (88.4%) and 11.5% African American.

FINDINGS

Sixty-seven percent reported that they had experienced some type of abuse.

IMPLICATIONS

The researchers concluded that the data validated that "runaway" youths are likely to come from abusive situations. They found that family violence within the home environment frequently induces youths to leave home and seek refuge elsewhere.

From "Self-Reported Experiences of Physical and Sexual Abuse among Runaway Youths," by J. K. Warren, F. Gary, and J. Moorhead, 1994, *Perspectives in Psychiatric Care, 30*(1), pp. 23–28.

NURSING TIP

Helping Caregivers Keep Kids Out of Gangs

If caregivers are able to meet the child's needs, the child will have less need to join a gang. Some important parenting skills include:

- Developing good communication with their children: Caregivers need to have frequent open lines of communication with their children that take on a positive tone. Children should not be condemned or put down, which will allow them to discuss any problem with the caregiver.

- Spending time with their children: Caregivers should spend time alone with their children; plan activities that the whole family can enjoy; and expose them to places outside the neighborhood: museums, beach, camping trips, and so on.

- Putting a high value on education: Caregivers should encourage their children to do the best they can in school and do everything possible to prevent them from dropping out.

- Occupying their children's free time: Caregivers should give their children responsibilities at home. They should get them involved in after-school sports, recreational activities, and other busy activities.

- Setting limits for their children: Caregivers should know what their children are doing. They should let their children, at an early age, know what is acceptable and unacceptable behavior. They should have a curfew and not allow their children to spend a lot of unsupervised time on the streets.

- Discouraging their children from hanging around with gang members: Caregivers should know their children's friends. They should talk to their children about gangs. Children should not be allowed to buy or dress in gang style clothing or write or use gang names or gang graffiti on their books, bodies, and so on (Gang Information, 1996).

cognitive abilities should be able to handle difficult family situations. Adults often blame adolescents when they respond to the parental abuse with mutual assault or verbal abuse (JAMA, 1993).

Adolescents who are incarcerated, homeless, runaways, involved in drug abuse, or have had an unwanted pregnancy during early adolescence are more likely to have a history of physical or sexual abuse. Their point of entry into the service system often determines how they are treated and what services are made available to them. Adolescents who are running away from home because of family violence are less likely to receive the physical and mental health care they need if they come to the attention of the juvenile justice system as opposed to being identified as abused by nurses or physicians in an emergency room (JAMA, 1993).

Community Violence

Community violence has reached epidemic proportions in many urban communities. Many children and teenagers living in these communities experience living

conditions similar to war zones. A recent survey found that 1 of every 10 children younger than age 6 attending the Boston City Hospital Pediatric Clinic had witnessed a shooting or stabbing. Half of the incidents took place in their home and the other half took place outside the home or in the street. According to the American Humane Association, 13 children are killed and 30 are wounded by guns every day. Since 1988 U.S. teenage boys are more likely to die from gunshot wounds than from all other causes combined (NCCAN, 1997).

Young people join gangs for a variety of individual, family, societal, and financial reasons. The factors that contribute to gang affiliation include ineffective parental skills, history of family gang involvement, and evidence of parental abuse and neglect. A dysfunctional family atmosphere affects the child's self-esteem and often leads to the child's having poor academic achievement, antisocial behavior, and associations with others experiencing similar social and personal problems. Children often are enticed to join a gang because it offers them a sense of belonging, status recognition, excitement, protection, and an opportunity to earn money for food, drugs, shelter, and other material goods. They also join to escape from an abusive home environment, to be free from their parents' rules, because of peer pressure and friendship, and because they are unemployed. Gang membership will shape their future (National Crime Prevention Council, 1996).

Gang affiliation extracts a terrible toll on children, families, and communities. Traditionally, gangs were structured along ethnic lines. Gang violence varies from individual assaults to drive-by shootings. Gangs gain power by fear and intimidation. They attempt to instill fear in their communities, intimidating rival gangs and citizens alike. When a gang seeks confrontation with rivals, the resulting violence often claims innocent victims. Today's street gangs have criminal operations that are sophisticated and claim as many as 400,000 members and cross state lines. They are engaged in high-stakes narcotic and weapons trafficking, gambling, kidnapping, motor vehicle thefts, robbery and murder, or other criminal activity for monetary gain. Local businesses suffer from property damage, graffiti, and loss of customers and employees (Gang Information, 1996).

The *L.A. Times* took an in-depth look at the 18th Street gang, which began more than 30 years ago in the impoverished L.A. neighborhood where the Santa Monica and Harbor freeways intersect, near 18th Street and Union Avenue ("An Inside Look at 18th Street's Menace," Nov. 17, 1996). The article claims that it is the biggest and deadliest street gang to rise in the nation's gang capital (L.A.). It has as many as 20,000 members in Southern California alone, about 60% of them illegal immigrants. The 18th Street gang breaks with gang tradition since its members come from all races. Veteranos oversee a loose-knit network of cliques. Its primary recruitment target is immigrant children, ages 11 to 13, who attend middle school and appear to be on the fringes of gang life. The gang scout method of recruiting them is to initially confront the children, instill fear in them, and then back off. The veteranos approach the children again, softening their approach, giving the impression of being friends and protectors. They promise action and excitement and make gang life appear glamorous by telling the children they will get money, guns, drugs, women, and protection. Once they join, many gang members believe that they are in *por vida*—for life. The 18th Street gang has become so influential in narcotics circles that it deals directly with Mexican and Colombian cartels and has ties to the Mexican Mafia prison gangs. It also rents street corners to nongang dope dealers who are forced to pay taxes (Connell & Lopez, 1996).

NURSING ALERT!

Indicators of Gang Membership

Caregivers should be aware of certain warning signs that indicate gang involvement. The following are indicators of gang membership (Gang Information, 1996; McNamara, 1994):

◆ An informal dress code (hats, scarves, jewelry, shoelaces, colors, tattoos, insignias, etc.)

◆ Street slang (nicknames, hand signs)

◆ Attitude changes or disinterest in family activities

◆ Solitary behavior

◆ Playing "gang" in the neighborhood

◆ Newly acquired and unexplained wealth often displayed or shared with peers

◆ Graffiti on personal property: book covers, notebooks, or clothing (initials, numbers, names, expressed racism, hatred of religious groups)

◆ Major and negative behavior changes (lower grades, staying out late without good reason, associating with known or suspected gang members, carrying weapons)

RAPE

Rape is a legal term, not a medical entity. It is a crime of violence. Rapists use sexual violence to dominate and degrade their victims and to express their own anger. It is not an act of lust or an overzealous release of passion done to satisfy a sexual urge.

According to Aguilera (1994, pp. 118–121), there are three basic types of rape: (1) people who know each other, for example, fathers and daughters, former and current friends (date rape), neighbors, partners and separated partners, prostitutes and dissatisfied clients; (2) gang rape; and (3) stranger-to-stranger rape. The latter, which women fear the most, follows an identifiable pattern. Such rapists look for women who are vulnerable, even though they differ on defining who is vulnerable. They might attempt to rape the elderly, people who are developmentally, physically, or mentally challenged, or intoxicated people. They might look for environments that are easy to enter and relatively safe (e.g., women's bedrooms) and where they will not be interrupted. They often select their victims long before they approach them and repeat the same pattern of victim selection over and over again. All types of rape can be an emotionally terrorizing experience for the survivors.

The following are definitions of rape and sexual assault, though states will vary on their legal definitions of sexual assault:

◆ **Rape** is an act of sexual intercourse in which the person does not give consent. It is accomplished against a person's will by means of force or fear of immediate and unlawful bodily injury or threats to retaliate in the future against the victim or other person (Sexual Assault Glossary of Terms, 1996, p. 1).

◆ **Criminal sexual assault** is any genital, anal, or oral penetration by a part of the perpetrator's body or by an object using force or without the victim's consent.

◆ **Aggravated criminal sexual assault** occurs when, in addition to the sexual assault, a weapon is used or displayed; the victim's life or someone else's is endangered or threatened; the perpetrator causes bodily harm to the victim; it occurs during the commission of another felony; or force is used to threaten or cause physical harm to the victim.

◆ **Forcible rape** is forced intercourse or penetration of a body orifice by a penis or other object by a perpetrator.

◆ **Statutory rape** is sexual activity with a person under the age of consent (in most states, under 16 years of age) and is considered to have occurred despite the apparent willingness of the underage person.

◆ **Sexual battery** occurs when a person touches an intimate part (sexual organs, groin, buttocks, breast) of another person, if that touching is against the will of the person touched and is for the purpose of sexual arousal, gratification, or abuse.

◆ **Acquaintance or date rape** is forcible rape or sexual battery that occurs by the victim's dates or acquaintances.

◆ **Spousal rape** is sexual intercourse against the victim's will by the spouse and is accompanied by force or fear of bodily harm or future retaliation.

◆ **Stranger rape** is generally aggravated criminal sexual assault, forcible rape, or sexual battery that is committed against a victim by persons not acquainted with the victim.

◆ **Gang rape** entails sexual acts that are proximate in time by multiple perpetrators who are either acquaintances of or strangers to the victim.

According to the U.S. Department of Justice's National Victimization survey, over 500,000 women and approximately 49,000 men *report* being sexually assaulted each year (AMA, 1995b). In 1995 for every 1000 persons age 12 and older there occurred two rapes or attempted rapes and two assaults with serious injury. Women age 12 and older annually sustained 5 million violent victimizations, the majority committed by persons who knew the victim. Women were about twice as likely as men to experience violence by a relative (U.S. Department of Justice, Bureau of Justice Statistics, 1997).

Estimating the incident rate for rape victims is difficult because the crime is vastly underreported by both women and men. The National Victim Center (NVC) (1996) estimates that 1871 rapes occur per day. A survey of those raped showed that 84% did not report the rape, 12% reported the rape within 24 hours, and 4% reported the rape after 24 hours. Twenty-nine percent of rapes were committed by acquaintances, 22% by strangers, 16% by other relatives, 11% by father/stepfather, 10% by boyfriend/ex-boyfriend, 9% by husband/ex-husband, and 3% not sure/refused to answer. Twenty-nine percent (29.3%) of victims were under the age of 11, 32.2% between the ages of 11 and 17, 22.2% between the ages of 18 and 24, 7.1% between 25 and 29, 6.1% over 29, and 3% were not sure or refused to answer (NVCS, 1996).

The AMA's Council on Scientific Affairs reported that at least 20% of adult women, 15% of college women, and 12% of adolescent girls have experienced sexual abuse and assault during their lifetimes. Estimates of rape for African American women are even higher. Children are the most at risk from sexual assaults by family members and other caretakers, whereas adolescent and young adult women are most at risk for acquaintance, date, or stranger rape. Both adult and older women are more vulnerable to sexual assaults by marital or ex-marital partners than rape by acquaintances, other family members, or strangers combined (AMA, Council on Scientific Affairs, 1992). It is estimated that approximately 14% to 25% of women experience forced sex at least once during their marriages. It may well be the most common form of sexual assault (Bergen, 1995).

Males are also raped, but there is little research about it. Only recently has sexual assault been legally defined in gender-neutral terms. Sexual assault against men in prison populations is significantly underestimated and underreported. One report estimates that as many as 130,000 adult males in prisons, 30,000 in jails, and 40,000 boys held in juvenile and adult facilities are victims of sexual assaults. Rape of males in prison differs from male rape in the community. It is generally open and accepted, if not condoned, by the prisoner subculture. It usually involves repeated sexual assaults following the initial rape. It may appear consensual to the casual observer, but the rape survivor needs protection from further massive assaults. The number of women sexually victimized by male guards is unknown (Stop Prisoner Rape, 1997).

Many women survivors of rape are inhibited from reporting this crime to either the police or health care professionals because of embarrassment, the perceived stigma, the belief that no purpose would be served in reporting the crime, the fear of retaliation, and the fear of court procedures. Male survivors of sexual assaults frequently do not seek help or report assaults for fear of being erroneously labeled homosexual or judged negatively or disbelieved by health care providers. The myths surrounding rape also inhibit survivors from reporting rape. Myths are associated with sociocultural beliefs about interpersonal violence, perceptions of male and female sex roles, and other social stereotypes. Table 24-1 discusses these myths.

Rape represents an immediate and disturbing crisis for the survivors and their families. Survivors generally experience a two-phase reaction to the crisis: initially an acute, highly confusing, and disorganized state followed by a long-term period in which survivors attempt to put their lives back into the order it had before the rape (Burgess, 1990). It is defined by the North American Nursing Diagnosis Association (NANDA) as the *rape-trauma syndrome*. The concept was first introduced in 1974 by Burgess and Holmstrom (1974). NANDA defines the *rape-trauma syndrome* as the forced, violent sexual penetration against the victim's will and consent. The trauma syndrome that develops from this attack or attempted attack includes an acute phase of disorganization of the victim's lifestyle and a long-term process of reorganization of lifestyle. NANDA classifies responses to rape in three categories: *rape-trauma, compound reaction*, and *silent reaction*; see the accompanying display.

The American Psychiatric Association has identified a specific syndrome similar to NANDA's, that rape survivors experience. Clients may be diagnosed with Acute Stress Disorder when the symptoms occur immediately after the rape or attempted rape and Post-Traumatic Stress Disorder when the symptoms are present for more than 1 month after the rape or attempted rape. Refer to the displays in the Nursing Diagnosis section for criteria used in making these diagnoses.

Medical problems that result from a sexual assault include acute injury, risk of pregnancy, and acquiring STDs. It affects the survivor's family and friends. Family members must deal with their own reactions as well as the psychological, medical, and behavioral changes in the victim. Following sexual assaults, survivors may avoid family and friends or they may cling to them (AMA, Nov. 1995a).

How clients cope when they are sexually assaulted will depend upon their developmental level, personal characteristics, and the reactions of significant others. A child will not react to being sexually assaulted by a parent in the same way an adult woman would if she were raped by a family friend. Whatever coping mechanisms clients use subsequent to the crisis precipitated by the sexual assault will probably not be adequate. Crisis counseling gives them a higher probability of full recovery. It offers them opportunities for emotional catharsis, reality testing for self-blame, active support on a short-term basis, and someone who will assist in identifying the situational supports available to them (Aguilera, 1994, p. 119).

The following excerpt illustrates that date rape is not sex or making love but a crime of violence and a desire by the rapist to dominate his victim, to feel powerful, and to express his anger. The story is of Elizabeth Mason, an attractive, talented college freshman who was raped by Jimmy Andrews, a handsome, athletic senior. She had

Table 24-1   Common Myths about Rape

MYTH	FACT
Rape is an isolated, infrequent event that only happens to certain kinds of people: attractive, young women or women who are promiscuous or provocative.	Anyone can be sexually assaulted. Research indicates that victims can range from infants to people in their nineties, lesbians/gays, people with disabilities, and people from every racial, ethnic, religious, economic, and social background (National Coalition Against Sexual Assault, 1997).
Rapists are strangers. *Real* rape only happens when a stranger attacks a woman or a man.	The vast majority of rapists are family members and acquaintances. It is not uncommon for a woman or a man to be raped by someone that she or he has been dating for a long time or by a former lover or a spouse. As many as 80% of sexual assaults are committed by someone the survivor knows.
Rapes are committed in out-of-the-way places.	Over 50% of sexual assaults occur in the home and as many occur during daytime as happen at night (National Coalition Against Sexual Assault, 1997).
Rape is motivated by sexual desire. Most rapists are oversexed and unable to control their urges.	Rape is an act of violence. It is motivated by anger and the desire for power and control.

Continued

Table 24-1 Common Myths about Rape *continued*

MYTH	FACT
Rape is provoked by women. They ask for it by the provocative way they dress, their seductive behaviors, and the places that they frequent. Only promiscuous women are raped. Women cannot be raped against their will. Rape can be avoided by resistance.	No one asks to be sexually assaulted. It is a misconception to assume that women can prevent the rape by dressing differently, avoiding certain social situations, or putting up a fight. Most women who were raped were in a situation that they considered safe. They knew the person assaulting them and were in a state of disbelief. They were not able to mobilize themselves to fight and hurt their assailants because they found it difficult to believe that someone they knew and trusted was raping them.
Women/men secretly desire to be raped.	It is a misconception to believe that women or men "secretly desire" to be raped or taken by force. Some people have fantasies about being overcome by their partners but they are in control of their fantasies, and that is different from being sexually assaulted.
Women often "cry rape" to get even with a man or to protect their reputations.	False reports about rape are no more likely than false reports of other felonies. The FBI reports that 2% of sexual assault reports are false accusations, which is a rate no higher than the rate of false reports for other crimes (AMA, Oct. 1995b, p. 23; National Coalition Against Assault, 1997). The fact is that 9 of 10 incidences of rape are never reported (National Coalition Against Sexual Assault, 1996, p. 2).
All victims of sexual assault are women. Men and boys do not get raped. If a man does not have an erection, rape cannot happen. Men can defend themselves. Male rape is homosexual rape. It only happens in prisons.	The majority of sexual assaults committed against both women and men are perpetrated by men. The FBI estimates that 1 of 10 men are victims of adult sexual assault. Researchers have found that 1 of 4–7 male children are sexually abused. Men are often attacked by gangs, assaulted with weapons, and taken by surprise. Physical strength is not always sufficient protection when faced with what is experienced as a life-threatening situation. Male rape is not an indicator of the sexual preference of either the survivor or the perpetrator. Most male survivors were raped as children or as adults who were never incarcerated (National Coalition Against Sexual Assault, 1997, p. 1). Women sometimes perpetrate sexual assaults against men and other women. Women who sexually assault men do so by intimidation and threat of violence rather than physical force. Penal erection can occur in response to extreme emotional states, such as anger, as well as sexual arousal.
If a woman or man consents to some sexual intimacy, it means that she or he is willing to have intercourse.	Agreeing to one form of sexual contact does not mean agreement to all forms of sexual contact. Men and women have a right to stop sexual activity whenever they want to. This is an underestimated problem in male homosexual relationships where the male who is penetrated may not have wanted it.
If the client is not a virgin, rape is not a traumatic event. If the client is not physically injured, recovery is quick. The best way for survivors to get over a sexual assault is to act as if it did not happen, to put it behind them, get on with their lives, and be "normal" again.	Rape is a devastating emotional experience. It can leave the survivor with emotional scars that can impede interpersonal and intimate relationships forever. Clients frequently experience post-trauma response after being sexually assaulted. Recovery becomes an ongoing process of healing, change, and empowerment.
Wives cannot be raped by their husbands.	Wives are raped by their husbands and are vulnerable to being repeatedly raped as part of domestic violence. According to the AMA, women from Hispanic backgrounds and some Middle Eastern and Asian countries and women who have immigrated from nations such as Vietnam, India, or Africa are more likely to believe that sexual abuse and assault are expected in marital relationships (AMA, Oct. 1995b, p. 23).
Prostitutes cannot be raped.	Prostitutes are frequently raped but seldom report the crime because they believe that they will not be believed by the police or the court system.

Adapted from AMA (1996). Council on Scientific Affairs (1992).

NANDA'S CHARACTERISTICS OF RESPONSES TO RAPE

RAPE-TRAUMA SYNDROME:

Acute Phase

Emotional reactions

◆ Anger

◆ Embarrassment

◆ Fear of physical violence and death

◆ Humiliation

◆ Revenge

◆ Self-blame

Multiple physical symptoms

◆ Gastrointestinal irritability

◆ Genitourinary discomfort

◆ Muscle tension

◆ Sleep pattern disturbance

Long-Term Phase

◆ Change in residence

◆ Dealing with repetitive nightmares and phobias

◆ Seeking family support

◆ Seeking social network support

RAPE-TRAUMA SYNDROME:

Compound Reaction

(in addition to the defining characteristics for rape-trauma syndrome)

Reactivated symptoms of such previous conditions, such as:

◆ Physical illness

◆ Psychiatric illness

◆ Reliance on alcohol and/or drugs

RAPE-TRAUMA SYNDROME:

Silent Reaction

◆ Abrupt changes in relationship with men

◆ Increase in nightmares

◆ Increased anxiety during interview: e.g., blocking of associations, long periods of silence, minor stuttering, physical distress

◆ Pronounced changes in sexual behavior

◆ No verbalization of the occurrence of rape

◆ Sudden onset of phobic reactions

From *NANDA Nursing Diagnoses: Definitions and Classification 1997–1998,* by North American Nursing Diagnosis Association, 1996, Philadelphia: Author.

thought that date rape could only happen to someone else, until one shattering night, while attending a fraternity party, she was raped. During the rape she expressed concern about her throat being damaged because she was a talented singer:

Prized Possessions

"This has been a truly lovely night, but now I have to go." She said this holding his wrist. He had not moved his hand away.

"How about a good night kiss, then?"

"One," she said, smiling.

"A good one," he responded.

They were still side by side, and as they kissed, he rolled on top of her. Quickly, so quickly and with such force she could not stop him, he moved his hand up under her skirt and inside her panties, his fingers pushing against her pubic hair, his middle finger inside her.

"No, Jimmy!"

She squirmed to get free of him, of his body, of his finger, but he had her pinned by the weight of his body, and she didn't have the arm strength to push him away from her. "You're wet. You're hot and wet for me."

"Jimmy, no! Please!"

He had moved his left arm across her chest to hold her down; his right hand worked at her vagina. She grabbed his wrist and tried to pull his hand away.

"You want it so bad."

"I beg of you—let me up."

"You want it."

"I don't! Stop!"

"You're going to love it. Don't fight it."

He continued to work at her with his finger. She screamed, "Help! Somebody help!"

He went to kiss her and she bit his lip.

"You bitch! You hurt me!"

Angrily, he grasped her throat.

"Help!" she screamed, but he pushed harder against her throat. "Please, don't hurt my throat."

She started to tremble and cry, and in so doing, lost her grip on his wrist, and he took the opportunity to slip his finger inside her again, while keeping the pressure on her throat.

"Don't hurt my throat. Please, Jimmy, my throat!" She called out to him, desperately.

He had the key. As long as he held her throat, she was defenseless. She went rigid with fear.

"You're so wet and hot for me," he murmured as he rubbed her inside and out. "You want it so much."

"No, no, stop. Please!"

While holding her down by the throat, with his free hand he expertly undid his pants and pulled them down.

"Help!" she screamed again.

She tried to punch his face, but she could not get leverage with his weight on her, and he applied more pressure to her throat.

"No, Jimmy, no, please."

"Please make love to me, you're saying."

"Don't!" she gasped.

"I know you really want it."

He pulled down her panties. Wedging his knees between her legs, he pushed them apart, continuing to hold her down by the throat. He was in her.

"You got a good rider here. Best in the west." Slowly he plunged inside her and pulled back and did it again. "In and out. And in and out." She was trembling, tears running down her face. "I'm a top stick man around these parts. How's that baby? And that! And that! And that!"

She remembered the time—she must have been seven; her brother was in a stroller—when her mother and father took her to the carousel in the park. She was wearing a party dress. She had been to a birthday party, and they came for her at the end of the party and walked through the park. Her father lifted her and placed her on the horse, and every time it came around they were standing there, waving, smiles on their faces, warm, loving smiles, and everyone was so happy . . .

"Sexually speaking, you're not a freshman anymore. . . ."

"I'll walk you back."

"You'll walk me back?"

"It's late."

"Why did you rape me?" she screamed, her eyes tearing with rage and despair, her entire body shaking.

"Bullshit!" he said. "I didn't rape you. You wanted it."

(Corman, 1991, pp. 57–59)

---

*Reprinted with the permission of Simon & Schuster from PRIZED POSSESSIONS by Avery Corman. Copyright ©1991 by Avery Corman, Inc.

⚙ *REFLECTIVE THINKING*

Rape

What are your thoughts about Elizabeth's being raped? Do you think she put herself in a vulnerable situation? Can you understand why Jimmy thought she might have wanted to have sex? Do you think he was in a power relationship with Elizabeth? Can you identify any coping strategies Elizabeth used when she was being raped? How do you anticipate she will cope with being raped? How would you feel interviewing Elizabeth? What advice would you give her?

DOMESTIC VIOLENCE

Spousal abuse was legal in the United States until 1824. A law allowed a husband to "chastise his wife with any reasonable instrument." The law was later modified to stipulate that the instrument he used could be "a rod not thicker than his thumb." The women's movement brought the seriousness of domestic violence to the public attention in the 1970s, but the O. J. Simpson arrest in 1994 and subsequent criminal and civil trials brought it from behind closed doors into unprecedented public scrutiny. The case put domestic violence in the national spotlight as never before, with the belief that it must be taken seriously in our homes, communities, and courts (Jezierski, 1994).

Domestic violence (often referred to as spousal/partner abuse or battering syndrome) is defined as intentional violent or controlling behavior by a person who is or has been intimate with the victim(s) and may or may not reside in the same household (Medical Education Group Learning Systems, 1995).

The Violent Crime Control and Law Enforcement Act of 1994 defines domestic violence as a felony or misdemeanor crime of violence committed by a current or former spouse, a person who is cohabiting with or has cohabited with the victim as a spouse, or a person similarly situated to a spouse of the victim under the domestic or family violence laws of that jurisdiction (U.S. Violent Crime Control and Law Enforcement Act of 1994, 1994).

Domestic violence occurs in relationships where intentional or controlling behavior is perpetrated by persons with whom a survivor has had or currently has an intimate relationship. The syndrome may include actual or threatened physical injury, sexual assault, psychological abuse, economic control, and/or progressive isolation (Medical Education Group Learning Systems, 1995).

It is estimated that 95% of abuse incidents are perpetrated by men against women (Jezierski, 1994; NCADV,

1995). The National Coalition Against Domestic Violence (NCADV) reports that at least 4 million women every year are survivors of domestic violence and that every 15 seconds a woman is battered in the United States by her husband, boyfriend, or live-in partner (NCADV, 1995). The National Coalition for the Homeless (NCH) reports that domestic violence is one of the leading causes of homelessness. They estimate that 40% of the sheltered homeless population is made up of abused family members and the majority of those families (in some areas more than 90%) are headed by women (NCH, 1995).

Many women report that they were first beaten when they were pregnant. Nursing research studies estimate that at least 15% of women who are pregnant are abused. Low-birth-weight and preterm infants have been associated with battering during pregnancy (Campbell et al., 1993; Thobaben, 1997).

According to the U.S. Department of Justice, Bureau of Justice Statistics (BJS), wives are the most frequent victims of fatal family violence. In a comprehensive study of more than 8000 homicides in large urban counties, the BJS found that 16% involved murder inside the family. A male was the assailant in about two-thirds of family murders. Most murders occurred at night, and nearly half of the killers had been drinking at the time of the family homicide (U.S. Department of Justice, 1994).

There continues to be debate whether domestic violence is linked to particular cultural or ethnic groups. For example, Kantor et al.'s research on Hispanic American families found that Hispanics (generically) do not significantly differ with Anglo Americans in wife assaults. The exception was that U.S.-born Mexican and Puerto Rican American wives had an increased risk of assaults by their husbands. They found that the presence of norms sanctioning wife assaults within any group, regardless of socioeconomic status, is a risk factor for wife abuse (Kantor, Jasinski, & Aldarondo, 1994).

⑤ RESEARCH HIGHLIGHT

Domestic Violence: Risk Factors and Outcomes

STUDY PROBLEM/PURPOSE

To identify risk factors for victims and perpetrators of domestic violence.

METHODS

Review of data from standardized interviews of 218 women who sought care from an emergency department for injuries due to domestic violence. Both victims and batterers were ethnically heterogeneous. The women ranged from ages 16 to 66. The age of the assailants ranged from 19 to 72 years.

FINDINGS

The victim was related to the batterer as a current or former girlfriend in 51% of cases or as a wife in 42%. The abuse often resulted in severe injury; 28% required admission to a hospital, and 13% required major surgical treatment. The typical presentation was injuries to the face, skull, eyes, extremities, and upper torso. A third of the cases involved a weapon, such as a knife, club, or gun. Ten percent of the women were pregnant and 10% reported that their children had also been abused by the batterer. Eighty-six percent had suffered at least one previous incident of abuse, and about 40% had previously required medical care for abuse.

IMPLICATIONS

Domestic violence occurs without respect to ethnicity or age. Nurses need to be aware of the most common injury sites and weapons used when performing a physical assessment to rule out domestic violence.

From "Domestic Violence: Risk Factors and Outcomes," by D. C. Berrios and D. Grady, 1991, *Western Journal of Medicine, 155*, pp. 133–155.

⑤ RESEARCH HIGHLIGHT

Culture and Domestic Violence

STUDY PROBLEM/PURPOSE

To examine the predictors of domestic violence.

METHODS

A sample of 60 immigrant Latinas, of whom 30 had sought assistance for abuse and 30 had sought other family services. Because of gender role rigidity and the "machismo" ethos highlight of power imbalance between genders, feminist theory suggested some clear and exciting insights into the possible causes of abuse among Latinos.

FINDINGS

The study did not support the hypothesis that a high endorsement of traditionally feminine attributes on the part of the women would result in increased levels of abuse.

IMPLICATIONS

The researchers recommend that more research is needed to understand the environment and dynamics of Latino families and couples, and for this more culturally relative and sensitive instruments must be developed.

From "Culture and Domestic Violence: The Ecology of Abused Latinas," by J. Perilla, R. Bakemann, and F. Norris, 1994, *Violence and Victims, 9*(4), pp. 325–339.

The research on the incidence of battering in gay and lesbian relationships is limited. Studies have indicated that abuse may occur in 25% to 48% of lesbian relationships (Coleman, 1994). It is thought to be underreported due to society's marginalization of gay and lesbian couples, resulting in a "conspiracy of silence." This places an additional burden on closeted gay or lesbian persons who are survivors of battering to disclose their sexual orientation to health professionals and law enforcement officials or family (Lynch & Ferri, 1997).

Domestic violence affects children. Children witness their mothers being abused by their fathers. They hear their mothers scream, crying, sounds of fists hitting flesh, glass breaking, cursing, and so on. They see their mothers' bruises, torn clothes, holes in the walls, and broken furniture. As violence against their mothers becomes more frequent and severe, children experience a 300% increase in physical abuse by their male parent. Studies indicate that these children suffer from anxiety and

depression. They have problems with poor health, low self-esteem, poor impulse control, sleep difficulties, and feelings of powerlessness. They are at risk for sexual acting out, alcohol and other drug abuse, running away from home, and suicide (NCADV, 1995).

Domestic violence occurs in relationships where conflict is the continuous result of power inequality between partners. One of the partners is afraid of and harmed by the other. This should not be confused with domestic arguments that are present in most relationships in which neither partner has more power or control than the other and thus neither is victim or abuser. Domestic arguments can be caused or made worse by many things, such as financial hardship, sexual infidelity, alcohol or other drug use, work pressure, jealousy, and difference in expectations about the relationship (W.I.S.E, 1997a).

Figure 24-1 illustrates the link between behaviors that, when taken together, form a pattern of violence. It shows how each seemingly unrelated behavior is an

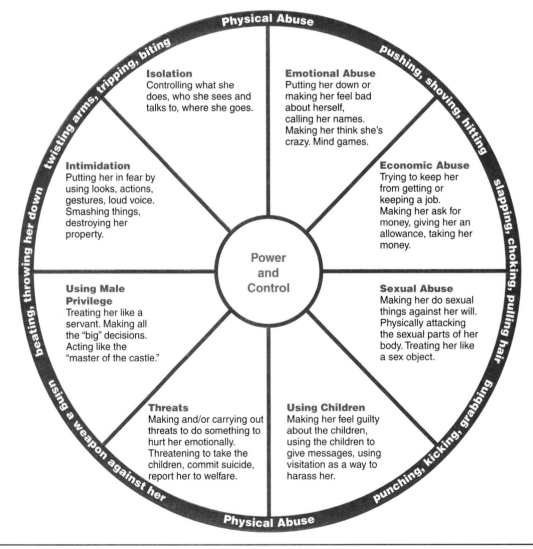

Figure 24-1   The Power and Control Wheel. *Courtesy of Minnesota Program Development, Inc., Domestic Abuse Intervention Project, Duluth, MN.*

important part of one person's overall effort to control another. Power and control are depicted as the axle of a wheel because they are the driving force of the behavior. The spokes are the tactics used by one person to maintain power and control over the other. The circular ring is the pervasive threat of physical harm that holds the wheel together. An example would be a husband who ridicules his wife's religious beliefs, intimidates her with a loud voice, calls her names, does not allow her to have access to their bank account or to visit her friends, makes her do sexual acts against her will, and threatens to take the children if she threatens to leave him.

The following nursery rhyme, published in 1916 but still repeated by children today, gives an illustration of the control one partner can have over the other:

The Pumpkin-Eater

Peter, Peter, pumpkin-eater,
Had a wife and couldn't keep her;
He put her in a pumpkin shell,
And there he kept her very well.

(The Real Mother Goose, *1916, p. 98)*

COMMON CHARACTERISTICS OF BATTERED WOMEN

COMMON CHARACTERISTICS

◆ Have low self-esteem

◆ Believe the myths about battering relationships

◆ Subscribe to the traditional feminine sex-role stereotype

◆ Accept responsibility for the batterer's actions

◆ Feel guilty and ashamed

◆ Deny the anger and terror they feel

◆ Have severe stress reactions and psychosomatic complaints

◆ Use sex as a way to establish intimacy

◆ View themselves as victims and believe no one can help them resolve their problems

◆ Rarely report incidents to the nurse, but instead seek care for psychosomatic conditions

◆ Repeatedly visit the doctor's office or emergency room

HEALTH SYMPTOMS OF BATTERED WOMEN

◆ Soft-tissue injuries to the head, chest, abdomen, buttocks, back

◆ Pain, especially chronic

◆ Psychosomatic complaints—chest pain, abdominal pain, GI disorders, pelvic pain, choking sensations

◆ History of being "accident prone"

◆ History of sexual abuse

◆ History of depression

◆ Self-destructive behavior

◆ Eating disorders

◆ Sleep disturbances

෨ම *REFLECTIVE THINKING*

Domestic Violence in Nursery Rhymes

How do you feel about the spousal relationship described in Peter the Pumpkin-Eater? How do you feel about Peter's isolating his wife? Do you think his wife has equal power in their relationship? What image does this nursery rhyme give children? How would you change it?

COMMON CHARACTERISTICS OF MEN WHO BATTER

◆ Have low self-esteem

◆ Believe the myths about battering relationships

◆ Believe in the stereotyped masculine sex role in the family; believe a woman's place is in the home and that men have the right to control women

◆ Blame others for their own actions

◆ Blame circumstances for their own problems

◆ Are pathologically jealous

◆ React to stress by using alcohol or other drugs and battering; behavior becomes worse when using drugs or alcohol

◆ Use sex as an act of aggression to enhance self-esteem

◆ Believe battering should not have negative consequences

◆ Always ask for a second chance; say they will change, that they will not do it again

◆ May seem charming, gregarious, gentle to nonfamily members

◆ May abuse their children

◆ Exhibit behavior that is unpredictable

There are common characteristics of people involved in domestic violence, both the survivors and the perpetrators. The accompanying displays include the types of personality characteristics that are common to battered women and battering men.

Myths about battering have perpetuated misunderstandings about it. They have been supported by society and often believed by those who are being abused. Table 24-2 describes the common myths associated with domestic violence.

Lenore Walker, a pioneer in the cause of women as survivors of violence, published her initial research in *The Battered Women* in 1979. She developed the Walker Cycle Theory Of Violence, which specifically addresses domestic violence. Her theory is based on Seligman's theory of learned helplessness (refer to Chapter 14, "The Client Experiencing Mood Disorder: Depression"), which helps explain the psychological dynamics of why women stay in abusive relationships. Women learn to become helpless as a result of being abused. They become anxious, depressed, and dependent upon the abuser and believe that they are unable to control or prevent their abuse. Their perception of helplessness becomes a reality.

Walker's theory describes battering as neither random nor constant but rather as occurring in repeated cycles. There is a common pattern of domestic violence. It

Table 24-2   Common Myths about Domestic Violence

MYTH	FACT
Domestic violence does not affect many people. It occurs primarily among those who hang out in bars, are poor, or are people of color.	Domestic violence is the leading cause of injury to women between the ages of 15 and 44 and the second leading cause of injury to women overall. Battering occurs at all levels of society and without regard for age, race, culture, status, education, or religion. It may be less prevalent among the affluent because they can find and afford more resources than the poor. The poor are more likely to come in contact with helping agencies.
Domestic violence does not occur in lesbian relationships since women do not batter other women. Gay and lesbian domestic violence is sadomasochistic sexual behavior; the victims actually like it.	Gay and lesbian partners experience violence for varied but similar reasons as heterosexual partners.
Men are never victims of domestic violence.	It is estimated that at least 5% of men are battered.
Pregnant women are protected against abuse.	Pregnant women are especially vulnerable to abuse and are more likely to suffer miscarriages and to give birth to babies with low birth weights.
Battered women are free to leave a relationship at any time. They can stop the abuse by divorcing or leaving the abuser.	The U.S. Department of Justice estimates that 75% of all spousal attacks occur between people who are separated or divorced. The risk of homicide is highest in the first 2 months after separation. The reasons women remain in relationships are very complex. There are many economic, societal, and emotional factors that operate to make it extremely difficult for a woman to leave her partner.
Battered women are mentally ill; otherwise, they would not remain in abusive relationships. They are masochistic and ask for and enjoy the abuse. They have some personality flaw or inappropriate behavior and deserve to be beaten.	Misconception focuses blame on the women and what could be wrong with them to cause the domestic violence. Women in violent relationships are not more psychiatrically or psychologically disturbed than other women. Many people fail to understand the difficulties faced by women who wish to leave a violent relationship and therefore assume that they stay in an abusive environment because they find pleasure or acceptance of abuse. Women have been socialized to believe that they are responsible for the battering.
Battering is only a momentary loss of temper. Battered women must have done something to deserve a beating.	This is a misconception that allows men to avoid taking responsibility for their acts of violence. Battering is the establishment of control and fear in a relationship through violence and other forms of abuse. The batterer uses acts of violence and a series of behaviors, including intimidation and threats, to coerce and control the other person.

Adapted from Chez, N. (1994). *Peace by Peace at Home.*

involves three phases: the tension-building phase, the acute battering incident, and the loving reconciliation. The first phase is characterized by an escalation of tension with verbal abuse and minor battering incidents. The woman senses the danger and attempts to cope by using techniques that may have been effective in the past. She engages in placating behavior since she is desperately trying to avoid serious incidents. If the house is dirty, she cleans it; she has dinner ready on time; and she tries to control the children's behavior. These tactics work for a while but only reinforce the woman's unrealistic belief that she can control his violent behavior. Because of her low self-esteem, she rationalizes that she is at fault and his behavior is justified. She denies being angry at him, but instead internalizes the anger and experiences depression, anxiety, and a sense of helplessness. She tries to maintain an equilibrium so that his violence will not increase in frequency or severity. She becomes fearful as the incidents increase and worsen over time. She may be reluctant to seek help because she feels ashamed and believes that others will blame her. The batterer knows that his behavior is inappropriate but denies it. He is afraid she will leave him. This increases his rage and his need to control her. This phase may last for weeks or even years, until the tension mounts to the breaking point. During this phase the woman suppresses the knowledge of the impending abuse from her partner.

Phase 2, the acute battering incident, is the outbreak of serious violence, which may last from 2 to 24 hours. The incident that sets off the man's violence may not be known or may be trivial. This often leaves the woman feeling helpless and confused. She may or may not fight back. She is powerless to affect the outcome of the second phase. She may call for help or try to escape. After the battering, she is in a state of shock. She may not even be aware of the seriousness of her injuries and may not get treatment. The batterer discounts the episode and underestimates his partner's injuries. He may not allow her to get medical treatment.

The third phase, often referred to as the honeymoon phase, may begin from a few hours to several days after the acute battering incident. There is a profound sense that the battering is over. The man is contrite and loving and promises to reform. He goes on a campaign to get her back. He may try to help her or take her to the hospital. The woman feels that this is her "real" man, and this behavior restores hope that he will change. She denies the inevitable reoccurrence of the abuse.

The cycle is progressive, and over time, the third phase occurs less often, leaving the woman trapped between the preoutburst tension and the battering episodes. During the tension-building phase the woman's anxiety is high, which often motivates her to seek help.

In the Tennessee Williams play *A Streetcar Named Desire*, Stella experiences the cycle of violence. In this play, conflicts and power struggles develop when Blanche

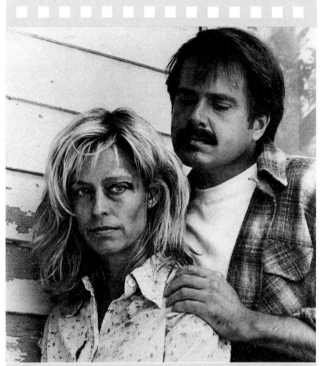

The Burning Bed. Source: NBC/Courtesy Kobal.

The movie *The Burning Bed* portrays the realities of domestic violence. The pattern of repeated cycles is presented, depicting the couple caught in violence, abuse, and family dysfunction.

DuBois visits her sister, Stella Kowalski, and brother-in-law, Stanley Kowalski. Stanley, the main male character, has many of the characteristics of a male batterer. He is controlled by his natural instincts, believes in the stereotypical masculine sex role in the family, is pathologically jealous, reacts to stress by using alcohol and battering, uses sex as an act of aggression to enhance his self-esteem, treats women as sexual objects, and is possessive of his wife and his possessions. Stella had been raised as an educated, refined, and sensitive person but marries a man of a lower class. She has many of the characteristics of a battered woman. She subscribes to the traditionalist sex-role stereotypes, denies being angry at being battered, and uses sex as a way to establish intimacy.

In the third scene, "The Poker Night," Stella is physically abused by Stanley. When Stella and Blanche return home from a show, Stanley is drinking and playing poker with friends. Stella reminds him that it is late, and he swats her on the rear and tells them to go into the other room until the game is over. (They live in a two-bedroom apartment.) Blanche turns on the radio and Stanley tells her to turn it off. He is upset because he is losing money in the poker game. She obeys. A few minutes later Blanche has a conversation with Mitch, one of Stanley's poker friends. She turns the radio on again and begins to waltz to the music to entice Mitch. Stanley is furious and charges into the bedroom and throws the radio out the window. Stella screams at Stanley and tells everyone to go home. Angrily, Stanley charges after Stella. His poker friends feebly tell him to take it easy. Stella reacts by saying:

You lay your hand on me and I'll—
(She backs out of sight. He advances and
disappears. There is a loud blow. Stella cries out.
Blanche screams and runs into the kitchen. The
men rush forward and there is grappling and
cursing. Something is overturned with a crash.)

(Williams, 1947, p. 63)

The men struggle with Stanley to stop him from continuing to physically abuse Stella. They are finally able to subdue him. Stella leaves with her sister to spend the night with her neighbor. When Stanley realizes that Stella has left, he becomes upset and starts screaming for her to return. Stella's neighbor tells him that he cannot beat a woman and then call her back. Within a few minutes, however, Stella returns to him and they have sex.

In scene 4, Blanche confronts Stella about returning to Stanley after being physically assaulted by him. Stella denies the seriousness of it and blames it on Stanley's drinking and the poker game. She describes Stanley as behaving like a lamb when she returned to him and being ashamed of himself. Blanche continues to confront Stella about the abuse by asking her if his remorse makes it all right. Stella tells her that it is not right, but people do it sometimes. Blanche continues to plead with Stella to leave Stanley. Stella tells her that she will not continue talking about it. She tells Blanche:

There are things that happen between a man
and a woman in the dark—that sort of make
everything else seem unimportant.

(Williams, 1947, p. 81)

⊂⊃ *REFLECTIVE THINKING*

Domestic Violence

What characteristics typical of battered women and men who batter do Stella and Stanley have? How would you apply the Walker Cycle Theory Of Violence to Stanley and Stella's relationship? What tactics does Stanley use to try to control Stella? If Stella were your client in the emergency room because of injuries caused by domestic violence, what thoughts would you have about her situation? How do you feel about working with women who endanger their lives and their children's by remaining in abusive relationships?

In scene 10, Stanley rapes Blanche while Stella is in the hospital delivering their baby. In scene 11, Stella is out of the hospital and Blanche tells her that Stanley has raped her. Stella tells one of her friends that she could not believe Blanche and continue living with Stanley. Her friend tells her:

Don't ever believe it. Life has got to go on. No
matter what happens, you've got to keep on going.

(Williams, 1947, p. 166)

As of March 1994, all but five states have laws that, to varying extents, require nurses to report cases of domestic violence. Most states have general laws that mandate health care providers report incidents when the injuries are caused by weapons (gun, knife, or other deadly weapon). Each state's statute has its definitions of terms, such as what constitutes "violence," "weapon," or "grave" injury, and when a health professional is mandated to report (Hyman, Schillinger, & Lo, 1995). Mandatory reporting laws have relieved some battered clients of the onus of reporting the batterers. However, some battered women are reluctant to seek medical care because they are afraid to admit their injuries have been caused by

✱ NURSING TIP

Exit Plan for Battered Women

A battered woman should have a carefully planned exit plan when she anticipates leaving a violent relationship. Advise her to do the following ahead of time:

◆ If injured, go to the emergency department or call the police.

◆ Know exactly where to go, how to get there, and arrange for transportation.

◆ Take house, car, and office keys.

◆ Obtain copies of medical records to help when filing charges with the district attorney's office (restraining orders, assault charges).

◆ Store clothes, toilet articles, medications, children's favorite toys, and so on, at a family member's or friend's house.

◆ Take identification, divorce papers, insurance papers, and any other legal papers that might be needed.

◆ Take the children's birth certificates and social security cards, and school records.

◆ Bring money, bankbooks, credit cards, and other important financial records.

From *Domestic Violence: The Facts*, by Peace At Home, Inc., 1995, Boston, MA: Author.

abuse. They are ashamed or fear their partners will retaliate against them. They are also reluctant to call the police because they do not believe it will help their situation or they fear retaliation from their partners after the police leave or the abusers are released from jail. When nurses are required to report abused women to law enforcement, they should inform clients of their legal obligations and try to ensure the women's safety.

Women' s safety may be in jeopardy as soon as their partners learn that their relationships may end. Women who leave their batterers are at 75% greater risk of being killed by the batterer than those who stay. Leaving requires a strategic plan and legal intervention to avert separation violence and to safeguard the woman and her children (NCADV, 1995).

Nurses must consider domestic violence when the assessment of the client includes injuries to the face, breasts, abdomen, and buttocks; nonspecific psychosomatic complaints; history of frequent injuries; old and new injuries; abdominal injuries during pregnancy; spontaneous abortion; and missed appointments. Women who are depressed, have low self-esteem, sleep disturbances, hypervigilance, and substance abuse may be suffering from domestic violence (Lynch & Ferri, 1997). Denial is the most common coping mechanism used by battered women. They deny the impending abuse, severity of injuries, and possibility of death. They may suffer from *anxiety* (NANDA) and Acute Stress Disorder (DSM-IV), or *post-trauma response* (NANDA) and Post-Traumatic Stress Disorder (DSM-IV). They may have also been raped and have the symptoms of *rape-trauma syndrome* (NANDA). Refer to displays later in this chapter for lists of the symptoms associated with these diagnoses.

Treatment for domestic violence begins with the nurse's conveying support and concern for the woman's predicament. The nurse should acknowledge the violence and inform the battered woman that the violence is illegal and not her fault. Her safety should be assessed. She should be provided with information about community resources and asked if she has a safe place to go.

It is not predictable when women will leave violent relationships. They are more likely to leave or seek assistance if some of the following circumstances exist (Carpenito, 1997, p. 285):

- They have been in the relationship for less than 5 years.
- Violence is frequent and severe and there is a sudden increase.
- They believe their situation will not improve.
- Emotional bonds with their partners have deteriorated.
- Injuries become visible or are witnessed by others.
- They are employed.
- They can confide in family or friends.

✦ NURSING TIP

Reasons Women Remain in Abusive Relationships

Women may choose to remain in abusive relationships because they (Hyman, Schilllinger, & Lo, 1995):

- Hope that the abuser will reform and that the abuse will stop
- Have no place to go and lack knowledge of community resources available to help them
- Believe children need their father or a two-parent family
- Have family, friends, and neighbors who are reluctant or refuse to help them or have isolated themselves from their families
- Believe that battering is normal for couples
- Are financially dependent or lack financial resources
- Fear the unknown
- Feel that divorce is shameful or against their religious beliefs
- Feel emotionally dependent on the abuser
- Fear reprisal from the abuser, including fear for her life and her children's lives

---

- Others identify their relationships as abusive and unjustified.
- They are knowledgeable of resources, such as shelters.

Domestic violence is complex without simple solutions for the survivors. Nurses can play a significant role in detecting domestic violence. Nursing interventions can make a critical difference in the lives of people who are battered.

ELDER ABUSE

Elder abuse became nationally recognized in 1981 after the House Select Committee on Aging issued its landmark report "Elder Abuse: An Examination of a Hidden Problem." The committee found that elder abuse was simply "alien to the American ideal." Because it is such a difficult concept to come to grips with, even the abused elderly are reluctant to admit their loved ones have abused them. The committee conducted a national study after receiving a letter about a paraplegic 80-year-old woman who had been sexually abused by her son-in-law. The letter stated that the son-in-law would threaten his mother-in-law with a hammer if she refused

☼ RESEARCH HIGHLIGHT

1981 National Study of Elder Abuse

STUDY PROBLEM/PURPOSE

To study the incidence and forms of elder abuse and effectiveness of state efforts.

METHODS

Questionnaire was mailed to the state Human Services Departments.

FINDINGS

Elder abuse was far from an isolated incident affecting only a few frail elderly and their pathological offspring. The victims of elder abuse were most likely to be women age 75 or older. The victims were generally in a position of dependency, that is, having to rely on others for care and protection. Physical violence, neglect, and financial abuse were the most common forms of abuse, followed by the abrogation of basic constitutional rights and psychological abuse. The profile of the abuser was a family member experiencing great stress. Alcoholism or other drug addictions, marital problems, and long-term financial difficulties all were factors that contributed to bringing the person to abuse his or her loved one. The son of the victim was the most likely abuser, followed by the daughter of the victim, and in many cases these adult children had been abused by the parent as a child. The state statutes were inadequate to fully meet the needs of the abused elderly.

IMPLICATIONS

The study highlighted the fact that research on elder abuse was in its infancy and needed to be expanded so that the problem could be addressed on a national level.

From *Elder Abuse (An Examination of a Hidden Problem)*, by U.S. House of Representatives, Select Committee on Aging, April 3, 1981, Washington, DC: U.S. Government Printing Office, Comm. Pub. No. 97-277.

☼ RESEARCH HIGHLIGHT

1990 National Study of Elder Abuse

STUDY PROBLEM/PURPOSE

To determine the nation's effectiveness in coming to grips with this national tragedy, the U.S. House of Representative's Committee on Aging, Subcommittee on Health and Long-Term Care, conducted another study of elder abuse a decade later.

METHODS

Questionnaire was mailed to the state Human Services Departments.

FINDINGS

The study found that the abuse of the elderly is increasing nationally. It is estimated that 5% of the nation's elderly may be victims of abuse from moderate to severe by family members or caregivers. This means about 1 out of every 20 older Americans, or more than 1.5 million persons, may be victims each year. The subcommittee found that elder abuse is far less likely to be reported than child abuse. It estimated that only 1 in 8 cases of elder abuse is reported, whereas 1 of 3 cases of child abuse is reported.

From *Elder Abuse: A Decade of Shame and Inaction*, by U.S. House of Representatives, Select Committee on Aging, Subcommittee on Health and Long-Term Care, April 1990, Washington, DC: U.S. Government Printing Office, Comm. Pub. No. 101-752.

◆ **Physical abuse** is conduct of violence that results in bodily harm or mental stress. It includes a spectrum of violence ranging from assault to murder.

◆ **Passive physical abuse**, or negligence, is conduct that is careless and a breach of duty that results in injury to the person or is a violation of rights. It includes the withholding of medication, medical treatment, food, and personal care necessary for the well-being of the elderly person.

◆ **Financial abuse** involves the theft or conversion of money or anything of value belonging to the elderly by their relatives or caregivers.

◆ **Psychological abuse** includes simple name calling and verbal assaults to a protracted and systematic effort to dehumanize the elderly, sometimes with the goal of driving the elderly to insanity or suicide. Psychological abuse usually exists in combination with one or more other abuses.

◆ **Sexual abuse** is threat of sexual assault or actual sexual battery, rape, incest, sodomy, oral copulation, penetration of genital or anal opening by a foreign object, coerced nudity, and sexually explicit photographing.

his sexual advances. The abuse had been going on for 6 years and was not likely to be reported by the elderly woman out of fear for her life (U.S. House of Representatives, 1990). The two accompanying Research Highlights give the findings of the 1981 House Select Committee on Aging's research on elder abuse and their follow-up study in 1990.

The House Select Committee on Aging (1981) defined the following types of elder abuse in their report *Elder Abuse (An Examination of a Hidden Problem)*: physical, passive physical, financial, psychological, sexual, and violation of rights.

Adult Children Who Abuse or Neglect Their Parents

The research highlights on elder abuse documented that some children abuse and neglect their parents. Family members are expected to care for elderly family members longer than in the past because of the ever-increasing life span. Yet, rarely are they prepared to cope with the long-term care of family members who have chronic and disabling conditions. There are limited options available for helping the abused elderly and the abuser.

Reflect on the following passage from the Old Testament. What are your thoughts about this passage when you think about children abusing their parents? Moses called together all the people of Israel and told them that the Lord our God had made a covenant, not only with our fathers but with all of us who are living today. He told them to listen to all the laws (the Ten Commandments) and learn them and obey them.

Deuteronomy 5:16

Honor thy father and thy mother, as the Lord thy God hath commanded thee; that thy days may be prolonged, and that it may go well with thee, in the land which the Lord thy God giveth thee.

(Holy Bible, *1913, p. 225*)

◆ **Violation of rights** occurs when the inalienable rights conferred by the U.S. Constitution and federal statutes are violated by a family member or caregiver. It includes such rights as not to have one's property taken without due process, the right to adequate appropriate medical treatment, and the right to freedom of assembly, speech, and religion (U.S. House of Representatives, 1981, pp. 3, 6, 13, 24, 26).

Elder abuse is grossly underreported. Abuse identification is rarely straightforward unless there is outright battering, and even then other excuses may be offered. Denial is often the first reaction to reports of abuse by the client, family, and nurses and other health care providers. Some nurses may never have had any education about the dynamics of family violence so they may find it difficult to believe that their older clients are being abused by family members. They may not detect that abuse is occurring since abused elders or their perpetrators rarely seek outside help or support specifically for abuse. They may have had a long-term relationship with the victims and their families and are unwilling to recognize the presence of abuse or neglect in these caregiving situations.

Abused elderly rarely report that they are being abused by family members. It remains hidden under the shroud of family secrecy. They may not want to jeopardize their current living situation because they are physically and/or financially dependent on their family. They may fear that if they report it, they will incite retaliation or be placed in a skilled nursing facility or other out-of-home facility. They may be ashamed that a family member that they had nurtured is abusing them. They believe they deserve the abuse because in the past they had been abusive to the family member who is abusing them. They may be isolated and feel hopeless or helpless about their situation and have no one to turn to for help.

Legislation

There is no federal legislation to protect elders from abuse, neglect, or exploitation. Forty-eight states, including the District of Columbia, have laws that offer some form of protection for the elderly or dependent adults. Adult abuse and protection laws are based on the legal premise that society (represented by the state) has the authority to act in a parental capacity for persons who are unable to care for and protect themselves and thus prevent them from suffering from abuse, neglect, or exploitation by those responsible for their care or from self-abuse. The purposes of adult protection service laws are to facilitate the identification of functionally impaired elders who are being abused, neglected, or exploited by others; to encourage expeditious reporting; and to extend protective services while protecting the rights of the abused. In most states, the adult protective services agency (APS) is the principal public agency that is designated to receive and investigate allegations of elder abuse and neglect. In most jurisdictions, the county departments of social services maintain the APS unit (Thobaben, 1989).

Forty-two states have adopted mandatory reporting provisions as part of their adult protective service statutes. Nurses need to be familiar with their state's laws, since there is wide variation. Intervening in cases of elder abuse will depend on whether clients accept assistance and if they are competent or incompetent. If they are incompetent and judged so by legal action, conservators or guardians can be appointed who have a legal right to make decisions on their behalf. If the conservators or legal guardians are abusing them, then legal action can be taken against them and the clients can be removed from their control. Competent clients are considered capable of making their own decisions and have a legal right to refuse health care. Incompetent clients can have interventions imposed upon them and be removed from an unsafe environment.

COMMON CHARACTERISTICS OF ABUSE OF ELDERS

PHYSICAL ABUSE AND NEGLECT

- Unexplained bruises and welts in various stages of healing, on the face, torso, arms, back, buttocks, thighs, clustered on the trunk, hidden under the breasts or on other areas of the body normally covered by clothing
- Unexplained burns, such as cigarette, especially on the soles, palms, back, buttocks; immersion, patterned, or rope burns
- Unexplained fractures to the skull or face in various stages of healing or multiple or spiral fractures
- Unexplained sprains, dislocations, and internal injuries or bleeding
- Sexual abuse, rape, copulation, incest: difficulty walking or sitting; unexplained STD; unexplained vaginal or anal bleeding; pain or itching in genital areas; torn, stained, or bloody underclothing; bruises around the breasts or genital area; cuts, lacerations, puncture wounds; elder's report of being sexually assaulted or raped
- Missing hair patches
- Dehydration and/or malnourishment without illness-related cause
- Inadequate or inappropriate administration of medication, over- or undermedication (chemical restraint), laboratory findings of medication overdose or underutilization of prescribed drugs
- Eye problems, retinal detachment
- Poor skin hygiene, decubiti, inappropriate clothing, fecal/urine smell, dirty, lice on person
- Constantly soiled clothing or bed
- Lack of necessary medical supplies, necessary appliances such as walkers, bedside commodes
- Restraint bruises or rope burns
- Locked in bedroom
- Lack of necessities—such as heat, food, water—and unsafe conditions
- Living in unsanitary and unclean living conditions (e.g., fleas, lice)
- Elder reports of being mistreated, hit, slapped, or kicked

PSYCHOLOGICAL ABUSE

- Sleep disturbance
- Being worried, anxious

- Seeming irritable, easily upset
- Change in eating habits
- Loss of interest in usual activities
- Fear of retribution
- Suicidal talk, wishes
- Frequent crying
- Extreme withdrawal
- Hesitation to talk openly, nonresponsiveness
- Displaying confusion or disorientation
- Displaying anger
- Denial
- Unusual behavior usually attributed to dementia (e.g., rocking, sucking)
- Elder reports of being verbally or emotionally mistreated

FINANCIAL ABUSE

- Sudden changes in bank account or banking practices, unusual activity in bank accounts, checks or other documents signed when the elder adult cannot write, the inclusion of additional names on an elder's bank signature card, unauthorized withdrawal of the elder's funds using the elder's ATM card
- Power of attorney given when the person is unable to comprehend the financial situation
- Discovery that an elder's signature was forged for financial transactions and for the titles of his or her possessions
- Abrupt changes in a will or other financial documents when the person is clearly incapable of making a will
- Elder's report of financial exploitation

CAREGIVER

- Treats the elderly person like an infant or gives the person the "silent treatment"
- Refuses to spend money on the care of the elder, with numerous unpaid bills and overdue bills, when family member is supposed to be paying the bills

Continued

Common Characteristics of Abuse of Elders, *continued*

- Refuses to buy the elderly person basic amenities (personal grooming items, appropriate clothing when the estate can well afford it)
- Has possession of elderly person's stolen personal belongings such as silverware and jewelry
- Refuses to allow visitors to see an elder alone and does not give the elderly an opportunity to speak
- Appears indifferent toward the elder

- Blames the elder (e.g., for being incontinent)
- Acts aggressive toward the elder (e.g., threatens, insults)
- Has a history of abusive behavior
- Gives conflicting accounts of incidents
- Inappropriately displays affection, flirtation, coyness (may indicate an inappropriate sexual relationship)

From *Elder and Dependent Adult Abuse Humboldt County Guidelines for Mandated Reporters*, by M. Thobaben, 1995, Eureka, CA: Northcoast Advocacy Services.

It can be difficult for nurses and other health professionals to interrupt an abusive cycle, but if they detect abusive situations sooner, interventions can be provided earlier. For nurses to be able to identify and intervene in cases of elder abuse, they must be able to recognize the common characteristics of abuse of elders. The accompanying display lists the common indicators of abuse of elders. The following is an actual case:

A woman in Missouri, age 77, who had suffered a recent stroke and was bedridden was left in the care of her only son, who was in his early 40s and on welfare. The son was a diabetic and suffered from asthma. The two people lived in a rowhouse confining themselves to the top floor bedrooms, cooking on a hot plate, and washing in the bathtub. Since the son had 20 to 30 cats, the house was extremely filthy and filled with cat feces. Although many agencies tried to intervene, the occupants would permit no one to visit or clean the house. The son was married about four or five years although he intimated that the marriage was never consummated. The daughter-in-law, who had since remarried, still visited her mother-in-law. The son owned two or three motorcycles and had an extensive gun collection plus a room full of World War II mementos. Occasionally, he worked as a drummer in a nightclub and was frequently known to become drunk and violent. He had often beaten his mother, who would contact the police when he did so. The police, who were aware of the family situation, were often able to calm the son. At other times, he threatened to kill her and stated he wished she were dead. Although she was frequently ill and required constant care, she had virtually no privacy. Health aides sent to the house were threatened by physical violence by the son and were afraid to return.

(U.S. House of Representatives, 1981, p. 29)

꩜ *REFLECTIVE THINKING*

Elder Abuse in the Home

How would you feel if you were requested to make a home visit to this family? Could you avoid blaming the son for abusing his mother? How would you know whether you had to report this situation to adult protective services? If you continued to make home visits to this family, how would you prioritize your nursing care?

NURSING PERSPECTIVES ON ABUSE AND NEGLECT

Nursing theories assist nurses in planning care for clients who are survivors of interpersonal violence and sexual assaults. The self-care deficit theory and crisis theory are especially helpful in planning nursing care for abused and neglected clients and rape survivors.

Self-Care Deficit Theory

As explained in Chapter 3, "Use of Theory as a Basis for Practice," and Chapter 14, "The Client Experiencing a Mood Disorder," Orem's (1991) Self-Care Deficit Theory views nurses' work as doing for the client that which he cannot do for himself. Clients who experience interpersonal abuse and sexual assaults are often in a crisis and unable to do for themselves. They may have severe physical injuries and psychological problems, such as depression and anxiety. They may need assistance in performing self-care activities that preserve and promote their health, life, and state of well-being. The ability of clients to provide for their own self-care activities Orem calls self-care agency. An abused or sexually assaulted client is likely to experience self-care deficit when the therapeutic self-care demand exceeds the clients' self-care agency. Nursing interventions are an appropriate way to address clients' self-care demands until they are able to take over that function for themselves. The nursing goal is to achieve clients' self-care agency by facilitating recovery from self-care deficit and promoting self-care ability. This involves the nurse's directly assisting the client to meet health care needs and enhancing the client's ability to carry on effectively without nursing intervention.

Crisis Intervention Theory

Interpersonal violence and sexual assaults often create a crisis for clients. (Refer to Chapter 9, "The Client Undergoing Crisis," for an in-depth explanation of the nature of crisis.) Crisis theory is a practical theory to use with clients experiencing a crisis. Aguilera (1994) has identified specific steps involved in the techniques of crisis intervention. Clients generally remain in treatment for 1 to 6 weeks.

The first phase is the assessment of the client and his problem. It includes an accurate assessment of the precipitating event and the resulting crisis that brought the client to seek professional help. If the client is a high suicidal risk, then a referral is made for consideration of hospitalization.

The second phase is the planning of therapeutic interventions. This phase is designed to restore the client to at least his precrisis level of equilibrium. The nurse needs to determine when the crisis occurred. Clients often do not seek help for 1 to 2 weeks after the crisis but may do so within the first 24 hours. The nurse needs to assess the extent to which the crisis has disrupted the client's life. She should assess his strengths, coping skills used successfully in the past but not being used presently, alternative coping skills that are not presently being used, and his support system. The effect the crisis is having on the client's significant others also needs to be assessed.

The third phase involves the nursing interventions, which include helping the client gain an understanding of the crisis and get in touch with his feelings, examining alternative ways of coping, and helping him utilize his support system.

The last phase is resolution of the crisis and anticipatory planning. The nurse assists the client in making realistic plans for the future and discusses ways in which the present experience may help in coping with future crises (Aguilera, 1994, pp. 20–21).

Orem's Self-Care Theory and Aguilera's Crisis Theory are complementary and ideal to use with clients who are survivors of interpersonal abuse and sexual assault. They promote self-reliance and advocate empowering clients to resolve their problems.

Nursing Responsibilities

To begin to adequately provide care to survivors of interpersonal abuse, nurses first need to deal with their own feelings and beliefs about it. It can take nurses time to work through their own thoughts and beliefs about interpersonal violence and sexual assault. They need to identify any stereotypical beliefs that they may have about abuse survivors and abusers. They need to become comfortable asking clients if they have been abused. They need to avoid "rescuer fantasies" that may interfere with their ability to assess the real needs of survivors and their families.

Nurses need to be knowledgeable about the dynamics of interpersonal violence. They need to keep in mind that the client they are caring for, regardless of the setting, may be in an abusive relationship. They need to develop skill in identifying survivors of interpersonal abuse and in working as a member of an interdisciplinary team.

Nurses need to know their state's legal requirements for reporting clients who are survivors of interpersonal violence and the specific requirements in their communities and agencies. Failure by a registered nurse to report actual or suspected abuse of clients of any age may constitute unprofessional conduct within the meaning of their state's Nursing Practice Act. In California, for example, the Board of Registered Nursing is mandated to take disciplinary action against registered nurses found guilty of unprofessional conduct, which includes the conviction of any offense substantially related to the functions and duties of a registered nurse (CABRN, 1996).

Nurses and other health professionals are mandated to report children who have experienced interpersonal violence and sexual assault to law enforcement or child protective services. If an adult client has been sexually assaulted, the report is made to law enforcement. In most states, if elderly clients are physically or sexually abused, a report is made to law enforcement or adult protective services.

In 1992 the Joint Commission on the Accreditation of Healthcare Organizations (JCAHO) adopted standards that require emergency and ambulatory care units to have written protocols regarding examining and treating clients who experience interpersonal violence and sexual assault. They must train their personnel in the criteria used to obtain client consent, identification of abused clients, and how to document the abuse in the clients' medical records. They must also educate their staff in the legal obligations of handling clients' evidentiary material and notifying and releasing evidence to the law enforcement officials. They must maintain and provide to victims a list of private and community family violence service agencies (Capezuti, Yurkow, & Goldberg, 1996).

All health care agencies need to educate nurses about the dynamics of interpersonal abuse. Survivors of abuse seek treatment not only for their immediate injuries but also for the health problems that result from interpersonal violence, such as stress-related illnesses (anxiety, sleep disturbance) and chronic health care problems (Campbell et al., 1993).

N U R S I N G   P R O C E S S

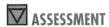 ## ASSESSMENT

There is no comprehensive assessment tool that offers conclusive evidence that interpersonal violence has occurred. Nurses will need to act like detectives when assessing clients, since clients or their abusers will rarely admit to abuse or violence. They will need to make direct observations of the client and family members. For example, does the child seem afraid of the caregiver? Does the caregiver hit the child? These observations are clues that more probing is necessary.

In order to properly assess survivors of abuse, nurses need to know the symptoms that are commonly seen in interpersonal violence and sexual assaults and the common characteristics of the abusers. Many of the symptoms are subjective, so the nurse and the health care team will need to piece together the evidence to determine if interpersonal violence has occurred or if clients are at risk for violence. Psychological abuse is a particularly difficult area to assess, as emotional relationships are very culture bound and words and emotions that may be harmful in one family are not necessarily so in another family.

The interview provides an opportunity for nurses to question clients about interpersonal violence. The type of questions the nurse asks survivors of interpersonal violence or sexual assault will depend upon the age of the survivor, the suspected type of abuse, and the situation.

Nurses will need to do a more extensive examination when the history or behavioral symptoms indicate

---

✴ NURSING TIP

Caring for the Abused Client

When questioning clients about the possibility of interpersonal violence or sexual assault, you need to quickly develop a rapport with clients and create an environment that indicates that their personal experiences are acceptable topics to discuss. This allows them an opportunity to express their fears and concerns. You can do this by:

- Treating them with dignity and concern
- Giving priority to them over nonemergency clients
- Placing them in quiet and private areas
- Not leaving them alone
- Speaking quietly in a nonjudgmental manner
- Using active and empathic listening skills
- Not acting shocked or surprised at the details of their experiences
- Reassuring them that it was not their fault
- Explaining any delays in treatment
- Asking permission to call family members, friends, or in the case of rape, rape crisis advocates
- Providing information about community resources

✴ NURSING TIP

Interviewing the Survivor of Abuse or Violence

The type of questions will depend upon the type of violence and whether survivors have told you they have been abused. If they have told you they have been abused, then you need to ask specific questions about the abuse. If they have not, then you need to ask more open-ended questions to allow them to disclose sensitive information to you. Generally speaking:

- Inform the client that it is necessary to ask some very personal questions.
- Use language appropriate for the age and developmental level of the survivor.
- Use conversational language or street language.
- Keep questions simple, nonthreatening, and direct.
- Pose questions in a manner that permits brief answers.
- Indicate sensitivity to and acceptance of the client's state of confusion.
- Avoid using leading statements that can distort the client's report.
- Do not criticize the client's family.
- Do not promise not to report the abuse; indicate you are required by law to report the abuse.

SAMPLE INTERACTIONS FOR CLIENTS INVOLVED IN ABUSE

CHILD

- "Who in your family has a bad temper?"
- "How does your mother/father act when he/she is (name a behavior, e.g., drinking)?"
- "Have you ever been hit with an object?" Do not focus on who is the abuser.
- "How do your parents punish you?"

ABUSING CAREGIVER

- "How do you discipline your child?"
- "What do you do when your child drives you crazy?"
- "What do you do when something is bothering you?"

ELDERS

- "Describe your relationship with your family."
- "Sometimes children (spouses) become frustrated taking care of their parents (wife) and do things they regret. Has this happened to you? Can you tell me about it?"
- "Have you ever been hit, kicked, or punched?"

DOMESTIC VIOLENCE

- "Describe your relationship with your partner."
- "Are you afraid of your partner?"
- "Are there situations where you feel unsafe?"
- "Did this injury arise as a result of someone's hitting or pushing you?"
- "Do you have a plan if your partner becomes abusive?"

SEXUAL ASSAULT SURVIVOR

- "Can you tell me what your attacker did to you?"

NURSE COMMENT TO THE SURVIVOR OF ABUSE

- "I am concerned about you."
- "(Name type of abuse) is never an acceptable behavior." Or "(Abuse) is illegal."
- "You are not to blame."

From Anderson (1995) and Feiner (1994).

⚡ NURSING ALERT!

Indicators of Abuse

When interviewing the client and family you need to be alert for behavioral signs of abuse, such as:

- A delay in seeking medical care and why the delay occurred
- An injury pattern inconsistent with the supposed cause of injury
- Inconsistent or suspicious explanations offered by the family members and the client, for example, "I fell down the stairs" or "He fell out of his crib"
- Discrepancies between what the client and the family members give in regard to dates, times, and causes of the injury or illness
- Interactions between clients and family members that indicate conflict might exist (caregiver screams at the child, blaming him for the injury)

✦ NURSING TIP

Documenting Interpersonal Violence and Sexual Assault Situations

Because interpersonal violence is a crime, the health care records of the victims can be subpoenaed and displayed in court. Medical and nursing records should *not* include any summary statements, inferences, or conclusions about the circumstances of the assault. The interpersonal violence or sexual assault should be carefully documented by including:

- The history of the incident that led to the injury or illness
- Conversations with client and family (if present) in exact quotes when possible
- Documentation that accurately reflects the extent of the force that was used
- Photographs of the client's physical injuries
- Specific and factual observations, not interpretations
- An objective evaluation of the findings of the injury or illness

interpersonal abuse. Clients will need to have physical examinations to assess the extent of their injuries and to collect forensic evidence to prove who assaulted them. A traumagram, or body map (a drawing of the front and back of a nude human figure), is generally used by the nurse or physician to mark on the figure the location of all visible injuries. Each state has legally mandated procedures for collecting evidentiary material, and nurses need to be sure that the legal "chain of evidence" pertaining to collection of forensic samples is unbroken. The medical record should document the injuries and nursing and medical treatment that may serve as legal evidence of the client's condition. Nurses need to know their state's requirements and their agency's protocol for collecting and documenting evidence (AMA, Oct. 1995b).

▽ NURSING DIAGNOSIS

When clients are seen soon after experiencing interpersonal violence or sexual assault, their nursing and medical examinations can add to their trauma. They may be experiencing *anxiety* (NANDA) and Acute Stress Disorder (DSM-IV) that may interfere with ability to cooperate with the nursing and medical examinations. They can disrupt the client's cognitive perceptions, rendering memory of events incomplete or inaccurate. If they are examined several weeks to months after the assaults, they may be experiencing symptoms of *post-trauma response* (NANDA) and Post-Traumatic Stress Disorder (DSM-IV). The accompanying displays list the symptoms associated with these diagnoses.

Other nursing diagnoses that may be applicable for clients who suffer from interpersonal violence or sexual assault will depend upon their injuries. The accompanying display lists NANDA nursing diagnoses that may be applicable in abusive cases.

NANDA CHARACTERISTICS OF ANXIETY

A vague, uneasy feeling exists whose source is often nonspecific or unknown to the individual. The defining characteristics are as follows:

SUBJECTIVE

Increased tension; apprehension; painful and persistent increased helplessness; uncertainty; fearful; scared; regretful; overexcited; rattled; distressed; jittery; feelings of inadequacy; shakiness; fear of unspecific consequences; expressed concerns due to change in life events; worried; anxious

OBJECTIVE

Sympathetic stimulation-cardiovascular excitation; superficial vasoconstriction; pupil dilation; restlessness; insomnia; glancing about; poor eye contact; trembling/hand tremors; extraneous movement (foot shuffling, hand/arm movements); facial tension; voice quivering; focus on self; increased wariness; increased perspiration

From *NANDA Nursing Diagnoses: Definitions and Classification 1997–1998*, by North American Nursing Diagnosis Association, 1996, Philadelphia: Author.

DSM-IV CRITERIA FOR ACUTE STRESS DISORDER

1. This disturbance lasts for a minimum of 2 days and a maximum of 4 weeks and occurs within 4 weeks of the traumatic event. Either while experiencing or after experiencing the distressing event, the individual has three (or more) of the following dissociative symptoms:

   ◆ A subjective sense of numbing, detachment, or absence of emotional responsiveness

   ◆ A reduction in awareness of his or her surroundings (e.g., "being in a daze")

   ◆ Derealization

   ◆ Depersonalization

   ◆ Dissociative amnesia (i.e., inability to recall an important aspect of the trauma)

2. The traumatic event is persistently reexperienced in at least one of the following ways:

   ◆ Recurrent images, thoughts dreams, illusions, flashbacks episodes, or a sense of reliving the experience

   ◆ Distress on exposure to reminders of the traumatic event

3. There is marked avoidance of stimuli that arouse recollections of the trauma (e.g., thoughts, feelings, conversations, activities, places, people).

4. There are marked symptoms of anxiety or increased arousal (e.g., difficulty sleeping, irritability, poor concentration, hypervigilance, exaggerated startle response, motor restlessness).

5. The disturbance causes clinically significant distress or impairment in the social, occupational, or other important areas of functioning or impairs the individual's ability to pursue some necessary task, such as obtaining necessary assistance or mobilizing personal resources by telling family members about the traumatic experience.

Reprinted with permission from the *Diagnostic and Statistical Manual of Mental Disorders*, Fourth Edition. Copyright 1994. American Psychiatric Association.

NANDA CHARACTERISTICS OF POST-TRAUMA RESPONSE

An individual experiences a sustained painful response to overwhelming traumatic event(s). The defining characteristics are as follows:

MAJOR CHARACTERISTICS

The characteristics include the reexperience of the traumatic event, which may be identified in cognitive, affective, and/or sensory motor activities, including:

◆ Flashbacks

◆ Intrusive thoughts

◆ Repetitive dreams or nightmares

◆ Excessive verbalization of the traumatic event

◆ Verbalization of survival guilt or guilt about behavior required for survival

MINOR CHARACTERISTICS

Psychic/emotional numbness:

◆ Impaired interpretation of reality

◆ Confusion

◆ Dissociation or amnesia

◆ Vagueness about a traumatic event

◆ Constricted affect

Altered lifestyle, self-destructiveness, such as:

◆ Substance abuse

◆ Suicide attempt or other acting-out behavior

◆ Difficulty with interpersonal relationship

◆ Development of phobia regarding trauma

◆ Poor impulse control/irritability

◆ Explosiveness

From *NANDA Nursing Diagnoses: Definitions and Classification 1997–1998*, by North American Nursing Diagnosis Association, 1996, Philadelphia: Author.

DSM-IV CRITERIA FOR POST-TRAUMATIC STRESS DISORDER

1. The duration of the disturbance is more than 1 month, and the disturbance causes clinically significant distress or impairment of important social, occupational, or other important areas of functioning. The symptoms may be acute or chronic or with delayed onset.

2. The person has been exposed to a traumatic event in which both of the following are present:

◆ The person experienced, witnessed, or was confronted with an event or events that involved actual or threatened death or serious injury or a threat to the physical integrity of self or others.

◆ The person's response involved intense fear, helplessness, or horror. In children, this may be expressed instead by disorganized or agitated behavior.

3. The traumatic event is persistently reexperienced in one (or more) of the following ways:

◆ Recurrent and intrusive distressing recollections of the event, including images, thoughts, or perceptions. In young children, repetitive play may occur in which themes or aspects of the trauma are expressed.

◆ Recurrent distressing dreams of the event. In children, there may be frightening dreams without recognizable content.

◆ Acting or feeling as if the traumatic event were recurring (includes a sense of reliving the experience, illusions, hallucinations, and dissociative flashback episodes, including those that occur on awakening or when intoxicated).

◆ Intense psychological distress at exposure to internal or external cues that symbolize or resemble an aspect of the traumatic event.

◆ Physiological reactivity on exposure to internal or external cues that symbolize or resemble an aspect of the traumatic event.

4. Persistent avoidance of stimuli associated with the trauma and numbing of general responsiveness (not present before the trauma) as indicated by three (or more) of the following:

◆ Efforts to avoid thoughts, feelings, or conversations associated with the trauma

◆ Efforts to avoid activities, places, or people that arouse recollections of the trauma

◆ Inability to recall an important aspect of the trauma

Continued

DMS-IV Criteria for Post-Traumatic Stress Disorder, *continued*

- Markedly diminished interest or participation in significant activities
- Feeling of detachment or estrangement from others
- Restricted range of affect (e.g., unable to have loving feelings)
- Sense of a foreshortened future (e.g., does not expect to have a career, marriage, children, or a normal life span)

5. Persistent symptoms of increased arousal (if not present before the trauma) as indicated by two (or more) of the following:
   - Difficulty falling or staying asleep
   - Irritability or outbursts of anger
   - Difficulty concentrating
   - Hypervigilance
   - Exaggerated startle response

Reprinted with permission from the *Diagnostic and Statistical Manual of Mental Disorders*, Fourth Edition. Copyright 1994. American Psychiatric Association.

NANDA DIAGNOSES RELATED TO ABUSE

CHOOSING
- *Ineffective individual coping*
- *Impaired adjustment*
- *Defensive coping*
- *Ineffective denial*
- *Ineffective family coping: disabling*
- *Ineffective family coping: compromised*
- *Noncompliance*
- *Ineffective management of therapeutic regimen: families*
- *Ineffective management of therapeutic regimen: individual*
- *Decisional conflict*

FEELING
- *Pain*
- *Chronic pain*
- *Dysfunctional grieving*
- *Anticipatory grieving*
- *Risk for violence: self-directed or directed toward others*
- *Risk for self-mutilation*
- *Post-trauma response*
- *Rape-trauma syndrome*
- *Rape-trauma syndrome: compound reaction*
- *Rape-trauma syndrome: silent reaction*
- *Anxiety*
- *Fear*

KNOWING
- *Knowledge deficit*
- *Impaired environmental interpretation syndrome*

- *Acute confusion*
- *Chronic confusion*
- *Altered thought processes*
- *Impaired memory*

PERCEIVING
- *Body image disturbance*
- *Self-esteem disturbance*
- *Chronic low self-esteem*
- *Situational low self-esteem*
- *Personal identity disturbance*
- *Unilateral neglect*
- *Hopelessness*
- *Powerlessness*

RELATING
- *Impaired social interaction*
- *Social isolation*
- *Risk for loneliness*
- *Altered role performance*
- *Altered parenting*
- *Risk for altered parenting*
- *Risk for altered parent/infant/child attachment*
- *Sexual dysfunction*
- *Altered family processes*
- *Caregiver role strain*
- *Risk for caregiver role strain*
- *Altered family process: alcoholism*
- *Parent role conflict*
- *Altered sexuality patterns*

VALUING
- *Spiritual distress*

From *NANDA Nursing Diagnoses: Definitions and Classification 1997–1998*, by North American Nursing Diagnosis Association, 1996, Philadelphia: Author.

▽ OUTCOME IDENTIFICATION

Outcomes for clients suffering from abuse and violence must be carefully and thoughtfully considered and developed in conjunction with the client. Nurses must be careful to avoid projecting their personal opinions and desires onto the client's situation and should focus energies instead on effecting changes that are realistic and achievable for the client. This may be particularly difficult to do, since cases of abuse and violence are often emotionally charged for all parties involved, and it may be a challenge for the nurse to identify outcomes that are in the best interests of the client and in line with the client's wishes. The nurse needs to remain as impartial as possible while being a client advocate and work to outline intermediate steps that can be taken toward reaching an ultimate goal.

▽ PLANNING/INTERVENTIONS

Planning care for survivors of abuse and their families will require input from the clients and a survey of their resources to ensure that the targeted care is in line with their expectations and commitments. Nursing interventions directed at primary prevention of interpersonal violence are those that reduce or control the causative factors associated with interpersonal violence and sexual assaults. Interventions directed toward potential abusers, survivors, and society in general are included. By identifying families at high risk for abuse, nurses can help the family plan efforts to modify those risk factors. This may

---

🕮 *REFLECTIVE THINKING*

Consider Your Life

◆ Were you abused as a child? By whom?

◆ Have you mistreated or abused your child, partner, or elderly parent?

◆ Are you currently or have you ever been in an abusive relationship?

◆ Have you been raped? Have friends or family members? How did you or they react? Did you or they seek counseling? Did you or they confide in anyone? Was the incident reported to the police? If so, what happened?

◆ Have you or a family member been victimized by a gang member?

◆ Would you care for your frail parent in your home? Have you considered the difficulties that doing so might present for you and your parent?

If you answered "yes" to any of the above, consider how these experiences might affect your interactions with survivors of abuse as you identify outcomes and plan nursing care.

---

include increasing the family's coping skills thus improving self-esteem and sense of competence. It may involve treating existing psychopathology or substance abuse, discussing developmental issues, and providing emotional support and relief from stress. It can include identifying and referring cases of child abuse and children of battered women for counseling since a major risk factor of partner abuse is growing up in a violent home.

Primary prevention includes empowering survivors of abuse by helping them learn to care for and protect themselves from the imposition by others. For example, children can be taught in health care settings or schools what to do if they are being abused. It also includes changing the family's perceptions of violence as an acceptable mode of conflict resolution (Clark, 1996).

Primary prevention also includes nurses giving clients anticipatory guidance. For example, by anticipating the challenges of toddlerhood, nurses can acknowledge that this can be a difficult period for parents and can provide practical advice about constructive discipline. They can teach college freshmen about date rape and to avoid vulnerable situations. They can encourage families with dependent elderly members to use respite care services and day care programs. The support and anticipatory guidance can enhance the family and clients' competency and diminish the likelihood of using violence or being abused.

Primary prevention directed toward society involves measures of advocacy and political activity. Nurses can advocate for state and national policies and programs that benefit children and families, the elderly, and battered women.

Secondary prevention involves early detection and treatment for interpersonal violence. The two major goals of secondary prevention are to protect the survivor from further abuse and to break the cycle of violence. This may require medical and mental health treatment for survivors of interpersonal violence, reporting the abuse (or suspected abuse) to authorities, and removing the survivor from the abusive situation. Promoting safety of the survivor may mean placement of an abused child in foster care or arranging for an abused spouse or elderly person to go to a temporary shelter. It may involve encouraging family members to seek counseling and treatment for substance abuse problems (Clark, 1996).

The goal of tertiary prevention is to provide appropriate supportive and rehabilitative services to violent families to prevent further abuse and neglect. High-risk families should receive follow-up care for ongoing supervision to prevent further abuse from occurring. Since many high-risk families are involved with multiple agencies, case management and agency collaboration are essential. When nurses care for abused clients, they need to coordinate their care with other community health and social service agencies. Their clients may be involved with their county department of social services, public health departments, battered women's shelters, legal assistance programs, and home health agencies.

A list of national organizations that may provide nurses or clients with additional information about interpersonal violence and sexual assaults is included at the end of this chapter.

▽ EVALUATION

Evaluation of the effectiveness of the nursing interventions and the plan of care will include assessment of the client and any changes in behavior, attitude, or family circumstances. Progress toward goals that were identified with the client (and family, as appropriate) should be considered, and any that were not met should be carefully reviewed for achievability within the time frame, appropriateness to client's developmental level, and realistic expectation given the circumstances. Coping mechanisms used by the client should be evaluated for their effectiveness, and the client should be redirected to strategies that may prove more effective.

Both nurses and clients need to keep in mind that progress toward achieving goals can be anywhere from very fast (removing a client from an immediate abusive situation) to painfully slow (changing attitudes toward abuse that have developed over a lifetime or changing responses and coping mechanisms used to deal with violent situations). As in identifying outcomes and planning care, the nurse must exercise caution in evaluating progress according to the client's needs, not the nurse's perception of what those needs may or should be.

CASE STUDY/CARE PLAN

Elizabeth is experiencing rape-trauma syndrome in an acute phase. She had been invited to a fraternity party, where she was raped by her date. After she was raped, she left the party alone. On the way back to her dorm she vomited in the street several times. The few people she saw on the way home did not approach her. She felt as if she looked like a coed who had had too much to drink. She said to herself, "I am meat. I am disgusting, violated meat." When she arrived at her dorm, she went into the bathroom before going to her room. She looked into the mirror and saw herself as ravaged, debased, her hair matted. She had vomit on her dress, legs, and shoes. The sight of herself made her sick again. She went into her room, where her roommate was sleeping. She put her clothes into a plastic bag and started crying. She douched and then showered for a half hour but still did not feel clean. She returned to her room and tried to sleep. She wept off and on for hours, reliving every moment of the evening. She concluded that she was naive and an ignorant fool for having wanted her date to like her because he was a senior and so poised and good-looking. She had had too much beer and had been too trusting. She felt humiliated and degraded. Her roommate heard Elizabeth crying and asked if she was all right. She was too humiliated and ashamed to tell her. She felt that she was in a nightmare.

If Elizabeth had been seen the next morning at the student health center, the following care plan would be appropriate.

ASSESSMENT

Elizabeth is experiencing classic symptoms of rape-trauma syndrome. Elizabeth has feelings of helplessness, anger, embarrassment, humiliation, and self-blame; gastrointestinal problems (nausea, vomiting, and anorexia); sleep pattern disturbance; and skeletal muscle tension. She felt responsible for the rape because she had been flattered that Jimmy asked her out.

NURSING DIAGNOSIS *Rape-trauma syndrome, acute phase,* related to forced intercourse, as evidenced by emotional reactions and physical symptoms

Outcomes	Planning/Interventions	Evaluation
◆ Elizabeth will acknowledge that she has been raped.	Assist Elizabeth in being able to accept that she has been raped by: ◆ Reassuring Elizabeth that she is in a safe environment ◆ Using active and empathetic listening skills ◆ Communicating unconditional acceptance of Elizabeth and her situation	Elizabeth stated that she trusted the nurse and felt safe at the health center. Elizabeth confided in the nurse that she had been raped. She admitted that she was having difficulty talking about the rape.

Continued

NURSING DIAGNOSIS *Ineffective individual coping*, related to situational crisis (rape), as evidenced by expression of anxiety and verbalization of inability to cope

Outcomes	Planning/Interventions	Evaluation
• Elizabeth will verbalize her feelings of anxiety, fear, and guilt.	• Encourage Elizabeth to discuss her reactions to the rape, including her feelings of anger, fear, guilt, rage, and helplessness.	Elizabeth acknowledged that how she was feeling and behaving was normal for someone who had been raped.
• Elizabeth will admit that she did not cause the rape.	• Provide Elizabeth with anticipatory guidance and discuss the common emotional and social reactions to rape.	Elizabeth admitted that she had begged Jimmy not to rape her and that she had tried to fight him off while he was raping her.
• Elizabeth will identify coping behaviors she used during the rape.	• Encourage Elizabeth to make her own decisions.	
	• Assist her in identifying her immediate concerns.	
• Elizabeth will seek support from family and friends to help her.	• Encourage her to confide in her parents and her roommate.	Elizabeth verbalized that she did not cause the rape but felt that she had put herself in a vulnerable situation.
• Elizabeth will verbalize an understanding of the rape-trauma syndrome.	• Obtain permission from her to talk with her parents and her roommate about he dynamics of the rape-trauma syndrome.	Elizabeth admitted that she had felt ashamed to call her family.
• Elizabeth will be actively involved in resolving her crisis.	• Advise her of the benefit of obtaining counseling to help her deal with the traumatic event.	Elizabeth consented to contacting her parents and telling them about being raped.
• Elizabeth will identify family and friends who will support her during this crisis.	• Provide her with a list of counselors who specialize in treating rape victims and strongly encourage her to seek therapy.	Elizabeth, with the help of the nurse, confided in her roommate that she had been raped.
• Elizabeth will return to and function at pre-rape level within a 6-week period.		Elizabeth's roommate helped her develop a plan so Elizabeth would feel safe attending her classes.
		Elizabeth verbalized the need for counseling to help her deal with her reactions to the rape.
		Elizabeth made an appointment with a rape crisis counselor before leaving the health center.

Continued

NURSING DIAGNOSIS *Body image disturbance*, related to psychosocial perception, as evidenced by verbalization of negative feelings about body and feelings of helplessness and powerlessness

Outcomes	Planning/Interventions	Evaluation
• Elizabeth will acknowledge how the rape has affected how she feels about herself. • Her self-esteem will be restored within 6 weeks.	• Help Elizabeth identify specific behaviors she used to prevent the rape. • Help Elizabeth feel less like a victim and more like a survivor of rape.	Elizabeth acknowledged that she felt better about herself after talking with the nurse. Elizabeth stated that she felt more in control of her emotions.

CRITICAL THINKING BAND

ASSESSMENT

What else should we take into account with Elizabeth?

NURSING DIAGNOSIS

Are there other diagnoses that might better manage Elizabeth's issues?

Outcomes	Planning/Interventions	Evaluation
What do you think that Elizabeth thought about these goals? Would they have to be mutual?	Could the same strategies that were used with Elizabeth work for other rape survivors? Where does the care need to be personalized?	What else should be considered with clients who have been raped? Do plans always work? How would we know if they did for Elizabeth? What do you think will work with other clients?

CASE STUDY/CARE PLAN

Vera is a survivor of domestic violence. She is married to Tom and they have two children. After the birth of their second child, Tom becomes jealous of the attention that Vera gives the baby. About a month after the birth of the baby, Vera is seen in the emergency room for physical injuries. Tom is with her and will not let her out of his sight. The nurse, suspecting that Vera has been abused, tells Tom to remain in the waiting room. She provides Vera a quiet, private examination room so she can have a private interview with her.

ASSESSMENT

Vera was seen in the emergency room for physical injuries related to her husband's hitting her and throw-

ing her against the wall. Vera told the nurse that the abuse was all her fault. She did not know what to do. She still had hope that Tom would change. She believed that their children needed him as a father. She stated that she felt blue. Vera stated that she was afraid that Tom would abuse her again. She stated that she was afraid that he would retaliate against her if the abuse were reported to law enforcement. Vera stated that she could not tell her family about the abuse. Her friends had told her that she should leave Tom, but they did not understand that he was not always bad. He loved her and the children. Vera stated that she was not familiar with the community resources.

Continued

NURSING DIAGNOSIS *Risk for injury*, as a result of physical abuse by her husband

Outcomes	Planning/Interventions	Evaluation
◆ Vera will develop a trusting relationship with the nurse.	◆ Interview Vera in a private place.	Vera stated that she felt safe the emergency room.
	◆ Reassure Vera that she was in a safe place.	Vera reported that she had been abused by her husband.
◆ Vera will admit her husband abused her.	◆ Interview Vera and be with her during the physical exam.	
◆ Vera will be treated for her injuries.	◆ Encourage Vera to discuss the battering incidents.	She was given a physical examination by the emergency room physician. She had no broken bones but did have old and new bruises on her face, abdomen, breasts, and upper extremities.
	◆ Obtain a history of her abusive relationship.	
		She was given treatment for her injuries.

NURSING DIAGNOSIS *Ineffective individual coping*, related to a situational crisis secondary to ongoing cycle of violence, as evidenced by inability to ask for help

Outcomes	Planning/Interventions	Evaluation
◆ Vera will verbalize her feelings, strengths, and needs.	◆ Provide crisis counseling.	Vera admitted that she did not deserve to be beaten by Tom.
	◆ Encourage Vera to express her feelings.	
◆ Vera will state that she does not deserve to be battered.	◆ Accept and acknowledge Vera's state of confusion.	She admitted that she was ashamed to contact her family.
	◆ Help Vera identify her strengths and help her reestablish feelings of control.	

NURSING DIAGNOSIS *Powerlessness*, related to lifestyle of helplessness, as evidenced by verbalization of fear for her safety and that of her children

Outcomes	Planning/Interventions	Evaluation
◆ Vera will verbalize alternatives she has available to her and her children.	◆ Offer Vera support but leave the final decision to stay or leave Tom to Vera.	Vera did not feel that her situation was bad enough to leave Tom.
	◆ Discuss with Vera her responsibility to report abuse.	The nurse and physician made a report to law enforcement. They informed Tom and Vera of their legal responsibilities to report the abuse.
◆ Vera will have thought through a safety plan.	◆ Consult with the physician to determine whether the nature of the injuries warrants reporting the abuse to authorities.	
		They discussed a safety plan with Vera.

Continued

NURSING DIAGNOSIS *Knowledge deficit*, related to unfamiliarity with information resources

Outcomes	Planning/Interventions	Evaluation
◆ Vera will identify resources and services that are available to her.	◆ Give Vera anticipatory guidance. ◆ Discuss available community resources available to Vera, such as shelters, social services, and job training programs.	Vera is more knowledgeable about available resources. She may consider contacting her family.

CRITICAL THINKING BAND

ASSESSMENT

Should the assessment of Vera's situation include an interview with Tom? Do you think his involvement would help or hinder Vera's progress and recovery?

NURSING DIAGNOSIS

What other psychosocial diagnoses might apply to Vera? Are additional diagnoses related to physical status appropriate?

Outcomes

Would Tom be likely to support those outcomes for Vera? How important do you think his support would be to Vera's progress?

Planning/Interventions

Do you think Vera will continue to respond as positively to the care plan once Tom is back in the picture?

Evaluation

How can you ensure Vera's continued commitment to protecting herself?

FUTURE DIRECTIONS

The U.S. Public Health Services identified violence as a critical public health problem. The United States ranks first among industrial nations in violent death rates. Violence is a health and social problem costing the U.S. society thousands of lives, millions of dollars, and untold physical and psychological morbidity (Cambpell et al., 1993). The federal government has begun a number of initiatives that are aimed at stopping interpersonal violence and sexual assault.

When Congress incorporated the Healthy People 2000 objectives into national legislation, it identified violent and abusive behavior as a national concern and a priority area. The Centers for Disease Control and Prevention is the lead agency for this objective. The specific objectives for this initiative include reversing the incidences of child abuse, physical abuse of women by male partners, rape and attempted rape, and physical fighting and weapon carrying among youth. Other objectives include improving emergency room protocols to enable staff to be able to identify, treat, and refer survivors of sexual assault and spouse, elder, and child abuse; improving child death review systems; evaluating and following up on abused children; and providing more emergency housing for battered women and their children (Healthy People 2000, 1997).

The Temporary Child Care for Children with Disabilities and Crisis Nurseries Act (TCCA) of 1988 provides federal funds for crisis nurseries. By 1996, the federal government had given out nearly 100 grants totaling more than $30 million. Communities in almost every state have started crisis nurseries that are designed to prevent child abuse by giving parents respite care for their children (Neighbours, 1996).

The National Center for the Prevention and Treatment of Child Abuse and Neglect was established in 1972 at the University of Colorado as a resource for issues of child abuse and neglect. It provides professional training, consultation, program development and evaluation, and research in all forms of child abuse and neglect (Kempe Center Programs, 1996–1997).

The American Academy of Child and Adolescent Psychiatry began an initiative, "Victory over Violence," to persevere in identifying and correcting the cause for the increase in interpersonal violence. One of the goals is to implement violence prevention in child and adolescent psychiatric training programs (Stone, 1997).

The Administration on Aging (AOA) and the Administration for Children and Families (ACF) are collaborating for the first time in funding an investigation of the national incidence of elder abuse. The study will examine abuse, neglect, and exploitation of elderly persons in domestic settings, including on Native American tribal reservations. Their objectives are to develop national information on the types and scope of elder abuse, neglect, and exploitation; to determine the characteristics of elder abuse victims and perpetrators; to determine elder abuse substantiation rates and types of elder abuse reporters; and to assess national trends in the incidence of elder abuse. The goal is to assist local program administrators in designing appropriate elder abuse prevention and treatment services nationwide (AOA, 1995).

The U.S. Department of Justice, Federal Bureau of Prisons, has established an inmate sexual assault prevention/intervention program. Its purposes are to provide specific guidelines to help prevent sexual assaults to inmates, to address the needs of inmates who have been sexually assaulted, and to discipline and prosecute inmates who sexually assault others (U.S. Department of Justice, Federal Bureau of Prisons, 1995).

All of these efforts indicate that U.S. society may finally be willing to do something besides give lip service to preventing interpersonal violence and sexual assault. Nurses need to be actively involved in community efforts to eliminate family violence from our society.

KEY CONCEPTS

◆ Violence in America is a major public health problem.

◆ Interpersonal violence includes child, partner, and elder abuse by family members; it involves clients'

being physically, psychologically, financially, or sexually abused.

◆ Domestic violence is usually abuse against women; it involves physical, emotional, financial, and frequently sexual abuse; it usually increases in severity and frequency and can escalate to homicide of either partner.

◆ Sexual assault is a crime of violence and power, not sexual passion.

◆ Nurses are in a position to assess and intervene in incidents of interpersonal violence and sexual assault; they need to understand the dynamics of violence to intervene effectively.

◆ Interpersonal survivors of violence may exhibit both physical and psychological signs and symptoms of abuse; the nurse should assess clients for both.

◆ Primary prevention is the single most important method of preventing interpersonal violence and sexual assaults.

◆ Secondary prevention of interpersonal violence is directed toward protecting the survivor and breaking the cycle of violence.

◆ Nurses are mandated by law to report known or suspected cases of child abuse and in some states elder abuse and sexual assault.

REVIEW QUESTIONS AND ACTIVITIES

1. Describe the types of interpersonal violence and sexual assaults.

2. What are your responsibilities in reporting child abuse, elder abuse, domestic violence, and sexual assaults?

3. How would Orem's Theory influence your interactions with clients?

4. What nursing interventions for an abused client are consistent with crisis theory?

5. What characteristics are seen in children, elders, and partners who are abused and their abusers?

6. Explain Walker's Theory of Violence.

7. What would you include in your assessment of an abused client?

8. Define the *rape-trauma syndrome*, *post-trauma response*, and *Post-Traumatic Stress Disorder*.

9. Describe nursing interventions that are used in primary, secondary, and tertiary prevention of interpersonal violence.

EXPLORING THE WEB

◆ Visit this text's "Online Companion™" on the Internet at **http://www.DelmarNursing.com** for further information on abuse, violence, and rape.

◆ What sources can you locate that deal with abuse, violence, and rape? Do these sites distinguish among child, elder, and spousal abuse?

◆ Check the sites of some of the major nursing and health care organizations, such as NANDA, NLN, and DSM (APA). Do they include pages or source information on abuse, violence, and rape?

◆ Do the resource organizations listed in this chapter also have Web sites? What types of information do they provide? Do they offer resources for both the abused and the abuser?

◆ Search government Web sites for information and support groups for survivors of violence or self-help programs for abusers. Is information available on line for any government research studies on violence and abuse?

REFERENCES

Administration on Aging: Elder abuse study to be conducted by AOA and ACF. AOA. (July 1995). http://www.aoa.ihhs.gov/aoa/pr/eldabuse.html.

Anderson, C. (1995). Childhood sexually transmitted diseases: One consequence of sexual abuse. *Public Health Nursing, 12*(1), 41–46.

Aguilera, D. C. (1994). Crisis intervention theory and methodology (7th ed.). St. Louis, MO: Mosby-Year Book.

American Academy of Child & Adolescent Psychiatry (AACAP). (11/1995). Child sexual abuse. Fact no. 9. *Facts for families.* http://www.ascap.org/fact Fam/sexabuse.htm. (March 3, 1997).

American Medical Association (AMA), Council on Scientific Affairs. (1992). Violence against women: Relevance for medical practitioners. *JAMA, 267*(23), 3184–3189.

American Medical Association (AMA). (Oct. 1995b). *Strategies for the treatment and prevention of sexual assault.* http://www.ama-assn.org/public/releases/assault/sa-guide.htm. (Jan. 14, 1997b).

American Medical Association (AMA). (Nov. 6, 1995a). *Sexual assault in America.* http://www.ama-assn.org/public/releases/assault/action.html. (Jan. 14, 1997a).

American Psychiatric Association *Diagnostic and Statistical Manual of Mental Disorders* Fourth Edition. Washington, DC: American Psychiatric Association, 1994.

American Public Health Association. (1991). *Healthy communities 2000: Model standards* (3rd ed.). Washington, DC: Author.

Bergen, R. K. (1995). Surviving wife rape: How women define and cope with the violence. *Violence Against Women*, (2), 117–138.

Berrios, D. C., & Grady, D. (1991). Domestic violence: Risk factors and outcomes. *Western Journal of Medicine, 155*, 133–155.

Biden, J. R. (1993). Violence against women: The congressional report. *American Psychologist, 48*(10), 1059–1061.

Burgess, A., & Holmstrom, L. (1974). Rape-trauma syndrome. *American Journal of Psychiatry, 131*(9), 981–985.

Burgess, A. W. (1990). Victims of rape. In *Psychiatric nursing in the hospital and the community* (5th ed.). East Norwalk, CT: Appleton & Lange.

CA Board of Registered Nursing (CABRN). (1995). BRN policy on registered nurse failure to report child abuse. Sacramento: State of CA Dept. of Consumer Affairs.

Campbell, J. C., Anderson, E., Fulmer, T. L., Girouard, S., McElmurry, P., & Raft, B. (1993). AAN working paper violence as a nursing priority: Policy implication. *Nursing Outlook, 41*(2), 83–92.

Campbell, J., & Humphreys, J. (1993). *Nursing care of survivors of family violence.* St. Louis, MO: Mosby-Year Book.

Capezuti, E., Yurkow, J., & Goldberg, E. (1996). Meeting the challenge of elder mistreatment. *Home Care Provider, 1*(4), 190–193.

Carpenito, L. J. (1997). *Nursing diagnosis application to clinical practice* (7th ed.). Philadelphia: JB Lippincott.

Carroll, L. (May 20, 1996). Sexual abuse tough to diagnose. *Medical Tribune News Service.* http://www.medscape.com/jobson/MedRibNew...96/may/20/SexualAbuseToughTo Diagnose.html. (April 5, 1997).

Chez, N. (1994). Helping the victim of domestic violence. *AJN,* 33–37.

Clark, M. J. (1996). Violence. In *Nursing in the Community* (2nd ed., pp. 839–875). Stamford: CT: Appleton & Lange.

Coleman, V. E. (1994). Lesbian battering: The relationship between personality and the perpetration of violence. *Violence and Victims, 9*(2), 139–152.

Connell, R., & Lopez, R. J. (Nov. 17, 1996). An inside look at 18th Street's menace. *L.A. Times.* http://www.latimes.com/18gang/18gang01.htm. (Nov. 25, 1996).

Feiner, B. (April 1994). It's none of my business . . . . *Emergency Medical Services.* p. 42.

Fontanarosa. (1995). The unrelenting epidemic of violence in America. *JAMA, 273*(22), 1792–1793.

Gang Information. (1996). *Is your child in a gang?* http://www.quiknet. com/spd/gangs.html. (Oct. 6, 1996).

Healthy people 2000 violent and abusive behavior resource list (Healthy People 2000). (1997). hppt://nhic.nt.health.org/nmp/hp2kpage/7vi2.htm. (Jan. 26, 1997).

Hyman, A., Schillinger, D., & Lo, B. (1995). Laws mandating reporting of domestic violence: Do they promote patient well-being? *JAMA, 273*(22), 1781–1787.

Jackson, L., & Miller, C. L. (1996). Nurses need to know signs of shaken baby syndrome. *Nurseweek, 9*(13), 10–11.

Jezierski, M. (1994). Abuse of women by male partners: Basic knowledge for emergency nurses. *Journal of Emergency Nursing, 20*, 361–368.

Journal of the American Medical Association (JAMA). (1993). Council report: Adolescents as victims of family violence. *JAMA, 270*(15), 1850–1856.

Kantor, G. K., Jasinski, J. L., & Aldarondo, E. (1994). Sociocultural status and incidence of marital violence in Hispanic families. *Violence and Victims, 9*(3), 207–222.

Kempe Center programs 1996–1997 and *Selected historical events of the C. Henry Kempe National Center for the Prevention and Treatment of Child Abuse and Neglect.* (1997). http://electricstores.com/kempe/history & programs.htm. (Jan. 15, 1997).

Lynch, M. A., & Ferri, R. S. (1997). Health needs of lesbian women and gay men. *Clinician Reviews, 7*(1), 85–112.

Medical Education Group Learning Systems. (1995). Domestic violence: A practical guide for physicians. http://www.cme.edu/phydom/domes.html. (Jan. 14, 1997).

McNamara, D. (1994). Gang violence and the street smart nurse. *Journal of Community Health Nursing, 11*(4), 193–200.

National Center on Child Abuse and Neglect (NCCAN). (1997). *Lessons learned: Introduction.* (1997). http://www.calif.com/nocanch/prevmonth/lessons/intro.htm. (April 5, 1997).

National Coalition Against Domestic Violence (NCADV). (1995). *Domestic violence fact sheet.* Washington, DC: Author.

National Coalition Against Sexual Assault. (1996). *About the sexual assault information page.* http://www.cs.utk.edu/~bartley/aboutSaInfoPage.html. (April 8, 1997).

National Coalition Against Sexual Assault. (1997). *Myths and facts about sexual violence.* http://www.achiever.com/freehmpg/ncas/facts.html. (April 8, 1997).

National Coalition for the homeless (NCH). (1995). *NCH fact sheet: Domestic violence and homelessness.* http://www2.ari.net/home/nch/domestic.html.

National Crime Prevention Council. (1996). *1-2-3—A parent's guide for preventing gangs.* Washington, DC: Author.

National Victim Center (NCV). (Dec. 27, 1996). *National victim center statistics.* http://pubwev.ucdavis.edu/Documents/RPEP/nvcstats.htm.

Neighbours, A. (Dec. 30, 1996). Crisis nurseries help parents in tough times. *Christian Science Monitor.* http://www.csmonitor.com/children/1230feat.3html. (Jan. 1, 1997).

North American Nursing Diagnosis Association. (1996). *NANDA nursing diagnoses: Definitions and classification 1997–1998.* Philadelphia: Author.

Olds, S. B., London, M. L., & Ladewig, P. W. (1996). Nursing care of the family in crisis: Child and domestic abuse. In *Maternal newborn nursing: A family centered approach* (5th ed., p. 185). Menlo Park, CA: Addison-Wesley Nursing, Benjamin/Cummings.

Orem, D. (1991). *Nursing: Concepts of practice* (4th ed.). New York: McGraw-Hill.

Peace at Home. (1995). *Domestic violence: The facts.* (1995). Boston: MA: Author.

Perilla, J., Bakemann, R., & Norris, F. (1994). Culture and domestic violence: The ecology of abused Latinas. *Violence and Victims, 9*(4), 325–339.

Polk-Walker, G. (1990). What really happened? Incidence and factor assessment of abused children and adolescents. *Journal of Psychosocial Nursing, 28*(11), 17–22.

Sedlak, A. J., & Broadhurst, D. D. (1996). *Executive summary of the third national incidence study of child abuse and neglect.* U.S. Department of Health and Human Services: National Center on Child Abuse and Neglect. http://www.calib.com/nccanch/data/nis3.txt (Feb. 1, 1997).

Sexual assault glossary of terms. (1996). http://pubweb.ucdavis.edu/Documents/RPEP/terms.ht. (Dec. 27, 1996).

Stone, L. A. (1997). The violence initiative: Violence & children: What we can do. *American Academy of Children and Adolescent Psychiatry.* http://www.aacap.org/health/humbpt.htm#TOP. (March 30, 1997).

Stop Prisoner Rape, Inc. (1997). What is "Stop Prisoner Rape"? http://www.igc.apc.org/spr/docs/whatis.html. (Jan. 14, 1997).

Tilden, V. P., Schmidt, T. A., Limandri, B. J., Chiodo, G. T., & Garland, M. J. (1994). Factors that influence clinicians' assessment and management of family violence. *American Journal of Public Health, 84*(4), 628–633.

Thobaben, M. (1989). State elder/adult abuse and protection laws. In R. Filinson & S. Ingman (Eds.), *Elder abuse practice and policy* (pp. 138–152). New York: Human Sciences.

Thobaben, M. (1995). *Elder and dependent adult abuse Humboldt county guidelines for mandated reporters.* Eureka, CA: Northcoast Advocacy Services.

Thobaben, M. (1996). Elder abuse and neglect. *Home Care Provider, 1*(5), 267–269.

Thobaben, M. (1997). In every midwife's caseload: Battered women. *Midwives, 110*(1317), 302–303.

United States Code Annotated, Title 42, The Public Health and Welfare, Chapter 67, Child abuse prevention and treatment and adoption reform; Subchapter 1, Child abuse prevention and treatment; Section 5102, Definitions; Title II, Victims of Child Abuse Act of 1990; Subtitle D, Federal victims' protection and rights; Section 226, Child abuse reporting. St. Paul, MN: West Publishing.

United States Violent Crime Control and Law Enforcement Act of 1994. Public Law 103-322, Sept. 13, 1994.

U.S. Department of Justice, Bureau of Justice Statistics. (1994). *Wives are the most frequent victims in family murders.* hppt://ncjrs.org71/0/4/3/2smurder.txt. (Jan. 10, 1997).

U.S. Department of Justice, Federal Bureau of Prisons. (1995). *BOP statement on sexual assault prevention/intervention.* http://www.igc.apc.org/spr/docs/bop.html. (Jan. 14, 1997).

U.S. Department of Justice, Bureau of Justice Statistics. (Jan. 5, 1997). *Statistics about crime and victims.* http://www.ojp.usdoj.gov/bjs/cvict.htm.#ncvs.

U.S. Department of Veterans Affairs (USDVA), National Center for Post-Traumatic Stress Disorder. (1997). *PTSD in children.* http://www.Dartmouth.Edu/dms/ptsd/Children.html.

U.S. House of Representatives, Select Committee on Aging, Subcommittee on Health and Long-Term Care. (April 1990). *Elder abuse: A decade of shame and inaction.* Washington, DC: U.S. Government Printing Office. Comm. Pub. No. 101-752.

U.S. House of Representatives, Select Committee on Aging. (April 3, 1981). *Elder abuse (an examination of a hidden problem).* Washington, DC: U.S. Government Printing Office. Comm. Pub. No. 97-277.

U.S. House of Representatives, Select Committee on Aging, Subcommittee on Retirement Income and Employment, Ninety-Seventh Congress, First Session. (April 3, 1981). *Physical and financial abuse of the elderly.* Washington, DC: U.S. Government Printing Office. Comm. Pub. No. 97-297.

Walker, L. E. (1979). *The battered woman.* New York: Harper & Row.

Warren, J. K., Gary, F., & Moorhead, J. (1994). Self-reported experiences of physical and sexual abuse among runaway youths. *Perspectives in Psychiatric Care, 30*(1), 23–28.

Whipple, E. E., & Finton, S. E. (1995). Psychological maltreatment by siblings: An unrecognized form of abuse. *Child and Adolescent Social Work Journal, 12*(2), 135–146.

Wiese, D., & Daro, D. (April, 1995). *Current trends in child abuse reporting and fatalities: The results of the 1994 Annual Fifty State Survey.* Chicago, IL: National Center on Child Abuse Prevention Research, a program of The National Committee to Prevent Child Abuse, Working Paper No. 808.

Women's Issues and Social Empowerment (WISE). (Feb. 27, 1997a). *The dynamics of domestic violence.* htttp://www.vicnet.net.au/~wise/DVDynamics.htm. (April 15, 1997).

Women's Issues and Social Empowerment (WISE). (April 14, 1997b). *Myths about domestic violence.* htttp://www.vicnet.net.au/~wise/DVMyths.htm#4.

World Congress Against Commercial Sexual Exploitation of Children. (Jan. 1, 1997). http://193.135.156.14/webpub/csechome/2262.htm.

≋ LITERARY REFERENCES

Corman, A. (1991). *Prized possessions.* New York: Simon & Schuster.

The Holy Bible. (1913). Cleveland, OH: World Syndicate Publishing (conformable to the edition of 1611, commonly known as the authorized or King James Version).

The Real Mother Goose. (1966/1916, 49th printing). Rand McNally & Co.

Williams, T. (1947). *A streetcar named desire.* New York: New Directions Publishing.

≋ SUGGESTED READINGS

Alexander, R. (1995). Recent legal trends in child sexual abuse cases: Direction for child protection workers. *Child and Adolescent Social Work Journal, 12*(3), 229–240.

American Medical Association. (1995). *Diagnostic and treatment guidelines on mental health effects of family violence.* Chicago: Author.

Burgess, A. W., Fehder, W. P., & Harman, C. R. (1995). Delayed reporting of the rape victim. *Journal of Psychosocial Nursing and Mental Health Services, 33*(9), 21–29.

Davidson, J. R. T., & Foa, E. B. (1993). *Post traumatic stress disorders, DSM-IV & beyond.* Washington, DC: American Psychiatric Press.

Denham, S. (1995). Confronting the monster of family violence. *Nursing Forum, 30*(3), 12–19.

Ellis, G. M. (1994). Acquaintance rape. *Perspectives in Psychiatric Care, 30*(1), 11–16.

Lynch, S. H. (1997). Elder abuse: What to look for, how to intervene. *AJN, 97*(1), 27–33.

Weaver, P. L., Filomena, F. V., Connors, R., & Regan-Kubinski, M. J. (1994). Adult survivors of childhood sexual abuse: Survivor's disclosure and nurse therapist's response. *Journal of Psychosocial Nursing, 32*(12), 19–24.

≋ RESOURCES

American Humane Association
Children's Division
63 Inverness Drive East
Englewood, CO 80112-5117
(303) 792-9900; (800) 227-4645

American Professional Society on the Abuse of Children (APSAC)
407 South Dearborn Ave., Suite 1600
Chicago, IL 60605
(312) 554-0166

Center for Women Policy Studies
2000 P Street, NW, Suite 508
Washington, DC 20036
(202) 872-1770

CSAP National Resource Center for the Prevention of Perinatal Abuse of Alcohol and Other Drugs
9302 Lee Highway
Fairfax, VA 22031
(703) 218-5600; (800)-353-8824

Healthy People 2000
Office of Disease Prevention and Health Promotion
U.S. Public Health Service
330 C St., SW, Room 2132
Washington, DC 20201
(202) 205-8583

Kempe National Center for the Prevention and Treatment of Child Abuse and Neglect
1205 Oneida St.
Dever, CO 80220
(303) 321-3963

National Association of State Victims of Child Abuse LAWS (VOCAL)
P.O. Box 1314
Orangevale, CA 95662

National Center for Education in Maternal and Child Health
2000 15th Street, North, Suite 701
Arlington, VA 22201-2617
(703) 542-7802

National Center for Missing and Exploited Children (NCMEC)
2101 Wilson Boulevard, Suite 550
Arlington, VA 22201-3052
(703) 235-3900; Hotline: (800) 843-5678

National Clearinghouse on Marital and Date Rape
2325 Oak St.
Berkeley, CA 94708
(510) 524-1582

National Clearinghouse for Alcohol and Drug Information (NCADI)
P.O. Box 2345
Rockville, MD 20847-2345
(800) 729-6686

National Clearinghouse on Child Abuse and Neglect
P.O. Box 1182
Washington, DC 20013-1182
(703) 385-7565; (800) FYI-3366

National Coalition Against Domestic Violence
P.O. Box 34103
Washington, DC 20043-4103
(202) 638-6388

National Coalition for the Homeless
National Headquarters
1612 K Street, N.W.
Washington, DC 20006
(202) 659-3310

National Coalition on Sexual Assault (NCASA)
912 N. 2nd St.
Harrisburg, PA 17102
(717) 232-7460

National Committee to Prevent Child Abuse
332 South Michigan Ave., Suite 1600
Chicago, IL 60604
(312) 663-3520

National Council on Child Abuse and Family Violence
1050 Connecticut Ave.
Washington, DC 20036
(202) 429-6695

National Council of Senior Citizens
925 15th St. N.W.
Washington, DC 20005
(202) 347-8800

National Institute on Aging Information Center
2209 Distribution Circle
Silver Spring, MD 20910

National Resource Center on Child Abuse and Neglect
63 Inverness Drive East
Englewood, CO 80112-5117
(303) 792-9900; (800) 227-5242

National Resource Center on Child Sexual
Abuse
2204 Whitezburg Drive, Suite 200
Huntsville, AL 35801
(800) 543-7006

National Victims Resource Center
Box 6000
Rockville, MD 20850-6000
(800) 627-6872

Older Women's League
1325 G. St. N.W.
Washington, DC 20001
(202) 783-6686

Parents Anonymous
520 South Lafayette Park
Suite 316
Los Angeles, CA 90057
Public Health Service

Centers for Disease Control and
       Prevention
Public Inquiries
1600 Clifton Road, NE
Mailstop A23
Atlanta, GA 30333
(404) 639-3534

Rape, Abuse & Incest National Network
       (RAIN)
252 10 Street NE
Washington, DC 20002
(202) 544-1034

Stop Prison Rape (SPR)
P.O. Box 2713, Manhattanville Station
New York, NY 10027-8817
(212) 663-5562

Women Against Rape
P.O. Box 02084
Columbus, OH 43202

HELP NUMBERS

800-I-AM-LOST	Child Find Hotline (parent reporting lost children)
800-4-A-Child	Child Help USA (for victims, offenders, and parents)
800-999-9999	Covenant House Hotline (for problem teens and runaways)
800-A-WAY-OUT	Hotline for parents considering abducting their children
800-843-5678	National Center for Missing and Exploited Children
800-231-6946	National Runaway Hotline
800-442-HOPE	National Youth Crisis Hotline
800-782-SEEK	Operation Lookout, National Center for Missing Youth
800-333-SAFE	Shelter Aid Hotline
800-HIT-HOME	Youth Crisis Hotline (reporting child abuse and help for runaways)

Unit

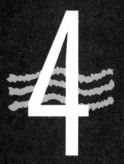

NURSING INTERVENTIONS AND TREATMENT MODALITIES

What drugs are prescribed to treat individuals suffering from psychiatric disorders? What are the doses and side effects of these medications? How can nurses participate in the individual care of persons with mental illness? How do nurses provide mental health care to families? What is the nurse's role in group therapy? How can nurses influence the mental health of communities? What unique or special therapies are available to people with mental illness?

These questions will be discussed in this unit entitled *Nursing Interventions and Treatment Modalities.*

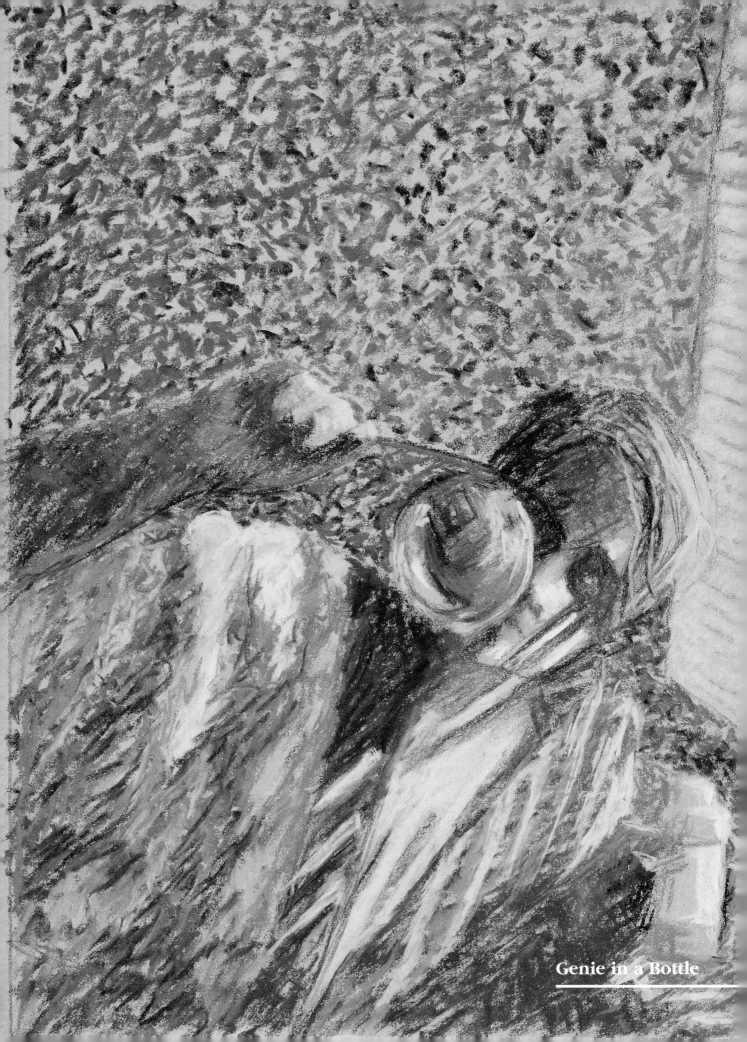

Genie in a Bottle

Chapter

25

PHARMACOLOGY
IN PSYCHIATRIC CARE

Lawrence E. Frisch

Wayne Wilson

Use of Medications in Psychiatric Care

Nurses must have current and accurate information regarding medications ordered for their clients. This chapter provides information on major groups of psychotropic drugs; however, every nurse needs to know where to find information on all drugs.

Consider the following:

◆ Do you know where to find drug information on the psychiatric unit where you are completing your student placement? Review the sources available there.

◆ Does your outpatient clinic have drug resources available to both staff and clients?

◆ Do you have a means of obtaining information through computer searching of a database?

◆ Have you already purchased a pharmacology book? A drug handbook?

Please review the sources of information available to you. Ensure that you have the means to obtain information when needed.

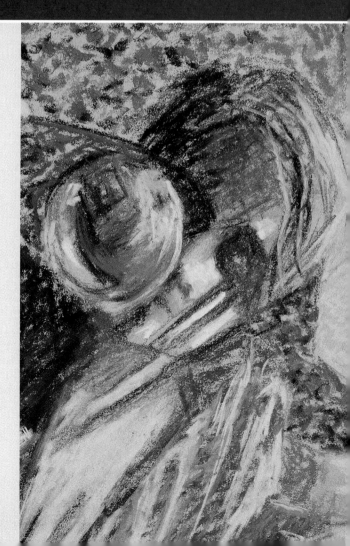

〰 CHAPTER OUTLINE

DRUGS FOR TREATING SUBSTANCE ABUSE AND DEPENDENCY

Substances with Little Role Outside Substance Abuse or Withdrawal

Methadone

Disulfiram

Nicotine Replacement

Opioid Receptor Antagonists

Other Medications of Use in Managing Substance Dependence

STIMULANT DRUGS

≋ COMPETENCIES

Upon completion of this chapter, the reader will have general reference information on the major psychotropic drugs related to:

◆ Antipsychotics

◆ Mood disorders

◆ Anxiety and sleep disorders

◆ Stimulants

◆ Drugs used to treat chemical dependency

≋ KEY TERMS

Akathisia Subjective sense of restlessness with a perceived need to pace or otherwise move continuously.

Antipsychotic Drugs Major tranquilizers administered to control symptoms of psychosis.

Blood-Brain Barrier Capillary barrier between blood and brain.

Dystonia Sustained, involuntary muscle spasms.

Half-Life Time for plasma concentrations of a drug to decrease to half of an initial value.

Neuroleptic Malignant Syndrome Disorder associated with sudden fever, rigidity, tachycardia, hypertension, and decreased levels of consciousness.

Oculogyric Crisis Reaction in which extraocular muscle spasm forces the eyes into a fixed, usually upward gaze.

Serotonergic Syndrome Drug reaction involving agitation, sweating, rigidity, fever, hyperreflexia, tachycardia, and hypotension.

Tardive Dyskinesia Neurological disorder characterized by involuntary movements, usually of the tongue and lips.

Therapeutic Window Time for peak effectiveness of a drug.

This chapter provides reference information on the major psychotropic drugs. While each of the chapters dealing with psychopathology discusses drugs that may be used for specific conditions, detailed information is presented in this chapter to provide a source of information on major drugs used in psychiatric care. The nurse will find discussion on the history of psychotropic medications, medications used to treat psychosis, medications used to treat mood disorders, medications for anxiety and sleep disorders, stimulants, and drugs used to treat chemical dependency.

HISTORY OF PSYCHIATRIC MEDICATION

The era of modern psychiatric drug treatment is less than 60 years old. Until very recently, only sedative/hypnotics (barbiturates, bromides, chloral hydrate) and stimulants (most commonly amphetamines) were used to affect individuals' moods, assist with sleep, and treat agitation or psychosis. Treatments were rarely effective, and unwanted side effects (including drug dependency) were common. Therapeutic options expanded rapidly beginning in the mid-20th century. While some kinds of drugs now in modern use were discovered or synthesized prior to the mid-20th century, virtually all the studies establishing modern drug effectiveness were carried out after 1950. The one exception to this description may be lithium: In 1886 John Aulde and Carl Lange recognized that lithium could be used to control symptoms of what was later called Bipolar Disorder (Schou, 1989). However, these early observations were forgotten, to be rediscovered by Cade and Schou in the mid-20th century (Schou, 1989).

The basic chemical structure underlying both tricyclic antidepressants and phenothiazine antipsychotics was initially synthesized in 1889. It was not until the early 1950s that pharmacological investigation led to modifications of this iminodibenzyl structure. These modifications produced both antidepressant and antipsychotic medications from remarkably similar underlying molecular structures. Benzodiazepine drugs for treatment of anxiety were first synthesized in the mid-1950s and released for clinical use in 1960. Carbamazepine (Tegretol) and divalproex (Depakote and others), used as alternatives to lithium in the management of Bipolar Disorder, were also brought into clinical practice as anticonvulsants at about this time. Much more recent pharmacological research has resulted in important therapeutic advances such as atypical antipsychotics (clozapine) and selective serotonin reuptake inhibitors [fluoxetine (Prozac) and others]. Current pharmacological treatments have serious deficiencies, of which the most important is that (as with many chronic diseases) they serve to control symptoms rather than to cure psychiatric disorders. Also, psychiatric drugs are not effective for, or tolerated by, a significant portion of affected individuals, often those with the most

REFLECTIVE THINKING

Serendipity and SAR

For many years, lack of knowledge of neuro-chemistry, neurophysiology, and ethical concerns led to the very slow development of psychiatric medications. Serendipity refers to the fortuitous discovery of an effect of a drug that was not expected. For example, chlorpromazine was discovered in a search for new antihistamines and sedatives. Imipramine was discovered to be an antidepressant while being tested for antipsychotic properties. For many years, most psychiatric medications were developed "accidentally" while searching for another property.

Structure-activity relationship (SAR) is a complicated way of saying that if two drugs are chemically and structurally similar, they probably will produce similar effects, but perhaps one will have fewer side effects or be more effective. This process has led to many more psychotropic medications than random searching for neurologically effective substances.

The rapid discovery of the many chemical receptors in the brain, along with the development of sophisticated biotechnology, has allowed the cloning of drug receptors and the more rational development of drugs that act specifically at a given receptor, thus reducing side effects and increasing efficacy. However, the function of many brain receptors remains unknown despite extensive investigation. New discoveries may lead to further dramatic changes in psychiatric care.

disabling symptoms. Despite these important limitations of current practice, the use of psychiatric medications offers great benefits to many clients. These benefits will continue to increase as ever more effective treatments are developed and brought into practice.

HOW AND WHY PSYCHIATRIC MEDICATIONS WORK

Understanding psychiatric medications requires a basic understanding of pharmacology and the concepts of administration, absorption, distribution, elimination, and metabolism. Many psychiatric medications are given orally (p.o.), and some are given parenterally, usually by the intramuscular (i.m.) route. Only rarely are psychiatric medications given intravenously (i.v.) or subcutaneously (s.c.). Rectal administration (p.r.) of psychiatric medications is now quite uncommon. Most drugs are absorbed quite predictably when given by a parenteral route, but oral administration may be significantly affected by foods, stomach acidity (often modified by antacids), and the nature of the drug itself. Once absorbed, drugs distribute

throughout the body depending on their solubility in water and fat and on their tendency to bind to proteins. Fat-soluble drugs tend to distribute widely in the body; protein-bound drugs may be very slow to diffuse out of the bloodstream. These characteristics affect drug actions. Once in the body, most drugs are eliminated by excretion (usually into the urine by the kidney or into the bile or feces by the liver). Prior to excretion, drugs are almost always metabolized, most often by the liver but occasionally by lungs or even skin. Some metabolic products are biologically inactive and are directly excreted; other metabolic products are even more active than are the original drugs. Many substances have pharmacological activity only after they have been metabolized into biologically active metabolites.

The potential effects of any drug are a complex balance of each of these factors: absorption, distribution, elimination, and metabolism. Another term for this balance is *pharmacokinetics*. In most cases, the goal of drug administration is the achievement of a "steady" pharmacokinetic state (often called steady state) in which the amount of drug absorbed is constantly balanced by the competing processes of distribution, elimination, and metabolism. It is often difficult to predict blood or tissue levels of a drug from the dose alone because pharmacokinetic relationships between absorption and steady state may not be linearly related to dose. Measurements of blood levels may be required to ensure appropriate dosing. Knowing something of a drug's half-life may help estimate pharmacokinetics, especially when combined with knowledge of absorption, distribution, and elimination/metabolism. The **half-life** is the time (typically in hours) that it takes for plasma concentrations of a drug to decrease to half of an initial value. After seven half-lives, less than 1% of a drug remains in the plasma. For a short-acting drug, such as triazolam, which has a half-life as short as 1.5 hours, seven half-lives may be very short (about 10 hours), whereas a long half-life drug such as fluoxetine (half-life of 3 days) may not be fully eliminated for several weeks.

While these pharmacokinetic factors are important for understanding the drug's steady state, nurses often want to know how long it takes a drug to act after administration. Most drug handbooks offer information on onset of action. Onset clearly varies with the mode of administration and is typically shorter for drugs given parenterally (especially intravenously) than for drugs given orally. Some psychiatric drugs are intended to have a significant effect after the first dose. Antipsychotic drugs, hypnotics, and anxiolytics most commonly have rapid single-dose effects. Other psychiatric drugs only work after a steady state has been achieved, typically several weeks after administration begins. The nurse studying psychopharmacology will need to understand which drugs are given for their acute effect and which are expected to work only after some days or weeks.

The concept of **blood-brain barrier** is also very important for understanding drug effects in psychiatric mental health nursing. Most psychiatric drugs act on the central nervous system and must therefore leave the bloodstream to enter the interstitial fluid, the cerebrospinal fluid (CSF), and/or the cells of the brain. The capillary blood vessels of the brain are uniquely resistant to the passage of large molecules (such as drugs) from the bloodstream to the central nervous system. Many drugs circulate in the blood bound to protein, and these protein-drug complexes are almost completely excluded by the capillary barrier between blood and brain. Fat-soluble drugs can often pass through capillary membranes, and many molecules are actively transported across capillary cell walls into the brain. Some drugs cannot cross the blood-brain barrier in an active form but will cross in an inactive form that is later changed into the active metabolite within the brain: Levodopa (L-dopa), used to treat parkinsonism, is metabolized to dopamine once it is transported across capillary walls.

NURSING ALERT!

Drug Risks in Pregnancy

Drugs are placed into one of four categories describing the risk during pregnancy:

Category A

Clinical studies have not demonstrated risk to the fetus during the first trimester of pregnancy; no risk has been demonstrated in later trimesters.

Category B

Animal studies indicate no adverse effects on the fetus, but there are no studies in humans, OR animal studies have demonstrated an adverse effect, but studies in pregnant women have not demonstrated a risk to the fetus during the first trimester of pregnancy and there is no evidence of risk in later trimesters.

Category C

Animal studies have shown an adverse effect on the fetus, and there are no human studies. Risk during pregnancy cannot be ruled out; the potential benefits of the drug may outweigh the potential risks.

Category D

There is positive evidence of risk to the human fetus if the drug is used during pregnancy. Potential benefits of the drug may outweigh the potential risks.

Category X

Studies in animals or humans demonstrate fetal abnormalities or adverse reactions that indicate fetal risk. The use of the drug in pregnancy is contraindicated; there is no potential benefit that outweighs the known risks.

Most drugs have their effect because they either bind to a specific brain receptor or because they have an effect on one or more brain neurotransmitter systems. For example, virtually all antipsychotic medications bind strongly to brain receptors for dopamine. In contrast, monoamine oxidase inhibitors disrupt the catabolism of monoamine neurotransmitters that are released at neural synapses. This effectively increases the concentration of a range of neurotransmitters throughout the brain (and other parts of the neuroendocrine system). While few psychoactive drugs have completely "pure" actions, receptor binding and/or neurotransmitter modification probably explain much of the success of contemporary psychopharmacology. Much research is currently being devoted to understanding basic mechanisms of drug action, and the actions of many psychoactive medications are as yet incompletely understood. New ideas of drug action may emerge from the evolving understanding of brain function and its relationship to psychiatric disorders.

ANTIPSYCHOTIC DRUGS

Antipsychotic drugs, also called "major tranquilizers," are administered to control the symptoms of psychosis such as hallucinations and bizarre or paranoid behavior. These drugs tend to produce a calming effect without significantly sedating the client or reducing alertness. A number of antipsychotic medications will be considered in this section. Among the most important are haloperidol (Haldol), chlorpromazine (Thorazine), thioridazine (Mellaril), fluphenazine (Prolixin), trifluoperazine (Stelazine), and clozapine (Clozaril).

Indications and Evidence for Effectiveness

Antipsychotic medications are effective treatment for psychoses whether caused by psychiatric or medical conditions. However, since many medically induced psychotic states are transient, treatment may not be necessary for brief or mild psychosis. The major psychotic disorders—schizophrenia and manic-depressive psychosis—respond well to antipsychotics. Symptoms for which antipsychotic treatment is often used include hallucinations, delusions, and disorganized thought processes, including paranoia. In the course of schizophrenic illness, such antipsychotic-responsive symptoms are termed "positive" symptoms because they result in socially disruptive behaviors. As emphasized in Chapter 11, the *negative symptoms* of schizophrenia (withdrawal, lack of initiative, failure to maintain hygiene) do not respond to classical antipsychotics, although they do sometimes improve after treatment with the "atypical" antipsychotic clozapine (Clozaril) (Pickar et al., 1992). While there is no evidence that any one of the commonly used antipsychotic drugs is more effective than the others, clozapine, often described as an "atypical antipsychotic, clearly offers therapeutic benefits not achieved by other medications" (Owens & Risch, 1995, p. 272). Not only are anti-

Neuroleptics and Antipsychotics

In the course of your professional duties, you may hear the term *neuroleptic* used in reference to a medication. This is an older term for the antipsychotics and is being used less to refer to a medication than to the neurological side effects nowadays. The preferred term is *antipsychotic*; it is clearer as to its use and more hopeful in its meaning. However, many physicians continue to use the terms interchangeably, and you should always consider what is meant when the term *neuroleptic* is used.

psychotics effective in controlling symptoms of acute psychosis, they have been shown by a number of carefully controlled studies to be effective in preventing relapse in individuals with chronic disorders. Current guidelines suggest 1 to 2 years of treatment following a first psychotic episode and at least 5 years of treatment following recurrent episodes (Kissling et al., 1991).

Pharmacology

There are nearly 20 antipsychotic drugs in clinical use in the United States. These drugs can be grouped in several ways:

Grouping by Chemical Class

Antipsychotic drugs can be classed as phenothiazines, thioxanthenes, butyrophenones, dibenzoxazepines, dihydroindolones, dibenzodiazepines, and benzisoxazoles. The phenothiazines, together with the next four categories (thioxanthenes, butyrophenones, dibenzoxazepines, and dihydroindolones), comprise the "classical" antipsychotic drugs, most of which have been in clinical use for several decades.

Because chemical names are complex, nurses and mental health professionals find it practical to classify antipsychotic drugs into two broad groups: (1) phenothiazines and other classical agents and (2) the newest drugs: risperidone (Risperdal) and clozapine (Clozaril). Risperidone (a benzisoxazole) is a relatively new medication that as yet has no clearly demonstrated advantage over classical antipsychotics. In contrast, clozapine is a dibenzodiazepine, which may be highly effective in persons not responding to other antipsychotics.

Grouping by Potency Class

Antipsychotic medications are commonly grouped by the amount of drug required to achieve an effect. Two phenothiazines—fluphenazine (Prolixin) and trifluoperazine (Stelazine)—and a butyrophenone—haloperidol (Haldol)—are classified as "high potency" because only a few milligrams have significant antipsychotic effects.

The "low-potency" drugs—chlorpromazine (Thorazine), thioridazine (Mellaril), and chlorprothixene (Taractan)—typically achieve effects comparable to a few milligrams of high-potency drugs with doses of approximately 100 mg. Beyond this 50-fold difference in absolute dose needed to achieve similar effects, there are some additional differences between potency classes. For example, the low-potency drugs are more sedating, whereas the high-potency drugs are more likely to produce certain troublesome complications (see discussion of adverse reactions below). The majority of drugs fall into an intermediate-potency range and also have intermediate sedative and adverse effects.

Grouping by Length of Action

The third major classification divides drugs into short- and long-acting preparations. Two drugs (fluphenazine decanoate and haloperidol decanoate) are given intramuscularly and have effects that last for several weeks. These drugs are compounded as decanoic acid esters so that their half-life may reach nearly 10 days. They are also available in much shorter acting forms with half-lives of only a few hours. An intermediate form of fluphenazine (fluphenazine enanthate) typically lasts 1 to 3 weeks. The nurse must use care in administering these drugs to ensure that the correct formulation is given. The remaining drugs, whether given orally or by injection, have clinically significant effects for 24 hours or less.

Non-Antipsychotic Drugs Commonly Used in the Treatment of Psychosis

Psychotic persons are often treated with benzodiazepines (discussed in the section on anxiety) and may be given antidepressants and/or lithium if they have psychosis due to or complicated by mood disorder. These latter drugs are occasionally useful in managing psychosis but are not antipsychotics. They are discussed below in the section on mood disorders. Many psychotic persons are treated simultaneously with antipsychotic drugs and with antiparkinsonian and/or anticholinergic agents. The antiparkinsonian and anticholinergic drugs are used to counteract antipsychotic medication side effects rather than for their specific effects on psychosis. These medications will be considered in a subsequent section describing adverse reactions to antipsychotic drugs.

As noted in Chapter 11, much current evidence suggests that schizophrenia (and perhaps other psychoses as well) involves excessive activation of brain D_2 dopamine receptors. (A more general discussion of the nature of receptors appears in chapter 3.) Antipsychotic drugs are all strong blockers of dopamine D_2 receptors in the brain. Clozapine blocks D_2 but also has effects on other dopamine receptors (D_1 and D_4) as well as several other neurotransmitter systems. This wider range of action may explain the enhanced effectiveness of clozapine, in comparison with other "classical" antipsychotics.

The phenothiazines, thioxanthenes, and dibenzoxazepines have a similar chemical structure, each with a central ring flanked on each side by two aromatic rings. The central ring is in turn linked to one of several longer chains, modifications of which may have a strong effect on drug potency. Because their chemical structure typically lacks highly polar regions, the antipsychotic drugs are not very water soluble, and as a result they have a high affinity for fatty tissues such as lung, brain, and adipose stores. Because of this fat affinity, lower doses may be required in very thin persons; however there are no standard recommendations to change dosage based on body weight or composition. This affinity affects how they are metabolized and excreted in the body. Figure 25-1 illustrates the chemical structure of selected antipsychotics.

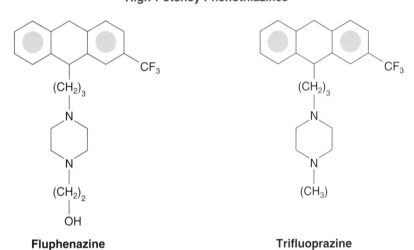

Figure 25-1   Chemical Structure of Selected Antipsychotics

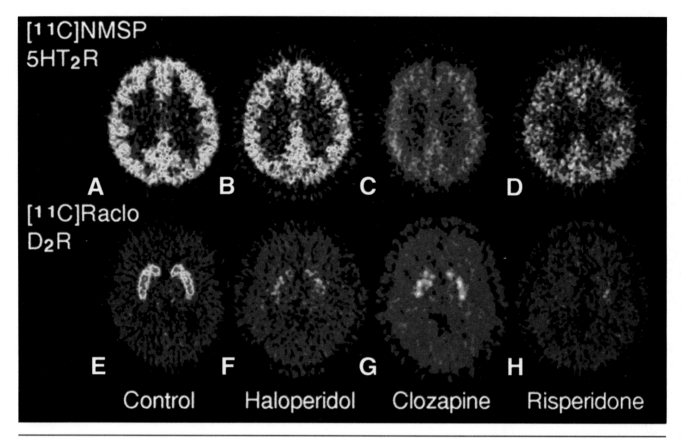

PET images of antipsychotic drug binding sites. PET studies can show how drugs bind to brain tissue. In this study, haloperidol does not seem to bind to serotonin receptors (compare control A with the haloperidol-treated B). However, clozapine and risperidone *do* bind to serotonin receptors (compare control A with treated patients C and D). All three drugs bind to dopamine$_2$ receptors (bottom images: F, G, H). Yellow and red/orange are PET images of receptors available to bind with drugs. As drug binds to receptors and they become unavailable, then the PET image changes to blue, green, or purple.
From "Chemical Brain Anatomy in Schizophrenia," by G. Sedvall and L. Farde, 1995, Lancet, *346(8977), p. 746.*

Dose/Administration

All of the currently available antipsychotic drugs are well absorbed when given either orally or by intramuscular injection. Injection typically produces significant clinical effects within 15 to 30 minutes, whereas oral administration more commonly takes 1 to 4 hours. Many of the antipsychotics are formulated as both pills and a liquid concentrate. Absorption of the liquid preparations is often somewhat faster than the pills. Oral absorption can be decreased by foods, coffee, smoking, and some other drugs. Many antipsychotic drugs are rapidly metabolized by the liver before they actually reach the bloodstream. Parenteral administration avoids both variable absorption and such "first-pass" metabolism. Consequently, parenterally administered medication not only works faster but also often has a greater clinical effect because of higher brain bioavailability.

The dosage of antipsychotics varies with the drug chosen and with the prescribing practice of the psychiatric clinician. In general, thioridazine (Mellaril), haloperidol (Haldol), and chlorpromazine (Thorazine) are the most commonly used preparations, accounting for nearly 70% of all prescriptions in one survey (Wysowski & Baum, 1989). Chlorpromazine and thioridazine dosages vary from 30 to 800 mg daily, whereas haloperidol doses range from 1 to 15 mg.

On arrival in the bloodstream following either oral or parenteral administration, most antipsychotic drugs are tightly bound to serum proteins. Only unbound drug—typically less than 10% of that circulating in the plasma—is available to cross the blood-brain barrier and exert an antipsychotic effect on the brain. Once in the bloodstream, antipsychotic drugs are metabolized and excreted by the liver. Free drug (i.e., drug not bound to serum protein) may pass rapidly into fatty tissues, finding its way to the liver only after some delay. This means both that long dosing intervals (single daily doses) are practical and that drug may remain in the brain (and body fat stores) far longer than measured serum levels would suggest. Since virtually all metabolism of antipsychotics occurs in the liver, genetic differences in the rate of hepatic metabolic processes may significantly affect blood and tissue levels (von Bahr et al., 1991). These differences may eventually be shown to have clinical relevance, but at present there is no practical way to detect such variations in hepatic metabolic rate.

As noted previously, some antipsychotic drugs have been specifically formulated to have a very long duration of action. These long-acting drugs are given by injection only and are manufactured as a preparation of drug dissolved in sesame oil. The sesame oil slows the diffusion of drug into adjacent muscle, and as a consequence absorption is significantly delayed. Once the drug diffuses out of the oil and reaches muscle, the antipsychotic medication is rapidly absorbed and becomes biologically active. Absorption from oil is so slow that it takes up to 3 months of weekly injections for a pharmacological steady state to be reached. After achieving steady state, a balance is attained between drug that reaches the brain and drug that is excreted by the liver. As a result, serum levels and clinical effects stabilize.

Drug Actions

The pharmacological actions of antipsychotics are complex. In general, these medications have two major characteristics: (1) They all bind to brain dopamine receptors, and (2) probably as a result of that binding, they produce a degree of indifference to both external and internal stressful stimuli. This indifference is associated with relatively little sedation or inhibition of pain responses. For example, animals conditioned to avoid electric shocks when a bell rings will ignore the bell after receiving antipsychotics, but they will still respond effectively on feeling the actual shocks (Baldessarini, 1990). These experiments show that the animals have not just been sedated or anesthetized. They respond appropriately to pain but otherwise ignore stimuli that in the absence of medication would lead to a reaction. Other medications that induce a degree of indifference to stress (e.g., narcotics and sedatives) produce sedation or a direct blockade of pain perception. Antipsychotics, in contrast, exert a calming effect without reducing alertness or sensitivity to pain. Narcotics and sedatives typically produce dependence and/or addiction after frequent or prolonged use. Dependency does not occur with antipsychotic medications, but clients should typically be tapered off these medications rather than stopped abruptly.

Drug Interactions

Because antipsychotic drugs are most commonly metabolized by the liver, other medications that affect the

rate of hepatic drug detoxification may have an effect on antipsychotic drug excretion. In recent years, psychiatrists have attempted to keep antipsychotic doses as low as possible so as to avoid common adverse effects. Interactions that further lower drug levels—the drug cimetidine (Tagamet) is an example—may reduce antipsychotic effects and lead to medication failure. The interaction between antipsychotics and cimetidine is particularly troublesome since cimetidine is widely promoted for dyspepsia and is available without prescription.

> ### NURSING ALERT!
> **Tagamet and Antipsychotics**
> Tagamet (cimetidine), an over-the-counter drug for dyspepsia, will lower the effectiveness of antipsychotics.

Some antipsychotic medications may themselves affect the way in which other medications are metabolized. Anticonvulsant medications, used either for seizure control or for mood stabilization, may lower plasma concentrations of antipsychotics. The commonly used mood stabilizer lithium also has a highly significant potential interaction with antipsychotics. This interaction occurs only rarely but may result in profound and permanent neurological impairment. While antipsychotics and lithium are frequently used together without problems, this combination requires close monitoring for signs of neurological disorder (Jeffries et al., 1984). Tricyclic antidepressants are also frequently combined with antipsychotics; this combination may increase serum antidepressant level and produce toxicity if levels are not monitored. Fluoxetine and other serotonin reuptake inhibitors may significantly increase antipsychotic drug levels and lead to serious adverse reactions; fortunately, this interaction is rare (Goff & Baldessarini, 1995). Some cardiac drugs (particularly quinidine, procainamide, and epinephrine) may interact with low-potency antipsychotics; the administration of epinephrine to persons taking medications such as chlorpromazine may result in severe hypotension. Very high levels of caffeine intake may worsen psychosis despite antipsychotic administration (Lucas et al., 1990). Antacids, especially those formulated as gels (Amphogel, Gelusil), may decrease oral antipsychotic drug absorption

> ### NURSING ALERT!
> **Epinephrine and Thorazine**
> Administration of epinephrine to persons taking phenothiazines [such as chlorpromazine (Thorazine)] may result in severe hypotension.

and should not be administered within 4 hours of an antipsychotic dose.

Use During Pregnancy/Lactation

There are no specific known contraindications to the use of antipsychotic medications in pregnancy, although most clinicians try to use the minimum possible dose and to avoid administration in early pregnancy and near the time of delivery (Cohen, 1989). Antipsychotic medications are excreted in breast milk so that breast feeding is contraindicated when these medications must be used following delivery.

Side Effects

Potentially troublesome side effects of antipsychotic medications include constipation, dry mouth, blurred vision, postural hypotension, urinary hesitancy or retention, weight gain, and sedation. Most of these are anticholinergic effects that may be minimized by choosing drugs with relatively lower anticholinergic action: for example, haloperidol (Haldol), trifluoperazine (Stelazine), and fluphenazine (Prolixin).

Adverse Effects

Antipsychotic medications have great potential for serious adverse affects. The classical agents such as thioridazine (Mellaril), haloperidol (Haldol), and chlorpromazine (Thorazine) frequently produce a variety of movement disorders. These include akathisia, dystonia, drug-induced parkinsonism, and tardive dyskinesia. Of these conditions, **akathisia** is the most common and consists of a subjective sense of restlessness with a perceived need to pace or otherwise move continuously. It is easy for the nurse to mistake akathisia for anxiety or agitation. (See the nursing tip on how to differentiate akathisia, anxiety, and agitation.) **Dystonia** consists of sustained, involuntary muscle spasms; these most commonly involve the head and neck but may occasionally occur in other muscle groups. One of the most dramatic dystonic reactions is **oculogyric crisis**, in which extraocular muscle spasm forces the eyes into a fixed, usually upward gaze. Parkinsonism results in tremor and an unsteady shuffling gait; the features of drug-induced parkinsonism may closely resemble those of true idiopathic parkinsonism. The distinction between these two conditions may occasionally be difficult, but idiopathic parkinsonism most commonly occurs in older individuals who have no history of antipsychotic drug use. In contrast, drug-induced parkinsonism is common and occurs in up to 30% of individuals who take long-term antipsychotic medications. These three conditions—akathisia, dystonia, and parkinsonism—usually respond rapidly to antipsychotic dosage reduction, anticholinergic drugs, or diphen-

---

> ### ✳ NURSING TIP
>
> ### Differentiating Akathisia, Anxiety, and Agitation
>
> #### *Akathisia*
> Assess for:
> - Describing "feeling antsy"
> - Inability to sit still
> - Pacing floor
> - Not being frightened
>
> #### *Anxiety*
> Assess for:
> - Expressing thoughts of worry or concerns
> - Having fears, even if unable to state the source of the worry
> - Often having somatic symptoms
>
> #### *Agitation*
> Assess for:
> - Exhibiting escalating anxiety and anger
> - Vocalizing concerns/complaints
> - Possibly demonstrating destructive behavior

---

hydramine (Benadryl). Parenteral diphenhydramine is usually given for acute dystonia, but akathisia is often treated by dosage reduction. Even without dose reduction, tolerance may eventually develop to akathisia.

The fourth movement disorder seen with antipsychotic drugs, tardive dyskinesia, is a more significant adverse effect because it may prove long-lasting despite withdrawal of antipsychotic medication. **Tardive dyskinesia** is a neurological disorder characterized by involuntary movements, most commonly of the tongue and lips. Grimacing, sucking movements, and lip smacking are among the most common tardive dyskinesias. When tardive dyskinesia affects the trunk and extremities, the result may be slow and irregular movements that diminish during relaxation and disappear during sleep. On occasion tardive dyskinesia may be so severe as to interfere with walking, eating, or even breathing. Tardive dyskinesia may improve or disappear when medications are stopped and may even improve with continued administration of classical antipsychotics (Marder & Van Putten, 1995, p. 257). Anticholinergic drugs are often used to treat medication-related movement disorders, but they are also frequently given along with antipsychotics in an effort to prevent the development of neurological symptoms. Common anticholinergic drugs include trihexyphenidyl (Artane) and benztropine (Cogentin). These drugs are usually given orally, but benztropine may be administered either orally or parenterally.

The oral dosage of trihexyphenidyl ranges from 5 to 15 mg daily, usually in two or more doses. The side effects of anticholinergics are predictable from their inhibition of the cholinergic nervous system: dry mouth, nasal congestion, urinary hesitancy, blurred vision, orthostatic hypotension, decreased sweating, constipation, and sedation. The anti-parkinsonian drug amantadine (Symmetrel) is also frequently used in treating drug-induced movement disorders. Amantadine is given only orally, typically in a dose of 100 to 200 mg twice a day. Side effects are common, particularly in the elderly, and may include drowsiness, confusion, depression, and toxic psychosis. Seizures may occasionally be precipitated, and anticholinergic side effects are not uncommon.

Tardive dyskinesia occurs in at least 5% of persons who continue on antipsychotic medications for more than a year, and its incidence increases significantly with longer durations of treatment. In an effort to reduce the prevalence of tardive dyskinesia, the American Psychiatric Association (1992) Task Force on Tardive Dyskinesia has recommended a set of basic guidelines for management of persons needing antipsychotic treatment:

1. Continue medication use only when there is objective evidence that antipsychotic medications are effective treatment for a given individual.

2. Use the lowest effective dose of antipsychotic medications.

3. Be very cautious in prescribing antipsychotic medications to individuals at highest risk of developing tardive dyskinesia: children, the elderly, and individuals with affective disorders.

4. Conduct regular physical examinations to seek evidence of tardive dyskinesia.

5. On diagnosis (or especially worsening) of tardive dyskinesia consider dosage reduction and substitution of other treatments. Utilize informed consent during antipsychotic administration.

Preliminary data suggest that relatively low-dose risperidone may be uniquely effective at controlling psychosis without producing movement disorders (Claus et al., 1992). Nonetheless, high doses of risperidone will also result in movement disorders. As noted below, clozapine has an exceedingly low incidence of associated movement disorders at any dose, but this advantage is counterbalanced by the risk of potentially fatal bone marrow suppression.

Neuroleptic Malignant Syndrome

This syndrome is yet another serious complication of antipsychotic medications. All of the antipsychotic medications, including clozapine, may occasionally result in **Neuroleptic Malignant Syndrome**. This unusual disorder is associated with sudden fever, rigidity, tachycardia, hypertension, and decreased levels of consciousness. Fever can rise to exceedingly high levels, and death may occur. These individuals are usually thought incorrectly to have an infectious condition, and unnecessary investigations and antibiotic treatment may delay diagnosis. Rapid treatment is required for survival, but this requires a high index of suspicion. Treatment includes discontinuation of antipsychotics and the potential administration of a variety of medications, including anti-parkinsonians, bromocriptine, dantrolene, and benzodiazepines. Neuroleptic Malignant Syndrome clinically resembles malignant hypothermia, a condition seen during surgical anesthesia in genetically predisposed individuals.

Not only is clozapine unique in its effectiveness, its adverse effects differ from those of other antipsychotics. Clozapine is only very rarely associated with movement disorders, including tardive dyskinesia. On the other hand, seizures occur in some persons, and 1% to 2% of persons on clozapine develop bone marrow suppression, which may progress to fatal agranulocytosis. Safe use of clozapine requires weekly monitoring of white blood cell counts with permanent discontinuation if the white cell count goes below 2000. Pharmacologists are currently trying to develop antipsychotic medications with the effectiveness of clozapine but without its potentially fatal adverse effects. Olanzapine (Zyprexa) is the first of such drugs to be released, and further experience may show that it truly does offer a safer alternative to clozapine.

Summary of Antipsychotics

Antipsychotic medications are frequently used in psychiatric nursing and in general medical practice. Chlorpromazine, long-acting fluphenazine, and haloperidol are included in the World Health Organization list of essential drugs for primary care (Wig, 1993). The nurse should be familiar with the indications, side effects, and adverse effects of both orally administered and parenteral antipsychotics. Table 25-1 presents a summary of selected antipsychotic drugs.

DRUGS FOR TREATING MOOD DISORDERS

Drugs for treating mood disorders are used either to treat depressed mood (antidepressants) or to treat mania (mood stabilizers). While these drugs rarely act quickly and are not invariably effective, they can greatly enhance clients' well-being and useful functioning.

Indications and Evidence for Effectiveness

Pharmacological treatment for mood disorders is most commonly indicated when both client and provider agree that modification of mood would lead to enhanced well-being and functioning. On rare occasions persons may be given mood-modifying medication against their

Table 25-1   Antipsychotic Medications

GENERIC NAME	TRADE NAME	MODE OF ADMIN- ISTRATION	SEDA- TION	EXTRA- PYRA- MIDAL	ANTI- CHOLIN- ERGIC	ORTHO- STATIC HYPO- TENSION	MAR- ROW SUPPRES- SION	DOSE RANGE (mg)	PLASMA LEVELS (mg/ml)
Phenothiazines									
Chlorpromazine	Thorazine	p.o., p.r., i.m., i.v.	3+	2+	2+	2+	0	30–800	30–500
Thioridizine	Mellaril	p.o.	3+	1+	3+	3+	0	150–800	—
Fluphenazine	Prolixin	p.o., i.m./s.c.	1+	3+	1+	1+	0	5–40	0.13–2.8
Trifluoperazine	Stelazine	p.o., i.m.	1+	3+	1+	1+	0	2–40	—
Thioxanthene									
Thiothixene	Navane	p.o., i.m.	1+	3+	1+	1+	0	8–30	2–57
Butyrephenone									
Haloperidol	Haldol	p.o., i.m.	1+	3+	1+	1+	0	1–15	5–20
Dibenzoxazepine									
Loxapine	Loxitane	p.o., i.m.	2+	3+	1+	2+	0	20–250	—
Dibenzodiazepines									
Clozapine	Clozaril	p.o.	3+	1+	3+	3+	4+	300–900	—
Olanzapine	Zyprexa	p.o.	3+	1+	3+	3+	0	5–10	—
Benzisoxazole									
Risperidone	Risperdal	p.o.	1+	3+	1+	1+	0	4–6	—

will, but such administration is invariably court ordered and given only to convicted criminals whose psychiatric hospitalization replaces a prison sentence.

Effectiveness data for antidepressants is well established for severe depression requiring hospitalization and for tricyclic medications. Tricyclic drugs tend to be less expensive than other antidepressants, and in public clinics or managed-care settings cost may be a major factor dictating medication choice. Both the cost and side effects profile of trazodone are midway between tricyclics and selective serotonin reuptake inhibitors (SSRIs); this makes trazodone a popular choice for many prescribers. Many clinicians favor SSRI antidepressants because they are probably safer in intentional overdose, a significant risk in depressed individuals. Concerns about safety are discussed at more length under "adverse effects" below.

Drugs for treating mood disorders generally fall into four categories: tricyclic (and related) antidepressants, SSRIs, monoamine oxidase inhibitors (MAOIs), and mood stabilizers. Each one of these categories will be discussed separately in the sections that follow. The tricyclic medications include imipramine (Tofranil), desipramine (Norpramin or Pertofrane), amitriptyline (Elavil), nortriptyline (Pamelor), clomipramine (Anafranil), trimipramine (Surmontil), doxepin (Sinequan), and protriptyline (Vivactil). Amoxapine (Asendin), a tetracyclic, and maprotiline (Ludiomil), a heterocyclic, are closely related to these in their structure and effects. Several other compounds—trazodone (Desyrel), bupropion (Wellbutrin), venlafaxine (Effexor), and nefazodone (Serzone)—are not chemically related to the tricyclics but are quite similar in their antidepressant effects; these will be discussed in the section on tricyclics and related antidepressants. The SSRIs include fluoxetine (Prozac), sertraline (Zoloft), paroxetine (Paxil), and fluvoxamine (Luvox). The MAOIs include phenelzine (Nardil) and tranylcypromine (Parnate). Mood stabilizers include lithium and several anticonvulsants: primarily valproic acid or divalproex (Depakote) and carbamazepine (Tegretol). Some clinicians use additional drugs in treating mood disorders; among these are the benzodiazepine alprazolam (Xanax), the antianxiety drug buspirone (Buspar), and stimulants such as amphetamines.

The neurobiology of depression is highly complex and is briefly reviewed in Chapter 12. A major current theory explaining depression states that depressed individuals have persistent abnormalities in the concentration and distribution of biogenic amines that serve as neurotransmitters within the brain. Most antidepressant medications in common use exert some measurable effect on levels of brain neurotransmitters, most commonly norepinephrine and/or serotonin. The SSRIs typically have negligible effects on norepinephrine systems but are quite specific moderators of brain serotonin levels.

Plasma norepinephrine levels are also linked to mania (Swann et al., 1990), but theories about causes of mania are less well developed than are those pertaining to depression. Nonetheless, lithium and other mood-stabilizing medications used in the treatment of bipolar disorder seem to affect the release of both norepinephrine, serotonin, and dopamine (another biogenic amine neurotransmitter) (Price et al., 1990).

Tricyclic and Related Antidepressants

Tricyclic and related drugs were the first antidepressants to come into clinical use, and these medications still have important roles in treating mood disorders. While many tricyclic and related antidepressants are available, there are relatively few highly significant differences among them. Imipramine was the first of the tricyclic drugs to be released, but no data demonstrate that any of the more recently introduced medications are more effective in treating depression. All of the cyclic antidepressants (tricyclic, tetracyclic, and heterocyclic) have a wide range of biochemical actions in the brain and elsewhere (Potter, Manji, & Rudorfer, 1995). These actions often result in side effects, and most choices among drugs are made in an effort to minimize such effects. These choices may be somewhat artificial since once in the body the liver modifies many of these drugs. For example, amitriptyline is converted by the liver to nortriptyline, and imipramine to desipramine. In general, imipramine or amitriptyline is used when sedation is a desired side effect, doxepin when both sedation and anxiety reduction are of primary importance, desipramine or nortriptyline when sedation is to be avoided, and protriptyline when some level of psychological stimulation is desired. Trazodone has a very different (and generally milder) spectrum of side effects when compared with tricyclic and heterocyclic antidepressants, but it may be less effective for the management of severe depression.

Dose/Administration

Antidepressants are only given orally, are typically well absorbed, and reach peak plasma concentrations in 2 to 6 hours. Sedation and side effects of antidepressants are seen within several hours of taking these medications: Clients often report improved sleep patterns from the first night. Antidepressant effect, as with virtually all the antidepressants, is usually significantly delayed, usually for at least 4 to 6 weeks after beginning treatment. Doses are usually begun quite low and increased gradually (typically at intervals of 1 to 4 weeks) until clinical improvement occurs (Potter et al., 1995). Cyclic antidepressants generally have half-lives of approximately 24 hours and can usually be given once daily. The half-lives of trazodone, amoxapine, bupropion, and venlafaxine are shorter, and these drugs should usually be given in divided doses. Total daily doses must be individualized based on response, side effects, and (occasionally) blood levels.

While assays for therapeutic (and toxic) blood levels are available for most of the tricyclic medications, they are of clear value only for nortriptyline, imipramine, and desipramine (Potter et al., 1995). Nortriptyline dose is generally 100 mg or less daily. The use of nortriptyline often requires careful monitoring of blood levels because antidepressant effects are not seen below 50 ng/ml or above 150 ng/ml. Therapeutic dosage ranges for most other medications are approximately 100 to 200 mg daily. Except in the elderly there is usually no need to measure levels until daily doses of 300 to 350 mg are exceeded. Clients with depression are commonly treated for at least 6 months. For many persons, maintenance treatment should be continued indefinitely. Those for whom long-term treatment should be considered include persons with profound depression, frequently recurring depression (two or more episodes of major depression probably justify long-term treatment), and suicidal ideation or attempts.

Drug Actions

Tricyclic and related antidepressants are usually, but not invariably, effective in relieving symptoms of depression. Individuals with relatively short duration of symptoms (less than a year) and with unipolar and/or melancholic depression are most likely to benefit from treatment. While some studies have suggested that trazodone is less effective than tricyclics in treating severe depression (usually defined as depression requiring hospitalization), its effectiveness for less severe forms of depression is well established (Schatzberg, 1987). Trazodone has a significant antianxiety effect in some individuals, and this effect is often seen well before depression improves. The nurse following a client receiving trazodone may observe less reported anxiety or may observe changes in the client's appearance or reaction to stressful situations. When antidepressant effects of trazodone and the cyclic antidepressants become evident after 2 to 4 weeks, the client will report improved mood, better and more restful sleep, and gradual loss of the primary depressive symptoms of anhedonia and dysphoria.

Tricyclic antidepressants have a number of indications beyond depression. Chief among these are the treatment of panic disorder (primarily with imipramine or nortriptyline), obsessive-compulsive disorder (with clomipramine), and psychotic depression with delusions (primarily with amoxapine, an antidepressant chemically related to antipsychotic medications).

Drug Interactions

Cyclic antidepressants have a large number of potential interactions with other drugs, but most of these are of doubtful significance (Ciraulo et al., 1994). Many of the cyclic drugs have significant anticholinergic side effects, and these may be enhanced to the point of toxicity by other anticholinergic drugs. This interaction is potentially most serious in the elderly and may be produced by antipsychotics, antihistamines, some general anesthetics and premedicating agents, and narcotic pain relievers, particularly meperidine. Norepinephrine may interact with some tricyclics, and even the small amount found in local anesthetics may potentially cause hypertension or arrhythmias if more than about 5 cc is injected (Yagiela, 1985). While the safety of oral sympathomimetics and inhaled bronchodilators is occasionally questioned, the combination of these medications with tricyclics seems to be safe (Ciraulo et al., 1994). Tricyclics may interact significantly with SSRIs and MAOIs; these interactions may produce significant elevations of tricyclic dosages and hypertensive crises, respectively. Cimetidine, available both by prescription and over the counter, may impair metabolism of tricyclic antidepressants and lead to elevated blood levels with resultant toxicity. Clients needing H_2 blockade should preferentially take an alternative medicine such as ranitidine (Zantac). Alcohol adds to central nervous system (CNS) depression that is produced by many antidepressant drugs (most cyclics and trazodone), and alcohol-related impairment may occur after fewer drinks in persons taking these medications. All clients should be informed of this potentially significant interaction.

NURSING ALERT!

Alcohol and Antidepressants

Alcohol adds to the CNS depression produced by antidepressants, and clients must be made aware that alcohol-related impairment occurs after fewer drinks than in persons not taking these medications.

Use During Pregnancy/Lactation

Cyclic antidepressants should generally not be taken during pregnancy. With the exception of maprotiline (Ludiomil), all of the cyclic drugs are classified in either risk category D (positive evidence of risk) or C (risk cannot be ruled out). Maprotiline is classified in category B (no evidence of risk in humans). The SSRIs are all in category B, though data on safety are limited. When the mother's well-being is judged to require antidepressant treatment, either an SSRI or maprotiline should probably be used. Antidepressants are generally excreted into breast milk, but little is known of real or potential risk from this source.

Side Effects

Cyclic antidepressants are sometimes called "dirty drugs" by psychiatrists and other mental health clinicians because they act on so many different receptor systems. Many of the actions of antidepressants on receptor systems probably have little or no direct relationship to antidepressant effects, but they are responsible for most drug side effects. While each of the cyclic medications has a different side effects profile, most have some effect on each of the following receptor systems: cholinergic (also called muscarinic), histaminergic, alpha-adrenergic, and dopaminergic. Anticholinergic effects include blurred vision, dry mouth, rapid heart rate, constipation, urinary retention, and perhaps impaired memory function. Antihistaminic effects include weight gain, sedation, hypotension, and interaction with other drugs that cause CNS depression. Alpha-adrenergic effects include postural hypotension, dizziness, and potential interaction with some antihypertensive medications. Antidopaminergic effects include movement disorders and endocrine changes (see under adverse effects below). Cyclic medications all have side effects in each of these categories, although desipramine and nortriptyline probably have the best side effects profile of this group of drugs. Trazodone has no anticholinergic effect, moderate alpha-adrenergic effect (typically manifested by postural hypotension), and very little antidopaminergic effect.

Adverse Effects

The most significant adverse effects of cyclic antidepressants are seen in accidental or intentional overdose. These drugs typically have a very limited therapeutic margin, and fatal overdose may occur with ingestion of only a few days' supply. Deaths have occurred with only 1000 mg of amitriptyline, and it is not uncommon for clients to take 150 to 300 mg daily. It is usually recommended that clinicians not dispense more than 1000 mg of these drugs at a time unless suicidal risk is judged completely absent. Symptoms of overdose include CNS depression, widening of electrocardiogram (EKG) QRS complexes with associated heart block, shock, seizures, and dangerous temperature elevations. There are some data suggesting that antidepressants may increase the risk of suicide, especially in persons with a history of impulsive or aggressive behavior (Charney, Miller, Licinia, & Salomon, 1995). Overdose is not necessary for tricyclic-associated fatalities to occur; occasional unexplained, and presumably drug-related, deaths in children taking tricyclics continue to be reported (Riddle, Geller, & Ryan, 1993).

Trazodone, along with most other non–cyclic antidepressants, is relatively free of direct cardiac side effects and probably safer in overdose than are cyclic medications. Nonetheless, trazodone may produce severe postural hypotension that, especially in the elderly, can cause falls, fractures, or perhaps even cardiovascular events such as stroke or myocardial infarction. Trazodone should probably be avoided in geriatric individuals. Trazodone may rarely cause priapism (sustained and painful erection) in men, usually in the first weeks of treatment. This

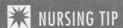

NURSING TIP

Monitoring the Use of Cyclic Antidepressants

◆ Antidepressants such as amitriptyline have a limited therapeutic margin.

◆ The therapeutic dose (300 mg/day) is such that a 3–4 day supply is equivalent to a lethal dose.

Nursing actions:

◆ Assess suicidal risk.

◆ Assess how often prescription is being refilled.

◆ Assess if the drug is being taken daily.

◆ May conduct pill counts to determine if the drug is being taken or stored.

◆ Blood levels of the drugs are indicated if there is a concern about dose.

complication may require surgical treatment and may result in permanent impotence. For this reason, and despite the rarity of priapism, many clinicians avoid the use of trazodone in men. Through their inhibition of dopaminergic pathways, tricyclics and occasionally other antidepressants may increase levels of the hormone prolactin. This may result in galactorrhea (leakage of milk from one or both breasts) in women and in loss of libido in both men and women. All of the cyclic antidepressants have a small chance of inducing seizures, even in persons who have not previously had epilepsy. Although remarkably free from other adverse effects, bupropion, a non–cyclic antidepressant, has had a reputation of being particularly likely to produce seizures. Some studies show that the risk of seizure production with bupropion is actually quite small (under 1%) and may actually not exceed that of tricyclics (Davidson, 1989).

Selective Serotonin Reuptake Inhibitors

In recent years a number of drugs have been developed whose actions primarily involve serotonin-related pathways. The tricyclic clomipramine was first among these, but in more recent years a series of selective serotonin reuptake inhibitors (SSRIs) has come into widespread clinical use. Chief among these are fluoxetine (Prozac), sertraline (Zoloft), paroxetine (Paxil), and fluvoxamine (Luvox). Several others are recently released or in development. As noted above, cyclic antidepressants and other closely related drugs show effects on a variety of brain neurotransmitters. These multiple actions are associated both with antidepressant effectiveness and with side and adverse effects. The SSRIs offer excellent antidepressant effect with relatively few short- and long-term side effects.

The SSRIs are generally regarded as first-line medications for depressed individuals, particularly outpatients with moderate depression. While studies have clearly established the effectiveness of SSRIs compared with placebo, no study has demonstrated any enhanced effectiveness of SSRIs over cyclic antidepressants. With the exception of fluoxetine's long metabolic effect after discontinuation, there are few clinical differences between SSRIs and no apparent pharmacological reason to select one SSRI over another.

The SSRIs are significantly more expensive than the older cyclic medications such as imipramine and trazodone. Wholesale costs for SSRIs typically exceed $50/month, compared with as little as $5 for amitriptyline or imipramine (Anonymous, 1995a). Since no data suggest SSRIs are more effective than tricyclics, they are often chosen because they are perceived to have fewer side effects and a greater margin of safety in overdose.

The SSRIs have been shown to be of value in a number of conditions other than depression. For example, SSRIs are clearly effective in treating Obsessive-Compulsive Disorder; fluoxetine and fluvoxamine are well documented to be of value in this condition. Fluoxetine and several other SSRIs have been shown to improve symptoms in bulimia. Data for Panic Disorder are less extensive but strongly suggest a valuable effect in some individuals. Premenstrual syndrome ("late luteal phase dysphoric disorder") has been shown to respond well to SSRIs in a number of patients. Other data suggest benefit in a variety of other conditions, including migraine, chronic pain, and alcohol dependency/abuse.

The SSRIs inhibit the reuptake of serotonin after it is released at the neuronal synapse. This means that serotonin is present for a longer time, and as a consequence its action is augmented. Because they augment or amplify the effect of serotonin released at synapses, SSRIs function as if they were directly stimulating brain serotonin pathways. In reality, that stimulation is brought about by naturally released serotonin because SSRIs increase the effect of an individual's own serotonin release. In most persons, such an increase in serotonergic effect is enough, after a period of time, to improve symptoms of depression.

Pharmacologically the various SSRIs are strikingly different in the degree to which they inhibit reuptake of both serotonin and several other neurotransmitters. Paroxetine seems to be among the strongest inhibitors of serotonin reuptake, but it also inhibits uptake of norepinephrine and dopamine. Sertraline is a bit less potent in its inhibition of serotonin reuptake but has even more inhibition of dopamine uptake than paroxetine. In contrast, fluvoxamine differs little from sertraline in its effects on serotonin reuptake, but it is strikingly ineffective in altering dopamine uptake (Boyer & Feighner, 1991). These differences among the various SSRIs are pharmacologically interesting, but there is as yet no evidence that they have any clinical importance. All of the SSRIs significantly alter serotonin effects at the synapse; the differences in their effects on other neurotransmitters so far seem relatively unimportant.

Dose/Administration

The SSRIs are all well absorbed after oral administration and are widely distributed throughout the body (including the brain). Dosage of SSRIs must be individualized and differs for each preparation. Compared with other antidepressants, most of the SSRIs have a fairly narrow therapeutic dose "window." Sertraline, for example, may be given in doses from 50 mg up to 200 mg, but effectiveness may decrease as dosage exceeds 200 mg (Tollefson, 1995). Blood levels of SSRIs have not been shown to be of clinical use in assessing nonresponse or toxicity. As with cyclic antidepressants, SSRIs take some time to work, typically at least a month, though some effect on depression may be seen after 10 to 14 days. Doses are rarely altered until after 3 to 4 weeks has elapsed, and there may be no benefit in raising dose for up to 8 weeks (Schweizer et al., 1990).

With the exception of fluoxetine, most SSRIs have elimination half-lives of about 24 hours. Fluoxetine's elimination half-life is somewhat longer, 24 to 72 hours, but unlike other SSRIs, fluoxetine has major metabolites that themselves have half-lives of up to 15 days. This means that in clinical use fluoxetine is uniquely long acting and has significant effects for many days after discontinuation. This characteristic is useful in preventing emergence of depressive symptoms if one or more doses are missed but may be a problem either when side effects require discontinuation or when it is necessary to switch to another medication (such as a tricyclic or an MAOI) that may interact with fluoxetine. A full 5-week "washout" period is recommended before starting a new medication. This may greatly delay effective treatment for individuals who do not respond to fluoxetine. The washout period for other SSRIs is generally 5 to 7 days. This washout is very critical and hence longer when moving from SSRI treatment to administration of an MAOI because MAOIs may interact dangerously with residual SSRIs long after the last dose has been given.

Drug Actions

All of the SSRIs effectively relieve symptoms of depression after 2 to 4 weeks. Clients report enhanced mood and decreased concern with thoughts or problems that would have upset or worried them previously. The SSRIs are often useful in management of Obsessive-Compulsive Disorder (though usually at higher dose than for the management of depression). As with depression, improvement of Obsessive-Compulsive Disorder is also delayed for some weeks. Many clients with depression also report significant anxiety, a symptom that generally decreases or disappears as medication brings depression under control. Symptoms of Panic Disorder also tend to resolve during treatment with SSRIs, although agoraphobia, commonly seen along with Panic Disorder, is less consistently improved.

Drug Interactions

As noted below, SSRI side and adverse effects are relatively mild; consequently drug interactions are relatively less important than with many of the cyclic antidepressants. Fluvoxamine and paroxetine interact with warfarin (Coumadin). Cimetidine (Tagamet) (available over the counter as well as by prescription) may raise SSRI concentrations by impairing hepatic metabolism. Some clinicians have combined SSRIs and tricyclics in an effort to utilize the latters' sedative qualities, but this practice may not always be safe because SSRI's may raise tricyclic blood levels and increase risk of toxicity. Monoamine oxidase inhibitors may interact significantly with SSRIs, and because of relatively long elimination half-lives, at least 2 weeks should be allowed for drug washout between stopping an SSRI and starting an MAOI (5 weeks for fluoxetine).

The SSRIs are less likely to increase the sedative or intoxicating potential of alcohol than are cyclic medications. While sertraline absorption is affected when taken with or near meals, other SSRIs are uninfluenced by food.

A rare and potentially serious drug interaction (usually with an MAOI) is called the **serotonergic syndrome** and resembles somewhat symptoms seen in intentional SSRI overdose. Symptoms include agitation, sweating, rigidity, fever, hyperreflexia, tachycardia, and hypotension. On occasion coma and even death may occur. The serotonergic syndrome is most commonly seen following drug interaction between an SSRI and an MAOI. As with overdose, treatment is largely supportive.

Use During Pregnancy/Lactation

The SSRIs are given a category B rating for pregnancy safety. Animal studies do not suggest harm, and there are no human data contraindicating use of the drug in pregnancy. These drugs do appear in breast milk in approximately the same concentration as serum. While no data suggest harm to infants from absorbing SSRIs during breast feeding, many clinicians counsel caution in combining breast feeding and SSRI administration.

Side Effects

Overall, the SSRIs are among the best tolerated antidepressants. In short-term trials 10% to 20% of patients have discontinued SSRIs because of side effects, compared with 30% to 35% taking tricyclic medications (Tollefson, 1995). Common side effects include anxiety, headache, and gastrointestinal disturbance (nausea, diarrhea). The SSRIs are particularly likely to interfere with sexual functioning (erection in men and orgasm in both men and women). Clients may not volunteer that they are experiencing these side effects, and so it is important for the nurse to inquire explicitly about any sexual dysfunction. Since depression is itself associated with decreased libido and sexual functioning, it may occasionally be difficult to be certain whether reported sexual dysfunction is due to the drug or to depression itself. The SSRIs, particularly fluoxetine, can cause akathisia, a symptom of restlessness discussed in this chapter as a side effect of antipsychotic medications.

Adverse Effects

The SSRIs are generally free of serious adverse effects, even in intentional overdose. Deaths have occurred following SSRI overdoses, particularly when taken in combination with alcohol. However, death is a rare complication of SSRI overdose, and most patients recover uneventfully with supportive care. Serotonergic syndrome, discussed earlier under drug interactions, may occasionally occur without known administration of any drug other than SSRIs. As noted earlier, symptoms include agitation, sweating, rigidity, fever, hyperreflexia, tachycardia, and hypotension. Treatment is largely supportive but must be given with vigilance to avoid a potentially fatal outcome.

Monoamine Oxidase Inhibitors

Monoamine oxidase inhibitors (MAOIs) are a group of drugs notable for their similar pharmacological actions, their good effectiveness in treatment of depression, and their potentially dangerous interactions with both drugs and foods. The MAOIs are useful "second-line" drugs for treating mood disorders but can only be used safely with careful monitoring in highly motivated clients.

Indications and Evidence for Effectiveness

The MAOIs have demonstrated effectiveness in depression, Panic Disorder, some other anxiety disorders (social phobia, Obsessive-Compulsive Disorder, Post-Traumatic Stress Disorder), and bulimia. The "classical" nonselective agents isocarboxazid (Marplan), phenelzine (Nardil), and tranylcypromine (Parnate) have generally been regarded as second- or third-line antidepressant medications, to be tried when tricyclics or SSRIs fail. A double-blind crossover study found phenelzine effective in the majority of clients who failed a trial of imipramine (McGrath et al., 1993). Many of these clients had atypical depression (see Chapter 12), a condition for which MAOIs and SSRIs are probably more effective than are tricyclic agents. Some data suggest that dysthymia (Chapter 13) may respond more effectively to MAOIs than to tricyclics, but as with atypical depression, most clinicians are likely to utilize SSRIs for these individuals. Elderly clients may respond particularly well to MAOIs.

As more selective reversible MAOIs are released, these medications may become even more widely used. Recently developed MAOIs seem to interact less significantly with foods and medications, have fewer side effects, and are probably at least as effective as the older MAOI agents. At the time of writing, none of these has been released for use in the United States.

Pharmacology

The MAOIs act by blocking an enzyme (monoamine oxidase) whose primary purpose is to metabolize three important brain neurotransmitters (norepinephrine, serotonin, dopamine) to biologically inactive forms. The inhibition of monoamine oxidase prevents the breakdown of the neurotransmitters and increases the concentration of these substances within neuronal cells. Over several weeks, this pharmacological effect results in changes in the number of cell-surface receptors for the involved neurotransmitters. Pharmacologists attribute the clinical usefulness of MAOIs both to this change in receptor levels and to increased amine levels. The MAOIs are commonly categorized by whether or not they fit into the following three groups: (1) those that belong to the chemical family of "hydrazines," (2) those that inhibit monoamine oxidase reversibly, and (3) those that are selective for one of the two forms of monoamine oxidase: MAO-A or MAO-B. The most frequently prescribed MAOI, phenelzine (Nardil) is a hydrazine that is a nonreversible inhibitor and is nonselective. Tranylcypromine (Parnate) is a similar nonhydrazine drug. Moclobemide remains unreleased in the United States, but it is both selective for MAO-A and reversible. Reversible inhibitors may be safer if food or drug interactions occur (see below). MAO-A affects primarily dopamine and norepinephrine metabolism, while MAO-B is relatively selective for serotonin. It seems highly likely that reversible MAO-A inhibitors offer clinical advantages and will soon be available in the United States. Pure MAO-B inhibitors are not in common clinical use, and there is little evidence to suggest that selective inhibitors offer any benefit over nonselective drugs. The MAO-B inhibitor selegiline is widely used in Parkinson's disease but in parkinsonian doses has not been found useful in treating depression.

Dose/Administration

The MAOIs are all given orally, are well absorbed, and reach peak plasma levels within approximately 1 hour. The half-life is about 12 hours, but because most of these drugs have long-acting metabolites, at least 2 weeks should elapse between stopping an MAOI and starting a different antidepressant. The MAOIs should be stopped gradually to avoid significant side effects.

Phenelzine is given three times per day with a rapid increase of dose from 15 to 20 mg. Total daily doses up to 90 mg are often used initially, but as the desired effects are seen, the dosage is often reduced to as little as 15 mg daily or every other day. Tranylcypromine is given two times per day at 15 mg/dose. Increases are made fairly slowly over 2 to 4 weeks. When desired response is achieved, dosage is also dropped to low levels: typically 10 to 20 mg daily.

Drug Actions

The MAOIs are used for depression of all degrees of severity. Tranylcypromine is somewhat more commonly employed in very severe depression and may have an effect sooner than other antidepressants, sometimes within 10 days. Tranylcypromine is chemically related to amphetamines (see the next general section on miscellaneous drugs for depression) and like amphetamines produces a stimulant effect that may contribute to drug effectiveness. Otherwise, like other categories of antidepressants, MAOIs take 3 to 4 weeks to improve symptoms of depression. As noted above, monoamine oxidase inhibition occurs quite rapidly, especially with irreversible inhibitors, but antidepressant effect typically takes some time to develop. This delay suggests that enzyme inhibition is only one of the effects that lead to improvement of depressive symptoms.

Drug Interactions

Significant drug interactions occur with MAOIs and may be quite serious. Since MAOIs inhibit the metabolism and detoxification of biogenic amines, ingestion of these substances or their analogues may result in prolonged and severe stimulation of nervous system pathways. The major drug interaction risks are other antidepressants (particularly SSRI), narcotic analgesics [especially meperidine (Demerol) and dextromethorphan, a common ingredient in nonprescription cough medications such as Robitussin-DM], and various preparations containing sympathomimetic drugs. The latter include a variety of decongestants and cold medications. The SSRIs are sometimes purposefully used with MAOIs, and many experts feel the risk have been exaggerated. Surgery is particularly dangerous for persons on MAOIs because of the potential inadvertent administration of meperidine to control postoperative pain. The interaction between meperidine and MAOIs

⚡ NURSING ALERT!

Demerol and MAOIs

◆ Demerol (meperidine) should not be given to persons taking MAOIs!

◆ There is a severe interaction between MAOIs and meperidine that produces fever, hypertension, and coma.

may result in coma, fever, and hypertension. Other drug-MAOI interactions may be dangerous and result in very high blood pressure, headache, sweating, and palpitations. Severe interactions may progress to decreased consciousness, extreme fever, intracranial hemorrhage, and death. Inadvertent medication interactions can be treated with a calcium channel blocker, typically nifedipine (Procardia). Usually a single oral dose will rapidly lower blood pressure and block the effects of drug interaction. When nifedipine is ineffective, phentolamine (Regitine) may be given intravenously. Sympathomimetic drugs pose somewhat uncertain and variable risks. In general, "direct" sympathomimetics such as epinephrine, norepinephrine, phenylephrine, isoproterenol, and methoxymine have the least serious interactions. "Indirect" sympathomimetics include amphetamine, methamphetamine, ephedrine, pseudoephedrine, phenylpropanolamine, and others. Many of these medications are available either as stimulant street drugs or as common ingredients in over-the-counter cough and cold treatments. Individuals on MAOIs must exercise great care to avoid these indirect sympathomimetics. Symptoms are similar to the meperidine interaction and include hypertension, agitation, fever, convulsions, and coma.

⚡ NURSING ALERT!

MAOIs and Robitussin (dextromethorphan)

Persons taking MAOIs must be alerted to the fact that over-the-counter medications with dextromethorphan, a common ingredient of cough medication, interact with MAOIs, producing hypertension, fever, and possibly coma.

Food and Alcohol Interactions

One of the major deterrents to the use of MAOIs is that a number of foods react strongly with these medications to produce serious reactions identical to those that accompany the interaction between MAOIs and sympathomimetics or meperidine. Most offending foods contain significant amounts of the amino acid tyramine, which is an indirect sympathomimetic agent. Individuals taking MAOIs must avoid foods containing more than 6 mg of tyramine. Intake between 6 and 10 mg provokes a moderate reaction: elevated blood pressure, headache, restlessness. Ingestion of 25 mg or more may result in severe symptoms requiring emergency treatment. Death may occasionally occur from such dietary indiscretions. Few if any foods have more than 25 mg of tyramine in a single serving, though some "strong" cheeses may have as much as 15 to 17 mg. Aged cheddar cheese (often labeled "sharp") contains 7.5 mg per slice, whereas Swiss gruyere has 1.9 mg. Salami has 5.6 mg per serving, whereas liver-

FOODS TO BE AVOIDED BY PERSONS TAKING MAO INHIBITORS

Foods to be completely avoided:

◆ Sharp (old) cheddar cheese

◆ Salami

◆ Sauerkraut

◆ Beer containing yeast

◆ Yeast extracts

◆ Wine containing yeast

◆ Avocados (overripe)

◆ Caviar

◆ Fava beans

Foods that can be consumed if used in moderation:

◆ Chocolate

◆ Coffee

wurst has only 0.1 mg. Sauerkraut has very high tyramine levels, and fairly high amounts are found in banana peels (though not in the fruit itself). Alcoholic beverages may interact with MAOIs, though not all experts agree on the potential seriousness of such interaction. Some imported beers have moderate tyramine concentrations; Guinness Extra Stout, for example, has slightly over a milligram per bottle. Red wines have small amounts of tyramine per 4-ounce serving, generally half a milligram or less. White wines, whiskey, gin, and vodka are probably safe in quantities up to 4 ounces. Even this restriction may be conservative since consuming a liter of Dubonnet would likely result in intake of less than 2 mg of tyramine (Ciraulo et al., 1994). Clearly, individuals on MAOIs must be carefully instructed on avoiding risky foods and beverages. Selecting foods that can be safely consumed is not difficult but requires vigilance, especially when eating in restaurants. When MAOIs are prescribed, the nurse will need to assist the client in acquiring the necessary skills to avoid dangerous medication or food interactions.

Use During Pregnancy/Lactation

The MAOIs are category C agents in pregnancy. Human data are sparse, and animal data suggest teratogenic potential for some agents. These drugs are usually avoided during pregnancy. Little data exist on use during lactation, and it is probably unwise to use these medications in lactating mothers.

Side Effects

Common side effects of nonselective MAOIs cause decreased heart rate, hypotension (which may lead to dizziness or syncope), and a variety of anticholinergic symptoms: dry mouth, blurred vision, and urinary hesitancy. Central nervous system symptoms occur on occasion and include agitation, anxiety, insomnia, and euphoria. Sexual dysfunction, weight gain, peripheral neuropathy, and impaired speech may sometimes occur as side effects. Newer MAOI agents such as moclobemide are remarkably generally free of these side effects but may occasionally cause nausea.

Adverse Effects

The most serious adverse effects of nonselective, nonreversible agents include syncope from hypotension, potentially resulting in physical injury and either hepatic abnormality or bone marrow suppression. Routine monitoring of liver functions or blood counts are usually not necessary. On occasion MAOIs can produce hypomania or full-blown psychosis. Clients with a history of mania or hypomania should generally be placed on mood stabilizers rather than antidepressants. When selective MAO-A inhibitors are released, they will probably come into fairly widespread usage because they are generally free of serious adverse effects. Table 25-2 presents a summary of MAOIs as well as the antidepressants.

Miscellaneous Antidepressant Drugs and Drug Combinations

Several medications have some utility in managing depression, although they are not usually considered to be first-line antidepressants. Among these are alprazolam (Xanax), amphetamines or other stimulant medications, and buspirone (BuSpar). Each of these drugs has other primary indications (anxiety and Panic Disorder for alprazolam, Attention-Deficit Disorder for amphetamines, and Generalized Anxiety for buspirone). While lacking Food and Drug Administration (FDA) approval for depression, each of these three medications has some demonstrated effectiveness for depression. Controlled studies, for example, show alprazolam to be as effective as tricyclics when given in the relatively high doses used for Panic Disorder (Warner et al., 1988). The data supporting use of stimulant drugs in refractory depression are much less convincing (Fawcett & Busch, 1995). Nonetheless, especially in combination with other antidepressants, case reports suggest that stimulant drugs can significantly increase both effectiveness and rapidity of onset of antidepressant effect. Buspirone has been shown effective in a number of trials, but quite large doses are required, often as high as 60 mg daily. Such high doses (two to four times the usual dose for treating anxiety) are very expensive, and although safe and relatively well tolerated, buspirone is unlikely to find wide use until it becomes less expensive.

Several additional drugs have shown promise in treating refractory depressive symptoms when combined with

Table 25-2   **Antidepressant Medications**

GENERIC NAME	TRADE NAME	ANTI-CHOLIN-ERGIC	SEDA-TION	ORTHO-STASIS	NOREPIN-EPHRINE BLOCKING ACTIVITY	SERO-TONIN BLOCKING ACTIVITY	HALF-LIFE (hours)	DOSE RANGE (mg/day)
Tertiary tricyclics								
Amitriptyline	Elavil	4+	4+	2+	2+	2+	31–46	25–300
Doxepin	Sinequan, Adapin	2+	3+	2+	11+	2+	8–24	25–300
Imipramine	Tofranil	2+	2+	3+	2+	4+	11–25	25–300
Trimipramine	Surmontil	2+	3+	2+	1+	1+	7–30	50–300
Secondary amines								
Amoxapine	Asendin	3+	2+	1+	3+	2+	8–30	50–600
Desipramine	Norpramin	1+	1+	1+	4+	2+	12–24	25–300
Nortriptyline	Pamelor	2+	2+	1+	2+	3+	18–44	30–100
Protriptyline	Vivactil	3+	1+	1+	4+	2+	67–89	15–60
Phenethylamines								
Venlafaxine	Effexor	0	0	0	3+	3+	5–11	75–375
Tetracyclic amines								
Maprotiline	Ludiomil	2+	2+	1+	3+	1+	21–25	50–225
Mirtazapine	Remeron	3+	2+	0	4+	2+	20–40	15–45
Phenylpiperazines								
Nefazodone	Serzone	1+	3+	3+	3+	3+	2–4	200–600
Trazodone	Desyrel	1+	3+	2+	0	3+	4–9	150–600
Aminoketones								
Bupropion	Wellbutrin	2+	2+	1+	1+	1+	8–24	200–450
SSRIs								
Fluoxetine	Prozac	0	0	0	1+	4+	>72	10–80
Fluvoxamine	Luvox	0	0	0	1+	4+	16–24	50–300
Paroxetine	Paxil	0	0	0	1+	4+	10–24	10–50
Sertraline	Zoloft	0	0	0	1+	4+	24	50–200
MAOIs								
Phenelzine	Nardil	0	0	0	0	0	6–8	45–90
Tranylcypramine	Parnate	0	0	0	0	0	6–8	30–60

other more standard medication regimens. Lithium may be given in combination with tricyclics, SSRIs, or MAOIs. These combinations may produce quite rapid antidepressant response (48 to 72 hours) in individuals who have failed other treatments, but it is more common for medications to take several weeks to improve symptoms. When combined with tricyclics for the treatment of unresponsive depression, thyroid hormone has been found to be as effective as lithium and significantly better than placebo (Joffe et al., 1993).

Mood Stabilizers

Mood-stabilizing medications are typically used to control the symptoms of mania and, once controlled, to prevent its recurrence. The most commonly utilized antimanic drugs are lithium (Lithobid, Eskalith), carbamaz-

epine (Tegretol), and two very closely related drugs: valproic acid (Depakene) and divalproex (Depakote). As noted earlier in this chapter, lithium has been used therapeutically for over a century. The other mood stabilizers are widely used as anticonvulsants but are equally effective in controlling mood. Valproic acid and divalproex are sufficiently similar that they will not be considered separately; compared with valproic acid, divalproex is more commonly used in psychiatric care.

Indications and Evidence for Effectiveness

Mood stabilizers are indicated for the management of mania. They can be used both to treat acute mania and to prevent the recurrence of mania in individuals who have a history of manic episodes. Antidepressants can provoke manic episodes in bipolar individuals (including those with Bipolar II Disorder where only hypomania has previously occurred). Prior treatment with mood stabilizers can prevent this somewhat unusual but undesirable outcome.

Numerous studies show that lithium is effective in the control and prevention of mania. About 80% of individuals respond to lithium, though response is typically delayed by at least 1 to 2 weeks. Lithium is generally effective in controlling depressive symptoms in individuals with Bipolar Disorder. Most of these persons do not need other antidepressants. The data for other mood stabilizers are less well established, but antimanic effects have been most convincingly shown for carbamazepine. Since 1978 more than 19 studies have been conducted that show that carbamazepine is more effective than placebo in the control of mania. Most of these studies are small, but the effectiveness of carbamazepine has probably been adequately established. Some data also suggest that certain types of mania, including rapid-cycling mania, may respond better to carbamazepine than to lithium (Delgado & Gelenberg, 1995). In general, lithium is used as primary treatment, with the other mood stabilizers employed only if lithium fails or is not tolerated. Divalproex may, however, be particularly effective in managing adolescents with mania or hypomania. In this group of clients it may frequently be the first mood stabilizer utilized.

Pharmacology

The neurobiology of mania is as yet incompletely understood, and perhaps as a result the precise mechanism of action of the mood stabilizers remains unknown. One of the extraordinary characteristics of lithium is that it has virtually no psychotropic effects in nonmanic individuals. Lithium is neither a sedative nor a depressant drug, and it appears not to affect mood in persons who do not have mania.

Lithium is well absorbed after an oral dose and is not metabolized in any way after absorption. Peak levels occur within 2 to 4 hours after ingestion of a single dose. Lithium is not bound to protein and is excreted almost completely by the proximal tubules of the kidney. Once in the circulation, lithium has a mean half-life of 18 hours; there is considerable range in this half-life (10 to 30 hours) so that lithium levels are often required to establish the appropriate dose. Individuals whose clearance of lithium is more rapid will have lower serum levels at a given dose, whereas those with slower clearance will have higher levels. Since lithium has a narrow **therapeutic window** (blood levels only a little above the therapeutic range may lead to serious adverse effects), blood levels can allow both effective and safe administration.

Carbamazepine (Tegretol) is most commonly used as an anticonvulsant but has become more widely used in the management of mania as well. Like lithium, carbamazepine is absorbed after oral dosage, but unlike lithium, it is metabolized by the liver and circulates in the plasma almost completely bound to protein. The absorption of carbamazepine is also somewhat delayed and is quite variable from individual to individual. Peak levels may not be reached until 24 hours after a dose. The half-life of carbamazepine is also variable and ranges from 10 to 20 hours in individuals who have taken the drug for some weeks. Carbamazepine has the property of inducing increased levels of the enzymes that metabolize it in the liver. As a result, the half-life is much longer in the first few days that the drug is taken or after a single dose.

Divalproex more closely resembles lithium in its absorption. Peak concentrations are reached after 1 to 4 hours, and the half-life is about 15 hours. Like carbamazepine, divalproex is strongly bound to plasma proteins and is metabolized in the liver (though by a different enzymatic pathway than the one that acts on carbamazepine).

Dose/Administration

Lithium dosage is typically 1800 mg (two 300-mg capsules or tablets given three times daily) for acute mania and 900 to 1200 mg total daily dose (typically in three divided doses) for maintenance. All lithium administration needs to be accompanied by careful monitoring of serum levels, but this is particularly true when high doses are utilized. Lithium levels are most commonly maintained between 0.6 and 1.2 mEq/l, though levels up to 1.5 mEq/l are sometimes required for control of acute symptoms. Levels much above 1.5 mEq/l are often associated with unacceptable symptoms of toxicity such as lethargy and dizziness. Very high levels may produce EKG changes and potentially fatal cardiac toxicity.

Carbamazepine is administered in divided doses with a total of 400 to 1200 mg given daily. Levels are frequently measured, and as in seizure control, the desirable levels are between 4 and 12 μg/ml. Divalproex is similarly given in doses of 500 to 1500 mg daily to achieve levels of 50 to 100 μg/ml.

Drug Actions

The specific antimanic pharmacological actions of lithium remain unknown. Chemically, lithium is a metallic element closely related to sodium and is chemically recognized as sodium in brain pathways. This substitution may affect the way that neurotransmitters react, and it certainly influences many of the aspects of lithium side effects and toxicity to be discussed later. Anticonvulsant drugs such as carbamazepine and divalproex (valproic acid) have effects on brain electrical functions. These effects reduce the brain's susceptibility to disorganized electrical activity, which produces seizure disorders, but their relationship to the control of mania remains incompletely understood.

Drug and Food Interactions

Since lithium interacts with body sodium metabolism, any drug that affects sodium levels may interact with lithium. Diuretics (often used to combat the lithium side effect of peripheral edema) may influence lithium effectiveness and safety by lowering serum sodium, reducing sodium clearance, and hence elevating lithium levels. Similarly, since lithium and sodium share the same pathways for renal excretion, a low-salt diet may result in decreased lithium excretion and therefore high lithium levels. Many nonsteroidal anti-inflammatory drugs, including a variety of nonprescription medications, can affect sodium excretion and increase lithium levels. This risk occurs with ibuprofen (Motrin, Advil), naproxen (Aleve), and probably ketoprofen (Orudis). A variety of prescription anti-inflammatory drugs can have similar effects: indomethacin (Indocin), piroxicam (Feldene), and phenylbutazone (Butazolodin). Haloperidol (potentially used to treat psychosis in Bipolar Disorder) may interact to produce a dangerous encephalopathic syndrome potentially leading to permanent CNS damage. Aminophylline, less commonly used for asthma than in past years but still relatively frequently prescribed, can decrease lithium doses and precipitate manic relapse.

Carbamazepine is strongly affected by interactions with the large number of drugs that affect the liver cytochrome system. Erythromycin may specifically interact with carbamazepine and raise blood levels, leading to toxicity. Cimetidine (Tagamet), widely used and available without prescription, can have similar effects.

Since divalproex and valproic acid are also metabolized by the liver, they have a number of potential interactions that may be of clinical importance. Each prolongs anticoagulant effects in clients treated with Coumadin and increases the effects of MAOIs.

Use During Pregnancy/Lactation

Lithium is potentially cardiotoxic and is usually not advised during pregnancy. Lithium teratogenicity is probably limited to the first trimester, and some psychiatrists will prescribe lithium for women in more advanced stages of pregnancy. Nonetheless, manic individuals may exhibit poor sexual decision making as part of their manic condition and as a consequence may not infrequently become pregnant while on lithium. They may also fail to seek prenatal care early in the first trimester and as a consequence may remain on lithium during the first 8 to 12 weeks in which important organ systems (particularly the vulnerable circulatory system) are undergoing morphogenesis. Fortunately, the teratogenic risk of lithium seems relatively low, and fetal malformation occurs only rarely. Carbamazepine and divalproex *may* have less risk during early pregnancy and are sometimes substituted for lithium. The management of mania during pregnancy is a difficult problem that should be undertaken with expert consultation.

Side Effects

Lithium has a spectrum of side effects that are often troubling to clients. Almost everyone who takes this medication develops thirst and polyuria because of the effect of lithium on the kidney. Another very common side effect is tremor, most noticeable in fine motor activities such as writing, buttoning clothes, and sewing. This tremor can be particularly troublesome to artistic individuals who need good fine motor coordination for their work. Weight gain is less common but does occur in up to 30% of individuals. A smaller percentage of persons experience chronic diarrhea, which can also be an early sign of toxicity and, when of recent onset, requires that blood levels be measured immediately. The nurse can assist clients to distinguish between nuisance side effects and those that, like diarrhea, can be warning signs for more serious adverse effects. Thyroid enlargement and even frank hypothyroidism may occur in persons taking lithium. Thyroid abnormality is less common than other side effects but does occasionally occur and may require treatment. Most individuals on lithium should have periodic measurements of their thyroid function [usually thyroid-stimulating hormone (TSH)].

Carbamazepine is generally better tolerated than is lithium, although occasional individuals may have dizziness, and drowsiness often occurs, at least initially. Unfortunately, carbamazepine may seriously affect bone marrow function and, occasionally, liver enzymes. Fatal agranulocytosis (loss of all functioning polymorphonuclear white blood cells) may result if blood counts are not carefully monitored. Agranulocytosis leads to serious infections and may not infrequently prove fatal. Persons beginning carbamazepine treatment generally require frequent (usually weekly) testing of blood counts and often of liver enzymes as well. The frequency of testing may decrease if results remain normal over time.

Divalproex is generally very well tolerated but has very rarely been associated with fatal liver damage. Individuals on divalproex need careful monitoring of liver functions to help avoid this catastrophic outcome. The nurse can assist clients to remember to get needed blood testing and to be alert for symptoms (loss of appetite, darkened urine, lightened stool, yellow color to skin, profound fatigue) that may indicate impending liver failure.

Adverse Effects

Divalproex and carbamazepine are relatively safer in overdose and with inadvertent high blood levels than is lithium. Lithium toxicity may be fatal as a result of cardiac arrhythmias. Individuals on lithium need to be alert for situations in which they may lose excess sodium, as in

Assessing for Lithium Toxicity

Symptoms: Depend on Serum Levels

Levels of 2 to 3 mEq/l:

- Agitation
- Ataxia
- Blurred vision
- Confusion
- Choreoathetoid movements
- Dysarthria
- Hyperreflexia
- Hypertonia
- Maniclike behavior
- Myoclonic twitching
- Slurred speech
- Tinnitus
- Incontinence
- Vertigo

Levels over 3 mEq/l:

- Arrhythmias
- Coma
- Hypotension
- Peripheral vascular collapse
- Seizures
- Spasticity
- Stupor
- Twitching of muscle groups

Treatment

- Early symptoms are treated by decreasing the dose or stopping treatment for 24 to 48 hours.
- Late symptoms are treated with gastric lavage, restoration of fluid and electrolyte balance, and increasing lithium excretion by giving aminophylline, mannitol, or urea.

Nursing Actions

- Observe carefully for symptoms of lithium toxicity.
- Report symptoms of toxicity whenever observed.
- Educate client to make own observations.
- Any situation where the client may lose excess sodium (as in heavy sweating during exercise) may produce lithium toxicity.

heavy sweating (such as occurs with vigorous physical exercise). Under such conditions, lithium toxicity may occur without any change in lithium intake. As noted previously, drug interactions (including interactions with drugs commonly available without prescription) may also result in dangerously high lithium levels.

Summary of Drugs for Treating Mood Disorders

Mood disorders may reflect either depressed or expansive (manic) abnormalities or a combination of both. While lithium is generally used to treat both depression and mania, the majority of drugs for mood disorders are targeted to either mood depression or mania. Drugs for depression fall into two categories: classical agents (most often tricyclics such as amitriptyline, imipramine, or related drugs such as trazodone), SSRIs (fluoxetine, sertraline, and paroxetine are among the most commonly used), and MAOIs (currently available nonselective MAOIs include phenylzine and tranylcypromine). Lithium, carbamazepine, and divalproex are commonly used to stabilize mood in persons with Mania or Bipolar Disorder. While mood stabilizers are most commonly prescribed by psychiatric specialists, antidepressants are widely used in general medical practice and frequently prescribed or furnished by nurse practitioners. Many of these drugs (in particular, amitriptyline, imipramine, lithium, carbamazepine, and divalproex) are included in the World Health Organization list of essential drugs for primary care (Wig, 1993). The nurse should be familiar with the indications, side effects, and adverse effects of the major classes of medications for mood disorders. The nurse who cares for persons taking lithium or MAOIs will need to combine expert knowledge of drug and food interactions with highly proficient client teaching skills; only through this combination can these valuable medications be administered without serious risk.

DRUGS FOR TREATING ANXIETY AND SLEEP DISORDERS

Symptoms of anxiety and insomnia are most commonly treated with benzodiazepines. Other medications useful on occasion include buspirone for generalized anxiety, antidepressants for Panic Disorder and Social Phobia, beta blockers for performance anxiety, and a variety of agents for insomnia. Antihistamines, antidepressants, barbiturates, and antipsychotics are sometimes prescribed for anxiety. Persons commonly self-medicate anxiety with a range of drugs, including ethanol and illegally acquired tranquilizers of many sorts. It is probable that self-medication occurs for other psychiatric disorders as well, but anxiety disorders cause such acute symptoms and respond so quickly to sedatives that self-medication is common.

Indications and Evidence for Effectiveness

While they have many clinical uses, benzodiazepines have been most distinctly shown to be effective for generalized anxiety and Panic Disorder. While all benzodiazepines may be equally effective for Panic Disorder, alprazolam (Xanax) was the first benzodiazepine approved for this treatment. There is no evidence that any other similar medication is more effective, but fairly high alprazolam doses are required: often 3 to 6 mg daily. Clinicians may use long half-life drugs [diazepam (Valium)] when daily administration is required but may prefer relatively shorter half-lives [i.e., lorazepam (Ativan)] when patients are more likely to benefit from intermittent symptom-driven treatment. The selection of hypnotic medications was discussed above and requires balancing onset of action, morning drowsiness, and rebound insomnia. Triazolam (Halcion) is particularly likely to produce rebound and may result in amnesia.

Pharmacology

The clinical effectiveness of benzodiazepines was first discovered in the mid-1950s. These medications have been in wide use since and remain among the most commonly prescribed drugs. Benzodiazepines are frequently diverted to street sales and are readily available for illicit purchase. Benzodiazepines may produce dependence and are not infrequently chosen as drugs of abuse, particularly in combinations with other agents (including alcohol). Subsequent research has shown that there is a benzodiazepine receptor in the mammalian brain and that this receptor is closely tied to the inhibitory neurotransmitter gamma aminobutyric acid (GABA). Benzodiazepines may increase the effectiveness of GABA but may also act separately by affecting brain metabolism of serotonin and norepinephrine (Ballenger, 1995). Zolpidem is a nonbenzodiazepine drug that nonetheless binds to benzodiazepine receptors and produces sleep induction with little effect on anxiety.

HISTORY AND DEVELOPMENT OF SOME PSYCHOTROPIC MEDICATIONS

Since the earliest times alcohol was known as an effective sedative and mood-altering agent. Laudanum, a mixture extracted from opium poppies, has been around since the 1700s, and herbals such as valerian have been used as sedatives for centuries. These three medications were probably the only truly effective sedative/psychotropic agents used medically until the 19th century. In the middle 19th century, a number of sedatives were discovered, including bromide salts, chloral hydrate (also known as a Mickey Finn, when placed in an alcoholic drink to produce unconsciousness for illicit purposes), paraldehyde, urethane, and sulfonal. Although these agents did sedate people, most had severe side effects and are now banned, with the exception of chloral hydrate, which is sometimes used as a sleep aid, and paraldehyde, which is still occasionally used for treating alcoholic withdrawal.

In 1903, barbital was discovered and found to be an effective, useful sedative without severe side effects. Phenobarbital came along in 1912 in a search for anticonvulsant agents and was discovered to be both effective for certain types of epilepsy and a useful sedative. Phenytoin and trimethadione, anticonvulsants still used today, were discovered at about the same time in the continuing search for antipsychotic sedatives. The 1950s and early 1960s were called the "age of the barbiturates." These drugs were widely and casually prescribed before their addiction potential and dangerous interaction with alcohol were known. Marilyn Monroe died of a combination of alcohol and a barbiturate. Amphetamines were also widely prescribed at this time, and many

people took a barbiturate to sleep and an amphetamine to wake up.

With the recognition of the dangers of these drugs, the FDA stepped in and regulated their prescribing, and physicians began to modify their attitudes toward these drugs as well.

In 1950, the first true anxyolytic agent was developed, meprobamate (Miltown). Sales of meprobamate skyrocketed, surprisingly enough, because Milton Berle was taking it and made frequent jokes and references about it on his very popular TV show, the most watched program at the time.

In 1957, a major advance occurred with the discovery of chlordiazepoxide (Librium), an anxiolytic with less sedative properties than the barbiturates, with fewer serious side effects, and in appropriate doses that allowed quite normal functioning. Beginning in 1961 the benzodiazepine era exploded, with over 3000 forms synthesized, 120 tested, and currently 35 in use worldwide. They serve a valid medical purpose in the short-term treatment of anxiety and as sleep aids and can also be used to calm agitated psychotic patients.

The benzodiazepines have largely displaced the barbiturates as drugs of choice due to their greater safety profile, though addiction and alcohol interaction remain problems.

Perhaps one of the most interesting developments in anxiolytic drugs is BuSpar. It appears to be nonaddictive, does not impair normal functioning, and is effective after 2 to 3 weeks. As time has passed, drugs have become more specific in their indications as well as more efficacious. The future development of psychotropic drugs is indeed promising.

Barbiturates, now primarily used for anesthesia induction and seizure control, also augment brain GABA inhibitory effects but through a somewhat different molecular mechanism than that of benzodiazepines. Alcohol probably also exerts its anxiolytic and sedative effects, at least in part through enhancement of GABA transmission (Nishinto, Mignot, & Dement, 1995).

All the benzodiazepines are readily absorbed after oral administration and often reach peak levels within an hour or less. Diazepam (Valium) acts particularly quickly after oral administration. Lorazepam and midazolam (Versed) can be given intramuscularly, and diazepam is frequently given intravenously (most commonly for seizures, but occasionally for anxiety). Nearly a dozen benzodiazepines are available for clinical use, and these vary most significantly in their half-lives. Triazolam, for example, has a half-life of only 6 hours and no clinically significant metabolites. As a result, triazolam is classified as a short-acting benzodiazepine. In contrast, diazepam has both a long half-life (nearly 24 hours) and active metabolites with similar long half-lives. The effect of metabolites can be quite important: flurazepam (Dalmane) itself has quite a short half-life (2 to 3 hours), but its major metabolite has a half-life of more than 2 days. As a result, this commonly used medication may prolong daytime drowsiness when used for treating insomnia.

Dose/Administration

Benzodiazepine doses are quite specific for the individual drugs chosen and vary over a rather wide range. Alprazolam (short to intermediate half-life) and clonazepam (long half-life) are perhaps the two most commonly used benzodiazepine medications for treating anxiety. Alprazolam (Ativan) daily doses range from 0.75 to 8 mg daily, with a common range of 1.5 to 3 mg. Clonazepam (Klonopin) is generally given in a dosage range of 1.5 to 10 mg daily.

Drug Actions

Benzodiazepines exert a significant effect on GABA-ergic CNS pathways and produce both sedation and a marked decrease in subjective anxiety. These drugs induce sleep, decrease frequency of awakenings, slightly decrease rapid eye movement (REM) sleep, and moderately decrease slow-wave or deep Stage 3 to 4 sleep. Individuals who take benzodiazepines for sleep generally report an increased subjective sense of sleep quality. Sleep latency (the time to fall asleep) is significantly decreased by short half-life benzodiazepines such as triazolam, but these medications frequently produce rebound insomnia on subsequent nights. Longer half-life benzodiazepines take somewhat longer to produce sleep and

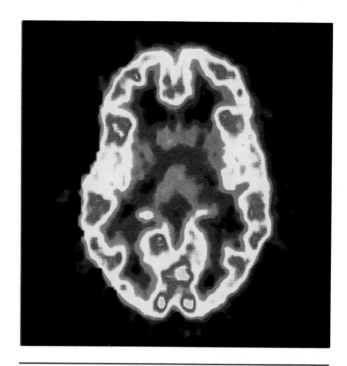

PET image of benzodiazepine receptors. Areas of high binding to benzodiazepines are represented as white, orange/red, and yellow. Note that almost all binding occurs in the cortex. Compare the degree of binding in the frontal lobes (lower part of the image) with the PET scan of opioid receptors (Chapter 15) and that for cocaine receptors (Chapter 15). These latter two images show very few frontal lobe binding sites. *From "Addiction: Brain Mechanisms and Their Related Implications," by D. J. Nutt, 1996,* Lancet, 347(8993), *pp. 33–35.*

cause some hangover the next day. Temazepam (Restoril) is a commonly prescribed hypnotic medication with an intermediate half-life and an onset of action within 2 to 3 hours.

Drug and Food Interactions

There are few benzodiazepine drug interactions of clinical significance. Alcohol is additive with the sedative effects of benzodiazepines and will produce increased drowsiness if taken along with these medications. The combination of alcohol and large amounts of benzodiazepines can produce fatal respiratory depression and coma. This is a particular problem since some clients find that combining alcohol with benzodiazepines, perhaps especially clonazepam, produces a desirable "high."

Use During Pregnancy/Lactation

Benzodiazepines are commonly prescribed to and self-administered by women of child-bearing age. There is little firm data on which to base recommendations for benzodiazepine use during pregnancy. Alcohol and barbiturates clearly cause fetal damage, but a "fetal benzodiazepine syndrome" has not been unequivocally defined. Only clonazepam is placed in pregnancy category C: Potential benefits may justify potential risk. Other benzodiazepines are in category D and are contraindicated during pregnancy. Risks during breast feeding are likely smaller, and in contrast to most other psychiatric medications, lower drug concentrations are found in milk than in plasma; consequently benzodiazepines are generally accepted as safe in lactating mothers.

Side Effects

Benzodiazepine side effects are largely limited to sedation, interference with safe driving, and occasional amnesia.

Adverse Effects

Severe adverse effects are rare, even in intentional overdose. Deaths have occurred in combination with alcohol and other substances but are unusual. The major adverse effects of benzodiazepines involve physical dependence. When given these medications over prolonged periods, many individuals have symptoms of increased anxiety and, rarely, seizures on abrupt withdrawal. Withdrawal should be accomplished slowly over several weeks and is most commonly a problem with alprazolam, a drug with relatively short half-life. When withdrawal from alprazolam is required, many clinicians first switch their patients from alprazolam to a longer acting drug such as diazepam or clonazepam and then proceed with a slow withdrawal.

Nonbenzodiazepine Drugs for Anxiety and Sleep Disorders

While the benzodiazepines are widely used for management of anxiety and insomnia, they are not the only medications of value for treating these conditions. Buspirone (BuSpar) is a unique antianxiety agent that has no effects on the benzodiazepine-GABA receptor. As a consequence, it produces relief of anxiety with virtually no sedation. Zolpidem (Ambien) does act on the benzodiazepine receptor, but it does not have the chemical structure of a benzodiazepine. As a consequence, zolpidem produces only sedation; it does not provide any relief from anxiety. Propranolol (Inderal), a beta blocker, has little demonstrated effect on anxiety, but it has proved useful when performance anxiety produces physical symptoms such as tremor or difficulty speaking. Administration of propranolol prior to activities such as public speaking or playing a musical instrument can sometimes improve performance by reducing tremor or other manifestations of

nervousness. There is some limited role for beta blockers in other anxiety disorders. Antidepressants (and very rarely antipsychotics) can sometimes be helpful for control of anxiety or insomnia. As noted previously, trazodone seems particularly anxiolytic and is often used to combat onset insomnia in anxious and/or depressed individuals.

Buspirone

Buspirone was released in 1986 as an anxiolytic drug. Pharmacologically, buspirone bears some resemblance to antipsychotic medications, but even in high doses it both lacks antipsychotic effects and fails to produce tardive dyskinesia or other movement disorders. There is no evidence for habituation to or dependency on buspirone. Buspirone is well absorbed orally and has a short half-life. Unlike benzodiazepines, which affect anxiety within minutes to hours, the effect of buspirone is delayed, often to as much as 7 weeks. While not all individuals respond to buspirone (some data suggest that those who have previously been treated with benzodiazepines may be more likely to be poor responders), when response does occur, buspirone is as effective as benzodiazepines in the management of Generalized Anxiety Disorder. Buspirone has few side effects and almost no drug interactions. Dizziness, headache, and nausea occur occasionally but frequently improve with continued administration. Because of the relatively short half-life, doses need to be given three times daily. This need for a multiple dosage regimen, slow onset of action, and buspirone's relatively high cost are its primary disadvantages. As noted above, buspirone in high doses is a very good antidepressant. It is not effective in Panic Disorder but may have some benefit in Social Phobia. Results in Obsessive-Compulsive Disorder remain ambiguous. Buspirone is safe in overdose, has no effect on alertness or other job-related functions, and is free of abuse potential. Despite this nearly ideal profile, buspirone is not used widely in psychiatric practice, probably because of its slow onset and its very high cost.

Beta Blockers

Beta blockers act peripherally to inhibit the beta-adrenergic receptor. They also have generalized CNS effects of sedation, fatigue, and occasionally depression. This sedative effect may produce some mild antianxiety effect, but beta blockers have at best only a minimal effect on generalized anxiety and probably no significant benefit in Panic Disorder. In contrast, there is some evidence to support the use of beta blockers in Social Phobia, especially, as noted earlier, when symptoms of autonomic arousal are debilitating. These symptoms include tremulousness, blushing, tachycardia, and subjective fear. Such symptoms are often mediated through peripheral beta-adrenergic stimulation and may be blocked with propranolol. Fear responds least well, and some studies have suggested no benefit of beta blockers on Social Phobia.

Obsessive-Compulsive Disorder does not respond to propranolol, but Post-Traumatic Stress Disorder may respond somewhat, particularly when symptoms of autonomic arousal are prominent.

Zolpidem

Zolpidem (Ambien) is a nonbenzodiazepine that nonetheless acts through the benzodiazepine receptor. Zolpidem has been marketed as a drug for treating insomnia, and in this use it may have some theoretical advantages over benzodiazepine hypnotics. Among these advantages are zolpidem's short half-life without rebound drowsiness. Long-acting benzodiazepines tend to produce early morning drowsiness whereas short-acting benzodiazepines may "wear off" in the middle of the night, leading to nocturnal wakefulness and daytime sleepiness. Zolpidem, in contrast, seems to produce restful sleep that lasts through the night. Unlike benzodiazepines, zolpidem appears also not to reduce the amount of REM sleep. It is thought to have little or no abuse or dependency potential, and it does not seem to affect next morning alertness or job performance. Zolpidem is quite expensive compared with benzodiazepines, and perhaps for this reason its use remains somewhat limited. Long-term usage of hypnotic drugs is generally discouraged, but where necessary, zolpidem would seem to be an appropriate medication for pharmacological management of chronic insomnia.

Antidepressants and Antipsychotics

Some clinicians use antidepressants to treat insomnia. Amitriptyline, doxepin, and trazodone are highly sedating and may help patients fall asleep. These medications are particularly useful when patients have coexisting insomnia and depression. It is generally regarded as atypical clinical practice to use antidepressants to treat insomnia in patients who do not meet DSM-IV criteria for depression. Some clinicians use highly sedating antipsychotics such as thioridazine for sleep disorders, especially in the elderly (Salzman, Satlin, & Burrows, 1995). In some cases the benefits of such treatment may outweigh the risks, but it is unlikely that antipsychotic drugs should be widely employed for this purpose.

Antihistamines

The sedating antihistamine diphenhydramine (Benadryl) has been approved for over-the-counter sales as a hypnotic. Diphenhydramine does produce drowsiness and probably decreases the time to sleep onset. Studies do not show improved sleep quality in persons taking diphenhydramine (Cole & Yonkers, 1995). The anticholinergic side effects of this drug may be significant, especially in the elderly. Such side effects include blurred vision, urinary hesitancy or obstruction, and impaired sweating and temperature regulation.

Summary of Antianxiety Drugs

As the reader of this book's chapter on anxiety disorders (Chapter 10) will recognize, anxiety causes profound human distress. Currently available medications can provide dramatic relief for clients suffering from symptoms of anxiety. Benzodiazepines are the most widely used and effective antianxiety drugs and are also effective for short-term management of insomnia. Long-term use of benzodiazepines may result in dependence and withdrawal symptoms. Buspirone is an effective but expensive and slow-acting antianxiety medication that does not carry any risk of habituation or dependence. Some anxiety disorders (Obsessive-Compulsive Disorder, Panic Disorder) are primarily treated with antidepressant medications, and some antidepressants, notably trazodone, are particularly effective anxiolytics. Anxiolytics are frequently used in psychiatric nursing and in general medical practice. Diazepam is included in the World Health Organization list of essential drugs for primary care (Wig, 1993). Table 25-3 provides a summary of antianxiety and hypnotic medications.

DRUGS FOR TREATING SUBSTANCE ABUSE AND DEPENDENCY

Substance abuse is discussed in some detail in Chapter 15. Medications have a useful role in bringing about withdrawal from substances that cause physical dependency. They may also be used to treat symptoms of physical withdrawal. Drugs may help maintain abstinence: either by directly substituting for the substance of abuse (methadone for heroin, nicotine by patch or gum for smoking) or through the unique aversive conditioning of disulfiram (Antabuse), which produces a highly unpleasant set of physical symptoms when alcohol is ingested. Many drugs used in managing substance-related conditions have other roles as antidepressants, antipsychotics, or antianxiety medications and have been discussed previously in this chapter. However, there are some agents used primarily or exclusively in managing substance abuse, dependency, and withdrawal.

Substances with Little Role Outside Substance Abuse or Withdrawal

This somewhat arbitrary classification of medications includes methadone, disulfiram, nicotine (for replacement in persons quitting smoking), and opioid receptor antagonists.

Methadone

Methadone is a relatively long-acting narcotic that is useful in both acute detoxification and in long-term main-

Table 25-3 **Antianxiety and Hypnotic Medications**

GENERIC NAME	TRADE NAME	MEDICATION TYPE	CLINICAL USE	DOSAGE (mg/day)	HALF-LIFE (hours)	SPEED OF ONSET (p.o.)
Alprazolam	Xanax	Benzodiazepine	Antianxiety	0.75–4	12–15	Intermediate
Chlordiazepoxide	Librium	Benzodiazepine		15–100	5–30	Intermediate
Clonazepam	Klonopin	Benzodiazepine	Antianxiety, anticonvulsant	1.5–20	18–50	Intermediate
Diazepam	Valium	Benzodiazepine	Antianxiety	5–40	20–80	Rapid
Lorazepam	Ativan	Benzodiazepine	Antianxiety	2–4	10–20	Intermediate
Flurazepam	Dalmane	Benzodiazepine	Hypnotic	15–30	2–3	Very rapid
Midazolam	Versed	Benzodiazepine	Sedative	i.m. or i.v., dosage usually based on weight	1–12	Very rapid
Temazepam	Restoril	Benzodiazepine	Hypnotic	15–30	8–15	Intermediate
Triazolam	Halcion	Benzodiazepine	Hypnotic	0.125–0.5	1.5–6	Rapid
Buspirone	BuSpar	Serotonin and dopamine agonist	Antianxiety	10–60	2–3	Slow (weeks)
Zolpidem	Ambien	Nonbenzodiazepine but binds to benzodiazepine receptors	Hypnotic	5–10	1.5–5	Very rapid

tenance of previously opioid-dependent individuals. A longer acting derivative of methadone, LAAM (L-α-acetylmethadol), is also in use for long-term maintenance.

Short-term use of methadone may reduce the intensity of withdrawal symptoms and allows detoxification using an easily administered oral regimen. Methadone doses for withdrawal are typically 40 mg or less given initially and then reduced by 10% to 20% daily until the individual is drug free after 1 to 2 weeks. Such a regimen may make withdrawal easier than suddenly stopping the intake of opioids. Such sudden stopping often leads to unpleasant symptoms (tearing, runny nose, nausea, agitation, and piloerection) and is frequently termed "cold turkey" withdrawal. Unlike alcohol withdrawal, which may occasionally be dangerous, cold turkey withdrawal from opioids, while distinctly uncomfortable, is not dangerous.

Long-term methadone maintenance is far more controversial since it substitutes oral methadone for injection drugs without any goal of eventually achieving a drug-free status. Advocates of methadone maintenance claim that it reduces criminality and (unless other injection substances are involved) should eliminate needle use—of immense importance in controlling spread of injection-associated infectious agents, notably HIV, hepatitis B, and hepatitis C. Methadone maintenance currently must be given through clinics specifically licensed for this purpose. Clients who "earn" the privilege of self-administration are typically given a week's supply of methadone and are subject to periodic urine testing to evaluate use of substances other than methadone. Other clients come to the clinic daily to receive their methadone. Relatively high doses of 60 to 80 mg are often given daily, and additional services of counseling and medical and psychiatric care are often provided. Regulations require that current physiological dependence be documented and that the individual have been opioid dependent for at least a year. Special rules apply to clients under 18 years of age. The LAAM allows individuals who cannot be trusted to self-administer methadone to receive clinic-administered medication as infrequently as three times weekly. Long-term methadone treatment remains a controversial but well-established approach to the management of opioid dependence.

Disulfiram

Disulfiram is an inhibitor of the enzyme alcohol dehydrogenase, which catalyzes a major step in the breakdown of alcohol. When the enzyme is inhibited and an individual drinks alcohol, blood concentrations of the toxic metabolite acetaldehyde increase significantly. Acetaldehyde produces unpleasant symptoms of flushing, tachycardia, nausea, vomiting, and hypotension. Especially in medically fragile individuals, these symptoms may rarely prove life threatening. Because of associated risks, disulfiram is used only with highly selected individuals who have good physical health and a high chance of remaining abstinent. Studies show that disulfiram maintenance can significantly reduce drinking (Fuller et al., 1986). The dose is typically 250 mg daily, though larger doses may be given, especially when dosing intervals exceed 1 day. The relatively long half-life of disulfiram ensures that several days must elapse between stopping medication and safely drinking alcohol; this long half-life probably decreases the likelihood of impulsive relapse. However, perhaps not surprisingly, the major difficulty with disulfiram as primary treatment for alcohol dependency is the difficulty in assuring long-term compliance with the medication. Such compliance may be enhanced by frequent clinic visits (including giving medication under observation every 3 to 4 days) and by enlisting others (visiting nurse, significant other) in ensuring compliance.

Nicotine Replacement

Smoking is an issue of particular concern to mental health nursing because of the high incidence of smoking among psychiatric patients. Alcohol abusers and schizophrenic individuals have especially high tobacco consumption. Depression and abuse of a variety of nonnicotine substances are also associated with tobacco abuse (Cornish, McNicholas, & O'Brien, 1995). Many individuals have nicotine dependency without any other diagnosable DSM-IV condition. Chemical replacement of nicotine may allow some highly dependent persons to quit more easily. Adhesive patches (Habitrol, Nicoderm, and others) supply a steady quantity of nicotine. Chewing gum (Nicorette) and patches have both shown enhanced 1-year abstinence rates compared with placebo (Anonymous, 1995b; Benowitz, 1993). These products may be purchased without prescription. Nicotine nasal spray is also available and may prove useful for some individuals. The nurse can assist clients in assessing their readiness to quit, in setting a "quit date," in assessing potential risks to successful quitting, and in finding a support group to enhance quitting success. In some settings, the nurse can serve as a resource when a client is having difficulties with nicotine abstinence.

Opioid Receptor Antagonists

Opioid receptor antagonists have been available for many years (naloxone, nalmefene, naltrexone, and others). These medications may be life saving when clients present with respiratory depression and coma due to narcotic agonists. Giving 0.4 to 0.8 mg of naloxone intravenously

will dramatically reverse symptoms of narcotic overdose but will often precipitate symptoms of withdrawal as clients awaken. The precipitation of withdrawal by injection of naloxone is sometimes used as a criterion for physical dependency (the establishment of which is required for entry into a methadone program). The long-acting receptor antagonist naltrexone is sometimes used for relapse prevention in a manner analogous to disulfiram. A single oral dose will block the subjective effects of administered opioids for up to several days. In contrast to disulfiram, no adverse reaction occurs if a person on naltrexone uses an opioid, but because of naltrexone receptor antagonism, there is no opioid "high" to rekindle a desire for continuing usage. (Such long-acting receptor blockade could theoretically pose difficulties if an acute injury or unexpected surgery required narcotic pain relief.) Naltrexone relapse prevention requires a higher level of motivation for abstention than is seen in most opioid-dependent individuals. This medication may work best for dependent professionals who have undergone detoxification and whose continuing licensure and maintenance of a (usually) prosperous livelihood require documented freedom from opioid use. Intriguingly, naltrexone has also been shown to be of some value in promoting abstinence from alcohol. Whether it will have long-term benefit for alcohol dependence is currently uncertain (Anonymous, 1995c).

Other Medications of Use in Managing Substance Dependence

Many of the drugs used in managing individuals dependent on a variety of substances have been discussed previously in this chapter in their roles as antidepressants, anxiolytics, and antipsychotics. Antidepressants, particularly imipramine, may be of value in reducing alcohol consumption in depressed individuals with alcohol dependency. Haloperidol and benzodiazepines are often used to manage excitement and toxic psychosis seen in acute phencyclidine (PCP) and stimulant drug intoxication. The vitamin thiamine is frequently given intravenously to alcoholics for prevention of Wernicke's encephalopathy, a serious complication that is most likely to occur when adequate nutrition is reestablished. Wernicke's encephalopathy (often called "Wernicke's syndrome") is characterized by confusion, memory loss, and abnormalities of cranial nerve function. Untreated, it can lead to death, permanent memory loss, or other neurological impairment. Early intravenous administration of glucose plus thiamine results in rapid, often complete, improvement in neurological functioning. Intravenous glucose (along with thiamine) is the treatment of choice for alcohol-induced hypoglycemia, and long-acting benzodiazepines [commonly diazepam and chlordiazepoxide (Librium)] are used in management and prevention of alcohol withdrawal. Clonidine (Catapres), an alpha-adrenergic agonist primarily employed to treat hypertension, has come to play a significant role in reducing symptoms of withdrawal from opioids and perhaps from nicotine as well. The antidepressant bupropion has demonstrated effectiveness in reducing symptoms of nicotine withdrawal.

⚡ NURSING ALERT!

Thiamine and Alcohol-Induced Hypoglycemia

When hydrating alcoholics, thiamine must also be given. The alcoholic person is hypoglycemic. When hydration increases glucose metabolism, the client uses up thiamine stores and there is an increased body requirement for thiamine. Failure to give thiamine prior to fluids and glucose may result in permanent neurological damage.

STIMULANT DRUGS

Clinically useful stimulant drugs include pemoline (Cylert), dextroamphetamine, and methylphenidate (Ritalin). Stimulant drugs (including these substances, but also cocaine, methamphetamine, and others) are major substances of abuse, but they also have significant benefits when used under clinical supervision. The use of stimulants as antidepressants was discussed previously in this chapter but remains controversial. These medications may work best in combination with other antidepressants and may be particularly useful in severely depressed, medically ill older individuals in whom rapid relief of symptoms is important to avoid suicide or physical deterioration. Stimulants may also be freer of significant side effects than other antidepressants.

Stimulant medications have their best-documented uses in the management of Narcolepsy and Attention-Deficit Disorder. There is little controversy surrounding stimulant use in Narcolepsy, a condition in which daytime sleepiness can make many common activities (notably driving) hazardous. Stimulant drugs reduce daytime sleepiness but must be given on a chronic basis, presumably for the individual's lifetime. Stimulants seem to be particularly effective for adult Attention-Deficit Disorder (Wender et al., 1985). Treatment of children with Attention-Deficit Disorder is somewhat more controversial. Many parents and clinicians are concerned about use of highly psychoactive controlled substances in young children, particularly since the demonstrated benefits, while consistent, are only modest and last only as long as the medication is given. Short-term benefits in behavior and learning have been clearly demonstrated, but prolonged administration of these drugs to children raises a number of serious issues involving safety, efficacy, and clinical wisdom (Schachar & Tannock, 1993).

✴ NURSING TIP

Nursing Implications in Pharmacotherapeutics

The nurse's role is to understand the reason that each medication is prescribed, to administer the medications safely, and to assess for untoward effects. Further, the nurse has an important role in client (and family) education, so that the client understands the drug, how to take it, and how to observe for side effects. For cross-reference, medications listed in this chapter are also described in chapters focusing on psychopathology, where the medication would be indicated in treatment of the condition.

◎ *REFLECTIVE THINKING*

The Drug-Receptor Hypothesis

For many years, the philosophy behind the use of a medication was "if it works, use it." Paul Ehrlich was the first scientist to see the possibility of targeting medicines at a specific cause or organism, sometimes referred to as the "magic bullet" hypothesis. As knowledge of drug actions increased, the mechanism of drug action, or exactly how they worked, began to be studied. It was primarily the work of Ehrlich that led to the concept that the effect of drugs is due to their interaction with specific receptors. Today, we have discovered receptors for benzodiazepines, morphine, serotonin, nicotine, and marijuana. This implies that the body produces substances naturally that act at these receptors. In the early 1970s, endorphins were discovered, naturally occurring peptides in the body that act at the morphine receptor. Acetylcholine acts at the nicotinic receptors, and amandamide and 2-arachidonyl-glycerol (2-AG) act at the so-called marijuana receptors. Scientists still do not know the biological functions of amandamide and 2-AG. Once a receptor is discovered, it can be cloned, receptor blockers synthesized, and function examined.

This drug receptor hypothesis can change the way one thinks about medications. What do you think the implications are of the statement that the body may produce substances that act at the receptors identified? How have plants "learned" to produce substances that act so strongly on our brain receptors?

≋ KEY CONCEPTS

◆ Psychotropic medications are an important and often an essential mode of treatment.

◆ Since the advent of modern pharmaceuticals, there have been many drugs developed as antipsychotic, antidepressant, and antianxiety medications.

◆ Each category of medication has helped us learn something about the etiology of mental disease.

◆ While medications help to alleviate symptoms, they do not cure the underlying problem or condition that causes the symptom.

≋ REVIEW QUESTIONS AND ACTIVITIES

1. Review the medications ordered for each client you care for during your psychiatric mental health nursing course.

2. Explain the following for each medication:
   a. Reason for drug to be ordered
   b. How you know if your client is on a therapeutic dose
   c. Side effects and adverse effects

3. For each of your clients, evaluate the level of compliance in taking drugs.

4. Describe specific activities you can do to increase compliance with the therapeutic regimen.

⚛ EXPLORING THE WEB

◆ Visit this text's "Online Companion™" on the Internet at **http://www.DelmarNursing.com** for further information on medications used in psychiatric care.

◆ Search **http://www.drugref.com** for information and updates on medications discussed in this chapter.

◆ Can you find any support groups or other information sources that families and support persons might consult with questions about the psychotropic medications?

≋ REFERENCES

American Psychiatric Association Task Force on Tardive Dyskinesia. (1992). Tardive dyskinesia: A task force report of the American Psychiatric Association. Washington, DC: American Psychiatric Press.

Anonymous. (1995a). Nefazodone for depression. *The Medical Letter, 37,* 33–34.

Anonymous. (1995b). Use of nicotine to stop smoking. *The Medical Letter, 37,* 6–8.

Anonymous. (1995c). Naltrexone for alcohol dependence, *The Medical Letter, 37,* 64–67.

Baldessarini, R. J. (1990). Drugs and the treatment of psychiatric disorders. In A. G. Gilman, T. W. Rall, A. S. Nies, & P. Taylor (Eds.), *Pharmacological basis of therapeutics* (8th ed., pp. 383–435). New York: Pergamon Press.

Ballenger, J. C. (1995). Benzodiazepines. In A. F. Schatzberg & C. B. Nereroff (Eds.), *The American Psychiatric Press textbook of psychopharmacology* (pp. 215–230). Washington, DC: American Psychiatric Press.

Benowitz, N. L. (1993). Nicotine replacement therapy: What has been accomplished—can we do better? *Drugs, 45,* 157–170.

Boyer, W. F., & Feighner, J. P. (1991). The efficacy of selective serotonin uptake inhibitors in depression. In J. P. Feighner & W. F. Boyer (Eds.), *Selective serotonin reuptake inhibitors* (pp. 89–108). Chichester, England: Wiley.

Charney, D. S., Miller, H., Licinia, J., & Salomon, R. (1995). Treatment of depression. In A. F. Schatzberg & C. B. Nemeroff (Eds.), *The American Psychiatric Press textbook of psychopharmacology* (pp. 587–588). Washington, DC: American Psychiatric Press.

Ciraulo, D. A., Creelman, W. L., Shader, R. I., & O'Sullivan, R. L. (1994). Antidepressants. In D. A. Ciraulo, R. I. Shader, D. J. Greenblatt, & W. L. Creelman (Eds.), *Drug interactions in psychiatry* (2nd ed.). Baltimore: Williams & Wilkins.

Claus, A., Bollen, J., De Cuyper, H., et al. (1992). Risperidone versus haloperidol in the treatment of chronic schizophrenic inpatients: A multicentre double-blind comparative study. *Acta Psychiatrica Scandinavia, 85,* 295–305.

Cohen, L. S. (1989). Psychopharmacology: Psychotropic drug use in pregnancy. *Hospital and Community Psychiatry, 40,* 566.

Cole, J. O., & Yonkers, K. A. (1995). Nonbenzodiazepine anxiolytics. In A. F. Schatzberg & C. B. Nereroff (Eds.), *The American Psychiatric Press textbook of psychopharmacology* (p. 231). Washington, DC: American Psychiatric Press.

Cornish, J. W., McNicholas, L. F., & O'Brien, C. P. (1995). Treatment of substance-related disorders. In A. F. Schatzberg & C. B. Nereroff (Eds.), *The American Psychiatric Press textbook of psychopharmacology* (p. 719). Washington, DC: American Psychiatric Press.

Davidson, J. (1989). Seizures and bupropion: A review. *Journal of Clinical Psychiatry, 50,* 256–261.

Delgado, P. L., & Gelenberg, A. J. (1995). Antidepressant and antimanic medications. In G. O. Gabbard (Ed.), *Treatments of psychiatric disorders* (pp. 1131–1168). Washington, DC: American Psychiatric Press.

Fawcett, J., & Busch, K. A. (1995). Stimulants in psychiatry. In A. F. Schatzberg & C. B. Nereroff (Eds.), *The American Psychiatric Press textbook of psychopharmacology* (pp. 417–435). Washington, DC: American Psychiatric Press.

Fuller, R. K., Branchey, L., Brightwell, D. R., et al. (1986). Disulfiram treatment of alcoholism: A Veterans Administration cooperative study. *Journal of the American Medical Association, 256,* 1449–1455.

Goff, B., & Baldessarini, R. J. (1995). Antipsychotics. In D. A. Ciraulo, R. I. Shader, D. J. Greenblatt, & W. L. Creelman (Eds.), *Drug interactions in psychiatry* (2nd ed., pp. 147–173). Baltimore: Williams & Wilkins.

Jeffries, J., et al. (1984). The question of lithium/neuroleptic toxicity. *Canadian Journal of Psychiatry, 29*, 601–605.

Joffe, R. T., Singer, W., Levitt, A. J., et al. (1993). A placebo controlled comparison of lithium and triiodothyronine augmentation of tricyclic antidepressants in unipolar refractory depression. *Archives of General Psychiatry, 50*, 387–393.

Keltner, N. L., & Folks, D. G. (1993). Drugs used for electroconvulsive therapy. In N. L. Keltner & D. G. Folks (Eds.), *Psychotropic drugs* (pp. 241–250). St. Louis: Mosby.

Kissling, W., Kane, J. M., Barnes, T. R., et al. (1991). Guidelines for neuroleptic relapse prevention in schizophrenia: Towards a consensus view. In W. Kissling (Ed.), *Guidelines for neuroleptic relapse prevention in schizophrenia* (pp. 155–163). Berlin: Springer-Verlag.

Knos, G. B., & Sung, Y. F. (1991). Anesthetic management of the high-risk medical patient receiving electroconvulsive therapy. In A. Stoudemire & B. S. Fogel (Eds.), *Medical psychiatric practice* (Vol. 1, pp. 99–144). Washington, DC: American Psychiatric Press.

Lucas, P. B., et al. (1990). Effects of the acute administration of caffeine to patients with schizophrenia. *Biological Psychiatry, 28*, 35.

Marder, S. R., & Van Putten, T. (1995). Antipsychotic medications. In A. F. Schatzberg & C. B. Nemeroff (Eds.), *The American Psychiatric Press textbook of psychopharmacology.* Washington, DC: American Psychiatric Press.

McGrath, P. J., Stewart, J. W., Nunes, E. V., et al. (1993). A double-blind crossover trial of imipramine and phenelzine for outpatients with treatment-refractory depression. *American Journal of Psychiatry, 150*, 118–123.

Nishinto, S., Mignot, E., & Dement, W. C. (1995). Sedative-hypnotics. In A. F. Schatzberg & C. B. Nemeroff (Eds.), *The American Psychiatric Press textbook of psychopharmacology* (p. 410). Washington, DC: American Psychiatric Press.

Owens, M., & Risch, S. C. (1995). Atypical antipsychotics. In A. F. Schatzberg & C. B. Nemeroff (Eds.), *The American Psychiatric Press textbook of psychopharmacology.* Washington, DC: American Psychiatric Press.

Pickar, D., Woen, R. R., Litman, R. E., et al. (1992). Clinical and biologic response to clozapine in patients with schizophrenia. *Archives of General Psychiatry, 49*, 345–353.

Potter, W. Z., Manji, H., & Rudorfer, M. (1995). Tricyclics and tetracyclics. In A. F. Schatzberg & C. B. Nemeroff (Eds.), *The American Psychiatric Press textbook of psychopharmacology* (p. 145). Washington, DC: American Psychiatric Press.

Price, L. H., Charney, D. S., Delgado, P. L., et al. (1990). Lithium and serotonin function: Implications for the serotonin hypothesis of depression. *Psychopharmacology (Berlin), 100*, 2–12.

Riddle, M. A., Geller, B., & Ryan, N. (1993). Another sudden death in a child treated with desipramine. *Journal of the American Academy of Child and Adolescent Psychiatry, 32,* 792–797.

Salzman, C., Satlin, A., & Burrows, A. B. (1995). Geriatric psychopharmacology. In A. F. Schatzberg & C. B. Nemeroff (Eds.), *The American Psychiatric Press textbook of psychopharmacology* (p. 812). Washington, DC: American Psychiatric Press.

Schachar, R., & Tannock, R. (1993). Childhood hyperactivity and psychostimulants: A review of extended treatment studies. *Journal of Child and Adolescent Psychopharmacology, 3,* 81–97.

Schatzberg, A. F. (1987). Trazodone: A 5 year review of antidepressant efficacy. *Psychopathology, 20,* (Suppl. 1), 48–57.

Schou, M. (1989). *Lithium treatment of manic-depressive illness* (4th ed., Rev.). Basel, Switzerland: Karger.

Schweizer, E., Rickels, K., Amsterdam, J. D., et al. (1990). What constitutes an adequate antidepressant trial for fluoxetine? *Journal of Clinical Psychiatry, 51,* 8–11.

Swann, A. C., Secunda, S. K., Stokes, P. E., et al. (1990). Stress, depression and mania; relationship between perceived role of stressful events and clinical and biochemical characteristics. *Acta Psychiatrica Scandinavia, 81,* 389–397.

Tollefson, G. D. (1995). Selective serotonin reuptake inhibitors. In A. F. Schatzberg & C. B. Nemeroff (Eds.), *The American Psychiatric Press textbook of psychopharmacology* (p. 167). Washington, DC: American Psychiatric Press.

von Bahr, C., et al. (1991). Plasma levels of thioridazine and metabolites are influenced by the debrisoquin hydroxylation phenotype. *Clinical Pharmacology Therapy, 49,* 234.

Warner, M. D., Peabody, C. A., Whiteford, H. A., et al. (1988). Alprazolam as an antidepressant. *Journal of Clinical Psychiatry, 49,* 148–150.

Wender, P. H., Reimherr, J., Wood, D., et al. (1985). A controlled study of methylphenidate in the treatment of attention deficit disorder, residual type, in adults. *American Journal of Psychiatry, 142,* 547–552.

Wig, N. N. (1993). Rational treatment in psychiatry, perspectives on psychiatric treatment by level of care. In N. Sartorius, G. de Girolamo, G. Andrews, G. A. German, & L. Eisenberg (Eds.), *Treatment of mental disorders* (pp. 423–441). Washington, DC: American Psychiatric Press.

Wysowski, D. K., & Baum, C. (1989). Antipsychotic drug use in the United States: 1976–85. *Archives of General Psychiatry, 46,* 929.

Yagiela, J. A., Duffin, S. R., & Hunt L. M. (1985). Drug interactions and vasoconstrictors used in local anesthetic solutions. *Oral Surgery Oral Medicine Oral Pathology, 59,* 565–571.

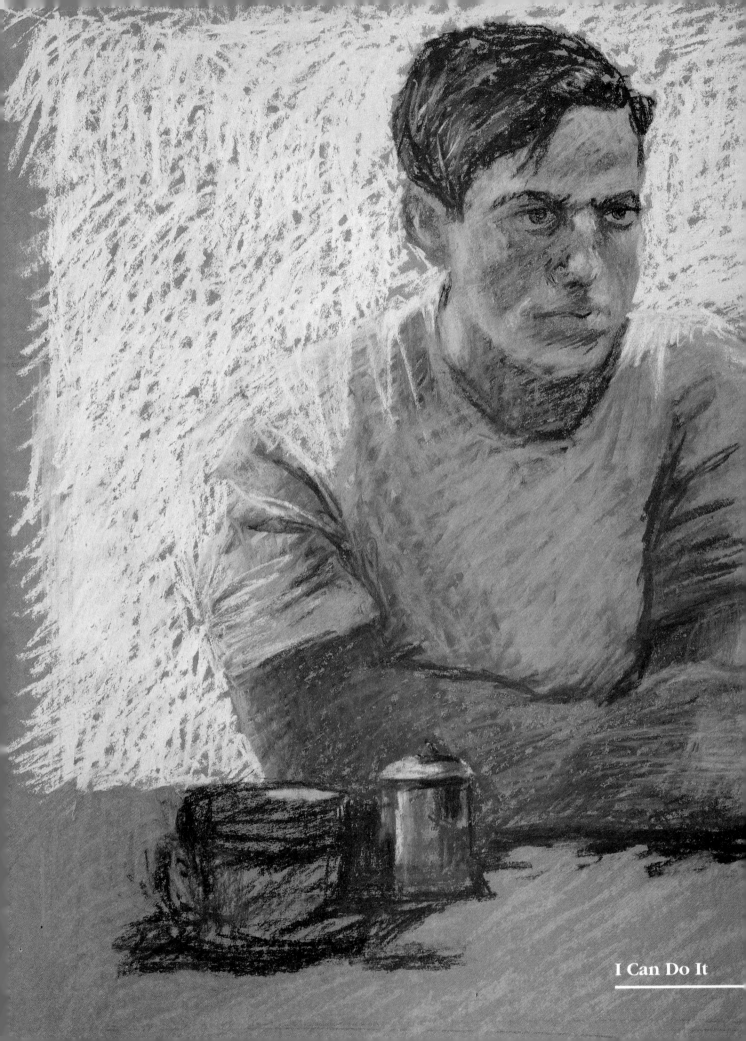

I Can Do It

Chapter 26

INDIVIDUAL PSYCHOTHERAPY

Noreen Cavan Frisch

Lawrence E. Frisch

Psychotherapy

Consider the reasons clients might seek individual therapy:
- ◆ Many persons seek a therapist during a time of crisis and change.
- ◆ Others seek therapy to deal with a specific issue (for example the breakup of a relationship) and then find there are other concerns that underlie the current issue.
- ◆ Still others seek therapy because their feelings and behaviors have impaired their ability to function effectively.

As you work with clients, consider the reasons that each is seeking care at this time and begin to evaluate how the motivation for treatment affects the type of therapy that will best meet the client's immediate needs.

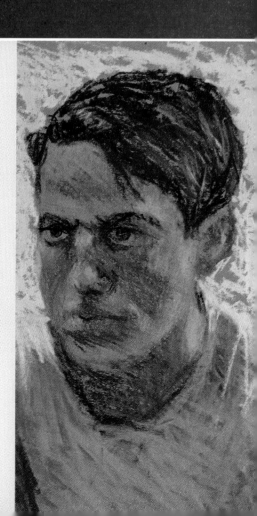

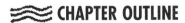 **CHAPTER OUTLINE**

PROVIDERS OF THERAPY

MAJOR APPROACHES TO PSYCHOTHERAPY

Insight-Oriented Therapy
    Psychoanalysis
    Psychodynamic Therapy
    Interpersonal Therapy

Task-Oriented Therapy

Experience-Oriented Therapy

RESEARCH BASE FOR PSYCHOTHERAPEUTIC INTERVENTIONS

PSYCHOTHERAPY AND CULTURAL SENSITIVITY

PSYCHOTHERAPY IN NURSING PRACTICE

Nursing Theory

Collaborative Interventions

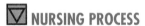 **NURSING PROCESS**

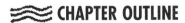 **COMPETENCIES**

Upon completion of this chapter, the reader should be able to:

1. Define psychotherapy.

2. Describe various approaches to therapy, including:
    ◆ Psychoanalysis
    ◆ Psychodynamic therapy
    ◆ Interpersonal therapy
    ◆ Cognitive-behavioral therapy
    ◆ Client-centered therapy

3. Suggest ways that psychotherapeutic approaches are used in nursing practice.

4. Relate major psychotherapeutic approaches to nursing theory.

5. Describe the research base of psychotherapeutic interventions.

≋ KEY TERMS

Catharsis Experience of release that occurs when unconscious thoughts are brought into consciousness.

Clarification Technique in which an analyst points out a behavior pattern that is not recognized by the client.

Client-Centered Therapy Process focused on bringing out individual internal resources and understanding.

Cognitive-Behavioral Therapy Short-term process that focuses on how the client thinks about himself and what he does. The therapy deals with beliefs and actions.

Confrontation Technique in which an analyst challenges a client's behavior or thought, with the goal of provoking a reaction and overcoming an emotional barrier to change.

Experience-Oriented Therapy Process focusing on the client's experiences as an agent for producing change.

Insight-Oriented Therapy Process focusing on helping an individual gain understanding of feelings and behaviors.

Interpersonal Therapy Process of gaining insight based on the recognition that psychological distress may occur in conjunction with disturbed human relationships.

Interpretation Technique in which an analyst offers an explanation of a client's unconscious behavior processes.

Manipulation Technique in which an analyst tries to influence a client's feelings about therapy, with the goal of enhancing the quality of the therapy.

Psychoanalysis Therapy focused on uncovering unconscious memories and processes.

Psychodynamic Therapy Brief process based on psychoanalytic principles, with the goal of improved functioning rather than personality reconstruction.

Psychotherapy Treatment of mental or emotional disorders through psychological rather than physical methods.

Repression Process in which painful memories, thoughts, or experiences are actively kept out of conscious awareness.

Suggestion Psychoanalytic technique in which the analyst interprets the client's thoughts, actions, or dreams.

Task-Oriented Therapy Process focused on helping an individual gain the tools needed to change behavior and feelings.

Psychotherapy is the treatment of mental or emotional disorders through psychological rather than physical methods (although it is often done in conjunction with somatic therapy, especially medications). Psychotherapy can be done with individuals or with groups (see Chapter 28). Individual psychotherapy is the use of psychological techniques applied in a one-on-one setting. The techniques are designed to help persons overcome mental distress and illness for the purpose of assisting those individuals to reach their optimum level of health. Psychotherapy has several characteristics that make it an important study for psychiatric nurses:

1. Data clearly establish the effectiveness of individual psychotherapy for a number of specific therapies targeted to specific disorders.

2. Many of the techniques of psychotherapy are of value to nurses in their daily work, both with psychiatric clients and with others.

3. Psychotherapy has potential relevance to all settings in which psychiatric nursing is carried out: inpatient, outpatient, and home care.

4. Relatively recent developments in psychotherapy have placed a strong emphasis on brief treatment techniques that differ significantly from past approaches to psychotherapy. It is important for nurses to understand how psychotherapies differ so that they can help clients choose appropriate treatment.

Only a few decades ago, individuals seeking counseling or therapy would have had few options: primarily lengthy, intensive psychoanalysis. Today, there are multiple approaches to therapy. Some of these approaches derive from psychoanalysis and rely on helping individuals gain insight into feelings and behaviors; these are known as **insight-oriented therapies**. Other therapies are **task-oriented**. They help individuals to gain tools that allow them to change behavior (and often feelings). Yet a third group of therapies is **experience-oriented**. These attempt to create an experience that will facilitate growth and personal development. The purpose of this chapter is to acquaint the nurse with major approaches to psychotherapy. However, because many different types of professionals offer psychotherapy, it is important to begin with a brief discussion of the identity and credentials of individuals who commonly offer psychotherapeutic services.

PROVIDERS OF THERAPY

Clients seeking therapy may be seen by a psychiatrist (an MD), a psychologist (a PhD), a nurse (an RN, MSN, or PhD), a social worker (an MSW), or a therapist/counselor. While the distinction between psychotherapy and counseling may be vague, psychotherapy is typically more intense and frequently more likely to be directed to persons with serious psychopathology. Counseling is more commonly sought by individuals experiencing acute situational crisis (see Chapter 9). Counselors are more often educated at the master's level and are less likely to have experience with seriously ill individuals.

Registered Nurses may provide counseling and client education related to crisis, stress, and mental health and may also provide referral to community sources for both therapy and counseling. In addition, experienced psychiatric nurses may provide client support and carry out interventions that are based on any of the psychotherapeutic approaches. In some settings, nurses in advanced practice roles (MSNs and/or PhDs) provide both counseling and psychotherapy; in some states, these practitioners may also perform physical examinations and prescribe medications.

MAJOR APPROACHES TO PSYCHOTHERAPY

Virtually all of the many varieties and schools of psychotherapy can be grouped into one of three categories: insight-oriented therapy, task-oriented therapy, and experience-oriented therapy. There are many specific types of therapy within each category, but if the nurse understands the principles underlying each major category, then he will be able to understand the principles of new or unfamiliar psychotherapeutic techniques.

Insight-Oriented Therapy

Psychoanalysis

Psychoanalysis is the oldest and best known of the insight-oriented therapies. It is derived from the Freudian view of psychosexual development (see Chapter 3). Psychoanalysis is a form of psychotherapy focusing on the uncovering of unconscious memories and processes: "Psychoanalysis is based on the observation that individuals are often unaware of many of the factors that determine their emotions and behavior. These unconscious factors may create unhappiness, sometimes in the form of recognizable symptoms and at other times as troubling personality traits, difficulties in work or in love relationships, or disturbances in mood and self-esteem. Because these forces are unconscious, the advice of friends and family, the reading of self-help books, or even the most determined efforts of will, often fail to provide relief" (American Psychoanalytic Association, 1997, Web page).

The goal of the psychoanalytic treatment is to demonstrate to the client how unconscious factors affect current relationship and behavior patterns. The treatment traces the patterns of behavior and relationships back to their origin in infancy or childhood. Through the process of reexperiencing life circumstances and interactions with the analyst, the client becomes both intellectually and emotionally aware of the underlying sources of diffi-

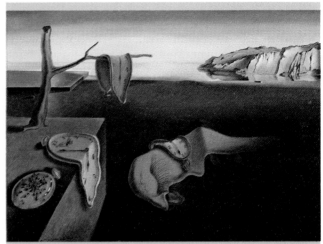

The Persistence of Memory by Salvador Dali (1931). Oil on canvas 9½×13" Given anonymously. Photograph © 1997 The Museum of Modern Art, New York. Source: The Museum of Modern Art, New York.

The landscape and subject evoke a dream or nightmare. Perhaps a pun on the distortion of time often experienced in dreams, the deformed watches may also be symbols from a frightening past—hence the title. This picture seems to demand a formal interpretation, but it is hard to believe that any would succeed short of detailed psychoanalysis of the painter himself. Painted during Freud's lifetime, this work strongly suggests the mysteries, and perhaps even the potential dangers, of deeply probing the unconscious self through psychoanalytic therapy.

culties. The client provides the analyst with clues to the unconscious sources of current difficulties: through identification of certain patterns of behavior, in the subjects that he finds hard to talk about, or in the ways he relates to the analyst. During the psychoanalytic process, the client grapples with insights, going over them again and again with the analyst, as well as repeatedly addressing these insights in daily life, in dreams, and in fantasies.

The process of psychoanalysis is highly individualized, and its course is dictated both by the nature of the presenting problem and by the personalities and backgrounds of both analyst and client. For this reason it is often hard to describe a "typical" psychoanalysis. Most psychoanalysts believe in the process of **repression**, in which painful memories, thoughts, or experiences are actively kept out of conscious awareness. These memories may have highly emotional content; for example, such memories may involve violence or sexual experiences. The analyst's goal is to uncover such unconscious experiences and to interpret them to a client who finds them painful and frightening.

Psychoanalytic theory assumes that clients actively resist coming to an understanding of repressed, unconscious thoughts or feelings. Because of this resistance, the

Table 26-1 Techniques Used in Psychoanalysis

TECHNIQUE	EXAMPLE
Suggestion: a technique in which the analyst tentatively interprets the client's thoughts, actions, or dreams.	Analyst states, "Your recurrent dreams about taking tests may be an indication of your worry about success."
Catharsis: the experience of release that occurs by bringing unconscious thoughts through to consciousness in efforts to cure psychological symptoms.	Client states, "I feel relieved, I can now see that the fearful figure in my dream is my father."
Manipulation: a technique where the analyst tries actively to influence the client's feelings about the therapy, with the goal of enhancing the quality of the therapy.	Analyst states, "You just think you can't remember your dreams. I'll bet if you write them down in the morning, as soon as you wake up, you'll be able to remember."
Confrontation: the analyst directly challenges the client's behavior or thought, usually intended to provoke a reaction from the client. Such reactions are intended to overcome emotional barriers to change.	Analyst states, "You are relating to your boss the same way you relate to your father."
Clarification: the analyst describes the client's behavior, pointing out a pattern that is not recognized by the client.	Analyst states, "You have a pattern of dealing with anger by laughing. That is an indirect means of expressing anger."
Interpretation: the analyst brings her understanding of the client's unconscious processes to explain behavior.	Analyst states, "You are angry with me because I'm telling you the same things your mother told you."

analyst must use specific therapeutic techniques that help the client grow in his willingness to accept uncomfortable conscious or unconscious thoughts and change dysfunctional behaviors. Some of these techniques are summarized in the Table 26-1. The accompanying display provides an example of a typical client-analyst interaction in a therapy session. In this session, the therapist is using the techniques of confrontation and clarification to assist the client to see that she is dealing with irritation and anger in a passive and indirect way. The purpose of the session would be to identify if the client has a longstand-

SAMPLE CLIENT-ANALYST INTERACTION IN THERAPY

Therapist: How do you feel when I indicate to you that you are passive?

Client: I don't like it. (The client is laughing, but it is quite evident that she is irritated.)

Therapist: But you are smiling.

Client: I know, Well . . . maybe that is my way of expressing my irritation.

Therapist: Then you are irritated?

Client: A little bit . . . yeah. . . .

Therapist: A little bit?

Client: Actually, quite a bit. (The client is laughing.)

Therapist: Let's look at what happened here. I brought to your attention your passivity, your noninvolvement. You got irritated and angry with me and the way you dealt with your irritation was by smiling.

From Short-term Dynamic Psychotherapy by H. Davanloo, 1980, p. 48 New York: Jason Aronson.

ing pattern of dealing with anger this way, to explore the origins of the pattern, and ultimately to gain insights that will permit the client to adopt more active and direct methods of dealing with anger: "Eventually the [client's] life—his or her behavior, relationships, sense of self—changes in deep and abiding ways" (American Psychoanalytic Association, 1997, Web page).

Psychoanalysis is inherently lengthy and, for this reason, quite costly. Clients have traditionally paid their analyst directly for psychotherapeutic services, although in recent years some insurance plans have included coverage for psychological treatment, including psychoanalysis. As the realities of managed care have become increasingly evident, there has been a growth of interest in therapeutic techniques that can provide needed psychological insights in a shorter and thus more cost-effective time. Prominent among these techniques is a psychotherapeutic technique called psychodynamic therapy.

REFLECTIVE THINKING

Psychoanalysis Techniques

Consider your own behavior and coping mechanisms. Do you find that you, intentionally or not, employ some of the techniques of psychoanalysis in your own behavioral strategies? What patterns can you recognize in your thoughts and behaviors?

Psychodynamic Therapy

Psychodynamic therapy is a "brief" therapy based on psychoanalytic principles and interpretations. Psychodynamic therapy attempts to replace full psychoanalysis with a process that focuses on selected therapeutic issues so as to get more rapidly to what the therapist perceives to be the core of the individual's psychological distress. The goal of psychodynamic therapy is improved functioning rather than complete personality reconstruction. Psychodynamic therapy may take place over a few months or weeks, rather than the years occupied by traditional psychoanalysis.

Both psychoanalysis and psychodynamic therapy begin with two assumptions: First, it is assumed that the client is seeking therapy and is trying as hard as possible to work with the therapist; second, it is assumed that the client has basic abilities of cognition and insight. These approaches to therapy may be difficult to carry out with individuals who have significant psychological problems, including psychosis, substance abuse, and personality disorders. Even less disabling problems such as phobia or obsessional symptoms may make a psychodynamic approach untenable (Worchel, 1990).

Interpersonal Therapy

Not all insight-based therapy is derived from the psychoanalytic perspective. **Interpersonal therapy**, also insight-based, is based on the recognition that psychological distress frequently occurs in conjunction with disturbed human relationships. Interpersonal therapy is based on the interpersonal theories of Sullivan and the related nursing theory of Peplau (see Chapter 3).

During interpersonal therapy, the client enters into a relationship with the therapist and is helped to examine patterns of relationships and interactions with others. It is assumed that the client can use the experience of a positive therapeutic relationship, coupled with insights about past relationships, to establish meaningful, positive relationships with others outside the therapy sessions. Whereas psychoanalysis and its less intense cousin, psychodynamic therapy, search for their insights deep within the individual's unconscious mind, interpersonal therapy seeks to provide its clients with insight into the processes of daily life and human interaction. As for all of the numerous insight-based therapies, the goal is enhanced self-understanding leading to enhanced personal and interpersonal success.

Task-Oriented Therapy

In recent years, the predominance of psychoanalytic methods has been giving way to a newer approach to the mind: cognitive-behavioral psychology. **Cognitive-behavioral therapy** is not about gaining insight into the presumed childhood origins of problems. It is not just about venting feelings or talking about problems. Rather, cognitive-behavioral therapy focuses on practical results. The main issue is not how an individual got to be the way he is; it is helping that individual make practical changes. Cognitive-behavioral therapy has several distinct characteristics:

1. It is result oriented. The therapy begins with assisting the client to define goals and will proceed to monitor progress toward those goals.
2. It is short term. For most clients, the goals of the therapy can be accomplished quickly, often within 5 to 20 sessions.
3. It is self-help oriented. The therapist is a coach or teacher who helps the client learn how to manage his own life better. The client learns new tools for living his life and dealing with life's challenges.

The major goals of cognitive-behavioral therapy are to provide cost-effective care for a wide range of problems; to alter clients' interpretations of themselves by changing their behavior, environment, or cognition directly; to increase clients' coping skills; and to increase the likelihood that gains made during therapy will be maintained once therapy is terminated (Wells & Giannetti, 1990).

Cognitive therapies are concerned with how the client thinks about himself. Behavioral therapies focus on precisely what the client does. Together, the cognitive-behavioral approach attempts to change both a client's beliefs and his behavior. The therapy rarely addresses why a client feels or acts in a certain way; it is sufficient to ascertain only that this feeling or action is undesirable. Often, the therapist will work with her client to determine specifically in what settings the undesired thoughts or behaviors occur. The therapist then helps the client focus on alternatives to the specific thoughts or actions and works to help the client feel that he can truly use these alternatives.

The therapy becomes task-oriented because the therapist gives the client "homework assignments" to complete in between therapy sessions. For example, a client

NURSING TIP

Sample Homework Assignments in Cognitive-Behavioral Therapy

- Reading: may include books, workbook material, or relevant articles
- Written assignments: keeping a journal or log of day-to-day events
- Experiential activities: planned activities that involve risk taking or trying out new behaviors in a safe setting

dealing with problems of anger and risk for violence may be asked to keep a journal detailing feelings of anger, situations bringing on angry feelings, and immediate behaviors following angry feelings. The therapist and the client will review the journal during the following therapy session to identify thoughts and behaviors that can be used to replace the patterns that are causing trouble for the client.

Cognitive-behavioral therapy is frequently used in the treatment of depression. From this standpoint, the therapy may be based on three principles:

1. Moods, feelings, and depression are created and maintained by one's thoughts and feelings. In this view, beliefs come first, feelings follow.

2. In depression, the majority of one's thoughts are negative; the individual has difficulty focusing on any positive aspects of a life situation.

3. In depression, one's negative thoughts and negativity are often irrational or distorted or bear little relationship to reality.

First, the client learns to recognize the presence of negative and disturbing thoughts. For example, a depressed person may think that his feelings of guilt derive from having done something bad, even if he has no idea what the bad deed may have been. Most depressed persons have such negative thoughts. One of the initial goals of therapy is to help such persons identify negative thoughts and to see these thoughts as harmful, abnormal, and the root cause of feelings of depression. The therapist may ask the client to write down all of the negative thoughts he experiences. Then, the client may be asked to analyze each thought and explain why it is irrational or exaggerated. Finally, the client is asked to substitute a nondepressed, positive thought in place of the negative one. Clients are coached in doing this until the substitution of the positive for negative thoughts becomes natural and automatic. Therapy actually teaches the client to recognize a series of specific thought distortions common in depression. The accompanying display summarizes some of these common thought distortions. Any of these thought distortions can be harmful and lead to continued depression. For exam-

---

COMMON THOUGHT DISTORTIONS ADDRESSED IN COGNITIVE-BEHAVIORAL THERAPY

◆ All-or-nothing thinking: seeing things only in absolutes

◆ Overgeneralization: interpreting every small setback as a never-ending pattern of defeat

◆ Dwelling on negatives: ignoring multiple positive experiences

◆ Jumping to conclusions: assuming that others are reacting negatively without definite evidence

◆ Pessimism: automatically predicting that things will turn out badly

◆ Reasoning from feeling: thinking that if one feels bad, one must be bad

◆ Obligations: living life around a succession of too many "shoulds," "shouldn'ts," "musts," "oughts," and "have-tos"

---

ple, a client who engages in "all-or-nothing" thinking will interpret life experiences to be either good or bad and see nothing in between. Thus, if the client finds fault with any part of a task he has performed, he will interpret the whole endeavor as bad. If, on the other hand, a client engages in "reasoning from feeling," he may think, for example, that if he has not slept well one night, he cannot either feel well or be well.

While cognitive-behavioral therapists most often treat depression, other problems that have been successfully addressed by cognitive-behavioral therapy include anxiety, anger, sexual dysfunction, chronic pain, substance abuse, and eating disorders. By its nature, cognitive-behavioral therapy requires that the client be intellectually intact. It is inappropriate to conduct cognitive-behavioral therapy with one who is psychotic or demented or unable or unwilling to cooperate actively with the therapist.

✆❂ REFLECTIVE THINKING

Sadness in Your Past

Remember a time when you felt sad or depressed. What thoughts or behaviors did you exhibit? At the time, did you view these thoughts as rational or irrational? Do you hold the same opinion now, after some time has passed? Do you feel that there were any interventions that might have changed these negative thoughts and behaviors?

Experience-Oriented Therapy

Experience-oriented therapy focuses on the client's experiences as an agent for producing change. The client's experience is facilitated by a therapist who has assessed the client and who directs experiences to produce a calculated change in behavior and feeling. Unlike insight-oriented therapy, experience-oriented processes do not emphasize the individual's discovery of unconscious knowledge, and unlike task-oriented therapy, the experience-oriented techniques do not require any "homework" or other efforts to consciously change thoughts and behaviors. Experience-oriented therapy engages the client in new interactions and in new ways-of-being within the therapy session.

Client-centered therapy (founded by Carl Rogers) is an example of experience-oriented therapy. Client-centered therapy is based on the idea that every individual has a store of internal resources and self-understanding and that these inner resources can be brought out when the therapist is open, nonjudgmental, and empathic. The therapist seeks to be uniformly supportive and kind. The therapist does not interpret client behaviors; rather the therapist attempts only to understand the client's inner feelings. The therapist offers respect and protection of the client's autonomy. The client is viewed as the expert about himself: The therapist is a supportive facilitator rather than an authority figure. The therapist will answer questions, give explanations, and shape experiments for the client to try. For example, the client may be asked to role-play with the therapist in a session. The therapist may play the client's boss, in an effort to bring an experience into the present, so that the client may interpret his emotions and actions.

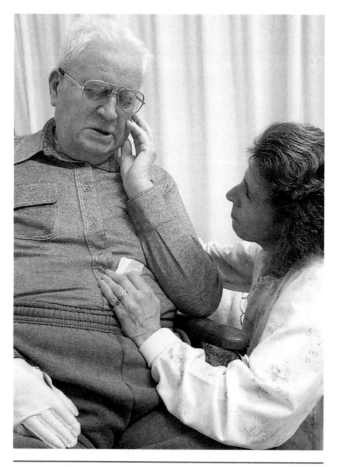

Figure 26-1 Clients undergoing individual therapy may become emotional as they recall significant personal life events. The nurse who embodies empathy, support, and caring will best be able to assist clients in dealing with the myriad emotions that surface during therapy sessions.

In contrast to psychoanalysis, in which the analyst attempts to overcome the client's repression of painful thoughts, this shaping of experiences is done gently, with the client's full cooperation. The client experiences therapy as a safe, empowering encounter with a kind and caring therapist. This encounter provides the grounding experience from which the client can try out new behaviors and grow interpersonally and emotionally. The therapy ideally results in the client's ability to see self differently and to promote self-growth and maturation.

RESEARCH BASE FOR PSYCHOTHERAPEUTIC INTERVENTIONS

Studies of insight-oriented therapies apply only to those individuals who are motivated enough to qualify for psychodynamic treatments. One psychodynamic therapist writes: "The therapy is not considered successful unless the patient is not only symptom free, but also the patient's maladaptive character defenses are replaced with adaptive character defenses. At the termination, the patient must have both cognitive and emotional insight into the structure of his pathology" (Worchel, 1990, p. 214). Studies have indicated that short-term psychodynamic treatments are of measurable value; however, there are significant differences among therapists in client outcomes (Crits-Cristoph, 1991).

Interpersonal therapy that addresses the specific interpersonal content surrounding episodes of psychological distress has been shown to be effective. Studies validate that short-term interpersonal therapy is highly effective in the management of major depression, particularly in young and middle-aged adults with unipolar symptoms. The combination of medication and interpersonal therapy has been shown to be more effective than either treatment alone in the management of major depression (Weissman, Klerman, Prusoff, Sholomskas, & Padian, 1981).

Many studies have established that task-oriented therapies, including cognitive and cognitive-behavioral therapies, are effective treatment for many psychological conditions. Cognitive therapy has been shown to be effective treatment for unipolar, and perhaps bipolar, depression (Hollon & Beck, 1994). This positive effectiveness seems to extend to both outpatient and inpatient treatment. One important study has suggested that cognitive therapy is less effective than medication for depression (Elkin, 1994), but most other studies have found the two treatments roughly comparable for the management of acute symptoms. There is some suggestion that cognitive therapy may decrease the risk of recurrence of depression, but this remains inconclusively proven (Evans et al., 1992).

In addition, cognitive therapies have been shown convincingly to be effective in the management of a range of anxiety disorders, including panic (Clark, 1986) and obsessive-compulsive disorder (see Chapter 10). Eating disorders, particularly bulimia, seem also to benefit from cognitive therapy (Wilson & Fairburn, 1993) (see also Chapter 18).

Experience-oriented and client-centered therapies are difficult to assess, and there are few if any studies on treatment outcome, perhaps largely because the therapist does not define the expected outcome prior to the start (or even conclusion) of therapy. The studies that have been done on client-centered therapy have focused on client feelings about the therapeutic process. Perhaps not surprisingly, therapists who score high on independent assessments of therapeutic empathy have clients who are more comfortable after their therapy sessions than before (Lafferty, Beutler, & Crago, 1991). The few outcome studies that have been done seem to support the philosophy of client-centered interactions. For example, assessment of therapist empathic ability is correlated very strongly with therapeutic efficacy in programs to treat alcoholism (Miller, Taylor, & West, 1980).

PSYCHOTHERAPY AND CULTURAL SENSITIVITY

There have been several studies done on the effectiveness of psychotherapy in persons from varied cultural and ethnic backgrounds. Because effectiveness of psychotherapy is related to multiple variables, such studies are difficult to conduct and findings may be inconclusive. However, the available research does seem to indicate that psychotherapy is effective in individuals, regardless of background (Stanley, Nolan, & Young, 1994). Most investigations further indicate that an ethnic match between client and therapist does not affect outcomes. However, there is some evidence of assessment bias that is related to the background of the therapist.

A classic 1980 study provides the best example of such biases. Li-Repac (1980) had white and Chinese-American therapists rate both white and Chinese-American clients. White clinicians rated the Chinese-American clients as "anxious," "awkward," "confused," "nervous," and "reserved," while the Chinese-American clinicians used words such as "alert," "dependable," "friendly," and

"practical" for the same clients. The Chinese-American clinicians rated the white clients as "active," "aggressive," and "rebellious," while the white clinicians rated the same clients as "affectionate," "adventurous," and "capable." These findings point out how easily the ethnic or cultural background of the therapist can influence therapy. Since much has been done since 1980 to increase awareness of and sensitivity to one ethnic and cultural group to the experiences and behaviors of other groups, it is possible that findings would be different if one replicated this study today (see also Chapter 6).

PSYCHOTHERAPY IN NURSING PRACTICE

In an era in which public and professional discussions often focus on the role of medication to treat mental distress and there is ever-increasing emphasis on the biological basis of mental disease, it is important to recognize that individual psychotherapy remains an important and well-validated therapeutic tool. Many clients are helped through processes that allow them to gain insight, to examine their thoughts and behaviors, and to try out new ways of relating to others.

Nurses in virtually any area of practice will encounter professional therapists who offer many different approaches to treatment. A 1997 Internet search resulted in a list of over 40 distinct approaches to therapy. Some of these therapies are relatively conventional (brief psychotherapy, psychoanalysis, client-centered therapy), while others may be viewed as unconventional (videotherapy, ritual therapy, or persuasion therapy). Each therapy has its strong proponents and clearly unique benefits. Clients may often seek the nurse's opinions regarding the value of specific therapeutic approaches.

Some nurses in advanced practice roles function as therapists, offering direct service to clients. These nurses have additional education in individual therapy, and many have experienced therapy themselves as a means to gain insight into their own professional and personal behaviors. Other nurses, however, may employ specific psychotherapeutic techniques to assist clients in all clinical settings. For example, a nurse may use the psychodynamic technique of interpretation to offer a suggestion of how she perceives the client is handling a crisis. The statement "While you are in the hospital, it seems difficult for you to take on the dependent role of client" offers an interpretation of the client's behavior, expresses empathy, and opens up areas for discussion between nurse and client. Techniques of cognitive-behavioral therapy that help the client look at his thought patterns may be used as well. For example, asking a client to identify something positive about his work performance, rather than dwelling on negatives, may be the first step for the client to reframe his thinking about himself. Lastly, principles of experiential therapies, with emphasis

---

✳ **NURSING TIP**

Psychotherapy and Cultural Sensitivity

To be an effective therapist, you must understand the experiences, the worldview, and the values of your clients. In an increasingly diverse society, you must be continually aware of potential areas of bias or misunderstanding.

DIFFERING KINDS OF THERAPIES

◆ Adventure therapy

◆ Analytical psychotherapy

◆ Art therapy

◆ Autogenic training

◆ Bibliotherapy

◆ Brief psychotherapy

◆ Client-centered therapy

◆ Cognitive-affective behavior therapy

◆ Cognitive-behavioral therapy

◆ Dance therapy

◆ Directed reverie therapy

◆ Dream therapy

◆ Ego state therapy

◆ Encounter group therapy

◆ Ethnocultural therapy

◆ Existential psychotherapy

◆ Experiential psychotherapy

◆ Expressive psychotherapy

◆ Family therapy

◆ Gestalt therapy

◆ Hypnotherapy

◆ Individual psychotherapy

◆ Insight therapy

◆ Logotherapy

◆ Marathon therapy

◆ Multimodal therapy

◆ Persuasion therapy

◆ Play therapy

◆ Primal therapy

◆ Process experiential psychotherapy

◆ Psychoanalysis

◆ Psychodrama

◆ Rational-emotive therapy

◆ Reality therapy

◆ Recreation therapy

◆ Relationship therapy

◆ Ritual therapy

◆ Self-psychology

◆ Short-term dynamic therapy

◆ Therapeutic writing

◆ Transactional analysis

◆ Videotherapy

on a caring, humanistic relationship, fit well in practice directed by nursing theory in which the goal is to provide a safe psychological environment for the client to explore the meaning of his life, his work, his illness, or his current circumstance.

Nursing Theory

Professional practice increasingly requires that nurses understand their care from a theory base. Thus, it is reasonable to ask how psychotherapeutic approaches fit with the philosophy of nursing theory.

Psychoanalysis and psychodynamic therapy are most consistent with nursing theories that emphasize human development and the influence of past experiences on present behaviors. Peplau's nursing theory is particularly compatible with a psychoanalytic and interpersonal therapy, and its development was directly influenced by the interpersonal theory and by concepts of psychoanalysis. Peplau identifies needs, frustrations, conflict, and anxiety as important factors that a nurse should explicitly evaluate in the context of a client's past history and present circumstances (Belcher & Fish, 1995).

Cognitive-behavioral therapy is consistent with nursing theories emphasizing adaptation, for example, Callista Roy's theory. Roy's theory assumes that behavior is adaptive and that changes in the environment (internal or external) can affect the client's feelings and behavior.

There is a very strong philosophical similarity between the nursing concept of human care and the client-centered approach of experience-oriented psychotherapy. In nursing, caring is a unique philosophy that emphasizes the nurse-client relationship and places value on positive regard, acceptance, human care, and nurturance. These qualities are an implicit part of the client-centered psychotherapeutic approach. Nurse theorists from Leininger to Watson to Erickson have repeatedly emphasized the caring aspects of nursing as the priority of focus. Nursing theories based on caring and client-centered psychotherapy seem to share a series of assumptions:

1. In contrast to therapeutic objectivity, caring within a nurse-client relationship maintains a therapeutic perspective, where feelings are acknowledged and integrated into a framework of understanding (Montgomery, 1993).

2. Caregivers can experience an existential or spiritual significance to their involvement with the client (Watson, 1988).

3. Nurses who are experienced in caring can respond to their own experiences and intuition to guide practice (Benner, 1984).

4. Self-disclosure of the therapist is acceptable when directed toward the goal of shared human experiences (Montgomery & Webster, 1994).

5. The therapist accepts the client's view of his world, and the client determines desired outcomes (Erickson, Tomlin, & Swain, 1983).

6. Instilling hope is an important aspect of caring (Montgomery & Webster, 1994).

These assumptions describe a therapeutic process that emphasizes humanistic caring with a focus on experiences shared between the client and nurse.

Collaborative Interventions

Like any area of nursing practice, psychiatric care is a discipline in which the nurse must work as a member of a treatment team composed of representatives of several professions. The team approach may dictate the nurse's style of intervention with his clients. For example, if the treatment team elects to use a psychodynamic approach, the nurse's interventions must be grounded in the principles of psychodynamic therapy. In contrast, if the treatment approach is cognitive-behavioral, the nurse must plan interventions consistent with identifying thoughts and changing behavioral outcomes. In such a collaborative setting, nurses must understand the treatment approaches selected for each client and then must ensure that nursing interventions are consistent with those of other team professionals.

NURSING PROCESS

When a nurse provides individual psychotherapy, the nurse is functioning as a therapist such that all professional actions are grounded in the theory or approach of the therapy. While therapists do make assessments of their clients and plan the therapy according to assessment data, therapists do not apply the nursing process. The nursing process requires assessment and analysis of data that result in a nursing diagnosis. Psychotherapy does not require a nursing diagnosis, and in some cases (for example, client-centered therapy), the therapist would not make a diagnosis of any kind. Analysis of data in psychotherapy is done according to the theory. For example, assessment of depressed emotions could be interpreted as anger toward self (psychodynamic therapy), as a manifestation of negative thinking (cognitive-behavioral therapy), or as the client's experience of his world (client-centered therapy). It is irrelevant to the therapy whether or not the client behaviors could be labeled according to a standard nursing diagnosis. The nursing process requires outcome identification as well, and in psychoanalytic, psychodynamic, and client-centered therapy, the therapist does not identify outcomes.

The nurse's role in individual psychotherapy reminds one that professional nurses do more than apply the nursing process and that the nursing process was never intended to document every activity a professional nurse provides. In some areas of advanced practice—psychotherapy as a prime example—the nurse is engaged in professional activities outside the nursing process.

🍥 *REFLECTIVE THINKING*

The Future of Individual Therapy

While there are numerous forms of individual therapy, to date no study has shown that one therapy is better than the others, though for some problems many evaluated therapies have been shown to be better than a placebo. In the near future, it is almost certain that the new therapies will be influenced by managed-care ideals that dictate outcome-based, cost-effective care. At this point, cognitive-behavioral approaches seem best suited to such a mandate. Some nurses using this approach have stated their philosophy: "Nurses, like other brief therapists, believe that being in the world is more important than being in therapy" (Shires & Tappan, 1992). Another group of nurses observe: "The traditional approach to mental health that we inherited from psychology and psychiatry has failed to meet the demands for affordable, accessible, and accountable mental health services" (Montgomery & Webster, 1994, p. 291).

◆ Do you agree with either of these statements?

◆ Given the cost-conscious health care environment, what do you feel the future of individual psychotherapy will be?

〰 KEY CONCEPTS

◆ Individual psychotherapy is the treatment of mental or emotional disorders through one-to-one encounters with a therapist/counselor.

◆ Therapies can be organized into three basic approaches: insight-oriented, task-oriented, and experience-oriented.

◆ Psychoanalysis and psychodynamic therapy are insight-oriented therapies grounded in Freudian theory.

◆ Interpersonal therapy is insight-oriented and based on the belief that psychological distress occurs in conjunction with disturbed human relationships.

◆ Task-oriented therapies focus on outcomes and give clients specific tasks or activities to assist them in achieving outcomes.

◆ Cognitive-behavioral therapy sets out to change a client's attitudes and behaviors.

◆ Experience-oriented therapy directs the client through specific experiences in a caring, therapeutic encounter.

◆ Nursing interventions may be grounded in any of the psychotherapeutic approaches.

◆ Psychotherapeutic approaches can be used within the framework of nursing theory.

◆ To date, no research has shown that one therapy is better than the others; all have benefit to clients.

◆ In a managed-care environment, the nursing challenge is to provide care that is affordable, accessible, and accountable.

REVIEW QUESTIONS AND ACTIVITIES

1. How do you distinguish between psychodynamic and interpersonal therapy?

2. Have you observed a client who has had cognitive-behavioral therapy? Describe the client's condition and how the approach was used.

3. Explain how experience-oriented therapy fits with Watson's nursing theory.

4. Do you think that the mandates of managed care will lead to an increased use of cognitive-behavioral therapy? Explain your answer.

5. What research is needed to expand our knowledge of psychotherapeutic approaches?

EXPLORING THE WEB

◆ Visit this text's "Online Companion™" on the Internet at **http://www.DelmarNursing.com** for further information on individual psychotherapy.

◆ Are there specific sites or resources on the Web dealing with psychoanalysis, psychodynamic therapy, interpersonal therapy, cognitive-behavioral therapy, and client-centered therapy?

◆ Are these sites geared toward the health care provider or toward the client?

REFERENCES

American Psychoanalytic Association. (1997). homepage, www.

Belcher, J. R., & Fish, L. J. B. (1995). Hildegard E. Peplau. In J. George (Ed.), *Nursing theories: The base for professional nursing practice* (4th ed., pp. 49–66). Norwalk, CT: Appleton & Lange.

Benner, P. (1984). *From novice to expert: Excellence and power in clinical nursing practice.* Menlo Park, CA: Addison-Wesley.

Clark, D. (1986). A cognitive approach to panic. *Behavioral Research Therapy, 24,* 461–470.

Crits-Cristoph, P. (1991). The efficacy of brief dynamic psychotherapy: A meta-analysis. *American Journal of Psychiatry, 149,* 151–158.

Davanloo, H. (1980). *Short-term dynamic psychotherapy.* New York: Jason Aronson.

Elkin, I. (1994). The NIMH treatment of the depression collaborative research program: Where we began and where we are. In A. Bergin & S. Garfield (Eds.), *Handbook of psychotherapy and behavior change* (pp. 114–139). New York: Wiley.

Erickson, H., Tomlin, E., & Swain, M. (1983). *Modeling and role-modeling: A theory and paradigm for nursing.* Englewood Cliffs, NJ: Prentice-Hall.

Evans, M., Hollon, S., DeRubeis, R., Plasecki, J., Grove, W., Garvey, M., & Tuason, V. (1992). Differential relapse following cognitive therapy and pharmacotherapy for depression. *Archives of General Psychiatry, 49,* 802–808.

Hollon, S. D., & Beck, A. T. (1994). Cognitive and cognitive-behavioral therapies. In A. Bergin & S. Garfield (Eds.), *Handbook of psychotherapy and behavior change* (pp. 428–465). New York: Wiley.

Lafferty, P., Beutler, L. E., & Crago, M. (1991). Differences between more and less effective psychotherapists: A study of select therapist variables. *Journal of Consulting and Clinical Psychology, 57,* 76–80.

Li-Repac, D. (1980). Cultural influences on clinical perception: A comparison between Caucasian and Chinese-American therapists. *Journal of Cross-Cultural Psychology, 11,* 327–342.

Miller, W. R., Taylor, C. A., & West, J. C. (1980). Focused versus broad-spectrum behavior therapy for problem drinkers. *Journal of Consulting and Clinical Psychology, 48,* 590–601.

Montgomery, C. L. (1993). *Healing through communication: The practice of caring.* Newbury Park, CA: Sage.

Montgomery, C. L., & Webster, D. (1994). Caring, curing, and brief therapy: A model for nurse-psychotherapy. *Archives of Psychiatric Nursing, VIII,* 291–297.

Shires, B., & Tappan, T. (1992). The clinical nurse specialist as brief psychotherapist. *Perspectives of Psychiatric Care, 28,* 15–18.

Stanley, S., Nolan, Z., & Young, K. (1995). Research on psychotherapy in culturally diverse populations. In A. Bergin & S. Garfield (Eds.), *Handbook of psychotherapy and behavior change* (pp. 783–817). New York: Wiley.

Watson, J. (1988). New dimensions in human caring theory. *Nursing Science Quarterly, 1,* 175–181.

Webster, D., Vaughn, K., Webb, M., & Player, A. (1995). Modeling the clients' world through brief solution-focused therapy. *Issues in Mental Health Nursing, 16,* 505–518.

Weissman, M. M., Klerman, G. L., Prusoff, B. A., Sholomskas, D., & Padian, N. (1981). Depressed outpatients: Results one year after treatment with drugs and/or interpersonal psychotherapy. *Archives of General Psychiatry, 38,* 51–55.

Wells, R., & Giannetti, V. (1990). *Handbook of the brief psychotherapies.* New York: Plenum.

Wilson, G. T., & Fairburn, C. G. (1993). Cognitive treatments for eating disorders. *Journal of Consulting and Clinical Psychology, 61*, 251–259.

Worchel, J. (1990). Short-term dynamic psychotherapy. In R. Wells & V. Giannetti (Eds.), *Handbook of the brief psychotherapies* (pp. 193–216). New York: Plenum.

≈≈ SUGGESTED READINGS

Baur, S. (1994). *Confiding: A psychotherapist and her patients search for stories to live by.* New York: Harper Perennial.

Beck, A. (1976). *Cognitive therapy and emotional disorders.* Philadelphia: Center for Cognitive Therapy.

Copeland, M. E. (1992). *The depression workbook.* Oakland, CA: New Harbinger.

Freud, S. (1953–1974). In J. Strachey (Ed.), *The standard edition of the complete psychological works of Sigmund Freud.* London: Hogarth Press and Institute for Psychoanalysis.

Peplau, H. (1952). *Interpersonal relations in nursing.* New York: Putnam.

Rogers, C. (1951). *Client-centered therapy.* Boston: Houghton Mifflin.

Sullivan, H. S. (1953). *The interpersonal theory of psychiatry.* New York: Norton.

Weinberg, G. (1996). *The heart of psychotherapy: A journey into the mind and office of the therapist at work.* New York: St. Martin's Griffin.

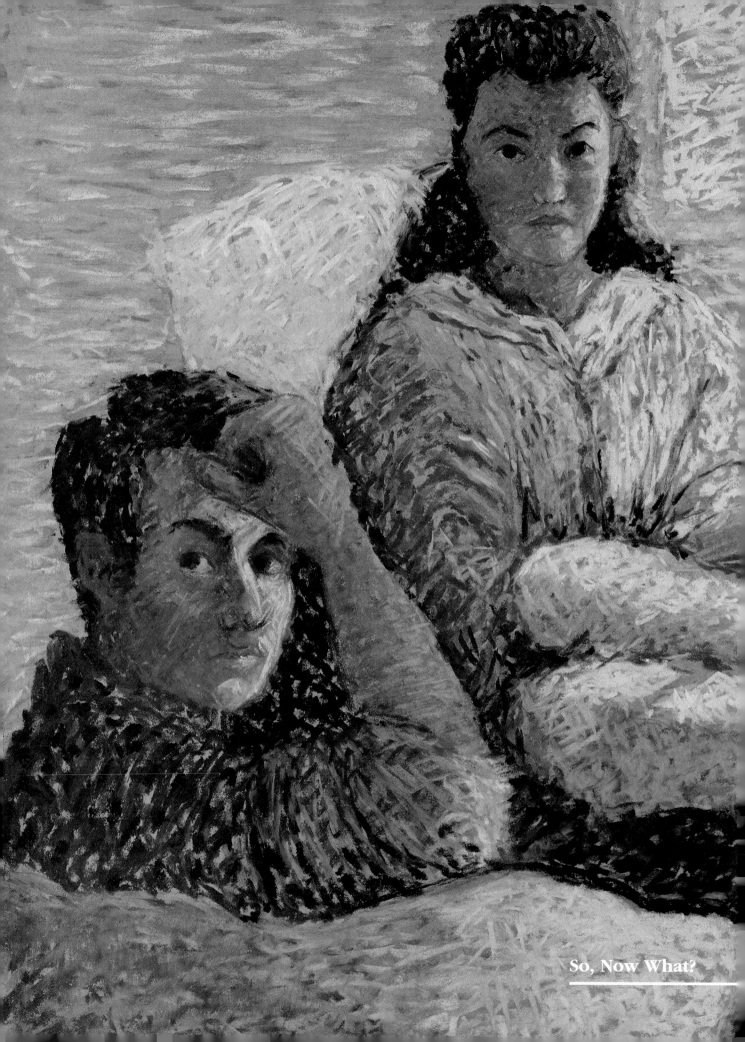

So, Now What?

Chapter

27

FAMILY THERAPY

Jane Kelley
Noreen Cavan Frisch

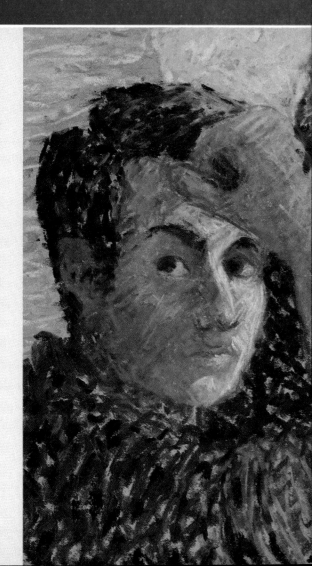

Your Family

You have been a member of a family all of your life. This is an area where you have much experience and expertise! Think about your family in two ways: First, think about your family as the context (background) of your growing up.

♦ Consider ways in which your family taught you how to understand others and society.

♦ Describe ways that your family offered you support or encouragement to do something, or ways that your family did not.

♦ Examine how your adult means of coping may have been learned from early experiences within your family household.

♦ If you have siblings, consider your similarities and differences, given that you were raised in the same environment.

Second, think about your family as a whole.

♦ Consider your own family as a group. Do you react or respond as one unit to others outside of the family?

♦ What stages of family development has your family gone through?

♦ What are the patterns of family behavior characteristic of your family as a whole?

As you begin this chapter consider two views of the family: as the context for care and as the focus of care. Use your experience within your own family to examine those situations in which one or the other approach is most appropriate.

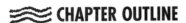 **CHAPTER OUTLINE**

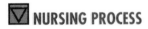
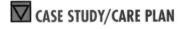
≋ **COMPETENCIES**

Upon completion of this chapter, the reader should be able to:

1. Define differing nursing approaches to working with families.
2. Apply the concepts of family development and family life cycle to assessments of families.
3. Describe Bowen's family theory, and make an assessment of family level of differentiation.
4. Explain structural family theory, and describe the nurse-therapist's role of entering into the family interactions and structure.
5. Use communication theory and the techniques of therapeutic communication to assist families in improving interfamilial communication.
6. Use the NANDA taxonomy to document family nursing diagnoses.
7. Complete family assessments using nursing assessment tools.
8. Use the nursing process to establish a plan of care for families in the psychiatric mental health setting.

〰 KEY TERMS

Circular Communication Predictable pattern of communication and response between two people.

Differentiation Process of unfolding, growth, and maturation, leading to a balance between emotional and intellectual components.

Ecomap Graphic depiction of family members' interactions with systems outside the family.

Emotional Cutoff Children's efforts to distance themselves from their families in order to achieve independence.

Family Social system composed of two or more persons who coexist within the context of some expectations of reciprocal affection, mutual responsibility, and temporal duration.

Family Attachment Diagram Representation of the reciprocal nature and quality of the affectional ties between family members.

Family Projection Process Situation in which adult family members deal with their own anxiety by projecting anxiety onto a child.

Genogram Graphic depiction of a family tree that records information over at least three generations.

Interventive Questions Circular questions used to uncover relationships and connections between individuals, events, ideas, and beliefs.

Multigenerational Transmission Process Situation in which patterns of dealing with anxiety are passed from one generation to the next.

Nuclear Family Emotional System Process by which a family manages anxiety.

Power Influences each family member has on the family processes and functioning.

Relativistic Thinking Process of understanding the contextual nature of the world from multiple perspectives.

Sibling Position Birth order of children.

Societal Regression Process of reversion in which anxiety leads to emotionally based decision making.

Triangulation Relational pattern among three members.

Nurses recognize that psychiatric and/or physical illnesses have great impact on families. The family can be the individual's first source of support and stability or it can become part of the problem that leads to ineffective coping. This chapter will explore the nature of nursing interventions with families, how nurses care for families, the various theories that guide nursing actions, and the interventions used by nurses with families in psychiatric mental health settings. The goals are to provide the reader with the background to give client care within the context of family and homelife and to provide care to the family as a unit, when appropriate.

WHAT IS A FAMILY?

To assess a family, the nurse must determine what constitutes a family. First, there is the family of origin, or the family of one's birth and the family of procreation. Some people think of a mother, father, and their children when they think of family. But in today's world, many different groups might be considered family. One way to decide which individuals make up a family is to limit family to those who live in the same household under the same roof. Another way to determine family is to include the nuclear family of mother, father, and their children, wherever they reside. But what about extended family members, such as grandparents, who may or may not reside in the same household? And what about blended families of couples with children of former marriages? Unmarried couples, gay and lesbian couples, persons living in communes, and other groupings of individuals that may consider themselves to be families?

Traditionally family was defined as relationships of blood, marriage, or adoption. But by the mid-1980s, family nursing moved to incorporate a broader definition believed to be more relevant to the times:

> The **family** is a social system composed of two or more persons who coexist within the context of some expectations of reciprocal affection, mutual responsibility, and temporal duration. The family is characterized by commitment, mutual decision making, and shared goals.
>
> (Department of Family Nursing, Oregon Health Sciences Center, 1985, quoted in Hanson & Boyd, 1996, p. 6)

Given the complexity of families, there is one relatively simple way to decide if a group of persons should be considered a family: Ask family members which individuals make up their family. When the family members agree on this point, the family is designated. In a case of disagreement, the nurse can note the disagreement and include as the designated family the persons who interact most often as the family unit.

Defining Families

Remember that it is the family members, not the nurse, who determine which individuals constitute their family unit. The family is who they say they are!

VIEWS OF THE FAMILY

Nurses have long recognized the importance of the family as a context for a client's illness and care, but an interest in incorporating the family as a unit into care has emerged more recently. The literature suggests that the client of the family nurse may be (Bomar & McNeely, 1996):

◆ The individual as client with the family as context

◆ The entire family unit as client

◆ The family interactional systems of dyads, triads, or other groupings as client

◆ Family aggregates (families sharing similar issues) as client

Figure 27-1 illustrates these four approaches.

Family as Context

In the family-as-context approach, the individual is the focus of care, and the family is part of the environment, serving as a base of support or stress for the client.

This approach to family nursing has had its roots in pediatric and maternal-child nursing (Hanson & Boyd, 1996). The impact and consequences of illness and treatment are considered in light of the family members' needs to adjust and/or adapt to changes. For example, changes in one person's diet will affect cooking and eating behaviors within the family. Further, from this perspective, changes in family structure (an obvious one being the birth of a baby) clearly have an impact on the family life. The nurse will assess the meaning and significance of each event, illness, stressor, or change to the family as a whole and will assist in whatever way possible to help the family make positive adjustments that promote health for each member. For nursing services provided under this framework, the nurse focuses on one family member as the "client" and views the family within the context of affecting the health, treatment, and management of the therapeutic regimen for the client.

Family as Client

In the family-as-client approach, the family itself is considered the focus of care. Here the "family is considered the sum of its individual members, and the focus is on every individual member" (Hanson & Boyd, 1996, p. 25). This approach to families is used often in primary care settings, where each person within the family is assessed for health needs and each client is known and understood in relation to the family group. Family nurse practitioners and family practice physicians commonly

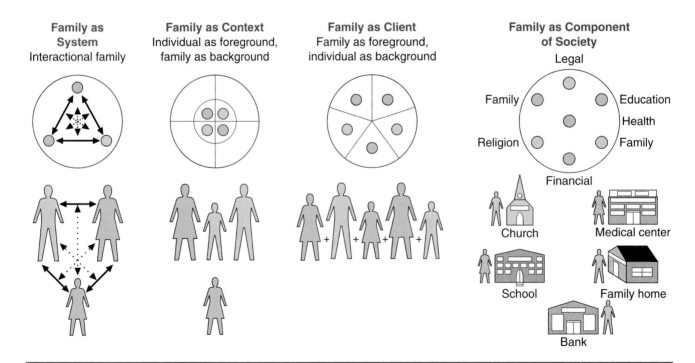

Figure 27-1 **Approaches to Family Nursing.** *From* Family Health Care Nursing: Theory, Practice & Research, *by S. Hanson & S. Boyd, 1996, Philadelphia: FA Davis.*

use this approach, making a clear distinction between care provided in primary care offices and care provided by physician specialists who see only individuals without knowing or assessing the family unit.

Family as System

In the family-as-system approach the family is viewed as more than the sum of its individual parts. If a significant event affects one family member, there is an impact on others. The nurse assesses both the individual members *and* the family group simultaneously. Systems theory suggests that the individuals within a family are emotionally connected such that any important event that affects one family member will have an effect on others as well. According to systems theory, when people are connected to each other in some meaningful way, events will necessitate a change or adjustment in all other parts of the system. It is helpful to think of the family as in balance. A family works to achieve a state of equilibrium. Then, if something happens to one member, the equilibrium is upset and the relationships, supports, and tasks of everyday living need to be readjusted (Frisch & Kelley, 1996). This family systems approach is used in mental health nursing, and the nurse focuses on the significant event, its impact on the individual, and its impact on the family unit. This family systems approach is also frequently used in family therapy.

Family as Component of Society

An emerging view of the family in nursing is to understand the family as a component of society (Hanson & Boyd, 1996). The family is one of many of society's institutions, understood by some to be the basic or primary unit. The family interacts with other social institutions (schools, churches, legal bodies, economic institutions) and either receives or provides communication or services. Social scientists have developed this interpretation of families, and the approach is being used by nurses in the community (Hanson & Boyd, 1996).

APPROACHES TO FAMILY NURSING

While discussions of family nursing suggest that nurses in one setting or specialty use one of the four approaches to family nursing, in mental health practice, psychiatric nurses use all of these perspectives. For example, when providing follow-up care to a client with Bipolar Disorder recently discharged to home, the nurse assesses the impact on the family as a whole of the client's illness, hospitalization, and need to be medicated on lithium. The family is viewed as the context in which continued treatment and management of the condition take place. In another setting or situation, the psychiatric nurse therapist will see a family in therapy as a group, viewing the family as an interactional system. In such a case, the nurse may focus on family interactions and how the family members can support one another to assist each member to meet the needs of the others. When dealing with major societal problems, such as those observed with youth drug addiction and violence, the psychiatric nurse must understand the family as a component of the larger society. Lastly, the family may be understood as the client by the community mental health nurse providing care to one member, understanding that care to each individual family member must be provided for each individual member to maintain health. Table 27-1 provides examples of each of the four approaches used in the psychiatric mental health setting. It is clearly not a situation in which one approach is "better" than another or one approach is more suitable to psychiatric nursing than the other. The nurse must have understanding of each approach to appropriately choose the strategy that will provide the best outcome for each individual situation. Further, the level of nursing education will dictate when the nurse will provide the care and when referral should be made to one with more specialized skill and expertise.

Table 27-1   Four Approaches to Family Nursing in Psychiatric Mental Health Care

APPROACH	USE IN PSYCHIATRIC MENTAL HEALTH	NURSE PREPARATION
Family as context	Individual is client. Management of individual care requires family support. Family needs education and/or explanation.	Undergraduate
Family as client	Each family member is known to the nurse. Care to individuals is part of care to the family unit. Family practice setting.	Nurse in primary care Nurse practitioner
Family as system	Use of therapeutic communication to enhance family communication. Family in therapy.	Undergraduate Graduate
Family as component of society	Family problems viewed from a public health and societal perspective.	Undergraduate and graduate

FAMILY THEORIES

As there are several distinct approaches to nursing of families, there are also several theories of families that influence and guide nursing practice. The following discussion provides background on the major theoretical approaches used in psychiatric nursing care. As will be seen, each theoretical approach provides a framework from which to understand families, and each provides guidance as to the nursing approach that will be most useful for the family unit.

Family Developmental Theory

Nurses are familiar with developmental theory to describe individual growth and development. Duvall's (1979) Family Development Theory is a similar model applied to families and incorporates eight chronological stages that include predictable tasks that families need to master before proceeding to the next stage. The stages are beginning family, child-bearing family, family with preschool children, family with teenagers, family launching young adults, families with middle-aged parents, and family in retirement. Family tasks include such challenges for the beginning family as adjusting to married life to make space for children and for the family with adolescents as shifting parent-child relationships to permit adolescents to move into or out of the family system (see Table 27-2). It is clear that Duvall's stages of family development are based on a traditional family structure and are defined by the ages of children. For use with modern families, other authors have suggested a Family Life Cycle Model that emphasizes typical transitions of most families that are connected to comings and goings of family members and require reorganization of roles and rules within the family (Wright & Leahey, 1994). In the Life Cycle Model, emphasis is placed

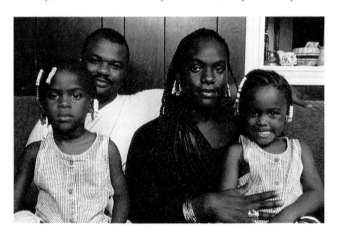

Figure 27-2   Families go through predictable growth stages as members are challenged to adapt to developmental transitions of the family unit combined with changing needs of individual members.

on family resources rather than deficits, on transitions rather than stages, and on the family's ability to integrate both stability and change. Assessment of family development evaluates "patterns of continuity, identity, and stability that can be maintained while new behavioral patterns are changing" (p. 59). Table 27-2 presents work that extends Duvall's theory to include family development for other than traditional families, life-cycle stages for three differing North American family types: (1) the traditional married couple with children; (2) the divorced or postdivorced family; and (3) the remarried couple with children.

Nursing Interpretations Based on Family Development

Assessing a family's stage in the family life cycle process aides the nurse in both identifying the level of anxiety the family might be experiencing and understanding the tasks the family is trying to accomplish. Many times family members are not fully aware of the complexities of the developmental or transitional tasks they face. For example, a new mother who expresses anxiety by wondering why it is so difficult to incorporate her infant into the family, return to work in 6 weeks, keep the house in order, and feel good about her physical appearance may need support that she and her family are facing one of the most difficult transitions for today's young families, that of joining child rearing, new roles of parenting, and meeting financial and household tasks. The nurse may give tremendous support to such a new mother by explaining some of the tasks typically associated with families with infants. Likewise, a couple going through divorce may seek out support from a nurse by asking what to expect of children, how to allay some of their anxiety. The nurse may explain that finding ways to continue effective parenting is difficult for all parents going through divorce and will offer continued support for the custodial parent and child. Thus, similar to using individual developmental theory to understand a person's anxiety going though life challenges, using family developmental theory helps a nurse by giving new dimension and depth to understanding families.

Bowen's Family Theory

Bowen's theory views each family as being within a multigenerational context and suggests that patterns of family interactions tend to repeat themselves over generations (Shepard & Moriarty, 1996). Eight interwoven concepts capture the familial and emotional interaction patterns: differentiation, triangulation, family projection process, multigenerational transmission process, nuclear family emotional system, sibling position, emotional cutoff, and societal regression (Bowen, 1978). Because of the centrality of the differentiation concept, key elements related to differentiation are described. A brief explanation of the other concepts follows.

Table 27-2   Family Life-Cycle Stages and Tasks for Three Types of Family Life Cycles

STAGE	TASK
I. Middle-Class North American Family Life Cycle	
1. Launching the single young adult	a. Differentiating self in relation to family of origin b. Developing intimate peer relationships c. Establishing self in relation to work and financial independence
2. Marriage: the joining of families	a. Establishing couple identity b. Realigning relationships with extended families to include spouse c. Making decisions about parenthood
3. Families with young children	a. Adjusting marital system to make space for child b. Joining in child-rearing, financial, and household tasks c. Realigning relationships with extended family to include parenting and grand-parenting roles
4. Families with adolescents	a. Shifting parent-child relationships to permit adolescents to move into or out of system b. Refocusing on midlife marital and career issues c. Beginning shift toward joint caring for older generation
5. Launching children and moving on	a. Renegotiating marital system as a dyad b. Developing adult-to-adult relationships between grown children and their parents c. Realigning relationships to include in-laws and grown children d. Dealing with disabilities and death of grandparents
6. Families in later life	a. Maintaining own and/or couple functioning and interest in the face of physiological decline: exploration of new familial and social role options b. Making room in the system for the wisdom and experience of the seniors c. Dealing with loss of spouse, siblings, and other peers and preparation for death
II. Divorce and Postdivorce Family Life Cycle	
1. Deciding to divorce	a. Accepting one's own part in the failure of the marriage
2. Planning the breakup of the system	a. Working cooperatively on problems of custody, visitation, and finances b. Dealing with extended family about the divorce
3. Separation	a. Mourning loss of nuclear family b. Restructuring marital and parent-child relationships and finances; adapting to living apart c. Realigning relationships with extended family; staying connected with spouse's extended family
4. Divorce	a. Retrieving hopes, dreams, and expectations from the marriage
Postdivorce: single-parent (custodial)	a. Making flexible visitation arrangements with ex-spouse and his or her family b. Rebuilding own financial resources c. Rebuilding own social network
Postdivorce: single-parent (noncustodial)	a. Finding ways to continue effective parenting relationship with children b. Maintaining financial responsibilities to ex-spouse and children c. Rebuilding own social network
III. Remarried Family Life Cycle	
1. Entering the new relationship; conceptualizing and planning the new marriage and family	a. Recommitting to marriage and to forming a family b. Developing openness and avoiding pseudomutuality in the new relationship c. Planning financial and coparental relationships with ex-spouse d. Planning to help children deal with fears, loyalty conflicts, and membership in two systems e. Realigning relationships with extended family to include new spouse and children f. Planning maintenance of connections for children with extended family of ex-spouse(s)
2. Remarriage and reconstitution of family	a. Restructuring family boundaries to allow for inclusion of new spouse-stepparent b. Realigning relationships and financial arrangements throughout subsystems to permit interweaving of several systems c. Making room for relationships of all children with custodial and noncustodial parents and grandparents d. Sharing memories and histories to enhance stepfamily integration

From *Family Nursing: Theory and Practice* (3rd ed., p. 82–105), by M. Friedman, 1992, Norwalk, CT: Appleton & Lange.

Differentiation is the process of unfolding, growth, and maturation, leading to a balance between emotional and intellectual components. Differentiation is the basis of Bowen's theory, and the goal of therapy is to increase the level of differentiation. A summary of key elements of the concept (Frisch & Kelley, 1996) notes that Bowen views persons as having both an emotional and an intellectual level of functioning. The emotional level is associated with lower brain centers and relates to feelings. The intellectual level is associated with the cerebral cortex or higher brain centers and relates to cognition. Bowen suggests that the emotional and intellectual systems of an individual are connected neurologically and the degree of connectedness varies among persons.

This degree of connectedness between emotional and intellectual systems of a person dramatically affects the person's functioning, especially in social circumstances such as family. The greater the balance between the intellectual process of thinking and the subjective process of feeling (a high differentiation of self), the better the individual (or family) is at managing anxiety, acting in a thoughtful, nonreactive manner, and having intimate relationships while maintaining a separate sense of self. The family whose adult members have a high level of differentiation is flexible in its interactions, seeks to support all members, understands each member as unique, and encourages members to develop differently from one another. Family roles are assigned on the basis of knowledge, skill, and interest.

Low Level of Differentiation

When there is a low level of differentiation, the person (or family) is governed by emotions, acts impulsively, has difficulty delaying gratification, cannot step back and analyze a situation before reacting, and cannot maintain intimate interpersonal relationships. Much like a 2-year-old child (developmentally at a low level of differentiation), the individual cannot give empathy, understanding, or love to another.

A 2-year-old child readily exhibits behaviors and actions consistent with a low level of differentiation. The child lives in the present, knows what he wants, and cannot understand the concept of delayed gratification. The child wants what he wants now! Emotions dominate actions. The child laughs or cries and experiences fear and anger, love and hate, all within a few moments. Intimate interpersonal relationships are not possible because the child cannot give empathy, understanding, or love to another. The child at this age is only able to accept and enjoy the attentions of another.

Young children are not the only individuals who exhibit low levels of differentiation. Many adults have not developed the connections between their emotional and intellectual components. These adults may be functioning well in other aspects of their lives; for example, they may be fully employed and successful in work roles. However, their emotions dominate relationships with others such that they are unable to form intimate relationships. They make decisions impulsively, on the basis of emotions. The adult functioning at this level is not able to step back from a situation and analyze what is happening and instead reacts emotionally to situations. Intense, short-term, often serial relationships are common.

Moderate Level of Differentiation

A person at this stage of development is less dominated by the emotional system. However, emotions dominate much of the person's relationships. Intellectually, the person tends to engage in dualistic thinking. The person views the world in terms of black and white. Things are either good or bad; people are either smart or stupid, loved or rejected. The person may have a closeness to another but finds that in a positive relationship he will "fuse" or enmesh with the other person. The goal of a relationship is to please the other person, and the individual loses himself.

People at this level form relationships, some of which last over periods of years. However, these people find that life becomes rule bound. They do "what is right" and stick to rules, commitments, and decisions. They expect others to do the same, and they are judgmental. Such an individual is unable to see the context of a situation or comprehend that an understanding of the context of a situation could lead to a different understanding of the event. A person at a moderate level of differentiation is unable to "step into another person's shoes" and cannot see the world from another's perspective.

High Level of Differentiation

People at a high level of differentiation have a balance between emotions and intellect. These people express emotions and understand them at the same time. They are able to feel anger and step back from that anger to understand what caused it. These people are able to temper anger by using intellectual functioning. They exhibit **relativistic thinking** and are able to understand the contextual nature of the world. This thinking enables them to understand events from multiple perspectives and to evaluate the circumstances and contexts of events. For individuals at this level of differentiation, the world is not a black-and-white place where decisions are grounded in rules. Decisions are not a matter of rules or a matter of doing what is right or doing what is expected; rather, decisions are made on the basis of the context, the impact, and the outcome. A person at this level of differentiation can form intimate relationships and appreciate the uniqueness of self and of others.

Family Dynamics and Level of Differentiation

Families take on a character that reflects the level of differentiation of the adult family members. Families whose adult members operate at a low level of differentiation exhibit impulsive patterns of interactions. They make decisions without thinking through the effects and consequences. They relate on an emotional level. They often will exhibit spousal abuse and other forms of violence, as they are unable to use intellectual powers to check an emotion as strong as anger. A family whose adult members have developed to a moderate level of differentiation exhibits rigid patterns of interactions. The family is bound by rules and order. Each family member is expected to have defined roles, and the family does not tolerate any variations in expected roles or behaviors.

In contrast, a family whose adult members have developed to a high level of differentiation is flexible in its interactions. The family actively seeks to support all of its members. Because the adults are able to see the world from another person's perspective, the family understands each member as unique and encourages family members to develop differently from one another. Family roles are assigned on the basis of knowledge, skill, and interest. Table 27-3 presents a summary of family patterns according to level of differentiation.

In addition to the concept of differentiation, there are seven major concepts from Bowen's theory. **Triangulation** is a relational pattern among persons. It is an emotional configuration involving three family members. One way of thinking about a triangle is "two people avoiding an issue by pulling in an outside person" (Shealy, 1988, p. 547). While triangles exist in all families, a pattern can be established where two persons avoid dealing with issues and closeness by using the third person to evade stress. For instance, a couple experiencing a stressful relationship may pull in the wife's mother or a child as a third person in the relationship, and the husband may react by withdrawing from his wife and involving himself in his work. Thus, the anxiety is diluted as it shifts to be borne by three instead of two. Because a triangle has much higher tolerance for anxiety than a relationship of two persons, most family relationships operate with triangles. The amount of interaction is usually relatively balanced, and shifts occur to maintain this balance. If one member withdraws, the other two move closer.

⊚ᗡ *REFLECTIVE THINKING*

The Multigenerational Projection Process

It is very difficult for people to believe the simple fact that every persecutor was once a victim. Yet it should be very obvious that someone who was allowed to feel free and strong from childhood does not have the need to humiliate another person (Miller 1983).

The **family projection process** describes the situation where adult family members deal with their own anxiety in relationships by projecting the anxiety onto a child. When this family projection process goes through successive generations, it is called the **multigenerational transmission process**. When the family projection process targets one child, that child is believed to have limited chances of reaching a high level of differentiation. Therefore, this child will likely choose a spouse or partner with a similarly low level of differentiation, and the family patterns will continue across generations.

The **nuclear family emotional system** describes how a family manages anxiety. Besides projecting the anxiety onto a child, the family may manage the anxiety through marital conflict or distance or through dysfunction of a spouse. **Sibling position**, or birth order of children, plays a role in analysis of expected behavioral characteristics based on birth order. When a child did not exhibit predicted behaviors, Bowen would examine if parental anxiety focused on this child. He noted a tendency for siblings in certain positions to assume certain roles and behaviors, such as an older child being responsible and taking on the role of caretaker of the other children, and sometimes taking on the role of adult family members as well.

Emotional cutoff is Bowen's term for the process of children's distancing themselves from their parents in order to become independent. In particular, children caught in

Table 27-3 Level of Differentiation and Family Patterns

PARAMETER	LOW DIFFERENTIATION	MODERATE DIFFERENTIATION	HIGH DIFFERENTIATION
Mode of operation	Emotions dominate relationships	Emotions dominate relationships; intellect plays a role	Emotions and intellect in balance
Anxiety level	High	Moderate	Low
Thought patterns	Live in present; will not think ahead	Dualistic thinking	Relativistic thinking
Family dynamics	Impulsive	Rigid	Flexible

From *Healing Life's Crises: A Guide for Nurses*, by N. Frisch and J. Kelley, 1996, Albany, NY: Delmar.

families with low to moderate levels of differentiation need to cut themselves off in order to achieve any autonomy. Finally, Bowen's concept of **societal regression** is used to describe the process of how intense anxiety leads to emotionally based decisions. In response to increasing and/or chronic anxiety, families' decisions become emotional rather than intellectual. Situations of extreme anxiety, such as during war or severe economic crises, produce such emotionally laden responses in virtually all families.

Nursing Interpretations Based on Bowen's Theory

Assessment of the family level of differentiation is the single most important aspect of understanding family dynamics. If a nurse knows the family's level of differentiation, the nurse also knows how the family thinks, what is important to the family, and how to communicate with the family on an appropriate level.

For example, knowing that a family is at a low level of differentiation, a nurse seeks to develop trust with the family and provide experiences that will help the adults develop cognitive skills to understand their emotions. The literature provides examples of how nurses and therapists help impulsive, violent persons deal with anger, and these are excellent examples of effective ways of dealing with persons with low differentiation. For example, one technique includes having a person keep an "anger journal," wherein the client keeps track of when the anger occurred and what brought it on. The person is taught to identify the anger and accept it as part of living. Further, the person is asked to remove himself from the situation so that escalation of the emotion cannot occur. Both drinking alcohol and driving must be avoided. The person learns to take time out by going for a walk or engaging in some other nonhurtful activity until the anger cools down. Thus, the person learns, in the instance of anger, how intellectual skills (that is, identifying the anger and using a contract to perform some nonhurtful activity) can be used to avoid negative expressions of the emotion. In this process, the person learns one method of using intellectual functioning to balance an emotion. For many clients, this is the first step in moving toward a higher level of differentiation. Here the nurse is working with an individual client using assessment of the family from Bowen's family theory and using the family as the context in which to provide care. Understanding that changes in one family member will affect the rest of the family, the nurse can predict changes in family health and dynamics by working with one family member.

In contrast, a family at a high level of differentiation needs nursing care that facilitates members' own abilities to feel emotions and understand events. The family members have many skills in dealing with their own situations but will often seek nursing care at a time of crisis or when facing a new and difficult task. The family will need help from the nurse, and the nurse recognizes that the adult family members are able to view their situation from one another's perspectives. The nurse may choose to see the family as a unit and focus on facilitating communication and problem solving.

Structural Family Theory

Structural family theory, developed by Minuchin (1974), posits that a family operates as a system such that a family with a dysfunction has some underlying structure that serves to maintain equilibrium in an unhealthy or dysfunctional way. Minuchin (1974) suggests that family structure creates an organization or foundation for the ways in which families interact. Therapy within this framework seeks to change the underlying family organization and structure, thus bringing about change in each family member's position within the group.

From this perspective, a person is seen as a social being, and each person's experience is based on his relationship with others in his environment. Family structures include two systems of constraints: a generic system, involving rules governing family organization, position, and power, and an idiosyncratic system, involving mutual expectations of family members (Minuchin, 1974).

Power has to do with the influences each family member has on the family processes and functioning. Some distribution of power is essential to maintain order. It is assumed that there is a power hierarchy such that parents have different levels of authority than do children. Optimally, parents have a sense of shared power, and children are given power on the basis of their level of maturity and responsibility.

Within a family, each member belongs to a number of subsystems. These subsystems can be formed by generation (parents and children and grandchildren), by sex (male and female family members), by interest (those who play music together), or by function (those who have jobs outside the home and those who do not). These subsystems are related to each other according to rules and patterns. Often, these rules develop in a family over time and are never articulated to family members. These rules can be taken for granted and may be unconscious. Often, it is only when a person outside the family sphere points out that the rules exist and dictate behavior that family members begin to see their own organization and learn that other families may not behave in a similar manner. Part of the nurse's role is to help the family understand its own structure and how its rules can positively or negatively affect its functioning.

Families that are dysfunctional will frequently have a "target" family member—the person with the problem that is causing the family to seek professional help. There may be a young child who cannot behave kindly toward others at preschool, or there may be a depressed teenager. When structural family theory is used as a basis for therapy, the goal of the therapy is to uncover the family structure, that is, its rules and organization, that allows the problem behavior to persist. For example, the preschooler may have learned he has more power within the family if he acts up at school and has to be taken home. The depressed teenager may be reacting to controls that will not allow him to become independent and competent. Only when the family members understand their rules and patterns are they able to make changes. Thus, structural family therapy deals with feedback between circumstances and the person(s) involved.

Different from other forms of therapy, structural family therapy is a therapy of action. The nurse using this approach joins the family in interactions with the goal of changing the family structure. The nurse's work is in the present, in interactions with the family as a whole. When the nurse joins the family system and participates in interactions, the interactions between and among all other family members are altered. Thus, the family members have a chance to experience new circumstances of interactions with each other and to see both themselves and one another in a new light.

Nursing Interpretations Based on Structural Family Theory

To use structural family theory as a therapist, the nurse must be trained as a therapist and will see the family members in sessions together. Advanced practice nurses may use this approach in both inpatient and outpatient psychiatric settings.

However, the theory may help a nurse who is not in an advanced practice role to understand a broader perspective on client problems than what is commonly discussed in many inpatient units. Minuchin (1992) provides an important description of a 10-year-old boy with a diagnosis of Attention-Deficit Disorder. The child had been hospitalized in a child psychiatric unit for 1 year of his life and had been placed on numerous medications. When Minuchin was called in to consult on the case, he received a detailed case history, on which he reflected: "The precision with which the ten people talking with me cover up the narrowness of their point of view impresses me" (p. 4). These professionals were looking at the child as a neurological system, completely devoid of life experiences. Minuchin's beginning approach with the family was to view the child in interaction with his family. Minuchin was the only professional to point out that the child would remain in the hospital as long as his mother could not control him. The problem is the fit between the mother and child, not simply the child. Expanding one's own views of family and "problem family members" will permit nurses to serve as client advocates and may open doors for referrals and services for those receiving nursing care and screening.

By way of example, consider another client situation. A mental health nurse working for the public schools is called because a 10-year-old girl, Gail, is acting out in class. She is not paying attention to her teacher, she is calling out to attract attention to herself, and she is making fun of some of the other children in the class. The nurse making an assessment from a structural family theory approach would first find out what is going on with the child's family and what reasons might explain the current change in the girl's behavior. Talking to the mother, the nurse learns that Gail's younger brother, Tommy, has been diagnosed with leukemia and that the family is experiencing a crisis situation in efforts to come to terms with his illness and to obtain appropriate care for him. Gail's behavior takes on a very different interpretation as the nurse assesses that Gail feels powerless and isolated as the family structure changes to meet the needs of her brother. Using structural family theory, the nurse can help the parents to understand Gail's anxiety and coping. Through a better understanding of the family structure and changes, the nurse, parents, and teacher can help to plan methods of returning power to Gail. The theory provides a means of helping the parents look further to the impact of Tommy's illness on each of them and the family as a whole. These understandings provide insights that assist in coping.

Communication Theory

Many theorists and therapists have focused on communication as the area within families needing attention and correction. Communication theorists have presented the view that verbal and nonverbal communication influence the behaviors of all family members (Shepard & Moriarty, 1996). Internationally known family therapist Virginia Satir intentionally focuses her work on communication. The goal of Satir's family therapy is to improve communication to the point of making all family communication clear, accurate, and meaningful (Satir, 1967).

Watzlawick, a communication theorist, presented four axioms, or rules, of communication that nurses have found useful in assisting communication within families. These axioms are (Watzlawick, Beavin, & Jackson, 1967):

1. All behavior, whether nonverbal or verbal, is communication and conveys a message.

2. All communication defines a relationship.

3. Persons communicate both verbally and nonverbally; the former presents more content whereas the latter informs more about the relationship.

4. All communication is either symmetrical (equality exists and either person is free to take the lead) or complementary (one leads and the other follows).

Satir (1967) emphasized nonverbal communication patterns. She identified roles that family members take on, for example, the placater (the one who fixes every problem), the blamer (the one who accuses others), and the computer (the nonemotional thinking person). She used these roles to help persons see themselves in relationship to others in their family. She identified an important goal for the family therapist as helping family members to see each other, not as bad or mean, but as people whose communications are not always clear.

Nursing Interpretations Based on Communication Theory

Nurses involved with families can use all of the skills of communication theory to help family members learn how to communicate their messages effectively. (Techniques of therapeutic communication are presented in this text in Chapter 5.) These techniques can be used by the nurse in sessions with all family members present to clarify communication, to affirm that messages are being heard and understood, and to provide a role model for effective listening and participation in the communication process. Nurses use these techniques in formal therapy sessions in an office and also in less formal situations such as during a home visit. In each of these cases, the nurse can view the family unit as the client.

Wright and Leahey (1994) provide an adaptation of communication theory to nursing through their work on the Calgary Family Assessment Model and the Calgary Family Intervention Model. They note that there is a pattern of circular communication in most relationships. **Circular communication** is a predictable pattern of communication and response between two people. Because the patterns are repeated again and again, the family members are often unaware of them. The nurse can point them out, resulting in surprise, awareness, and then ability to change. A common negative circular communication is described in the following example: An angry wife is criticizing her husband; the husband's response is to feel anger and to withdraw; the wife becomes angrier and criticizes more; the husband becomes angrier and withdraws further. Each sees the other person as the problem. A nurse pointing out the communication as circular, unending, and negative is able to help the couple see themselves differently and thus make a decision to change.

NURSING PROCESS

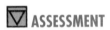 **ASSESSMENT**

Family assessment involves interviewing, observing, and creating diagrams of information for pattern analysis. The nurse must begin with assessment designed to obtain information about the family as well as its individual members. While several assessment tools exist and may be helpful, the Family Assessment Tool is suggested as a means of obtaining detailed information about a family and its members' views of their own strengths and problems. The tool was modified on the basis of the work of several family nursing experts. A brief outline of the Family Assessment Tool is presented in Table 27-4 (the complete version is given at the end of this chapter) and is modified only slightly from the Calgary Family Assessment Model developed by Wright and colleagues.

In addition to recording basic assessment information in narrative form, there are three diagrams that can be used to depict large amounts of information about the families in a graphic form. The three diagrams are the genogram, the attachment or interaction diagram, and the ecomap.

The **genogram** is a graphic depiction of a family tree that records information about family members and their relationships for at least three generations (McGoldrick & Gerson, 1985). There are various ways to construct genograms, and each will provide a tangible illustration of family information. A genogram helps the nurse to keep the whole family in mind as a unit, even if the nurse is

caring for one family member at a time. A genogram can be constructed during the first encounter with a family and can be kept as part of the clinical record.

Inasmuch as families repeat behaviors and patterns across generations, a genogram presents a representation of family patterns. A genogram depicts the family tree, with information on pertinent health history (most notably, major illnesses and cause of death) and social history (births, deaths, marriages, separations, divorces). The information is obtained from the family members themselves, and the genogram can be shared with the family members. Often, patterns emerge that were unnoticed by the family members. For example, in a family where parents and grandparents had a history of multiple separations and divorces, a family may see that there is a tendency toward ending marriage. Other families may have a history of persistent and chronic health problems that create stress and difficulty across generations. Many nurses find that a genogram can be used as a basis for discussion with families and that the information opens up areas for prevention and risk management. Figure 27-3 provides a basic form for a three-generation genogram. The case study at the end of this chapter provides an example of a completed genogram.

A **family attachment diagram** is a representation of the reciprocal nature and quality of the affectional ties between the family members. Some authors suggest that the family interaction pattern symbols be inserted into the genogram (McGoldrick & Gerson, 1985); however, because

Table 27-4 Family Assessment Tool: Brief Version

I. Identifying data

II. Graphic family diagrams
   A. Genogram
   B. Family attachment diagram
   C. Ecomap

III. Family structure
   A. Internal structure
      1. Family composition
      2. Gender
      3. Rank order
      4. Subsystems
      5. Boundaries
      6. Power structure
   B. External structure
      1. Extended family
      2. External systems
   C. Context
      1. Race/ethnicity
      2. Social class
      3. Religion
      4. Environment

IV. Family development/life cycle
   A. Stages
   B. Tasks
   C. Attachments

V. Family function
   A. Instrumental functioning
      1. Activities of daily living
   B. Affective and socialization functioning
      1. Affective
      2. Socialization
   C. Expressive functioning
      1. Emotional communication
      2. Verbal communication
      3. Nonverbal (and paraverbal) communication
      4. Circular communication
      5. Problem solving
      6. Roles
      7. Alliances/coalitions
      8. Influence
         a. Instrumental
         b. Psychological
         c. Corporal
   D. Health care functioning
      1. Beliefs (about health care)
      2. Health practices

From *Nurses and Families: A Guide to Family Assessment and Interventions*, by L. Wright and M. Leahey, 1994, Philadelphia: FA Davis, with minor additions from *Family Nursing: Theory and Practice* (3rd ed.), by Friedman, 1992, Norwalk, CT: Appleton & Lange. Modified with permission.

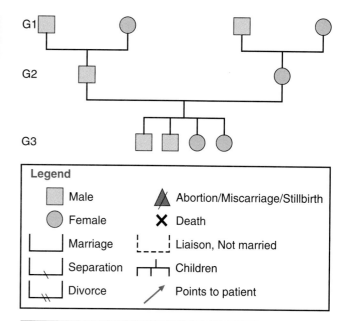

Figure 27-3 Basic Genogram Form

of confusion that can occur when too many symbols are used in a genogram, the attachment diagram is presented separately in this text. Figure 27-4 illustrates the symbols used in such a diagram. The case study at the end of this chapter illustrates the application of a family attachment diagram.

Lastly, the **ecomap** depicts the family members' interactions with systems outside the family. The diagram is similar to the attachment diagram in that it depicts the nature of the family members' relationships with institutions, agencies, and significant people outside the group designated as immediate family. The strength and positive or conflictual nature of relationships with such groups as the extended family, neighbors, friends, work, school, and the health care system are diagrammed.

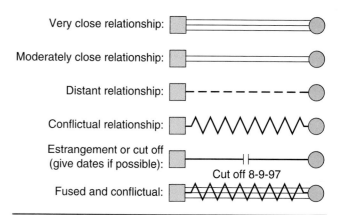

Figure 27-4 Symbols Used in an Attachment Diagram. *From* Genograms in Family Assessment, *by Monica McGoldrick and Randy Gerson. Copyright © 1985 by Monica McGoldrick and Randy Gerson. Reprinted with permission of W.W. Norton & Company, Inc.*

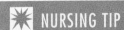 **NURSING TIP**

Family Assessment

Keep in mind that family assessment is also in a sense family intervention, as the assessment process requires communication and information gathering from different family members.

In construction of an ecomap, the immediate family is put in a center circle. The significant individuals, organizations, or agencies with which the family members interact are put in circles surrounding the center circle. The nature of the relationship between the family member and the outer circle is represented by straight lines (strong communication), number of lines (more lines indicate a stronger relationship), dotted lines (tenuous connection), and zig-zag lines (stressful connection). Further, arrows may be placed on the lines to indicate flow of energy and resources. Figure 27-5 depicts the symbols and form used in an ecomap. See the case study at the end of the chapter for an illustration of the application of an ecomap in family assessment.

In addition to their value in family assessment, the

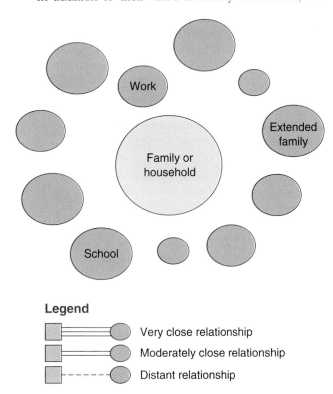

Figure 27-5   Symbols and Form Used in a Family Ecomap. *From Hartman, A.* Finding Families: An Ecological Approach to Family Assessment and Adoption. *Copyright © 1979 by Sage Publications. Reprinted by permission of Sage Publications.*

construction of the diagrams serves as an intervention with the family. When the nurse shares the diagrams with the family members, new insights are drawn as patterns are noted.

 NURSING DIAGNOSIS

In work with families, the NANDA taxonomy of nursing diagnoses provides a language to identify nursing concerns regarding the family unit. There are diagnoses specifically dealing with the family unit, and through the development of axes to the existing diagnoses, there is opportunity to identify any diagnosis as pertaining to the family as a whole. (Chapter 4 of this text provides a detailed description of the NANDA diagnoses.)

There are diagnoses specifically pertaining to families; these are related to family processes, family coping, and home maintenance management (NANDA, 1996). Each of these diagnoses may be used to describe the various nursing roles in problem intervention, preventive care, and promotion of wellness. These are used extensively by nurses in psychiatric and community settings who document care under a nursing model. Each will be discussed below, after a brief summary of the trifocal model of nursing diagnoses, which gives language to nursing work in wellness, prevention, and problem intervention.

Trifocal Model

For far too long in the nursing community, nurses assumed that a diagnostic label meant (as in the "medical model") that the nurse was diagnosing a problem situation and providing interventions that would serve to cure or eliminate the problem. The current model of nursing diagnoses is to use diagnostic language to document the full nursing role in client care (Kelley, Frisch, & Avant, 1995). This role includes more than dealing with problems and generally is believed to cover three levels of care: wellness, prevention, and problem intervention. In all cases, the same nursing diagnosis is addressed; the level of care and the level of need are different. Language that describes these nursing roles is presented in Table 27-5. It can be seen that for each level of care the diagnosis remains the same; the level of nursing intervention changes. These terms and the trifocal model are further described in Chapter 4. The trifocal model will be used to discuss each of the family nursing diagnoses.

Family Processes

Family processes is a phrase that refers to family functioning. A family that normally functions well and experiences a crisis or change leading to a disruption of family processes is considered to have *altered family*

Table 27-5 **Language of Nursing Roles**

ROLES	NURSING LANGUAGE
Wellness	Opportunity to enhance family processes
	Opportunity to enhance family nutritional status
Prevention	Risk for altered family processes
	Risk for altered family nutrition
Problem intervention	Altered family processes
	Altered family nutrition

processes (NANDA, 1996). A family with the diagnosis *altered family processes* is unable to meet the physical, emotional, or spiritual needs of its members. This family requires support to find a new adjustment or equilibrium in order to regain its function. Often, a family undergoing a maturational change or experiencing the death of a member or birth of a baby will demonstrate *altered family processes*. A nursing role is to identify with the family when and how the new event or situation affected their typical family functioning and to work with the family in finding a suitable resolution. This diagnosis, however, may be used either to prevent a problem (if there is reason to suspect risk) or (if the family wants) to examine and make changes in how they function.

Typical uses of this diagnosis to illustrate the three nursing roles are given in the following examples:

1. A nurse in a community geriatric day care center is called upon to make home visits to a family. One of the center's clients, Mr. Lawrence, a 68-year-old man with dementia, has just moved in with his daughter and her family. The client has reached a point where he is unable to safely care for himself, and the family believes that the best care could be provided by having him move into their home. The family unit consists of the client's daughter and her husband, their 25-year-old son who lives with his own family 5 miles away, and an 18-year-old daughter living at home and going to school. The wife does not work outside the home and is ready to accept the role of caregiver to her father. The nurse obtains a family history that indicates the family has functioned well in the past and that the family members all view themselves as close and supportive. With this information, the nurse may use the diagnosis of *altered family processes* related to family adjustments dictated by changed living arrangements and the need for Mr. Lawrence to receive care from his daughter. In using this diagnostic statement, the nurse is identifying that the family is facing changes, these changes will put them in a state

of imbalance, and they will have to change many of their family patterns.

2. While talking with a woman who has brought her child in for a school athletic physical, a nurse in a primary care clinic discovers that the family is about to move to another city, about 200 miles away. The family will face changes in jobs (both parents are professionals who have already secured employment in the new location), and all three school-aged children will be in a new elementary school. This nurse may use the diagnosis of *risk for altered family processes* related to the upcoming change and inevitable adjustment to a new living situation.

3. A school nurse is talking with the mother of a 10-year-old with asthma about the child's medications and activity level when the mother states that she is expecting her second child. The mother begins to ask the nurse questions regarding how a new baby in the home may affect her 10-year-old child and also relates that both parents have begun to give some thought to the changes that will occur in their home once the new baby arrives. This nurse uses the diagnosis of *opportunity to enhance family processes* to indicate that there is an opening for her to initiate work with the family to promote wellness and a positive adjustment.

Family Coping

Family coping refers to the family's patterns of interactions that have to do with its ability to provide sufficient and effective support, encouragement, or assistance to its members facing illness or threats to well-being.

Ineffective family coping refers to the situations where the family has insufficient coping patterns to deal with a new challenge. The nurse is usually called in to assist the family because there is a target event (for example, an incidence of spousal abuse) that draws attention to the ineffective family patterns. In situations where the family as a whole, or one of its members, expresses willingness to change their means of interactions, the nurse may use the wellness diagnosis label of *opportunity to enhance family coping*. For example, a situation where one family member states he will seek therapy to assist himself and the family to support one another in a more positive way exhibits an admission that the current coping patterns are not adequate and expresses, both by actions and words, a desire to make changes.

Home Maintenance Management

Home maintenance management refers to the family's ability to independently maintain a safe and growth-promoting immediate environment for its members.

Defining characteristics include the subjective expression from the family for help in the area of home maintenance and objective data of a disorderly home environment, accumulation of dirt and waste, and overtaxed family members who do not have the resources (emotional, physical, or financial) to provide for a safe and supportive home environment.

Community nurses may make this diagnosis when it is clear that a family requires services or supports to maintain a desirable environment. For example, consider a nurse visiting the home of a new mother with a 5-day-old baby who assesses that the mother is undergoing significant postpartum depression. The nurse will first take appropriate steps to see that the mother is evaluated and treated for her condition. Second, the nurse will also assess the home environment and may well observe that the young mother and her family have been unable to meet the basic needs of providing and keeping food in the home, caring for the baby, and maintaining a clean, safe environment. The nurse could make a diagnosis of *impaired home maintenance management* and work with the family to find community resources to assist until the mother and other family members have sufficient resources to maintain the household. In another situation, the same community nurse may visit a young, single mother who is doing well with her new baby—both physically and emotionally—but finds that the new mother is asking the nurse for assistance in organizing and maintaining her apartment now that the baby has arrived. The nurse could make a diagnosis of *opportunity to enhance home maintenance management* while providing care to this mother.

Other Nursing Diagnoses

It is increasingly important for nurses to direct their attention to the ongoing needs of families who become the caregivers of members who, by the nature of their psychiatric illness, are unable to safely care for themselves. *Caregiver role strain* is an identified nursing diagnosis (NANDA, 1996) and is one that may be underutilized in community mental health. One nurse author has documented that families of persons with severe mental illness often live in anguish because of stressors of the caregiving role (Parker, 1993). Nurses should assess for emotional distress, including signs of grief, guilt, anger, powerlessness, and fear. The family providingcare needs to be included as part of the team that is caring for the client. Parker warns that "many families have been deeply wounded by being given the role of caregiver to persons with severe mental illness, without any preparation or support. Mental health providers must redress this wrong" (p. 21). Parker goes on to recommend that families be provided with education regarding the illness of their family member and suggests that family self-help groups are a viable source of support in many communities.

In addition to identifying specific diagnoses addressing families, nurses using nursing diagnoses have suggested that any nursing diagnosis can be used, with the unit of analysis being an individual, family, or community group (Hoskins, 1991; Warren, 1991). The thinking behind this idea is that there could be an introduction of axes into the taxonomy such that the nurse could identify the appropriate unit receiving nursing care (see Chapter 4). Thus, potentially any diagnosis on the NANDA-approved list can be applied to family nursing. For example, diagnoses such as *powerlessness, altered nutrition,* or *decisional conflict* could be made to underscore that the problem the nurse is seeing has to do with underlying familial patterns and/or structures. The nursing role could be to treat individual members of the family with these nursing concerns; however, it is often most appropriate to see the family as a whole and to provide care at the level of the family. Thus, the axis indicating that the diagnosis pertains to the family group along with interventions such as family therapy or communication counseling is an important way to indicate the family nursing role.

▼ OUTCOME IDENTIFICATION

When a nurse diagnoses a family problem, the nurse and family together must define outcomes. Often the family members will simply say, "We don't want to feel so frustrated," or "Things have got to change . . . this family is no fun anymore." Only as the nurse works with the family over time will the nurse and family begin to identify real, achievable outcomes. In the beginning it is enough to state that the family wishes to work with the nurse to effect a change.

Outcomes will be dictated by the theoretical approach. For example, if a nurse were using communication theory to effect change, the outcome would be that the family members would state a change in communication and a new understanding of each other's communications. In another example, if a nurse used Bowen's concept of differentiation, a goal of interventions for a family at a low level of differentiation would be that the family members would learn to step back from problem situations and think or talk about them before reacting emotionally.

▼ PLANNING/INTERVENTIONS

Once assessments have been completed and outcomes identified, the nurse will plan needed care and interventions. Nursing interventions may be directed toward an individual within the context of the family or toward the family as a unit. Current nursing interventions include family therapy on a structural or systems model and family therapy directed at improving communication. Such therapy will be based on the theoretical perspectives previously described.

Nurses who are not functioning as nurse-therapists typically provide interventions in the areas of:

1. Educating and informing families of their illnesses, resources, and treatment regimens and working with members to provide effective management of illness

2. Using techniques of therapeutic communication to assist families to improve their interfamily communication

3. Assisting families to modify their home environment to provide a supportive environment for safety, interaction, and health

4. Serving as case manager and/or resource person to help families obtain services and referrals

These interventions may be considered supportive, in that they assist the family members to make the best adjustments possible to the situations in which they find themselves. These interventions focus on the human response to health problems, the nursing role becoming one of supporting the family's adjustment (Hanson & Boyd, 1996).

A differing approach to family nursing interventions is presented by the Calgary Family Intervention Model (CFIM). This model is based on several theoretical foundations, concepts, and components (Wright & Leahey, 1994) and focuses on "promoting, improving, and/or sustaining effective family functioning in three domains: cognitive, affective and behavioral" (p. 99). Using this model, the nurse begins interventions by determining the predominant domain of family functioning (cognitive, affective, or behavioral) that needs changing. Recommended interventions are selected from two categories: interventive questions (which are a specific form of therapeutic communication) and other interventions.

Interventive questions are circular questions used to uncover the explanations of the problem to understand and discover relationships and connections between individuals, events, ideas, and beliefs (Wright & Leahey, 1994, pp. 101–102). Four types of circular questions are described: difference questions (exploring differences between people, relationships, time, ideas, and belief); behavioral effect questions (exploring the effect of one person's actions on another); hypothetical or future-oriented questions (questions that explore outcomes, the what-if questions); and triadic questions (questions posed to a third person about the relationship between two others). These four types of circular questions can be used to trigger exploration and change in any of the family functional domains. Table 27-6 illustrates examples of circular questions in the domain of family functioning.

ꙮ RESEARCH HIGHLIGHT

Family Therapy versus a Relatives' Group for Schizophrenia

STUDY PROBLEM/PURPOSE

To compare relapse rates for clients receiving family therapy and those receiving relatives' therapy, which excluded the client.

METHODS

A two-year trial of family sessions in the home (including the clients) versus a relatives' group (excluding clients).

FINDINGS

Researchers found that relapse rates for clients whose families were in either group were significantly lower than for clients whose families offered no help. Specifically, the relapse rates for clients in the family therapy group were 33% and for the relatives' group were 36%. Combining these data with results of a previous trial, the researchers report that families who obtained social interventions had a relapse rate of 40%, compared with 75% for those families without social interventions. Researchers noted that family members' critical comments and hostility diminished during the first 9 months of the trial, and family members' overinvolvement also reduced steadily throughout the trial.

IMPLICATIONS

Relatives' groups in conjunction with family sessions in the home are recommended for families whose members are at risk for relapse.

From "A Trial of Family Therapy versus a Relatives' Group for Schizophrenia: Two-Year Follow-Up," by J. Leff, R. N. Berkowitz, N. Shavit, A. Strachan, I. Glass, and C. Vaughn, 1990, *British Journal of Psychiatry, 157*, pp. 571–577.

Table 27-6 Examples of Circular Questions to Invite Change in Family Functioning

DOMAIN OF FAMILY FUNCTIONS	DIFFERENCE	BEHAVIORAL EFFECT	HYPOTHETICAL/ FUTURE-ORIENTED	TRIADIC
	Explores differences between people, relationships, time, ideas, beliefs	Explores connections between the effect of one family member's behavior on another	Explores family options and alternative actions or meanings in the future	Question posed to a third person about the relationship between two other people
COGNITIVE Offer new ideas, opinions, information, education	*To mother*—What is the best advice you have been given about managing your daughter's eating disorder? *To mother*—Who would benefit most from more information?	*To mother*—How do you make sense of your husband's refusal to discuss your daughter's condition?	*To daughter*—What do you think will happen if you begin to believe the prescribed diet will not make you fat?	*To mother*—If your daughter begins to regain her weight, what will your husband think about it?
AFFECTIVE Reduce or increase intense emotions	*To daughter*—Who in the family is most worried about your eating disorder?	*To daughter*—How does your mother show her concern for your health?	*To mother*—If your daughter begins to eat the prescribed diet, what do you think her mood will be? Sad? Mad? Resigned?	*To daughter*—When your dad gets angry with you, how does your mother feel?
BEHAVIORAL Assist to behave differently toward one another	*To mother*—Who in the family is best at getting your daughter to take her medicine?	*To daughter*—What could your father do that would indicate to your mother that he understands her fears?	*To mother*—How long do you think it will take before your husband opens himself to your daughter's need for treatment?	*To daughter*—If your father were willing to share his feelings with your mother, what do you think he would say?

From *Nurses and Families: A Guide to Family Assessment and Interventions*, by L. Wright and M. Leahey, 1994, Philadelphia: FA Davis. Adapted with permission.

Other interventions cited by Wright and Leahey are similar to those described by others; they are interventions aimed at offering support, education, encouragement, and hope. Table 27-7 presents examples of other interventions.

▽ EVALUATION

Evaluation of a nurse's work with any family depends, of course, on the stated outcomes. Families often want to feel better about themselves, about their shared lives. The nurse will not be able to change the family's life circumstances but may significantly change the family's reactions to it.

When terminating with a family because the work of the nurse is accomplished, one means of assisting the family to maintain a new level of functioning is to ask a question about what each will do to maintain the change. Thus, in terminating, the nurse helps the family members to continue their positive work.

Table 27-7 Nursing Interventions with Families

DOMAIN	INTERVENTIONS
Cognitive	Commending family and individual strengths
	Offering information/opinions
	Reframing
	Offering education
	Externalizing the problem
Affective	Validating/normalizing emotional responses
	Drawing forth family support
Behavioral	Encouraging family members as caregivers
	Encouraging respite

Note: Interventions do not pertain to only one domain, but dividing by domains may start the process of thinking through how they can be used.

From *Nurses and Families: A Guide to Family Assessment and Interventions*, by L. Wright and M. Leahey, 1994, Philadelphia: FA Davis. Adapted with permission.

CASE STUDY/CARE PLAN

Caroline Milton is a 20-year-old college student from an affluent family. She attends a small, private college. She has distinguished herself in her academic courses and in tennis, as well as in her role as a campus leader. She is noted for her peacemaking skills and her desire to please. She is soft spoken and quite beautiful, except that she is somewhat thin even for the fashion norm of her age. Caroline and her family are referred to the family nurse by her physician when her mother and the physician determine that there is a strong likelihood that Caroline is developing an eating disorder. At the initial interview, the nurse discovers that the parents believe that Caroline has always been the "perfect child," never causing any trouble, always following the rules, and making the family proud. They cannot understand her desire to lose so much weight, and they worry about her health.

The father, William, is head of a successful business that he inherited from his father, John. The mother, Marie, is very active in various volunteer organizations. The family places high value on serving the community and strictly following the rules of their Protestant religion.

Caroline has become very thin and is still losing weight, and her mother is very concerned about the possibility that Caroline has an eating disorder. The father is less concerned and believes that Caroline is beautiful, even if a bit thin, and that if she would just start eating more of the "right things" she would be fine again. He states that he does not have time to attend family sessions with the nurse at this time of the business year but may attend later.

ASSESSMENT

The Milton family identifies Caroline's eating pattern as the presenting problem.

Genogram

The nuclear family consists of 47-year-old William, his wife, Marie, who is 45 years old, a son, Charles (25 years old), Caroline (20 years old), and another son, David (19 years old). William is the first-born son to survive, following a miscarriage, and has one younger brother. William's father was also an oldest son with one younger brother. Marie is the younger sister of an older brother. Marie's father's first wife died giving birth to a stillborn baby. See Figure 27-6.

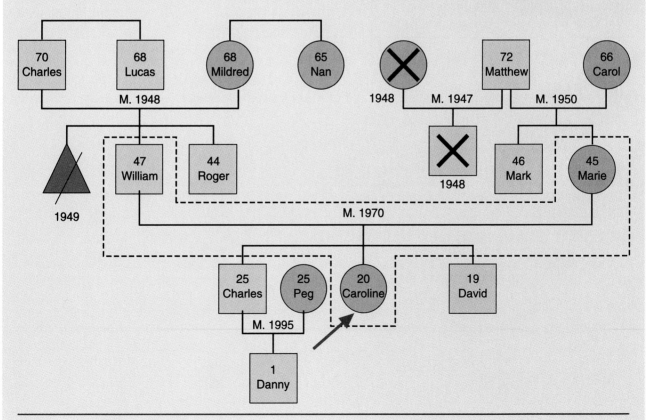

Figure 27-6   Milton Family Genogram

Continued

Family Attachments

The parents describe the home life as "normal" and harmonious. Caroline has two brothers, Charles, who graduated from college with honors and now works with his father, and David, who became rebellious in high school, dropped out of college, and now lives on a commune out West. The parents say that they cannot understand David and guess that he will "come to his senses" someday—soon they hope. While describing the family interactions when David was at home, the family reveal that Caroline would try to make peace between the parents and her brother. The mother would spend much time talking with Caroline about the situation, but the father would become angry with the mother and Caroline, withdraw, and spend more and more time at work and with the older son. Since Caroline has been at college, her father has expressed high expectations for her success, attends many ceremonies, and on occasion takes her to dinner to celebrate. See Figure 27-7.

Ecomap

The ecomap reveals that William is enmeshed with his work, spends time with Marie mostly at business and community social gatherings, and spends time with Charles at work or discussing work-related matters. Marie spends much of her time with her community volunteer efforts as well as with friends shopping and planning events and visiting her parents and inviting them to dinner regularly. She and Caroline have lunch out, or Caroline comes home for dinner and to do her laundry twice a week. Caroline studies many hours and is very involved in a sorority and in her campus leadership activities. She practices tennis daily for one and a half hours, except Sundays. She visits one set of grandparents every 2 weeks, making sure that she distributes her time equally between the couples. She communicates with David through letters and occasional telephone calls and sees Charles and his

wife and baby at her parent's home for occasional dinners. See Figure 27-8.

Interpretation of Family Assessment Data

The Milton family perceives itself to be both a nuclear family and a multigenerational family whose members all reside in the same city, except for David, who has been essentially cut off from the family for over a year. Gender roles have been traditional, with men working outside the home and bearing the financial responsibility for the family and women, although educated, investing their time in volunteer and social activities.

Family Development/Life Cycle

The Milton family is in the "launching of young adults" stage. Marie and William have invested little time in the tasks of the parental life-cycle stage of launching children and moving on as a couple.

Level of Differentiation

The family is at a moderate level of differentiation. There seems to be a suppression of emotion. Emotions, or the suppression thereof, tend to dominate personal relationships. There is evidence of dualistic thinking, and there are rigid patterns of interactions that are bound by rules and order. Neither Charles nor Caroline has differentiated self from the family; David has physically removed himself from the family, and it is not known if he has resolved the emotions and allowed himself to be autonomous emotionally.

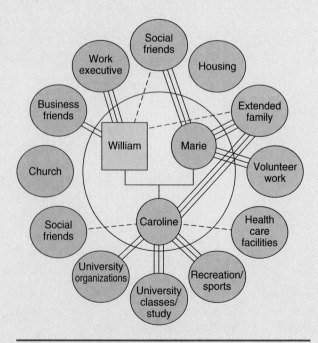

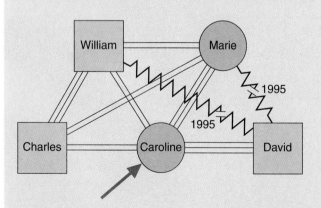

Figure 27-7 Milton Family Attachment Diagram

Figure 27-8 Milton Family Ecomap

NURSING DIAGNOSIS   *Altered family processes*, related to daughter's eating disorder, as evidenced by inability or unwillingness to express feelings

Outcomes	Planning/Interventions	Evaluation
◆ Within 1 month of weekly sessions with the nurse, family members will begin to identify that change in communication patterns would help them to understand each other and deal with Caroline's eating disorder.	◆ Use interventive questions, across each domain, to stimulate reflection. ◆ Encourage the family to participate in therapy as a unit, especially the father, who previously was unwilling to commit time to therapy.	Within 1 month, Marie was beginning to recognize that she had fears related to Caroline's eating and Caroline's becoming an adult that she had not expressed. Caroline expressed ambivalence about being required to spend so much time with her family members rather than her peers. Both women began to see the men in the family as distant and requested that William make the time to become involved in the sessions.

NURSING DIAGNOSIS   *Family coping: potential for growth*, related to goals of self-actualization, as evidenced by Caroline's moving toward a health-promoting lifestyle to optimize wellness

Outcomes	Planning/Interventions	Evaluation
◆ Within 1 month, Caroline will state, with the support of her family, that her eating patterns need attention in order to maximize her health.	◆ Initiate family sessions in which family dynamics and expectations are discussed as related to Caroline's eating habits (e.g., desire to please, desire to succeed, expectations of perfection).	After several weeks, Caroline agrees with her family's assessment that her weight loss is not healthy. She admits to feeling pressure from her family, especially her father, to succeed effortlessly at all she does, including looking good and healthy. She agrees, with her family's help, to begin monitoring her eating patterns in an effort to identify problem areas and behaviors.

Continued

CRITICAL THINKING BAND

ASSESSMENT

What other family issues should be considered as possibly having an impact on Caroline's health and family position? Do you think sibling position is relevant in this case? What about the fact that Caroline is the first female born into her father's family in over three generations? Do you think this fact brings with it certain expectations, given the nature of this family?

NURSING DIAGNOSIS

Why did the nurse choose communication as the priority diagnosis? What would happen if another diagnosis were selected?

Outcomes

How do you know if outcomes selected were appropriate? What would you tell the family if you believed family members could enhance their communication with each other? Are there other ways you could draw attention away from Caroline's eating and on to other issues?

Planning/Interventions

Examine the questions presented in Table 27-6. Provide examples of other interventive questions you might use.

Evaluation

Once the family members have begun to see their own patterns of communication, what do you think the nurse can do to clarify and support each member? Do you think reflective questions are appropriate? Does this approach include collaboration with the family members?

〰 KEY CONCEPTS

◆ Nurses provide care to families using four approaches: (1) viewing the family as the context for care of an individual, (2) viewing the family as a unit, (3) viewing the family as a system, and (4) viewing the family as a component of society.

◆ Family theories give a framework for understanding and interpreting family patterns.

◆ Bowen's theory is founded on the concept of differentiation.

◆ Structural theory emphasizes family rules and organization.

◆ Communication theory stresses family communication patterns and focuses on assisting family members with clear, honest, and open communication.

◆ Family assessment includes evaluation of family patterns and identification of stressors and strengths.

◆ The NANDA nursing diagnoses give the nurse a means of documenting the need for family care under a nursing model.

◆ Nursing interventions with families include providing information/education, serving as facilitator of effective communication, working as a family therapist, providing assessment and referrals to social agencies, and evaluating and treating actual and potential family health problems, enhancing the family functioning when a window of opportunity exists.

◆ Evaluation of outcomes depends on goals set by the nurse and family members. Initially, specific outcomes may not be identified, but over time, the nurse and family should identify specific, measurable goals.

≈ REVIEW QUESTIONS AND ACTIVITIES

1. Provide case examples of nurses' work in the following:
   a. The family as context
   b. The family as a unit
   c. The family as a system
   d. The family as a unit of society

2. Which care settings lend themselves to each of the above (a–d)?

3. Examine a family you know well from the perspective of each of the family theories discussed (Bowen, structural, and communication).

4. Describe a nursing focus with a family having to do with each nursing role: wellness, prevention, and problem identification.

5. Familiarize yourself with family nursing assessment tools by completing one on a family.

6. Complete a genogram, a family attachment diagram, and an ecomap on your own family. Identify patterns.

⚛ EXPLORING THE WEB

◆ Visit this text's "Online Companion™" on the Internet at **http://www.DelmarNursing.com** for further information on family therapy.

◆ Are there specific sites or resources on the Web offering information on family therapy? Are these sites geared toward the health care provider or toward the family?

◆ What organizations can you think of that might offer family counseling information on the Internet: For instance, does Alcoholics Anonymous have a site?

≈ REFERENCES

Bomar, P., & McNeely, G. (1996). Family health nursing role: Past, present and future. In P. Bomar (Ed.), *Nursing and family health promotion* (2nd ed., pp. 3–21). Philadelphia: Saunders.

Bowen, M. (1978). *Family therapy in clinical practice.* New York: Jason Arsonson.

Duvall, E. (1979). *Marriage and family development* (5th ed.). Philadelphia: JB Lippincott.

Friedman, M. (1992). *Family nursing: Theory and practice* (3rd ed.). Norwalk, CT: Appleton & Lange.

Frisch, N., & Kelley, J. (1996). *Healing life's crises, a guide for nurses.* Albany, NY: Delmar.

Hanson, S. M. H. (1996). Family assessment and intervention. In S. M. H. Hanson & S. T. Boyd (Eds.), *Family health care nursing, theory, practice and research* (pp. 147–172). Philadelphia: FA Davis.

Hanson, S. M. H., & Boyd, S. T. (1996). Family nursing: An overview. In S. M. H. Hanson & S. T. Boyd (Eds.), *Family health*

care nursing, theory, practice and research (pp. 4–37). Philadelphia: FA Davis.

Hartman, A. (1979). *Finding Families: An ecological approach to family assessment in adoption.* Thousand Oaks, CA: Sage Publications.

Hoskins, L. M. (1991). What is the focus of Taxonomy II? Nursing diagnosis axes. In R. M. Carroll-Johnson (Ed.), *Classification of nursing diagnoses: Proceedings of the ninth conference* (pp. 35–37). Philadelphia: JB Lippincott.

Kelley, J., Frisch, N., & Avant, K. (1995). A trifocal model of nursing diagnosis: Wellness reinforced. *Nursing Diagnosis, 6,* 123–128.

Leff, J., Berkowitz, R., Shavit, N., Strachan, A., Glass, I., & Vaughn, C. (1990). A trial of family therapy versus a relatives' group for schizophrenia. Two-year follow-up. *British Journal of Psychiatry, 157,* 571–577.

McGoldrick, M., & Gerson, R. (1985). *Genograms in family assessment.* New York: Norton.

Miller, A. (1983). *Unintentional cruelty hurts, too. For your own good: Hidden cruelty in child-rearing and the roots of violence* (pp. 247–253). New York: Farrar, Straus, Giroux.

Minuchin, S. (1974). *Families and family therapy.* Cambridge, MA: Harvard University Press.

Minuchin, S. (1992). *Family healing.* New York: Free Press.

North American Nursing Diagnosis Association (NANDA). (1996). *Nursing diagnoses: Definitions and classification 1997–98.* Philadelphia: Author.

Parker, B. A. (1993). Living with mental illness: The family as caregiver. *Journal of Psychosocial Nursing and Mental Health Services, 31,* 10–21.

Satir, V. (1967). *Conjoint family therapy.* Palo Alto, CA: Science and Behavior Books.

Shealy, A. H. (1988). Family therapy. In C. Beck, R. Rawlins, & S. Williams (Eds.), *Mental health-psychiatric nursing, a holistic life-cycle approach* (pp. 543–557). St. Louis: Mosby.

Shepard, M. P., & Moriarty, H. J. (1996). Family mental health nursing. In S. M. H. Hanson & S. T. Boyd (Eds.), *Family health care nursing, theory, practice and research* (pp. 302–375). Philadelphia: FA Davis.

Warren, J. (1991). Implications of introducing axes into a classification system. In R. M. Carroll-Johnson (Ed.), *Classification of nursing diagnoses: Proceedings of the ninth conference* (pp. 38–44). Philadelphia: JB Lippincott.

Watzlawick, P., Beavin, J., & Jackson, D. (1967). *The pragmatics of human communication.* New York: Norton.

Wright, L., & Leahey, M. (1994). *Nurses and families: A guide to family assessment and interventions.* Philadelphia: FA Davis.

≈ SUGGESTED READINGS

Friedman, M. (1992). *Family nursing: Theory and practice* (3rd ed). Norwalk, CT: Appleton & Lange.

Hanson, S., & Boyd, S. (1996). *Family health care nursing.* Philadelphia: FA Davis.

Mischke-Berkey, K., & Hanson, S. M. H. (1991). *Pocket guide to family assessment and intervention.* St. Louis: Mosby-Year Book.

Wright, L., Watson, W., & Bell, J. (1996). *Beliefs: The heart of healing in families and illness.* New York: Basic Books.

≈ RESOURCE: FAMILY ASSESSMENT TOOL (Complete Version)

I. IDENTIFYING DATA

A. Family name

B. Address, telephone

C. Identified individual client (if any)
   client's presenting problem

D. Family's presenting problem

II. GRAPHIC FAMILY DIAGRAMS

A. Genogram

B. Family attachment diagram

C. Ecomap

III. FAMILY STRUCTURE

A. Internal structure

   1. Family composition (see genogram)

     a. Family type (nuclear, single parent, three generational, etc.)

     b. Who does the family consider to be family?

     c. Changes in family composition. Has anyone recently moved out or in?

   2. Gender
   (questions to ask the family members)

     a. What are expected behaviors for men? For women?

     b. How should a man behave toward a woman?

     c. How should a woman behave toward a man?

     d. Should men express emotion?

     e. Should women be competitive?

     f. What effect has your parents' ideas had on your views about masculinity and femininity?

     g. Would you like your child to believe differently about masculinity and femininity?

   3. Rank order (position of the individual within the family in terms of age and gender) (refer to genogram)

     a. How many siblings do you have? Are you the oldest? Youngest? Middle?

     b. Are you an older/younger sister/brother?

     c. Is your spouse an older/younger sister/ brother?

     d. Are the spouses' birth rank orders likely to be complementary (e.g., older brother, younger sister) or competitive (e.g., older brother, older sister)?

     e. How many children do you have?

     f. Do any patterns appear when the genogram and family attachment diagram are examined for rank order?

   4. Subsystems (refer to family attachment diagram)

     a. Are there any family subgroups with close emotional ties? Subgroups who do activities together?

     b. What do the women do as a group without the men? The men without the women?

     c. How do you feel when a subgroup does things together without you?

   5. Boundaries

     a. Does the family boundary tend to be diffuse, rigid, or permeable?

     b. Are family members enmeshed? Disengaged? Is this true for all members? Only in special situations?

     c. Is there someone outside/inside the family you would talk to if you felt sad or stressed? Happy? Would anyone in the family not like your talking to that person?

   6. Power structure

     a. Who makes decisions within the family?

     b. Who handles family finances?

     c. Who disciplines the children?

     d. Who decides family activities?

     e. In a disagreement, who has the last say?

     f. Are family members satisfied with the present power structure?

     g. On a family power continuum, does the family seem more chaotic (no leader), egalitarian, or dominated by an individual? If dominated, by whom?

B. External structure

   1. Extended family (see genogram, family attachment diagram, and ecomap)

     a. Is the extended family significant to the family's functioning?

     b. Are extended family members available when needed to support the family?

   2. External systems (e.g., work, social agencies, health facilities) (see ecomap)

     a. What relationship is there between the family and external systems?

     b. How regularly do they interact?

     c. Are external systems overinvolved or underinvolved with the family?

     d. If the family is seeking help from an agency, do the family and agency agree on the problem definition and proposed solution?

C. Context

   1. Race/ethnicity

     a. If immigrants, what is the country of origin? Length of time in the U.S.?

     b. Language spoken in the home? In the neighborhood? Level of facility with English?

     c. What is the family's ethnicity (self-identified)?

     d. Does the family live in a neighborhood of the same ethnicity?

e. Is the family's social network of the same ethnicity? Exclusively, or are persons of other ethnicity included, too?

f. How traditional are the family's practices regarding dress, diet, home life? Regarding family roles and power structure? Regarding illness and health care?

g. Does the family have more than one ethnic or racial makeup?

h. What difference can you notice between practices of relatives of different ethnic/racial origins and your own?

2. Social class

a. Into what social class would the family be classified (based on cultural, social, and economic factors)?

b. How does the family classify themselves with respect to social class?

c. Does the family consider their income to be adequate?

d. Does the family receive financial assistance? From what source(s)?

3. Religion

a. Are there obvious signs of religious influence (in the home, on persons)?

b. Do family members identify an affiliation with religious organization(s)?

c. Are religious controversies a source of problems within the family?

d. Who most actively participates in religious activities?

e. Who is considered to be the most spiritual among the family members?

f. Do family members find their spiritual beliefs to be a resource for them?

4. Environment

a. Characteristics of the residence (if assessed)

(1) Is the residence adequate and safe for the family's needs?

(2) How satisfied is the family with their housing arrangements?

b. Characteristics of the neighborhood

(1) Neighborhood type (rural, farm, urban, suburban, inner city, industrial, residential)

(2) Neighborhood condition (cleanliness, age, how well maintained, how safe)

(3) Neighborhood and community demographics

(4) How available and accessible are community agencies and resources?

c. Family/neighborhood interactions

(1) Family's geographic mobility. How long in this neighborhood? This residence?

(2) Does the family have a social support system within the community?

(3) Which family members use what community services or agencies? How frequently? (refer to ecomap)

(4) How satisfied is the family with the community and its resources?

(5) Is the family aware of most community resources?

IV. FAMILY DEVELOPMENT/LIFE CYCLE

A. States

1. What is (are) the present family life-cycle stage(s)?

Designate present family life-cycle stage(s):
Middle-class North American
Divorce and postdivorce
Remarried
Professional
Low income
Adoptive

B. Tasks

1. How well is the family fulfilling developmental tasks appropriate to the present family life-cycle stage?

2. Does the family describe a balance between satisfaction and stress drawn from the developmental tasks?

C. Attachments

1. Does the pattern of attachments (see family attachment diagram) reflect the tasks of the present life-cycle stage?

V. FAMILY FUNCTION

A. Instrumental functioning

1. How well is the family able to carry out routine activities of daily living, such as eating, sleeping, preparing meals?

2. Does a family member's illness affect any of the family's daily activities?

3. Is the family able to meet caregiving needs of an ill family member?

B. Affective and socialization functioning

1. Affective

a. Do family members perceive and respond to the needs of other members?

b. Are family members' needs being met by the family?

c. Do family members provide mutual support and nurturance to each other?

d. Is there a sense of closeness and intimacy among family members?

e. How does the family deal with separateness and connectedness of its members?

2. Socialization

a. Are the family's child-rearing practices appropriate for healthy socialization of the children?

C. Expressive functioning
  1. Emotional communication
   a. Do all family members express a broad range of emotion (e.g., happiness, sadness, anger, affection)?
   b. Does one group (e.g., parents) express an emotion (e.g., anger) while another group (e.g., children) does not?
   c. Are family members' verbal messages congruent with nonverbal messages?
   d. Do family members firmly and clearly express their feelings and needs?
   e. Do family members seek or discourage feedback to their ideas and behaviors?
   f. Do family members listen attentively to one another?
   g. Do members react negatively to messages from other members?
   h. Do members respond on the basis of unclarified assumptions and make judgmental statements?
   i. How are emotional messages communicated within the family?
   j. Are there areas that are closed off for discussion within the family?

  2. Verbal communication
   a. Is there a pattern of direct communication, or are messages displaced onto others?
   b. Are verbal messages clearly stated, or is meaning distorted and masked?

  3. Nonverbal (and paraverbal) communication
   a. Do nonverbal communications match verbal content of messages?
   b. What can be inferred from other family members' nonverbal behaviors when one member is talking?
   c. What effect does the nonverbal behavior of one family member have on another (e.g., sadness expressed nonverbally by daughter to mother's discussion of nearing death)?

  4. Circular communication
   a. Is a pattern of circular communication evident (negative or adaptive)?

  5. Problem solving
   a. Is the family generally able to solve its own problems effectively?
   b. Are problems usually identified by someone within the family or by someone from outside? If within, by whom?
   c. What are the family's solution patterns? From whom is help sought?

  6. Roles
   a. What formal roles are fulfilled by individual family members? By subgroups?
   b. Are these roles acceptable to the family and consistent with family expectations?
   c. How competently do family members fulfill these roles?
   d. Is there flexibility in role performance when needed?
   e. What informal or covert roles exist in the family?
   f. What purpose do these covert roles serve?
   g. Is there a transgenerational pattern of dysfunctional covert roles?
   h. Who were the role models for family members?

7. Alliances/coalitions

   a. Are two-person relationships within the family complementary and symmetrical?

   b. Is there evidence of triangles in the three-person relationships within the family?

   c. Are there cross-generational patterns of coalitions?

8. Influence (instrumental, psychological, corporal)

   a. What objects or privileges, if any, are used to reinforce behaviors (e.g., money, television watching, candy, vacation)?

   b. What psychological methods are used to reinforce behaviors (e.g., praise, approval, criticism, guilt induction)?

   c. Is corporal control used (e.g., hugging, spanking, other forms of physical contact)?

   d. Is the influence method most used by the family consistent? Based on encouragement or punishment?

D. Health care function

  1. Beliefs (about a health problem)

   a. What do the family members believe about the etiology, treatment, and prognosis of a health problem, the role of health care professionals, the role of the family, and the level of control the family has relative to the health problem?

   b. Are the family members' beliefs congruent, or do they disagree?

   c. What does the family believe about the availability and usefulness of resources, medication, and treatment?

   d. What influence does the family believe the health problem has on the family?

   e. What strengths does the family believe it has at present for coping with the health problem?

   f. What concerns does the family have related to its ability to handle the health problem?

  2. Health practices

   a. Are the family's dietary practices healthy for the family members?

   b. Do factors such as finances, knowledge of nutrition and food safety, or cultural practices serve as a source of risk to family dietary practices?

   c. What function do mealtimes serve for the family?

   d. Are family sleep and rest habits meeting family needs?

   e. Are family exercise and recreation patterns adequate and healthy to meet family members' needs?

   f. What is the pattern of drug and substance use in the family?

   g. Does the family encounter unsafe levels of environmental hazards?

   h. Are the family's cleanliness and hygiene practices within the limits of safety?

   i. Do family members practice dental hygiene and preventive care?

   j. What is the three-generational pattern of family health? Are illness or behavior patterns evident?

From *Nurses and Families: A Guide to Family Assessment and Interventions*, by L. Wright and M. Leahey, 1994, Philadelphia: FA Davis. With modifications based on information from Friedman (1992). Adapted with permission.

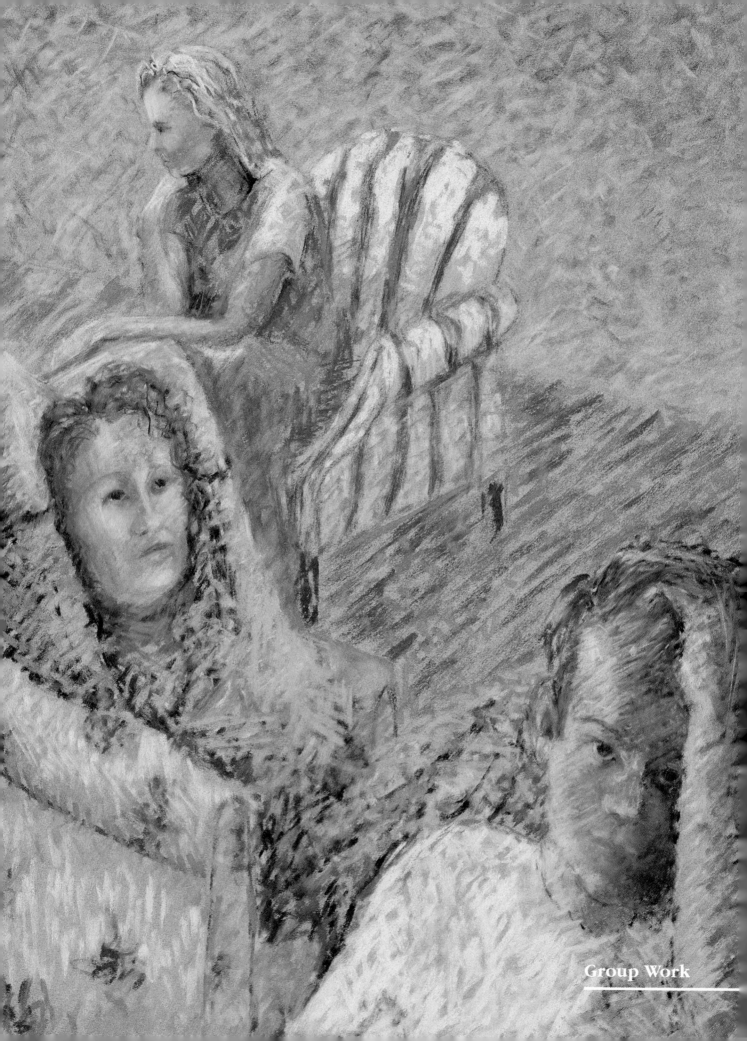

Group Work

Chapter

28

GROUP THERAPY

Noreen Cavan Frisch

Reflections on Groups

Try to remember situations in which:

◆ Other students in a class asked the very question you were thinking about asking.

◆ Someone with whom you were socializing expressed a feeling that was the same as yours, for example, "That movie scared me!"

◆ Another person reached out to you and demonstrated empathy, such as another nurse at work, saying, "You must be tired today because your baby is sick at home. Can I help you with your work?"

How did your feelings about the situation change when you realized that someone else shared the same thoughts as you or empathized with your position?

Consider how you have been helped by persons whose relation to you is that you and they are part of a group—a class, a social group, or a work group. Purposeful use of groups allows a nurse to offer help to clients in a similar way.

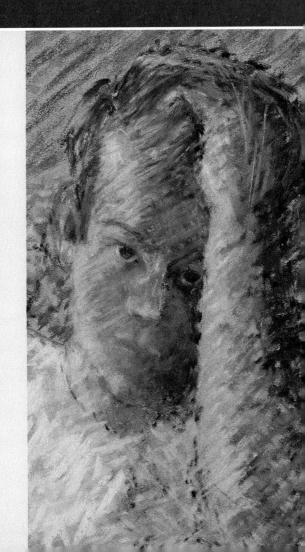

〰️ CHAPTER OUTLINE

GROUPS

PHASES OF GROUP WORK

Orientation Phase

Working Phase

Termination Phase

GROUP DYNAMICS, GROUP CONTENT, AND GROUP PROCESS

Preparation of Group Leaders/Facilitators

Number of Group Leaders

APPROACHES TO THERAPY GROUPS

Psychoanalytic Approach

Interpersonal Groups

Existential Groups

Cognitive-Behavioral Groups

Psychodrama

APPROACHES TO SUPPORTIVE GROUPS

Socialization Groups

Recreation Groups

Educational Groups

Reality Orientation Groups

Reminiscence Groups

Self-Help Groups

NURSING PROCESS

Case Example

Case Example

Case Example

〰️ COMPETENCIES

Upon completion of this chapter, the reader should be able to:

1. Outline the three phases of group work: orientation phase, working phase, and termination phase.
2. Explain the terms *group dynamics*, *group content*, and *group process*.
3. Analyze the dynamics of a group session.
4. Define nursing roles with groups in the psychiatric mental health nursing setting.
5. Explain major theoretical approaches used in group therapy.
6. Explain the nursing role in supportive groups.
7. Compare and contrast different types of groups (socialization, recreation, educational, reality orientation, reminiscence, and self-help) in terms of purpose, nursing interventions, and evaluation.

〰️ KEY TERMS

Closed Group Meeting with a defined number of participants that is not open to new members.

Group Collection of persons who come together in some way that makes them interdependent.

Group Content Specific problems, topics, or conditions addressed by a group.

Group Dynamics Underlying forces working to produce behavior patterns in groups.

Group Leader/Facilitator Person who invites or selects group members and identifies the purpose and goals of the group.

Group Process Interaction (verbal and nonverbal) between and among group members.

Open Group Meeting in which participants are free to come and go, depending on their individual needs.

Self-Help Group Persons coming together who are facing a common difficulty.

Supportive Group Persons coming together to offer support, education, socialization, and/or recreation.

Therapy Group Persons coming together to receive psychotherapy.

In an increasing number of situations, nurses are called upon to work with groups of clients, and in psychiatric mental health care, the nurse has many different roles in the group setting. For example, a nurse may see a group of clients in therapy sessions; facilitate a support group for persons who share a particular problem; plan and carry out recreational activities for a client group that has a need to socialize; or provide patient education information to a client group. The purpose of this chapter is to give the reader descriptive background information on the nature of group work in mental health nursing and to provide knowledge about different types of groups and different approaches to working with a client group. A nurse with knowledge of group process and group dynamics can increase her effectiveness in work with many kinds of clients.

GROUPS

A **group** is a collection of persons who come together in some way that makes them interdependent. A group, therefore, may be a client group who come together for mutual support and therapy once a week or a group of persons admitted to a chemical dependency unit who are a group by nature of being on the unit at the same time. For purposes of this chapter, two types of groups will be discussed: **therapy groups**—groups of persons that come together to receive psychotherapy in a group setting—and **supportive groups**—groups of persons that come together for the primary purpose of offering support, education, and/or socialization/recreation.

The members of a group are usually strangers coming

BENEFITS OF GROUP INTERVENTIONS

Benefits for client:

◆ Able to learn from others' experiences

◆ Able to observe others in social interaction; others are role models

◆ Able to try out new ways of interaction in a supportive environment

◆ Have a place to belong; a group identity

Benefits for the group leader:

◆ Able to serve several clients at once; cost and time effective

◆ Able to provide additional social and supportive interactions to clients

◆ Can draw on strength and ideas of group to arrive at creative solutions

---

together for some purpose. There is a **group leader** or **facilitator**, the person who invites or selects group members according to what the group can accomplish and who helps to identify the purpose and goals of the group. A group is referred to as open or closed. An **open group** is one where participants may come and go, depending on their individual needs. In an open group, participants may come for as many sessions as they perceive they need; these groups are common on inpatient units and as self-help groups. In contrast, a **closed group** begins with a certain number of participants and is not open to new members. Closed groups are often found in outpatient settings and often have a focus on psychotherapy. Some groups are ongoing, that is, they meet indefinitely, while others meet only for a certain period of time.

PHASES OF GROUP WORK

Whatever the kind of group, virtually all groups go through phases of work identical to those described in chapter 5 relating to the nurse-client relationship: the orientation phase, the working phase, and the termination phase (Table 28-1).

Table 28-1 Three Phases of Group Work

PHASES	GROUP TASKS	ROLE OF GROUP LEADER
Orientation	Get to know each other	Help to make members comfortable and feel welcome
	Set out rules and expectations	
	Build cohesion	Ensure expectations are clear
		Set atmosphere of respect and trust
Working	Actively accomplish purposes of the group	Keep group on task
		Support individual members accomplishing goals
Termination	Prepare for separation	Describe how purposes have (or have not) been accomplished
	Help each other plan for the future	Acknowledge contributions of each member
		Acknowledge the group experience

Orientation Phase

In a group, the orientation phase is the time during the initial meetings of the group when the leader/facilitator introduces the reason for bringing the individuals into the group. In the orientation phase the participants begin to get to know each other, and the group members set the stage for the group work that will come later. It is essential in every group that the participants establish a level of trust with one another. Therefore, there are rules of group behavior that must be made explicit at the outset. For example, participants are asked to agree to treat one another in a respectful manner and to try to understand and value each member. Further, participants agree that information shared in the group sessions is confidential, so that no one member need fear that personal disclosure would or could result in gossip or discussion with others outside of the session. Other group rules or expectations may include regular attendance (indicating a commitment to the group), encouragement of verbal expression, and participation of all group members.

The group leader/facilitator has the responsibility to ensure that all members of the group know and agree to the rules of behavior, and this is an essential step in establishing trust. Further, the group leader/facilitator has the responsibility to ensure that all members know and agree to any requirements for payment of fees and such matters as shared responsibility for setting up rooms, putting chairs away, and the like. Sometimes group rules are formalized with a written contract; sometimes a verbal agreement is all that is needed.

The orientation phase is a time of give and take, often a time of testing to see if the group is really accepting, or nonjudgmental, or to see if the group notices and cares about such matters as one participant's absence. Particularly during the orientation phase, participants feel anxiety, and there are frequently long pauses of silence. The group leader/facilitator must permit the silences to occur, allowing the group participants to deal with their own feelings. The leader/facilitator will use techniques of therapeutic communication to draw out members who are silent and withdrawn and to ensure that one or two persons do not take over the entire discussion. The goal for this phase is that the participants develop a sense of belonging to the group. This sense of belonging occurs over time and only when the participants get to know and trust each other. Group members feel a sense of cohesion and a sense of belonging once the orientation phase is complete.

Working Phase

The working phase refers to the time when the participants are actively accomplishing the purposes of the group: They may share their feelings and fears with one another; they may try out new behaviors; they may confront similar problems; and they may point out behavior patterns to one another. The group participants learn to rely on one another for honest feedback, for support, and to be there to listen and care. The leader/facilitator serves to guide the group to achieve its goals by keeping discussions related to group goals, by ensuring that each participant is having his or her needs met, and by serving as a role model for behaviors such as showing respect, listening, responding honestly, and providing nonjudgmental support.

If and when counterproductive behaviors such as ignoring or monopolizing occur, the group leader/facilitator will point out the behavior, explain why it is counterproductive, and let the group participants develop their own skills in working together. For example, if one group member spends all of his time talking and does not permit others to join in or respond, the leader might say, "I notice that you, Howard, have a lot to say tonight, but maybe someone else also has something to say; let's give time for others to speak." In another situation, if one group member has expressed an idea and there is no response, the other group members might go on to a different topic. The leader might say, "Vera expressed a thought a few minutes ago, and I didn't hear a response to her. Let's go back and consider what Vera said." Thus, the working phase of the group provides the participants with a safe place to learn about their behaviors and to achieve their own goals related to the group, which often include trying out new behaviors in a supportive and kind environment.

Termination Phase

Termination of a group occurs when it is a time-limited, closed group and the number of sessions comes to an end or when an open group no longer needs to meet because the purposes have been met. Termination brings about inevitable feelings of change, often including loss or sadness of parting. The group members may want to provide support to one another during parting, and the leader/facilitator can serve as a resource. For many groups, a ritual celebration is an important way to mark the event. This celebration may be as simple as

---

✦ NURSING TIP

Guidelines for Behavior of Group Members

- ◆ Ensure that all statements made in group are confidential.
- ◆ Allow other group members time to speak.
- ◆ Consider the needs of each group member.
- ◆ Provide other group members with your respect and attention.
- ◆ Contribute to the group by sharing your opinions, experiences, and feelings whenever you are comfortable doing so.

bringing food to share with one another during the last meeting or as elaborate as providing each member with a written remembrance of his or her contribution or something that resembles a "graduation" ceremony. Each type of ritual provides a way for members to meet the transition of stepping into a new role. The leader/facilitator may be in a position to help the participants consider alternatives in marking the last group meeting as a significant event in their life and work. The leader/facilitator also helps each participant to see that participation in the group has benefited him or her in some way, by stating how each member has taken a step toward achieving some individual goal in the process of helping one another.

GROUP DYNAMICS, GROUP CONTENT, AND GROUP PROCESS

Group dynamics refers to the underlying forces that work to produce behavior patterns within groups. The group dynamics include both the group content and the group processes. **Group content**, as implied by its name, refers to the specific problems, topics, or conditions addressed by the group as a whole. **Group process** refers to the interaction (verbal and nonverbal) between the group members. Process also refers to all of the factors that contribute to the group purposes. The role taken by each individual and the resultant behaviors in the group are part of the group process. For example, the group leader/facilitator is the person "in charge" of the group. One person may take on the role of being friendly and agreeable within the group; another person may seem unfriendly and may frequently disagree with the group. Or, in a different situation, one person may take on the role of being timid and unable to answer questions; another person may "come to her rescue" and answer questions for her. When a scenario such as the one involving a timid participant is played out in the group, it is the responsibility of the group leader to notice the process and comment on it. For example, the group leader might say, "I notice that Maria seems to answer the questions for Joe. Joe, do you want to answer for yourself?" In doing so, the leader makes explicit the interactions between the two individuals and may challenge the timid person to take on a more active or direct role. The group leader also may comment and respond to the group content; however, it is the group process that brings forward many unconscious and unnoticed means of interaction. Attention to process is the factor most likely to stimulate growth in group participants. Refer to Figure 28-1 for a sample sequence of group dynamics for the first few minutes of a group session.

> ✳ **NURSING TIP**
>
> **Group Management**
>
> In situations where a group seems unproductive, the group leader can redirect the group most readily by making a comment on the group process, for example:
>
> ◆ "We're talking about what was on TV last night, as a group we are not focusing on what brought us here. Let's get back to the topic at hand."
>
> OR
>
> ◆ "I noticed that Tanya has become the spokesperson for the group. She presents opinions and feelings for all our members. Does everyone agree with this direction?"

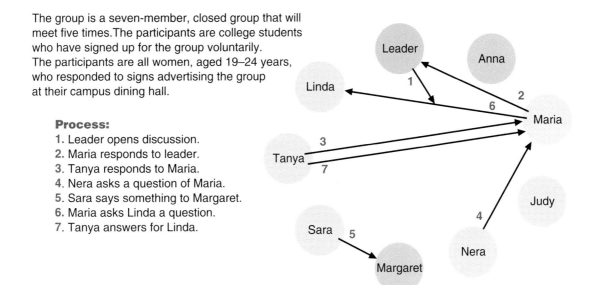

The group is a seven-member, closed group that will meet five times. The participants are college students who have signed up for the group voluntarily. The participants are all women, aged 19–24 years, who responded to signs advertising the group at their campus dining hall.

Process:
1. Leader opens discussion.
2. Maria responds to leader.
3. Tanya responds to Maria.
4. Nera asks a question of Maria.
5. Sara says something to Margaret.
6. Maria asks Linda a question.
7. Tanya answers for Linda.

Figure 28-1 Sample Group Dynamics: Assertiveness Training Group

ROLES GROUP MEMBERS MAY TAKE

◆ Problem solver: one who tries to work through situations and reach a resolution of issues

◆ Controller: one who tries to direct group conversation and activities

◆ Talker: one who talks more than others, frequently dominating discussions

◆ Silent one: one who is shy and retiring, who does not participate (or rarely participates) in discussions

◆ Nay sayer: one who predicts negative outcomes

◆ Supporter: one who attempts to be kind and helpful to all

◆ Intimidator: one who takes over, who scares off others

◆ Devil's advocate: one who finds fault with seemingly everyone and everything

Table 28-2   Nursing Roles in Groups, with Associated Educational Preparation

ROLE	EDUCATIONAL PREPARATION
Nurse therapist	Graduate
Cotherapist	Graduate
Facilitator, socialization or recreation group	Undergraduate
Leader, support group for clients with specific illness, such as breast cancer	Undergraduate, with continuing preparation in group dynamics and the content of the group
Leader, educational group	Undergraduate, with preparation in the content area
Facilitator/resource person to self-help groups	Undergraduate

Preparation of Group Leaders/Facilitators

The educational and experiential background for group leaders will be dictated by the purpose of a group. If the group is a therapy group, using a distinct psychological/psychiatric theoretical approach, the nurse functioning as group therapist will need graduate-level education and experience in group therapy. On the other hand, if the group is primarily an educational group, providing clients with information about medication and assisting them in establishing methods of compliance with medication and food regimens, the nurse will be appropriately prepared at the undergraduate level. If the group is dealing with issues related to recovery from chemical addiction, the nurse will need preparation at the undergraduate level along with extensive continuing education in the areas of drug and alcohol abuse. Table 28-2 provides examples of commonly occurring nursing roles in group settings and suggests the appropriate educational level. It is important to note that the American Nurses Association (ANA) Statement on Scope and Standards of Practice for Psychiatric/Mental Health Clinical Nursing Practice requires that nurses functioning as group therapists be master's-prepared clinical nurse specialists (1994). The ANA guideline is in keeping with the criteria for membership in the American Group Psychotherapy Association (AGPA), which also requires at least a master's level preparation.

Typical personal characteristics of group leaders include being sociable, friendly, and comfortable in small-group situations. Styles of group leaders do vary: Some may be more reflective, others may be more spontaneous and talkative. However, all successful group leaders will have well-developed techniques of therapeutic communication, observation, and listening. Further, successful group leaders will be comfortable with silences.

Number of Group Leaders

In establishing a group, the nurse will consider whether the groups will be led or facilitated by one or two persons. Traditionally, there is always one leader for a group. However, a number of group therapists have suggested there are real benefits of having two leaders (Shaffer & Galinsky, 1989). Two leaders provide a perspective on group process and dynamics from two points of view, and this always adds to the analysis of group activities. Further, there will be fewer interruptions in the actual group session, for if one person is needed away from the session or to provide individual counseling or support, one of the leaders may go and the other can stay with the group. Group participants have the opportunity to observe a collaborative and positive relationship between the two group leaders, and this interaction may serve as the only role model some clients have for adult-to-adult collaboration. At times, when one of the leaders is male and the other female, the ability to relate equally well to group members of both genders becomes easier. A nurse setting up a group, then, will consider the possible benefits of coleaders and may decide to invite another to collaborate.

APPROACHES TO THERAPY GROUPS

There are several theoretical approaches to group therapy currently used in practice. Major approaches will be discussed following.

Psychoanalytic Approach

Psychoanalysis was developed as a therapy for individual clients (see Chapter 26). Only after the development of a kind of systems approach in which any small group could be viewed as a whole could psychoanalytic techniques be applied in a small-group setting. Typically, a therapist using this approach in group work is providing individual therapy to all of the group members and brings the persons together for the group to achieve additional benefits that only a group can provide.

Psychoanalysis is described in Chapter 26 of this text and emphasizes the client's growth through the uncovering of the client's unconscious self and awareness of past experiences. These discoveries provide insight into current patterns and difficulties. Concepts such as *resistance*, *transference*, and *working through* are central to the theory of psychoanalysis. It is expected that the client will exhibit resistance, or opposition, to attempts to draw out unconscious and unrecognized patterns. Transference is the result of the client's either distorting or misperceiving the behaviors of another (typically the therapist), due to unconsciously viewing the therapist as someone from his past. Understanding one's own resistance and transference is central to growth. Working through is the process of taking new insights and using them for change.

Some goals of psychoanalytic therapy are very well achieved in group settings. Some examples are provided by Shaffer and Galinsky (1989):

1. The client may learn that other people can disclose their problems openly and that they gain some relief in doing so.

2. The client learns that he is not alone in having problems and others have similar difficulties.

3. The client may reexperience early family relationships in a setting that is emotionally safe.

4. The client may be able to see and understand his own transferential relationships with both the therapist and other group members.

5. The client may gain more direct and immediate feedback as to the ways in which others perceive his style and defenses than is possible in normal social life or in individual therapy.

Further, the use of group therapy from a psychoanalytic perspective permits the client to wean himself from a prolonged, excessively soul-searching, and sometimes dependent relationship on the therapist that often may occur in individual psychoanalysis (Shaffer & Galinsky, 1989) and allows the client to get on with the business of making life changes and moving effectively back into the world. Thus, the psychoanalytic approach is an effective approach for client groups, particularly when the clients are at a point in their therapy where they can benefit from interactions with others rather than remaining only in individual therapy.

Interpersonal Groups

The interpersonal theory of Sullivan (1953) and the interpersonal psychiatrists forms the basis for working with groups (see Chapter 26). According to this approach, group members examine their interactions. The therapist's goal is to help the client identify interpersonal difficulties and to encourage more successful styles of relating to others. While interpersonal theory can be used in individual therapy, the group setting offers a good context in which to assist the client to develop differing interpersonal styles.

Peplau, the nursing theorist whose work is grounded in interpersonal theory, believed that the closeness of a therapeutic relationship can build trust, empathy, and growth toward healthy behaviors (Belcher & Fish, 1995). Group therapy can provide this kind of therapeutic relationship with others in the group. A positive group experience will put the client in a situation where he is accepted by others and begins to experience satisfying relationships with others. The focus of the group and the therapist is to provide a place where all group members are accepted, where they can interact with one another openly and honestly, where they can identify with others as "belonging," and where they receive honest and constructive feedback regarding relationship styles.

Existential Groups

Based on the work of existential philosophers, an existential approach to therapy emerged in the 1950s and 1960s that shifted attitudes away from a "scientific" approach to human experience (as exemplified in Freudian psychology and causality) toward an approach that emphasized human subjective experience. Existential psychology includes beliefs in the ideas that each person has a need to give meaning to his life, and in so doing there is an inevitable fear of death; each person's unconscious contains forces for courage and creativity as well as for violence and cruelty; and in a therapeutic relationship the therapist and client are more equal than unequal because each has to reconcile the same problems of existence (Shaffer & Galinsky, 1989). The existential approach also requires the therapist to "let the patient be" (Keen, 1970, p. 169), meaning that the therapist accepts all aspects of the client, including the client's freedom to resist treatment.

In nursing, theories of human becoming and human care (Parse, 1996; Watson, 1988) have been clearly influenced by existential thought. These theories emphasize the relationship between nurse and client, strive for mutuality and spontaneity, are grounded in the notions of human care, and attend to the importance of the client's subjective experience of his life.

From an existential perspective, in group therapy the group leader may be seen as the person in the group most experienced in the search to understand the meaning of existence and striving to live a life of authenticity and honesty. The group becomes a place where individuals can experience each other, seek to establish relationships based on equality and mutuality, and explore and ultimately give up self-confirmations based on others' notions of what they should be. The group members provide strong support for all participants who strive to relate to each other from an "authentic" base.

Cognitive-Behavioral Groups

Like a cognitive-behavioral approach to individual therapy (see Chapter 26), a cognitive-behavioral approach to group work is concerned with the thought processes and the behavioral patterns of the clients. Unlike other approaches that focus on the "why" of behavior, this approach focuses on the attitudes. The cognitive-behavioral therapists assume that negative attitudes or negative thinking will result in an interpretation that the world is "bad," and this thinking will result in maladaptive behavior patterns. Believing that if one part of a system changes the other parts of the system will change allows these therapists to reason that changing the negative attitudes and thoughts into positive ones will result in changed behavior and better adjustment (Lonergan, 1994).

An example of this approach is as follows: If a person is depressed, he may spend his whole day thinking that the world is a destructive place and that he should just "give up" and not try to achieve anything. A cognitive approach to therapy would have this man acknowledge his negative thinking, and the therapist would try to help him see how his views are destructive. The therapist might suggest that he consciously stop the negative thinking and put a more positive idea in its place. This would be rather like seeing a glass as half-full instead of seeing it as half-empty. Positive affirmations and making positive statements about self ("I am able to take this test today") represent one technique often used to assist persons to develop a more positive way of thinking. Also a technique of reframing is used to assist a client to reframe an event into its most positive light. For example, "I lost this job, but the next one may be even better" would be a means of reframing a bad situation into a more positive and hopeful one.

Cognitive-behavioral groups work with clients to assist all to monitor negative thoughts, recognize the connections between their thoughts and actions, and substitute reality-based interpretations of life events. Group members gain support from one another as they examine their own attitudes and behaviors and observe others doing the same.

Psychodrama

Psychodrama is a group therapy approach that encourages expression of feelings that underlie personal problems through use of spontaneous, dramatic role-play

(Shaffer & Galinsky, 1989). The dramatic acting out of situations and scenes significant to the client is important in allowing the client to "relive" events, to feel the emotions as if the event were happening once again, but in the psychodrama, the client has the ability to reformulate the problems. The psychodrama functionally puts the client back into the situation, rather than simply encouraging one to talk about the situation. The client uses other members of the group to play roles of persons in the drama. This technique forces the client to "show" other group members how persons in the drama/life situation would respond by taking on various roles to demonstrate. Thus, the client must be able to take on roles of significant persons (boss, mother, father, siblings, etc.) and, for at least a short while, to speak from their perspective and take on their worldview.

The technique originated with the work of Moreno (1970), and the concept has now been in existence for over 25 years. Some psychodrama groups are held in "theaters" expressly designed for this purpose; others are held in more typical group therapy rooms, where the center of the group becomes the "stage."

The emphasis in psychodrama is on the "here and now." If a group member is disturbed about something that happened yesterday or 10 years ago, that situation is brought into the present in a drama, and its impact on the

---

✇ RESEARCH HIGHLIGHT

Groups for Inpatients with Bipolar Disorder

STUDY PROBLEM/PURPOSE

To describe content and process of short-term group therapy for individuals with Bipolar Disorder.

METHODS

The study reports use of content analysis procedures to describe the content and process issues in 40 short-term group psychotherapy sessions attended by 65 inpatients with Bipolar Disorder.

FINDINGS

Five core categories emerged from the content: understanding of the disorder, relating with others, managing daily life, relating with self, and living in society. Guidance, universality, and self-understanding were identified as the group events most significant to the group members.

IMPLICATIONS

Researchers recommend that therapy and education be provided to this population through a topic-oriented group model.

From "Content Analysis of Groups for Inpatients with Bipolar Disorder," by L. E. Pollack, 1993, *Applied Nursing Research, 6,* pp. 19–27.

RESEARCH HIGHLIGHT

Effects of Group Interventions on Cognition and Depression in Nursing Home Residents

STUDY PROBLEM/PURPOSE

To evaluate group techniques on cognition and depression among elderly.

METHODS

Seventy-six depressed nursing home residents who had a mild to moderate cognitive decline participated in one of three groups: cognitive-behavioral group therapy, focused visual imagery (a technique requiring that persons imagine situations, given cues), and education-discussion groups. The group sessions were 24-week, nurse-led meetings based on protocols.

FINDINGS

After the first 8 weeks in group, those subjects in the cognitive-behavioral and the visual imagery groups showed improvement in cognition. There were no observed changes in residents' depression, hopelessness, and measures of life satisfaction.

IMPLICATIONS

The researchers suggest that cognitive-behavioral and visual imagery groups may have positive impact on cognition in this population.

From "Effects of Group Interventions on Cognition and Depression in Nursing Home Residents," by I. L. Abraham, M. M. Neundorfer, and L. J. Currie, 1992, *Nursing Research, 41*, pp. 196–202.

client's here-and-now behavior is explored. The psychodrama is a powerful technique, in that there are no means of hiding behind feelings or leaving emotions unfinished or without closure. The drama puts the client into the situation such that a resolution must be found. The psychodrama occurs within a very supportive environment in which the client may explore past events, relive uncomfortable emotions in a safe, secure, and helpful environment, and try out new means of handling similar situations in the present life.

APPROACHES TO SUPPORTIVE GROUPS

A nurse does not have to be in an advanced practice role to provide care to a client group, for there are many situations where nurses apply the nursing process and give care to a group. Some are discussed below: socialization groups, recreation groups, education groups, reality orientation groups, reminiscence groups, and self-help groups. The reader is encouraged to identify additional situations where a nurse might intervene with a group in

practice settings. The following discussion serves as a guide to the kind of group activities common in psychiatric mental health nursing.

Socialization Groups

For many mental health clients, there is a need for increased socialization and social contacts. Some persons have never developed basic skills of conversation with others; other persons specifically express the need and desire to have friends; some persons are affected by the negative symptoms of schizophrenia and have need for support in social activities. Socialization groups are group activities aimed at providing clients with experiences in social situations and assisting them to learn methods of interaction with others.

Typically, such groups are common on inpatient psychiatric units and in outpatient clinics. A group of persons comes together with a facilitator to interact with one another. The atmosphere in such a group is informal. Often, participants will sit in a lounge (with couches and comfortable chairs) rather than in a room designed for "group therapy." Clients are encouraged to talk about events that happened to them that day, plans for weekend activities, and the like, so that interaction between any given client and others is increased. There is no goal to provide in-depth therapy or analysis: The purpose is to increase interactions and develop social skills. One nurse author emphasizes the use of storytelling as a means to reduce social isolation and promote a connection between individuals (Wenckus, 1994).

Recreation Groups

The recreation group is an extension of the socialization group. The purpose is to plan and experience activities for enjoyment, camaraderie, and socialization. Participants come together with a facilitator to plan activities such as picnics, fishing trips, trips to the movies, and the like, so that a group of otherwise isolated clients who might stay in their rooms is able to participate in a structured activity. Over time, persons who participate in recreation groups develop a repertoire of activities, some of which they find enjoyable. The overall purpose is to introduce clients to activities that they might choose to continue outside of the group and also to encourage movement, interaction, and travel to places within the community.

Educational Groups

Nurses are quite familiar with the need for client education. Whenever a nurse brings a group of clients together who have similar needs for health education, that nurse is engaged with the group as his client. There are two main purposes for providing education in group settings: (1) It is more cost effective to teach a group of people together than it is to provide education on a one-to-one basis, and (2) bringing the group together provides the benefits of universality (each client learns he is not alone and that other people have the same or similar needs and difficulties). Clients may benefit by listening to the questions and concerns raised by other group members. Further, bringing a group of clients together provides them with some socialization with one another, although this may not be the express purpose of the education group.

Reality Orientation Groups

In situations where mental health clients, nursing home residents, or residents of board-and-care facilities are out of touch with reality, the reality orientation group serves to reorient the client to time, place, and season and to provide information of current events of note. These groups are often conducted in inpatient settings in rooms where groups of clients may be gathered for another purpose, such as a day room or dining room. The facilitator of the group will state the place, date, and time to provide basic orientation. Frequently, the facilitator or one of the participants will read from a daily newspaper to orient the group to current events. Participants in the group may be asked to comment on news events. Often, important personal events may be announced, for example, birthdays, anniversaries, visits by family members, and the like. The purpose of such groups is orientation as well as promoting social interaction and involvement in daily activities and current events.

Reminiscence Groups

Groups for the elderly that are specifically aimed at permitting reminiscence or life review are considered helpful when a person is at a developmental stage where he is feeling he has completed his life and has a need to look back over significant events. These groups are particularly effective at encouraging socialization and self-esteem. Strategies used in reminiscence groups include sharing photos of important life events, storytelling around a theme (e.g., "what school was like when I was in eighth grade" or "when I played football"), or describing family gatherings at holiday times. These groups are discussed in Chapter 23 of this text.

Self-Help Groups

The 1990s may well be the age of the self-help group. **Self-help groups** are groups of persons coming together who are facing a common difficulty. They purposefully seek out others so that they may give and receive support with others whose experience is very similar to theirs. Often, persons attending self-help groups explain that others in their lives who do not face their problems

cannot really understand what they are going through. Alcoholics Anonymous (AA) is probably the best known and largest self-help group (see Chapter 15). Other self-help groups include groups for persons who are facing a life-threatening illness, groups for persons with a specific medical diagnosis (e.g., breast cancer), women's support groups, men's support groups, groups for parents of children with particular problems, groups for caregivers of family members requiring physical care in the home, and mother's groups for women with infants and pre-schoolers. These groups may be organized and facilitated by group members; however, in many situations, nurses or other professionals serve as facilitators. In such cases, the nurse may have identified the need for such a supportive group in her community and taken steps to set up the group (i.e., securing a meeting room, helping with publicity, and providing support to those persons who wish to meet in a group). Often, as in the case of a group for women with breast cancer, the nurse will attend the group and serve as a facilitator and resource person to the women coming together for mutual support.

The self-help group is empowering to those who attend, because participants learn they are not alone, and they can provide help to one another. Further, they develop a sense of camaraderie and support, often supplying each other with personal telephone numbers and support outside of the group.

In the age of computer technology, there are several self-help groups emerging "on-line" where persons from around the country can join a discussion group over the Internet (Frisch, 1996). This is a new means of persons' reaching out to learn of others' experiences and provides an increased means of support, particularly to persons who are facing a relatively rare physical health problem or individuals who are homebound. Over time, the number of self-help discussion groups over the Internet will continue to increase. Persons can find such self-help groups through a search engine of the Internet, for example, a Netscape search under the name of a particular illness will usually provide a link to a self-help group, if one exists.

NURSING PROCESS

As in individual psychotherapy (see Chapter 26), a nurse therapist conducting a therapy group does not apply the nursing process per se. The nursing process requires the steps of assessment, analysis and diagnosis, outcome identification, planning/interventions, and evaluation. While a therapist will assess group members and apply strategies to assist clients toward healthful outcomes, a therapist is guided by the psychotherapeutic theory. A therapist's assessment will be in terms of that specific theory and will not lead to a nursing diagnosis. Further, in some approaches to group therapy (the existential group, for example), the therapist will not identify outcomes, but rather will focus the experience in the present. Thus, the nurse functioning as group therapist is in a different role than the nurse applying the nursing process to clients in supportive groups.

In working with supportive groups, the nurse will apply the nursing process, much as in any other area of nursing. The nurse will complete an assessment of needs, and these assessment data of individuals may indicate that a group of persons, known to the nurse, could benefit from group interactions. Areas of need are identified (nursing diagnoses), and target outcomes are established and outlined. Then, planning the group itself is a nursing intervention aimed at meeting a group of clients' individual needs. Assessments and evaluation of individual client outcomes are also important in documenting the nursing role in client care.

The following case examples are presented to illustrate the nursing role in establishing, implementing, and evaluating group interventions, highlighting the emphasis on the supportive group roles that undergraduate-prepared nurses are expected to carry out.

∞ *REFLECTIVE THINKING*

Group Therapy

The nurse has the skills and the license to assess and provide care for clients as a group in many settings. Psychiatric mental health nursing is a specialty where the nurse frequently may combine personal expertise in group process and dynamics, experience in client education, and personal creativity to establish and manage supportive groups. Consider the client population currently under your care. How would you approach assessing the need for group interventions? What benefits can you envision to a group approach to providing care to your client population? How could you initiate group activities? What checkpoints would you outline to monitor the group's progress toward the goals you have established?

CASE EXAMPLE *The Socialization Group on an Inpatient Unit*

Nurse Bob is working on an inpatient psychiatric unit for persons who require hospitalization over a period of 1 month or longer. Most of the clients on the unit carry a DSM-IV diagnosis of Schizophrenia, although others on the unit may be hospitalized for Bipolar Disorder, Major Depression, or other diagnoses.

ASSESSMENT

Bob notices that there are five persons on the unit who rarely leave their rooms unless specifically asked to go somewhere or when told it is time for meals. These clients have a program of activities that includes recreational and occupational activities and individual therapy. Bob believes that each of these persons could benefit from a socialization group.

Bob begins with an assessment of each of the five individuals. May, a 60-year-old woman who has had repeated psychiatric hospitalizations, was admitted to the unit 5 days ago from a board-and-care home because she was hallucinating. May is having her medication evaluated and has been encouraged to participate in unit activities. May, however, spends her time alone. She interacts with Bob on a one-to-one basis and says she has "no one to talk to." Joe is a 25-year-old man who has had a history of paranoid ideations. He has been on the unit for 2 weeks. He is not actively hallucinating now, keeps to himself, but interacts with others who approach him. Sharon is a 30-year-old

housewife who was finding herself unable to carry out daily activities at home. She expresses feeling "depressed" and "tired." She was hospitalized for evaluation of major depression/psychosis. She appears in touch with reality, is withdrawn, and keeps herself isolated from others. Ed is a long-time client in Bob's unit. He is hospitalized frequently for schizophrenia due to noncompliance with medications. Ed was found by neighbors last week wandering in the streets, out of touch with reality, and unable to give his name to his neighbor. He is hospitalized for his own protection and to evaluate his need for medication and supervision upon hospital discharge. Susan is a 40-year-old woman with much the same history as Ed. She is on Bob's unit awaiting placement in a board-and-care home where she will receive supervision.

NURSING DIAGNOSIS

The nursing diagnoses that Bob has identified are *social isolation; impaired social interaction;* and *risk for loneliness.*

OUTCOME IDENTIFICATION

The expected outcome for the group is to increase social contact among the five persons on the unit. Bob will serve as facilitator, bringing the clients together and helping to initiate conversation and discussion.

Continued

PLANNING/INTERVENTIONS

Bob concludes that a structured socialization group would be indicated for all of these five persons. The purpose of the group would be to provide an activity each morning wherein the group participants would be encouraged to interact with each other. Bob has developed a rapport with each client as an individual and believes they would attend a morning session after breakfast at his urging. He explains his assessment and treatment plan at a unit team meeting, and others agree that Bob should set up a one-half-hour socialization group to meet each morning. Bob discusses the group with each individual client and plans to have the first meeting tomorrow.

EVALUATION

Bob will evaluate the degree to which each person in the group increases social contact. He will first observe and evaluate if each person contributes to the group meetings by talking and listening to others. Further, he will observe the clients on the unit outside of the group sessions and evaluate if the number of social contacts increases.

CASE EXAMPLE *The Reality Orientation Group in a Geriatric Day Care Facility*

Two student nurses, Mario and John, are assigned to work each Wednesday morning at a geriatric day care center where frail elderly come for meals, activities, physical therapy, and nursing care. Mario and John have noticed that there are several clients who have trouble remembering the day of the week, and a few have sometimes been confused about where they are. Comments such as "What is the name of this place?" and "Am I at home?" and "Will my daughter be here?" have indicated to Mario and John that at least some of the clients could benefit from daily reality orientation.

ASSESSMENT

Further assessment of the clients indicates to Mario and John that, of 25 clients, at least 15 have had some difficulty with orientation in the past. The average age of the clients at the facility is 78 years, with the range being 64 to 96 years. Mario and John discuss their plans with their nursing instructor and with the day care staff. All agree some form of orientation group is indicated. Mario and John plan for such a daily group and conduct the group themselves on Wednesdays; center staff agree to conduct the group when Mario and John are not there.

NURSING DIAGNOSIS

The nursing diagnosis that Mario and John have identified is *impaired environmental interpretation syndrome:* reality orientation.

OUTCOME IDENTIFICATION

Mario and John expect that with initiation of the orientation sessions each client at the center will show signs of progress in being oriented to person, place, and time every morning; use of the calendar is designed to serve as a reminder to clients throughout the day. Further, their use of a local newspaper should serve to keep participants informed regarding local and national issues.

PLANNING/INTERVENTIONS

The group will meet for a 15-minute session every morning at 10 AM when the clients at the facility have a morning snack. The facilitator of the group introduces himself and gives the month, day, and year and places an X on a large calendar on the wall of the meeting room. Then, the facilitator discusses activities to be done at the center that day. Next, the facilitator reads selected items from a local newspaper, emphasizing current local and national events. The participants are asked to comment on the news items. Discussion may last for up to 10 minutes.

EVALUATION

Mario and John will evaluate the degree to which the clients demonstrate improvement in reality orientation. They will observe how well clients are oriented to person, place, and time. They will listen for client discussion of current events. Further, Mario and John will observe if the clients refer to the calendar on the wall at any time later in the day.

CASE EXAMPLE   *An Educational Group for Parents/Support Persons of Young Adults Diagnosed with Schizophrenia*

Tara is a community mental health care nurse who is making follow-up home visits to clients served by a community outpatient mental health clinic. She identifies six young adults (aged 17 to 25 years) on her caseload who have been diagnosed with schizophrenia within the past 6 months. She understands that management of their illness requires support from family members. Each of these young adults is living with relatives, four with their parents, one with an aunt, and one with his older brother. During a home visit, she identified the person who is serving as the primary support person to each of the clients and plans an educational group to meet once a week for 2 months to provide information to the caregivers/support persons.

ASSESSMENT

Tara assessed that each identified family member requires further information on the disease of schizophrenia, its management, its genetic base, and the meaning of their loved one's living with the illness. Further, each family member requires information on medications used to treat the condition and the role of therapy. All require information on community services and what to do if their family member becomes sick, threatening, or potentially violent. Families have each disclosed to Tara that they live in fear that their family member will go "out of control" and they will not know what to do.

NURSING DIAGNOSIS

The nursing diagnoses Tara is addressing are *knowledge deficit* related to the therapeutic management and support of a family member with schizophrenia, and *risk for caregiver role strain* related to being in a setting of caring and supporting a family member with a chronic psychiatric illness.

OUTCOME IDENTIFICATION

Tara believes that the educational group will not only provide these family members with needed information, it will also serve to let each know he is not alone, will provide a support network for families facing similar difficulties, and will engage the families as an active part of the treatment team who will be caring for these clients in years to come.

PLANNING/INTERVENTIONS

Tara has planned educational sessions to meet once a week for 2 months, covering the topics of the disease of schizophrenia, including what is known about the genetic base of the disease, its pharmacological management, and the meaning of negative symptoms. Further, Tara has planned 15 to 20 minutes at the end of her teaching session for discussion of topics relevant to each family member. Tara also will provide a box where any participant may write down a question and leave it for her to cover in one of the following sessions. She uses this technique to encourage questions one might feel too shy to ask but that are important enough for group discussion.

EVALUATION

Tara will evaluate the success of the group in two ways. First, she will determine through individual contacts with the families if the information provided was understood and is being applied in the home setting. Second, she will observe the level of interaction and support the participants give one another during and after the sessions. She will observe for informal communication and spontaneous discussion of common issues.

KEY CONCEPTS

◆ There are two types of groups with which nurses are involved: therapeutic and supportive.

◆ All groups go through the three phases of relationship: orientation, working, and termination.

◆ Therapy groups are conducted on the basis of identified theoretical frameworks.

◆ Supportive groups are designed to meet specific client needs.

◆ Supportive groups are conducted within the framework of the nursing process.

REVIEW QUESTIONS AND ACTIVITIES

1. Describe the difference between a therapy group and a supportive group.

2. Observe a group therapy session (if at all possible) and document the group dynamics.

3. Identify which of the major approaches to group therapy might be most useful for a specific group of clients you know.

4. Describe how you could set up a supportive group to meet client needs you have identified.

EXPLORING THE WEB

◆ Visit this text's "Online Companion™" on the Internet at **http://www.DelmarNursing.com** for further information on group therapy.

◆ Are there specific sites or resources on the web dealing with groups on socialization, recreation, reality orientation, or reminiscence?

◆ Self-help is always a popular topic. What sites can you locate that are geared toward the health care provider? Toward the client? Toward the family?

≈ REFERENCES

Abraham, I. L., Neundorfer, M. M., & Currie, L. J. (1992). Effects of group interventions on cognition and depression in nursing home residents. *Nursing Research, 41,* 196–202.

American Nurses Association (ANA). (1994). *Statement on scope and standards of practice for psychiatric/mental health clinical nursing practice.* Washington, DC: Author.

Belcher, J., & Fish, L. (1995). Hildegard E. Peplau. In J. George (Ed.), *Nursing theories: The base for professional nursing practice* (4th ed., pp. 49–66). Norwalk, CT: Appleton & Lange.

Frisch, N. (in press). When physical illness becomes a crisis. *Home Health Care Management and Practice, 9,* 56–60.

Keen, E. (1970). *Three faces of being: Toward an existential clinical psychology.* Englewood Cliffs, NJ: Prentice-Hall.

Lonergan, E. C. (1994). Using theories of group therapy. In H. S. Barnard & K. R. MacKenzie (Eds.), *Basics of group psychotherapy* (pp. 189–216). New York: Guillford.

Moreno, J. L. (1970). *Psychodrama* (3rd ed.). New York: Beacon House.

Parse, R. (1996). *Theory of human becoming.* New York: National League for Nursing.

Pollack, L. E. (1993). Content analysis of groups for inpatients with bipolar disorder. *Applied Nursing Research, 6,* 19–27.

Porter, K. (1994). Principles of group therapeutic technique. In H. S. Barnard & K. R. McKenzie (Eds.), *Basics of group psychotherapy* (pp. 100–122). New York: Guillford.

Shaffer, J., & Galinsky, M. D. (1989). *Models of group therapy.* Englewood Cliffs, NJ: Prentice-Hall.

Sullivan, H. S. (1953). *Interpersonal theory of psychiatry.* New York: Norton.

Watson, J. (1988). *Nursing science of human care.* New York: National League for Nursing.

Wenckus, E. M. (1994). Storytelling: Using an ancient art to work with groups. *Journal of Psychosocial Nursing and Mental Health Service, 32,* 30–32.

Wolf, A., & Schwartz, E. K. (1962). *Psychoanalysis in groups.* New York: Grune & Straton.

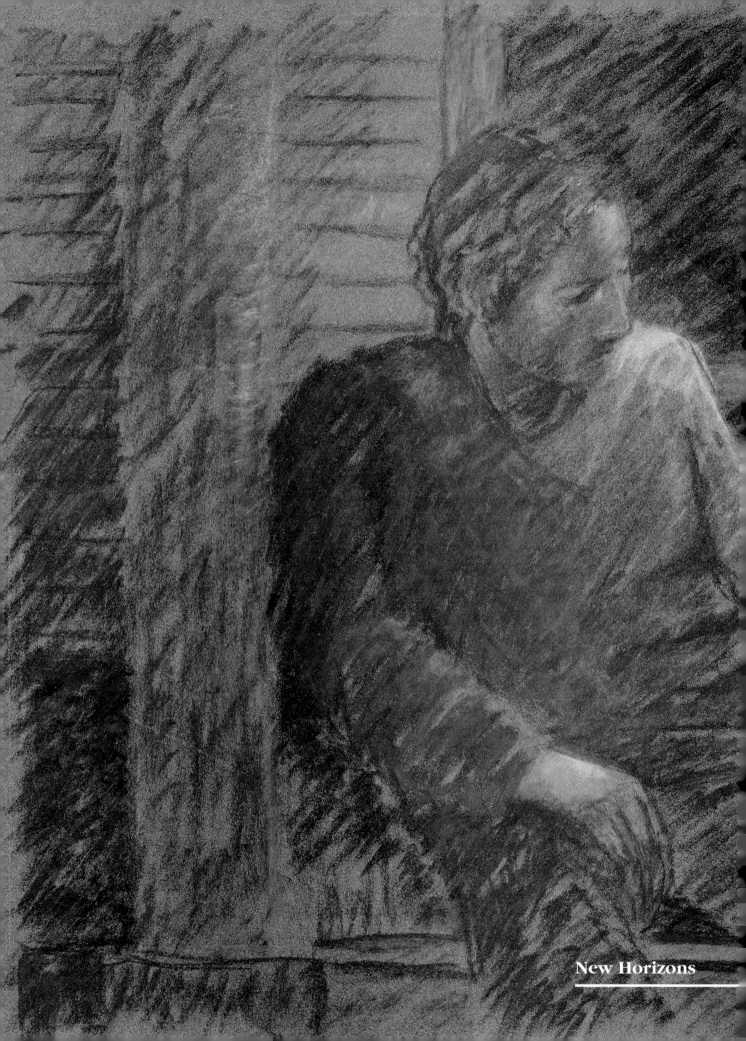

New Horizons

Chapter

29

COMMUNITY MENTAL HEALTH NURSING

Genevieve M. Bartol

Considering Community Health Nursing

◆ What is the relationship between community health nursing, public health nursing, and home health nursing?

◆ How is the focus of mental health care changing?

◆ What is meant by a community-based, population-focused approach to planning, delivering, and evaluating nursing care?

◆ What are the goals of community-based mental health care?

◆ What is the nurse's role in designing, managing, monitoring, and evaluating systems of care that address mental health problems experienced by aggregates (population groups)?

Consider these questions as you read this chapter.

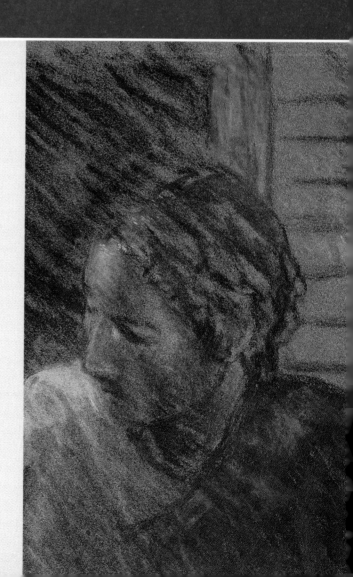

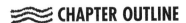 **CHAPTER OUTLINE**

THE CHANGING FOCUS OF CARE

FEDERAL GOVERNMENT IN MENTAL HEALTH CARE

Deinstitutionalization

Case Management

CONSUMER INVOLVEMENT

MODELS FOR COMMUNITY MENTAL HEALTH NURSING

Client-Centered Model

Case Management Model

Capitation and Managed-Care Models

Public Health Model

FUTURE DIRECTIONS

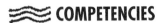 **COMPETENCIES**

Upon completion of this chapter, the reader should be able to:

1. Describe the changing focus of care in the field of mental health.

2. Explain a conceptual framework for nursing practice with aggregates (population groups).

3. Explain selected strategies that can be used to improve the health status of aggregates (population groups).

4. Describe nursing practice with aggregates (population groups).

KEY TERMS

Aggregate Population or defined group.

Capitation Funding mechanism in which all defined services for a specified period of time are provided for an agreed-upon single payment.

Case Management Constellation of services that includes screening, assessment, care planning, arranging for service delivery, monitoring, reassessment, evaluation, and discharge, for the purpose of ensuring continuity of care.

Community Health Nursing Synthesis of nursing and public health practice to promote, maintain, and conserve the health of population aggregates in the community.

Community Mental Health Synthesis of community nursing and public health practice to promote, maintain, and conserve the health of population aggregates in the community, with particular emphasis on mental health.

Community Support System (CSS) Organized network of people committed to helping persons with severe mental illness meet their needs and move toward independence.

Deinstitutionalization Movement of clients and mental health services from state mental hospitals into community settings.

Home Health Nursing Delivery of health services in the home under the direction of a health care agency.

Managed Care Prepaid health plan in which an identified intermediary is given authority to manage the means and the source from which the client may obtain services.

Population Aggregate of persons in the community who share a common characteristic, such as age or diagnosis.

Primary Prevention Activities directed at reducing the incidence of mental disorder within a population.

Program for Assertive Community Treatment (PACT) Model providing a full range of medical, psychosocial, and rehabilitation services by a community-based, multidisciplinary team.

Prospective Payment System Reimbursement mechanism based on predetermined payment for a specific period or diagnosis.

Public Health Nursing Field of nursing that addresses the social, economic, and environmental conditions that influence health.

Secondary Prevention Activities directed at reducing the prevalence of mental disorders by shortening the duration of a sufficient number of established cases.

Tertiary Prevention Activities directed at reducing the residual defects that are associated with mental disorders.

The terms *public health nursing* and *community health nursing* are sometimes used interchangeably. Public health nursing was first used by Lillian Wald in 1893 (Figure 29-1). Wald realized that individual nursing care was not sufficient for the people she served. Clients who lived in squalid conditions and could not buy nourishing food would not get well without proper housing and food. According to Wald, nurses working in the community who addressed social, economic, and environmental conditions that influenced health engaged in **public health nursing** (Bradshaw, 1997).

By the 1960s many nurses were practicing in the community but not necessarily practicing public health. The term *community health nursing* was coined to describe nurses who practice in community settings. Over time, community health nursing was viewed by some nurses as a broad term that applies to all nurses working in community settings. Some nurses insist that public health nursing does not fit under the umbrella of community health nursing. **Community health nursing** is defined by this author as the synthesis of nursing and public health practice to promote, maintain, and conserve the health of population aggregates in the community. **Population** refers to an aggregate of persons in the community who share a common characteristic, such as age or a diagnostic category. **Aggregate** refers to a population or defined group.

Still, the debate about the proper use of these terms continues today and is further confounded by the advent of home health nursing. **Home health nursing** refers to the delivery of health services in the home under the direction of a health care agency. Home health services are an outgrowth of shortened hospital stays in an era of cost containment. Sometimes hospitals establish home health programs to quickly move clients from hospitals to the community. Some psychiatric nurses engaged in private practice provide home health services. Private home care agencies are also beginning to serve psychiatric clients. Psychiatric home care, which may include help with housework and companionship, is considered a major factor in maintaining clients in the home (Morris, 1996). The use of these terms is not simply a semantic question but may well shape the role of nurses in health care (Bradshaw, 1997). In this chapter, **community mental health** is viewed as a synthesis of community health nursing and public health with particular emphasis on mental health (though not to the exclusion of physical health).

THE CHANGING FOCUS OF CARE

Before 1840 people who were mentally ill were generally placed in prisons, asylums, and county homes. Only the wealthy could afford the luxury of a private hospital. The purpose for placement in any of these settings was to protect the ill person from harming others or being harmed, neither of which was ensured by the arrangement.

In 1841, Dorothea Dix, a former school teacher who was distressed by the poor care given to the mentally ill, personally crusaded for enlightened treatment. Dix insisted that each state assume responsibility for its own mentally ill residents. Her efforts led to the establishment of 32 state mental hospitals throughout the United States. Most of the hospitals were built in rural areas, where the environment was considered healthful and clients could be removed from the communities who feared them. Consequently, the people who entered the state psychiatric hospitals left their communities at the door and were often forgotten by those they left behind (Stanhope & Lancaster, 1996).

By 1900 the state hospitals were overcrowded and understaffed. The construction of new hospitals had not kept pace with the growing population. Once again concern arose as the conditions in state hospitals deteriorated. Adolf Meyers took up the crusade initiated by Dix and recommended that clinics for the mentally ill be established in communities. Meyers's efforts marked the beginning of the movement of mental health care back to the community (Stanhope & Lancaster, 1996).

The move to the community received a major impetus in 1908 with the publication of Clifford Beers's book *A Mind That Found Itself.* In this book, Beers graphically describes his experiences as a client in a psychiatric hospital and advocates for better treatment for the mentally ill. He is credited with the establishment of the Connecticut Society for Mental Hygiene, whose purpose was to educate the public about mental illness. In 1909, the National Committee for Mental Hygiene was founded. Within the next 10 years, 19 state mental hygiene societies were formed (Stanhope & Lancaster, 1996). Consumer interest in mental health steadily increased thereafter.

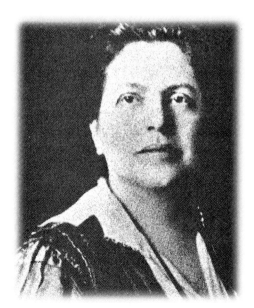

Figure 29-1   Lillian D. Wald. *Courtesy American Nurses Association.*

FEDERAL GOVERNMENT IN MENTAL HEALTH CARE

The shift in responsibility for mental illness from states to the federal government began with the passage of the Social Security Act in 1935. This change was based on the concept that if local communities could not effectively care for their ill members, the federal government should take responsibility (Stanhope & Lancaster, 1996).

World War II brought additional attention to the problem of mental illness. Almost 6% of draftees were barred from service because of existing mental illness (Stanhope & Lancaster, 1996). As a nation, we had to acknowledge that mental illness was a major problem.

A significant increase in the government's involvement in mental health followed the war. The National Mental Health Act of 1946 was passed in an attempt to improve care for the growing number of psychiatric patients. The U.S. government awarded grants to the states to develop mental health programs outside state hospitals. Psychiatric units and outpatient psychiatric services were set up in general hospitals. In 1949, the National Institute of Mental Health (NIMH) was established and charged with the responsibility for mental health in the United States (Beers, 1921). Legislation was designed to apply a community health approach to promoting mental health and preventing mental illness. In actuality, the medical model, with its emphasis on individual psychotherapy, remained dominant because adequate funding for community services was not provided with the legislation (Stanhope & Lancaster, 1996).

In 1955, the Joint Commission on Mental Health and Illness was established by Congress to survey the nation's mental health needs and to recommend new approaches to improve mental health care (Stanhope & Lancaster, 1996). This commission, made up of representatives of 36 organizations and agencies selected by NIMH, published their report in 1961. Their historic document, *Action for Mental Health*, emphasized the need for better training for caregivers, early and intensive treatment for the acutely ill, and improvements in education and research of mental illness. President Kennedy appointed a cabinet-level committee to review the report and to make recommendations for federal action. In 1963, Kennedy called for a new approach that would return mentally ill clients to their local communities. The concept of the comprehensive community mental health center was born. Community mental health centers were constructed through the joint efforts of federal and state governments (Stanhope & Lancaster, 1996).

In 1963, Public Law 88-164, the Mental Retardation Facilities and Community Mental Health Centers Construction Act, was passed. This act was designed to provide comprehensive mental health services to all residents in a specific area. The designated service area usually included about 75,000 to 200,000 people and was referred to as a catchment area. Each center was required to provide five essential services to qualify for funding. The

---

SERVICES INCLUDED IN COMPREHENSIVE MENTAL HEALTH CENTERS

ESSENTIAL SERVICES

◆ Inpatient care for patients requiring short-term hospitalization
◆ Partial hospitalization incorporating day and night care
◆ Outpatient treatment
◆ Twenty-four-hour emergency help
◆ Consultation/education for the community

SUGGESTED ADDITIONAL SUPPLEMENTARY SERVICES

◆ Diagnostic services
◆ Vocational counseling
◆ Research
◆ Evaluation

---

five services included inpatient care for clients requiring short-term hospitalization, partial hospitalization incorporating day and night care, outpatient treatment, 24-hour emergency help, and consultation/education for the community. Additional supplementary services, such as diagnostic services, vocational counseling, research, and evaluation were encouraged. Money, based on a declining formula of federal support over a 51-month period, was allocated to the states to launch the centers. The plan did not work where state and/or local funds did not increase sufficiently to compensate for the declining federal support, and the services provided were uneven. Clients in states using this mental health center model again suffered neglect (Stanhope & Lancaster, 1996).

Deinstitutionalization

The movement of clients beginning in the late 1960s toward community care was spurred on by the increased availability of psychotropic medications and the promise of saving money (Bartol, Moon, & Linton, 1994). Many psychiatric hospital beds were eliminated, and clients were returned to families or placed in supervised nursing homes, rest homes, and apartments. This shift of clients and mental health services from state mental hospitals to community settings is referred to as **deinstitutionalization**. It was believed that the mentally ill would be better cared for in their home communities surrounded by those who were not mentally ill. Unfortunately, adequate support services were not in place in many communities, and a decreased quality of life for the mentally ill resulted (Francell, Conn, & Gray, 1988). Clients were often returned to hospitals, stabilized, and discharged again in a cycling pattern (sometimes described as the "revolving door") (Burns & Santos, 1995). Some discharged clients did not return to the hospital and became homeless (Report of the Federal Task Force on Homelessness and Severe Mental Illness, 1992) (see Chapter 20).

In 1974, NIMH began to study the problems resulting from deinstitutionalization. Consumers, family members, and mental health professionals were asked for input about the services needed. The concept of an organized network of people committed to helping persons with severe mental illness meet their needs and move toward independence, known as the **community support system** (CSS), resulted. Returning the mentally ill to large, isolated hospitals was no longer considered a viable option. The CSS concept comprises an entire array of treatment, life-support, and rehabilitation services.

It is the community mental health centers that have the primary responsibility for developing and implementing CSS for their catchment areas. The essential components of CSS include client identification and outreach, mental health treatment, health and dental care, crisis response services, protection and advocacy, rehabilitation, family and community support, peer support, income support, and entitlement and housing (NIMH, 1987). (See Figure 29-2.)

Coordinating Agency

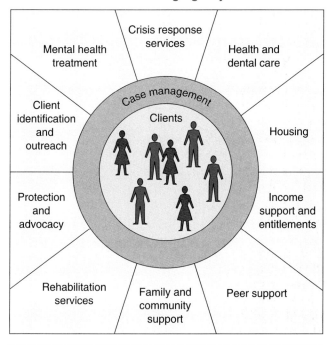

Figure 29-2 Components of a Community Support System (CSS). *From* Toward a Model Plan for a Comprehensive, Community-Based Mental Health System, *by the National Institute of Mental Health, 1987, Rockville, MD: US Public Health Service, Alcohol, Drug Abuse, and Mental Health Administration, Division of Education and Service System Liaison.*

Legislation known as the Amendments of 1975 (Pubic Law 94-63) provided a more stable funding for community mental health centers to develop CSSs. Monies were provided for specialty areas, including child care, aging, court screening, care for discharged clients, transitional services, and substance abuse counseling. Funding was extended in 1977. Legislative mandates and incentives facilitated the movement toward a community-based system of care (Bentley, 1994).

The efforts to improve services for the mentally ill continued despite financial difficulties because of the strong advocacy movements (Bentley, 1994; Donley, 1997). Research, moreover, demonstrated that community-based care was cost effective. The CSS, which includes components of other human services, such as housing support and coordination across the fragmented human service system, was promoted. In 1985, for example, the Robert Wood Johnson Foundation, in collaboration with the U.S. Department of Housing and Urban Development, sponsored a $100 million program for communitywide projects that would consolidate and expand services for the long-term mentally ill. The Social Security Administration (SSA) sent SSA workers into mental health settings to improve the process of determining disability. Health services, social services, and housing and income needs for the mentally ill require coordination and cooperation to provide successful community-based care. The CSS model was viewed as the most appropriate model for caring for the mentally ill in the community (NIMH, 1987). Philosophically, the community is believed to have an abundant source of resources for mental health consumers and their families (Bentley, 1994). The CSS model is designed to help clients assess those resources.

Of course, there are also forces resisting the movement to community-based care (Bentley, 1994). The concern of state hospital employees for their jobs, families' anxiety about long-term care requirements, public fear and discrimination, state and federal battles over authority, and inadequate support services for clients in the community exert significant pressure for a return to inpatient care. Moreover, insurance companies often will provide reimbursement for inpatient services but not for outpatient services.

Case Management

Case management is a constellation of services that includes screening, assessment, care planning, arranging for service delivery, monitoring, reassessment, evaluation, and discharge for the purpose of ensuring continuity of care. As Figure 29-2 shows, case management is integral to the CSS. Case managers, a position often held by nurses, help seriously mentally ill persons build skills and access supports so they can function as independently as possible. Six activities form the core of case management: identification and outreach, assessment, service planning, linkage with needed services, monitoring service delivery, and advocacy. See Table 29-1 for examples of case management activities.

The major goal of case management is to help the mentally ill person remain in the community. Case management services for the seriously mentally ill is the key component of CSS that coordinates all the other services and ensures that needed services are received.

High-quality, general case management programs are effective. The case manager plans and brokers services and advocates on behalf of clients in a community support system as described above. Case managers are mobile and provide crisis services. A single case manager, however, is typically responsible for about 25 to 30 clients. Case managers, therefore, cannot always provide enough individualized help. Some seriously mentally ill clients need the help of a more intensive program, known as the **Program for Assertive Community Treatment (PACT)** (Drake & Burns, 1995). This model provides a full range of medical, psychosocial, and rehabilitation services by a community-based, multidisciplinary team that operates 7 days a week, 24 hours a day and is responsible for only about 10 to 12 clients. The model presumes that bringing care to the client will more effectively develop needed skills and eliminate problems associated with missed appointments. For example, medications could be administered to the patient in a timely manner, which would prevent exacerbation of symptoms. The accompanying display shows the services offered by PACTs.

Table 29-1 Examples of Case Management Activities

ACTIVITY	EXAMPLE
Identification and outreach	Identifying a client who is missing appointments for medication checks and providing additional services to ensure proper treatment
Assessment	Calling the client who missed an appointment to determine why the appointment was missed
Service planning	Holding a care conference for a client who is having difficulty adjusting to a job situation
Linkage with needed services	Making an appointment for a client with a vocational rehabilitation counselor
Monitoring service delivery	Making a follow-up call to find out if the client kept the appointment with the vocational counselor and received help
Advocacy	Speaking to a client's landlord to arrange for necessary repairs

⑤ RESEARCH HIGHLIGHT

Effectiveness of PACT Services

STUDY PROBLEM/PURPOSE

To determine the effectiveness of services for clients admitted to PACTs.

METHODS

Two hundred clients at risk for readmission to psychiatric hospitals were assessed on admission and at 6-month intervals for a total of 18 months. Data were collected on rehospitalization, quality of life, and level of functioning.

FINDINGS

The results showed that rehospitalization was reduced by one-third and the number of inpatient days by 50% after client admission to a PACT. Improvements were progressive and continuous over the 18-month study. Quality-of-life measures as measured by staff also showed progressive improvement. Staff report that clients demonstrated improved family and social support, increased self-reliance and independence, and improved daily living skills.

IMPLICATIONS

Results of the study support the effectiveness of assertive community treatment and suggest that PACTs be widely included in services for persons with serious mental illness.

From "A Multisite Study of Client Outcomes in Assertive Community Treatment," by J. H. McGrew, G. R. Bond, L. Dietsen, M. McKasson, and L. D. Miller, 1995, *Psychiatric Services, 46*(7), pp. 696–701.

◎◎ *REFLECTIVE THINKING*

PACT Services

◆ Which psychiatric clients would most likely benefit from a PACT?

◆ What are the expected benefits for the clients who are enrolled in a PACT?

◆ How can PACT teams be cost effective when they provide such intensive services?

DESCRIPTION OF PACT SERVICES

1. Medication support
   - Order medications from pharmacy.
   - Deliver medications to clients.
   - Educate about medication.
   - Monitor medication compliance and side effects.

2. Rehabilitative approach to daily living skills
   - Do grocery shopping and cooking.
   - Purchase and maintain clothing.
   - Facilitate access to transportation.
   - Foster social and family relationships.
   - Educate about legal rights.

3. Family involvement
   - Provide crisis management.
   - Do counseling and psychoeducation with family and extended family.
   - Coordinate with family service agencies.

4. Work opportunities
   - Give support in finding volunteer and vocational opportunities.
   - Serve as liaison with and educator for employers.
   - Serve as job coach for clients.

5. Entitlement
   - Assist with documentation.
   - Accompany clients to entitlement offices.
   - Manage food stamps.
   - Assist with redetermination of benefits.

6. Health promotion
   - Provide preventive health education.
   - Conduct medical screening.
   - Schedule maintenance visits.
   - Act as liaison for acute medical care.
   - Provide reproductive counseling and sex education.

7. Housing assistance
   - Find suitable shelter.
   - Secure leases and pay rent.
   - Purchase and repair household items.
   - Develop relationships with landlords.
   - Improve housekeeping skills.

8. Financial management
   - Plan budget.
   - Troubleshoot financial problems, e.g., disability payments.
   - Assist with bills.
   - Increase independence in money management.

9. Counseling
   - Encourage problem-solving approach.
   - Facilitate integration into continuous work.
   - Orchestrate goals addressed by all team members.
   - Develop communication skills.
   - Coordinate a comprehensive rehabilitative approach.

Adapted from *Hospital without Walls*, by Duke University Medical Center: Division of Social and Community Psychiatry, Department of Psychiatry, 1993 (Study guide accompanying video *Hospital without Walls*).

CONSUMER INVOLVEMENT

Advocacy for the mentally ill is still needed. As late as 1980 a federal law was passed because mentally ill persons were still found to be subject to abuse and neglect. For example, clients were being unnecessarily secluded or restrained. The Mental Health System Act (MHSA, 1980) adopted into law a Bill of Rights for persons receiving mental health treatment services.

Consumer groups are a primary force in changing mental health care from a provider-driven to a consumer-driven delivery system (Francell et al., 1988). The National Alliance for the Mentally Ill (NAMI) educates, advocates, and lobbies on behalf of primary (current or former clients) and secondary (family members and significant others) consumers. Local chapters of NAMI serve as a forum for members to tell their stories and gain support and advice. As a result, consumers who once felt frustrated and helpless about their particular situations are beginning to recognize their right to information about mental illness and the options for treatment. Consumers are increasingly claiming their right to collaborate with health care providers in planning their care.

Also, NAMI is a major force for legislative changes on a state and national level and for programmatic changes on the local level. Members of NAMI channel their energies into positive, constructive efforts to improve the lot for the mentally ill. For example, NAMI struggles to eliminate stigmatization of the mentally ill by fighting the use of disempowering labels. Through their efforts the terms we use changed from chronically mentally ill to long-term mentally ill and eventually to seriously mentally ill. These

BILL OF RIGHTS FOR CLIENTS

1. The right to appropriate treatment in settings and under conditions most supportive and least restrictive to personal liberty

2. The right to an individualized written treatment plan, periodic review of treatment, and revision of plan

3. The right to ongoing participation in the planning of services and the right to a reasonable explanation of general mental condition, treatment objective, adverse effects of treatment, reasons for treatment, and available alternatives

4. The right to refuse treatment except in an emergency or as permitted by law

5. The right not to participate in experimentation

6. The right to freedom from restraint or seclusion

7. The right to a humane treatment environment

8. The right to confidentiality of records

9. The right to access to records except data provided by third parties or unless access would be detrimental to health

10. The right of access to telephone use, mail, and visitors

11. The right to know these rights

12. The right to initiate grievances when rights are infringed

13. The right to referral when discharged

From Mental Health System Act, 1980, 96th Congress, Public Law 96-398, Section 9501, Amendment to Senate Bill 1177, September 23, 1980.

⑤ RESEARCH HIGHLIGHT

Caregiving Burden

STUDY PROBLEM/PURPOSE

To examine the experiences of siblings of persons with mental illness and the factors contributing to the experience of subjective burden.

METHODS

Survey of a sample of 164 siblings of persons with serious mental illness.

FINDINGS

Findings revealed that the well sibling's experience of burden was consistently related to the symptomatology of the ill sibling. Furthermore, siblings who saw the ill sibling's behavior as outside his or her control exhibited lower levels of subjective burden in comparison to those who viewed the behavior as within the sibling's control.

IMPLICATIONS

The findings of this study suggest that the experience of subjective burden is probably related to the ill sibling's symptoms and not the caregiving demands. The role of siblings as caregivers for their mentally ill sibling will increase as the population ages, so nurses will need to consider this in their plan of care.

From "Factors Associated with Subjective Burden in Siblings of Adults with Severe Mental Illness," by J. S. Greenber, H. W. Kime, and J. R., Greenley, 1997, *American Journal of Orthopsychiatry, 67*(2), pp. 231–240.

changes in wording spawn hope that mental illness, though serious, can be cured and emphasize the view that mental illness is a brain disease for which a definitive cure may be found (Stanhope & Lancaster, 1996).

Consumer empowerment is also a goal of the CSS concept. Therefore, NIMH funds consumer organizing activities. The National Ex-Patient Teleconference and the National Mental Health Consumer Self-Help Clearinghouse and Alternatives, an annual consumer conference, are examples of collaborative projects funded by NIMH and consumer groups. In the past families were often blamed for their members' illness. Now it is recognized that successful community-based care requires united efforts of clients, their families, caregivers, and society (Lefley, 1997; Stanhope & Lancaster, 1996).

Families play a major role in the client's health status. Members of the family movement (e.g., NAMI) advocate for protection, clinical services, and basic research. The health consumer movement emphasizes autonomy for the client. Nevertheless, both groups see optimal autonomy as a therapeutic goal. Evidence suggests that the feelings of emotional burden experienced by family members are directly related to the severity of stressors generated by the ill member. Moreover, it appears that emphasis on autonomy for the client may be the most effective way of relieving the family burden. Research on families of clients with severe mental illness indicates that the caregiving burden can be significant (Lefley, 1997).

Legislation continues to advocate for the mentally ill even when it is not solely directed to the mentally ill. The Americans with Disabilities Act of 1990 (Public Law 101-336), for example, prohibited discrimination based on disability, including mental disability. Haimowitz (1991) notes that such legislation establishes a mandate to bring all persons with disabilities into the social and economic mainstream and may influence the way the community thinks about mentally ill people (Bentley, 1994).

In 1991, NIMH and the National Advisory Mental Health Council (NAMHC) published a national plan of research to improve services for persons with severe mental disorders. The plan represents a systematic review of knowledge about the best ways to provide care for the severely and persistently mentally ill. Gaps in knowledge were identified and important questions formulated. The goal of finding ways to improve the quality of care provided to the mentally ill remains. The task is further complicated by the growing diversity of the population and the need to design culturally sensitive approaches. What works in some instances may not be appropriate in others.

Still, progress is slow and uneven. Deregulation legislation during the Reagan and Bush presidencies reduced federal authority and funding and shifted responsibility for health care back to the states: "Deregulation, price control and competition became the tools of cost reduction" (Donley, 1997, p. 294). Fewer community-based public health programs and clinics served the poor as a result of the decrease in federal regulation and spending. Price control and competition were encouraged, and diagnostic-related grouping (DRG) was devised through amendments to the Social Security Act and the Medicare program (Nunnery, 1997). The DRG is a construct that groups diagnoses into categories that require similar levels of resources. Payment for services is linked to a flat rate for each category. If the costs of treatment exceed the DRG payment allotted in that category, the provider is required to absorb the extra costs. While mental health did not initially come under the threat of DRGs, "the writing was on the wall," and concerns about cost increasingly guided treatment decisions. More attention was also directed to demonstrating the cost effectiveness of specific treatments.

In 1992, a report of the Federal Task Force on Homelessness and Severe Mental Illness noted that one out of every three homeless persons in the United States suffers from a severe mental illness. The task force stated that any successful effort to end homelessness among the seriously mentally ill must be pluralistic. Federal, state, and local governments as well as providers, family members, voluntary organizations, and mental health consumers must take part in the effort. The recommendations of the task force emphasize the need for integration in care delivery systems that serve the mentally ill. Nevertheless, community-based mental health care has been clearly pronounced as a national goal (Bentley, 1994). Even the growth of home health nursing underscores the shift in the locus of care from hospitals to the community.

MODELS FOR COMMUNITY MENTAL HEALTH NURSING

Client-Centered Model

As noted above, community mental health nursing incorporates community nursing and public health nursing. Community nursing refers to nursing practice in the community (the emphasis is on the locus of the practice). Community nursing, as presently practiced, is client centered and eclectic in its approach. Case management and PACT described above are interventions that would fit into the category of client-centered care.

Case Management Model

As noted above, some clients do not fit into one service system but require multiple systems simultaneously. For example, clients who have a dual diagnosis, such as a substance abuse problem and a psychiatric disorder, would require services from multiple providers. Some clients suffering from depression who attempt to self-treat their depression with alcohol, for example, may become addicted. Such clients will probably need the services of a psychiatrist, psychiatric nurse, social worker, substance abuse counselor, and perhaps even a vocational rehabilitation counselor. A case manager orchestrates the necessary services. Clients with mental illness who also have acquired immunodeficiency syndrome/human immunodeficiency virus (AIDS/HIV) need services from the general health sector as well as psychiatric services. Again, a case manager could take responsibility for coordinating all those services. Nurses, because of their unique preparation in a medical framework with a holistic orientation, are often best prepared to serve as a case manager for clients with complex problems.

Clients who are seriously mentally ill and/or homeless mentally ill may require the more intense services offered by PACT. These services would be directed toward maintaining such clients at their highest level of functioning in a community setting. Nurses are valuable members of such teams.

Capitation and Managed-Care Models

Reimbursement mechanisms that favor cost containment are influencing the patterns of service delivery in community mental health. Capitation and managed care, which are increasingly evident in the general health sector, are examples of prospective payment systems. **Prospective payment systems** provide a predetermined payment for a specific period of time or diagnosis for an individual client. Both these models have as their goal providing effective care at the lowest possible cost and include prospective payment systems.

Capitation is a funding mechanism in which all defined services for a specified period of time are provided for an agreed-upon single payment. The payment is tied to the care of a particular client or group of clients. The provider contracts in advance to accept the risk for costs exceeding the agreed-upon amount (Malloch, 1997).

Managed care is not the same as case management even though the terms are often used interchangeably and they share a similar historical development (Buchda, 1997). **Managed-care** programs are prepaid health plans in which an identified intermediary is given authority to manage how and from whom the client (patient) may obtain services. When managed-care programs include mental health services in their benefit package, the services provided are under the constraints of whatever group provides payment (Malloch, 1997). As efforts are made to contain the rising costs of health care, capitation and managed-care programs will have increasing influence in health care delivery.

Public Health Model

Caplan (1964) developed the guiding principles for community mental health nursing in the early years of the community mental health movement. In this model the client is the community rather than the individual, and the focus of practice is the factor that promotes or inhibits mental health. Caplan (1964) focused on preventive psychiatry and introduced three important terms: primary prevention, secondary prevention, and tertiary prevention.

Primary prevention refers to activities directed at reducing the incidence of mental disorder within a population. Population is defined as a collection of individuals who share one or more personal or environmental characteristics.

Primary prevention is a community concept. Aggregates (population groups) at risk of developing the identified mental disorder and environmental factors that may contribute to that risk are targeted. Population-focused practice refers to the target population to which the intervention is directed. Primary prevention does not seek to prevent a specific person from developing a mental disorder. Rather, it reduces the risk for aggregates within a population through health promotion. Examples of primary prevention activities engaged in by nurses are (a) teaching classes on stress management to factory workers, (b) conducting support groups for children moving from a small local elementary school to a large consolidated high school, and (c) teaching parenting skills to single, teenage mothers.

Secondary prevention refers to activities directed at reducing the prevalence of mental disorders by shortening the duration of a sufficient number of established cases. This reduction is achieved by encouraging early referrals, decreasing barriers to early diagnosis, and pro-

Prevention Levels

There has been a rash of "copycat" suicides among 15- to 18-year-old persons in your catchment area in the past year. You notice that many of the suicides occurred during the spring term in two high schools. You are meeting with a group of concerned health professionals to define the problem, identify the major factors, and appraise the strategies that may reduce the incidence of suicide in the target aggregate. Which of the following interventions are representative of (a) primary prevention activities, (b) secondary prevention activities, and (c) tertiary prevention activities?

- Ongoing assessment of students who are receiving failing grades in school
- Teaching concepts of stress management at Parent-Teacher Association meetings
- Sending crisis teams into the schools when a suicide has occurred
- Monitoring effectiveness of follow-up appointments in community mental health centers
- Operating a suicide hotline
- Writing an article on teenage suicide for the local newspaper
- Making referrals to support services (e.g., Big Brothers or Sisters) as indicated for teens who are seen at the community mental health center for depression
- Establishing a support group for teens dealing with the divorce of their parents
- Teaching the school nurse to identify signs of physical, sexual, and emotional abuse in students
- Supporting legislation for a recreational center for teens in a poor neighborhood.
- Teaching parenting skills to prospective parents
- Conducting stress reduction classes for high school students

viding effective treatment. Examples of secondary prevention activities engaged in by nurses are (a) staffing rape crisis centers, (b) operating shelters for abused women and their children, and (c) screening clients with debilitating chronic disease who are at high risk for developing depression.

Tertiary prevention activities are aimed at reducing the residual defects that are associated with mental disorders. Examples of tertiary prevention activities engaged in by nurses are (a) teaching social skills to clients enrolled in partial hospitalization programs, (b) monitoring the effectiveness of after-care services with follow-up appointments in community mental health centers, and (c) conducting medication groups for clients in group homes or other transition housing programs.

The services provided in the public health model are based on a community needs assessment. Descriptive statistics found in public records and reports provide social indicators that are highly correlated with mental health problems. Income level, marital status, population density, and crime statistics are examples of social indicators that may be used.

Epidemiological studies that examine the incidence and prevalence of mental disorders in a specific catchment area are also used. Chapter 7 in this text describes several major epidemiological studies that were conducted to assess the needs of large groups. Data from such studies often serve as the basis of the work done by task forces composed of experts from several disciplines who come together to explore the information and make recommendations for addressing the problems noted. An example of such a task force is given in the Report of the Federal Task Force on Homelessness and Severe Mental Illness (1992). *Healthy People 2000* (U.S. Department of Health and Human Services, 1991) is another example.

In addition, local community mental health centers regularly collect data on the people they serve. Aggregate data are used for the purposes of evaluation of local programs, for reports to funding sources, and to compile the statistics for government agencies.

In the public health model, the role of the nurse is largely collaborative. The nurse, functioning as part of a team of health professionals, (a) assesses the needs of the community, (b) identifies and determines priorities for high-risk aggregates (population groups), and (c) designs, implements, and evaluates appropriate interventions. Few nurses function primarily in this model partly because basic nursing education seldom prepares nurses adequately for this role. Instead, social workers and psychologists dominate administrative and managerial positions in the public health model. As nurses become better educated in community interventions, it can be surmised that nurses will return to exercise their original role in the community, and not be limited to tasks such as administering medications, and care for the chronically mentally ill.

FUTURE DIRECTIONS

Nurses are sometimes valued in community mental health because of their traditional nursing skills, which are well known and readily accepted by psychiatrists. In the client-centered model nurses take responsibility for medication management and participate in outreach programs,

such as family support groups. The variable educational preparation of nurses, however, complicates the situation. When salary scales are based on the number of years of basic preparation, nurses with associate degrees or diplomas compare unfavorably with psychologists and social workers with baccalaureates or master's degrees. At the same time, the salary scale for nurses working in hospitals is generally higher in contrast to that of nurses working in community mental health centers. Psychiatric nurses working in inpatient settings are developing an awareness of the need for rehabilitation services for clients who experience long-term mental illness. With the advent of managed care, more nurses will move to rehabilitation-oriented community-based settings, some of which may be under the auspices of the psychiatric inpatient unit

✿ RESEARCH HIGHLIGHT

Culturally Competent Care

STUDY PROBLEM/PURPOSE

To describe the mental health beliefs and practices of Chinese-American immigrant women.

METHODS

The qualitative portion used a focus group ($N=14$) and key informant interviews ($N=2$) to learn about the beliefs, practices, and knowledge about mental health of Chinese-American immigrant women. The quantitative portion consisted of a convenience sample of 72 women who completed a set of questionnaires, including demographic questions, a culture and work subscale, and the mental health portion of the Health Behavior Scale of the Survey of Chinese American Mental Health.

FINDINGS

The cultural value placed on the avoidance of shame, the use of both Western and traditional Chinese practitioners and treatments, and the inadequacy of Western-type services provided act as barriers to appropriate care. Higher levels of acculturation are related to greater use of mental health services.

IMPLICATIONS

Language and cultural misunderstandings may become barriers to effective care. Demonstrates the need to address cultural beliefs in the delivery of mental health care.

From "Mental Health Beliefs, Practices, and Knowledge of Chinese American Immigrant Women," by B. L. Tabora and J. H. Flaskerud, 1996, *Issues in Mental Health Nursing, 18,* pp. 173–189.

(Furlong-Norman, Palmer-Erbs, & Jonikas, 1997). Community health nurses in a managed-care system will need to be prepared to serve clients who have mental health problems as well as other health problems (Ehrhardt & Furlong, 1996). Nurses in all settings will need to expand beyond their traditional roles and take their place as members of interdisciplinary teams. Nurses will need to overcome personality and turf barriers to provide adequate care for clients (Polivka, Kennedy, & Chaudry, 1997). Moreover, collaboration among all agencies is essential to providing quality care to the mentally ill.

Nurses for the 21st century will need to provide mental health care to an increasingly diverse society. An understanding of culture as a group of persons with common race or ethnicity and shared values, norms, and behaviors is not sufficient. There is increasing diversity within such groupings. A cultural assessment, one's own as well as that of one's client, is needed to provide culturally congruent mental health care. Efforts to reconcile the differences between the two cultural perspectives are required to design effective interventions. The acknowledgment of an emerging global perspective is essential to be a culturally competent nurse (Tuck, 1996).

KEY CONCEPTS

◆ There are commonalities and differences among community health nursing, public health nursing, and home health nursing.

◆ Despite unevenness, the focus of mental health care is moving steadily toward community-based care.

◆ Community mental health centers strive to meet their goals of providing accessible, comprehensive mental health services, but fluctuation in funding is a continuing challenge.

◆ Deinstitutionalization of seriously mentally ill clients has dramatically altered the services provided by nurses working in community mental health centers.

◆ Consumers and their families are important collaborative partners in planning mental health care.

◆ Case management requires an understanding of the special needs of the target population, the individual, and community resources.

◆ Capitation and managed care are increasingly affecting services provided by community mental health centers.

◆ Nurses have skills that uniquely prepare them to work with the high-risk populations served by community mental health centers.

REVIEW QUESTIONS AND ACTIVITIES

1. Describe the changing focus of mental health care, and explain the major factors that influenced the change in focus.

2. What is meant by a community-based, population-focused approach to planning, delivering, and evaluating nursing care?

3. What are the goals of community-based mental health care?

4. Explain two models for practice for community mental health nursing.

5. What is the nurse's role in designing, managing, monitoring, and evaluating systems of care that address mental health problems experienced by aggregates?

6. Relate the process of community mental health planning for a specific aggregate.

7. Explain three selected strategies that can be used to improve the health status of a target aggregate (population group) in your community.

8. Name an intervention activity for each of the following categories: primary prevention, secondary prevention, and tertiary prevention.

EXPLORING THE WEB

◆ Visit this text's "Online Companion™" on the Internet at **http://www.DelmarNursing.com** for further information on community mental health nursing.

◆ Search the Web for sites and resources on managed care and case management.

◆ Can you locate information through government sites dealing with deinstitutionalization or capitation?

◆ What do you find when you search under different topic headings, such as public health, community health, or home health? Do the major nursing organizations, such as the National League for Nursing and the American Nurses Association, have chat rooms in these areas?

REFERENCES

Bartol, G. M., Moon, E., & Linton, M. (1994). Nursing assistance for families of patients. *Journal of Psychosocial Nursing*, 27–29.

Beers, C. W. (1921) *A mind that found itself.* Garden City, NY: Doubleday.

Bentley, K. J. (1994). Supports for community-based mental health care: An optimistic review of federal legislation. *Health and Social Work, 19*(4), 288.

Bradshaw, T. W. (1997). Nursing in the community. In R. K. Nunnery (Ed.), *Advancing your career: Concepts of professional nursing* (pp. 348–359). Philadelphia: FA Davis.

Buchda, V. L. (1997). Managing and providing care. In R. K. Nunnery (Ed.), *Advancing your career: Concepts of professional nursing* (pp. 244–258). Philadelphia: FA Davis.

Burns, B. J., & Santos, A. B. (1995). Assertive community treatment: An update of randomized trials. *Psychiatric Services, 46*, 669–674.

Caplan, G. (1964). *Principles of preventive psychiatry.* New York: Basic Books.

Donley, R. (1997). Health care agenda and reform. In R. K. Nunnery (Ed.), *Advancing your career: Concepts of professional nursing* (pp. 289–303). Philadelphia: FA Davis.

Drake, R. E., & Burns, B. J. (1995). Special section on assertive community treatment: An introduction. *Psychiatric Services. 46*(7), 667–668.

Duke University Medical Center, Division of Social and Community Psychiatry, Department of Psychiatry. (1993). *Hospital without walls.* Study Guide for distribution with videotape. Author.

Ehrhardt, P. M., & Furlong, B. (1996). Integrating mental health into community health nursing. *Nurse Educator, 21*(3), 33–36.

Francell, C. G., Conn, V. S., & Gray, D. P. (1988). Family perspectives of burden of care for chronically mentally ill. *Hospital and Community Psychiatry, 39*, 1296–1300.

Furlong-Norman, K., Palmer-Erbs, V. K., & Jonikas, J. (1997). Exploring the field: Strengthening psychiatric rehabilitation nursing practice with new information and ideas. *Journal of Psychosocial Nursing and Mental Health Services, 35*, 35–39.

Greenber, J. S., Kime, H. W., & Greenley, J. R. (1997). Factors associated with subjective burden in siblings of adults with severe mental illness. *American Journal of Orthopsychiatry, 67*(2), 231–240.

Haimowitz, S. (1991). Americans with Disabilities Act of 1990: Its significance for persons with mental illness. *Hospital and Community Psychiatry, 42*, 23–24.

Heller, T., Roccoforte, J. A., Hseih, K., Cook, J. A., & Pickett, S. A. (1997). Benefits of support groups for families of adults with severe mental illness. *American Journal of Orthopsychiatry, 67*(2), 187–196.

Lefley, H. P. (1997). The consumer recovery vision: Will it alleviate family burden? *American Journal of Orthopsychiatry, 67*(2), 210–219.

Malloch, K. (1997). Health-care economics. In R. K. Nunnery (Ed.), *Advancing your career: Concepts of professional nursing* (pp. 320–332). Philadelphia: FA Davis.

McGrew, J. H., Bond, G. R., Dietzen, L., McKasson, M., & Miller, L. D. (1995). A multisite study of client outcomes in assertive community treatment. *Psychiatric Services, 46*(7), 696–701.

Mental Health System Act. (1980). 96th Congress. Public Law 96-398, Sec. 9501, Amendment to Senate Bill 1177, September 23.

Morris, M. (1996). Patients' perceptions of psychiatric home care. *Archives of Psychiatric Nursing, 10*, 176–183.

National Institute of Mental Health (NIMH). (1987). *Toward a model plan for a comprehensive, community-based mental health system.* Rockville, MD: US Public Health Service, Alcohol, Drug Abuse, and Mental Health Administration, Division of Education and Service System Liaison.

National Institute of Mental Health and National Advisory Mental Health Council. (1991). *Caring for people with severe mental disorders: A national plan of research to improve services.* Washington, DC: Author (ADM 91-1762).

Nunnery, R. K. (1997). *Advancing your career: Concepts of professional nursing.* Philadelphia: FA Davis.

Pew Health Professional Commission. (1991). *Healthy American: Practitioners for 2005.* Durham, NC: Pew Health Foundation.

Polivka, B. J., Kennedy, C., & Chaudry, R. (1997). Collaboration between local public health and community mental health agencies. *Research in Nursing and Health, 20*, 153–160.

Report of the Federal Task Force on Homelessness and Severe Mental Illness. (1992). *Outcasts on main street.* Washington, DC: Author (ADM 92-1904).

Stanhope, M., & Lancaster, J. (1996). *Community health nursing* (4th ed.). St. Louis: Mosby.

Tabora, B. L., & Flaskerud, J. H. (1997). Mental health beliefs, practices, and knowledge of Chinese American immigrant women. *Issues in Mental Health Nursing, 18*, 173–189.

Tuck, I. (1997). The cultural context of mental health nursing. *Issues in Mental Health Nursing, 18*, 269–281.

U.S. Department of Health and Human Services. (1991). *Healthy People 2000.* Washington, DC: U.S. Government Printing Office.

〜〜〜 **SUGGESTED READINGS**

Chafetz, L. (1996). The experience of severe mental illness: A life history approach. *Archives of Psychiatric Nursing, 10*, 24–31.

Cornwell, C., & Chiverton, P. (1997). The psychiatric advanced practice nurse with prescriptive authority: Role development, practice issues and outcomes measurement. *Archives of Psychiatric Nursing, 11*(2), 57–65.

Eggert, L. L., Thompson, E. A., Herting, J. R., & Nicholas, L. J. (1994). Prevention research program: Reconnecting at-risk youth. *Issues in Mental Health Nursing, 15*(2), 107–135.

Godin, P. (1996). The development of community psychiatric nursing: A professional project? *Journal of Advanced Nursing, 23*, 925–934.

Gorman, D. (1997). Psychiatric nursing with Australia's multicultural patients. *Issues in Mental Health Nursing, 18*(3), 259–268.

Tuck, I., du Mont, P., Evans, G., & Shupe, J. (1997). The experience of caring for an adult child with schizophrenia. *Archives of Psychiatric Nursing, 11*(3), 118–125.

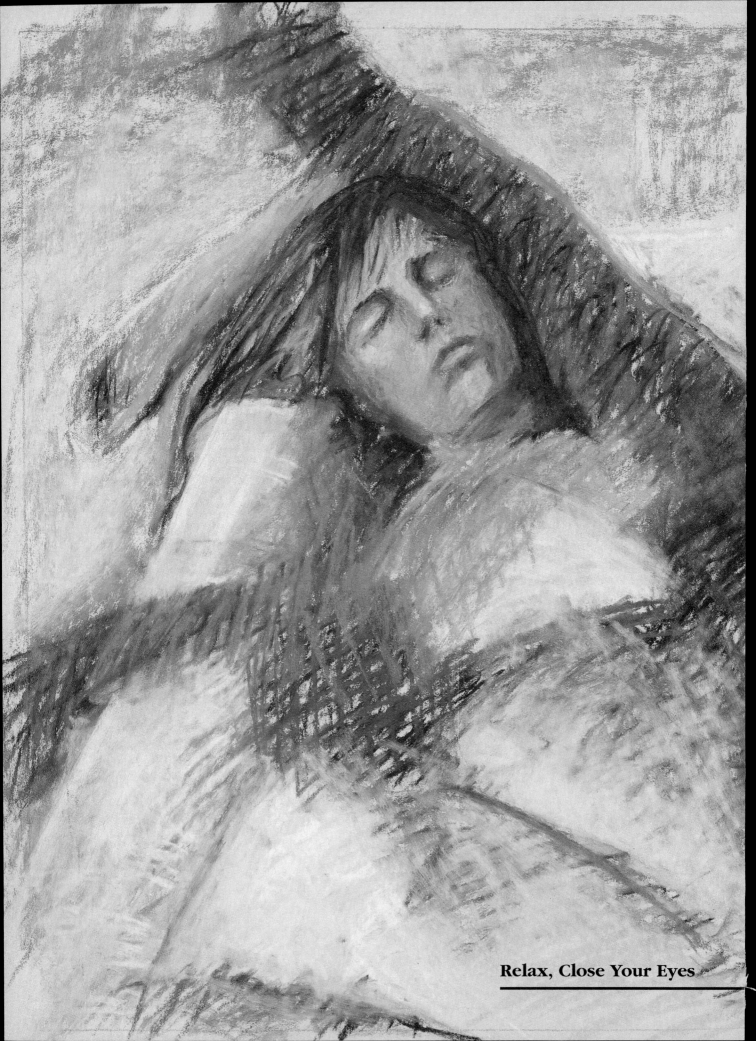

Relax, Close Your Eyes

Chapter

30

COMPLEMENTARY AND SOMATIC THERAPIES

Noreen Cavan Frisch

Using Complementary Therapies in Daily Life

Different people deal with stress and tension in various ways. What do you do to relax? Do you take a warm bath or soak your feet? Sit under a tree? Fantasize? Play a sport or do some physical exercise?

- ◆ Try practicing guided imagery informally to help you manage stressful situations. Close your eyes, and imagine that you are in your favorite place. Involve as many of your senses as you can (sight, smell, touch, hearing, etc.). Do you experience any changes in your level of relaxation as a result of completing this exercise?

- ◆ Have you ever used music as a form of emotional outlet, perhaps to relieve stress or to help deal with painful emotions such as sadness or loneliness? What type(s) of music do you find to be uplifting in such situations?

- ◆ Think about the role of physical touch in your own life. Do you come from a family background where expression of comfort and support through physical touch is encouraged or discouraged? As a nursing professional, how comfortable would you be with using appropriate physical touch with a client?

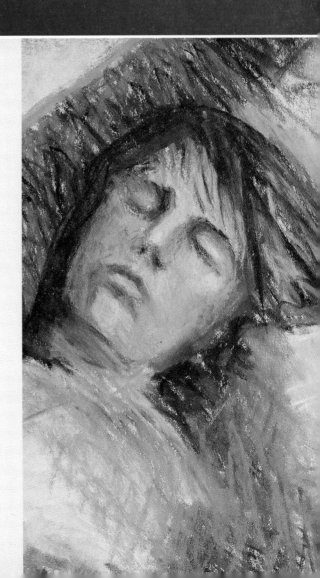

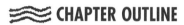 **CHAPTER OUTLINE**

COMPLEMENTARY MODALITIES

Relaxation

Guided Imagery

Hypnotherapy

Massage and Touch

Energy-Based Modalities
    Therapeutic Touch
    Healing Touch

Energy-Based Modalities in Psychiatric Mental Health Care

Music Therapy

Pet-Assisted Therapy

NURSING ROLE IN SOMATIC INTERVENTIONS

Anger Control Assistance
    Physical Restraints
    Seclusion
    Reentry of the Client to the Unit

Light Therapy

COLLABORATIVE INTERVENTIONS IN PSYCHIATRIC SOMATIC TREATMENTS

Electroconvulsive Therapy
    Pharmacological Aspects of ECT
    Nursing Care

COMPETENCIES

Upon completion of this chapter, the reader should be able to:

1. Describe the use of six complementary modalities as nursing interventions in psychiatric mental health care: relaxation and guided imagery, hypnosis, massage, energy-based modalities (therapeutic touch and healing touch), music therapy, and animal-assisted therapy.

2. Intervene to control escalating anger in a client.

3. Describe the use of physical restraints and seclusion in control of violent behavior.

4. Describe the use of light therapy for treatment of seasonal affective disorder (SAD).

5. Describe the current indications for electroconvulsive therapy (ECT), and provide nursing care to a client undergoing the procedure.

≋ KEY TERMS

Anger Control Assistance   Nursing intervention aimed at facilitation of the expression of anger in an adaptive and nonviolent manner.

Animal-Assisted Therapy   Use of animals to provide attention, affection, diversion, and/or relaxation.

Complementary Modalities   Those modalities being used as an adjunct to medical care and psychiatric treatment that are thought to have effects on stress, sleep disturbance, anxiety, and/or other emotions.

Electroconvulsive Therapy (ECT)   Passage of an electrical stimulus to the brain to produce a seizure.

Energy-Based Modalities   Techniques for healing grounded in the notion of the human energy field.

Guided Imagery   An unconditional process in which the practitioner leads the subject with specific words, suggestions, symbols, or images to elicit a positive response.

Healing Touch   Systematic approach to healing using several energy interventions that incorporate a variety of therapeutic maneuvers.

Hypnosis   Assisting the client to an altered state of consciousness to create an awareness and a directed-focus experience.

Light Therapy (Phototherapy)   Provision of artificial indoor lighting, 5 to 20 times brighter than ordinary lighting, to the environment of a person with Seasonal Affective Disorder (SAD).

Massage   Stimulation of the skin and underlying tissues for the purposes of increasing circulation and inducing a relaxation response.

Music Therapy   Use of specific kinds of music and its ability to effect changes in behavior, emotions, and physiology.

Relaxation   A psychophysiological state characterized by parasympathetic dominance involving multiple visceral and somatic symptoms, including the absence of physical, mental, and emotional tension.

Seclusion   State of a client being put in an isolated room or cell.

Somatic Therapies   Interventions used in the management of psychiatric symptoms, for example, use of seclusion or physical restraints in control of anger.

Therapeutic Imagery   The ability to take one's natural thought processes and to direct those thoughts in a creative way, potentiating a positive outcome.

Therapeutic Massage   Extension of massage techniques, involving deep tissue and advanced massage techniques.

Therapeutic Touch (TT)   Five-step process of touch that involves centering; assessing the client's energy field; smoothing, or "unruffling," the field; modulating or transferring energy; and knowing when to stop.

The purpose of this chapter is to provide the reader with information on the use of a rather wide range of interventions currently being used in psychiatric mental health nursing. Some of these interventions are defined as **complementary modalities**—those modalities being used as an adjunct to medical care and psychiatric treatment that are thought to have effects on stress, sleep disturbance, anxiety, and/or other emotions. Other of these interventions, known as **somatic therapies**, have long been used in the management of psychiatric symptoms, for example, use of seclusion or physical restraints in control of anger. Each of these interventions has a role in modern-day nursing care, and all are listed in the second edition of the Nursing Interventions Classification (NIC) (discussed in Chapter 4). Each intervention is presented along with practice examples to give the reader illustrations of recommended and appropriate use. In addition, there is a section on nursing collaborative interventions for specific psychiatric somatic therapies to provide information on the nursing care required for the client undergoing specific procedures. The goal of the chapter is to broaden the reader's knowledge of the scope of nursing practice relevant to psychiatric mental health care. The chapter is divided into two sections: one on complementary modalities and the other on somatic interventions.

COMPLEMENTARY MODALITIES

There are several complementary modalities used in psychiatric mental health care. Table 30-1 provides a summary of the complementary modalities discussed in this section and indicates when the modality is most useful in psychiatric mental health care. Each of these modalities is discussed below to provide the reader with basic information about the modality and its use in psychiatric mental health care. The purpose of this discussion is neither to provide details on how to apply each of the modalities nor to make the reader a practitioner of any of the modalities. Each of the modalities and techniques described requires further study and, in many cases, certification as a practitioner to incorporate into practice. Interested readers are referred to the resource list at the chapter's end for contact information regarding further study.

Relaxation

Relaxation is defined as a psychophysiological state characterized by parasympathetic dominance involving multiple visceral and somatic symptoms including the absence of physical, mental, and emotional tension (Kolkmeier, 1988). Relaxation permits a person to quiet himself, retreat mentally from his surroundings, and decrease tension, anxiety, and/or pain.

Table 30-1 Complementary Modalities in Psychiatric Mental Health Care

MODALITY	DEFINITION	USE IN PSYCHIATRIC MENTAL HEALTH CARE
Relaxation	Use of techniques to elicit a relaxation response	Antidote to stress/anxiety
Guided imagery	Use of sensory images to enhance relaxation and healing	Helpful in reducing depression and overcoming addictions
Hypnosis, hypnotherapy	Assisting the client to an altered state of consciousness	Adjunct to psychotherapy; helpful in overcoming addictions
Massage	Stimulation of the skin and underlying tissues	Produces relaxation; helpful to induce sleep; meets client's need for "safe" touch
Energy-based modalities	Nursing interventions based on the concept of the human energy field	Helpful in reducing anxiety/stress, working through grief, and assisting in addictions recovery
Music therapy	Use of music to alter behavior, emotions, and/or physiology	Reduces anxiety; promotes sleep
Pet-assisted therapy	Use of animals to provide affection, attention, diversion, and relaxation	Decreases feelings of loneliness; increases socialization; provides diversional activities

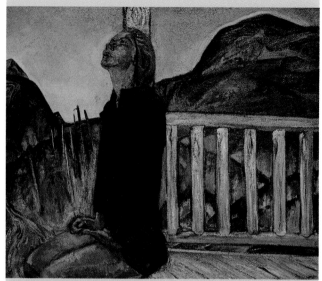

Dhârâna by Frederick H. Varley (1932). Source: Art Gallery of Ontario, Gift from the Albert H. Robson Memorial Subscription Fund, 1942. Reproduced courtesy Estate of Kathleen McKay.

While never abandoning his strong Christian beliefs, Varley was deeply attracted to Eastern thought and to the mysteries of nature revealed in the remote Canadian wilderness. (See his painting of Arctic icebergs in Chapter 7.) *Dhârâna* combines his appreciation of nature and of the spirit in one powerful vision of deep meditation.

The term *relaxation response* was first used by Herbert Benson when referring to the psychophysiological state where muscles are relaxed; tension is released; blood pressure, heart rate, and respiratory rate are decreased; the brain is in the alpha state; and the parasympathetic nervous system is activated. When the parasympathetic system is activated, the person feels calm (as opposed to the sympathetic system associated with the fight-or-flight response); the alpha brain wave state is a deepened state of relaxation. Assisting a client to achieve a relaxation state is an "antidote to stress" and helps the client to access inner resources that may have been obscured by the anxious state (Shames, 1996).

There are several techniques used by nurses to activate the relaxation response. All begin by starting in a quiet, relaxed area, breathing deeply, and concentrating on quiet and calm. Progressive muscle relaxation (PMR) is a technique of alternately tensing and relaxing muscle groups throughout the body to become aware of tensions and the contrast between muscle tension and relaxation. Persons undergoing PMR are led through sessions by the nurse, who coaches them to assume a comfortable position and suggests the process of tensing and releasing major muscle groups (working from the feet to the head):

The client is first encouraged to take several deep breaths and relax. He is then advised to feel his feet on the floor. Next he is told to squeeze the muscles in his feet and perhaps scrunch his toes and tighten his feet until his feet feel small, perhaps round. Then, the client is told to relax those muscles. This technique serves to focus attention on body parts, one by one, and to make the client very aware of what it feels like when that part is tense, and how it feels to relax that same part.

(Shames, 1996, p. 74)

Persons receiving PMR as a treatment are able to get in touch with tensions and become aware of how these tensions are affecting their physical body (Frisch & Kelley, 1996). For clients completing this technique, there is frequently a sense of relief and a subjective sense of letting go of the tensions.

Other relaxation techniques include "countdown" and eye muscle tightening and relaxing. Countdown is a technique in which the client is advised to count down slowly from 10 to 0 and to feel both refreshed and relaxed when he reaches 0. Eye muscle tightening and relaxing is done while the client is in a comfortable position with his eyes open. He is instructed to focus intently on an object, which results in a certain amount of eye muscle tightening and fatigue. He is then instructed to relieve the fatigue by closing his eyes. Shames (1996) states: "The juxtaposition of the tightening followed by the relaxation encourages the onset of a relaxed state" (p. 75).

Many clients will learn that they can induce their own relaxation response at home after practicing the techniques and sometimes with the addition of an audiotape that leads them through the process of PMR. The purpose of using relaxation techniques in nursing practice is to help the client first acknowledge the degree to which he feels tension and anxiety, to provide a contrast to the daily experience of tension by teaching relaxation, and to give the client the ability to use relaxation therapy as a self-help intervention.

Guided Imagery

A technique that goes hand in hand with relaxation, guided imagery builds on the relaxation response and adds visual or other sensory images to enhance the relaxation and/or to present an image for the client that is one of healing. **Therapeutic imagery** is defined as the ability to take one's natural thought processes and to direct these thoughts in a creative way, potentiating a positive outcome. Shames (1996) defined **guided imagery** as an "unconditional process in which the practitioner leads the subject with specific words, suggestions, symbols, or images to elicit a positive response" (p. 71).

One example of a simple guided imagery technique is a "pleasant memory technique" in which a client who is comfortable and relaxed is told to close his eyes and is given the suggestion to think back to an enjoyable event. Thinking of a pleasant event can bring many positive sensations to the client, as he will remember sights, sounds, and smells of a joyful time. For example, one client might remember being in his grandmother's kitchen, smelling and eating home-made bread; another might remember walking in an attractive park, with sounds and smells of being in the woods. This technique can be extended to ask the client to think of a "special place" or a "safe place" where he has positive memories. A client can use his

imagination to remember a place and experience being there. This technique has been useful when nurses are working with clients who will be undergoing medical procedures that are uncomfortable and/or scary. The nurse can suggest that the client return to the pleasant place brought up in his memory and think about being there rather than in the medical office, dentist's chair, or other similarly negative situation. The nurse will assist the client in developing the scene by asking questions like: "How does it look?" "What does it smell like?" "What does it feel like?" The nurse chooses words or phrases that convey positive images and may suggest sensations like floating, releasing, washing away the pain/discomfort, and so on. To end a guided imagery session, the nurse will encourage the patient to express thoughts and feelings about the experience to whatever degree the client is comfortable disclosing his personal experiences.

Relaxation and guided imagery techniques have great use in nursing practice. As mentioned above, there is use

---

⑨ RESEARCH HIGHLIGHT

Use of Guided Imagery with Depressed Children

STUDY PROBLEM/PURPOSE

An experimental design was used to study the effects of guided imagery as an independent nursing intervention for depressed, hospitalized, school-aged children. The researcher hypothesized that children who received guided imagery would show a lower posttest score on the Child Depression Inventory (CDI) and would demonstrate improvement on variables pertaining to sleep, appetite, self-esteem, coping skills, and social interaction.

METHODS

The experimental group received ten 30-minute guided imagery sessions, while the control group received ten 30-minute play sessions.

FINDINGS

Results were that the experimental group had a statistically significant improvement on the CDI, whereas the control group did not. Further, data indicate improvement among children in both the experimental and control group on all variables measured.

IMPLICATIONS

The researcher concluded that guided imagery is effective in reducing depression in children.

From *Classification of Nursing Diagnoses: Proceedings of the tenth conference* (p. 371), by G. Bufe, 1994, Philadelphia: JB Lippincott.

in preparing clients to go through procedures, but there are other documented uses as well. Relaxation and imagery have long been used in maternity care for preparation for and management of labor and childbirth. One nurse researcher has documented the use of guided imagery in hospitalized, depressed children and found it is an effective technique in reducing measured depression (refer to the Research Highlight on the use of guided imagery) (Bufe, 1994). Many nurses have documented the use of guided imagery as beneficial for patients undergoing chemotherapy and cancer treatments (Troesch, Rodehaver, Delaney, & Yanes, 1993; Sloman, 1995). Others have documented a positive role of imagery in assisting clients to overcome addictions (Wynd, 1992; Zimmerman, 1989). These techniques, however, have not been as helpful for clients with severe anxiety disorders; for example, a client experiencing panic attacks will not be able to concentrate on the relaxation exercises and may in fact become more anxious when asked to do so. However, in situations where the client is undergoing stress, relaxation and imagery are two nursing interventions that give nurses tools to use in a highly stressful world. They are noninvasive techniques that can assist the client to regain control, both for the moment as in using imagery while undergoing a procedure or in the long term as in using imagery to give up an addiction such as cigarette smoking.

The nurse is cautioned, however, that imagery is never recommended for use with clients who are psychotic or who have a background of schizophrenia: "It is generally considered that these people are often bombarded with too many images already, and are unable to differentiate between those they choose to envision and those that plague their mental processes involuntarily" (Shames, 1996, p. 95). The therapeutic use of imagery demands an ability to sustain one's focus and concentration, and clients who are psychotic and/ or schizophrenic are usually unable to maintain these components.

The processes of relaxation and guided imagery are discussed here for nursing practice at the elementary level. These interventions are both listed and described in the NIC (McCloskey & Bulechek, 1996). Both of these techniques, however, can be practiced at an intermediate and advanced level for those who seek out additional education. The technique called interactive guided imagery was developed by the faculty at the Academy for Guided Imagery in Mill Valley, California. Interactive guided imagery is described as "a powerful modality for helping a patient/client connect with the deeper wellsprings of what is true for them at cognitive, affective, and somatic levels" (Shames, 1996, p. 32). This use of imagery requires education, and the reader is referred to the list of resources at this chapter's end for further information.

⚙ NURSING ALERT!

When Imagery Is Contraindicated

Guided imagery is contraindicated for persons who are psychotic or who have a history of schizophrenia.

Hypnotherapy

Hypnosis is defined as "assisting the client to an altered state of consciousness to create an awareness and a directed focus experience" (McCloskey & Bulechek, 1996, p. 326). The word *hypnosis* actually refers to the induction of sleep. In practice, hypnosis is a technique in which the practitioner is quite active in directing the client and the client is suggestible and in a very relaxed state. Hypnosis has been used in health care to varying degrees of success for centuries. Many anthropologists believe that some form of hypnosis, or trance state, has been used among all known primitive cultures. Its use in modern health care began in the late 1950s, when the technique was used to treat soldiers suffering from postwar traumas of World Wars I and II. The British Medical Society endorsed the practice of hypnosis in medical school education in 1955, and the American Medical Association (AMA) followed (Shames, 1996). Since then, the technique has been used in many areas of medical, dental, and nursing practice. Frequently, hypnosis is used to assist a client to gain relief from pain, which can be either acute (as in childbirth) or chronic (as in arthritis). Recent reports in nursing literature indicate that hypnosis can be successfully used in several areas of reproductive health, including sexual dysfunction, urinary incontinence, chronic pelvic pain, hyperemesis gravidarum, and pain relief during labor and delivery (Baram, 1995; Letts, Baker, Ruderman, & Kennedy, 1993). Other studies indicate a positive effect in pain management (Spira & Speigel, 1992). The next Research Highlight provides data from a study on the use of hypnosis in a psychiatric liaison service (Kaye & Schindler, 1990). Hypnosis has also been used to alter physiological processes and to assist in changing behaviors such as smoking. For advanced practitioners, hypnotherapy—the use of hypnosis to achieve resolution of psychic trauma and distress—is used along with other forms of psychotherapy.

In nursing practice, the use of hypnosis is governed by licensure laws in each state. Nurses are advised to consult with their State Board of Nursing or their licensing body regarding regulation governing their locality. In all cases, nurses who practice hypnotherapy must have formal training in the use of the modality. Most often this training is accompanied by a graduate degree and always by a period of supervised work with a faculty member who is an advanced practitioner.

✺ RESEARCH HIGHLIGHT

Use of Hypnosis in a Psychiatric Liaison Service

STUDY PROBLEM/PURPOSE

The researchers report a study on the use of hypnosis as a adjunct modality to traditional medical and psychologic treatment.

METHODS

Subjects were 29 women and 8 men from 24 to 75 years of age who were hypnotized for management of depression, pain, anxiety, or side effects from chemotherapy. Subjects were given tapes for autohypnosis to use for reinforcement.

FINDINGS

Researchers report excellent results, with total to almost total relief of symptoms in 68% of the patients, moderate relief of symptoms in 22%, little relief of symptoms in 11%. There were no differences among the results for various conditions.

IMPLICATIONS

Researchers conclude that hypnotherapy can be useful in a psychiatric liaison setting.

From "Hypnosis on a Consultation Liaison Service," by J. M. Kaye and B. A. Schindler, 1990, *General Hospital Psychiatry, 12*, pp. 379–383.

Massage and Touch

Massage is the stimulation of the skin and underlying tissues for the purposes of increasing circulation and inducing a relaxation response. Massage and the use of touch have long been a part of nursing practice. Massage techniques include the back rub, a very traditional part of care, frequently given to patients on bedrest, confined to wheelchairs, and before the hours of sleep. Also, techniques of stimulating the skin to increase circulation during bathing are massage techniques. These basic massage techniques are taught to student nurses and are included in texts of fundamentals of nursing skill (Perry & Potter, 1994; Smith & Duell, 1996). Nurses are skilled in the basic massage movements of *effleurage* (long, soothing strokes) to increase circulation and *tapotement* (stimulating rapid percussive movements) and *petrissage* (kneading motions) for stimulation.

Therapeutic massage is an extension of massage techniques involving deep tissue and advanced massage techniques. Nurses providing therapeutic massage have received advanced education in massage, and many have become certified as massage therapists. The National Association of Nurse Massage Therapists (NANMT) is a resource for nurses wishing to obtain information on advanced education in therapeutic massage. Massage has obvious benefits in inducing relaxation, in assisting with sleep disturbances, and in offering the client contact involving touch. For those in advanced massage practice, massage techniques can also assist in healing/repair of muscle trauma.

Simple touch—reaching out to physically contact another—is a therapy too often neglected in busy nursing practice. Simpler than massage, touch is accessible to all nurses. Keegan (1988) writes that touch "is perhaps one of our most highly used, yet least applauded of the five recognized senses" (p. 337). Touch is one mechanism of communicating caring, support, and nurturing to clients who may feel isolated and fearful. For example, reaching out to take a client's hand is a way to communicate caring and support. Often, touching a client on the shoulder is a means of letting the person know that the nurse is present and cares about the client.

Studies have documented that the elderly in particular have a need to be touched (Rozema, 1986). One study on the utilization of touch by health care personnel found that patients in the age range of 66 to 100 years received the least amount of touch, when compared with younger patients (Barnett, 1972). Clients in geriatric institutions place great importance and value on the smallest gesture of touch (Burnside, 1973). Keegan (1988) reports a study that documented that the less mobile nursing home residents were, the more positively they responded to touch.

✺ RESEARCH HIGHLIGHT

Use of Massage in Hospice

STUDY PROBLEM/PURPOSE

Researchers studied the effects of slow-stroke back massage on measures of relaxation in 30 hospice clients.

METHODS

Measures included systolic and diastolic blood pressure, heart rate, and skin temperature. Measurements were taken before the treatment, immediately after massage, and again after 5 minutes of resting. The sequence was repeated again 24 hours later.

FINDINGS

There were statistically significant changes in all variables measured.

IMPLICATIONS

The researchers conclude that slow-stroke back massage can elicit relaxation.

From "Effect of Slow Stroke Back Massage on Relaxation in Hospice Clients," by S. S. Meek, 1993, *Image, 25*, pp. 17-21.

In mental health practice, massage has been found helpful in decreasing agitation in persons with dementia (Synder, Egan, & Burns, 1995) and decreasing stress for seriously ill inpatients who have unfulfilled needs for safe touch, that is, touch that is perceived as supportive and caring rather than invasive (Hilliard, 1995). In an experimental study, slow-stroke back massage was found to induce relaxation in hospice clients (Meek, 1993), as indicated by the preceding Research Highlight.

Touch, of course, has many personal connotations to both nurses and their clients. The interpretation of touch is both culturally and familially derived. The nurse should never assume that any individual client wants to be touched, must assess the client's individual needs and desires before implementing any form of massage, and should never offer touch in situations where the client is uncomfortable with it. The best means of determining how the client feels is, for example, to state, "Here, you can hold my hand if you like while the procedure is being done" or "I'll put my hand on your shoulder, if you like, while you talk about yesterday's experiences in the group."

Energy-Based Modalities

For purposes of this chapter, **energy-based modalities** refer to techniques for healing grounded in the notion of the human energy field. The reader will remember that Martha Rogers, the nurse theorist who developed the theory of nursing called the Science of Unitary Human Beings, defined the person as a unified whole possessing individual integrity that is more than and different from the sum of the parts (Rogers, 1970). From this perspective, the human being is an energy field that is in constant interactions with the environmental fields. Rogers (1991) wrote that "the concept of the field provides a means of perceiving people and their respective environments as irreducible wholes" (p. 27).

With the perspective of a human energy field, the nurse can be viewed as an integral part of the client's environmental field. Thus, healing interventions can be performed where the "nurse uses his or her hands as a mediating focus in the continuing patternings of the mutual patient-environmental energy field process" (Meeham, 1990, p. 74). The best-known nursing intervention using the human energy field perspective is Therapeutic Touch. However, there are several other techniques and approaches based on the same or similar ideas of working within the client's energy field to balance the energy through interaction with the nurse. Figure 30-1 is an illustration of human interaction seen as an energy exchange of two energy fields. In energy-based work, the nurse develops skills to assess the balance of the client's field and effect changes through the nurse's own energy patterning.

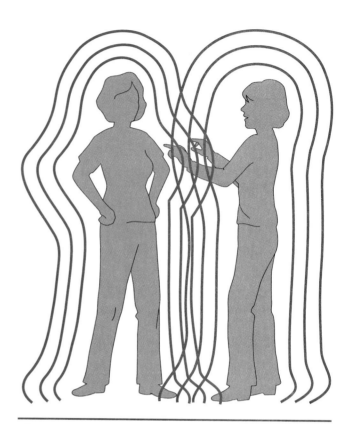

Figure 30-1   Human Interaction as an Exchange of Energy between Two Fields

Therapeutic Touch

Therapeutic Touch (TT) is a specific technique developed in the 1970s by Dolores Krieger (1979) at New York University. Therapeutic Touch is a five-step process of centering; assessing the client's energy field; smoothing, or "unruffling," the field; modulating or transferring energy; and knowing when to stop. Krieger describes TT as "a contemporary interpretation of several ancient healing practices. These practices consist of learned skills for consciously directing or sensitively modulating human energies" (Krieger, 1993, p. 11). This five-step procedure is often referred to as the Krieger-Kunz method of Therapeutic Touch, in acknowledgment of Krieger's work and that of her colleague, Dora Kunz.

The technique of TT has been widely investigated by nurses, beginning with Krieger herself. In 1988, Quinn published a review article of the state of TT research from the time period 1974 to 1986. Since then, research on the use of TT in varied settings continues, and Scandrett-Hibdon (1996) presents a current review of research on TT. The findings of these studies have shown TT to have a positive and consistent effect in producing a relaxation response. In some situations, TT has been effective in controlling headache pain (Keller & Bzdek, 1986), reducing anxiety and stress (Gange & Toye, 1994; Olson & Sneed, 1995; Quinn, 1981, 1983), and promoting accelerated wound healing (Wirth, Richardson, Eidelman, &

O'Malley, 1993). While an extensive review of the research literature on TT is beyond the scope of this chapter, the reader is referred to the review articles cited and to the organization Nurse Healer's Professional Associates (listed in the chapter's end) for detailed information on the topic. Therapeutic Touch is currently listed in the NIC as a nursing intervention that involves "directing one's own interpersonal energy to flow though the hands to help or heal another" (McCloskey & Bulechek, 1996, p. 564).

Healing Touch

Healing Touch is a program of study that involves a "systematic approach to healing using several energy interventions that incorporate a variety of therapeutic maneuvers" (Scandrett-Hibdon, 1996, p. 27). Some of these interventions include full-body techniques, where the maneuvers are used over the entire body to complete balancing of the entire energy field. Other techniques are localized to effect a specific clinical outcome, for example, a "mind clearing" technique used for relaxation and to focus the mind (Mentgen, 1996). These healing touch techniques all involve work with the energy field and are based on the assumptions described above. All of the healing touch techniques have been published and are available for the student wishing further information on the subject (Hover-Kramer, 1996a).

✿ RESEARCH HIGHLIGHT

Therapeutic Touch Used on an Adolescent Inpatient Psychiatric Unit

STUDY PROBLEM/PURPOSE

The effect of using therapeutic touch (TT) on adolescents was studied.

METHODS

Seven hospitalized adolescent psychiatric inpatients received a total of 31 therapeutic touch sessions and were interviewed about their experiences.

FINDINGS

Two overarching themes emerged from the clients' experiences: the therapeutic relationship with the nurse and the connection of body and mind. The adolescents enjoyed the experience of receiving therapeutic touch and wanted more of it.

IMPLICATIONS

Nurses noted that the adolescents seemed able to achieve a calmer state after the TT sessions.

From "Therapeutic Touch with Adolescent Psychiatric Patients," by P. Hughes, R. Grochowski, and C. Harris, 1996, *Journal of Holistic Nursing, 14*, pp. 6–23.

Energy-Based Modalities in Psychiatric Mental Health Care

Hover-Kramer (1996b) describes several uses of energy-based techniques in mental health care. She indicates that emotional distress, such as that seen during grief, depression, anxiety, and stress, causes imbalances in the energy field. When a psychotherapist is able to work with the energy field at the same time that he is working with the subjective and verbal expression of the distress, he is able to offer the client an additional powerful technique to help the client to restore harmony and balance. Hover-Kramer (1996b) suggests the usefulness of these techniques in working through the grief process, treating anxiety and stress, working with hyperactivity in children, and assisting in addictions recovery.

Music Therapy

The arts provide the nurse with an opportunity to work with clients in avenues that do not require verbal expression or the rational, cognitive processes. There are many times when the client is unable or unwilling to express emotion (particularly negative emotion) through words. Visual and expressive arts are a means of communication that circumvent the need for talk and permit the client and nurse to interact on emotional and intuitive levels. There is ample evidence that use of the arts can be highly therapeutic and of significant benefit in mental health practice.

Music therapy is concerned with the use of specific kinds of music and its ability to effect changes in behavior, emotions, and physiology (Guzzetta, 1988). The form of music therapy used primarily by nurses is providing music for the client that will help to achieve a specific change in behavior or feeling (McCloskey & Bulechek, 1996).

Guzzetta (1988) warns that the nurse is not to confuse music as therapy with music as entertainment or diversion. One hears music for enjoyment at a concert, and one hears music as diversion while being placed "on hold" on a telephone answering system. To be therapy, the goal is the reduction of psychophysiological stress, pain, anxiety, or isolation. According to Guzzetta (1988), music therapy has been shown to help clients relax, develop a sense of self-awareness, improve learning, and cope with a variety of psychophysiological dysfunctions. The healing capabilities of music are intimately bound to the personal experience of inner relaxation (Hamel, 1979).

Music can be used as a catalyst to facilitate mental suggestion and to enhance the client's self-healing. Music has been used in birthing rooms, in operating rooms, during massage therapy sessions, during counseling sessions, on psychiatric inpatient units, and during addictions treatment. It is believed that music therapy offers a response because music produces alterations in physiology: "Soothing music can produce a hypometabolic response characteristic of relaxation in which autonomic, immune, endocrine, and neuropeptide systems are altered" (Guzzetta, 1988, p. 268). There is, likewise, a psychological response in that there is a reduction of tensions, anxiety, and fear.

There is a skill in selecting music to be played for therapy. Certain types of music have been shown to produce physiological benefits consistently, regardless of the clients' ages, cultural backgrounds, and musical preferences, and these are Baroque, classical, and New Age music (Harvey, 1987). These forms of music usually have a beat that is slower than the human heart rate. Music for therapy is not necessarily the music a client would choose to hear for entertainment; however, there is always a matter of personal preference that must be assessed. Researchers have demonstrated that playing music has a desired effect in reducing anxiety in surgical patients (McClelland, 1979; Moss, 1988) and in assisting clients having sleep disturbances to sleep (Mornhinweg & Voignier, 1995).

RESEARCH HIGHLIGHT

Use of Music Therapy for Sleep Disturbance in the Elderly

STUDY PROBLEM/PURPOSE

Researchers conducted a study on the effect of listening to tape recorded music as an intervention to promote sleep in 25 elderly, community-based subjects who had volunteered for the study.

METHODS

Subjects were visited by the researcher in their homes and were given tape recorders, headphones, and tapes of both Baroque and New Age music. Subjects were instructed to continue with typical bedtime rituals and to listen to the tapes if unable to fall asleep. If subjects had problems waking earlier than the desired time, they were instructed to listen to the tapes at that time.

FINDINGS

Twenty-four of the 25 subjects reported that their sleep problems were at least somewhat reduced by the music. A majority believed that the music helped them to fall asleep, return to sleep quicker if awakened during the night, or sleep longer in the morning. Both types of music appeared to assist the subjects with their sleep problems.

IMPLICATIONS

Music appears to be an effective, noninvasive, and self-administered, nonpharmacological intervention for sleep disturbances in the elderly.

From "Music for Sleep Disturbance in the Elderly," by G. C. Mornhinweg and R. R. Voignier, 1995, *Journal of Holistic Nursing, 13,* pp. 248–254.

Pet-Assisted Therapy

The idea that pets can provide companionship, affection, and comfort is not new. In health care settings, however, the notion of bringing animals into agencies for the express purpose of providing therapy is still somewhat new. **Animal-assisted therapy** is the purposeful use of animals to provide affection, attention, diversion, and/or relaxation (McCloskey & Bulechek, 1996). The concept is based on a growing knowledge of benefits that animals can provide to the sick, the elderly, and the isolated (Barba, 1995). Pets, particularly dogs, puppies, and cats, have been shown to decrease feelings of loneliness. One investigation suggests that visiting volunteers and pets to a nursing home re-create "an aura of domesticity for residents who had been cut off from home and families by age and illness" (Savishinsky, 1992, p. 1325). In one hospice program, the introduction of a resident miniature poodle appeared to have facilitated staff-client interactions, eased client-visitor relations, and improved staff and client morale on a situational basis (Chinner & Dalziel, 1991). In another setting, the presence of a dog facilitated socialization among nursing home residents attending a socialization group (Fick, 1993). In addition, animals may be brought into a facility to meet the clients' need for diversional activity (Rantz, 1991). In these situations, the clients are encouraged to play with the animals,

RESEARCH HIGHLIGHT

Presence of a Dog in a Socialization Group

STUDY PROBLEM/PURPOSE

Researchers report a study to determine if presence or absence of a dog would have an observed effect on the frequency and types of social interaction among nursing home residents during a socialization group.

METHODS

A group of 36 residents was evaluated under two conditions: one with a dog and one without.

FINDINGS

A significant difference in verbal interactions occurred with the dog present.

IMPLICATIONS

The researchers conclude that these findings are consistent with prior work in the subject and state that animal-assisted therapy programs are "an effective medium for increasing socialization among residents in long-term care facilities."

From "The Influence of an Animal on Social Interactions of Nursing Home Residents in a Group Setting," by K. M. Fick, 1993, *American Journal of Occupational Therapy, 47,* pp. 529–534.

feed them, and groom them. The use of animals for therapy is still being investigated, but there seems to be evidence that, at least for some clients, introduction of pets into the care facility has positive effects on emotions, socialization, and adjustment.

NURSING ROLE IN SOMATIC INTERVENTIONS

Anger Control Assistance

Control of anger and escalating violence is an important part of psychiatric care. In inpatient units, one expects to be in contact with clients who are hospitalized because they are unable to control their own behaviors and are assessed to be a risk either to themselves or to others. Similarly, nurses in emergency departments should be prepared to interact with both clients and family members who are experiencing anger and at risk for losing control.

Anger control assistance is defined as a nursing intervention aimed at facilitation of the expression of anger in an adaptive and nonviolent manner (McCloskey & Bulechek, 1996). For the psychiatric nurse, anger control includes establishing a basic level of trust and rapport with the client and using a calm and reassuring manner. The nurse should use every means possible to learn from the client (or his family/friends) what situations are likely to bring on anger. Further, the nurse should encourage the client to let the nursing staff know when he is feeling tension. While the nurse has a responsibility to help the client learn to deal with his anger, she also has a clear duty to assess for inappropriate aggression and intervene before it is expressed.

Some of the techniques used in anger control include limiting access to frustrating situations, providing physical outlets for expression of anger or tension [such as punching bags, large motor activities (sports), and use of anger journals], and ensuring that a client for whom anger is a

---

NURSING TIP

Assessing for Risk of Violence

- Be aware of those clients with past history of violence and poor impulse control.

- Observe the client's body language: Notice changes in behavior, words, or dress.

- Assess for aggressive behaviors, increasing tensions, clenched fists, loud or angry tone of voice, narrowed eyes, and pacing.

    Remember that hostility tends to be contagious. Do not reciprocate with anger and hostility!

---

problem is given enough personal space that he does not have to feel encroached upon by others when he is unable to tolerate environmental stimuli. However, even when all of the techniques available are used to assist the client to remain in control, there are times when the client must be physically stopped from harming himself or others.

There are two commonly used interventions for situations where the client is out of control: use of physical restraints and use of seclusion. These external controls may be used only when there is no other option for protecting the client and/or others.

Physical Restraints

Physical restraints, usually leather straps, are used to immobilize a person who is clearly dangerous to self or others and there is sufficient risk of harm. Physical restraints may be applied only under the direction and supervision of a Registered Nurse and must comply with state laws regarding their use. In almost all cases, there must be a physician's order to apply the restraints, and there must be clearly documented evidence that the restraints were needed. Some of the observable behaviors indicating that restraints are necessary include increased motor activity, verbal and/or physical threats, overresponsiveness to stimuli, and actual physical assault.

To be effective, application of physical restraints must be done quickly, as soon as the decision is made that they are needed. Sufficient numbers of staff persons must be present to restrain the client, to maintain privacy from other patients during the process, and to maintain the client's dignity. The staff members should carry out the restraining procedure in a matter-of-fact, nonemotional manner and never give the indication that the restraints are being used as punishment. The reason for the restraints must be given to the client, for example, "We are going to restrain you now, because you are not in control of yourself. You will be restrained so that you can regain your control."

While in restraints, the client must be observed, and he cannot be left alone. The restraints are padded to avoid circulation problems and skin breakdown; however, these potential problems must be assessed. The nurse should ensure that the client is restrained in a position of anatomical alignment, that his vital signs are checked, that he is observed for any sign of circulatory impairment, and that a staff person is available to talk to the client. Basic needs for food, fluid, and elimination must be met. The client should not be restrained any longer than is absolutely necessary. In general, if the client requires restraints for longer than 2 hours, the restraints must be removed for at least 5 minutes every 2 hours, so that the extremity can be assessed. The nurse should always check the institutional guidelines and policies for specific expectations.

Seclusion

Seclusion is the process of confining a client to a single room. The room may be locked or unlocked, and it may have furnishings or it may not. The purpose of seclusion is to provide security, to remove the client from a situation of escalating anger and violence, and to remove the client who is hypersensitive to environmental stimuli from the stimulation of a hospital unit. Seclusion, like the use of physical restraints, can be used only when all other avenues for control have been exhausted. The client must be told what is happening and why. He must not be left alone; a staff member should be assigned to observe the client, usually from the doorway. Seclusion is an enforced "time out" where the client is removed from the situation only long enough that he can calm down, regain a sense of control, and then reenter the unit. It should be noted that a general policy in many institutions is that suicidal clients should not be secluded; they may harm themselves, even if the staff have removed potentially dangerous objects and clothing. As in the case of physical restraints, there must be a physician's order to use seclusion, there must be clear documentation of the indications for seclusion, and there must be a record of staff observations and nursing care provided during the seclusion period.

Reentry of the Client to the Unit

When the client is ready to come out of restraints or seclusion, the nurse must reassure the client that the staff will assist him in learning how to deal with anger in a non-violent way and take steps to help him. The nurse should establish the clear expectation that the client can and will learn to control his behavior. Some interventions that are useful are to help the client identify what makes him angry, assist him to plan strategies to prevent the escalation of the anger, help the client to learn of calming measures (such as taking a "time out"), and provide role models of persons who can appropriately deal with anger. In all situations where anger has been handled appropriately, the nurse should provide positive reinforcement (McCloskey & Bulechek, 1996).

Light Therapy

Light therapy (or **phototherapy**) is a treatment for individuals with Seasonal Affective Disorder (SAD) (described in Chapter 12), a nonpsychotic depression experienced during winter months. Seasonal Affective Disorder is a cyclical illness, and in most cases, episodes begin in fall or winter and remit in spring. The prevalence of winter-type SAD appears to vary with latitude, age, and sex. Prevalence increases with higher latitudes, younger persons are at higher risk than older adults, and women comprise 60% to 90% of persons with the illness (American Psychiatric Association, 1996).

Light therapy is an intervention that provides artificial lighting, brighter than indoor lighting, to the environment of an individual experiencing SAD. It relieves symptoms in about 75% of persons with SAD. Light therapy needs to be administered by a knowledgeable professional and consists of exposing clients to artificial therapeutic lighting, which is about 5 to 20 times brighter than indoor lighting. Lights with a set of broad-spectrum fluorescent bulbs have been designed to produce the intensity and color of outdoor daylight. Persons with SAD sit in their homes with such lights and engage in their usual activities—eating, reading, and so on. A newer device, a "light visor" or "light goggle," has been developed so that a person can wear the device about the head. The advantage of such devices is that the person may walk about while receiving treatment. The amount of light required to achieve remission of symptoms seems to vary with individuals and with the intensity of the light. In general, the brighter the light, the more effective the treatment.

Light therapy seems to have positive effects on depressive symptoms within 1 week of initiating treatment. While the mechanism of action is unknown, it is clear that light therapy is based on biological rhythms and provides the equivalent of bright outdoor light to persons living in dark winter climates. The nurses' role is to explain the treatment, assist the person to obtain and set up light sources in the home, and support their use. Light therapy is an important alternative to drug treatment for the nearly 15 million Americans who experience SAD.

COLLABORATIVE INTERVENTIONS IN PSYCHIATRIC SOMATIC TREATMENTS

Electroconvulsive Therapy

Electroconvulsive Therapy is a somatic treatment that, while rarely used in current psychiatric settings, has a role in the management and control of symptoms otherwise unresponsive to therapy and medication. **Electroconvulsive therapy (ECT)** is the passage of an electrical stimulus to the brain to produce a seizure. It has been used for more than a century, and, as a therapy, it has had its critics and its supporters. Electroconvulsive therapy emerged as a treatment in the 1930s at a time when psychiatrists believed that schizophrenia and epilepsy were incompatible (Keltner & Folks, 1993). Early advocates of ECT thought this treatment would result in dramatic cures for many disorders. And while there was a clearly documented effect for some conditions, the treatment did not prove to be the cure early advocates had hoped for. Although ECT was used for a wide range of disorders, it became increasingly clear that it was most effective in treatment of depressive illness and mania (Bolwig, 1993). Still, the reasons for its outcomes are not clear.

During the 1960s and 1970s, ECT came under harsh criticism, and its use declined dramatically. In the ensuing years, the actual procedure for administering the treatment was changed, such that ECT is currently modified by brief anesthesia, relaxation with succinylcholine, and ventilation with oxygen. Further, there is careful estimation of the seizure threshold, whereby the physician can administer a precise amount of current with few unwanted effects on cognitive function (Bolwig, 1993). As a treatment, ECT is considered safe and has fewer side effects and risks than many medications. In the 1980s, the use of ECT increased once again but only in highly selected cases. Currently, the indications for ECT include cases of major depression that have not responded to other treatments, severe suicidal tendencies, acute mania, and catatonia.

ECT has been used for years, but the technique has been modified such that the client does not experience a full grand mal seizure, as in years past. For the client today there is passage of an electrical current for 0.5 to 2 seconds only; the resulting seizure lasts between 20 and 120 seconds (Keltner & Folks, 1993). Those who read past accounts of ECT must remember that there is a clear distinction between the "old" ECT and its current use and that the descriptions found in novels are examples of the old procedure.

Pharmacological Aspects of ECT

Modern ECT is administered under highly controlled settings and is quite safe, even for medically ill individuals (Knos, Sung, Cooper, & Stoundenine, 1990). In some settings an anesthesiologist always participates in ECT, whereas in others the psychiatrist serves to monitor anesthesia as well as to supervise shock administration. The ECT anesthesia typically involves a short-acting barbiturate [methohexital (Brevital)] followed by succinylcholine to produce muscle paralysis. As for many surgical procedures, premedication with atropine (usually 0.4 to 0.6 mg intramuscular or subcutaneous) is given an hour before ECT. Mechanical ventilation with 100% oxygen is provided prior to inducing electrical seizure activity and until the effects of succinylcholine paralysis wear off and the client is able to breathe on his or her own, typically about 5 minutes (Keltner & Folks, 1993).

Nursing Care

As for any procedure, a consent form must be signed. The client will receive nothing by mouth from midnight the night before the treatment, and preprocedure medications such as atropine must be given as ordered. The client should be asked to urinate before the treatment; hairpins, dentures, and so on should be removed. Vital signs should be taken and recorded. During the procedure the nurse will assist in monitoring the vital signs and electroencephalography. Postprocedure, the nurse will monitor for respiratory difficulties and will continue to assess vital signs. Electroconvulsive therapy causes confusion, so the nurse will need to reorient the client and observe for level of confusion/orientation after each treatment and during a series of treatments.

≋ KEY CONCEPTS

◆ Complementary modalities, such as guided imagery, hypnosis, relaxation, massage, therapeutic touch, music therapy, and pet-assisted therapy, are nursing interventions that are being used as an adjunct to medical care and psychiatric treatments that are thought to have effects on stress, sleep disturbance, anxiety, and/or other emotions.

◆ Each of the complementary modalities addressed in this chapter is included in the Nursing Interventions Classification and is being researched by nurses.

◆ Anger control assistance requires that the nurse develop a sense of trust with the client and carefully observe any signs of escalating anger.

◆ Use of physical restraints and/or seclusion is appropriate when there are no other means to ensure safety.

◆ Light therapy is a useful treatment for Seasonal Affective Disorder (SAD) and involves bringing high-intensity lighting into the homes and environments of affected individuals.

◆ Electroconvulsive therapy (ECT) is a treatment involving an electrical shock to the brain and is indicated in highly specific situations.

≋ REVIEW QUESTIONS AND ACTIVITIES

1. For each of the complementary modalities listed, describe a client population for whom the intervention would be appropriate:

    a. Relaxation and guided imagery

    b. Hypnosis

    c. Massage

    d. Energy-based modalities

    e. Music therapy

    f. Pet-assisted therapy

2. Describe a situation where you observed escalating anger in a client.

3. Identify four things you can do to assist a client to gain control of his anger.

4. Describe the indications for physical restraints and seclusion. Examine the policy at your own facility.

5. Suggest ways you could support a client undergoing light therapy for SAD in his home.

6. Review the indications for ECT and the nursing responsibilities.

⚛ EXPLORING THE WEB

◆ Visit this text's "Online Companion™" on the Internet at **http://www.DelmarNursing.com** for further information on complementary and somatic therapies

◆ Try searching the Web using the phrases "psychiatric treatment and complementary therapies" and "psychiatric treatment and somatic therapies."

◆ What resources are listed for complementary and somatic therapies and health care professionals?

◆ What organizations or professional journals could you search for information on nursing and complementary and somatic therapies?

◆ What other key terms might you search (e.g., guided imagery, therapeutic massage, energy-based modalities, music therapy)?

〰 REFERENCES

American Psychiatric Association *Diagnostic and Statistical Manual of Mental Disorders*, Fourth Edition. Washington, DC: American Psychiatric Association.

Baram, D. A. (1995). Hypnosis in reproductive health care: A review and case reports. *Birth, 22*, 37–42.

Barba, B. E. (1995). The positive influence of animals: Animal-assisted therapy in acute care. *Clinical Nurse Specialist, 9*, 199–202.

Barnett, K. (1972). A survey of the current utilization of touch by health team personnel with hospitalized patients. *International Journal of Nursing Studies, 9*, 195–209.

Bolwig, T. G. (1993). Biological treatments other than drugs. In N. Sartorius, G. de Girolamo, G. Andrews, G. A. German, & L. Eisenberg (Eds.), *Treatment of mental disorders: A review of effectiveness* (pp. 91–128). Washington, DC: American Psychiatric Press.

Bufe, G. (1994). Guided imagery with depressed children. In R. M. Carroll-Johnson (Ed.), *Classification of nursing diagnoses: Proceedings of the tenth conference* (p. 371). Philadelphia: JB Lippincott.

Burnside, I. M. (1973, December). Touch is talking. *American Journal of Nursing*, pp. 2060–2066.

Chinner, T. L., & Dalziel, F. R. (1991). An exploratory study on the viability and efficacy of a pet-facilitated therapy project within a hospice. *Journal of Palliative Care, 7*, 13–20.

Fick, K. M. (1993). The influence of an animal on social interactions of nursing home residents in a group setting. *American Journal of Occupational Therapy, 47*, 529–534.

Frisch, N., & Kelley, J. (1996). *Healing life's crises: A guide for nurses*. Albany, NY: Delmar.

Gange, D., & Toye, R. C. (1994). The effects of therapeutic touch and relaxation therapy in reducing anxiety. *Archives of Psychiatric Nursing, 8*, 184–189.

Guzzetta, C. (1988). Music therapy: Healing the melody of the soul. In L. Keegan, B. Dossey, C. Guzzetta, & L. Kolkmeier (Eds.), *Holistic nursing practice* (p. 288). Rockville, MD: Aspen.

Hamel, P. M. (1979). *Through music to the self*. Boulder, CO: Shambala Press.

Harvey, A. (1987, December 17). Music and health. *USA Today*, pp. 9–12.

Hilliard, D. (1995). Massage for the seriously mentally ill. *Journal of Psychosocial Nursing and Mental Health Services, 33*, 29–30.

Hover-Kramer, D. (1996a). *Healing touch: A resource for health care professionals*. Albany, NY: Delmar.

Hover-Kramer, D. (1996b). Interrelationships with psychotherapy. In D. Hover-Kramer (Ed.), *Healing touch: A resource for health care professionals* (pp. 189–199). Albany, NY: Delmar.

Hughes, P., Grochowski, R., & Harris, C. (1996). Therapeutic touch with adolescent psychiatric patients. *Journal of Holistic Nursing, 14*, 6–23.

Kaye, J. M., & Schindler, B. A. (1990). Hypnosis on a consultation liaison service. *General Hospital Psychiatry, 12*, 379–383.

Keegan, L. (1988). Touch: Connecting with the healing power. In L. Keegan, B. Dossey, C. Guzzetta, & L. Kolkmeier (Eds.), *Holistic nursing practice* (pp. 331–355). Rockville, MD: Aspen.

Keller, E., & Bzdek, V. M. (1986). Effects of therapeutic touch on tension headaches. *Nursing Research, 35*, 101–105.

Keltner, N., & Folks, D. (1993). *Psychotropic drugs*. St. Louis: Mosby.

Knos, G. B., Sung, Y. F., Cooper, R. C., & Stoundenine, A. (1990). Electroconvulsive therapy-induced hemodynamic changes unmask unsuspected coronary artery disease. *Journal of Clinical Anesthesia, 2*, 37–41.

Kolkmeier, L. (1988). Relaxation: Opening the door to change. In L. Keegan, B. Dossey, C. Guzzetta, & L. Kolkmeier (Eds.), *Holistic nursing practice* (pp. 195–222). Rockville, MD: Aspen.

Krieger, D. (1979). *Living the therapeutic touch: Healing as a lifestyle*. New York: Dodd, Mead.

Krieger, D. (1993). *Accepting your power to heal*. Santa Fe, NM: Bear and Co.

Letts, P. J., Baker, P. R. A., Ruderman, J., & Kennedy, K. The use of hypnosis in labor and delivery: A preliminary study. *Journal of Women's Health, 2*, 335–341.

McClelland, D. C. (1979). Music in the operating room. *AORN Journal, 29*, 252–260.

McCloskey, J. C., & Bulechek, G. M. (1996). *Nursing Interventions Classification (NIC)* (2nd ed.). St. Louis: Mosby.

Meeham, T. C. (1990). The science of unitary human beings and theory-based practice: Therapeutic touch. In M. Barrett (Ed.), *Visions of Rogers' science-based nursing*. New York: National League for Nursing.

Meek, S. S. (1993). Effect of slow stroke back massage on relaxation in hospice clients. *Image, 25*, 17–21.

Mentgen, J. (1996). Specific interventions for identified problems. In D. Hover-Kramer (Ed.), *Healing touch: A resource for health care professionals* (pp. 141–153). Albany, NY: Delmar.

Mornhinweg, G. C., & Voignier, R. R. (1995). Music for sleep disturbance in the elderly. *Journal of Holistic Nursing, 13,* 248–254.

Moss, V. A. (1988). Music and the surgical patient. *AORN Journal, 40,* 64–69.

Olson, M., & Sneed, N. (1995). Anxiety and therapeutic touch. *Issues in Mental Health Nursing, 16,* 97–108.

Perry, A. G., & Potter, P. A. (1994). *Clinical nursing skills and techniques* (3rd ed.). St. Louis: Mosby.

Quinn, J. (1981). An investigation of the effect of Therapeutic Touch done without physical contact on the state of anxiety of hospitalized cardiovascular patients. Unpublished doctoral dissertation, New York University.

Quinn, J. (1983). Therapeutic touch as energy exchange: Testing the theory. *Advances in Nursing Science, 6,* 42–49.

Quinn, J. (1988). Building a body of knowledge: Research on Therapeutic Touch 1974–1986. *Journal of Holistic Nursing, 6,* 37–45.

Rantz, M. (1991). Diversional activity deficit. In M. Maas, K. Buckwalter, & M. Hardy (Eds.), *Nursing diagnosis and interventions for the elderly* (pp. 299–312). Redwood City, CA: Addison-Wesley.

Rogers, M. E. (1970). *An introduction to the theoretical basis of nursing.* Philadelphia: FA Davis.

Rogers, M. E. (1991). Nursing science and the space age. *Nursing Science Quarterly, 5,* 27–34.

Rozema, H. (1986, September/October). Touch needs of the elderly. *Nursing Homes,* pp. 42–43.

Savishinsky, J. S. (1992). Intimacy, domesticity and pet therapy with the elderly: Expectation and experience among nursing home volunteers. *Social Science and Medicine, 34,* 1325–1334.

Scandrett-Hibdon, S. (1996). Research foundations. In D. Hover-Kramer (Ed.), *Healing touch: A resource for health care professionals* (pp. 27–42). Albany, NY: Delmar.

Shames, K. (1996). *Creative imagery in nursing.* Albany, NY: Delmar.

Sloman, R. (1995). Relaxation and the relief of cancer pain. *Nursing Clinics of North America, 30,* 697–709.

Smith, S. F., & Duell, D. J. (1996). *Clinical nursing skills, basic to advanced skills.* Stamford, CT: Appleton & Lange.

Spira, J. L., & Speigel, D. (1992). Hypnosis and related techniques in pain management. *Hospice Journal, 8,* 89–119.

Synder, M., Egan, E. C., & Burns, K. R. (1995). Efficacy of hand massage in decreasing agitation behaviors associated with care activities in persons with dementia. *Geriatric Nursing, 16,* 60–63.

Troesch, L. M., Rodehaver, C. B., Delaney, E. A., & Yanes, B. (1993). The influence of guided imagery on chemotherapy-related nausea and vomiting. *Oncology Nurses Forum, 20,* 1179–1185.

Wirth, D., Richardson, J. T., Eidelman, W. S., & O'Malley, A. C. (1993). Full-thickness dermal wounds treated with non-contact therapeutic touch: A replication and extension. *Complementary Therapies in Medicine, 1,* 127–132.

Wynd, C. A. (1992). Personal power imagery and relaxation techniques used in smoking cessation programs. *American Journal of Health Promotion, 6,* 184–189, 196.

Zimmerman, M. L. (1989). Using principles of relaxation, visualization, and guided imagery in the care of persons recovering from addictions. *Addictions Nursing Network, 1,* 9–11.

≋ SUGGESTED READINGS

Dossey, B. (1997). *Core curriculum for holistic nursing.* Gaithersburg, MD: Aspen.

Dossey, B., Keegan, L., Guzzetta, C., & Kolkmeier, L. (1995). *Holistic nursing: Handbook for practice.* Gaithersburg, MD: Aspen.

≋ RESOURCES

American Holistic Nurses Association
2733 E. Lakin Dr, Ste 2
Flagstaff, AZ 86004-2130

Colorado Center for Healing Touch
198 Union Blvd. #204
Lakewood, CO 80228

Academy for Guided Imagery
PO Box 2070
Mill Valley, CA 94942

National Association of Nurse Massage Therapists
PO 1173
Abita Springs, LA 70420

Nurse Healers Professional Associates
PO Box 444
Allison Park, PA 15101-0444

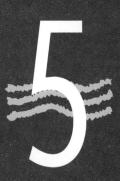

5

CARING FOR THE NURSE

Psychiatric nursing can often be demanding and stressful. How can the nurse protect herself against stress and burnout? What are some movies to watch that illustrate the experience of mental illness?

These questions are answered in the content of this unique unit, *Caring for the Nurse*.

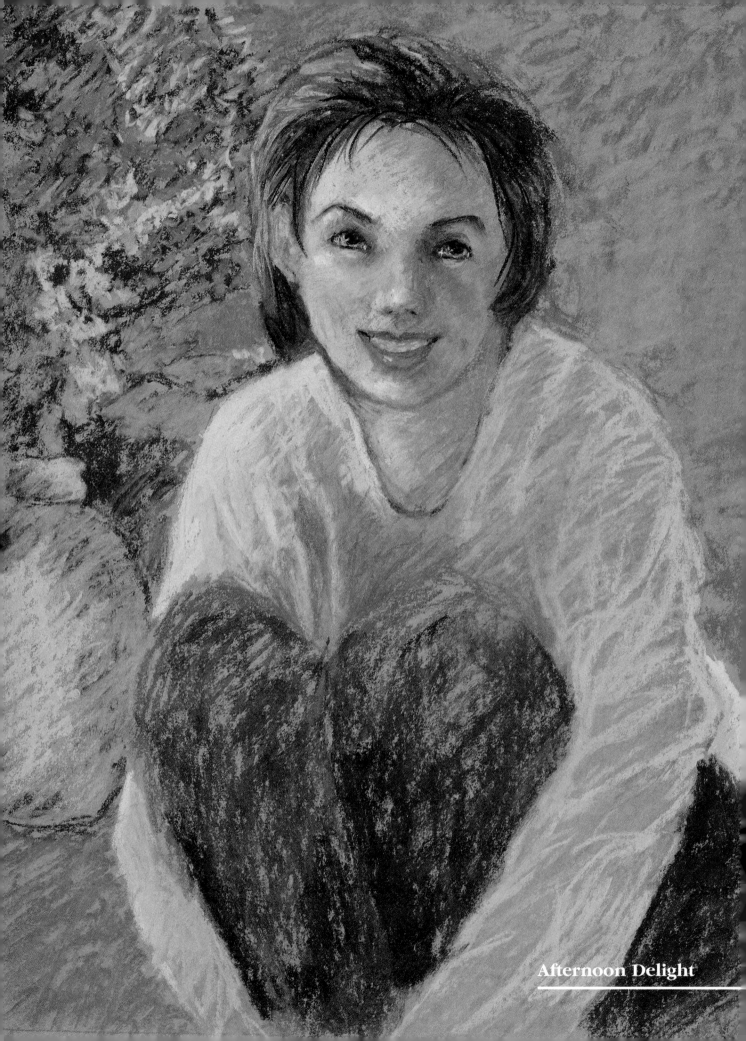

Afternoon Delight

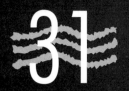

Chapter

31

SELF-CARE MODALITIES

Karilee Halo Shames
Dorothea Hover-Kramer

Who Cares for the Caregiver?

Have you ever felt, after a difficult day at work, that you had
nothing left to give? That you were drained? That you were
depleted?

Did you ever wish you had learned in your academic training:
- How to use your mind to heal your body?
- How self-hypnosis could make you more effective in
  your nursing work?
- The health benefits of traveling mentally to a peaceful,
  inner place?
- The value of support groups and how to create them?
- The role that humor plays in the healing process?
- How to balance and center yourself?

At first, these questions may appear unusual or perhaps
unrelated to nursing. As you think about them, you will
recognize how caring for your own health and emotional
well-being opens a whole new avenue for the further
development of your professional life and chosen career.
In psychiatric nursing, especially, we are exposed to mental
aberrations and severe emotional distresses that can lead to
rapid professional burnout. This can be avoided through
effective self-care interventions.

This chapter focuses on the role of the nurse as self-healer,
presenting techniques and tools to support your healthy
professional development.

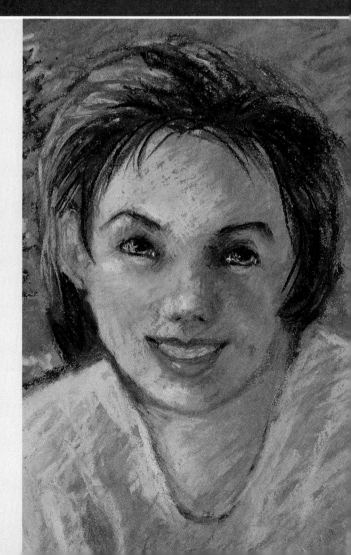

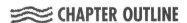 **CHAPTER OUTLINE**

SELF-CARE: A NEW MODALITY FOR PSYCHIATRIC NURSES

Attitudes

Behaviors

Practices

SELF-CARE MODALITIES

Imagery

Relaxation through Meditation

Self-Hypnosis

Energy Balancing/Centering

Humor

Support Groups

NURSING SELF-CARE PROCESS

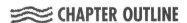 **COMPETENCIES**

Upon completion of this chapter, the reader should be able to:

1. Define meditation, imagery, and self-hypnosis.
2. Describe the differences among these three self-help modalities.
3. Explain the importance of self-help for psychiatric caregivers.
4. Describe a few means by which support groups can develop.
5. Identify three ways in which humor promotes healing.
6. Employ the use of relaxation and imagery for self-care.
7. Identify two reasons for centering prior to entering a psychiatric care unit.
8. Use the nursing self-care process to achieve a higher level of personal wellness as a caregiver.

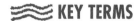 **KEY TERMS**

Burnout Description for caregivers who find themselves unable to provide the quality of care that is desirable; characterized by depletion of energy, decreased ability to concentrate, and a sense of hopelessness.

Circadian Rhythm Biorhythm that determines human responses to the environment; refers to attention span in relation to the presence or absence of daylight.

Parasympathetic System Response Nervous system response that works in opposition to the sympathetic nervous system, bringing about a decrease in heart and respiratory rates, dilation of peripheral blood vessels, muscle relaxation, lowered blood pressure, and increased flow of endorphins.

Sympathetic System Response Nervous system responses to stress that include increased heart rate, breathing, and blood pressure; constriction of peripheral blood vessels; muscle tension; gastric hyperacidity; release of adrenaline; and formation of cortisol.

Victim Consciousness Belief that one is at the mercy of circumstances beyond one's control.

Throughout this text, we have explored various aspects of psychiatric nursing. We have examined mental health nursing, as well as clients, students, institutions, diagnostic systems, nurse-client relationships, psychiatric disorders, and treatment modalities. We have had the opportunity to consider how various psychiatric diagnoses are viewed by the people experiencing them. We have observed emotional instability, whether it is reflected in a chronic state of low energy, as in depression, or in a fluctuating mood disorder, such as in bipolar illness. In all of these situations, the caregiver is challenged to bring a sense of balance and wholeness to an otherwise unstable situation. We can rightly conclude that providing psychiatric care can be extremely intense for the professional, demanding a vast amount of mental and emotional resourcefulness.

The natural question follows: How does the nurse maintain a sense of balance in the midst of mental chaos? Is it possible to hold on to one's composure, to be centered, while working with emotional instability and tension? How do we, as caregivers, recharge our own supply of energy and health?

In her book *Caregiver, Caretaker* (1992), nurse Caryn Summers describes a concept she calls "the chase." She proposes that nurses often gravitate to areas that, somehow, feel comfortable, like our home environments. In other words, as nurses, we might choose specialty areas representative of environments we have endured, and even survived, in our developmental years. Her concept of the chase might lead us to look more closely at our reasons for choosing psychiatric nursing as a specialty. It is possible that many of us are drawn to professional practices in psychiatric units for reasons outside of our conscious awareness. These areas of subconscious motivation require our full attention, lest we succumb to older, less desirable behavior patterns learned in our childhood experiences.

Another nurse writes about her involvement with clients' emotional needs, appropriately calling her work *I'm Dying to Take Care of You* (Snow & Willard, 1989). She lists the many ways that nurses, because of their caring attributes, become victims to their own dependency needs. The pattern of putting others' requirements ahead of our own is both a gift and a great liability. We risk losing our sense of boundaries and seeking approval to validate our good intentions; we may be unduly affected by stress created by those around us. To use a psychological term, we may act in a codependent fashion, enabling ourselves to be abused. The very nature of the organizations within which most of us work further supports this distortion of our healing intentions. The sociologist Anne Wilson Schaef suggests that American organizations, including managed care, hospitals, home care, and health maintenance groups, are addictive in nature (Schaef & Fassel, 1988). The very fabric of our society seems to undervalue the caregiver and emphasize the administrative,

financial aspects of organizational structures.

Nurses who have not faced addictive challenges might find it even more difficult to find ways of coping in environments filled with emotionally needy individuals, some of whom are acting out and exhibiting bizarre behavior. This chapter supports the nurse in learning to be the calm within the storm, to use her heart and head to work with people in need, even when the maladies are not visible to the untrained eye.

SELF-CARE: A NEW MODALITY FOR PSYCHIATRIC NURSES

Nurses have long been considered the keepers of health, guardians of physical welfare for persons in need. Recent changes in the way we practice our art have led to increasingly less time for the application of our humanistic skills and have demanded that we work more effectively and efficiently.

Nursing as a profession has witnessed the phenomenon known as **burnout**, whereby caregivers find themselves unable to provide the quality of care that is desirable. Nurses experiencing burnout may feel a depletion of energy, decreased ability to concentrate, and a sense of hopelessness. They feel pressed and burdened, functioning automatically to meet the demands of an impossible schedule. The constant pressure of the work situation causes many caregivers to become physically, emotionally, or mentally sick. For many, the joy of their work is lost in the chaos, and they need to seek new ways to rejuvenate and redefine their roles.

Presently, the nurse is continually challenged by the crisis orientation prevalent in hospitals and other facilities.

ༀ *REFLECTIVE THINKING*

Health Care Trends and Self-Care

Financial concerns of institutions often translate into:

◆ Shorter stays for clients, meaning nurses have less interaction and relationship-building time with clients and often will see only the acute phase of illness, not the recovery phase

◆ Downsizing or replacement of trained staff with lesser skilled workers, which leads nurses to question their job security

What impact do you think these general trends in health care have on the mental health of nurses? Have you felt the impact of these trends? Have they led you to reflect on the value of being a nurse, or have they underscored for you the importance of caring first for yourself as a means of being an effective caregiver to others?

Many institutions are offering lower salaries, eliminating benefits, and expecting more from the remaining staff. Those nurses who survive have developed attitudes, behaviors, and practices that support their sense of balance and well-being in their work. These self-caring attributes were described extensively in studies of caregivers who maintained high vitality in the workplace (Mabbett, 1989; Hover-Kramer, Mabbett, & Shames, 1996). Exploring the three major areas identified in this research will convey new ideas that empower nurses to make choices that are healthy for themselves while they provide effective client care.

Attitudes

When we feel beaten down, we have little left to offer to our clients. If our self-esteem is missing, we cannot empower others. If we feel unsupported, we may need to examine how we helped to create such a situation and find remedies. We need to decide that we can not only survive but also actually thrive, despite stressful working environments.

Many nurses seem to feel that they have no power. Yet, when we explore this myth, it becomes readily apparent that power comes from within; it is an internally generated strength. From this inner strength comes ability to effect change. We are actually in a pivotal position, particularly if we understand that responsibility is not a burden, but rather encompasses our full ability to respond and be effectively in charge of our lives. When we look from this vantage point, we have the ability to respond in many powerful ways to meet and surpass the demands of daily caregiving.

Nursing is a unique art and science, and if we are to be effective and powerful, we need to reclaim our strength. We must be willing to acknowledge our gifts and limitations and to honor those who work alongside us as equal partners. To do this, we need to give up the **victim consciousness**, or belief that one is at the mercy of circumstances beyond one's control, that has burdened nursing for far too long and replace it with a renewed understanding of our unique strengths and talents (Shames, 1993).

Our license grants us the privilege to use our hands, and hearts, for the betterment of our clients. We can arrive at new understandings of ourselves as caregivers: To be truly effective in working with others, we need to be healthy and powerful, individually and collectively. Therefore, we see how the concept of the nurse as healer embraces self-care, encouraging us to help ourselves. When we have the ability to see work-related stress in a new way, we can make healthy decisions for care of ourselves and others.

Historically, nursing has emphasized caring for others at the expense of self-care, beginning with church-affiliated hospices in the 13th century (Donahue, 1985). This attitude certainly requires rethinking if we are to move into the 21st century as leaders and role models of health. We might look to the past to review the attitudes that have served and nurtured us and those that have detracted from our strengths.

We will also need to understand that the maximal benefit to our clients will be derived from a partnership, one in which physician, nurse, other professionals, and clients work collaboratively, each powerful from his or her own perspective. Nurses, while not the only caregivers, may be in the best position to take time to be deeply connected with clients, to hear the soft words of their hearts, and to articulate a plan of care to the remaining members of the health care team. Physicians have a different, unique, and viable contribution. In the midst of this, we must remember that our clients are truly healers of themselves. Our work, as Florence Nightingale stated clearly (in Calabria & Macrae, 1994), is to inspire clients to move beyond their challenges by helping to create an environment for their self-healing.

How can we best accomplish this? One method might well be to embrace an attitude of openness in our own lives, to actualize ourselves as models of physical and emotional health, and to empower these qualities through our living example. This leads to a discussion of the ways in which we might modify our behaviors to bring about healthy changes.

Behaviors

A direct reflection of improved, healthy attitudes will be our ability to work from a different mental framework. Rather than believing that we exist solely for the benefit of the client, we will need to see nursing as an art, one that needs to be approached with the commitment and creativity of an artist.

Each situation calls forth a different response from us. A nurse who is alert and empowered can respond to each request with expectations of the best possible outcomes. To do this, the nurse needs to respond in new ways: Behaviors demonstrate an understanding of the interconnectedness between thinking, feeling, and action. To be effective role models for those entrusted to our care, we need to act professionally and from a position of strength. We need to understand, on very deep levels, that caring for ourselves not only benefits the client but also is the very behavior that makes healing possible.

Consider, as an example, the following passage written by a nurse who was preparing to work with a hostile client who was dying of acquired immunodeficiency syndrome (AIDS). The nurse exhibits self-caring behaviors that are noteworthy as we move into a deeper understanding of how the word *responsibility* actually becomes her "ability to respond" with creative flexibility.

The Nightingale Conspiracy

"First, I went into the laundry to take a quiet moment. I did some slow, deep breathing, became aware of any feelings and tension in my body, and consciously released them. I prayed and asked for help and guidance in caring for Mr. Smith. I asked to be granted the perfect words and thoughts to join my soul with him in total harmony, and to be protected from any disease.

Next, I waited until I felt a peaceful calm envelop me, and I had a vision of an angel hovering near, smiling. I emerged back into the hall, feeling eager to be with Mr. Smith.

When I entered, he was belligerent initially. When he felt my calm presence, he quieted immediately, and was soon resting. I sat near his bedside, maintaining loving thoughts and sending peaceful energy into the space we shared. His breathing was labored, and I knew he would be leaving the Earth soon. Suddenly, I felt honored to be with him. . . ."

Jeannette said that at that moment, without the least hesitation, she found herself surrounding him in her arms and cradling him. . . . He burst out in deep sobs, and she rocked him for a long tender while. Finally, his sobs subsided gradually, and she felt his body relax and go limp. She had helped usher him to another plane. His peaceful smile and energy let her know that he was fine, and she felt humbled and deeply grateful for the opportunity to share in his transition.

(Shames, 1993, p. 181)

It is evident that Jeannette seized the moment to center, or balance herself, in preparation for her encounter. What she described apparently took a brief amount of time yet enabled her to be present with her client in a very real and meaningful way.

Nurses today are rushed, short of time, and sometimes unable to make the best decisions on their client's behalf. When we take the time to evaluate our role, we can more easily acknowledge that a part of our job is to handle each situation with our full, careful attention.

It may seem that we cannot afford to "waste" time in centering ourselves. Yet, when we are thinking clearly, it becomes apparent that we are not doing our job well if we are not acting in the best interests of the client. We are, after all, the client's advocate, and in order to be the compassionate presence in the midst of confusion, we

need to demonstrate healing activities such as centering before interacting with a client.

We also need to evaluate realistically how much time is wasted when we are not fully attentive. For example, when we speak improperly or impatiently to co-workers or clients, we find ourselves in the uncomfortable position of having to clarify misconceptions and to make amends. We spend valuable time and energy trying to undo problems that result from hasty actions. From this perspective, it is much more energy efficient to take the time to be well prepared in advance, rather than being burdened later by having to repair damage.

With understanding that behaviors affect every aspect of our work life, we now move on to a discussion of commitment to daily practices that will support optimum self-care and well-being.

Practices

There are a great number of specific practices that can support us as psychiatric nurses. Beyond preventing professional burnout, we want to thrive and be vital, effective, and resourceful. The holistic, integrative framework allows us to address our entire energy system: by paying attention to the needs of the *physical* body, by increasing awareness of our *emotional* selves, by developing positive *mental* patterns, and by enhancing our sense of *spiritual* connectedness.

Beginning with the physical dimension, then, we want to be attentive to the need for rest as well as for movement. Often, when the body is tired, and we are more prone to accidents and errors, it is because we have exceeded the natural circadian rhythm for optimum attentiveness, which is 90 to 120 minutes in most people. **Circadian rhythm** is a biorhythm that determines human responses to the environment; specifically, it refers to attention span in relation to the presence or absence of daylight (i.e., some people are most alert in the morning, others in the afternoon or evening). Breaks at work, therefore, are not only pleasant but essential for the physical body to revive itself and for the mind to return to full alertness. In addition, movement that allows the body to stretch to full ranges of motion is a daily requirement for maintenance.

While most of us know we need to eat regularly, we may not be attentive enough to know which foods truly nourish our bodies. Especially when we are rushed or under pressure, we may stuff food into the mouth as quickly as possible without much thought of its effects. For example, sugar, carbohydrates, and caffeine give a seeming boost in energy levels that is usually short-lived and followed by a drop in energy, while protein eaten several times during a day sustains the sense of vitality. It is crucial to keep the physical body in shape through proper exercise and diet. Regular cardiovascular exercise coupled with sensible dietary habits allow for a well-oiled machine, one that enables us to rise in meeting the demands of everyday life.

Similar to the physical, the emotional body needs nurturing and cycles of activity and rest. Attention to what goes into our emotional being allows us to sort out the feelings we enjoy from the ones that require releasing. Tension and anger in the workplace as well as in personal life, for example, need quick clearing out in a safe way. When something is amiss, we need to ask who owns the problem. Teamwork issues require resolution at the collegial level; organizational issues belong to management settings; and personal issues or shortcomings require our attention and willingness to learn from mistakes. Emotional support through friendship circles, specialty groups, and personal counseling allows us to grow and move forward rather than to feel distressed, discouraged, or stuck. An excellent resource for nurses learning to heal on mental/emotional levels is *STAT: Special Techniques in Assertiveness Training* by Melodie Chenevert (Mosby, St. Louis, MO, 1994).

The mental dimension equally deserves our attention. Thought patterns can be destructive when they are limiting or excessively negative. For instance, patterns of blaming others and saying we are helpless while waiting for others to take charge significantly limit our sense of viable choices. Even before considering our actions, we need to look at the thoughts that precede the action and ask, "Is this the best choice for me? Are there other options? How can I find more resources for myself or for the situation at hand?"

To open more fully to the spiritual dimension, we may just need to be silent and let intuition come to us. In the busy activity of our daily lives, there is usually little room for contemplation or time to connect with the true goal and purpose of our lives. The perspective that allows us to extend awareness beyond our personal selves to the Higher Self or the transpersonal dimension is a valuable ally in directing and facilitating all that we do. Seeing our temporary situations as human dilemmas within the context of a much larger picture—our soul's journey toward wholeness—lifts and transforms us (Hover-Kramer, 1989).

To assist with our work in psychiatric care settings, we now move our focus from the broad areas of physical, emotional, mental, and spiritual domains to six specific modalities that are directly helpful in maintaining ourselves as counselors. These are the use of imagery, relaxation skills, self-hypnosis, balancing/centering, humor, and meeting in support groups. Any of these modalities lend themselves to application in a wide variety of settings. It is also helpful to remember that nursing is an art as well as a science: Revitalizing the artist on a daily basis allows for the flow of creativity so that genuine caregiving can occur.

SELF-CARE MODALITIES

Imagery

Imagery is a nursing tool that has been steadily growing in popularity over the past decade (Achterberg, Dossey, & Kolkmeier, 1994; Shames, 1996). It involves the use of internal pictures, sounds, or sensations to evoke our personal healing responses.

As defined in dictionaries, an image is a mental picture, or representation of something, that can be either real or imagined. We experience emotional and physiological responses to images. We might also think of images as a thought with a sensation attached. Not everyone sees visual pictures in the mind's eye, but most people have sensory responses to external symbols.

Consider, for example, the image of a rose. As you read the word *rose*, you may begin to make some mental associations, such as a color, a shape, a smell, a bush on which a rose grows. To continue, you may recall the last time you held a rose in your hand, the person who gave it to you, or feeling the prick of a rose thorn. Now, if we ask you to imagine a lemon, a very tart, juicy lemon, you may begin to salivate. Your response is not to an actual piece of fruit but simply to the thought and sensation attached to the word.

Images are extremely powerful and can be used to evoke a wealth of internal experiences, including a sense of health and well-being. When working with our clients, we can help them to feel more relaxed by speaking softly and encouraging them to picture a scene that is peaceful. They might envision themselves lounging comfortably in a favorite place, by the ocean or in a special setting where they would like to be. It does not matter that they are actually in a treatment facility. At that moment, they have actually traveled to a different, more healing place. When we are using such therapeutic imagery, we are helping clients to direct their minds toward a beneficial outcome, rather than repeating patterns of anxiety.

The following exercises are suggestions for self-care of the nurse using imagery. As you read them, allow yourself to take time to step into each experience as fully as possible and begin to experience the benefits of imagery for well-being.

EXERCISES

The Release Balloon

Sitting comfortably in a quiet place, allow yourself to release the breath, letting all the stress and tension of the day flow out as you exhale. Do this several times to further unburden yourself. Imagine a pile forming in front of you of specific issues that bother you. Make a symbol of something that is especially annoying to you (e.g., an imposing stack of papers to symbolize paperwork). Let the pile attract many issues like a magnet. Put the pile into the basket of a big, colorful hot air balloon. When the basket is full, gradually untie the lines that hold the balloon. Watch it rise. Drift above the treetops— above the clouds—until it is out of sight. Take several deep breaths and feel lighter and freer.

The Safe Place

Sitting comfortably in a quiet place, think of the most peaceful place in which you have ever been. It may be a picture that you have seen or a place that you remember. After selecting the site, allow your imagery to develop. See the colors of this safe place. See the surroundings. Hear the sounds associated with this special place. Smell the air of this place. Feel the safety and comfort. If someone is with you, hear the person's soothing words or feel the person's breath. Let your whole body sense the peace of this place. Enjoy the full experience of this safe haven. Gently, come back to full awareness, feeling refreshed and renewed, knowing that you can return to this sensation any time that you choose.

The Image of Health and Wholeness

Sitting comfortably in a quiet place, release the breath and note areas of discomfort in your body. Image a screen in front of you that shows your body to you with exact detail of the uncomfortable, stressed areas. You may note that the areas that are stressed are tighter and darker, while the healthy areas are warmer and brighter. Gradually, let each area of grayness fill in with a healing color, or sunlight, gently washing away the distress as you breathe into each area. See the whole body filled with light, warmed by your loving breath, filling with health and wholeness. Now, embrace the picture, let it become a part of you. Experience your whole being filling with light and caring. Breathe fully and deeply before moving forward to your next task.

With these understandings, we can proceed to a brief exploration of how imagery can be incorporated into work settings. The following excerpt shows how a moment with imagery promoted a priceless experience of healing:

Dying Peacefully

A nurse was working with an agitated dying client who had always wanted to go to Europe. It was apparent that the wish would never be fulfilled. The nurse took ten minutes of relaxation with the client, mentally escorting him to a quiet place where he felt comfortable and had no pain. The nurse gently guided the client by asking questions such as "Where would you like to go?"; "What would you like to do?"; and "How does that feel?" When she looked over, the client was crying and said he really felt that he had gone to Europe, and that it was wonderful. Within two days, the client died peacefully.

(Shames, 1996, p. 98)

We see imagery as an easily used, effective tool that can be applied any time, any place. It involves the ability of the nurse to assist the client in imagining something more pleasant than the current dilemma. It can allow the client who is upset or in pain an opportunity to escape, perhaps only for a few moments, from his disturbing reality. This brief respite may be all that is needed for the client to become more relaxed or for the person to reconnect to his internal resources, making better decisions for self-healing.

Active use of the imagination, however, may not always be appropriate with psychiatric clients. There are times that using the mind to escape is not appropriate, for instance, when working with psychotic people who cannot distinguish between reality and fantasy. In these instances, the nurse must help the client to relax and "escape" within the parameters of the existing environment, perhaps by focusing on something pleasant in the room, such as a picture or a vase of flowers.

Nurses who use imagery in their daily lives often attest to being more focused, present, and powerful in their interactions. Whereas many other modalities require larger blocks of time, imagery can be amazingly effective in a minute time span. The nurse can go into a laundry room and calm herself by envisioning a peaceful scene, then step out and move into the client environment with a positive outlook. It has often been said that the mind is the builder and the physical a result. If this is so, then it is important for us to use the mind to build healthier, happier surroundings, one thought at a time.

While imagery may not always be the best tool for psychiatric clients, it is certainly always an appropriate and helpful tool for the psychiatric nurse. Our clients may be emotionally unstable or mentally confused, but we can influence their care through our own focused presence.

Relaxation through Meditation

Throughout human history the concept of quieting the busy mind has been celebrated as the art of the developed, wise person. The word *meditation* simply means to focus one's thoughts, to bring the mind to a state of contemplation and reflection. The effects of setting aside time for contemplation range from calming of the physical body to awareness of our hidden emotions to increased mental clarity and new heights of spiritual enlightenment.

We begin with the physical effects of relaxation, which were described in detail by Hans Selye over 40 years ago (1956) and more recently by Herbert Benson at Harvard Medical School (1987). In Eastern traditions, meditation had been known to have positive physical and emotional benefits, but it was not until the effects were extensively studied in the West that the benefit of a meditative practice was fully appreciated. Consider the physiology of our response to stress, which activates a **sympathetic system response** that includes increased heart and breathing rates, increased blood pressure, peripheral blood vessel constriction, muscle tension, gastric hyperacidity, release of adrenaline, and over time the harmful cortisol, to name a few. In short, we have activation of the body's fight-or-flight mechanisms that may be repeated hundreds of times until the body literally goes into overdrive and develops stress-related illness. The effects of calming oneself through meditative practice stimulate the neurons of the autonomic nervous system, which are oppositional to the stress response: **Parasympathetic system response** activation brings about decreases in heart and respiratory rates, dilation of peripheral blood vessels, muscle relaxation, lowered blood pressure, and increased flow of endorphins, the body's own chemicals that increase a sense of well-being. Benson coined the term *relaxation response* to describe these extensive physiological shifts, which can be activated readily through our own willingness to learn ways of relaxing ourselves.

The activation of the relaxation response, then, is one of the most direct benefits of a meditative practice. Other benefits are the deepening of our relationship with our inner selves by connecting with suppressed feelings and thoughts on a regular basis. In working with emotionally disturbed persons, the need to experience our own center is even more crucial than in more mechanically oriented professions, such as working with computer technologies.

In the *Miracle of Mindfulness* Thich Nhat Hanh (1987, p. 11) describes mindfulness as "keeping one's consciousness alive to the present reality." If our minds are very cluttered, being present to our inner reality means to experience the clutter and acknowledge it. Mental overloading is well-known in the Buddhist tradition, in which it is called the state of the monkey mind. Observing the present state of reality, even one that seems unpleasant at first, opens a path to greater self-understanding.

Below are three examples of meditative practices that build on awareness of the breath, awareness of the body, and awareness of thought patterns. As you read the exercises, allow yourself to take time to recognize an aspect of yourself that may be new to you. Enjoy the discovery of meeting your own best friend!

EXERCISES

Focusing with the Breath

Sit or lie comfortably, stretching a few times to release any tension. Exhale fully, letting the breath flow out slowly, as if you are blowing out a candle. Repeat two more times, blowing out even more slowly and deliberately. Note that the inhalations are becoming deeper as well. Now count as you exhale, 1, 2, 3, 4. . . . Wait a moment before inhaling. As you inhale, count slowly, 1, 2, 3, 4. . . . Again, wait a moment as if wondering when the exhale will naturally come. Repeat several times until you get a sense of a natural flow, a cycle of bringing in and releasing—filling and letting go. Just bring your mindful awareness to the breath, aware of the miracle of its flow. In 5 to 10 minutes of this gentle mindfulness practice you will feel calmer and more relaxed.

Learning from the Body

Sitting or lying down comfortably, relax a few times with the breath. Then, follow the path of your body's circulation with your mind's eye. Beginning with the lungs, feel the exchange of air as carbon dioxide is exhaled and fresh oxygen is taken in. Watch the nourished blood from the vessels in the lungs move to the heart pump and through it to the aorta. Watch the flow of nourishing blood to the head, helping the brain to function well. See bright, red blood flowing to the arms and shoulders. Feel the flow in the internal organs, stomach, pancreas, liver, spleen, intestines, kidneys, bladder. Sense the flow of nourishing blood to the pelvis, thighs, legs, and feet. See the return flow through the tiny capillaries to veins and back to the heart. Feel the continuous flow of support and nourishment in the miracle of your own body. Bring your mindful attention to any part of the body that needs extra nourishment, oxygen, or love. Feel the area fill with the miracle of your mindfulness. Gently, come back to full present awareness so that you can move forward, feeling refreshed and replenished.

Learning from the Mind

Sitting or lying down comfortably, let your mind wander while you pay attention to its meanderings. As you have a pleasant thought, note to yourself, "This is a pleasant thought." As you have an unpleasant thought, note to yourself, "This is an unpleasant thought." Without any judgment or criticism, just notice how your thoughts roam around—sometimes pleasant, sometimes unpleasant. Maybe you have a tendency to get a little stuck on the unpleasant thoughts, so as soon as you notice one, let yourself move on to a more pleasing thought. Let yourself be both the mind and the observer of the mind—back and forth, just noticing, just bringing the quality of mindfulness to the experience. And, if you wish, imagine that you place the unpleasant thoughts on the back of a little monkey. Let it scamper around, perhaps running up and down a tree, as you feel more quiet and calm. After 10 to 15 minutes, let yourself come back to ordinary awareness, noting what you have learned.

Any task that is repetitive gives an opportunity for activating the relaxation response. For, example, if you wash dishes, or clean the house, you might do it in a hurry while you are thinking about your next task or you may take time to be fully present to the moment. Set aside a period of time for self-discovery. Pick up each dish slowly, hold it to the light, feel the water, the soap, and so forth. Experience joy and peace in every moment of this time. Most important, do not get overly ambitious or demanding of yourself:

Create an Inner Calmness

In the first six months, try only to build up your power of concentration, to create an inner calmness and serene joy. . . . You will be refreshed and gain a broader, clearer view of things, and deepen and strengthen the love in yourself. And you will be able to respond more helpfully to all around you.

(Thich Nhat Hanh, 1987, p. 42)

Self-Hypnosis

The ability to tap the healing potential of the human mind has been explored for thousands of years. Hypnosis, originally a term related to facilitating sleep or inducing a trancelike state, has come to be understood as a way of using mental suggestions to bring about relaxation and a change in thought patterns. As a tool for personal care, giving ourselves helpful suggestions, through self-hypnosis, is another valuable resource for us as nurse healers. Self-hypnosis further expands and builds on the self-awareness that is developing through our use of imagery and meditative relaxation states.

Using the mind to heal itself is a powerful expansion of the idea of self-healing. For our discussion self-hypnosis can be viewed as the creative use of relaxation with mindfulness and specific meaningful imagery. Thus, we are combining the concepts presented in the previous two sections into integrative exercises that can powerfully enhance your sense of personal identity and emotional health.

EXERCISES

The Equivalent of an Hour of Sleep

Since the mind is very flexible, the suggestion of an hour of sleep can actually create the sensation of having experienced an hour of sleep. Needless to say, this is not a replacement for actual sleep, but the exercise can be very helpful when a mental rest is needed.

Set aside at least 10 minutes in an undisturbed place with a timer that will ring after 8 minutes.

Sitting or lying down comfortably, use any of the previous exercises, with imagery or the breath, to relax the body and release emotional tension. Then, let yourself be in the peaceful place that you have selected. Let yourself see, hear, smell, and feel the comfort and safety of the place. Tell yourself, "I will now have the equivalent of an hour of sleep until I hear the wake-up bell." Continue to sense the comfort and peace of your favorite place. Nothing else is important. Experience every aspect of the peaceful place as fully as possible.

When the alarm rings, turn it off and tell yourself, "I have now had the equivalent of an hour of sleep." Allow yourself to stretch as you would upon waking and move forward, ready to face the world.

Helping the Body to Heal Itself

Sitting or lying comfortably, notice a part of the body that hurts or is in need of healing. Surround the body part with your love and bring the light of caring to the area. Take several deep breaths to release tension in the area and to facilitate the flow of blood to the area. Imagine the breath cleansing and nourishing the affected cells. Give yourself the suggestion, "I now bring the light of healing to

_____ (name the body part). I now fill _____ with love from the unlimited supply of energy in the universe. With every breath I enhance my healing potential and my desire to heal my _____." Feel the breath steady and surge as you repeat the affirmations. Bring your mindful compassion to the body part in need of your care. After 5 to 10 minutes, complete your work, affirming it is so and returning to ordinary awareness.

Letting Problem Solutions Come to You

Sitting or lying down comfortably, set aside at least 15 minutes to speak with your inner friend and resource about a specific problem that seems to be recurring in your life. Increase your relaxation with the breathing release, and then mentally go down a spiral staircase, noting each step carefully and knowing that you will be in a special place for healing resources when you arrive at the bottom of the steps. Count backward slowly: 10, 9, . . . , 1. There is a very comfortable chair for you to sit in and a sophisticated computer at your fingertips. See the details of this "resource place." Now, see or type in the name of the problem you have identified. Let the screen go blank, rest for a moment, taking some more deep breaths. See the possible solutions come on the screen. Some may be funny or unusual; remember not to censor them in any way, just let them pop up in front of you, one by one. Number them until you have at least three to five possibilities. Thank your inner resources for their time and suggestions. Depart from the room, knowing you can return whenever you wish. Move up the stairs, counting from 1 to 10, feeling lighter and stronger with each step. When you are fully at the top, write down what you received and evaluate the possible solutions for implementation.

A word of caution is always in order when we work with the powerful forces of the mind to heal itself. Just as the suggestion of an hour of sleep is no substitute for regular sleep, neither is the suggestion of physical healing a substitute for appropriate medical care. As an adjunct or complement to medical treatment, however, self-hypnosis can be exceedingly useful.

Similarly, coming up with our own problem solutions is no substitute for professional help in problem solving or psychotherapy when you are dealing with severe issues. In fact, the idea of getting help may be one that comes to you as you work with your inner healer. When we take stock of the dilemmas our clients are facing because they did not get appropriate help soon enough, we are inspired to receive help as soon as we become aware of issues that exceed our coping skills.

Energy Balancing/Centering

Nurses in psychiatric settings are especially exposed to the effects of mental confusion and emotional anxiety. We might speak of feeling energetically drained by the distress that surrounds us, of being fragmented or scattered, and of feeling pulled in many directions. We correctly sense that we need to "get it together," to "recharge our batteries," and to gain a sense of our own center. These descriptions of our energy levels correctly describe conditions in the human energy field. Seeing our interactions with others as the movement between human energy fields gives us an enhanced way of understanding what really occurs in nurse-client exchanges.

The well-recognized nurse theorist Martha Rogers researched quantum physics extensively. She noted how fields surrounding matter create an effect on surrounding particles. This can be seen readily with a magnet and the path scattered metal pieces will make to align with the invisible energy field of the magnet. The effects of energy fields can also be seen in schools of fish and the ways birds in flight hold together in a pattern as if they were one unit. Rogers expanded the concept of energy fields from physics to conceptualize the interconnectedness of all human interactions with each other and with the environment. Of special relevance to her were nurse-client interrelationships, the foundation of her theory of unitary human beings (Rogers, 1980).

Using Rogers's model, we see that one person, who is an energy field, influences other fields nearby. Our focused intent can help to expand and balance our personal energy field. However, if we are scattered, fragmented, and unaware, our field can become very depleted; we may even unwittingly begin to take on some of the pain that is present in our clients' fields. Thus, we see the importance of being centered, especially in the midst of chaos, stress, and confusion.

According to the work of Rogers and related theorists, we can calm the disturbed energies around us by effecting change in our own energy fields. It is as if focusing our thoughts and intentions creates a vibrational pattern that emanates outward, creating a higher frequency in the client's depleted field through resonance. Conversely, if we are not fully focused or intent on creating a sense of calm, our field can be influenced toward chaos from our challenging surroundings. In psychiatric nursing, then, we use our minds as well as our energy fields to restore a sense of balance and wholeness.

Figure 31-1 provides a basic understanding of human energy field interaction, showing how we may assist the client's energy field by allowing energy to flow from our fuller, more balanced field to the diminished field of the client, in the way water flows from a fuller area in a hose

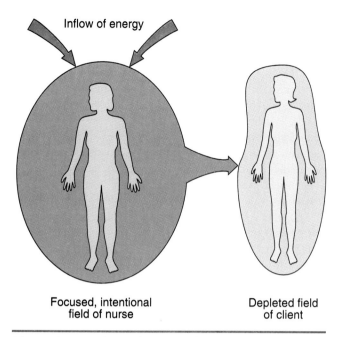

Inflow of energy

Focused, intentional field of nurse

Depleted field of client

Figure 31-1   Flow of Energy from Nurse to Client

to an emptier one. The image again underscores the importance of engaging in on-going self-care, in order to be sure our field is restored before, during, and after each stressful interaction, whether with clients, co-workers, or superiors.

The three exercises that follow give beginning steps in working with your energy field. A number of courses especially designed for nurses and other health care professionals are available to learn energy-oriented healing, such as Transformational Pathways, Therapeutic Touch, and Healing Touch (see Chapter Resources).

EXERCISES

Centering

This practice, once established, should take only 30 to 60 seconds to accomplish, so that you can recenter continuously throughout the workday, especially before approaching a client or doing something new, difficult, or unknown.

Release tension quickly with several deep breaths and full exhalations. Feel the earth under your feet supporting you and enhancing your energy field. Set your intent for the work you are about to do, deciding to be fully present to your client at this time. If needed, review the steps of what you hope to accomplish in the interaction with your client. Ask that whatever occurs be for the highest good of the client, even when you have no idea what the most desirable outcome would be. Affirm that you are fully present with your compassionate intuition and knowledge.

Sensing the Protective Layers in Your Field

Any time you are feeling vulnerable or unprotected, take a moment to sense your human energy field. The major layers of the field extend out about as far as your arms can comfortably reach in all directions around your body, the sides, the front, and the back.

Use your mind's eye to visualize your energy field as a protective egg of golden light that shines out from your inner center. If you wish, move your arms around you to strengthen the sense of your field, releasing and brushing out any tension. (If it is not appropriate to do this in your work environment, imagine brushing down your arms and releasing tension so your field is unencumbered.) If you are in need of strong boundaries around a difficult individual, let the protective layers build slowly and become thicker to form an invisible shield. If you want to make sure you can receive good messages from the other person, think of the field as a selective semipermeable membrane that lets positive qualities in and bars the harmful vibrations. Reinforce the sense of your confident, protective field throughout the workday.

Filling with Energy from the Universal Energy Field

The supply of energy in the universe is literally unlimited. The actual physical nature of the sun, generating the visible light that has nurtured all life on this planet for over 10 billion years, is a good metaphor. Even when we cannot see the sun, its energy is present and we can tap into our internal image of its power.

Sitting or lying down comfortably, release tension with the breath and access the sense of inner peace that may come by being in your favorite place. Let yourself be surrounded by the warmth and nurturing of the sun as well as any other force in nature that is especially meaningful to you. With the breath, bring golden sunlight into your body, let it flow to each major body organ, let it flow with the bloodstream, the immune system, the endocrine system, and so forth. Let each body organ glow with an inner smile as it receives the nurturing warmth. Feel the sunlight accumulating in the energy field's storage area, the solar plexus. Note that this stored energy will be available to you in dark or difficult times. If you wish, place your hands over the solar plexus to feel the continued support of the unlimited supply of energy from the universal energy field. Gently return to full daytime awareness, feeling relaxed and refreshed.

Humor

Nurse-humorist Patty Wooten (1996) describes humor as "a quality of perception that enables us to experience joy even when faced with adversity" (p. 49). She reminds us that the environments in which nurses function are particularly stress filled and that we need to remember to protect ourselves to remain balanced and healthy.

Laughter seems to be the perfect antidote to stress. For many years, she has been addressing health care providers, offering her own particular, delightful blend of humor and data about the healing effects of laughter. She presents data about the interrelationship between laughter and lowered serum cortisol, activated T lymphocytes, natural killer cells, and T cells with helper/suppressor receptors. She explains how the growing field of psycho-neuroimmunology defines communication links between emotional experience and immune response. In other words, there are messages continually sent back and forth between the nervous system and brain and the immune system. When we are distressed, the messages weaken immune response, whereas when we are relaxed and joyful, our vitality is enhanced.

Humor enables us to feel better for a variety of reasons. Physiologically, humor and laughter produce changes in blood chemistry. In exploring the research, we see that humor stimulates immune function. Furthermore, our cells are continually changing, occasionally forming cancerous cells. When the immune system is strong, it can mobilize natural killer cells to destroy the abnormal ones. Also, the emotions can trigger release of neurotransmitters from brain neurons, which bond in receptor sites on the surface of the immune cell, altering metabolism positively or negatively.

The ground-breaking work of Norman Cousins (1979) awakened health caregivers to the potential thera-peutic effects of laughter. Cousins, suffering from a life-threatening illness, practiced laughing and focusing on positive and humorous events to inspire joy, hope, and love. He based this idea on the belief that if negative emotions could destructively affect his health, then perhaps positive emotions could beneficially affect his health. His last decade was devoted to researching this relationship at the University of California, Los Angeles Medical School, Department of Behavioral Medicine, where he established the Humor Research Task Force. This project was able to coordinate and support clinical research on humor throughout the world.

Research further indicates that when we engage in humorous activities and responses, we gain a greater sense of mastery. Though we cannot always control events in the external world, we can learn to relax and release positive chemicals such as endorphins and enkephalins, thus having more control over our inner environment.

To have more laughter in our lives, we need to learn to laugh at ourselves more, seek out people with naturally developed sense of humor, read uplifting and humorous material, and stay in touch with our "inner child," the part that knows intuitively how to laugh at life's events.

However, we might also keep in mind that what often passes for humor is based on making fun of certain people or groups, which can actually be destructive and hurtful. The use of appropriate humor requires a certain level of professional maturity.

There are times when individuals resort to humor to avoid facing painful situations. Humor can be a defense mechanism, covering the deep layers of painful memories or feelings stored beneath the immediate consciousness. Certain individuals develop patterns of injecting humor at tense moments to avoid feeling the immediate pain of the situation. Some people also laugh when anxious or nervous, confusing those in their presence. This response is often a result of pent-up emotion, but it can result in hurt feelings when others are attempting to deal with the gravity of a dire situation. For these individuals, some stress-relieving maneuvers coupled with opportunities to talk about painful situations can lead to a more appropriate effect over time.

For most of us, we can consider humor as a balm to life's constant challenges. Consider a balanced diet between stressful or negative intake and positive, humorous intake. For example, reading the newspapers regularly and watching daily news in graphic detail can be stressful, activating corticosteroid production, which has an immunosuppressive effect. Consider, instead, the health benefits of reading more humorous material and watching less violent, stressful television.

Remember, we are constantly receiving and processing information. Be sure your energy field has enough laughter and fun to sustain a joyfulness as you undertake a day's work in stress-filled environments. Have you had your laughter fix for the day?

✳ NURSING TIP

Use of Humor

Though humor can be useful in most situations, there are certain times when it would not be helpful or appropriate to attempt to introduce humor. If a person has just received severely distressing news, such as a terminal diagnosis or notification of the death of a loved one, no attempt at humor is appropriate. Similarly, humorous responses can be confusing in serious situations or when important decisions must be made. Humor is inappropriate with individuals who are already challenged to understand, as may occur when communicating with culturally diverse populations, or with individuals who are imbalanced in their psychological orientation. In general, one must be well attuned to the individuals and the situation to inject humor.

Thus, it is important to relax and remember the lighter side of life, even when life is stressful. For example, consider the following entry written by a breast cancer client:

Standard Procedure:

Whatever the prognosis is
For better or for worse,
For updating: see the doctor
For uplifting: see the nurse.

(Wooten, 1994, p. 37)

In another example, written by the mother of a child with cancer, we also see how humor helps people to cope:

Humor

Humor is what got all of us through the clinic visits, the hospital stays, the blood tests, the loss of hair and weight. There is always something on the light side if you can look for it. I'm sure people think "How can he laugh when he has cancer?" Our human nature is such that we can't feel terribly bad all the time.

(Wooten, 1994, p. 172)

Each of these statements serves to exemplify how people use humor to adapt to the challenges of life. For some, there is more occurring than simply accepting; some people, through maintaining a sense of humor, actually seem to rise above a situation, transforming it for themselves and for everyone around them. This is only one of the many ways in which we can inspire and support each other.

Support Groups

Nurses are making healthy changes, but no one can change a system alone. In addition to our endeavors to be healthier, we need to join forces in order to support each other in making healthy changes in our environments.

Napoleon Hill (1960), in his book *Think and Grow Rich*, left us a legacy with his explanation of a "mastermind." He explained that a mastermind group, where many minds join forces in synergistic action or mutual energy exchange, allows us to transcend the limitations of the individual mind and access the largest wisdom, what Jung called the collective unconscious.

When nurses join forces, they are able to give each other exactly what is needed for empowerment. The ingredients needed for true empowerment include skills, tools, information, and support. Nursing has long been rich in the first three, but support has been our weakest link. We can affect our entire profession by recognizing the value of joining forces and supporting each other's goals. United we thrive.

Support does not mean we have to listen sympathetically to each other's stressful stories or that we should help others to the detriment of ourselves and our own personal or professional well-being. However, support might mean that we lend our wisdom, and intent, toward creating healthier environments and working conditions.

There are many ways to initiate formal or informal support groups for nurses. One of the simplest is to listen to our colleagues with an open heart. Many of us, facing challenging situations, find that we need to talk about our experiences, however painful, and to be heard and honored. The act of intentional listening can make all the difference during a difficult time, providing a fair witness to pain and thus releasing previously pent-up emotions that might have been weighing heavily upon the soul.

In addition to hearing each other, we can also offer suggestions that might empower our colleagues. Rather than giving advice, the suggestions might best center around reflective listening, where we reflect exactly what we are hearing the person say. Sometimes we can best hear our own wisdom with this approach. We might realize how we sound, and hearing our words affirmed can give impetus to healthy changes.

At times, it might be appropriate to offer suggestions. An example of this might be when Chandra, a night nurse, spends a long time complaining to you about the condition she found a client in after the evening shift. Rather than getting caught up in the politics or personality issues, you might suggest, "Have you spoken to Irma (the evening nurse) about this?" This act can remind Chandra that she needs to go directly to the source for positive action, rather than complain and talk *about* one person to someone else.

A support group can be a meeting between only two nurses, established purely for the purpose of support. Rather than allowing it to turn fully into a griping session, provide some intentional listening; then, at an appropriate point, offer simple suggestions by relating what has worked for you in a similar situation. Consider the following situation:

Wilma spends the first 10 or 15 minutes venting, then catches herself and realizes that she wants some help, rather than to complain. Or, after 20 minutes, Connie decides she needs to intervene to support Wilma's strength in meeting the challenge. Connie suggests, "I had a similar situation last month when working with Dr. Agrwal. Let me tell you how we resolved that. Perhaps you will get some new ideas from this story." In this manner, rather than supporting Wilma's victimized state, Connie is presenting a powerful example of how to handle such a situation.

Many nurses have tried forming support groups only

to find that they become gripe sessions with no relief. It might be helpful, in forming a positive group, to elect someone to monitor the energy, perhaps reflecting what has been happening and suggesting a progression toward resolution.

For example, the nurses on Unit C have agreed to meet regularly to discuss their challenges and arrive at policies they all agree with for handling situations. Mary is monopolizing the conversation, groaning about her husband and home problems. Doris, the elected group energy monitor, may step in: "Thank you for sharing what's going on with you, Mary. We will all do whatever we can to support you here. Are there any issues on Unit C we can help you with?"

Hopefully, an intervention like this is all that will be needed to redirect the group's focus. Some groups have found it helpful to limit each person's time to talk so it is even for all members. Each group is a unique composition of individuals and may require special handling, but ultimately people working together discover ways that work for them, within their beliefs and framework, and eliminate things that do not work well in their experience.

A good source for information on groups is *Peace and Power: Building Communities for the Future* (Chinn, 1995), which was written by a group of nurses working together for an extended period. The group came up with a framework that supported each individual, allowed each person to feel safe in telling her story, and explored what a true cooperative model might look like. In the beginning of this book, one nurse explains their mission:

Swimming Upstream

We are tired to death of swimming upstream alone; we want to feel grounded, connected, to be able to touch the earth and put down roots. We are searching for simplicity and balance in our lives, for comradeship and challenge in our work and our relationships. We feel a need for hope, for possibilities in the midst of despair, for integrity and wholeness in the struggle against alienation, for stability in place of rootlessness, for nurturing and closeness based on equality and respect, not on obligation and exploitation. These needs dictate the journey that leads us to community.

(Chinn, 1995, p. xv)

To create community, this group explored its purpose, collective values and beliefs, personal values, expectations, and goals. The depth of their joining is witnessed by the integrity evident in their collective writings. It is a beautiful testament to the power of nurses when they join together. Each group created will differ; some will be loosely structured around the simple purpose of sharing support, while others might be highly organized in terms of structure, purpose, and function.

What is most crucial is that each member be willing to have it be a safe place for every other member, that confidentiality and respect are provided for every member, and that each person be committed to speaking her truth with compassion and clarity. With these guidelines, a support group can be a place of tremendous growth and learning.

NURSING SELF-CARE PROCESS

Through ongoing support, each nurse can create goals for her personal healing journey and can utilize the nursing process to meet those goals. We can assess ourselves honestly, with the added positive support from our colleagues, and create a plan of action that is realistic for our complex lifestyles, with change built into the system in small increments. True change takes time, patience, and support as well as perseverance.

Once we establish a proactive plan, we can implement the plan, evaluate its results with supportive feedback, and move accordingly in the direction of a greater and greater sense of well-being. This ongoing process allows us to evolve individually and collectively toward a new model of nurse-healer. With healthy support, nursing can redefine its purposes, goals, and vision, and each nurse can be an instrumental part of the process. To be effective, however, we need to start with ourselves.

Remember, we are all in the process of creating new models for nursing. We do not have to reinvent the wheel, for there have been many before us who have undertaken similar work. Let us commit to learning from them, sharing our heartfelt desires and wisdom, and supporting other nurses with the same loving care and compassion that we would offer to our clients.

≋ KEY CONCEPTS

- ◆ Nurses can inspire healing in others through modeling health.
- ◆ Nurses are challenged to heal themselves.
- ◆ Nurses can provide models of inspiration to those entrusted to their care by allowing themselves to create the support they need.
- ◆ Nurses must engage in adequate self-care to remain centered and balanced—the "calm in the storm."

◆ There are a multitude of pathways to wholeness: imagery, relaxation, meditation, self-hypnosis, centering our energy fields, humor, and support groups.

◆ Healthy nursing care is a tremendous gift, one that can best be provided by starting with ourselves.

REVIEW QUESTIONS AND ACTIVITIES

1. Consider the following situation: Lucy is a psychiatric nurse who has been coordinating an inpatient unit in a county facility for 12 years. Lately, she has been feeling exhausted and drained of all enthusiasm while at work. Her staff is similarly depleted, and she would like some new tools for supporting their sense of well-being and empowerment. She would like to feel better, enjoy her work more, and contribute to an elevation in enthusiasm on her unit.

a. How could you describe the importance of self-care to Lucy?

b. What would you tell her about the role of attitude and behaviors?

c. What daily practices could you recommend?

d. What would you tell her about the use of meditation, self-hypnosis, and imagery?

e. Could you tell Lucy about the beneficial aspects of humor?

f. How would you help her to create nurse support groups?

2. What aspects of your professional life would you like to explore to enhance your self-healing endeavors?

3. How might support groups enhance your healing journey?

4. Provide an example of how you might use the nursing self-care process to support your healing goals.

EXPLORING THE WEB

◆ Visit this text's "Online Companion™" on the Internet at **http://www.DelmarNursing.com** for further information on self-care modalities.

◆ Do the resource organizations listed in this chapter also have Web sites? What types of information do they provide?

◆ What additional sites can you find that support self-care for nurses? Discussion groups? Chat room? Hotlines?

◆ Is there a listing of books, videos, or other media on self-care for nurses available on the Internet? Are these resources available in your local library or through purchase over the Web?

REFERENCES

Achterberg, J., Dossey, B., & Kolkmeier, L. (1994). *Rituals of healing: Using imagery for health and wellness.* New York: Bantam Books.

Benson, H. (1987). *Your maximum mind.* New York: Random House.

Calabria, M., & Macrae, J. (Eds.). (1994). *Suggestions for thought by Florence Nightingale.* Philadelphia, PA: University of Pennsylvania Press.

Chenevert, M. (1994). *STAT: Special techniques in assertiveness training for women in the health professions* (4th ed.). St. Louis: Mosby.

Chinn, P. (1995). *Peace and power.* New York: National League for Nursing Press.

Cousins, N. (1979). *Anatomy of an illness.* New York: WW Norton.

Donahue, M. P. (1985). *Nursing: The finest art.* St. Louis: Mosby.

Hill, N. (1960). *Think and grow rich.* New York: Ballantine Books.

Hover-Kramer, D. (1989). Creating a context for self-healing: The transpersonal perspective. *Holistic Nursing Practice, 2, 3.*

Hover-Kramer, D., Mabbett, P., & Shames, K. H. (1996). Vitality for caregivers. *Holistic Nursing Practice, 10, 2.*

Jung, C. G. (1964). *Man and his symbols.* London: Aldus Books.

Mabbett, P. (1989). Maintaining vitality. Unpublished doctoral dissertation, University of Humanistic Studies, Del Mar, CA.

Rogers, M. (1980). Nursing: A science of unitary man. In J. Riehl & C. Roy (Eds.), *Conceptual models for nursing practice.* New York: Appleton-Century-Crofts.

Schaef, A. W., & Fassel D. (1988). *The addictive organization.* San Francisco, CA: Harper & Row.

Selye, H. (1956). *The stress of life.* New York: McGraw-Hill.

Shames, K. H. (1993). *The Nightingale conspiracy.* Montclair, NJ: Enlightenment.

Shames, K. H. (1996). *Creative imagery in nursing.* Albany, NY: Delmar.

Snow, C., & Willard, D. (1989). *I'm dying to take care of you.* Redmond, CA: Professional Counselor Books.

Summers, C. (1992). *Caregiver, caretaker.* Mt. Shasta, CA: Commune-a Key Publishing.

Thich Nhat Hanh. (1987). *The miracle of mindfulness.* Boston, MA: Beacon.

Wooten, P. (1996). Humor: An antidote to stress. *Holistic Nursing Practice, 10*(2), 49–56.

LITERARY REFERENCES

Chinn, P. (1995). *Peace and power.* New York: National League for Nursing Press.

Shames, K. H. (1993). *The Nightingale conspiracy.* Montclair, NJ: Enlightenment.

Shames, K. H. (1996). *Creative imagery in nursing.* Albany, NY: Delmar.

Thich Nhat Hanh. (1987). *The miracle of mindfulness.* Boston, MA: Beacon.

Wooten, P. (1994). *Heart, humor, & healing.* Mt. Shasta, CA: Commune-a-Key Publishing.

≋ SUGGESTED READINGS

Chopra, D. (1989). *Quantum healing.* New York: Bantam Books.

Dossey, B., Keegan, L., Guzzetta, C., & Kolkmeier, L. (1995). *Holistic nursing: A handbook for practice* (2nd ed.). Gaithersburg, MD: Aspen.

Hover-Kramer, D., & Shames, K. (1997). *Energetic approaches to emotional healing.* Albany, NY: Delmar.

Rossman, M. (1987). *Healing yourself: A step-by-step program to better health through imagery.* New York: Walker & Co.

≋ RESOURCES: SELF-CARE PROGRAMS FOR NURSES

The following organizations sponsor programs especially designed for nurses and related health care professionals:

American Holistic Nurses Association (AHNA) sponsors Certificate Program in Holistic Nursing, local networking, and regional and national conferences for nurses. Contact AHNA at 2733 E. Lakin Dr., Suite 2, Flagstaff, AZ

86004-2130. Telephone: 1-800-278-AHNA. Certificate Program in Holistic Nursing can be reached directly at P.O. Box 307, Shutesbury, MA 01072. Telephone: (413) 253-0443.

Holistic Alliance of Professional Practitioners, Entrepreneurs, and Networkers, Inc. (HAPPEN) sponsors the Transformational Pathways program leading to national certification in multidimensional healing. Contact at 1031 N.W. Sixth St., Suite F-I, Gainesville, FL 32601. Telephone: (352) 337-1185.

Nurse Healers Professional Associates Inc. sponsors Therapeutic Touch courses for health professionals. Contact at 175 Fifth Ave., Suite 2755, New York, NY 10010.

Colorado Center for Healing Touch sponsors Healing Touch courses leading to certification in Healing Touch for non-professionals and professionals. Contact at 198 Union Blvd., Suite B., Lakewood, CO 80228.

Nurses Certificate Program in Interactive Imagery sponsors program in Interactive Imagery in cooperation with The Academy for Guided Imagery. Contact at P.O. Box 8177, Foster City, CA 94404-3004. Telephone: (415) 570-6157.

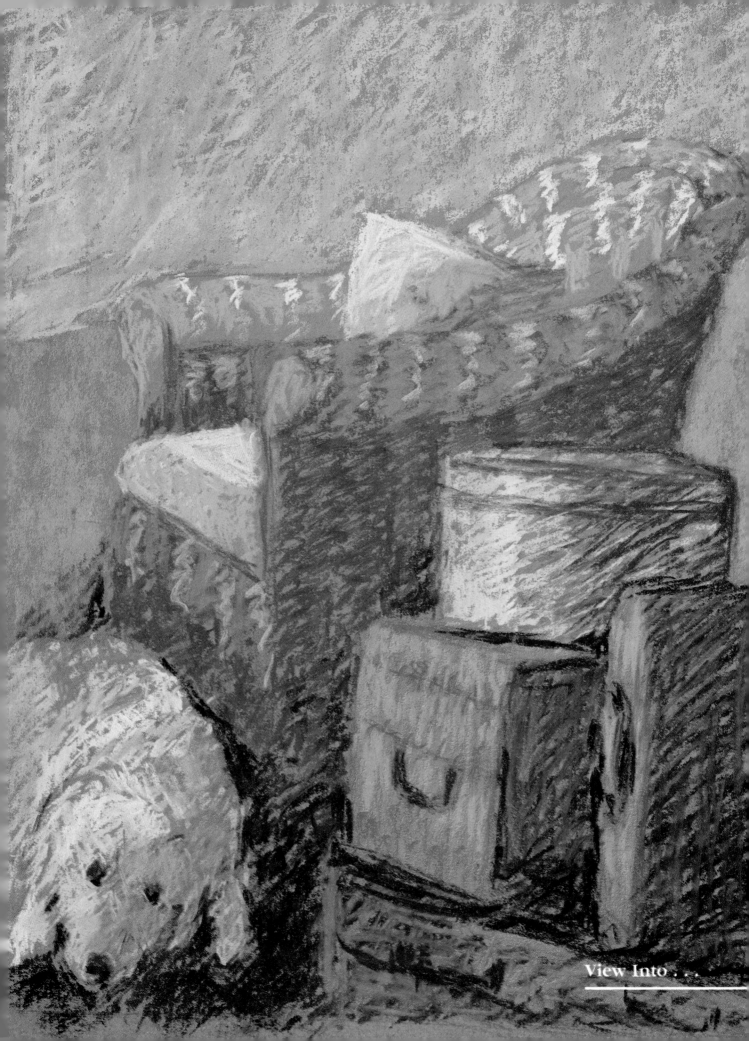

View Into . . .

FRIDAY NIGHT AT THE MOVIES

Lawrence E. Frisch

Psychiatric Disorders: A Cinematic View

Many of the films in this chapter vividly capture the human experience of emotional distress. As you view each film, consider the following questions:

- ◆ Do the characters in the movies you are watching exhibit any traits of a specific psychiatric disorder?
- ◆ What societal or cultural attitudes are reflected in the depiction of mental illness, its treatment, and the role of the nurse?
- ◆ What ethical questions have arisen in the movies you are watching?
- ◆ How do you react to the characters in each film? Does your knowledge of the field of psychiatric nursing change your response to the film or to its characters?
- ◆ How would you use the film to help clients, families, populations, or health care staff to better understand mental illness or its treatment?

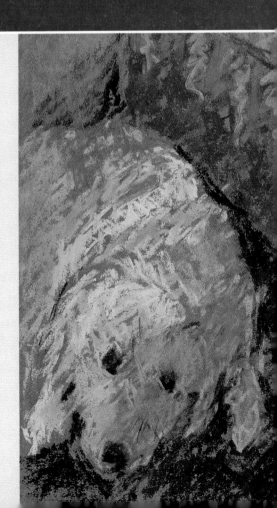

≈≈≈ CHAPTER OUTLINE

UNIT 1: FOUNDATIONS FOR PRACTICE

Chapters 1, 2, and 6: Psychiatric Institutions, Psychiatric Care, Cultural Considerations
- One Flew Over the Cuckoo's Nest
- Marat Sade
- The Madness of King George
- Down to Earth
- Day at the Races
- A Man Facing Southeast
- King of Hearts
- Titticut Follies
- Kids in the Hall: Brain Candy

UNIT 2: CLIENTS WITH PSYCHIATRIC DISORDERS

Chapter 9: The Client Undergoing Crisis
- Cleo from 5 to 7
- On the Beach

Chapter 10: The Client Experiencing Anxiety
- The Onion Field
- Vertigo
- High Anxiety
- The Fear Inside
- Copycat

Chapter 11: The Client Experiencing Schizophrenia
- Clean, Shaven
- Angel Baby
- I Never Promised You a Rose Garden
- David and Lisa
- Mine Own Executioner
- The Story of Adele H.
- Through a Glass Darkly
- El: This Strange Passion
- Sorry, Wrong Number
- The Tenant
- They Might Be Giants
- Don Juan de Marco

Chapter 12: The Client Experiencing Depression
- The Bell Jar
- Despair
- Face to Face
- The Fire Within

Chapter 13: The Client Experiencing Mania
- Mr. Jones
- A Fine Madness
- How to Get Ahead in Advertising
- Mosquito Coast
- Animal House

Chapter 14: The Client Who Is Suicidal
- The Big Chill
- Harold and Maude
- It's a Wonderful Life
- Ordinary People
- Whose Life Is It Anyway?
- Vincent and Theo

Chapter 15: The Client Who Abuses Chemical Substances
- Days of Wine and Roses
- Educating Rita
- I'll Cry Tomorrow
- Long Day's Journey into Night
- The Lost Weekend
- The Verdict
- Clean and Sober
- Trainspotting
- I'm Dancing as Fast as I Can
- The Man with the Golden Arm
- Panic in Needle Park
- Postcards from the Edge

Chapter 16: The Client with a Personality Disorder
- Heavy
- Stuart Saves His Family
- A Clockwork Orange
- Rebecca
- Pee Wee's Big Adventure
- A Canterbury Tale
- Henry: Portrait of a Serial Killer
- Gypsy
- The Secret Life of Walter Mitty
- Gone with the Wind

Dissociative Disorders (Multiple Personalities)
- Dr. Jekyll and Mr. Hyde
- Sybil
- The Three Faces of Eve

COMPETENCIES

This chapter is provided for the student to experience learning while enjoying a movie!

Remember, learning is possible in many situations: Invite your friends to watch with you, keep up your skills in observation, and don't forget the popcorn.

One of the most important concepts of this textbook is that mental health nursing is a core discipline for all of nursing practice. While only some nurses will practice exclusively in psychiatric settings, all will work closely with clients to help each achieve his or her optimum physical, emotional, and spiritual well-being. The subject of mental health nursing is human psychological makeup and variation—the normal varieties and the abnormal extremes of the human response to life events. Grief, loss, depression, anxiety, disordered thought, substance use and abuse, these are among the essential human experiences, experiences not just of the psychiatrically disturbed but also of many individuals at some time in their lives. The nurse who learns to listen to, understand, empathize with, and provide help for the emotional aspects of a client's life and illness will have at his or her disposal some of the most powerful tools of a skilled healer. The core of psychiatric mental health nursing involves the understanding of human experience, an understanding also sought by writers and, in recent decades, by makers of films. The editors and authors of this book feel strongly that there is no better way to understand nursing clients and their varied psychiatric conditions and diagnoses than by entering into their lives through reading literature *or* by turning down the lights and experiencing the magic world of film. The purpose of this chapter is to offer summary descriptions of more than 100 films, each available on VHS video, that complement the various sections of the text. Some of these films were made for television and may be difficult to find in video rental stores, while others are among the most famous classic films. Some were made decades ago, and others are as recent as this textbook itself. No attempt has been made to censor this list, and many viewers may find the violence or sexuality in a few of the films to be disturbing. The authors have tried to indicate which films should be viewed selectively, and it should be possible to choose films from the given list that are consistently appropriate for adult viewers. Your "Friday Night at the Movies" need not be Friday, nor does it have to be every week. We think, however, that the more of these films you are able to watch, the more we will achieve our goal of communicating to you something of the *experience* of human transitions and human distress.

UNIT 1: FOUNDATIONS FOR PRACTICE

Chapters 1, 2, and 6: Psychiatric Institutions, Psychiatric Care, Cultural Considerations

The films in this section provide an introduction to psychiatric care and its special challenges both in the contemporary United States and at other times and places.

One Flew Over the Cuckoo's Nest
(1975) United Artists

A very fine film produced at the height of the de-institutionalization movement. A sane but personality disordered patient meets his match in the person of Big Nurse. This film defined a whole generation's view of mental health facilities and personnel. Its negative view of the abuse of medical and nursing authority contributed to public and legislative enthusiasm for the downsizing of mental health institutions. *One Flew* is regarded by many as among the greatest films of the last 25 years.

Marat Sade
(1966) United Artists

An imagining of the 18th-century insane asylum

where the infamous Marquis de Sade was housed for many years as a (probably thoroughly sane) threat to French public morals. In this film—as he did in real life—the Marquis produces a play with his fellow patients as actors. The film is intriguing, and it provides a somewhat fanciful view of the care of the mentally ill in another country and another era.

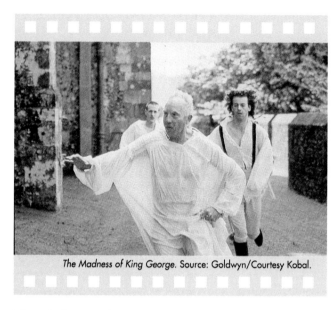

The Madness of King George. Source: Goldwyn/Courtesy Kobal.

The Madness of King George
(1994) Samuel Goldwyn Company

Another view of madness in a distant country and time, but this time the madness of King George III, the ruler of England at the time of the American Revolution. It is currently believed that George suffered from hereditary porphyria, a metabolic disorder that produces episodic abdominal pain and psychosis. In the movie George is odd, if not psychotic, and his caretakers give some insight into competing 18th-century views of psychiatric management.

Down to Earth
(1917) Douglas Fairbanks Pictures

A remarkable silent-era film starring the great Douglas Fairbanks as the "liberator" of a mental institution in which his girlfriend has been placed. The film offers a marvelous view of a now-distant institutional world through the camera skills of a (then) young Victor Fleming, who went on to direct two immortal films: *Gone with the Wind* and *The Wizard of Oz*.

Day at the Races
(1937) MGM

In this Marx Brothers farce Groucho plays a veterinarian who, through a series of not entirely accidental misunderstandings, becomes chief psychiatrist at an institution for the mentally ill. While neither a lifelike portrayal of an earlier era's mental institutions nor one of the Marx Brothers' greatest, this film is still an amusing spoof on psychiatry and the definition of sanity in a bureaucratic society.

A Man Facing Southeast
(1986) Cinaquanon

A film from Argentina about an unexpected visitor to an institution for the mentally ill. The movie describes a psychologist's attempt to determine if the visitor is truly insane or if, as he claims, he is really an alien from another world. The movie offers insights into mental health care in another culture and raises intriguing questions about the nature of sanity.

King of Hearts
(1966) Compania Cinamatografica Montoro

A notable film about a war-torn French town repopulated by inhabitants of the local institution for the mentally ill. While decidedly odd in some ways, the society created by these "sick" individuals seems abundantly more sane than that of the world around them. This is a memorable film of great warmth, charm, and humanity.

Titticut Follies
(1964) Bridgewater Film Productions

This film is now almost impossible to obtain, though some libraries may have copies. *Titticut Follies* is a true-life documentary about the squalor and degradation experienced by patients at a large public mental institution near Boston. The public outcry that director Frederick Wiseman's film generated on its release gave great impetus to deinstitutionalization. The film is highly disturbing in its shocking depiction of dehumanization but is a "must see" if it can be located.

Kids in the Hall: Brain Candy
(1996) Paramount Pictures

Most of the films reviewed in this chapter are serious attempts to depict and understand the human experience of mental illness. *Brain Candy* is the exception: a (more or less) comic story about the invention of a new anti-depressant medication. While highly successful in reversing depression, the new drug, "Gleemonox," turns out to eventually cause irreversible coma in its users. The film turns improbable, but with a disturbing hint of truth, when the drug's promoters attempt to market the comatose state as a desirable outcome. *Brain Candy* is far from an accurate portrayal of depression, antidepressants, or even the ethical problems of postmarketing drug side effects. It *is* sometimes funny and would make a good Friday night break from studies.

UNIT 2: CLIENTS WITH PSYCHIATRIC DISORDERS
Chapter 9: The Client Undergoing Crisis

The films in this section depict real or (in the case of *On the Beach*) imagined physical or psychological crises and the human reactions that follow them.

Cleo from 5 to 7
(1962) Rome-Paris Films

This French film follows Cleo's wanderings through Paris while she waits to learn whether or not she has cancer. A well-respected film from the 1960s, *Cleo* realistically portrays the stress that comes from uncertainty about illness.

On the Beach
(1959) United Artists

An antiwar movie about life after a nuclear holocaust. A remarkable cast—Gregory Peck, Anthony Perkins, Ava Gardner, Fred Astaire—portrays one extreme of possible human crises.

Chapter 10: The Client Experiencing Anxiety

Anxiety is one of the commonest and most distressing human experiences. Many films powerfully depict anxiety in its various forms.

The Onion Field
(1979) Columbia Pictures

A violent and disturbing film about the kidnapping and murder of a policeman and the effects on his police partner, who proves unable to help and (barely) escapes with his life. The film portrays post-traumatic stress disorder and the power that anxiety can have to destroy a strong, healthy individual who faces terror and death without any power to intervene. Adapted from a true story.

Vertigo
(1958, 1997) Paramount Pictures

A classic Alfred Hitchcock film (spoofed in Mel Brooks's *High Anxiety* discussed below) in which the hero's fear of heights leads to the death of a friend and (perhaps) to the death of a mysterious woman who returns to haunt his days and nights. Anticipates by 20 years some of the themes in *The Onion Field*. A great dramatic portrayal of two anxiety diagnoses: fear of heights and post-traumatic stress disorder. *Vertigo*, re-released in a much improved 1997 version is widely acknowledged as one of the greatest of all motion pictures.

High Anxiety
(1977) 20th Century Fox

In this film, comic director Mel Brooks (*Blazing Saddles*) spoofs both fear of heights and some of Alfred Hitchcock's most famous thriller films. The leading character is a psychiatrist who is afraid of heights and gets caught up in solving a murder mystery that requires him to visit a number of very scary high places. Since such "exposure therapy" has been shown to be of value for persons with phobias, this otherwise whacky film contains a core of serious psychological truth.

The Fear Inside
(1992) Viacom Pictures

Agoraphobia makes the heroine of this film deathly afraid of the world outside her home. The strength of this movie is the realistic sense of ungrounded fear that it conveys. Not one of the all-time greats, but a good portrayal of a common anxiety disorder.

Copycat
(1995) Warner Brothers

In this film, Sigourney Weaver plays a criminologist whose near murder leads to a profound post-traumatic agoraphobia. From the seclusion of her apartment she is able to help a trusting detective (Holly Hunter) find a vicious serial killer. Serial killers generally have antisocial personality disorder, but the movie is not an extraordinary example of this psychiatric diagnosis. It does convey fairly accurately the terror that keeps persons with agoraphobia out of situations in which they feel exposed and threatened. Few persons become agoraphobic because, like Sigourney Weaver, they have been assaulted and suffer from post-traumatic stress disorder. However, if you can tolerate gratuitously violent movies, you will come away from *Copycat* with a better understanding of the experience of agoraphobia.

Chapter 11: The Client Experiencing Schizophrenia

Film makers have been powerfully attracted to stories involving schizophrenia and other psychotic states. The results have been a number of powerful and fairly accurate portrayals of both the experience of schizophrenia and a number of other psychotic—primarily delusional—states.

Clean, Shaven
(1993) Good Machine

It is hard to imagine a better, and more disturbing, movie about the experience of schizophrenia. This is a film starring Peter Greene (also seen in *Pulp Fiction*) as a young man with schizophrenia trying to survive in a confusing and sometimes terrifying world. While the film's soundtrack reflects seemingly random noise and disconnected speech, the camera brilliantly details Peter's obsessions and his fearful encounters with daily reality. The plot is loosely about Peter's search for a daughter from his preillness life and about the way schizophrenia robs him, but not completely, of the ability to love and be loved. Shocking, touching, unnerving, *Clean, Shaven* is *the* movie about psychosis. Not easy to watch, it should not be missed.

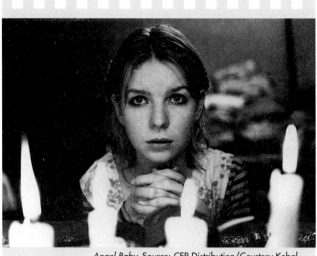

Angel Baby. Source: CFP Distribution/Courtesy Kobal.

Angel Baby
(1995) Cinepix Film Properties

An unforgettable movie, *Angel Baby* describes the ultimately tragic love affair between two persons with schizophrenia who meet in therapy. Harry hears voices but on medication is functional enough to write computer software. Kate is more seriously disturbed and has a complex delusional system. When Kate becomes pregnant, she decides to stop her antipsychotic medication to avoid potential fetal damage. Harry stops his as well, and their ensuing psychoses spiral to a catastrophic conclusion. While both Harry and Kate are somewhat atypical in having almost exclusively "positive" schizophrenic symptoms of delusions and hallucinations, they are portrayed with great sensitivity. This film joins *David and Lisa*, *Clean, Shaven*, and the hard-to-find *I Never Promised You a Rose Garden* as our pick for the best films about living with psychosis.

I Never Promised You a Rose Garden
(1977) New World

A film version of the popular 1960s book of the same name that portrays the development and treatment of schizophrenia in an adolescent woman. Realistic and touching but very hard to find in most video stores. The book is just as good and much easier to come by.

David and Lisa
(1962) Continental Distributing

A classic film about psychotic mental illness. David and Lisa are institutionalized adolescents who fall in love and, as a consequence, pose immense problems for their paternalistic caretakers. A beautiful and touching movie.

Mine Own Executioner
(1947) London Films

In this preneuroleptic film, schizophrenia combines with post-traumatic stress disorder to complicate the lives of both patient and (not completely sane) therapist.

The Story of Adele H.
(1975) Les Productions Artistes Associes

A young French woman becomes psychotic after her betrayal and rejection by an English soldier. She lives out her last years in an institution, writing letters in an indecipherable code. Captures the experience of psychosis as well as any film that has been made. Sad, but not as depressing as most other films about mood and thought disorders. Beautifully photographed and directed by François Truffaut—a "must see." (French, with English subtitles.)

Through a Glass Darkly
(1961) Svensk Filmindustri

One of Ingmar Bergman's most somber films; about a young schizophrenic woman, her husband, her family, and a remote Swedish island. A visually remarkable film by one of the 20th-century's great film makers. The title derives from the *New Testament* metaphor about the human inscrutability of God's ways. A dark film that seeks existential truth perhaps more than mere psychological accuracy.

El: This Strange Passion
(1952) Nacional Film

A film about delusion. The hero, convinced his wife is unfaithful, becomes obsessed and in his jealousy increasingly loses touch with reality. A good portrayal of the progressive development of delusional psychosis. Directed by the famous Spanish director Luis Bunuel. (Spanish with English subtitles.)

Sorry, Wrong Number
(1948) Columbia Pictures

Another film about delusions, this time with a who-done-it subplot. A woman thinks she overhears her husband plotting a murder, and her growing paranoia leads them both into an exciting series of suspenseful complications. Remade in 1989, but the original starring Barbara Stanwyck and Burt Lancaster is the better of the two versions.

The Tenant
(1976) Paramount

The previous tenant committed suicide; the present one becomes more and more certain that his neighbors are plotting to kill him. A study in paranoia, directed in 1976 by Roman Polanski (*Knife in the Water, Rosemary's Baby*); stars Polanski, Jo van Fleet, and Shelley Winters. Film is of more psychological than dramatic interest.

They Might Be Giants
(1971) Universal Pictures

This film can be hard to find but makes a good antidote to the extreme seriousness of films such as *Through a Glass Darkly*. Starring Joanne Woodward as a psychiatrist who treats actor George C. Scott for delusions of grandeur: He believes he is Sherlock Holmes. If he is pronounced insane and committed, Scott's money goes to another character, so Woodward is under a lot of pressure. Parts of this film are very funny, and it serves as a good introduction to grandiose delusions.

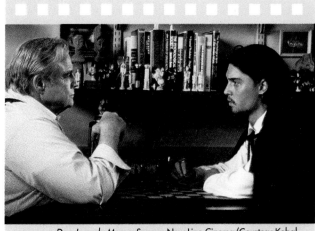

Don Juan de Marco. Source: New Line Cinema/Courtesy Kobal.

Don Juan de Marco
(1995) New Line Cinema

Yet another film about grandiosity. This hero is convinced he is truly Don Juan, the famous seducer of women immortalized in Mozart's opera *Don Giovanni*. An enjoyable recent treatment of delusions of grandeur.

Chapter 12: The Client Experiencing Depression

Loss and depression are nearly universal human experiences that a number of excellent films have explored sensitively.

The Bell Jar

(1979) AVCO Embassy Pictures

Not a particularly great film and not particularly easy to find (probably for that reason). The book of the same name (see Chapter 14) is much better, but if you can find this video, it is worth seeing.

Despair

(1978) NF Geria

Aptly titled. Features three greats: the two screenwriters (novelist Vladimir Nabokov and playwright Tom Stoppard) along with director Werner Fassbinder. A tragic story of a German factory owner whose increasing depression and madness parallel the simultaneous rise of Hitler and Nazi power. Full of despair but remarkably funny in parts.

Face to Face

(1976) Paramount

First we see *through a glass darkly* and then *face to face*, so the New Testament tells us. Ingmar Bergman's *Face to Face* followed his *Through a Glass Darkly* (see films under Chapter 11 above) by 15 years, but it is no more cheerful. Liv Ullmann plays a psychiatrist who becomes increasingly depressed and psychotic until her suicide attempt brings both help and (some) hope. Not as dark as *Through a Glass* but heavy going. A good evocation of severe depression. See it with a cheerful friend.

The Fire Within

(1963) Nouvelles Editions de Films

As depressing as movies come. The hero, despondent and alcoholic, becomes increasingly depressed after his psychiatric hospitalization. He gives up hope and calmly makes plans to kill himself. A realistic evocation of the very depths of despair. Based on the true story of the life of a well-known French writer.

Chapter 13: The Client Experiencing Mania

Movies are particularly useful for understanding mania because, unlike depression, which we all feel at some time, mania is an unusual experience of extraordinary intensity. Several films do a remarkable job of portraying this seriously disruptive mood disorder.

Mr. Jones

(1993) Columbia Tri-Star

There is much to dislike about this movie, perhaps its ending and especially its love affair between the manic-depressive patient (Mr. Jones) and his psychiatrist. While psychiatrists do continue to become emotionally involved with their clients, outside a Hollywood movie any romantic involvement is considered unethical and can lead to loss of licensure. Although actor Richard Gere is thoroughly convincing at both poles of his bipolar disorder, no other film we know of gives such a great portrayal of mania. Seeing this film, you may wish the psychiatrist would give Mr. Jones a little less attention and a little more lithium, but you will have a great understanding of what it means to be manic.

A Fine Madness

(1966) Warner Brothers

A probably manic poet cavorting through the fairly pleasant New York of the 1960s. (See this film along with *The Fisher King*, which shows an equally manic Robin Williams in a far more threatening modern New York.)

How to Get Ahead in Advertising

(1989) Handmade Films Ltd.

Is this guy obsessive-compulsive or manic (or both)? Although the hero works selling acne cream, it is hard to believe that his own pimples would *really* talk back to him (certainly an unusual form of auditory hallucination). However, no one could see this film and doubt that both the hero and the whole world of commercial advertising are thoroughly mad. A funny satire on defining one's life and sanity through selling things that people do not need.

Mosquito Coast

(1986) Warner Brothers

Not a particularly successful film, but probably evokes something of the spirit of mania. The hero moves his family to a remote jungle location. He battles to overcome a range of obstacles that seem more interesting in the book (by Paul Theroux) than they do in the movie.

Animal House

(1978) Universal Pictures

A movie whose tone is abundantly manic. So, it might seem, was John Belushi, who stars in *Animal House* and went on to a number of equally zany acting roles before his untimely death. The film's subject is fraternity life (or some fictional view of what fraternity life could be at its very worst); it includes moviedom's grossest foodfight. Primarily a cult film, but it does give a good sense of the energy that gives rise to manic behavior.

Chapter 14: The Client Who Is Suicidal

The Big Chill

(1983) Columbia Pictures

A friend's suicide leads to the reunion of a group of college friends who recall his life and its intermingling with their own. A beautiful and touching film about friendship, death, and changing eras and values.

Harold and Maude
(1971) Paramount Pictures

A 1970s cult classic that looks wryly at youth, old age, and love. A suicidally depressed 20-some-year-old and an 80-year-old fall improbably in love; the result is at times very funny and often very touching. *Harold and Maude* is perhaps a bit dated, and its view of depression may be more theatrical than realistic, but this is an often remarkable "must see" film.

It's a Wonderful Life
(1946) RKO Pictures

This is a 1940s "feel good" film that evokes a postwar Hollywood view of optimism and hope. The hero, played by James Stewart, is saved from suicidal depression by an unlikely visit from a (heavenly) angel who shows him the love and warmth that truly surrounds his life. This film is sugary and far from an accurate depiction of the suicidal depths of depression. Few nonpsychotic individuals are saved from suicide by a celestial visitor, but this is otherwise vintage Hollywood at its best. *It's a Wonderful Life* would probably have walked away with all of the Oscars for 1946, but it was released the same year as the even greater *The Best Years of Our Lives*. See them together to understand how deeply the stresses of war affected American life 50 years ago.

Ordinary People
(1980) Paramount Pictures

A powerful story about how death and suicide can stress the limits of a not completely functional family. This film garnered four Oscars in 1980, including best picture. Directed by Robert Redford and starring Mary Tyler Moore and Donald Sutherland.

Whose Life Is It Anyway?
(1981) MGM

A funny movie that raised important questions about assisted suicide of the severely ill long before such questions reached wide public attention. Richard Dreyfuss plays a sculptor who becomes paraplegic and wants to die. The acting is excellent, and the issues remain contemporary many years after the film's release.

Vincent and Theo
(1990) Arena Films

This textbook includes reproductions of a number of paintings by the great 19th-century artist Vincent van Gogh, who is the subject of this exquisite film about art, mental illness, and the love of friends and brothers. This is a beautiful and touching film that (despite Vincent's tormented life and eventual suicide) is probably more about art and love than mental illness.

Chapter 15: The Client Who Abuses Chemical Substances

It sometimes seems hard to find a film that *does not* depict excessive drinking or other substance use. Some films, however, do an extraordinary job of portraying the experience of substance dependence and addiction.

Days of Wine and Roses
(1962) Warner Brothers

A convincing dramatization of the development of alcoholism in an upwardly mobile couple. Originally made for television, this film was one of the first realistic portrayals of middle-class alcohol abuse. Now almost 40 years old and dated, but still worth seeing.

Educating Rita
(1983) Columbia Pictures

A warm and optimistic film about a somber subject, this film suggests that love, hope, and a sense of vocation can help overcome addiction. The movie offers a particularly realistic portrayal of alcoholism by Michael Caine.

I'll Cry Tomorrow
(1955) MGM

One of Susan Hayward's great 1950s films about an actress's struggle with alcoholism. This movie features a variety of notable period songs.

Long Day's Journey into Night
(1962) Ely Landau (Republic Pictures)

There are several film adaptations of the Eugene O'Neill play about a family's struggles with alcoholism, other substance use, and self-destruction. Katharine Hepburn's 1962 version is probably the best. This play and film were shocking at the time for their strikingly realistic portrayals of the underside of American life. Both the play and film remain among the great accomplishments of 20th-century American arts and letters.

The Lost Weekend
(1945) Paramount Pictures

One of Hollywood's all-time great films and a stunning depiction of alcoholic denial. This film won four Oscars in 1945, including best picture. It remains eminently worth seeing despite a less than realistic ending.

The Verdict
(1982) 20th Century Fox

Many regard actor Paul Newman as a model of social responsibility for his many financial contributions to the physical and mental health of children. In this 1982 film, Newman plays an alcoholic lawyer who struggles to recover from his addiction. This is Newman at his very best.

Clean and Sober
(1988) Warner Brothers

Morgan Freeman turns in a fine supporting performance as Michael Keaton plays a substance-abusing real estate salesman who struggles to kick his habit. A tough film that effectively captures some of the desperation behind addiction and substance abuse.

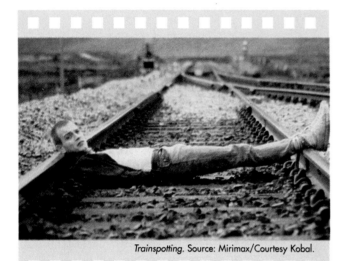

Trainspotting. Source: Mirimax/Courtesy Kobal.

Trainspotting
(1996) Mirimax Films

A violent and "in your face" movie about heroin abuse. This film is tough, disturbing, and sometimes hard to understand with its strong Scottish accent. Nonetheless, it is one of the best modern films about the culture of addiction.

I'm Dancing as Fast as I Can
(1982) Paramount Pictures

Not a great film, but a fairly realistic 1980s portrayal of prescription drug abuse, a problem that often seems less visible than the abuse of street drugs. Based on a true story.

The Man with the Golden Arm
(1955) United Artists

A great Frank Sinatra movie about heroin addiction. While 1955 audiences found this film shocking, it may seem somewhat melodramatic today. Realistically portraying many aspects of addict life, this is a film in the same spirit as William Burroughs's heroin memoirs (see chapter 15).

Panic in Needle Park
(1971) 20th Century Fox

Al Pacino's first major film, *Panic in Needle Park* is a realistic portrayal of substance abuse, crime, and prostitu-

tion. While crack cocaine has significantly changed the culture of addiction, this film still gives an accurate picture of the desperate lives of many substance abusers. Far less violent than Pacino's later films (*The Godfather, Scarface*), *Panic* is not for the easily depressed.

Postcards from the Edge
(1990) Columbia Pictures

An amazing cast, including Meryl Streep, Shirley MacLaine, Gene Hackman, and Richard Dreyfuss. Drug dependence (Meryl Streep) is only part of this story about an aspiring actress. Perhaps not one of Streep's all-time greats, but a fast-paced and captivating movie worth seeing on a Friday night.

Chapter 16: The Client with a Personality Disorder

With the exception of the antisocial personalities who flourish in *film noir* and inhabit most of Hollywood's most violent movies, few directors set out to depict any specific DSM-IV personality disorder. However, elements of both the dramatic and the eccentric personality categories are frequently and effectively depicted in numerous films.

Heavy
(1995) Columbia Tri-Star Home Video

Victor is an obese young man with a severe personality disorder that keeps him from all but the most limited forms of social relationships. His transformation through falling in love with a younger woman is touchingly unbelievable. A good introduction to odd and eccentric characters.

Stuart Saves His Family
(1995) Paramount Pictures

Adapted from a *Saturday Night Live* routine, this movie depicts a decidedly eccentric character whose family background includes nearly every imaginable psychiatric pathology. While Stuart saves neither his family nor the movie itself (which is not always funny), he does represent a striking "antihero" with charm and humanity.

A Clockwork Orange
(1971) Warner Brothers

This 1971 classic vividly portrays antisocial personality disorder. While many find the violence and sadism of *Clockwork Orange* repellant, others regard the film as director Stanley Kubrick's greatest; one of the outstanding films of the past three decades.

Rebecca

(1940) Selznick International Pictures

This classic Alfred Hitchcock movie is richly suggestive of several personality disorders in its leading characters. This is the only film that won Hitchcock a best picture Oscar (1940), and it remains an excitingly suspenseful movie whose character studies are only part of its appeal.

Pee Wee's Big Adventure

(1985) Warner Brothers

Pee Wee is too charming to be schizoid, too socially committed to be avoidant, and probably too unique to have a clearly diagnosable personality disorder. Still, it would be hard to find a movie that gives a more sympathetic view of the problematic interaction between ordinary society and a distinctly "odd" personality. A great introduction to the topic of personality disorders and a delightful not-to-be-missed movie experience.

A Canterbury Tale

(1944) Eagle Lion

This film about England during World War II is included here because it includes a character, "the Glue Man," with an eccentric personality disorder manifesting itself as an obsession with English history and female purity. In order to prevent young women from being seduced by soldiers on leave, the Glue Man pours glue on their heads (resulting in a 1940s version of dreadlocks), presumably to make the women unattractive to the GIs. Better than it sounds, but hard to find.

Henry: Portrait of a Serial Killer

(1990) Maljack

X-rated because of extreme violence, this film is definitely not for the faint hearted. However, for those who can stomach its real-life blood and gore, *Portrait* offers a minimally fictionalized view of antisocial personality disorder. The film is based on the real life and violent deeds of a convicted serial killer.

Gypsy

(1962) Warner Brothers

A musical adaptation of the Broadway play about (among other matters) histrionic personality disorder. See the 1962 version starring Rosalind Russell and Natalie Wood, although there is a 1993 remake with Bette Midler in the title role.

The Secret Life of Walter Mitty

(1947) RKO

Danny Kaye starred in this cheerful adaptation of James Thurber's story about avoidant personality disorder.

Unlike Ashley in *Gone with the Wind*, Mitty does not worry much about his pattern of avoiding conflict and involvement. Instead, he withdraws into his own life of fantasy.

Gone with the Wind

(1939) Selznick International Films

On nearly anyone's list of all-time great movies, *Gone with the Wind* is far more than a study of Ashley Wilkes's avoidant personality disorder. This immortal Hollywood epic runs to nearly four hours, and Ashley's avoidant personality is central to the story.

Dissociative Disorders (Multiple Personalities)

The concept of multiple personalities has captured popular imagination for many years. How real or common this abnormality is remains controversial among experts, but this has not stopped film makers from producing at least three well-known films.

Dr. Jekyll and Mr. Hyde

(1911, 1920, 1932, 1941, 1968, 1973) 1932—Paramount Pictures

The Robert Louis Stevenson classic of split personality has been filmed at least six times. The 1932 version is arguably the best.

Sybil

(1976) NBC/Lorimar

A television production about a woman who seems to have had 16 separate personalities. While dissociative disorder is not a major topic of this book, the film makes for excellent drama and a good introduction to the somewhat controversial diagnosis.

The Three Faces of Eve

(1957) 20th Century Fox

A 1957 drama starring Joanne Woodward (see *They Might Be Giants*, Chapter 11) as a psychologically distressed woman who turns out to have three distinct personalities. Not as many faces as *Sybil*, but a far better film.

Chapter 17: The Client with a Psychosomatic Illness

The Barretts of Wimpole Street

(1934) MGM

Few films feature somatization disorders, but this 1934 movie takes on the real-life story of 19th-century poets Robert Browning and Elizabeth Barrett. Until she met and married Browning, Elizabeth was confined to bed with a succession of ill-defined sicknesses. Somatization disorder may today present somewhat differently, but this film emphasizes what a profound effect somatization may have on an individual's life. While Freud attributed many of the symptoms of hysteria to repressed sexuality, falling in love is rarely the cure that it was for Elizabeth Barrett Browning.

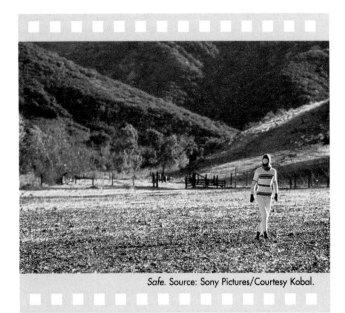

Safe. Source: Sony Pictures/Courtesy Kobal.

Safe
(1995) Sony Pictures Classics

Safe is the story of a Los Angeles woman who becomes profoundly ill, perhaps as a result of exposure to chemical fumes and odors in her home environment. The illness progresses dramatically, and she receives little help from traditional medical or psychiatric care. Her search for healing in a highly unconventional and probably exploitive "therapeutic environment" highlights the complex interaction between physical and emotional factors in illness. The film portrays its heroine's illness as primarily somatic, but because "environmental sensitivity" is a highly controversial medical diagnosis, many psychiatrists would probably give Conversion Disorder as an alternative. A good introduction to the complexities of the somatoform disorders as well as some of their unusual medical mimics.

Chapter 18: The Client with Disorders of Self-Regulation: Sleep Disorders, Eating Disorders, Sexual Disorders

Film makers have frequently portrayed individuals who live "at the edge" of society and social norms. The disorders of regulation are not infrequently depicted in films and documentaries.

The Best Little Girl in the World
(1981) ABC

A fine 1980s TV movie about anorexia nervosa. This film can often be found in video-rental stores and, if available, should not be missed.

Superstar: The Karen Carpenter Story
(1987) Iced Tea Productions

In real life, Karen Carpenter was a highly successful 1960s popular singer who died at age 32 from complications of anorexia nervosa. This extraordinary 43-minute film features no human actors after the opening depicting Karen's death, but only "barbie dolls" playing the roles of Karen and the often uncaring people around her. This film can be hard to locate but is so unusual that it should definitely be seen as an introduction to eating disorders and the way in which society's expectations about behavior and appearance influence the way women live and die.

Life Is Sweet
(1990) Film Four International

An English movie about obsessive eating. More accurately, a movie about middle-class English life in which eating plays a disproportionately important role. While not a clinical study of bulimia, this movie offers realistic portrayals of binging and purging behaviors and how they are hidden from friends and family.

The Hairdresser's Husband
(1990) TF1 Film Productions

A film about paraphilia: The hero has a "hair fetish" and finds happiness married to a woman who cuts others' hair. An unusual film about an unconventional subject, but overall pleasant entertainment despite a sad ending.

Le Cri de la Soie
(1996) Mimosa Productions

An odd but touching movie about a woman who is hospitalized because she has a fetish for silk and cannot resist stealing swatches of it from fabric stores. She is treated by a sympathetic doctor who, it turns out, is also a silk fetishist. Silk fetish is rare enough that the probability of such an encounter between therapist and client is highly unlikely. "The Scream of the Silk" is an attractive evocation of World War I France, but it also makes a particularly useful introduction to understanding paraphilia.

The Mark
(1961) 20th Century Fox

A study of pedophilia, this film effectively presents scenes from the life of a convicted child molester on his release from prison. From the early 1960s, but still a convincing portrayal and a moving film.

The Offence
(1973) United Artists

Sean Connery (*Goldfinger, Indiana Jones*) plays a policeman whose lethal violence toward an arrested child molester derives from his own repressed childhood experiences. A useful study of repression as well as pedophilia.

Dreamchild
(1985) Universal Pictures

Lewis Carroll (his real name was Charles Dodgson) wrote *Alice in Wonderland*, but he also photographed naked young girls (amazingly, with their mothers' permission) and likely today would have been diagnosed as having pedophilia. This is a fictional movie about the "real" Alice, who, more than 70 years after her encounter with Carroll, remains haunted by his memory and the fictional creations of his imagination. *Dreamchild* is a beautiful movie about childhood reflected in old age; it features dream sequences filled with stunning Muppet characters. Only partly about pedophilia, it suggests how disturbing but "forgotten" childhood experiences can remain as subconscious images through an entire lifetime.

Witman Fiuk
(1997) MTM Kommunikacio

A disturbing but not overtly graphic story about two adolescent brothers who develop necrophilia (attraction to dead persons and animals) after their father dies. Necrophilia is not a pleasant subject at best, and this Hungarian film is only for those with strong stomachs.

UNIT 3: SPECIAL POPULATIONS

Chapter 19: The Physically Ill Client Experiencing Emotional Distress

A few films have explored the human response to illness with great sensitivity.

Beaches
(1988) Touchstone Pictures

Bette Midler stars in this film about friendship and dying. A touching story about the healing role of relatedness in life's crises.

The Elephant Man
(1980) Paramount Pictures

A somewhat fictionalized account of a man afflicted with a grotesquely deforming hereditary skin disease, probably neurofibromatosis. Based on a real story, this film boldly illustrates the rejection that deformed persons face in conventional society. Recent popular films have tended to offer generous and colorful portrayals of Victorian and turn-of-the-century British life; this film uses stark black-and-white images to detail Victorian upper class intolerance.

Parting Glances
(1986) Rondo Pictures

An early account of two gay men coming to personal understanding of the tragedy of AIDS. Less flamboyant than the Oscar-winning 1993 film *Philadelphia*, but, for many, *Parting Glances* may be a more moving film experience.

The Pride of the Yankees
(1942) RKO Pictures

The great New York Yankees baseball player Lou Gehrig died young of the devastating neuromuscular disease amyotrophic lateral sclerosis. This 1942 Gary Cooper film tells his story vividly and movingly. For a more modern view of another extraordinary man's battle with this same neurological disorder, see *A Brief History of Time*, a biographical study of a great modern physicist confronting the same neurological handicap that felled Gehrig over 50 years before.

Passion Fish
(1992) Atchafalaya

This film may not always avoid sentimentality, but it offers a touching and realistic portrayal of the difficulties posed by catastrophic spinal cord injury. A vigorous New York actress becomes paralyzed and returns to her home in the rural South. The film portrays her efforts to find personal fulfillment in her newly dependent role.

The Shadow Box
(1980) ABC/The Shadowbox Film Company

This film may be difficult to find, but it is a fine movie version of the prize-winning theater production excerpted in Chapter 9 of this textbook. A film that takes place in a hospice and explores the impending cancer death of three residents. Another powerful film starring Joanne Woodward (*The Three Faces of Eve*) and directed by Paul Newman (*The Verdict*).

Awakenings
(1990) Columbia Pictures

Awakenings is a dramatization of Oliver Sacks's book about the (temporary) effectiveness of the drug L-Dopa in restoring responsiveness to persons "frozen" by postencephalitic parkinsonism. Sacks's book reminds us that persons who seem unaware and even unconscious can sometimes be remarkably in touch with their environment. A decent movie with several Oscar nominations, *Awakenings* is worth seeing, especially if you cannot read the book. Robin Williams stars as a character based on Oliver Sacks himself, and the movie features Robert De Niro as one of the patients who "awaken" after L-Dopa treatment. More about neurology than psychiatry, but an attractive film about the potential for modern pharmacology to change the lives of physically and mentally ill individuals.

Chapter 20: Forgotten Populations: The Homeless and Incarcerated

Prison inmates are frequently depicted in modern films, but neither prisoners nor the homeless are frequently given sympathetic hearings. A few films have approached these special populations with sensitivity.

The Saint of Fort Washington
(1993) Carrie Productions, Inc.

A film about homelessness that also gives a fairly convincing portrait of schizophrenia and of post-traumatic stress disorder. Most of us look the other way when confronted by the reality of homelessness and the mental illness that often accompanies it. This film allows us to hide behind the camera and look fairly accurately at a world we might not otherwise see. At times the film focuses too much on the "drama" of physical violence and exploitation; it is probable that the day-to-day experience of homelessness involves far more "quiet desperation" than violence, but desperation does not sell movies.

The Fisher King
(1991) Columbia Pictures

A somewhat surrealistic film mostly about bipolar (manic-depressive) psychosis. Some will find the psychedelic portrayals of psychosis unconvincing, but this remarkable Robin Williams (*Dead Poets' Society, Mrs. Doubtfire*) film excels above all in capturing the desperation and squalor in which America's homeless live.

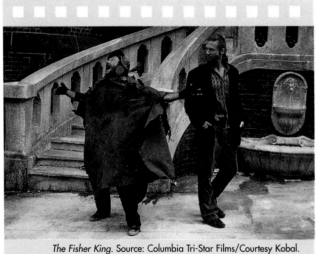

The Fisher King. Source: Columbia Tri-Star Films/Courtesy Kobal.

Dead Man Out
(1989) HBO

A convicted murderer becomes insane while waiting on Death Row. Can he be cured so that his execution can take place? Does society—and his psychiatrist—have a moral responsibility to return him to sanity for the purpose of facing his death sentence? An intriguing, thought-provoking, and exciting film. Also an excellent film to see while reading about the ethics of mental health care.

Short Eyes
(1977) Short Eyes Entertainment

More a film about the harshness of prison life than pedophilia, this film describes the prison persecution of a convicted child molester. A highly realistic view of New York penal life, with excellent acting.

Chapter 21: The Child

Children frequently appear in films, but movies about mentally ill children are relatively rare. The French director François Truffaut had a particular fondness for children and a remarkable vision of the bittersweet nature of childhood.

The 400 Blows
(1959) Les Films du Carosse

One of the great movies of the 20th century, *The 400 Blows* attempts to capture the complexities of early adolescence as seen through the eyes of a 12-year-old boy. There is little explicitly about mental health in this film of growing up in France, but few artists have managed to convey the joys and trials of childhood with as little sentimentality as does François Truffaut in this semi-autobiographical movie.

Small Change
(1976) Les Films du Carosse

Another Truffaut movie made almost 20 years after *The 400 Blows, Small Change* celebrates childhood—despite deprivation and parental neglect—as a golden time. More sentimental than its famous predecessor, *Small Change* is still a heartwarming film about the everyday lives of children.

Lorenzo's Oil
(1992) Universal Pictures

This film describes one family's real-life struggles to find a cure for their child's rare neurological disorder. This is a good film for health professionals to watch because it portrays hospitals, doctors, and nurses as they too often appear to anxious families in need: unhelpful, impersonal, and uncaring.

Chapter 22: The Adolescent

Adolescents suffer from most of the same psychiatric disorders that affect adults, but their responses to these disorders are powerfully influenced by their developmental status. Some remarkable films have captured some of the poignancy of adolescent experience with mental illness and psychological distress.

Mouchette
(1967) Parc Films

Mouchette can be difficult to find and for some is difficult to watch. The story of a lonely, depressed adolescent, this film ends in her suicide. This film has a very Catholic viewpoint and, despite its somber story, can serve as an important reminder of the importance of spiritual values in a healthy life.

My Left Foot
(1989) Palace/Ferndale Films

This movie won two Oscars (plus three additional nominations) for its portrayal of Christy Brown's triumph over devastating neurological impairment from cerebral palsy. The acting is superb, and the film, based on a true story, is a testimony to a mother's faith in her child's potential. A must-see.

Gaby: A True Story
(1987) Columbia Tri-Star

A similar story to *My Left Foot* but not as successful (no Oscars) or as emotionally powerful. With the aid of her supportive family, a young woman battles cerebral palsy to become a successful author.

Wildflower
(1991) The Polone Company

A highly emotional film about physical illness (epilepsy, hearing loss) and child abuse, *Wildflower* suggests that friendship and goodwill can occasionally overcome the severest of human handicaps. This film raises important questions about families and social responsibility. It also serves as a reminder of the potential for adolescence as a time for growth and caring.

Chapter 23: The Elderly

Old age is inevitably a time of loss, of either friends or personal capabilities or of both. It is also a time for growth, wisdom, and sometimes great joy. All of these attributes of elder life have been depicted in a number of fine films.

Age Old Friends
(1989) Central Independent Television Plc.

A touching film about the effects of dementia on friendship and family ties. This movie features marvelous acting and highly realistic subject matter. A wonderful introduction to the special concerns and needs of the elderly and their children.

Driving Miss Daisy
(1989) Warner Brothers

One of the most celebrated recent movie portrayals of aging, *Driving Miss Daisy* won a best picture Oscar in 1989. This film perhaps treats issues of race prejudice more directly than those of aging, but Jessica Tandy's portrayal of Daisy is particularly memorable.

Harry and Tonto
(1974) 20th Century Fox

A wonderful film about the travels of 70-something Harry and his cat Tonto. Art Carney stars in this film, which serves as a forceful reminder that aging need not lead to a loss of vitality or the ability to care deeply for others—human and animal alike. This film also reminds viewers that the quality of life can sometimes be greatly improved by slowing down its pace.

Gin Game
(1984) RKO

A celebrated film about love in a nursing home starring Jessica Tandy (*Driving Miss Daisy*) and Hume Cronyn (*Age Old Friends*). Two wonderful actors in a warm and touching story.

Kotch
(1971) Kotch Company Productions

A fine film starring Walter Matthau and directed by Jack Lemmon about the relationship between aging parents and their children.

The Last Laugh
(1922) Fox Film Corporation

A silent film about how in upper class European society aging leads inevitably to loss of position and status. An influential film because of its technical innovations, but also a moving portrayal of the triumph of human dignity in the face of prejudice.

Children of Nature
(1991) Northern Arts Entertainment

A warm movie from a very cold country, this film in Icelandic (with English subtitles) is a charming tale of romance involving two nursing home residents.

A Woman's Tale
(1991) Illumination Films

A film about the last days of a vital 78-year-old. Wonderful acting by Sheila Florence, who herself died of cancer soon after the film was completed. A very special movie about the richness of a fully lived life.

Chapter 24: Survivors of Violence or Abuse

It seems hard for many parents and moviegoers to find a film that is *not* about violence. The film world has been relatively slow to address intrafamilial violence and sexual abuse, but some excellent movies have treated these and related topics.

Judgment
(1990) HBO

This made-for-cable-television film dramatizes a true case of child sexual abuse perpetrated by a parish priest. An important truth in this story is that many parents know of their children's molestation but remain silent. Such "conspiracy of silence" is not an infrequent finding when children have been sexually abused, especially when the perpetrator is a parent.

Sleeping with the Enemy
(1991) 20th Century Fox

One of the better recent films about intrafamilial violence, this movie emphasizes the real danger and abject fear that affect many abused women's lives.

Murmur of the Heart
(1971) NEF Filmproduktion

There are few films about incest. *Murmur* portrays an adolescent coming of age in France and depicts an episode of mother-son incest that apparently occurs without much consequence for either. Not a terribly realistic view of a typical incestuous relationship: more commonly involving both a daughter and some element of physical coercion or intimidation.

UNIT 4: NURSING INTERVENTIONS AND TREATMENT MODALITIES

Few directors set out to write films about psychiatric treatment modalities, but some films seem to help us understand better what treatments can "work" and occasionally why. Others have looked with interest at popular or controversial psychiatric treatments such as psychotherapy or electroshock therapy.

Shall We Dance?
(1996) Mirimax Films

A marvelous Japanese movie that can be seen as a metaphor for the cognitive-behavioral therapy of depression. The hero is a middle-aged businessman who lives his life without pleasure from work, family, or social interaction. Walking down the street at night he is captivated by the image of a woman standing in a second-floor dance studio. Taken by her beauty, he conquers his shyness, physical ineptness, and the strong social disapproval of dancing in traditional Japanese culture. Practicing his steps as he works and walks, he begins to dance with the beautiful dance-studio instructor. Their relationship is limited to dancing, but it transforms his life into one of fullness and joy as dancing meets and overcomes dysthymia. (If you have missed *Strictly Ballroom*, see both of these films for a dancing treat!)

Freud
(1962) U-1 Films

Freud has fallen a bit from intellectual favor in some circles, and this film may be difficult to find. Worth seeing if it can be located.

The Dream Team
(1989) Universal Pictures

A sometimes charming comedy about therapy, murder, and insanity, *The Dream Team* depicts four mentally ill individuals who leave their psychiatric unit on a furlough and, losing their psychiatrist escort to an act of random violence, find themselves wandering freely (and off medication) in New York City. This movie offers a nice depiction of Axis II obsessive-compulsive personality disorder (probably combined with delusions of

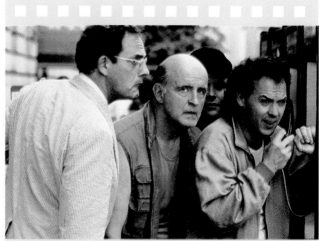

The Dream Team. Source: Universal/Courtesy Kobal.

grandeur). Three of the "escapees" are also interesting and well-cast "odd personalities" who may or may not truly be candidates for inpatient psychiatric care. The plot (preventing their psychiatrist's murder by the mob) is a bit far-fetched, but the movie is a worthy exercise in understanding and sympathizing with four unusual men trying to accomplish good against physical and psychological odds.

Secrets of a Soul
(1926) Neumann-Filmproduktion

A silent film about psychoanalysis and the interpretation of dreams. Beautiful film work, especially in the dream sequences, and a relatively painless introduction to the theory and practice of psychoanalytic therapy. Produced when Freud's influence and reputation were particularly strong.

Spellbound
(1945) Selznick International Pictures

Another Freudian movie featuring both psychoanalysis and the interpretation of dreams. This film is an Alfred Hitchcock great starring Gregory Peck and Ingrid Bergman. The dream scenes were designed by the artist Salvador Dali, and the plot, involving murder and amnesia, offers its share of excitement and unexpected developments. This film received multiple Oscars, including best picture of 1945.

Lilith
(1964) Columbia Pictures

Warren Beatty, playing a young psychotherapist, experiences countertransference as he falls in love with his patient and nearly loses his own sanity. This film raises more than just ethical questions and is worth seeing for its often realistic exploration of the difficult relational issues that can arise during intense therapy.

Pressure Point
(1962) United Artists

Another intense film on the troubled relationship between therapist and client. The great actor Sidney Poitier plays a psychiatrist who must treat an imprisoned Nazi and racist. Based on a true story, this film dramatically addresses the difficulties that arise in therapy when personal values and beliefs separate therapist and patient.

Prince of Tides
(1991) Columbia Pictures

A psychiatrist (played by Barbra Streisand) helps two troubled twins sort out deeply troubled lives. This film is at times not a fully realistic portrait either of mental illness or of psychiatry, but it is a fine story and a beautifully filmed movie. It received multiple Oscar nominations in 1991, including best picture and best actor.

Frances
(1982) Brooks Films

A moving and tragic account of the mental illness of actress Frances Farmer, whose depression, substance abuse, and seemingly atrocious mental health care led to disaster. Frances ultimately had a prefrontal lobotomy, and the movie offers a dramatic portrayal of the worst effects of surgery for psychiatric conditions. Excellent acting by Jessica Lange keeps this film from being a melodrama about inept psychiatric treatment.

REVIEW QUESTIONS AND ACTIVITIES

1. Consider how you might provide nursing care to one of the characters in the movies you saw. Write a nursing care plan for the character (include assessment questions, nursing diagnoses/DSM diagnoses, desired outcomes, and nursing interventions).

2. As a nursing professional, you may be caring for people with many of the psychiatric disorders you have seen depicted in these films. Consider what you can do to foster in yourself an attitude of understanding, empathy, and respect toward these people.

3. Our past personal experiences, family backgrounds, and relationships can affect our attitudes toward people with certain psychiatric disorders. Think about your reaction (either positive or negative) to one of the characters in the films you watched who remind you of someone you know. Did your past experience cause you to react more strongly to this character? If so, how might this affect your interaction with a client who has a similar disorder?

4. Think about the ethical questions that arose in one or more of the films you viewed. Were there nursing actions that you might handle differently? How would you treat a client experiencing that particular psychiatric disorder?

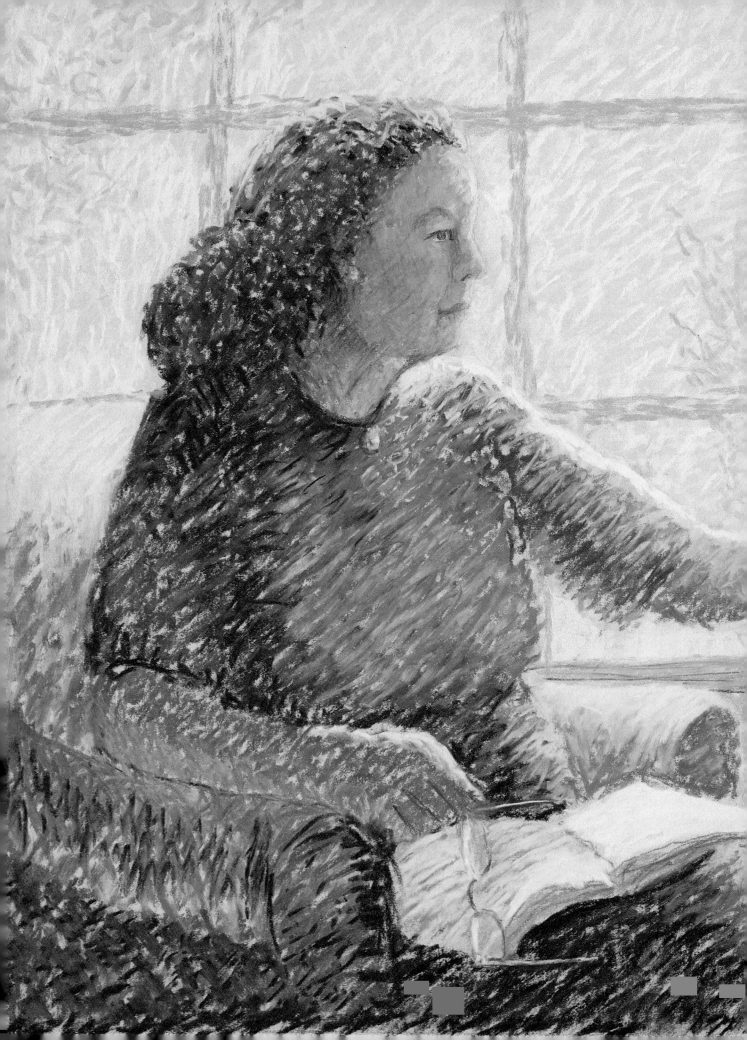

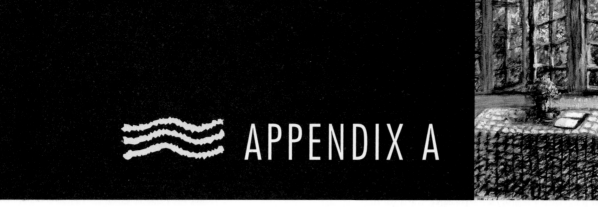
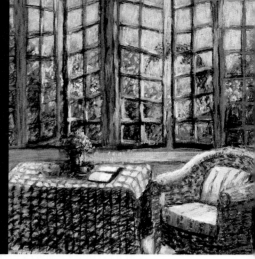

APPENDIX A

Standards of Psychiatric-Mental Health Clinical Nursing Practice

STANDARDS OF CARE

Standard I. Assessment

The psychiatric-mental health nurse collects client health data.

Standard II. Diagnosis

The psychiatric-mental health nurse analyzes the assessment data in determining diagnoses.

Standard III. Outcome Identification

The psychiatric-mental health nurse identifies expected outcomes individualized to the client.

Standard IV. Planning

The psychiatric-mental health nurse develops a plan of care that prescribes interventions to attain expected outcomes.

Standard V. Implementation

The psychiatric-mental health nurse implements the interventions identified in the plan of care.

Standard Va. Counseling

The psychiatric-mental health nurse uses counseling interventions to assist clients in improving or regaining their previous coping abilities, fostering mental health, and preventing mental illness and disability.

Standard Vb. Milieu Therapy

The psychiatric-mental health nurse provides, structures, and maintains a therapeutic environment in collaboration with the client and other health care providers.

Standard Vc. Self-Care Activities

The psychiatric-mental health nurse structures interventions around the client's activities of daily living to foster self-care and mental and physical well-being.

Standard Vd. Psychobiological Interventions

The psychiatric-mental health nurse uses knowledge of psychobiological interventions and applies clinical skills to restore the client's health and prevent further disability.

Standard Ve. Health Teaching

The psychiatric-mental health nurse, through health teaching, assists clients in achieving satisfying, productive, and healthy patterns of living.

Standard Vf. Case Management

The psychiatric-mental health nurse provides case management to coordinate comprehensive health services and ensure continuity of care.

Standard Vg. Health Promotion and Health Maintenance

The psychiatric-mental health nurse employs strategies and interventions to promote and maintain mental health and prevent mental illness.

From American Nurses Association. (1994). A statement on psychiatric-mental health clinical nursing practice and standards of psychiatric-mental health clinical nursing practice. Washington, DC: Author.

Advanced Practice Interventions Vh–Vj

The following interventions (Vh–Vj) may be performed only by the certified specialist in psychiatric-mental health nursing.

Standard Vh. Psychotherapy

The certified specialist in psychiatric-mental health nursing uses individual, group, and family psychotherapy, child psychotherapy, and other therapeutic treatments to assist clients in fostering mental health, preventing mental illness and disability, and improving or regaining previous health status and functional abilities.

Standard Vi. Prescription of Pharmacological Agents

The certified specialist uses prescription of pharmacologic agents in accordance with the state nursing practice act to treat symptoms of psychiatric illness and improve functional health status.

Standard Vj. Consultation

The certified specialist provides consultation to health care providers and others to influence the plans of care for clients, and to enhance the abilities of others to provide psychiatric and mental health care and effect change in systems.

Standard VI. Evaluation

The psychiatric-mental health nurse evaluates the client's progress in attaining expected outcomes.

STANDARDS OF PROFESSIONAL PERFORMANCE

Standard I. Quality of Care

The psychiatric-mental health nurse systematically evaluates the quality of care and effectiveness of psychiatric-mental health nursing practice.

Standard II. Performance Appraisal

The psychiatric-mental health nurse evaluates own psychiatric-mental health nursing practice in relation to professional practice standards and relevant statutes and regulations.

Standard III. Education

The psychiatric-mental health nurse acquires and maintains current knowledge in nursing practice.

Standard IV. Collegiality

The psychiatric-mental health nurse contributes to the professional development of peers, colleagues, and others.

Standard V. Ethics

The psychiatric-mental health nurse's decisions and actions on behalf of clients are determined in an ethical manner.

Standard VI. Collaboration

The psychiatric-mental health nurse collaborates with the client, significant others, and health care providers in providing care.

Standard VII. Research

The psychiatric-mental health nurse contributes to nursing and mental health through the use of research.

Standard VIII. Resource Utilization

The psychiatric-mental health nurse considers factors related to safety, effectiveness, and cost in planning and delivering client care.

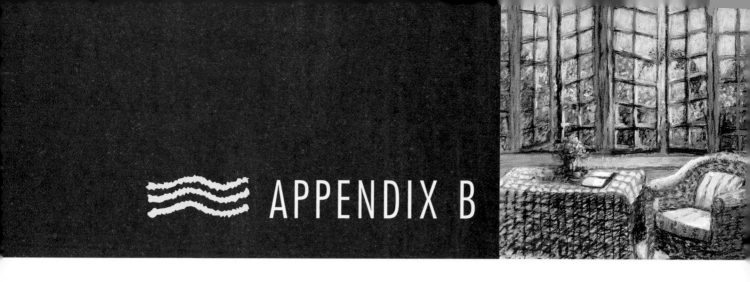

APPENDIX B

Canadian Standards of Psychiatric and Mental Health Nursing Practice

INTRODUCTION

The purpose of the Canadian Standards of Psychiatric and Mental Health Nursing Practice is to provide a basis for the evaluation of nursing practice in any setting in which the promotion of *mental health* and/or the psychiatric care of a *client* is a focus. This purpose is in accordance with the profession's obligation to maintain and improve the quality of nursing care. As standards for a specialized field of nursing practice, they complement the Canadian Nurses Association's Standards for Nursing Practice (1980).

Standards are meant to reflect the current state of knowledge and understanding of a discipline and are, therefore, conditional, dynamic and subject to change. The manner in which the individual psychiatric and mental health nurse will achieve the accepted performance levels will be determined by the conceptual model of nursing utilized. It is recognized, as well, that the social, cultural, economic and political environments of health care will influence every nurse's practice (Health and Welfare Canada, 1988).

The Standards presented here are written within a "domains of practice" framework. Benner (1984) identified seven practice domains in clinical nursing through research examining nurses' descriptions of their caregiving: the helping role, the diagnostic and monitoring function, the administering and monitoring of therapeutic interventions, effective management of rapidly changing situations, the teaching/coaching function, monitoring and ensuring the quality of health care practice and organizational and work role competencies. The use of these domains as an organizing framework permits an encompassing description of psychiatric and mental health

nursing performance. The nursing process, which has provided the framework for most nursing standards of practice in the past, has been subsumed here. Though important as a problem-solving approach within practice, the nursing process was not found to be a sufficient structure for a rich description of psychiatric and mental health nursing.

If nursing competency is conceptualized on a continuum that ranges from the novice level through levels of advanced beginners, competent, and proficient to the level of expert, it is the competent level of practice that is described by these Standards. This is the level of practice typified by a nurse who has two to three years of experience in this specialty area. This document includes a statement of beliefs about psychiatric and mental health nursing, standards of practice, and a glossary.*

BELIEFS ABOUT PSYCHIATRIC AND MENTAL HEALTH NURSING

Psychiatric and mental health nursing is a specialized area of nursing that focuses on the promotion of mental health and the care of clients experiencing *mental health problems* and *mental disorders*. As described in *Mental Health for Canadians: Striking a Balance* (1988), mental health and mental disorders are conceptualized as belonging to separate continuums. The poles of the mental health continuum are optimal and minimal mental health respectively. Mental disorders are represented by poles of severity and absence of symptoms.

The psychiatric and mental health nurse works with clients in institutional and community settings. Clients may be unique in their vulnerability as, in this area of nursing practice, they can be involved involuntarily and can be

---

From Canadian Federation of the Mental Health Nurses. (1995). *Canadian standards of psychiatric and mental health nursing practice.* Ottawa, Ontario: Canadian Nurses Association.

*Words in italics are defined in this appendix glossary.

committed to an institution under the law. Furthermore, if found incompetent, they can receive treatment against their will. This fact affects the nature of the nurse-client relationship and often raises complex ethical dilemmas.

Our practice is founded on the *therapeutic use of self* which means that nurse-client interactions are purposeful and directed at promotion of mental health. We are particularly concerned with fostering the *functional status* of our clients. The psychiatric and mental health nurse understands how the disease process, the recuperative powers, and the level of mental health are affected by *contextual factors*. This understanding is used in interactions with clients toward optimizing their level of mental health. Constant advances in knowledge (for example, the current increase in understanding of the biological basis of mental disorders and of the sociological determinants of behavior) require that psychiatric and mental health nurses continually incorporate new findings into their practice. We are striving to make our practice research-driven, and we acknowledge a responsibility to promote research within this specialty area.

We share with other mental health disciplines a body of knowledge based on theories of human behavior. We collaborate closely with these other disciplines and, in fact, in some settings there may be an overlapping of roles. We recognize that we are accountable to society for both the discrete and shared functions of our practice.

STANDARDS

   I The Helping Role
  II The Diagnostic and Monitoring Function
 III The Administering and Monitoring of Therapeutic Interventions
 IV Effective Management of Rapidly Changing Situations
  V The Teaching-Coaching Function
 VI Monitoring and Ensuring the Quality of Health Care Practices
VII Organizational and Work-Role Competencies

STANDARD I: THE HELPING ROLE

The helping role is fundamental to all nursing practice. In psychiatric and mental health nursing the nurse achieves this role within a *therapeutic relationship* with the client. This client may be an individual, a family, a group, or a community. The centrality of psychiatric and mental health nursing is the promotion of mental health and in this sense, our practice within nursing is unique.

The nurse:

1. Offers the client a therapeutic relationship.
2. Helps the client identify therapeutic goals.
3. Uses therapeutic communication techniques—verbal and nonverbal.
4. Uses *therapeutic empathy.*

5. Recognizes and responds appropriately to therapeutic impasses.
6. Understands the influences of the nurse's own beliefs, values, and life experiences on the therapeutic use of self
7. Acknowledges cultural differences in human interaction, recognizes the impact of culture on the therapeutic process, and modifies nursing practice accordingly.
8. Understands and interprets human responses to distress, such as fear, anger, anxiety, grief, humor, helplessness, hopelessness.
9. Guides the client through behavioral, emotional, and developmental change while affirming and promoting the client's responsibility, participation, and choice in his or her own recovery.
10. Understands that the client exists in a social system that may influence the onset, duration, and cause of illness and the level of mental health.
11. Supports client's coping abilities by supporting and augmenting the client's sense of self-esteem, power, and hope.
12. Provides supportive care to the client's significant others.

STANDARD II: THE DIAGNOSTIC AND MONITORING FUNCTION

Effective diagnosis and monitoring is dependent upon knowledge of mental disorders and psychiatric and mental health nursing principles. This knowledge, integrated with the nurse's conceptual model of nursing practice, provides a framework for processing client data. The nurse makes clinical judgments regarding the relevance and importance of this data.

The nurse:

1. Collects meaningful data from a variety of available resources (client, significant others, health care professionals, medical records) through observation, examination, interviewing, and consultation, while being attentive to issues of confidentiality.
2. Assesses the functional status of the client.
3. Documents and analyzes baseline data to identify functional status, health care deficits, potential for danger to self and others, alterations in thinking, perceiving, communicating, and decision-making abilities.
4. Formulates and documents a plan of care in collaboration with the client, recognizing variability in the ability to participate in the process. This plan is consistent with the overall treatment goals.
5. Assesses and documents significant change in the client's status, comparing new data with the baseline assessment.

6. Anticipates problems in the future course of the client's functional status (e.g., shifts in mood indicative of change in potential for self-harm).

7. Assesses the client's response to and perception of nursing interventions.

STANDARD III: ADMINISTERING AND MONITORING THERAPEUTIC INTERVENTIONS

There are unique practice issues confronting the psychiatric and mental health nurse in administering and monitoring therapeutic interventions that result from the nature of mental health problems and mental disorders. The nurse needs to know about potential for risk in particular disorders. Safety in psychiatric and mental health nursing has unique meaning because many clients are at risk for self-harm and/or self-neglect. Clients may not be legally competent to participate in decision-making. The psychiatric and mental health nurse needs to be alert to adverse reactions as clients' ability to self-report may be impaired. Therapeutic interventions are undertaken in collaboration with the client to the greatest possible extent.

The nurse:

1. Monitors effectiveness of therapeutic use of self by evaluating client responses to therapeutic processes.

2. Actively shapes a *therapeutic milieu.*

3. Monitors client safety, minimizing risk (e.g., use of observation levels, seclusion, need for hospitalization).

4. Administers medications accurately and safely, monitoring therapeutic responses, reactions, untoward effects, toxicity, and incompatibilities.

5. Makes discretionary clinical decisions, using knowledge of client's unique responses and *paradigm cases* as the basis for the decision (e.g., provision of as-needed medication, frequency of client contact in the community).

6. Participates in the treatment of clients requiring *somatic therapies.*

7. Uses crisis intervention.

8. Assists client when deficits in activities of daily living (ADLs) occur in response to mental health problems or mental disorders.

9. Uses contracting for goal attainment.

10. Uses therapeutic elements of group process and can lead structured group activities.

11. Incorporates knowledge of family dynamics in the provision of care (e.g., consequences of abusive relationships on self-esteem, appropriate discharge planning).

12. Collaborates with the client, health care providers, and others to access and coordinate resources.

STANDARD IV: EFFECTIVE MANAGEMENT OF RAPIDLY CHANGING SITUATIONS

The effective management of rapidly changing situations is essential in critical circumstances that may be termed *psychiatric emergencies.* These situations include self and other assaultive behaviors and *rapidly changing mental health states.*

The nurse:

1. Knows resources required to manage potential emergency situations and plans access to these resources.

2. Uses continual assessment to detect early changes in client status.

3. Commences critical procedures in an institutional setting (e.g., suicide precautions, emergency restraint, elopement precautions, when necessary). In a community setting, uses appropriate community support systems (e.g., police, ambulance services). Invokes Mental Health Act provisions as necessary.

4. Coordinates care to prevent errors and duplication of efforts where rapid response is imperative.

5. Considers the legal and ethical implications of responses to rapidly changing situations.

6. Evaluates the effectiveness of the rapid responses and modifies critical care plans as necessary.

7. Explores with the client the precipitants of the critical incident and makes plans to minimize risk of recurrence.

8. Participates in debriefing process with team and other services providers (e.g., review of critical incidents).

STANDARD V: THE TEACHING-COACHING FUNCTION

All nurse-client interactions are potentially teaching/learning situations. In psychiatric and mental health nursing the client's mental health and well-being is the major focus. The nurse attempts to understand the life experience of the client and uses this understanding to support and promote learning related to health and personal development.

The nurse:

1. Provides the client with an interpretation of the client's health condition in consultation with the other members of the health care team.

2. Explains psychiatric nursing procedures and treatment procedures provided to the client.

3. Acknowledges the impact of the client's mental health problem or mental disorder on readiness to learn and plans teaching times and strategies accordingly.

4. Plans and implements, with the client, health education in accordance with functional health assessment.

5. Provides anticipatory guidance regarding the client's situational needs (e.g., assists client in identifying changes in daily living requirements created by a transition from hospital to community care).

6. Coaches the client in finding ways of integrating the implications of mental illness, chronic illness, recovery, or improved functioning into lifestyle.

7. Creates opportunities for the client to learn experientially whenever possible.

8. Provides relevant information and guidance to the client's significant others.

9. Documents the teaching/learning process (assessment, plan, implementation, client involvement, and evaluation).

10. Evaluates and validates with the client the effectiveness of the educational process.

STANDARD VI: MONITORING AND ENSURING THE QUALITY OF HEALTH CARE PRACTICES

Because of the nature of mental health problems and mental disorders, our clients may be particularly vulnerable as recipients of health care. Mental health care is conducted under the provisions of provincial Mental Health Acts and related legislation. It is essential for the psychiatric and mental health nurse to be informed regarding the interpretation of relevant legislation and its implications for nursing practice. This nurse has a responsibility to advocate for the client's right to receive the least restrictive form of care and to respect and affirm the client's right to pursue individual goals of equality and justice.

The nurse:

1. Identifies limitations in the workplace or care setting that interfere with the nurse's ability to perform with skill, safety, and compassion; takes appropriate action.

2. Expands knowledge of innovations and changes in mental health and psychiatric nursing practice to ensure safe care.

3. Uses current mental health and psychiatric nursing research findings in practice.

4. Ensures and documents ongoing review and evaluation of psychiatric and mental health nursing care activities.

5. Asserts the necessity for the psychiatric and mental health nurse to understand and question the interdependent functions of the team within the overall plan of care.

6. Follows agency/institutional procedures when dissatisfied with the safety of a treatment plan and/or management interventions of other mental health care providers.

7. Advocates for the client within the context of institutional, professional, family and community interests.

8. Maintains and monitors confidentiality of client information.

STANDARD VII: ORGANIZATIONAL AND WORK-ROLE COMPETENCIES

The psychiatric and mental health nursing role is assumed within an organizational structure particular to the provision of health care. As mental health care in Canada tends to be provided using a multidisciplinary approach, the psychiatric and mental health nurse needs to be skilled in collaborative decision-making and teamwork.

The nurse:

1. Collaborates in the formulation of mental health promotion activities and overall treatment plans and decisions.

2. Recognizes and addresses the impact of the dynamic of the treatment team on the therapeutic process.

3. Actively participates in the development of policy by reviewing and responding to agency/institutional documentation.

4. Acts as a role model for nursing students and the novice nurse in the provision of psychiatric and mental health nursing care.

GLOSSARY

These definitions apply for the purposes of this document.

Client The person(s) to whom nursing activities are directed. May be an individual, family, a group, or community. Synonymous terms may be patient, beneficiary, recipient, resident.

Contextual factors The individual, interpersonal and environmental variables that comprise a person's unique life experience.

Functional status A client's adaptive levels associated with a change in mental health or the acuity of mental disorder. Nurses are concerned with the impact of a client's mental disorder or changes in mental health status on social relationships, occupational functioning and physical health.

Mental disorder A recognized medically diagnosable illness that results in the significant impairment of an individual's cognitive, affective or rational abilities. Mental disorders result from biological, developmental, and/or psychosocial factors (Health and Welfare Canada).

Mental health The capacity of the individual, the group and the environment to interact with one another in ways that promote subjective well-being, the optimal development and use of mental abilities (cognitive, affective and relational), the achievement of individual and collective goals consistent with justice and the attainment and preservation of conditions of fundamental equality (Health and Welfare Canada).

Mental health problem A disruption in the interactions between the individual, the group and the environment. Such a disruption may result from factors within the individual, including physical or mental illness, or inadequate coping skills. It may also spring from external causes, such as the existence of harsh environmental conditions, unjust social structures, or tensions within the family or community (Health and Welfare Canada).

Paradigm case A composite case that emerges from knowledge and experience and serves as a guide for practice.

Rapidly changing mental health states Severe impairments of thought and judgment, constituting a medical emergency, which can occur in association with acute psychosis (a clinical syndrome that may be caused by a variety of disorders such as mania, schizophrenia, drug abuse).

Somatic therapies Therapy in which the physical body of the client is the initial focus of the treatment intervention. The most common somatic therapies include psychotropic chemotherapy, electroconvulsive therapy, activity therapy and use of physical constraint.

Therapeutic empathy The ability to know and understand the subjective experience of the client; to communicate this understanding to the client; to use it in the provision of care.

Therapeutic milieu An environment manipulated in a systematic manner for therapeutic purposes, e.g., for the promotion of optimal functioning in activities of daily living or for the improvement of interpersonal skills.

Therapeutic relationship An alliance between a client and a professional caregiver with the goal of helping the client.

Therapeutic use of self Use of the self in the nurse-client relationship for therapeutic purposes. The nurse is aware of his/her personal impact on others and combines self-awareness with theoretical and experiential knowledge of therapeutic relationships.

REFERENCES

Aguilera, D. & Messick, J. (1990). *Crisis intervention: Theory and methodology* (6th ed.). St. Louis, Missouri: Mosby.

American Psychiatric Association. (1987). *Diagnostic and statistical manual of mental disorders* (3rd ed., revised). Washington, DC: Author.

Benner, P. (1984). *From novice to expert: Excellence and power in clinical nursing practice.* Don Mills, Ontario: Addison-Wesley.

Health & Welfare Canada. (1988). *Mental health for Canadians: Striking a balance* (Cat. H39-128/1988E). Ottawa, Ontario: Minister of Supply and Service Canada.

Canadian Nurses Association. (1987). *A definition of nursing practice. Standards for nursing practice.* (ISBN 0-919108-51-2). Ottawa, Ontario: Author.

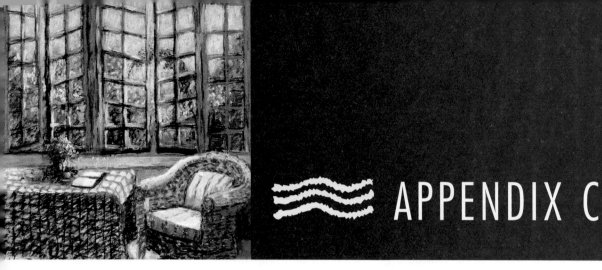

APPENDIX C

DSM-IV Classification

NOS = Not Otherwise Specified.

An *x* appearing in a diagnostic code indicates that a specific code number is required.

An ellipsis (. . .) is used in the names of certain disorders to indicate that the name of a specific mental disorder or general medical condition should be inserted when recording the name (e.g., 293.0 Delirium Due to Hypothyroidism).

If criteria are currently met, one of the following severity specifiers may be noted after the diagnosis:
Mild
Moderate
Severe

If criteria are no longer met, one of the following specifiers may be noted:
In Partial Remission
In Full Remission
Prior History

DISORDERS USUALLY FIRST DIAGNOSED IN INFANCY, CHILDHOOD, OR ADOLESCENCE

Mental Retardation

Note: *These are coded on Axis II.*
317 Mild Mental Retardation
318.0 Moderate Mental Retardation
318.1 Severe Mental Retardation
318.2 Profound Mental Retardation
319 Mental Retardation, Severity Unspecified

Learning Disorders

315.00 Reading Disorder
315.1 Mathematics Disorder

315.2 Disorder of Written Expression
315.9 Learning Disorder NOS

Motor Skills Disorder

315.4 Developmental Coordination Disorder

Communication Disorders

315.31 Expressive Language Disorder
315.31 Mixed Receptive-Expressive Language Disorder
315.39 Phonological Disorder
307.0 Stuttering
307.9 Communication Disorder NOS

Pervasive Developmental Disorders

299.00 Autistic Disorder
299.80 Rett's Disorder
299.10 Childhood Disintegrative Disorder
299.80 Asperger's Disorder
299.80 Pervasive Developmental Disorder NOS

Attention-Deficit and Disruptive Behavior Disorders

314.xx Attention-Deficit/Hyperactivity Disorder
  .01 Combined Type
  .00 Predominantly Inattentive Type
  .01 Predominantly Hyperactive-Impulsive Type
314.9 Attention-Deficit/Hyperactivity Disorder NOS
312.8 Conduct Disorder
    Specify type: Childhood-Onset Type/Adolescent-Onset Type
313.81 Oppositional Defiant Disorder
312.9 Disruptive Behavior Disorder NOS

Based on information from the *Diagnostic and Statistical Manual of Mental Disorders*, Fourth Edition. Copyright 1994, American Psychiatric Association.

Feeding and Eating Disorders of Infancy or Early Childhood

307.52   Pica
307.53   Rumination Disorder
307.59   Feeding Disorder of Infancy or Early Childhood

Tic Disorders

307.23   Tourette's Disorder
307.22   Chronic Motor or Vocal Tic Disorder
307.21   Transient Tic Disorder
         Specify if: Single Episode/Recurrent
307.20   Tic Disorder NOS

Elimination Disorders

——.–   Encopresis
787.6   With Constipation and Overflow Incontinence
307.7   Without Constipation and Overflow Incontinence
307.6   Enuresis (Not Due to a General Medical Condition)
         Specify type: Nocturnal Only/Diurnal Only/Nocturnal and Diurnal

Other Disorders of Infancy, Childhood, or Adolescence

309.21   Separation Anxiety Disorder
         Specify if: Early Onset
313.23   Selective Mutism
313.89   Reactive Attachment Disorder of Infancy or Early Childhood
         Specify type: Inhibited Type/Disinhibited Type
307.3   Stereotypic Movement Disorder
         Specify if: With Self-Injurious Behavior

313.9   Disorder of Infancy, Childhood, or Adolescence NOS

DELIRIUM, DEMENTIA, AND AMNESTIC AND OTHER COGNITIVE DISORDERS

Delirium

293.0   Delirium Due to . . . *[Indicate the General Medical Condition]*
——.–   Substance Intoxication Delirium *(refer to Substance-Related Disorders for substance-specific codes)*
——.–   Substance Withdrawal Delirium *(refer to Substance-Related Disorders for substance-specific codes)*
——.–   Delirium Due to Multiple Etiologies *(code each of the specific etiologies)*
780.09   Delirium NOS

Dementia

290.xx   Dementia of the Alzheimer's Type, With Early Onset *(also code 331.0 Alzheimer's disease on Axis III)*
   .10   Uncomplicated
   .11   With Delirium
   .12   With Delusions
   .13   With Depressed Mood
         Specify if: With Behavioral Disturbance
290.xx   Dementia of the Alzheimer's Type, With Late Onset *(also code 331.0 Alzheimer's disease on Axis III)*
   .0   Uncomplicated
   .3   With Delirium
   .20   With Delusions
   .21   With Depressed Mood
         Specify if: With Behavioral Disturbance
290.xx   Vascular Dementia
   .40   Uncomplicated
   .41   With Delirium
   .42   With Delusions
   .43   With Depressed Mood
         Specify if: With Behavioral Disturbance
294.9   Dementia Due to HIV Disease *(also code 043.1 HIV infection affecting central nervous system on Axis III)*
294.1   Dementia Due to Head Trauma *(also code 854.00 head injury on Axis III)*
294.1   Dementia Due to Parkinson's Disease *(also code 332.0 Parkinson's disease on Axis III)*
294.1   Dementia Due to Huntington's Disease *(also code 333.4 Huntington's disease on Axis III)*
290.10   Dementia Due to Pick's Disease *(also code 331.1 Pick's disease on Axis III)*
290.10   Dementia Due to Creutzfeldt-Jakob Disease *(also code 046.1 Creutzfeldt-Jakob disease on Axis III)*
294.1   Dementia Due to . . . *[Indicate the General Medical Condition not listed above] (also code the general medical condition on Axis III)*
——.–   Substance-Induced Persisting Dementia *(refer to Substance-Related Disorders for substance-specific codes)*
——.–   Dementia Due to Multiple Etiologies *(code each of the specific etiologies)*
294.8   Dementia NOS

Amnestic Disorders

294.0   Amnestic Disorder Due to . . . *[Indicate the General Medical Condition]*
         Specify if: Transient/Chronic
——.–   Substance-Induced Persisting Amnestic Disorder *(refer to Substance-Related Disorders for substance-specific codes)*
294.8   Amnestic Disorder NOS

Other Cognitive Disorders

294.9   Cognitive Disorder NOS

MENTAL DISORDERS DUE TO A GENERAL MEDICAL CONDITION NOT ELSEWHERE CLASSIFIED

293.89   Catatonic Disorder Due to . . . *[Indicate the General Medical Condition]*

310.1   Personality Change Due to . . . *[Indicate the General Medical Condition]*
Specify type: Labile Type/Disinhibited Type/ Aggressive Type/Apathetic Type/Paranoid Type/ Other Type/Combined Type/Unspecified Type

293.9   Mental Disorder NOS Due to . . . *[Indicate the General Medical Condition]*

SUBSTANCE-RELATED DISORDERS

[a]*The following specifiers may be applied to Substance Dependence:*

With Physiological Dependence/Without Physiological Dependence

Early Full Remission/Early Partial Remission/Sustained Full Remission/Sustained Partial Remission

On Agonist Therapy/In a Controlled Environment

The following specifiers apply to Substance-Induced Disorders as noted:

[I]With Onset During Intoxication/[W]With Onset During Withdrawal

Alcohol-Related Disorders

Alcohol Use Disorders

303.90   Alcohol Dependence[a]
305.00   Alcohol Abuse

Alcohol-Induced Disorders

303.00   Alcohol Intoxication
291.8   Alcohol Withdrawal
Specify if: With Perceptual Disturbances
291.0   Alcohol Intoxication Delirium
291.0   Alcohol Withdrawal Delirium
291.2   Alcohol-Induced Persisting Dementia
291.1   Alcohol-Induced Persisting Amnestic Disorder
291.x   Alcohol-Induced Psychotic Disorder
   .5   With Delusions[I,W]
   .3   With Hallucinations[I,W]
291.8   Alcohol-Induced Mood Disorder[I,W]
291.8   Alcohol-Induced Anxiety Disorder[I,W]
291.8   Alcohol-Induced Sexual Dysfunction[I]
291.8   Alcohol-Induced Sleep Disorder[I,W]

291.9   Alcohol-Related Disorder NOS

Amphetamine (or Amphetamine-Like)–Related Disorders

Amphetamine Use Disorders

304.40   Amphetamine Dependence[a]
305.70   Amphetamine Abuse

Amphetamine-Induced Disorders

292.89   Amphetamine Intoxication
Specify if: With Perceptual Disturbances
292.0   Amphetamine Withdrawal
292.81   Amphetamine Intoxication Delirium
292.xx   Amphetamine-Induced Psychotic Disorder
   .11   With Delusions[I]
   .12   With Hallucinations[I]
292.84   Amphetamine-Induced Mood Disorder[I,W]
292.89   Amphetamine-Induced Anxiety Disorder[I]
292.89   Amphetamine-Induced Sexual Dysfunction[I]
292.89   Amphetamine-Induced Sleep Disorder[I,W]

292.9   Amphetamine-Related Disorder NOS

Caffeine-Related Disorders

Caffeine-Induced Disorders

305.90   Caffeine Intoxication
292.89   Caffeine-Induced Anxiety Disorder[I]
292.89   Caffeine-Induced Sleep Disorder[I]

292.9   Caffeine-Related Disorder NOS

Cannabis-Related Disorders

Cannabis Use Disorders

304.30   Cannabis Dependence[a]
305.20   Cannabis Abuse

Cannabis-Induced Disorders

292.89   Cannabis Intoxication
Specify if: With Perceptual Disturbances
292.81   Cannabis Intoxication Delirium
292.xx   Cannabis-Induced Psychotic Disorder
   .11   With Delusions[I]
   .12   With Hallucinations[I]
292.89   Cannabis-Induced Anxiety Disorder[I]

292.9   Cannabis-Related Disorder NOS

Cocaine-Related Disorders

Cocaine Use Disorders

304.20   Cocaine Dependence[a]
305.60   Cocaine Abuse

Cocaine-Induced Disorders

292.89   Cocaine Intoxication
Specify if: With Perceptual Disturbances
292.0   Cocaine Withdrawal
292.81   Cocaine Intoxication Delirium
292.xx   Cocaine-Induced Psychotic Disorder
   .11   With Delusions[I]
   .12   With Hallucinations[I]

292.84 Cocaine-Induced Mood Disorder[I,W]
292.89 Cocaine-Induced Anxiety Disorder[I,W]
292.89 Cocaine-Induced Sexual Dysfunction[I]
292.89 Cocaine-Induced Sleep Disorder[I,W]

292.9 Cocaine-Related Disorder NOS

Hallucinogen-Related Disorders

Hallucinogen Use Disorders

304.50 Hallucinogen Dependence[a]
305.30 Hallucinogen Abuse

Hallucinogen-Induced Disorders

292.89 Hallucinogen Intoxication
292.89 Hallucinogen Persisting Perception Disorder (Flashbacks)
292.81 Hallucinogen Intoxication Delirium
292.xx Hallucinogen-Induced Psychotic Disorder
   .11   With Delusions[I]
   .12   With Hallucinations[I]
292.84 Hallucinogen-Induced Mood Disorder[I]
292.89 Hallucinogen-Induced Anxiety Disorder[I]

292.9 Hallucinogen-Related Disorder NOS

Inhalant-Related Disorders

Inhalant Use Disorders

304.60 Inhalant Dependence[a]
305.90 Inhalant Abuse

Inhalant-Induced Disorders

292.89 Inhalant Intoxication
292.81 Inhalant Intoxication Delirium
292.82 Inhalant-Induced Persisting Dementia
292.xx Inhalant-Induced Psychotic Disorder
   .11   With Delusions[I]
   .12   With Hallucinations[I]
292.84 Inhalant-Induced Mood Disorder[I]
292.89 Inhalant-Induced Anxiety Disorder[I]

292.9 Inhalant-Related Disorder NOS

Nicotine-Related Disorders

Nicotine Use Disorder

305.10 Nicotine Dependence[a]

Nicotine-Induced Disorder

292.0 Nicotine Withdrawal

292.9 Nicotine-Related Disorder NOS

Opioid-Related Disorders

Opioid Use Disorders

304.00 Opioid Dependence[a]
305.50 Opioid Abuse

Opioid-Induced Disorders

292.89 Opioid Intoxication
   Specify if: With Perceptual Disturbances
292.0 Opioid Withdrawal
292.81 Opioid Intoxication Delirium
292.xx Opioid-Induced Psychotic Disorder
   .11   With Delusions[I]
   .12   With Hallucinations[I]
292.84 Opioid-Induced Mood Disorder[I]
292.89 Opioid-Induced Sexual Dysfunction[I]
292.89 Opioid-Induced Sleep Disorder[I,W]

292.9 Opioid-Related Disorder NOS

Phencyclidine (or Phencyclidine-Like)–Related Disorders

Phencyclidine Use Disorders

304.90 Phencyclidine Dependence[a]
305.90 Phencyclidine Abuse

Phencyclidine-Induced Disorders

292.89 Phencyclidine Intoxication
   Specify if: With Perceptual Disturbances
292.81 Phencyclidine Intoxication Delirium
292.xx Phencyclidine-Induced Psychotic Disorder
   .11   With Delusions[I]
   .12   With Hallucinations[I]
292.84 Phencyclidine-Induced Mood Disorder[I]
292.89 Phencyclidine-Induced Anxiety Disorder[I]

292.9 Phencyclidine-Related Disorder NOS

Sedative-, Hypnotic-, or Anxiolytic-Related Disorders

Sedative, Hypnotic, or Anxiolytic Use Disorders

304.10 Sedative, Hypnotic, or Anxiolytic Dependence[a]
305.40 Sedative, Hypnotic, or Anxiolytic Abuse

Sedative-, Hypnotic-, or Anxiolytic-Induced Disorders

292.89 Sedative, Hypnotic, or Anxiolytic Intoxication
292.0 Sedative, Hypnotic, or Anxiolytic Withdrawal
   Specify if: With Perceptual Disturbances
292.81 Sedative, Hypnotic, or Anxiolytic Intoxication Delirium
292.81 Sedative, Hypnotic, or Anxiolytic Withdrawal Delirium
292.82 Sedative-, Hypnotic-, or Anxiolytic-Induced Persisting Dementia

292.83 Sedative-, Hypnotic-, or Anxiolytic-Induced Persisting Amnestic Disorder

292.xx Sedative-, Hypnotic-, or Anxiolytic-Induced Psychotic Disorder
  .11 With Delusions[I,W]
  .12 With Hallucinations[I,W]

292.84 Sedative-, Hypnotic-, or Anxiolytic-Induced Mood Disorder[I,W]

292.89 Sedative-, Hypnotic-, or Anxiolytic-Induced Anxiety Disorder[W]

292.89 Sedative-, Hypnotic-, or Anxiolytic-Induced Sexual Dysfunction[I]

292.89 Sedative-, Hypnotic-, or Anxiolytic-Induced Sleep Disorder[I,W]

292.9 Sedative-, Hypnotic-, or Anxiolytic-Related Disorder NOS

Polysubstance-Related Disorder

304.80 Polysubstance Dependence[a]

Other (or Unknown) Substance-Related Disorders

Other (or Unknown) Substance Use Disorders

304.90 Other (or Unknown) Substance Dependence[a]
305.90 Other (or Unknown) Substance Abuse

Other (or Unknown) Substance–Induced Disorders

292.89 Other (or Unknown) Substance Intoxication
  Specify if: With Perceptual Disturbances

292.0 Other (or Unknown) Substance Withdrawal
  Specify if: With Perceptual Disturbances

292.81 Other (or Unknown) Substance–Induced Delirium

292.82 Other (or Unknown) Substance–Induced Persisting Dementia

292.83 Other (or Unknown) Substance–Induced Persisting Amnestic Disorder

292.xx Other (or Unknown) Substance–Induced Psychotic Disorder
  .11 With Delusions[I,W]
  .12 With Hallucinations[I,W]

292.84 Other (or Unknown) Substance–Induced Mood Disorder[I,W]

292.89 Other (or Unknown) Substance–Induced Anxiety Disorder[I,W]

292.89 Other (or Unknown) Substance–Induced Sexual Dysfunction[I]

292.89 Other (or Unknown) Substance–Induced Sleep Disorder[I,W]

292.9 Other (or Unknown) Substance–Related Disorder NOS

SCHIZOPHRENIA AND OTHER PSYCHOTIC DISORDERS

295.xx Schizophrenia

The following Classification of Longitudinal Course applies to all subtypes of Schizophrenia:

Episodic With Interepisode Residual Symptoms (*specify if:* With Prominent Negative Symptoms)/Episodic With No Interepisode Residual Symptoms

Continuous (*specify if:* With Prominent Negative Symptoms)

Single Episode In Partial Remission (*specify if:* With Prominent Negative Symptoms)/Single Episode In Full Remission

Other or Unspecified Pattern

  .30 Paranoid Type
  .10 Disorganized Type
  .20 Catatonic Type
  .90 Undifferentiated Type
  .60 Residual Type

295.40 Schizophreniform Disorder
  Specify if: Without Good Prognostic Features/With Good Prognostic Features

295.70 Schizoaffective Disorder
  Specify type: Bipolar Type/Depressive Type

297.1 Delusional Disorder
  Specify type: Erotomanic Type/Grandiose Type/Jealous Type/Persecutory Type/Somatic Type/Mixed Type/Unspecified Type

298.8 Brief Psychotic Disorder
  Specify if: With Marked Stressor(s)/Without Marked Stressor(s)/With Postpartum Onset

297.3 Shared Psychotic Disorder

293.xx Psychotic Disorder Due to . . . *[Indicate the General Medical Condition]*
  .81 With Delusions
  .82 With Hallucinations

——.— Substance-Induced Psychotic Disorder *(refer to Substance-Related Disorders for substance-specific codes)*
  Specify if: With Onset During Intoxication/With Onset During Withdrawal

298.9 Psychotic Disorder NOS

MOOD DISORDERS

Code current state of Major Depressive Disorder or Bipolar I Disorder in fifth digit:

1 = Mild
2 = Moderate
3 = Severe Without Psychotic Features
4 = Severe With Psychotic Features
    Specify: Mood-Congruent Psychotic Features/Mood-Incongruent Psychotic Features
5 = In Partial Remission
6 = In Full Remission
0 = Unspecified

The following specifiers apply (for current or most recent episode) to Mood Disorders as noted:

[a]Severity/Psychotic/Remission Specifiers/[b]Chronic/[c]With Catatonic Features/[d]With Melancholic Features/[e]With Atypical Features/[f]With Postpartum Onset

The following specifiers apply to Mood Disorders as noted:

[g]With or Without Full Interepisode Recovery/[h]With Seasonal Pattern/[i]With Rapid Cycling

Depressive Disorders

296.xx	Major Depressive Disorder,	
.2x	Single Episode[a,b,c,d,e,f]	
.3x	Recurrent[a,b,c,d,e,f,g,h]	
300.4	Dysthymic Disorder	

Specify if: Early Onset/Late Onset
Specify if: With Atypical Features

311   Depressive Disorder NOS

Bipolar Disorders

296.xx Bipolar I Disorder,
  .0x   Single Manic Episode[a,c,f]
      Specify if: Mixed
  .40   Most Recent Episode Hypomanic[g,h,i]
  .4x   Most Recent Episode Manic[a,c,f,g,h,i]
  .6x   Most Recent Episode Mixed[a,c,f,g,h,i]
  .5x   Most Recent Episode Depressed[a,b,c,d,e,f,g,h,i]
  .7   Most Recent Episode Unspecified[g,h,i]
296.89 Bipolar II Disorder[a,b,c,d,e,f,g,h,i]
      Specify (current or most recent episode): Hypomanic/Depressed
301.13 Cyclothymic Disorder
296.80 Bipolar Disorder NOS

293.83 Mood Disorder Due to . . . *[Indicate the General Medical Condition]*
      Specify type: With Depressive Features/With Major Depressive–Like Episode/With Manic Features/With Mixed Features
——.— Substance-Induced Mood Disorder *(refer to Substance-Related Disorders for substance-specific codes)*
      Specify type: With Depressive Features/With Manic Features/With Mixed Features
      Specify if: With Onset During Intoxication/With Onset During Withdrawal

296.90 Mood Disorder NOS

ANXIETY DISORDERS

300.01 Panic Disorder Without Agoraphobia
300.21 Panic Disorder With Agoraphobia
300.22 Agoraphobia Without History of Panic Disorder
300.29 Specific Phobia
      Specify type: Animal Type/Natural Environment Type/Blood-Injection-Injury Type/Situational Type/Other Type

300.23 Social Phobia
      Specify if: Generalized
300.3   Obsessive-Compulsive Disorder
      Specify if: With Poor Insight
309.81 Posttraumatic Stress Disorder
      Specify if: Acute/Chronic
      Specify if: With Delayed Onset
308.3   Acute Stress Disorder
300.02 Generalized Anxiety Disorder
293.89 Anxiety Disorder Due to . . . *[Indicate the General Medical Condition]*
      Specify if: With Generalized Anxiety/With Panic Attacks/With Obsessive-Compulsive Symptoms
——.— Substance-Induced Anxiety Disorder *(refer to Substance-Related Disorders for substance-specific codes)*
      Specify if: With Generalized Anxiety/With Panic Attacks/With Obsessive-Compulsive Symptoms/With Phobic Symptoms
      Specify if: With Onset During Intoxication/With Onset During Withdrawal
300.00 Anxiety Disorder NOS

SOMATOFORM DISORDERS

300.81 Somatization Disorder
300.81 Undifferentiated Somatoform Disorder
300.11 Conversion Disorder
      Specify type: With Motor Symptom or Deficit/With Sensory Symptom or Deficit/With Seizures or Convulsions/With Mixed Presentation
307.xx Pain Disorder
  .80   Associated With Psychological Factors
  .89   Associated With Both Psychological Factors and a General Medical Condition
      Specify if: Acute/Chronic
300.7   Hypochondriasis
      Specify if: With Poor Insight
300.7   Body Dysmorphic Disorder
300.81 Somatoform Disorder NOS

FACTITIOUS DISORDERS

300.xx Factitious Disorder
  .16   With Predominantly Psychological Signs and Symptoms
  .19   With Predominantly Physical Signs and Symptoms
  .19   With Combined Psychological and Physical Signs and Symptoms
300.19 Factitious Disorder NOS

DISSOCIATIVE DISORDERS

300.12 Dissociative Amnesia
300.13 Dissociative Fugue
300.14 Dissociative Identity Disorder
300.6   Depersonalization Disorder
300.15 Dissociative Disorder NOS

SEXUAL AND GENDER IDENTITY DISORDERS

Sexual Dysfunction

The following specifiers apply to all primary Sexual Dysfunctions:

Lifelong Type/Acquired Type
Generalized Type/Situational Type
Due to Psychological Factors/Due to Combined Factors

Sexual Desire Disorders

302.71   Hypoactive Sexual Desire Disorder
302.79   Sexual Aversion Disorder

Sexual Arousal Disorders

302.72   Female Sexual Arousal Disorder
302.72   Male Erectile Disorder

Orgasmic Disorders

302.73   Female Orgasmic Disorder
302.74   Male Orgasmic Disorder
302.75   Premature Ejaculation

Sexual Pain Disorders

302.76   Dyspareunia (Not Due to a General Medical Condition)
306.51   Vaginismus (Not Due to a General Medical Condition)

Sexual Dysfunction Due to a General Medical Condition

625.8   Female Hypoactive Sexual Desire Disorder Due to . . . *[Indicate the General Medical Condition]*
608.89   Male Hypoactive Sexual Desire Disorder Due to . . . *[Indicate the General Medical Condition]*
607.84   Male Erectile Disorder Due to . . . *[Indicate the General Medical Condition]*
625.0   Female Dyspareunia Due to . . . *[Indicate the General Medical Condition]*
608.89   Male Dyspareunia Due to . . . *[Indicate the General Medical Condition]*
625.8   Other Female Sexual Dysfunction Due to . . . *[Indicate the General Medical Condition]*
608.89   Other Male Sexual Dysfunction Due to . . . *[Indicate the General Medical Condition]*
——.–   Substance-Induced Sexual Dysfunction *(refer to Substance-Related Disorders for substance-specific codes)*
Specify if: With Impaired Desire/With Impaired Arousal/With Impaired Orgasm/With Sexual Pain
Specify if: With Onset During Intoxication

302.70   Sexual Dysfunction NOS

Paraphilias

302.4   Exhibitionism
302.81   Fetishism
302.89   Frotteurism
302.2   Pedophilia
Specify if: Sexually Attracted to Males/Sexually Attracted to Females/Sexually Attracted to Both
Specify if: Limited to Incest
Specify type: Exclusive Type/Nonexclusive Type
302.83   Sexual Masochism
302.84   Sexual Sadism
302.3   Transvestic Fetishism
Specify if: With Gender Dysphoria
302.82   Voyeurism
302.9   Paraphilia NOS

Gender Identity Disorders

302.xx   Gender Identity Disorder
    .6   in Children
    .85   in Adolescents or Adults
Specify if: Sexually Attracted to Males/Sexually Attracted to Females/Sexually Attracted to Both/Sexually Attracted to Neither
302.6   Gender Identity Disorder NOS

302.9   Sexual Disorder NOS

EATING DISORDERS

307.1   Anorexia Nervosa
Specify type: Restricting Type; Binge-Eating/Purging Type
307.51   Bulimia Nervosa
Specify type: Purging Type/Nonpurging Type
307.50   Eating Disorder NOS

SLEEP DISORDERS

Primary Sleep Disorders

Dyssomnias

307.42   Primary Insomnia
307.44   Primary Hypersomnia
Specify if: Recurrent
347   Narcolepsy
780.59   Breathing-Related Sleep Disorder
307.45   Circadian Rhythm Sleep Disorder
Specify type: Delayed Sleep Phase Type/Jet Lag Type/Shift Work Type/Unspecified Type
307.47   Dyssomnia NOS

Parasomnias

307.47   Nightmare Disorder
307.46   Sleep Terror Disorder

307.46   Sleepwalking Disorder
307.47   Parasomnia NOS

Sleep Disorders Related to Another Mental Disorder

307.42   Insomnia Related to . . . *[Indicate the Axis I or Axis II Disorder]*
307.44   Hypersomnia Related to . . . *[Indicate the Axis I or Axis II Disorder]*

Other Sleep Disorders

780.xx   Sleep Disorder Due to . . . *[Indicate the General Medical Condition]*
    .52   Insomnia Type
    .54   Hypersomnia Type
    .59   Parasomnia Type
    .59   Mixed Type
——.—   Substance-Induced Sleep Disorder *(refer to Substance-Related Disorders for substance-specific codes)*
            Specify type: Insomnia Type/Hypersomnia Type/Parasomnia Type/Mixed Type
            Specify if: With Onset During Intoxication/With Onset During Withdrawal

IMPULSE-CONTROL DISORDERS NOT ELSEWHERE CLASSIFIED

312.34   Intermittent Explosive Disorder
312.32   Kleptomania
312.33   Pyromania
312.31   Pathological Gambling
312.39   Trichotillomania
312.30   Impulse-Control Disorder NOS

ADJUSTMENT DISORDERS

309.xx   Adjustment Disorder
    .0   With Depressed Mood
    .24   With Anxiety
    .28   With Mixed Anxiety and Depressed Mood
    .3   With Disturbance of Conduct
    .4   With Mixed Disturbance of Emotions and Conduct
    .9   Unspecified
            Specify if: Acute/Chronic

PERSONALITY DISORDERS

Note: *These are coded on Axis II.*
301.0   Paranoid Personality Disorder
301.20   Schizoid Personality Disorder

301.22   Schizotypal Personality Disorder
301.7   Antisocial Personality Disorder
301.83   Borderline Personality Disorder
301.50   Histrionic Personality Disorder
301.81   Narcissistic Personality Disorder
301.82   Avoidant Personality Disorder
301.6   Dependent Personality Disorder
301.4   Obsessive-Compulsive Personality Disorder
301.9   Personality Disorder NOS

OTHER CONDITIONS THAT MAY BE A FOCUS OF CLINICAL ATTENTION

Psychological Factors Affecting Medical Condition

316   . . . *[Specified Psychological Factor]* Affecting . . . *[Indicate the General Medical Condition]*
            Choose name based on nature of factors:
            Mental Disorder Affecting Medical Condition
            Psychological Symptoms Affecting Medical Condition
            Personality Traits or Coping Style Affecting Medical Condition
            Maladaptive Health Behaviors Affecting Medical Condition
            Stress-Related Physiological Response Affecting Medical Condition
            Other or Unspecified Psychological Factors Affecting Medical Condition

Medication-Induced Movement Disorders

332.1   Neuroleptic-Induced Parkinsonism
333.92   Neuroleptic Malignant Syndrome
333.7   Neuroleptic-Induced Acute Dystonia
333.99   Neuroleptic-Induced Acute Akathisia
333.82   Neuroleptic-Induced Tardive Dyskinesia
333.1   Medication-Induced Postural Tremor
333.90   Medication-Induced Movement Disorder NOS

Other Medication-Induced Disorder

995.2   Adverse Effects of Medication NOS

Relational Problems

V61.9   Relational Problem Related to a Mental Disorder or General Medical Condition
V61.20   Parent-Child Relational Problem
V61.1   Partner Relational Problem
V61.8   Sibling Relational Problem
V62.81   Relational Problem NOS

Problems Related to Abuse or Neglect

V61.21   Physical Abuse of Child
         (code 995.5 if focus of attention is on victim)
V61.21   Sexual Abuse of Child
         (code 995.5 if focus of attention is on victim)
V61.21   Neglect of Child
         (code 995.5 if focus of attention is on victim)
V61.1   Physical Abuse of Adult
         (code 995.81 if focus of attention is on victim)
V61.1   Sexual Abuse of Adult
         (code 995.81 if focus of attention is on victim)

Additional Conditions That May Be a Focus of Clinical Attention

V15.81   Noncompliance With Treatment
V65.2   Malingering
V71.01   Adult Antisocial Behavior
V71.02   Child or Adolescent Antisocial Behavior
V62.89   Borderline Intellectual Functioning
         Note: *This is coded on Axis II.*
780.9   Age-Related Cognitive Decline
V62.82   Bereavement
V62.3   Academic Problem
V62.2   Occupational Problem

313.82   Identity Problem
V62.89   Religious or Spiritual Problem
V62.4   Acculturation Problem
V62.89   Phase of Life Problem

ADDITIONAL CODES

300.9   Unspecified Mental Disorder (nonpsychotic)
V71.09   No Diagnosis or Condition on Axis I
799.9   Diagnosis or Condition Deferred on Axis I
V71.09   No Diagnosis on Axis II
799.9   Diagnosis Deferred on Axis II

MULTIAXIAL SYSTEM

Axis I   Clinical Disorders
           Other Conditions That May Be a Focus of
             Clinical Attention
Axis II   Personality Disorders
           Mental Retardation
Axis III   General Medical Conditions
Axis IV   Psychosocial and Environmental Problems
Axis V   Global Assessment of Functioning

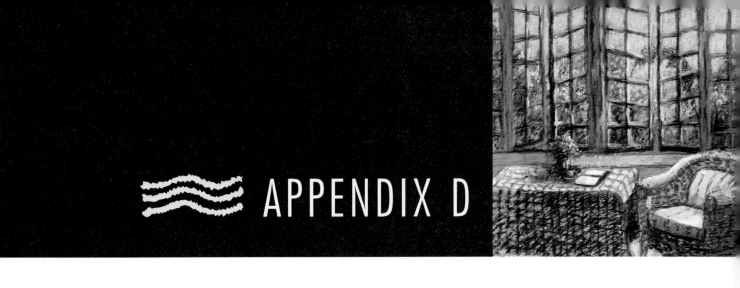

APPENDIX D

NANDA Approved Nursing Diagnoses

PATTERN 1: EXCHANGING

1.1.2.1	Altered Nutrition: More Than Body Requirements
1.1.2.2	Altered Nutrition: Less Than Body Requirements
1.1.2.3	Altered Nutrition: Risk for More Than Body Requirements
1.2.1.1	Risk for Infection
1.2.2.1	Risk for Altered Body Temperature
1.2.2.2	Hypothermia
1.2.2.3	Hyperthermia
1.2.2.4	Ineffective Thermoregulation
1.2.3.1	Dysreflexia
1.3.1.1	Constipation
1.3.1.1.1	Perceived Constipation
1.3.1.1.2	Colonic Constipation
1.3.1.2	Diarrhea
1.3.1.3	Bowel Incontinence
1.3.2	Altered Urinary Elimination
1.3.2.1.1	Stress Incontinence
1.3.2.1.2	Reflex Incontinence
1.3.2.1.3	Urge Incontinence
1.3.2.1.4	Functional Incontinence
1.3.2.1.5	Total Incontinence
1.3.2.2	Urinary Retention
1.4.1.1	Altered (Specify Type) Tissue Perfusion (Renal, cerebral, cardiopulmonary, gastrointestinal, peripheral)
# 1.4.1.2.1	Fluid Volume Excess
# 1.4.1.2.2.1	Fluid Volume Deficit
1.4.1.2.2.2	Risk for Fluid Volume Deficit
# 1.4.2.1	Decreased Cardiac Output
1.5.1.1	Impaired Gas Exchange
1.5.1.2	Ineffective Airway Clearance
# 1.5.1.3	Ineffective Breathing Pattern
1.5.1.3.1	Inability to Sustain Spontaneous Ventilation
1.5.1.3.2	Dysfunctional Ventilatory Weaning Response (DVWR)
1.6.1	Risk for Injury
1.6.1.1	Risk for Suffocation
1.6.1.2	Risk for Poisoning
1.6.1.3	Risk for Trauma
1.6.1.4	Risk for Aspiration
1.6.1.5	Risk for Disuse Syndrome
1.6.2	Altered Protection
1.6.2.1	Impaired Tissue Integrity
1.6.2.1.1	Altered Oral Mucous Membrane
1.6.2.1.2.1	Impaired Skin Integrity
1.6.2.1.2.2	Risk for Impaired Skin Integrity
1.7.1	Decreased Adaptive Capacity: Intracranial
1.8	Energy Field Disturbance

PATTERN 2: COMMUNICATING

2.1.1.1	Impaired Verbal Communication

PATTERN 3: RELATING

3.1.1	Impaired Social Interaction
3.1.2	Social Isolation
3.1.3	Risk for Loneliness
3.2.1	Altered Role Performance
3.2.1.1.1	Altered Parenting
3.2.1.1.2	Risk for Altered Parenting
3.2.1.1.2.1	Risk for Altered Parent/Infant/Child Attachment
3.2.1.2.1	Sexual Dysfunction
3.2.2	Altered Family Processes
3.2.2.1	Caregiver Role Strain
3.2.2.2	Risk for Caregiver Role Strain
3.2.2.3.1	Altered Family Process: Alcoholism
3.2.3.1	Parental Role Conflict
3.3	Altered Sexuality Patterns

Reprinted with permission from NANDA (1996). *Nursing diagnoses: Definitions & classification 1997–1998.* Philadelphia: Author.

PATTERN 4: VALUING

4.1.1   Spiritual Distress (Distress of the Human Spirit)
4.2   Potential for Enhanced Spiritual Well-Being

PATTERN 5: CHOOSING

\# 5.1.1.1   Ineffective Individual Coping
5.1.1.1.1   Impaired Adjustment
5.1.1.1.2   Defensive Coping
5.1.1.1.3   Ineffective Denial
\# 5.1.2.1.1   Ineffective Family Coping: Disabling
\# 5.1.2.1.2   Ineffective Family Coping: Compromised
5.1.2.2   Family Coping: Potential for Growth
5.1.3.1   Potential for Enhanced Community Coping
5.1.3.2   Ineffective Community Coping
5.2.1   Ineffective Management of Therapeutic Regimen (Individuals)
5.2.1.1   Noncompliance (Specify)
5.2.2   Ineffective Management of Therapeutic Regimen: Families
5.2.3   Ineffective Management of Therapeutic Regimen: Community
5.2.4   Effective Management of Therapeutic Regimen: Individual
5.3.1.1   Decisional Conflict (Specify)
5.4   Health Seeking Behaviors (Specify)

PATTERN 6: MOVING

6.1.1.1   Impaired Physical Mobility
6.1.1.1.1   Risk for Peripheral Neurovascular Dysfunction
6.1.1.1.2   Risk for Perioperative Positioning Injury
6.1.1.2   Activity Intolerance
6.1.1.2.1   Fatigue
6.1.1.3   Risk for Activity Intolerance
6.2.1   Sleep Pattern Disturbance
6.3.1.1   Diversional Activity Deficit
6.4.1.1   Impaired Home Maintenance Management
6.4.2   Altered Health Maintenance
6.5.1   Feeding Self Care Deficit
6.5.1.1   Impaired Swallowing
6.5.1.2   Ineffective Breastfeeding
6.5.1.2.1   Interrupted Breastfeeding
6.5.1.3   Effective Breastfeeding
6.5.1.4   Ineffective Infant Feeding Pattern
6.5.2   Bathing/Hygiene Self Care Deficit
6.5.3   Dressing/Grooming Self Care Deficit
6.5.4   Toileting Self Care Deficit
6.6   Altered Growth and Development
6.7   Relocation Stress Syndrome
6.8.1   Risk for Disorganized Infant Behavior
6.8.2   Disorganized Infant Behavior
6.8.3   Potential for Enhanced Organized Infant Behavior

PATTERN 7: PERCEIVING

7.1.1   Body Image Disturbance
\# 7.1.2   Self Esteem Disturbance
\# 7.1.2.1   Chronic Low Self Esteem
\# 7.1.2.2   Situational Low Self Esteem
7.1.3   Personal Identity Disturbance
7.2   Sensory/Perceptual Alterations (Specify) (Visual, Auditory, Kinesthetic, Gustatory, Tactile, Olfactory)
7.2.1.1   Unilateral Neglect
7.3.1   Hopelessness
7.3.2   Powerlessness

PATTERN 8: KNOWING

\# 8.1.1   Knowledge Deficit (Specify)
8.2.1   Impaired Environmental Interpretation Syndrome
8.2.2   Acute Confusion
8.2.3   Chronic Confusion
\# 8.3   Altered Thought Processes
8.3.1   Impaired Memory

PATTERN 9: FEELING

\# 9.1.1   Pain
\# 9.1.1.1   Chronic Pain
\# 9.2.1.1   Dysfunctional Grieving
\# 9.2.1.2   Anticipatory Grieving
\# 9.2.2   Risk for Violence: Self-Directed or Directed at Others
9.2.2.1   Risk for Self-Mutilation
9.2.3   Post-Trauma Response
9.2.3.1   Rape-Trauma Syndrome
9.2.3.1.1   Rape-Trauma Syndrome: Compound Reaction
9.2.3.1.2   Rape-Trauma Syndrome: Silent Reaction
9.3.1   Anxiety
9.3.2   Fear

\# Diagnoses revised by small work groups at the 1994 Biennial Conference on the Classification of Nursing Diagnoses; changes approved and added in 1996.

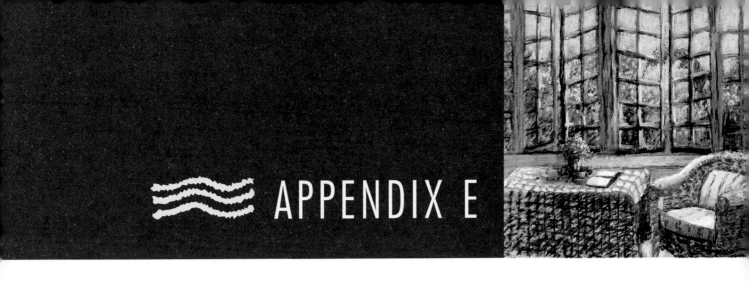

Critical Pathway for a Client Experiencing Depression

HEALTH CARE TEAM MEMBERS AND THEIR RESPONSIBILITIES

Physician   Directs the client's medical care.

Registered Nurse (RN)   Provides skilled observation and assessment. Performs nursing procedures as needed. Teaches client and family how to maintain health at home. Plans and coordinates care with the physician. Registered nurses are available 24 hours daily.

Physical Therapists   Teach strengthening exercises to increase physical independence.

Occupational Therapists   Help the client return to her previous lifestyle with aids to daily living.

Speech Therapists   Evaluate communication problems and work with the client and family to improve communication.

Nursing Assistants   Provide services under the direction of a Registered Nurse. They assist client and family to achieve independence in daily activities. They also assist with personal hygiene.

Social Workers   Assist with family or financial problems.

OVERALL GUIDELINES FOR THE NURSE

Guidelines for the nurse providing education to the depressed client in home health:

◆ Client will make a written agreement with the nurse to seek help prior to acting on suicidal thoughts. Agreement will be renewed each visit.

◆ Client verbalizes the importance of eating 60% of meals three times a day.

◆ Client verbalizes the importance of sleeping at least six hours per night.

◆ Client is able to demonstrate at least three relaxation techniques.

◆ Client will name each medication, identify the purpose, when it is to be taken, and be able to list two potential side effects caused by each.

◆ Client will verbalize the importance of compliance with medication.

◆ Client will verbalize the importance of compliance with follow-up care.

◆ Client will demonstrate increased energy and motivation by attending one meeting or social function per week.

◆ Client will increase activity by one activity each week.

Developed by Wanda Horn, RNC, Southeast Missouri Hospital, Psychiatric Unit.

Critical Pathway for a Client Experiencing Depression

DRG <u>426</u>   Anticipated LOS <u>3 months</u>   Admit Date _____   Discharge Date _____

DSM-IV Diagnosis _____

Psychiatrist/Physician _____   Consultants _____

_____

Problem: **Suicide Risk**

Nursing Diagnosis: *High risk for self directed violence* r/t depressed mood, feelings of hopelessness, worthlessness.

Date Initiated _____   Modified _____   Resolved _____

Expected Outcome: 1. Client will not harm herself while in the home environment.

2. Client will comply with taking medications as prescribed.

3. Client will report suicidal thoughts to nurse, counselor, or physician prior to taking action.

Nursing Assessment/
Interventions
(practice standards)

1. Establish a therapeutic rapport with client.

2. Establish a contract with client that she will not harm self & if thoughts of self harm occur, client will inform family, counselor, nurse, or physician prior to acting on such thoughts.

3. Assess safety of environment.

Problem: **Weight Loss, Lack of Energy**

Nursing Diagnosis: *Altered nutrition: less than body requirements* r/t decreased energy levels, poor appetite, lack of motivation to prepare and consume food.

Date Initiated _____   Modified _____   Resolved _____

Expected Outcome: 1. Client will eat at least 60% of three meals daily.

2. Client will maintain current weight.

3. Client will demonstrate increased energy and motivation to prepare and consume meals.

Nursing Assessment/
Interventions
(practice standards)

1. Weigh client every visit.

2. Assess ability of client to prepare meals.

3. Assess client's motivation to consume meals.

Problem: _____

Nursing Diagnosis: _____

Date Initiated _____   Modified _____   Resolved _____

Expected Outcome: 1. _____

Nursing Assessment/
Interventions
(practice standards)

1. _____

2. _____

3. _____

Path and discharge goals explained to the client/significant other with mutual agreement.

Date _____   RN Signature _____

Critical Pathway for a Client Experiencing Depression

	Admission VISIT #1	VISIT #2	VISIT #3
Therapeutic Rapport	Prior to visit, call and make an appointment. Arrive on time. Establish trust. Allow time to talk prior to physical assessment. Establish ground rules of the relationship. Encourage client participation in forming plan of treatment. Set mutual goals.	Maintain trusting relationship. Actively listen; clarify; repeat; allow time for client to verbalize feelings. Offer encouragement and support. Promote: positive thinking; increased self esteem; increased sociability.	Maintain trusting relationship. Actively listen; clarify; repeat; allow time for client to verbalize feelings. Offer encouragement and support. Promote: positive thinking; increased self esteem; increased sociability.
Mental Status	**Anxiety Level:** ☐ Moderate ☐ Severe ☐ Panic **Mood:** ☐ WNL ☐ Labile ☐ Angry ☐ Hopeless ☐ Depressed ☐ Euphoric ☐ Guilt ☐ Worthless ☐ Incongruent **Thought Processes:** ☐ Incoherent ☐ Preoccupied ☐ Disorganized **Insight/Judgment:** ☐ WNL ☐ Poor ☐ Dangerous/Reckless **Suicide Potential:** ☐ Yes ☐ No ☐ Plan ☐ Physician Notified **Appearance:** ☐ Clean ☐ Unkempt ☐ Dirty **Behavior:** ☐ Friendly ☐ Evasive ☐ Indifferent **Speech:** ☐ Rate ☐ Cadence ☐ Tone **Orientation:** ☐ Month ☐ Day ☐ Year ☐ Time	**Anxiety Level:** ☐ Moderate ☐ Severe ☐ Panic **Mood:** ☐ WNL ☐ Labile ☐ Angry ☐ Hopeless ☐ Depressed ☐ Euphoric ☐ Guilt ☐ Worthless ☐ Incongruent **Thought Processes:** ☐ Incoherent ☐ Preoccupied ☐ Disorganized **Insight/Judgment:** ☐ WNL ☐ Poor ☐ Dangerous/Reckless **Suicide Potential:** ☐ Yes ☐ No ☐ Plan ☐ Physician Notified **Appearance:** ☐ Clean ☐ Unkempt ☐ Dirty **Behavior:** ☐ Friendly ☐ Evasive ☐ Indifferent **Speech:** ☐ Rate ☐ Cadence ☐ Tone **Orientation:** ☐ Month ☐ Day ☐ Year ☐ Time	**Anxiety Level:** ☐ Moderate ☐ Severe ☐ Panic **Mood:** ☐ WNL ☐ Labile ☐ Angry ☐ Hopeless ☐ Depressed ☐ Euphoric ☐ Guilt ☐ Worthless ☐ Incongruent **Thought Processes:** ☐ Incoherent ☐ Preoccupied ☐ Disorganized **Insight/Judgment:** ☐ WNL ☐ Poor ☐ Dangerous/Reckless **Suicide Potential:** ☐ Yes ☐ No ☐ Plan ☐ Physician Notified **Appearance:** ☐ Clean ☐ Unkempt ☐ Dirty **Behavior:** ☐ Friendly ☐ Evasive ☐ Indifferent **Speech:** ☐ Rate ☐ Cadence ☐ Tone **Orientation:** ☐ Month ☐ Day ☐ Year ☐ Time
Physical Assessment	☐ Past Health History Dietary Needs Met? ☐ Yes ☐ No Wt _____ Fluid Intake _____ N/V_____ LBM_____ **Vital Signs:** BP____ R____ P____ T____ ☐ Apical Pulse ☐ Lung Sounds ☐ Skin Integrity ☐ Bowel Sounds ☐ Mobility ☐ Edema ☐ Pulses of Extremities ☐ Sleep	Dietary Needs Met? ☐ Yes ☐ No Wt _____ Fluid Intake _____ N/V_____ LBM_____ **Vital Signs:** BP____ R____ P____ T____ ☐ Apical Pulse ☐ Lung Sounds ☐ Skin Integrity ☐ Bowel Sounds ☐ Mobility ☐ Edema ☐ Pulses of Extremities ☐ Sleep	Dietary Needs Met? ☐ Yes ☐ No Wt _____ Fluid Intake _____ N/V_____ LBM_____ **Vital Signs:** BP____ R____ P____ T____ ☐ Apical Pulse ☐ Lung Sounds ☐ Skin Integrity ☐ Bowel Sounds ☐ Mobility ☐ Edema ☐ Pulses of Extremities ☐ Sleep
Complete Assessment	☐ Safety ☐ MSW ☐ ADLS		

Critical Pathway, Visits 1–3 continues

	VISIT #1 Admission (continued)	**VISIT #2** (continued)	**VISIT #3** (continued)
Self Care		☐ WNL ☐ Needs Assist	☐ WNL ☐ Needs Assist
Diagnostic Studies	☐ Obtain Labs PRN	☐ Obtain Labs PRN	☐ Obtain Labs PRN
Medications	☐ How are you taking your medications? ☐ Have you missed any doses? ☐ Have you had any problems with the medications? ☐ Provide information regarding adverse effects & benefits of meds. ☐ Fill medication box. ☐ Aims	☐ How are you taking your medications? ☐ Have you missed any doses? ☐ Have you had any problems with the medications? ☐ Provide information about side effects & benefits of meds. ☐ Fill medication box. ☐ Aims	☐ How are you taking your medications? ☐ Have you missed any doses? ☐ Have you had any problems with the medications? ☐ Provide information about side effects & benefits of meds. ☐ Fill medication box. ☐ Aims
Discharge Planning	**Assess:** Self management of medication regime; caregiver's ability to manage medications; willingness of caregiver; motivation and ability to keep appointments for follow up. **Teach:** The importance of medication compliance. **Refer:** Support groups; community resources.	**Assess:** Self management of medication regime; caregiver's ability to manage medications; willingness of caregiver; motivation and ability to keep appointments for follow up. **Teach:** The importance of medication compliance. **Refer:** Support groups; community resources.	**Assess:** Self management of medication regime; caregiver's ability to manage medications; willingness of caregiver; motivation and ability to keep appointments for follow up. **Teach:** The importance of medication compliance. **Refer:** Support groups; community resources.
Expected Outcomes	Client will maintain a therapeutic relationship with the HH nurse. Client will be oriented to the benefits of home health care. Client will be able to maintain safety while in a home environment. Client will provide a written contract with nurse to seek help prior to acting on suicidal thoughts. Client will comply with taking medications as ordered by the physician. Client will maintain adequate diet. Client will sleep 6 hours per night. Client will report suicidal thoughts prior to acting on them. Client will keep all follow-up appointments.	Client will be able to maintain safety while in a home environment. Client will comply with taking medications as ordered by the physician. Client will maintain adequate diet. Client will sleep 6 hours per night. Client will report suicidal thoughts prior to acting on them. Client will be able to describe medication regime.	Client will be able to maintain safety while in a home environment. Client will comply with taking medications as ordered by the physician. Client will maintain adequate diet. Client will sleep 6 hours per night. Client will report suicidal thoughts prior to acting on them. Client will list 3 side effects of medications and how to manage them.
Variances			

	VISIT #4	**VISIT #5**	**VISIT #6**
Therapeutic Rapport	Maintain trusting relationship. Actively listen; be empathetic; redefine; allow time for client to verbalize feelings. Offer encouragement & support. Promote: positive thinking; increased self esteem; increased sociability.	Maintain trusting relationship. Actively listen; be genuine; be nonjudgmental; allow time for client to verbalize feelings. Offer encouragement & support. Promote: positive thinking; increased self esteem; increased sociability.	Maintain trusting relationship. Actively listen; be honest; offer hope; allow time for client to verbalize feelings. Offer encouragement & support. Promote: positive thinking; increased self esteem; increased sociability.
Mental Status	**Anxiety Level:** ☐ Moderate ☐ Severe ☐ Panic **Mood:** ☐ WNL ☐ Labile ☐ Angry ☐ Hopeless ☐ Depressed ☐ Euphoric ☐ Guilt ☐ Worthless ☐ Incongruent **Thought Processes:** ☐ Incoherent ☐ Preoccupied ☐ Disorganized **Insight/Judgment:** ☐ WNL ☐ Poor ☐ Dangerous/Reckless **Suicide Potential:** ☐ Yes ☐ No ☐ Plan ☐ Physician Notified **Appearance:** ☐ Clean ☐ Unkempt ☐ Dirty **Behavior:** ☐ Friendly ☐ Evasive ☐ Indifferent **Speech:** ☐ Rate ☐ Cadence ☐ Tone **Orientation:** ☐ Month ☐ Day ☐ Year ☐ Time	**Anxiety Level:** ☐ Moderate ☐ Severe ☐ Panic **Mood:** ☐ WNL ☐ Labile ☐ Angry ☐ Hopeless ☐ Depressed ☐ Euphoric ☐ Guilt ☐ Worthless ☐ Incongruent **Thought Processes:** ☐ Incoherent ☐ Preoccupied ☐ Disorganized **Insight/Judgment:** ☐ WNL ☐ Poor ☐ Dangerous/Reckless **Suicide Potential:** ☐ Yes ☐ No ☐ Plan ☐ Physician Notified **Appearance:** ☐ Clean ☐ Unkempt ☐ Dirty **Behavior:** ☐ Friendly ☐ Evasive ☐ Indifferent **Speech:** ☐ Rate ☐ Cadence ☐ Tone **Orientation:** ☐ Month ☐ Day ☐ Year ☐ Time	**Anxiety Level:** ☐ Moderate ☐ Severe ☐ Panic **Mood:** ☐ WNL ☐ Labile ☐ Angry ☐ Hopeless ☐ Depressed ☐ Euphoric ☐ Guilt ☐ Worthless ☐ Incongruent **Thought Processes:** ☐ Incoherent ☐ Preoccupied ☐ Disorganized **Insight/Judgment:** ☐ WNL ☐ Poor ☐ Dangerous/Reckless **Suicide Potential:** ☐ Yes ☐ No ☐ Plan ☐ Physician Notified **Appearance:** ☐ Clean ☐ Unkempt ☐ Dirty **Behavior:** ☐ Friendly ☐ Evasive ☐ Indifferent **Speech:** ☐ Rate ☐ Cadence ☐ Tone **Orientation:** ☐ Month ☐ Day ☐ Year ☐ Time
Physical Assessment	Dietary Needs Met? ☐ Yes ☐ No Wt _____ Fluid Intake _____ N/V _____ LBM _____ **Vital Signs:** BP____ R____ P____ T____ ☐ Apical Pulse ☐ Lung Sounds ☐ Skin Integrity ☐ Bowel Sounds ☐ Mobility ☐ Edema ☐ Pulses of Extremities ☐ Sleep	Dietary Needs Met? ☐ Yes ☐ No Wt _____ Fluid Intake _____ N/V _____ LBM _____ **Vital Signs:** BP____ R____ P____ T____ ☐ Apical Pulse ☐ Lung Sounds ☐ Skin Integrity ☐ Bowel Sounds ☐ Mobility ☐ Edema ☐ Pulses of Extremities ☐ Sleep	Dietary Needs Met? ☐ Yes ☐ No Wt _____ Fluid Intake _____ N/V _____ LBM _____ **Vital Signs:** BP____ R____ P____ T____ ☐ Apical Pulse ☐ Lung Sounds ☐ Skin Integrity ☐ Bowel Sounds ☐ Mobility ☐ Edema ☐ Pulses of Extremities ☐ Sleep
Self Care	☐ WNL ☐ Needs Assist	☐ WNL ☐ Needs Assist	☐ WNL ☐ Needs Assist
Diagnostic Studies	☐ Obtain Labs PRN	☐ Obtain Labs PRN	☐ Obtain Labs PRN

Critical Pathway, Visits 4–6 continues

	VISIT #4 (continued)	VISIT #5 (continued)	VISIT #6 (continued)
Medications	☐ How are you taking your medications? ☐ Have you missed any doses? ☐ Have you had any problems with the medications? ☐ Provide information regarding adverse effects & benefits of meds. ☐ Fill medication box. ☐ Aims	☐ How are you taking your medications? ☐ Have you missed any doses? ☐ Have you had any problems with the medications? ☐ Provide information regarding adverse effects & benefits of meds. ☐ Fill medication box. ☐ Aims	☐ How are you taking your medications? ☐ Have you missed any doses? ☐ Have you had any problems with the medications? ☐ Provide information regarding adverse effects & benefits of meds. ☐ Fill medication box. ☐ Aims
Discharge Planning	**Assess:** Self management of medication regime; caregiver's ability to manage medications; willingness of caregiver; motivation and ability to keep appointments for follow up. **Teach:** Importance of medication compliance. **Refer:** Support groups; community resources.	**Assess:** Self management of medication regime; caregiver's ability to manage medications; willingness of caregiver; motivation and ability to keep appointments for follow up. **Teach:** Importance of medication compliance; relaxation techniques. **Refer:** Support groups; community resources.	**Assess:** Self management of medication regime; caregiver's ability to manage medications; willingness of caregiver; motivation and ability to keep appointments for follow up. **Teach:** Importance of medication compliance; coping strategies. **Refer:** Support groups; community resources; financial support.
Expected Outcomes	Client will maintain a therapeutic relationship. Client will be able to maintain safety while in a home environment. Client will comply with taking medications as ordered by the physician. Client will keep all follow-up appointments. Client will maintain adequate diet. Client will sleep 6 hours per night. Client will report suicidal thoughts prior to acting on them.	Client will maintain a therapeutic relationship. Client will be able to maintain safety while in a home environment. Client will comply with taking medications as ordered by the physician. Client will keep all follow-up appointments. Client will maintain adequate diet. Client will sleep 6 hours per night. Client will report suicidal thoughts prior to acting on them. Client will verbalize 3 benefits of taking medications.	Client will maintain a therapeutic relationship. Client will be able to maintain safety while in a home environment. Client will comply with taking medications as ordered by the physician. Client will keep all follow-up appointments. Client will maintain adequate diet. Client will sleep 6 hours per night. Client will report suicidal thoughts prior to acting on them. Client will demonstrate 1 relaxation technique other than medication. Client will attend 1 support group during the week.
Variances			

	VISIT #7	VISIT #8	VISIT #9
Therapeutic Rapport	Maintain trusting relationship. Actively listen; clarify; be empathetic; allow time for client to verbalize feelings. Offer encouragement & support. Promote: positive thinking; increased self esteem; increased sociability.	Maintain trusting relationship. Actively listen; be nonjudgmental; offer hope; allow time for client to verbalize feelings. Offer encouragement & support. Promote: positive thinking; increased self esteem; increased sociability.	Maintain trusting relationship. Actively listen; clarify; be accepting; allow time for client to verbalize feelings. Offer encouragement & support. Promote: positive thinking; increased self esteem; increased sociability.
Mental Status	**Anxiety Level:** ☐ Moderate ☐ Severe ☐ Panic **Mood:** ☐ WNL ☐ Labile ☐ Angry ☐ Hopeless ☐ Depressed ☐ Euphoric ☐ Guilt ☐ Worthless ☐ Incongruent **Thought Processes:** ☐ Incoherent ☐ Preoccupied ☐ Disorganized **Insight/Judgment:** ☐ WNL ☐ Poor ☐ Dangerous/Reckless **Suicide Potential:** ☐ Yes ☐ No ☐ Plan ☐ Physician Notified **Appearance:** ☐ Clean ☐ Unkempt ☐ Dirty **Behavior:** ☐ Friendly ☐ Evasive ☐ Indifferent **Speech:** ☐ Rate ☐ Cadence ☐ Tone **Orientation:** ☐ Month ☐ Day ☐ Year ☐ Time	**Anxiety Level:** ☐ Moderate ☐ Severe ☐ Panic **Mood:** ☐ WNL ☐ Labile ☐ Angry ☐ Hopeless ☐ Depressed ☐ Euphoric ☐ Guilt ☐ Worthless ☐ Incongruent **Thought Processes:** ☐ Incoherent ☐ Preoccupied ☐ Disorganized **Insight/Judgment:** ☐ WNL ☐ Poor ☐ Dangerous/Reckless **Suicide Potential:** ☐ Yes ☐ No ☐ Plan ☐ Physician Notified **Appearance:** ☐ Clean ☐ Unkempt ☐ Dirty **Behavior:** ☐ Friendly ☐ Evasive ☐ Indifferent **Speech:** ☐ Rate ☐ Cadence ☐ Tone **Orientation:** ☐ Month ☐ Day ☐ Year ☐ Time	**Anxiety Level:** ☐ Moderate ☐ Severe ☐ Panic **Mood:** ☐ WNL ☐ Labile ☐ Angry ☐ Hopeless ☐ Depressed ☐ Euphoric ☐ Guilt ☐ Worthless ☐ Incongruent **Thought Processes:** ☐ Incoherent ☐ Preoccupied ☐ Disorganized **Insight/Judgment:** ☐ WNL ☐ Poor ☐ Dangerous/Reckless **Suicide Potential:** ☐ Yes ☐ No ☐ Plan ☐ Physician Notified **Appearance:** ☐ Clean ☐ Unkempt ☐ Dirty **Behavior:** ☐ Friendly ☐ Evasive ☐ Indifferent **Speech:** ☐ Rate ☐ Cadence ☐ Tone **Orientation:** ☐ Month ☐ Day ☐ Year ☐ Time
Physical Assessment	Dietary Needs Met? ☐ Yes ☐ No Wt _____ Fluid Intake _____ N/V _____ LBM _____ **Vital Signs:** BP ___ R ___ P ___ T ___ ☐ Apical Pulse ☐ Lung Sounds ☐ Skin Integrity ☐ Bowel Sounds ☐ Mobility ☐ Edema ☐ Pulses of Extremities ☐ Sleep	Dietary Needs Met? ☐ Yes ☐ No Wt _____ Fluid Intake _____ N/V _____ LBM _____ **Vital Signs:** BP ___ R ___ P ___ T ___ ☐ Apical Pulse ☐ Lung Sounds ☐ Skin Integrity ☐ Bowel Sounds ☐ Mobility ☐ Edema ☐ Pulses of Extremities ☐ Sleep	Dietary Needs Met? ☐ Yes ☐ No Wt _____ Fluid Intake _____ N/V _____ LBM _____ **Vital Signs:** BP ___ R ___ P ___ T ___ ☐ Apical Pulse ☐ Lung Sounds ☐ Skin Integrity ☐ Bowel Sounds ☐ Mobility ☐ Edema ☐ Pulses of Extremities ☐ Sleep
Self Care	☐ WNL ☐ Needs Assist	☐ WNL ☐ Needs Assist	☐ WNL ☐ Needs Assist
Diagnostic Studies	☐ Obtain Labs PRN	☐ Obtain Labs PRN	☐ Obtain Labs PRN

Critical Pathway, Visits 7–9 continues

	VISIT #7 (continued)	**VISIT #8** (continued)	**VISIT #9** (continued)
Medications	☐ How are you taking your medications? ☐ Have you missed any doses? ☐ Have you had any problems with the medications? ☐ Ask client to provide information regarding adverse effects & benefits of meds. ☐ Discuss medication names as client fills medication box. ☐ Aims	☐ How are you taking your medications? ☐ Have you missed any doses? ☐ Have you had any problems with the medications? ☐ Request information regarding adverse effects & benefits of meds. from client. ☐ Assist as client fills medication box. ☐ Aims	☐ How are you taking your medications? ☐ Have you missed any doses? ☐ Have you had any problems with the medications? ☐ Ask client to verbalize information regarding benefits & adverse effects of meds. ☐ Observe as client fills medication box. ☐ Aims
Discharge Planning	**Assess:** Self management of medication regime, caregiver's ability to manage medications; willingness of caregiver; motivation and ability to keep appointments for follow up. **Teach:** Importance of medication compliance; relaxation techniques. **Refer:** Support groups; community resources.	**Assess:** Self management of medication regime; caregiver's ability to manage medications; willingness of caregiver; motivation and ability to keep appointments for follow up. **Teach:** Importance of medication compliance; relaxation techniques. **Refer:** Support groups; community resources.	**Assess:** Self management of medication regime; caregiver's ability to manage medications; willingness of caregiver; motivation and ability to keep appointments for follow up. **Teach:** Importance of medication compliance; relaxation techniques. **Refer:** Support groups; community resources.
Expected Outcomes	Client will maintain a therapeutic relationship. Client will be able to maintain safety while in a home environment. Client will comply with taking medications as ordered by the physician. Client will keep all follow-up appointments. Client will maintain adequate diet. Client will sleep 6 hours per night. Client will report suicidal thoughts prior to acting on them. Client will demonstrate medication regime. Client will identify 3 ways of coping with side effects of medications.	Client will maintain a therapeutic relationship. Client will be able to maintain safety while in a home environment. Client will comply with taking medications as ordered by the physician. Client will keep all follow-up appointments. Client will maintain adequate diet. Client will sleep 6 hours per night. Client will report suicidal thoughts prior to acting on them. Client will exhibit increased energy level by cleaning house. Client will identify 3 ways of decreasing medication side effects.	Client will maintain a therapeutic relationship. Client will be able to maintain safety while in a home environment. Client will comply with taking medications as ordered by the physician. Client will keep all follow-up appointments. Client will maintain adequate diet. Client will sleep 6 hours per night. Client will report suicidal thoughts prior to acting on them. Client will demonstrate 2 relaxation techniques other than medication.
Variances			

	VISIT #10	**VISIT #11**	**VISIT #12**
Therapeutic Rapport	Maintain trusting relationship. Actively listen; redefine; repeat for clarification; allow time for client to verbalize feelings. Offer encouragement & support. Promote: positive thinking; increased self esteem; increased sociability.	Maintain trusting relationship. Actively listen; offer hope; be genuine; allow time for client to verbalize feelings. Offer encouragement & support. Promote: positive thinking; increased self esteem; increased sociability.	Maintain trusting relationship. Actively listen; be empathetic; nonjudgmental; allow time for client to verbalize feelings. Offer encouragement & support. Promote: positive thinking; increased self esteem; increased sociability.
Mental Status	**Anxiety Level:** ☐ Moderate ☐ Severe ☐ Panic **Mood:** ☐ WNL ☐ Labile ☐ Angry ☐ Hopeless ☐ Depressed ☐ Euphoric ☐ Guilt ☐ Worthless ☐ Incongruent **Thought Processes:** ☐ Incoherent ☐ Preoccupied ☐ Disorganized **Insight/Judgment:** ☐ WNL ☐ Poor ☐ Dangerous/Reckless **Suicide Potential:** ☐ Yes ☐ No ☐ Plan ☐ Physician Notified **Appearance:** ☐ Clean ☐ Unkempt ☐ Dirty **Behavior:** ☐ Friendly ☐ Evasive ☐ Indifferent **Speech:** ☐ Rate ☐ Cadence ☐ Tone **Orientation:** ☐ Month ☐ Day ☐ Year ☐ Time	**Anxiety Level:** ☐ Moderate ☐ Severe ☐ Panic **Mood:** ☐ WNL ☐ Labile ☐ Angry ☐ Hopeless ☐ Depressed ☐ Euphoric ☐ Guilt ☐ Worthless ☐ Incongruent **Thought Processes:** ☐ Incoherent ☐ Preoccupied ☐ Disorganized **Insight/Judgment:** ☐ WNL ☐ Poor ☐ Dangerous/Reckless **Suicide Potential:** ☐ Yes ☐ No ☐ Plan ☐ Physician Notified **Appearance:** ☐ Clean ☐ Unkempt ☐ Dirty **Behavior:** ☐ Friendly ☐ Evasive ☐ Indifferent **Speech:** ☐ Rate ☐ Cadence ☐ Tone **Orientation:** ☐ Month ☐ Day ☐ Year ☐ Time	**Anxiety Level:** ☐ Moderate ☐ Severe ☐ Panic **Mood:** ☐ WNL ☐ Labile ☐ Angry ☐ Hopeless ☐ Depressed ☐ Euphoric ☐ Guilt ☐ Worthless ☐ Incongruent **Thought Processes:** ☐ Incoherent ☐ Preoccupied ☐ Disorganized **Insight/Judgment:** ☐ WNL ☐ Poor ☐ Dangerous/Reckless **Suicide Potential:** ☐ Yes ☐ No ☐ Plan ☐ Physician Notified **Appearance:** ☐ Clean ☐ Unkempt ☐ Dirty **Behavior:** ☐ Friendly ☐ Evasive ☐ Indifferent **Speech:** ☐ Rate ☐ Cadence ☐ Tone **Orientation:** ☐ Month ☐ Day ☐ Year ☐ Time
Physical Assessment	Dietary Needs Met? ☐ Yes ☐ No Wt _____ Fluid Intake _____ N/V _____ LBM _____ **Vital Signs:** BP ___ R ___ P ___ T ___ ☐ Apical Pulse ☐ Lung Sounds ☐ Skin Integrity ☐ Bowel Sounds ☐ Mobility ☐ Edema ☐ Pulses of Extremities ☐ Sleep	Dietary Needs Met? ☐ Yes ☐ No Wt _____ Fluid Intake _____ N/V _____ LBM _____ **Vital Signs:** BP ___ R ___ P ___ T ___ ☐ Apical Pulse ☐ Lung Sounds ☐ Skin Integrity ☐ Bowel Sounds ☐ Mobility ☐ Edema ☐ Pulses of Extremities ☐ Sleep	Dietary Needs Met? ☐ Yes ☐ No Wt _____ Fluid Intake _____ N/V _____ LBM _____ **Vital Signs:** BP ___ R ___ P ___ T ___ ☐ Apical Pulse ☐ Lung Sounds ☐ Skin Integrity ☐ Bowel Sounds ☐ Mobility ☐ Edema ☐ Pulses of Extremities ☐ Sleep
Self Care	☐ WNL ☐ Needs Assist	☐ WNL ☐ Needs Assist	☐ WNL ☐ Needs Assist
Diagnostic Studies	☐ Obtain Labs PRN	☐ Obtain Labs PRN	☐ Obtain Labs PRN

Critical Pathway, Visits 10–12 continues

	VISIT #10 (continued)	VISIT #11 (continued)	VISIT #12 (continued)
Medications	☐ How are you taking your medications? ☐ Have you missed any doses? ☐ Have you had any problems with the medications? ☐ Have client list benefits & adverse effects of meds. ☐ Observe as client fills medication box. ☐ Aims	☐ How are you taking your medications? ☐ Have you missed any doses? ☐ Have you had any problems with the medications? ☐ Ask client to name each medication. ☐ Ask client to verbalize 2 adverse effects of medications. ☐ Observe client as she fills medication box. ☐ Aims	☐ How are you taking your medications? ☐ Have you missed any doses? ☐ Have you had any problems with the medications? ☐ Ask client to name each medication. ☐ Ask client to list 2 side effects of medications. ☐ Observe client as she fills medication box. ☐ Ask client to verbalize when each medication is due.
Discharge Planning	**Assess:** Self management of medication regime; caregiver's ability to manage medications; willingness of caregiver; motivation and ability to keep appointments for follow up. **Teach:** Importance of medication compliance; relaxation techniques. **Refer:** Support groups; community resources.	**Assess:** Self management of medication regime; caregiver's ability to manage medications; willingness of caregiver; motivation and ability to keep appointments for follow up. **Teach:** Importance of medication compliance. **Refer:** Support groups; community resources.	**Assess:** Self management of medication regime; caregiver's ability to manage medications; willingness of caregiver; motivation and ability to keep appointments for follow up. **Teach:** Importance of medication compliance. **Refer:** Support groups; community resources.
Expected Outcomes	Client will maintain a therapeutic relationship. Client will be able to maintain safety while in a home environment. Client will comply with taking medications as ordered by the physician. Client will keep all follow-up appointments. Client will maintain adequate diet. Client will sleep 6 hours per night. Client will report suicidal thoughts prior to acting on them. Client will demonstrate increased energy by attending 2 social activities during the week.	Client will maintain a therapeutic relationship. Client will be able to maintain safety while in a home environment. Client will agree not to discontinue or add medications without consulting the physician. Client will verbalize methods of decreasing side effects of medications such as hard candy for dry mouth, drink water, exercise to decrease constipation. Client will keep all follow-up appointments. Client will maintain adequate diet. Client will sleep 6 hours per night. Client will deny suicidal thoughts. Client will demonstrate 1 relaxation technique other than medication.	Client will maintain a therapeutic relationship. Client will be able to maintain safety while in a home environment. Client will be able to list medications and verbalize purpose for each. Client will keep all follow-up appointments. Client will maintain adequate diet. Client will sleep 6 hours per night. Client will report no suicidal thoughts. Client will demonstrate 1 relaxation technique other than medication. Client will attend at least 3 social functions per week. Client will verbalize community resources available for assistance.
Variances			

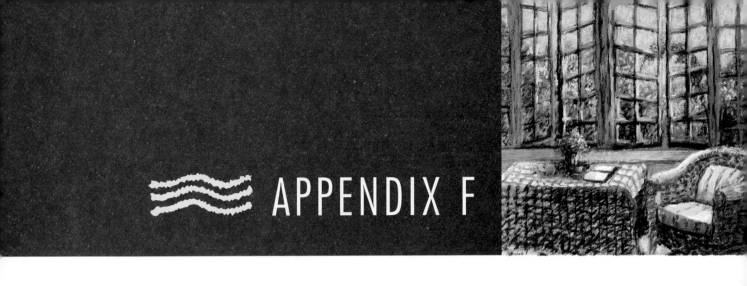

APPENDIX F

Psychological Tests in Common Use

Psychological tests are assessment tools that provide information to the clinician regarding either the intellectual or cognitive abilities of the client. Psychological tests can also provide an assessment of personality. Formal psychological tests are designed to be administered and scored by a professional psychologist or psychometrician. They are different from brief screening tools or questionnaires of the sort that clinicians frequently use in diagnosis or client follow-up. Examples of screening tools include the CAGE interview, the Michigan Alcohol Screening Test, the Beck Depression Inventory, and the Mini Mental Status Test. These screening tools have been validated in multiple study populations, but they are typically used to suggest diagnoses or to monitor the severity of conditions on repeat visits. In contrast, formal psychological testing is generally used for diagnostic purposes, often in conjunction with psychiatric interview data and direct observations of client behaviors. Because DSM-IV criteria form the basis for most current psychiatric diagnoses, formal testing may be less frequently used than in the past. The following should prove useful when an unfamiliar test is encountered in clinical practice. Formal psychological tests may be of three types: projective tests, objective tests, and intelligence tests (the latter is a variety of objective test designed to assess specific cognitive abilities).

PROJECTIVE TESTS

A projective test uses unstructured stimuli to measure relevant psychological attributes.

Draw-a-Person Test

The client is given a blank piece of paper and asked to first draw any person, then specifically a person of the opposite sex.

Interpretation: There are standardized norms for interpreting the results. This test assesses factors related to self-esteem, body image, and interpersonal relationships.

In children, the draw-a-person test can provide important clues to level of psychomotor development.

Rorschach Test

The Rorschach test presents a client with 10 standardized "ink-blot" images. The client is asked to describe what she sees in these black and white forms.

Interpretation: Each image has a set of potential responses, and the test is scored in accord with what the client describes seeing. The results are closely tied to psychoanalytic theories of personality development.

Thematic Apperception Test (TAT)

The client is presented with a standardized series of 30 ambiguous pictures and asked to make up a story about each picture.

Interpretation: Scoring is standardized. The person's responses reveal personality dynamics and issues of importance to the client.

Sentence Completion Test (SCT)

The client is presented with 75 to 100 incomplete sentences and asked to complete these sentences with the first idea that comes into his mind, no matter how odd or inappropriate it may seem. An incomplete sentence might be "The nursing student is . . . ." (This sentence is not part of the SCT, but you might want to imagine how you would complete it.)

Interpretation: The test is standardized and can help identify the client's preoccupations, fears, or goals.

OBJECTIVE TESTS

Objective tests present the client with a series of multiple-choice questions regarding values, attitudes, or descriptions of situations for which responses have been normed, so that the individual's responses can be compared to those of others.

Minnesota Multiphasic Personality Inventory (MMPI)

This lengthy test has 567 items designed to measure aspects of personality such as hypomania, paranoia, hypochondriasis, depression, schizophrenia, psychopathic deviation, and degree of masculinity/femininity. The test questions were empirically constructed based on clinical observations. This is one of the most common psychological tests given to adults.

Interpretation: Scores for each scale are compared to norms. Client tendencies for specific behaviors and psychiatric conditions/diagnoses are reported.

California Personality Inventory

This test has 17 separate scales and focuses on factors that seem to reflect personality.

Interpretation: Standardized norms provide indications of personality characteristics and traits, such as responsibility or socialization.

INTELLIGENCE TESTS

Intelligence tests are a type of objective test that provides information about intelligence, normed against a subset of the population. The WAIS and WISC are divided into verbal and nonverbal scales. While all intelligence tests are culturally biased toward the group from which the norms were calculated, intelligence tests may provide information about a client's strengths or weaknesses. The WAIS has an important role in assessing persons with mental retardation and other developmental disorders presenting in adulthood. It has less value in the assessment of dementia where clinical screening (including the Mini Mental Status Examination) is used more often. The WISC is exceedingly important in evaluating developmental problems in children and adolescents.

Wechsler Adult Intelligence Scale (WAIS)

This is a test with subscales covering vocabulary, comprehension, information, similarities, digit span, arithmetic, picture arrangement, picture completion, object assembly, block design, and digit symbol.

Interpretation: Scores yield a measure of intelligence expressed as IQ (intelligence quotient).

Wechsler Intelligence Scale for Children (WISC)

A version of the WAIS that is appropriate for children ages 5 to 15 years.

Interpretation: Scores yield a measure of intelligence expressed as IQ, normed for children.

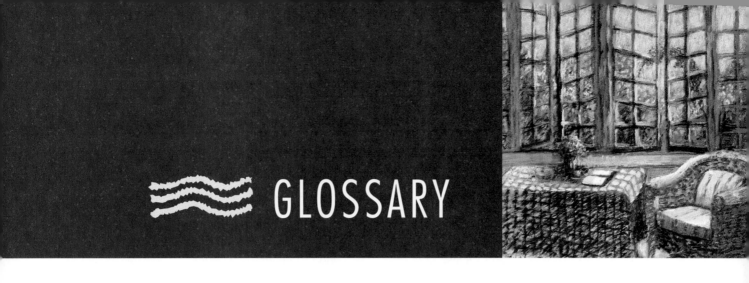

GLOSSARY

Abandonment Negligence in which a client is left in need without alternatives for treatment.

Acquaintance (or Date) Rape Forcible rape or sexual battery that occurs by the victim's dates or acquaintances.

Adaptive Energy Individual's ability to respond to a stressor.

Adaptive Potential Capacity of the person to respond to stressors—to utilize resources to cope.

Adaptive Potential Assessment Model Erickson and colleague's model describing three states of coping potential: arousal, equilibrium, and impoverishment.

Addiction Inability to abstain from drug use, accompanied by drug tolerance and withdrawal.

Adversity Measure of the strength of a given stimulus for anxiety.

Aggravated Criminal Sexual Assault Criminal sexual assault in which a weapon is used or displayed; the victim's life or someone else's is endangered or threatened; the perpetrator causes bodily harm to the victim; the assault occurs during the commission of another felony; or force is used to threaten or cause physical harm to the victim.

Aggregate Population or defined group.

Agoraphobia Fear of going out in public places.

Akathisia Subjective sense of restlessness with a perceived need to pace or otherwise move continuously.

Akinesia Reaction involving loss of movement.

Alcoholism Compulsion to drink alcohol.

Alogia Tendency to speak very little and use brief and seemingly empty phrases.

Anger Control Assistance Nursing intervention aimed at facilitation of the expression of anger in an adaptive and nonviolent manner.

Anhedonia Persistently depressed mood and loss of interest or pleasure in almost all activities; inability to find enjoyment in daily activities.

Animal-Assisted Therapy Use of animals to provide attention, affection, diversion, and/or relaxation.

Anorexia Nervosa Psychological eating disorder characterized by profound disturbance in body image, failure to maintain minimum weight, and obsession with weight, despite underweight status.

Antipsychotic Drugs Major tranquilizers administered to control symptoms of psychosis.

Antisocial Personality Disorder Behavior pattern characterized by violence, impulsiveness, dishonesty, carelessness, and irresponsibility.

Anxiety State where a person has strong feelings of worry or dread, where the source is non-specific or unknown.

Aphasia Difficulty or inability to recall words.

Arousal Stress state in which an individual possesses coping resources.

Asylum Large public hospital of the 18th century that provided for the treatment of the insane.

Autonomy Individual's right to self-determination and independence.

Avoidant Personality Disorder Behavior pattern characterized by social inhibition, feelings of inadequacy, and shyness.

Avolition Lack of motivation for work or other goal-oriented activities.

Beneficence Belief that all treatments must be for the client's good.

Bipolar Depression Mood disorder characterized by up and down swings.

Bipolar Disorder Mood disorder characterized by cyclic experiences with both mania and depression.

Blinded Clinical Trial Study in which subjects do not know whether they are receiving an active treatment or a placebo.

Blood-Brain Barrier Capillary barrier between blood and brain.

Borderline Personality A personality disorder characterized by a pervasive pattern of instability of interpersonal relationships, self-image, and objects, and marked impulsivity.

Borderline Personality Disorder Behavior pattern characterized by unstable interpersonal relationships and self-image, efforts to avoid being abandoned, and impulsive actions.

Brief Dynamic Therapy Short-term psychotherapy that focuses on resolving core conflicts that derive from personality and living situations.

Brown Report A 1948 report authored by Esther Lucille Brown on the future of nursing. This report advised that psychiatric hospitals be used as agencies for affiliation in teaching of nurses.

Bulimia Nervosa Psychological eating disorder characterized by fasting, binging, purging, by either self-induced vomiting or misuse of laxatives, diuretics, or enemas, and lack of extreme weight loss.

Burnout Description for caregivers who find themselves unable to provide the quality of care that is desirable; characterized by depletion of energy, decreased ability to concentrate, and a sense of hopelessness.

Capitation Funding mechanism in which all defined services for a specified period of time are provided for an agreed-upon single payment.

Case-Control Study Study comparing two groups: the cases (all members have the given disease or condition) and the controls (all members are free of the disease or condition).

Case Group *See* Experimental Group.

Case Management Constellation of services that includes screening, assessment, care planning, arranging for service delivery, monitoring, reassessment, evaluation, and discharge for the purpose of ensuring continuity of care.

Cataplexy Sudden loss of muscle power at times of sudden emotion.

Catastrophic Reaction Severe overreaction out of proportion to the stimulus.

Catatonia Behavior disorder marked by a decrease in reactivity to the environment, sometimes reaching an extreme degree of complete unawareness.

Catharsis Experience of release that occurs when unconscious thoughts are brought into consciousness.

Child Abuse Any physical or mental injury, sexual abuse, exploitation, negligent treatment, or maltreatment of a child by a parent or caregiver.

Child Molestation Sexual involvement with a child, such as oral-genital contact, genital fondling and viewing, or masturbation in front of a child.

Child Pornography Sexually explicit reproduction of a child's image.

Chronic Grief Unresolved bereavement.

Circadian Rhythm Biorhythm that determines human responses to the environment; refers to attention span in relation to the presence or absence of daylight.

Circular Communication Predictable pattern of communication and response between two people.

Civil Commitment Period of hospitalization requested by a mental health provider following an emergency hospitalization.

Clarification Technique in which an analyst points out a behavior pattern that is not recognized by the client.

Classification System of categorization that allows useful distinctions to be established.

Client-Centered Therapy Process focused on bringing out individual internal resources and understanding.

Closed Group Meeting with a defined number of participants that is not open to new members.

Code of Ethics Positive statements and guidelines of what persons should do.

Codependence Behaviors exhibited by significant others of a substance-abusing individual that serve to enable and protect the abuse at the exclusion of personal fulfillment and self-development.

Cognition Process by which a person "knows the world" and interacts with it.

Cognitive Behavior Therapy Treatment approach aimed at helping clients identify stimuli that cause their anxiety, develop plans to respond to those stimuli in a nonanxious manner, and problem-solve when unanticipated anxiety-provoking situations arise.

Cognitive Therapy Short-term psychotherapy that focuses on removing symptoms by identifying and correcting perceptual biases in client's thinking and correcting unrecognized assumptions.

Cohort Study *See* Longitudinal Study.

Community Crisis Threat of proportion that affects an entire group of people.

Community Health Nursing Synthesis of nursing and public health practice to promote, maintain, and conserve the health of population aggregates in the community.

Community Mental Health Synthesis of community nursing and public health practice to promote, maintain, and conserve the health of population aggregates in the community, with particular emphasis on mental health.

Community Support System (CSS) Organized network of people committed to helping persons with severe mental illness meet their needs and move toward independence.

Competency to Stand Trial Judgment that an individual is able to understand the nature of legal proceedings and is able to tell his or her own story to an attorney and the court.

Complementary Modalities Those modalities being used as an adjunct to medical care and psychiatric treatment that are thought to have effects on stress, sleep disturbance, anxiety, and/or other emotions.

Compulsion Repetitive behavior or act, the goal of which is to prevent or reduce anxiety or distress.

Concept Basic building blocks of a theory.

Conceptual Framework Group of concepts that are linked together to provide a way of organizing or viewing something.

Confabulation Intentional efforts to cover up memory losses or gaps.

Confrontation Technique in which an analyst challenges a client's behavior or thought, with the goal of provoking a reaction and overcoming an emotional barrier to change.

Confusion Multidimensional phenomenon incorporating changes in both cognition and behavior.

Conservative-Withdrawal State Psychological response to stress; stage of exhaustion.

Conservator Person appointed to handle the estate of another person who is judged incompetent.

Continuous Cycling Recurrent movement from mania to depression without an intervening normal period.

Control Group Persons receiving no treatment or being free of a given condition or disease under study.

Controlled Clinical Trials Evaluations in which neither the clients nor their caregivers are allowed to know exactly what treatment is being given.

Conversion Disorder Condition in which an individual exhibits physical symptoms that cannot be explained by any medical or neurological conditions.

Craving Strong, overpowering urge for drugs felt by an individual who abuses or is dependent on drugs.

Created Environment Mobilization of all system variables.

Criminal Sexual Assault Genital, anal, or oral penetration by a part of the perpetrator's body or by an object using force or without the victim's consent.

Crisis Stressor or life challenge that requires an individual to adjust to the unexpected and to adapt to an unpredicted situation or event.

Cultural Blindness Attempt to treat all persons fairly by ignoring differences and acting as though the differences do not exist; misguided attempt to achieve "fairness" by ignoring real cultural differences.

Cultural Care Facets of culture that deal with individual and group health and well-being, including efforts to improve upon the human condition or to deal with illness, handicaps, or death.

Cultural Care Accommodation/Negotiation Nursing actions and decisions that involve reshaping the way in which care values are enacted so the actions will better support well-being, dealing with handicaps, recovering from illness, or facing death.

Cultural Care Preservation/Maintenance Nursing actions and decisions that help people of a cultural group keep or preserve those care values that are applicable to the current situation to maintain well-being, deal with handicaps, recover from illness, or face death.

Cultural Care Repatterning/Restructuring Change in culturally based care practices.

Cultural Crisis Situation of shock resulting from an individual's adaptation to a new culture or return to a previously experienced culture; also known as culture shock.

Cultural Facilitator/Broker Person who can interpret the language, culture, and health care culture of another as a means to bridging the communication barriers between people from different cultures.

Culture Values, beliefs, norms, and lifeways that are learned and shared within a particular group.

Culture Shock State in which a person is overwhelmed or even immobilized by cultural differences in expectations, communication, and general habits between an individual's culture of origin and a new culture to which the individual is trying to assimilate. (*See also* Cultural Crisis)

Cyclothymic Pattern Cycle of an individual's mood changing back and forth between hypomanic and melancholic states.

Defense Mechanisms Unconscious responses used by individuals to protect themselves from internal conflict and external stress.

Deinstitutionalization Movement of clients and mental health services from state mental hospitals into community settings.

Delayed Grief Bereavement that is not accomplished at the time of the loss, and remains with the individual.

Delirium Acute change in a person's level of consciousness and cognition that develops over a short period of time.

Delusion False belief that misrepresents either perceptions or experiences.

Dementia Gradual onset of multiple cognitive changes in memory, abstract thinking, judgment, and perception often results in a progressive decline in intellectual functioning and decreased capacity to perform daily activities.

Deontology Theory founded on human duties to others and the principles on which these duties are based.

Dependent Personality Disorder Behavior pattern characterized by clinging and submissiveness.

Depression State in which an individual feels very sad and despondent and has no energy or sense of future.

Derailment Speech that gets off the point or subject.

Descriptive Study Survey to determine the incidence and prevalence of a disease or condition.

Differentiation Process of unfolding, growth, and maturation, leading to a balance between emotional and intellectual components.

Disability Impairment in one or more important areas of functioning.

Distress Negative response to stimuli that are perceived as threatening.

Domestic Violence (Often referred to as spousal/partner abuse or battering syndrome.) Intentional violent or controlling behavior by a person who is or has been intimate with the victim(s) and may or may not reside in the same household.

Double-Blinded Trial Study in which neither subjects nor persons evaluating the outcome know whether subjects are receiving treatment or a placebo.

Drug Dependence Condition occurring when individuals exhibit a set of behaviors associated with inability to control use of a drug.

Drug Use Any taking of a drug.

DSM-IV *Diagnostic and Statistical Manual*, 4th edition: classification system for mental disorders.

Dyssomnia Condition where there is an abnormality in the amount, quality, or timing of sleep.

Dystonia Reaction manifested by painful muscle spasms lasting from a few seconds to several days.

Echolalia An involuntary, parrotlike repetition of words spoken by others.

Ecomap Graphic depiction of family members' interactions with systems outside the family.

Ego Conscious mind governed by the reality principle; controls the impulses of the id.

Electroconvulsive Therapy (ECT) Passage of an electrical stimulus to the brain to produce a seizure.

Emergency Hospitalization Power of states to detain a person in an emergency situation for a limited time until further evaluation and court proceedings can occur.

Emotional Cutoff Children's efforts to distance themselves from their families in order to achieve independence.

Endemic Descriptor for a disease or condition that is constantly or regularly found in the population.

Energy-Based Modalities Techniques for healing grounded in the notion of the human energy field.

Epidemic Descriptor for a disease or condition that spreads or circulates within a population.

Epidemiology Study of the causes and distribution of injuries and diseases in a population.

Equilibrium State of balance following a stress state.

Ethics Branch of philosophy that considers how behavioral principles guiding human interactions can be analyzed and set.

Ethnicity Identification with a socially, culturally, and politically constructed group that holds a common set of characteristics not shared by others with whom its members come in contact (Lipson, 1996b, p. 8).

Ethnocentrism Perception that one's worldview is the only acceptable truth and that the beliefs, values, and behaviors sanctioned by one's culture are superior to all others.

Euthanasia Act of killing or permitting a death for reasons of mercy.

Exaggerated Grief Bereavement that is overwhelming.

Exhibitionism Exposing one's genitals to a stranger.

Experience-Oriented Therapy Process focusing on the client's experiences as an agent for producing change.

Experimental Group Persons receiving treatment or having a given condition or disease under study; also known as case group.

External Environment Forces, factors, and influences that occur outside the boundaries of a system.

Extrapersonal Stressor Stimuli from outside the system boundary at a great distance.

Factitious Disorder Condition marked by physical or psychological symptoms that are intentionally and knowingly produced by an individual in order to gain attention; also known as Munchausen's Syndrome.

Family Social system composed of two or more persons who coexist within the context of some expectations of reciprocal affection, mutual responsibility, and temporal duration.

Family Attachment Diagram Representation of the reciprocal nature and quality of the affectional ties between family members.

Family Projection Process Situation in which adult family members deal with their own anxiety by projecting the anxiety onto a child.

Fear State where a person feels a strong sense of dread focused on a specific object or event.

Feedback Response of a receiver of a message to the communicator.

Fetishism Sexual arousal occurring from contact with a nonliving object, often an article of clothing.

Fidelity Individual's obligation to honor commitments and contracts.

Fight-Flight Response Psychological response to stress; state of high anxiety and energy.

Financial Abuse Theft or conversion of money or anything of value belonging to the elderly by their relatives or caregivers.

Fixation Preoccupation with pleasures associated with a previous developmental stage.

Flattened Affect Loss of expressiveness.

Folk System Culturally based acts that respond to apparent or anticipated needs related to living, health, well-being, handicaps, or death.

Forcible Rape Forced intercourse or penetration of a body orifice by a penis or other object by a perpetrator.

Foreclosure One of four identity statuses; refers to the adolescent's lack of thoroughly exploring alternatives before making a commitment to an adult identity.

Frotteurism Recurrent sexual touching of a nonconsenting individual, usually a stranger and usually in a crowded public place.

Gang Rape Sexual acts that proximate in time by multiple perpetrators who are either acquaintances of or strangers to the victim.

Gender Dysphoria Condition existing when an individual has a strong desire to live as the opposite sex.

Gender Identity An individual's subjective feeling associated with being male or female.

Gender Identity Disorder Condition in which an individual feels him- or herself to be a member of the opposite sex and desires gender change.

Gender Role Learned expressions of femaleness and maleness; public recognition of one's gender assignment as male or female and the individual's expression of appropriate social behaviors related to that assignment.

General Adaptation Syndrome Specific, predictable, physiological response to stress involving an alarm reaction, a resistance stage, and an exhaustion stage.

Generalized Anxiety Disorder Psychiatric illness characterized by excessive anxiety or dread.

Genetic Marker Identifiable patterns of DNA structure that can be readily confirmed by laboratory analysis.

Genogram Graphic depiction of a family tree that records information over at least three generations.

Genome Entire complement of heritable information.

Grandiose Delusion Perception of importance, special powers, or religious significance that is not in line with reality.

Grief Healthy expression of bereavement.

Group Collection of persons who come together in some way that makes them interdependent.

Group Content Specific problems, topics, or conditions addressed by a group.

Group Dynamics Underlying forces working to produce behavior patterns in groups.

Group Leader/Facilitator Person who invites or selects group members and identifies the purpose and goals of the group.

Group Process Interaction (verbal and nonverbal) between and among group members.

Guided Imagery An unconditional process in which the practitioner leads the subject with specific words, suggestions, symbols, or images to elicit a positive response.

Half-Life Time for plasma concentrations of a drug to decrease to half of an initial value.

Hallucination State in which an individual hears voices or sees images of things that others cannot hear or see.

Healing Touch Systematic approach to healing using several energy interventions that incorporate a variety of therapeutic maneuvers.

Histrionic Personality Disorder Behavior pattern characterized by excesses of emotional expression and a desire to be the center of attention.

Home Health Nursing Delivery of health services in the home under the direction of a health care agency.

Homelessness Condition of being without shelter or a permanent place to live.

Hypnosis Assisting the client to an altered state of consciousness to create an awareness and a directed-focus experience.

Hypoactive Sexual Desire Disorder Significant distress or disturbance in interpersonal relationships when the sexual desire is truly less than would be normal for an individual.

Hypochondriasis Condition marked by preoccupation with fear of having a serious disease, based on misinterpretation of bodily symptoms or functions.

Hypomania Mild form of mania (elevated mood) that lasts for only 4 days.

ICD International Classification of Diseases: a comprehensive listing of clinical diagnoses, each associated with a unique numerical code.

Id Unconscious mind; the reservoir of psychic energy or libido.

Identity Achievement One of the four identity statuses in which an adolescent makes a commitment to an adult identity after a period of exploring alternatives.

Identity Diffusion One of the four identity statuses in which an adolescent avoids making a full commitment to an adult identity and does not reach his or her potential; often associated with restricted emotional expression or detachment from others.

Identity Formation An adolescent's process of finding a place within the larger society beyond the boundaries of the family.

Impoverishment Stress state in which an individual's coping resources are depleted.

Incarcerated Condition of being in jail or other correctional institution.

Incest Sexual relations between children and blood relatives or surrogate family members.

Incidence Number of new cases of an illness, condition, or injury that begin within a certain time period.

Incoherence Speech that is not logically connected.

Incompetence State of an individual with a mental disorder that causes inability to make judgments and renders the person unable to handle his or her own affairs.

Insight-Oriented Therapy Process focusing on helping an individual gain understanding of feelings and behaviors.

Insomnia Sleep disorder characterized by difficulty in initiating or maintaining sleep.

Internal Environment Forces, factors, and influences that occur completely within the boundaries of a system.

Interpersonal Stressor Stimuli from outside the system boundary but proximal to the system.

Interpersonal Therapy Process of gaining insight based on the recognition that psychological distress may occur in conjunction with disturbed human relationships.

Interpretation Technique in which an analyst offers an explanation of a client's unconscious behavior processes.

Interrater Agreement Accord on diagnosis between individuals evaluating the same condition.

Interrater Reliability Accord on diagnosis between different evaluators on the same examination.

Interventive Questions Circular questions used to uncover relationships and connections between individuals, events, ideas, and beliefs.

Intrapersonal Stressor Stimuli from within the system boundary.

Intrarater Reliability Accord on diagnosis on different examinations by the same evaluator.

Justice Principle ensuring fairness, equity, and honesty in decisions.

Least Restrictive Alternative Legal principle requiring that clients be treated with the least amount of constraint of liberty consistent with their safety.

Liaison Psychiatry/Liaison Psychiatric Nursing Practice concerned with the study, diagnosis, treatment, and prevention of psychiatric illness in the physically ill and of psychological factors affecting physical conditions.

Light Therapy (Phototherapy) Provision of artificial indoor lighting, 5 to 10 times brighter than ordinary lighting, to the environment of a person with SAD.

Longitudinal Study Population-based study conducted over a period of time, typically years; also known as cohort study.

Malingering Fabrication of symptoms with the intent of achieving some objective goal.

Malpractice Negligence in the medical field that results in harm.

Managed Care Prepaid health plan in which an identified intermediary is given authority to manage the means and the source from which the client may obtain services.

Mania Psychiatric condition characterized by excess energy, abnormal excitability, and an exaggerated sense of well-being.

Manic Episode Distinct period of abnormally and persistently elevated, expansive, or irritable mood, lasting at least 1 week.

Manipulation Technique in which an analyst tries to influence a client's feelings about therapy, with the goal of enhancing the quality of the therapy.

Marital Therapy Short-term psychotherapy that attempts to resolve problems that occur within a marriage.

Masked Grief Bereavement that is hidden by either a physical symptom or a maladaptive behavior; the individual is unaware of the connection to the grief or loss.

Massage Stimulation of the skin and underlying tissues for the purposes of increasing circulation and inducing a relaxation response.

Maturational Crisis Stage in an individual's life requiring adjustment or adaptation to new responsibilities or life patterns.

Mental Disorder Behavior or psychological syndrome or pattern associated with distress or disability or increased risk of suffering, death, pain, or loss of freedom.

Mental Health State in which a person has knowledge of self, meets basic needs, assumes responsibility for behavior and self-growth, integrates thoughts and feelings with actions, resolves conflicts, maintains relationships, respects others, communicates directly, and adapts to change in the environment.

Mental Illness State in which an individual shows deficits in functioning, cannot view self clearly or has a distorted image of self, is unable to maintain personal relationships, and cannot adapt to the environment.

Mental Injury Harm to a child's psychological or intellectual functioning; manifested as severe anxiety, depression, withdrawal or outward aggressive behavior, or a combination of these behaviors.

Meta-Analysis Statistical analysis that combines the results of several separate clinical studies.

Mind-Modulation Processes by which thoughts, feelings, attitudes, and emotions are converted by the brain into neurohormonal messenger molecules.

M'Naghten Test Legal definition of lack of guilt of a crime by virtue of insanity.

Modeling Assessment with the goal of understanding the client's world from the client's perspective.

Mood Disorder Pattern of mood episodes that result in difficulty functioning in family, work, and social affairs.

Mood Episode Experience of a strong emotion of depression, mania, or a mixture of both for a period of at least 2 weeks.

Moratorium One of the four identity statuses in which an individual delays making a decision about adult identity while exploring various alternatives during adolescence.

Morbid Ideation Thinking of matters of a gruesome or unwholesome nature.

Multigenerational Transmission Process Situation in which patterns of dealing with anxiety are passed from one generation to the next.

Munchausen's Syndrome Also known as Factitious Disorder.

Munchausen's Syndrome by Proxy Form of child abuse marked by a caregiver falsely giving reports of a child's illness and resulting in unnecessary medical investigations or treatments.

Music Therapy Use of specific kinds of music and its ability to affect changes in behavior, emotions, and physiology.

Mutuality Client involvement in the therapeutic relationship.

NANDA North American Nursing Diagnosis Association prepared a taxonomy of nursing diagnoses, which are statements of the phenomena of concern to nurses.

Narcissistic Personality Disorder Behavior pattern characterized in part by lack of empathy for others and a grandiose sense of self-importance.

Narcolepsy Sleep disorder characterized by frequent irresistible urges for sleep, hallucinatory dreamlike states, and episodes of cataplexy.

National Mental Health Act Provided federal funds for research and education in all areas of psychiatric care. Act was passed in 1946. Established NIMH.

Negligence Behaving in a way in which a prudent individual would *not* have behaved or failing to use the diligence and care expected of a reasonable individual in similar circumstances.

Negligent Treatment Failure of a parent or caregiver to provide, for reasons other than poverty, adequate food, clothing, shelter, or medical care, which may lead to serious endangerment of the physical health of the child.

Neologistic Word Invented word, often used by persons suffering from schizophrenia.

Neuroleptic Malignant Syndrome Disorder associated with sudden fever, rigidity, tachycardia, hypertension, and decreased levels of consciousness.

Neurotransmitter Chemical messenger.

NIC Nursing Interventions Classification: outlines list of nursing interventions designed to identify activities that nurses perform to assist client status or behavior.

Nightmare Exceedingly vivid dreams from which the sleeper wakens in fear, often sweating and with heart racing, and is able to recall the dream.

NIMBY Literally "not in my backyard." Condition of persons or groups who state support for services for the homeless or underprivileged groups, but refuse to have such services in their own neighborhood.

NMDS Nursing Minimum Data Set: grouping that identifies the minimum information necessary to meet information demands of nursing practice.

Nonmaleficence Belief that care providers must do no harm.

Nonverbal Communication Messages sent by means other than oral or written.

Normal Sexual Behavior Any sexual act that is consensual, lacks force, is mutually satisfying to both partners, and is conducted in private. [In adults]

Normative Ethics Guidelines and procedures useful in establishing moral decisions and actions.

Norms Learned behaviors that are perceived to be appropriate or inappropriate in a culture.

Nuclear Family Emotional System Process by which a family manages anxiety.

Nurse Agency Nursing activities required to compensate for the client's inability to meet his own self-care needs (Orem's Theory).

Nursing Learned humanistic and scientific profession focused on human care phenomena and activities in order to assist, support, facilitate, or enable individuals or groups to maintain or regain their well-being in culturally meaningful and beneficial ways or to help people face handicaps or death.

Nursing Agency Characteristic that allows nurses to act for others in meeting therapeutic self-care demands.

Nursing Situation Context in which nursing occurs.

Obsession Recurrent thought, image, or impulse that is experienced as intrusive and inappropriate and that causes marked anxiety or distress.

Obsessive-Compulsive Personality Disorder Behavior pattern characterized by preoccupation with order, cleanliness, control, and perfectionism.

Oculogyric Crisis Reaction in which extraocular muscle spasm forces the eyes into a fixed, usually upward gaze.

Open Group Meeting in which participants are free to come and go, depending on their individual needs.

Orientation Phase First stage of a relationship during which the nurse and client get to know one another, establish trust, and outline goals and boundaries.

Panic Disorder Psychiatric illness characterized by discrete episodes of intense anxiety (panic attacks) that begin abruptly and peak within 10 minutes.

Paranoid Personality Disorder Behavior pattern characterized by persistent yet unfounded fear of exploitation or harm by others.

Paraphilia Disorder of sexual interest, arousal, and orgasm.

Parasomnia Condition in which the person suffers from profoundly disturbed sleep, most commonly nightmares, sleep terrors, or sleepwalking.

Parasympathetic System Response Nervous system response that works in opposition to the sympathetic nervous system, bringing about a decrease in heart and respiratory rates; dilation of peripheral blood vessels; muscle relaxation; lowered blood pressure; and increased flow of endorphins.

Passive-Aggressive Personality Disorder Behavior pattern characterized by pervasive negativity with passive resistance to social/occupational demands, procrastination, and stubbornness.

Passive Physical Abuse (or Negligence) Conduct that is careless and a breach of duty that results in injury to the person or is a violation of rights; includes the withholding of medication, medical treatment, food, and personal care necessary for the well-being of the elderly person.

Pedophilia Sexual interests directed primarily or exclusively toward children.

Persecutory Delusion Paranoid perception that others are "out to get me."

Personality Habitual patterns and qualities of behavior expressed by physical and mental activities and attitudes; the distinctive individual qualities of a person.

Personality Disorder Pervasive and inflexible pattern of behavior demonstrating unhealthy characteristics that limit the individual's ability to function in society.

Personality Trait Qualities of behavior that make a person unique.

Phobia Persistent fear of a specific object or situation.

Physical Abuse Conduct of violence that results in bodily harm or mental stress; includes a spectrum of violence ranging from assault to murder.

Physical Injury Lacerations, fractured bones, burns, internal injuries, severe bruising, or serious bodily harm.

Physical Restraint Use of an apparatus that significantly inhibits mobility.

Placebo Treatment that has no intended effect on the expected outcome of a trial.

Play Therapy Therapeutic technique using games and toys to help children express their feelings, explore relationships, and attempt new solutions to problems.

Population Aggregate of persons in the community who share a common characteristic, such as age or diagnosis.

Positron Emission Tomography (PET) Scan   Tool to accurately measure blood flow patterns in the brain.

Post-Traumatic Stress Disorder   Anxiety disorder resulting from a frightening event such as a crime, accident, or battle.

Power   Influences each family member has on the family processes and functioning.

Presence   Activity of being physically present with another person that begins with the nurse's genuine commitment to caring and nurturing the potential of the client.

Prevalence   Number of persons in a population who are living with a disease or disorder at any time; includes both new and old cases.

Primary Hypersomnia   Severe daytime sleepiness despite normal nighttime sleep patterns that interferes with daily activities; a condition that cannot be explained by any other sleep, medical, or pharmacological cause.

Primary Insomnia   Condition in which an individual can fall asleep easily and remain asleep for several hours but does not feel rested upon waking.

Primary Prevention   Activities directed at reducing the incidence of mental disorder within a population.

Probate Proceedings   Judicial hearing to determine the competence of an individual to manage personal affairs.

Process Recording   Verbatim account of a communication, with interpretation of techniques used and their effectiveness.

Professional System   Acts based on formal preparation for dealing with health, illness, and wellness.

Program for Assertive Community Treatment (PACT)   Model providing a full range of medical, psychosocial, and rehabilitation services by a community-based, multidisciplinary team.

Prospective Payment System   Reimbursement mechanism based on predetermined payment for a specific period or diagnosis.

Psychiatric Mental Health Advanced Practice Registered Nurse   A licensed nurse educationally certified at the masters or doctoral level who is nationally certified as a clinical specialist in psychiatric and mental health nursing.

Psychiatric Mental Health Nurse   A licensed nurse who has passed a certification exam and is thereby certified within a specialty.

Psychoanalysis   Therapy focused on uncovering unconscious memories and processes.

Psychodynamic Therapy   Brief process based on psychoanalytic principles, with the goal of improved functioning rather than personality reconstruction.

Psychological Abuse   Simple name calling and verbal assaults in a protracted and systematic effort to dehumanize the victim, sometimes with the goal of driving the victim to insanity or suicide; usually exists in combination with one or more other abuses.

Psychological Development   Continuum of milestones from infancy through adulthood showing evolution of personal history.

Psychosis   State in which an individual has lost the ability to recognize reality.

Psychotherapy   Treatment of mental or emotional disorders through psychological rather than physical methods.

Psychotic   Mental state involving the loss of rational thought and/or loss of ability to accurately interpret the environment.

Public Health Nursing   Field of nursing that addresses the social, economic, and environmental conditions that influence health.

Quasi-Experimental Study   Analytical study in which a population is studied before and after a given event; usually includes both a case and a control set.

Rape   Act of sexual intercourse in which the person does not give consent; accomplished against a person's will by means of force or fear of immediate and unlawful bodily injury or threatening to retaliate in the future against the victim or other person.

Rapid Cycling   Four or more episodes of mania in a year.

Referential Delusion   Perception that common events refer specifically to the individual.

Regression   Reversion to pleasures of a previous developmental stage.

Relativistic Thinking   Process of understanding the contextual nature of the world from multiple perspectives.

Relaxation   A psychophysiological state characterized by parasympathetic dominance involving multiple visceral and somatic symptoms including the absence of physical, mental, and emotional tension.

Reliability   Measurement of reproducibility of a testing instrument.

Repression   Process in which painful memories, thoughts, or experiences are actively kept out of conscious awareness.

Risk Factors   Traits that predispose an individual to a disease.

Role-Modeling   Developing an individualized plan of care based on the client's world model.

Schizoaffective Disorder   Condition characterized by elements of schizophrenia and manic-depressive disorder.

Schizoid Personality Disorder   Behavior pattern characterized by lack of emotion and close friendships and detachment from persons and events in the immediate environment.

Schizophrenia   Mental disorder characterized by disordered thoughts, hallucinations, and delusions.

Schizotypal Personality Disorder   Behavior pattern characterized by inability to form close relations and a pattern of cognitive and perceptual distortions and eccentricities.

Seclusion State of a client being put in an isolated room or cell.

Secondary Prevention Activities directed at reducing the prevalence of mental disorders by shortening the duration of a sufficient number of established cases.

Self-Awareness Perception of oneself in relation to others and relative to society's expectations.

Self-Care Activities that humans perform for themselves.

Self-Care Agency Ability to perform self-care in light of gender, age, socioeconomic status, developmental level, health, family, environment, living patterns, and availability of resources (Orem's Theory).

Self-Care Deficit State that occurs when an individual's therapeutic self-care demand is greater than the capacity to meet that demand.

Self-Efficacy Ability to organize and manage individual responses to the demands of the environment.

Self-Help Group Persons coming together who are facing a common difficulty.

Serotonergic Syndrome Drug reaction involving agitation, sweating, rigidity, fever, hyperreflexia, tachycardia, and hypotension.

Sexual Abuse (child) Employment, use, persuasion, inducement, enticement, or coercion of a child to engage in or assist another person to engage in sexually implicit conduct; includes rape, molestation, prostitution, or other forms of sexual exploitation of children or incest with children.

Sexual Abuse (elder) Threat of sexual assault or actual sexual battery, rape, incest, sodomy, oral copulation, penetration of genital or anal opening by a foreign object, coerced nudity, and sexually explicit photographing.

Sexual Battery Activity of a person touching an intimate part (sexual organs, groin, buttocks, breast) of another person if that touching is against the will of the person touched and is for the purpose of sexual arousal, gratification, or abuse.

Sexual Dysfunction Condition existing when a person experiences a change with any aspect of sexuality that is viewed as unsatisfying, unrewarding, or inadequate.

Sexual Exploitation Child pornography, sexually explicit reproduction of a child's image, or child prostitution.

Sexual Masochism Disorder characterized by sexual excitement resulting from fantasies or behaviors about being the recipient of physical abuse or humiliation.

Sexual Sadism Disorder characterized by sexual excitement resulting from persistent fantasies or behaviors involving infliction of suffering on others.

Sexually Explicit Conduct Actual or simulated sexual intercourse, bestiality, masturbation, lascivious exhibition of the genitals of a person or animal, or sadistic or masochistic abuse.

Sibling Position Birth order of children.

Situational Crisis Event that poses a threat or challenge to an individual.

Sleep Hygiene Specific activities that assist many persons to achieve restful sleep.

Sleep Latency Time it takes to fall asleep.

Sleep Paralysis Sensation of being unable to move, speak, or breathe during sleep.

Sleep Terrors Parasomnia in which there is *no recall* of the sleep-related event.

Sleepwalking Pattern of sleep behavior usually including getting out of bed, walking around in the bedroom, or on occasion outside of the bedroom, and then returning to bed.

SNOMED Systematized Nomenclature of Medicine: coding system that includes nursing diagnoses, nursing interventions, multiple axes that identify causative factors of illness, and related functional deficits and social factors.

Social Competence Degree to which significant others rate an individual as successful at performing expected social tasks.

Societal Regression Process of reversion in which anxiety leads to emotionally based decision making.

Sodomy Anal intercourse.

Somatic Therapies Interventions used in the management of psychiatric symptoms, for example, use of seclusion or physical restraints in control of anger.

Somatization Disorder Somatoform disorder in which there are multiple physical complaints without an apparent physiological cause.

Somatoform Disorder Psychiatric condition manifested in physical rather than psychological symptoms.

Spousal Rape Sexual intercourse against the victim's will by the spouse; accompanied by force or fear of bodily harm or future retaliation.

Status Style used by an adolescent in resolving issues of adult identity.

Statutory Rape Sexual activity with a person under the age of consent (in most states, under 16 years of age) and considered to have occurred in spite of the apparent willingness of the underage person.

Stereotyping Assumption that people sharing certain characteristics will think and act similarly.

Stranger Rape Aggravated criminal sexual assault, forcible rape, or sexual battery that is committed against a victim by persons not acquainted with the victim.

Stress Stimulus that an individual perceives as challenging or harmful.

Substance Abuse Maladaptive pattern of use of a drug in situations of real or potential harm.

Suggestion Psychoanalytic technique in which the analyst interprets the client's thoughts, actions, or dreams.

Suicidal Ideation Thoughts of taking one's life.

Suicide Purposefully taking one's own life.

Suicide Potential Person's risk level for completing a suicide.

Suicide Survivor Friends and family of individuals who die from suicide.

Superego Conscious mind, governed by conscience and ego ideal.

Supportive-Educative Role Nursing activities that focus on enhancing the client's ability both to carry on effectively without nursing support and to rise above the feelings of depression (Orem's Theory).

Supportive Group Persons coming together to offer support, education, socialization, and/or recreation.

Switch Process Mood changes between mania and depression.

Sympathetic System Response Nervous system responses to stress that include increased heart rate, breathing, and blood pressure; constriction of peripheral blood vessels; muscle tension; gastric hyperacidity; release of adrenaline; and formation of cortisol.

Synapse Structure formed where axons and dendrites come together.

Tangentiality Speech marked by failure to reach a goal or stick to the original point.

Tarasoff Duty to Warn Legal obligation of health care professionals to advise potential victims of violence so that they may seek protection.

Tardive Dyskinesia Movement disorder characterized by repetitive motions such as chewing or grimacing.

Task-Oriented Therapy Process focused on helping an individual gain the tools needed to change behavior and feelings.

Termination Phase Third stage of a relationship during which the nurse and client evaluate the progress made toward reaching goals and determine that the client is ready to move forward independently of the nurse.

Tertiary Prevention Activities directed at reducing the residual defects that are associated with mental disorders.

Therapeutic Communication Purposeful use of dialogue to bring about the client's insight, control of symptoms, and healing.

Therapeutic Imagery The ability to take one's natural thought processes and direct these thoughts in a creative way, potentiating a positive outcome.

Therapeutic Massage Extension of massage techniques, involving deep tissue and advanced massage techniques.

Therapeutic Self-Care Demand Activities needed to meet self-care requisites to fulfill self-care agency.

Therapeutic Touch (TT) Five-step process of touch that involves centering; assessing the client's energy field; smoothing, or "unruffling," the field; modulating or transferring energy; and knowing when to stop.

Therapeutic Window Time for peak effectiveness of a drug.

Therapy Group Persons coming together to receive psychotherapy.

Tolerance Acquired resistance to the effects of a drug.

Trait Anxiety Personality characteristic reflecting susceptibility to anxiety.

Transvestic Fetishism Cross dressing or fantasies about cross dressing.

Triangulation Relational pattern among three members.

UMLS Unified Medical Language System: thesaurus of all terms included in existing taxonomies.

Unipolar Depression Disorder in which mood swings are always in one direction, either up or down.

Utilitarianism Theory based on the principle that an ethical decision serves to produce the greatest good for the greatest number of persons.

Validity Measurement of accuracy of a testing instrument.

Values Learned beliefs about what is held to be good or bad in a culture.

Victim Consciousness Belief that one is at the mercy of circumstances beyond one's control.

Violation of Rights Abuse that occurs when the inalienable rights by the U.S. Constitution and federal statutes are violated by a family member or caregiver; includes such rights as not to have one's property taken without due process, the right to adequate appropriate medical treatment, and the right to freedom of assembly, speech, and religion.

Voyeurism Observing or fantasizing about observing others disrobing, naked, or involved in sexual activity.

Withdrawal Condition occurring when stopping use of a drug results in a drug-specific set of symptoms that would be relieved by additional doses of the drug.

Word Salad Speech marked by a group of disconnected words.

Working Phase Second stage of a relationship during which the nurse and client implement interventions designed to bring about the outcomes identified during the orientation phase.

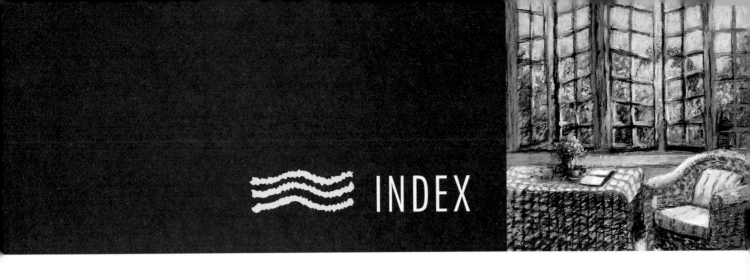

INDEX

Note: Page numbers in *italics* indicate artwork and film clips; page numbers followed by "t" indicate tables; page numbers followed by "b" indicate boxed material.